BLUEPRINTS

Obstetrics & Gynecology

SEVENTH REVISED EDITION

Obstetrics & Gynecology

SEVENTH REVISED EDITION

Tamara L. Callahan, MD, MPP, FACOG

Associate Professor
Quality and Patient Safety Director
Department of Obstetrics and Gynecology
Division of Gynecologic Specialties
Vanderbilt University Medical Center
Nashville, Tennessee

Aaron B. Caughey, MD, MPP, MPH, PhD

Professor and Chair
Department of Obstetrics and Gynecology
Oregon Health & Science University
Portland, Oregon

Philadelphia • Baltimore • New York • London
Buenos Aires • Hong Kong • Sydney • Tokyo

Acquisitions Editor: Matt Hauber
Product Development Editor: Andrea Vosburgh
Editorial Coordinator: Katherine Burland
Marketing Manager: Michael McMahon
Production Project Manager: Bridgett Dougherty
Design Coordinator: Stephen Druding
Manufacturing Coordinator: Margie Orzech
Prepress Vendor: S4Carlisle Publishing Services

Seventh revised edition

Copyright © 2018 Wolters Kluwer.

Copyright © 2013 Lippincott Williams & Wilkins, a Wolters Kluwer business. All rights reserved. This book is protected by copyright. No part of this book may be reproduced or transmitted in any form or by any means, including as photocopies or scanned-in or other electronic copies, or utilized by any information storage and retrieval system without written permission from the copyright owner, except for brief quotations embodied in critical articles and reviews. Materials appearing in this book prepared by individuals as part of their official duties as U.S. government employees are not covered by the above-mentioned copyright. To request permission, please contact Wolters Kluwer at Two Commerce Square, 2001 Market Street, Philadelphia, PA 19103, via email at permissions@lww.com, or via our website at lww.com (products and services).

9 8 7 6 5 4 3 2 1

Printed in China (or the United States of America)

Library of Congress Cataloging-in-Publication Data

ISBN-13: 978-1-9751-3487-7
ISBN-10: 1-9751-3487-7

Cataloging-in-Publication data available on request from the Publisher.

This work is provided "as is," and the publisher disclaims any and all warranties, express or implied, including any warranties as to accuracy, comprehensiveness, or currency of the content of this work.

This work is no substitute for individual patient assessment based upon healthcare professionals' examination of each patient and consideration of, among other things, age, weight, gender, current or prior medical conditions, medication history, laboratory data and other factors unique to the patient. The publisher does not provide medical advice or guidance and this work is merely a reference tool. Healthcare professionals, and not the publisher, are solely responsible for the use of this work including all medical judgments and for any resulting diagnosis and treatments.

Given continuous, rapid advances in medical science and health information, independent professional verification of medical diagnoses, indications, appropriate pharmaceutical selections and dosages, and treatment options should be made and healthcare professionals should consult a variety of sources. When prescribing medication, healthcare professionals are advised to consult the product information sheet (the manufacturer's package insert) accompanying each drug to verify, among other things, conditions of use, warnings and side effects and identify any changes in dosage schedule or contraindications, particularly if the medication to be administered is new, infrequently used or has a narrow therapeutic range. To the maximum extent permitted under applicable law, no responsibility is assumed by the publisher for any injury and/or damage to persons or property, as a matter of products liability, negligence law or otherwise, or from any reference to or use by any person of this work.

shop.lww.com

Contributing Editors

Allison Allen, MD
Fellow, Maternal-Fetal Medicine
Department of Obstetrics and Gynecology
Oregon Health & Science University
Portland, Oregon

Alison Barlow, WHNP
Assistant Professor
Department of Obstetrics and Gynecology
Division of Midwifery and Advanced Practice Nursing
Vanderbilt University Medical Center
Nashville, Tennessee

Howard Curlin, MD
Assistant Professor
Department of Obstetrics and Gynecology
Division of Gynecologic Specialties
Vanderbilt University Medical Center
Nashville, Tennessee

Jeff Davis, DO
Assistant Professor
Department of Obstetrics and Gynecology
Division of General Obstetrics and Gynecology
Vanderbilt University School of Medicine
Nashville, Tennessee

Jessica Heft, MD
Fellow, Female Pelvic Medicine and Reproductive Surgery
Department of Obstetrics and Gynecology
Division of Female Pelvic Medicine and Reconstructive Surgery
Vanderbilt University School of Medicine
Nashville, Tennessee

William J. Kellett, DO
Associate Professor
Department of Obstetrics and Gynecology
Division of General Obstetrics and Gynecology
Vanderbilt University Medical Center
Nashville, Tennessee

Tamara Keown, MSN, WHNP-BC
Assistant Professor
Department of Obstetrics and Gynecology
Division of Midwifery and Advanced Practice Nursing
Vanderbilt University Medical Center
Nashville, Tennessee

Dineo Khabele, MD, FACOG, FACS
Director, Division of Gynecologic Oncology
The University of Kansas Cancer Center
Professor, Obstetrics and Gynecology
The University of Kansas School of Medicine
Kansas City, Kansas

Lucy Koroma, MSN, WHNP-BC
Assistant Professor
Department of Gynecology and Obstetrics
Division of Minimally Invasive Gynecology
Johns Hopkins University School of Medicine
Baltimore, Maryland

Erica E. Marsh, MD, MSCI
Associate Professor and Chief Division Director
Department of Obstetrics and Gynecology
Division of Reproductive Endocrinology and Infertility
University of Michigan Medical School
Ann Arbor, Michigan

Christina Megli, MD, PhD
Fellow, Maternal-Fetal Medicine
Department of Obstetrics and Gynecology
University of Pittsburgh Medical Center
Pittsburgh, Pennsylvania

Melinda New, MD
Associate Professor and Vice Chair of Education
Department of Obstetrics and Gynecology
Division of Gynecologic Specialties
Vanderbilt University Medical Center
Nashville, Tennessee

Rachel Pilliod, MD
Fellow, Maternal-Fetal Medicine
Department of Obstetrics and Gynecology
Oregon Health & Science University
Portland, Oregon

Jessica Pippen, MD
Fellow, Maternal-Fetal Medicine
Department of Obstetrics and Gynecology
Ohio State University College of Medicine
Columbus Ohio

Erica Robinson, MD, FRCSC
Assistant Professor
Department of Obstetrics and Gynecology
Division of Gynecology
Wake Forest School of Medicine
Winston-Salem, North Carolina

Bethany Sabol, MD
Fellow, Maternal-Fetal Medicine
Department of Obstetrics and Gynecology
Washington University
St. Louis, Missouri

Stacey Scheib, MD, FACOG
Assistant Professor
Director, Multidisciplinary Fibroid Center
Department of Gynecology and Obstetrics
Division of Minimally Invasive Gynecology
Johns Hopkins University School of Medicine
Baltimore, Maryland

Katherine A. Smith, MD
Fellow, Minimally Invasive Gynecologic Surgery
Department of Obstetrics and Gynecology
Mayo Clinic
Jacksonville, Florida

May Thomassee, MD
Assistant Professor
Department of Obstetrics and Gynecology
Division of Gynecology
University Hospitals and Clinics of Lafayette
Louisiana State University School of Medicine
Lafayette, Louisiana

Laurie Tompkins, WHNP
Assistant Professor
Department of Obstetrics and Gynecology
Division of Midwifery and Advanced Practice Nursing
Vanderbilt University Medical Center
Nashville, Tennessee

Ashley M. Van Wormer, MD
Resident
Department of Obstetrics and Gynecology
Louisiana State University School of Medicine
New Orleans, Louisiana

Jessica L. Young, MD
Assistant Professor
Department of Obstetrics and Gynecology
Division of General Obstetrics and Gynecology
Vanderbilt University Medical Center
Nashville, Tennessee

Contributing Editors from Previous Editions

Marisa Adelman, MD
Assistant Professor
Department of Obstetrics and Gynecology
Division of General Obstetrics and Gynecology
University of Utah
Salt Lake City, Utah

Jeff Andrews, MD, FRCSC
Executive Editor-in-Chief, Journal of Lower
  Genital Tract Disease
Worldwide Medical Director of Women's
  Health & Cancer
BD Life Sciences
BD Diagnostic Systems
Sparks, Maryland

Lisa Bayer, MD
Assistant Professor, Family Planning
Department of Obstetrics and Gynecology
Oregon Health & Science University
Portland, Oregon

Stephanie Beall, MD, PhD
Department of Obstetrics and Gynecology
Division of Reproductive Endocrinology and
  Infertility
Shady Grove Fertility
Columbia, Maryland

Daniel H. Biller, MD, MMHC
Associate Professor
Department of Obstetrics and Gynecology
Division of Urogynecology and Female
  Pelvic Medicine
Vanderbilt University Medical Center
Nashville, Tennessee

Lynne Black
Research Coordinator
Department of Obstetrics and Gynecology
Vanderbilt University Medical Center
Nashville, Tennessee

Nicole S. Carroll, MD
Department of Obstetrics and Gynecology
Wilmington Health
Wilmington, North Carolina

Annette Chen, MD
Department of Obstetrics and Gynecology
Division of Gynecologic Oncology
Kaiser Permanente
Oakland, California

Yvonne W. Cheng, MD, PhD
Director
Maternal-Fetal Medicine
California Pacific Medical Center
San Francisco, California

Bruce B. Feinberg, MD
Assistant Professor
Department of Obstetrics and Gynecology
Division of Maternal-Fetal Medicine
Columbia University Medical Center
New York, New York

Karen P. Gold, MD, MSCI
Interim Chair and Residency Program Director
Department of Obstetrics and Gynecology
Division of Urogynecology-Female Pelvic
  Medicine and Reconstructive Surgery
University of Oklahoma-Tulsa
Tulsa, Oklahoma

Linda J. Heffner, MD, PhD
Professor
Department of Obstetrics and Gynecology
Division of Maternal-Fetal Medicine
Boston University School of Medicine
Boston, Massachusetts

Celeste O. Hemingway, MD, MHPE
Assistant Professor and Residency Director
Department of Obstetrics and Gynecology
Division of General Obstetrics and Gynecology
Vanderbilt University Medical Center
Nashville, Tennessee

Nariman Heshmati, MD
Department of Obstetrics and Gynecology
The Everett Clinic
Everett, Washington

Beth Colvin Huff, MSN, NP
Editorial Board, Journal of Lower Genital
  Tract Disease
Previous Board of Directors
American Society for Colposcopy and
  Cervical Pathology

Sarah E. Little, MD, MPH
Assistant Professor
Maternal-Fetal Medicine
Department of Obstetrics and Gynecology
Brigham and Women's Hospital
Boston, Massachusetts

Sara Newmann, MD, MPH
Associate Clinical Professor
Department of Obstetrics, Gynecology and
  Reproductive Sciences
University of California San Francisco
San Francisco General Hospital
San Francisco, California

Erin Rebele, MD
Assistant Professor
Department of Obstetrics and Gynecology
Division of General Obstetrics and Gynecology
Vanderbilt University Medical Center
Nashville, Tennessee

Brian L. Shaffer, MD
Director
Department of Obstetrics and Gynecology
Fetal Diagnosis & Treatment Center
Associate Professor
Oregon Health & Science University
Portland, Oregon

Christopher M. Sizemore, DO
Assistant Professor
Department of Obstetrics and Gynecology
Division of General Obstetrics and Gynecology
Vanderbilt University Medical Center
Nashville, Tennessee

Merielle M. Stephens, MD
Assistant Professor
Department of Obstetrics and Gynecology
Tufts University School of Medicine
Boston, Massachusetts

Susan H. Tran, MD
Associate Professor, Maternal-Fetal Medicine
Department of Obstetrics and Gynecology
Oregon Health & Science University
Portland, Oregon

Jing Wang Chiang, MD
Chief
Division of Gynecologic Oncology
Department of Obstetrics and Gynecology
Santa Clara Valley Medical Center
Santa Clara, California

Keenan Yanit, MD
Assistant Professor
Department of Obstetrics and Gynecology
Oregon Health & Science University
Portland, Oregon

Amanda Yunker, DO
Associate Professor
Department of Obstetrics and Gynecology
Division of Minimally Invasive Gynecology
Vanderbilt University Medical Center
Nashville, Tennessee

Preface

In 1997, the first five books in the Blueprints series were published as board review for medical students, interns, and residents who wanted high-yield, accurate clinical content for USMLE Steps 2 and 3. Twenty years later, we are proud to report that the original books and the entire Blueprints brand of review materials have far exceeded our expectations.

The feedback we have received from our readers has been tremendously helpful and pivotal in deciding what direction the seventh revised edition of the core books would take. To ensure that the seventh revised edition of the series continues to provide the content and approach that made the original Blueprints a success, we have expanded the text to include the most up-to-date topics and evidence-based research and therapies. Information is provided on the latest changes in the management of cervical dysplasia and cervical cancer screening, abnormal uterine bleeding, hypertension in pregnancy, cervical insufficiency, prenatal diagnosis, and preterm labor. The newest and future techniques in contraception and sterilization and menopausal hormone therapies are covered, as are contemporary treatment options for uterine fibroids and ovarian cysts.

The succinct and telegraphic use of tables and figures was highly acclaimed by our readers, so we have redoubled our efforts to expand their usefulness by adding updated and improved artwork, including the section of color plates. In each case, we have tried to include only the most helpful and clear tables and figures to maximize the reader's ability to understand and remember the material.

We have likewise updated our bibliography to include evidence-based articles as well as references to classic articles and textbooks in both obstetrics and gynecology. These references are now provided in electronic format. It was also suggested that the review questions should reflect the current format of the boards. We are particularly proud to include new and revised board-format questions in this edition with full explanations of both correct and incorrect options provided in the answers. In particular, we have added a section of case-based clinical vignettes questions at the end of each chapter to facilitate review of the topics and practice for the boards.

That said, we have also learned from our readers that Blueprints is more than just board review for USMLE Steps 2 and 3. Students use the books during their clerkship rotations, sub-internships, and as a quick refresher while rotating on various services in early residency. Residents studying for USMLE Step 3 often use the books for reviewing areas outside their specialty. Students in physician assistant, nurse practitioner, and osteopath programs use Blueprints as a companion to review materials in their own areas of expertise.

When we first wrote the book, we had just completed medical school and started residency training. Thus, we hope this new edition brings both that original viewpoint and our clinical experience garnered over the past 20 years. However, you choose to use Blueprints, we hope that you find the books in the series informative and valuable to your own continuing education.

Tamara L. Callahan, MD, MPP, FACOG
Aaron B. Caughey, MD, MPP, MPH, PhD

Acknowledgments

I would like to express my sincere and deep appreciation to my coauthor, Dr. Caughey, and to the OB/Gyn residents and faculties at Harvard and Vanderbilt who gave liberally of their time and expertise to make this book something of which we can all be proud. Without the extraordinary talent and commitment of these physicians and providers, this project would not have been possible. This accomplishment is also credited in no small part to an incredible core of family and friends who lovingly and selflessly allow me to follow my passion for education and women's health. And to my children, Connor and Jaela, being your mother has been an indescribable honor and an immeasurable joy—a blessing which I try to earn each and every day. I would also like to acknowledge my mentors, Dr. William F. Crowley, Jr., Dr. Janet Hall, Dr. Linda J. Heffner, Dr. Nancy E. Oriol, Dr. Robert Barbieri, and Dr. Nancy Chescheir whose strength, insight, leadership, and drive are exemplary of what it means to be an active contributor to academic medicine and women's health. Lastly, I'd like to thank the many medical students and residents who have shared their input and enthusiasm with us along this exciting journey. Their support has been paramount to the success of this project and to our quest to make this book the very best it can be. It has truly been a privilege to be a small part of their never-ending learning experience.

Tamara L. Callahan, MD, MPP, FACOG

I would like to acknowledge and extend my thanks to everyone involved in the seventh revised edition of our book, most importantly my coauthor, Dr. Callahan, as well as all of those who contributed to the first six editions, particularly Dr. Chen, Dr. Feinberg, and Dr. Heffner, and the staff at both Blackwell and LWW. I would also like to thank my colleagues and mentors for the supportive environment in which I work, in particular, the residents and faculty in the department of Obstetrics and Gynecology at OHSU as well as my mentors, Dr. Washington, Dr. Norton, Dr. Ames, Dr. Repke, Dr. Blatman, Dr. Macones, Dr. Robinson, and Dr. Norwitz. I would also like to acknowledge the suggestions and critiques from medical students around the country and particularly those at Harvard, UCSF, and OHSU who keep pushing us to produce better editions of this work. I would also like to thank my parents, Bill and Carol, for their support for all these years. To my wife, Susan, thank you for your patience and support during all of my projects. To my children, Aidan, Ashby, Amelie, and, Atticus—you are my inspiration to work harder every day, but also to take the time to enjoy this journey we are on. I love you all so very much.

Aaron B. Caughey, MD, MPP, MPH, PhD

Contents

Contributing Editors v
Contributing Editors from Previous Editions vii
Preface ix
Acknowledgments x
Abbreviations xiii

PART I: OBSTETRICS — 1

1. Pregnancy and Prenatal Care — 1
2. Early Pregnancy Complications — 15
3. Prenatal Screening, Diagnosis, and Treatment — 27
4. Normal Labor and Delivery — 46
5. Antepartum Hemorrhage — 72
6. Complications of Labor and Delivery — 92
7. Fetal Complications of Pregnancy — 112
8. Hypertension and Pregnancy — 133
9. Diabetes During Pregnancy — 145
10. Infectious Diseases in Pregnancy — 157
11. Other Medical Complications of Pregnancy — 181
12. Postpartum Care and Complications — 199

PART II: GYNECOLOGY — 215

13. Benign Disorders of the Lower Genital Tract — 215
14. Benign Disorders of the Upper Genital Tract — 229
15. Endometriosis and Adenomyosis — 249

16	Infections of the Lower Female Reproductive Tract	262
17	Infections of the Upper Female Reproductive Tract and Systemic Infections	279
18	Pelvic Organ Prolapse	291
19	Urinary Incontinence	302
20	Puberty, the Menstrual Cycle, and Menopause	320
21	Amenorrhea	336
22	Abnormalities of the Menstrual Cycle	350
23	Hirsutism and Virilism	367
24	Contraception and Sterilization	379
25	Termination of Pregnancy	406
26	Infertility and Assisted Reproductive Technologies	417
27	Vulvar and Vaginal Neoplasia	435
28	Cervical Neoplasia and Cervical Cancer	445
29	Endometrial Cancer	463
30	Ovarian and Fallopian Tube Tumors	473
31	Gestational Trophoblastic Disease	487
32	Benign Breast Disease and Breast Cancer	502

Questions 524
Answers 546
Index 571

Abbreviations

3β-HSD	3β-hydroxysteroid dehydrogenase	CKC	cold-knife conization (biopsy)
5-FU	5-fluorouracil	CMV	cytomegalovirus
17α-OHP	17α-hydroxyprogesterone	CNS	central nervous system
ACTH	adrenocorticotropic hormone	CPD	cephalopelvic disproportion
AD	autosomal dominant	CRS	congenital rubella syndrome
ADH	antidiuretic hormone	CSF	cerebrospinal fluid
AED	antiepileptic drug	CT	computed tomography (CAT scan)
AFE	amniotic fluid embolus	CVA	cerebrovascular accident
AFI	amniotic fluid index	CVAT	costovertebral angle tenderness
AFLP	acute fatty liver of pregnancy	CVD	collagen vascular disorders
AFP	α-fetoprotein	CVS	chorionic villus sampling
AGC	atypical glandular cells	CXR	chest X-ray
AIDS	acquired immunodeficiency syndrome	DA	developmental age
ALT	alanine transaminase	D&C	dilation and curettage
AMA	advanced maternal age	D&E	dilation and evacuation
AMH	anti-Mullerian hormone	DCIS	ductal carcinoma in situ
APA	antiphospholipid antibody	DES	diethylstilbestrol
AR	autosomal recessive	DEXA	dual-energy X-ray absorptiometry
ARDS	adult respiratory distress syndrome	DHEA	dehydroepiandrosterone
ART	assisted reproductive technology	DHEAS	dehydroepiandrosterone sulfate
ASC	atypical squamous cells	DHT	dihydrotestosterone
ASC-H	atypical squamous cells—cannot exclude high-grade squamous intraepithelial lesion	DIC	disseminated intravascular coagulation
ASC-US	atypical squamous cells of undetermined significance	DMPA	depot medroxyprogesterone acetate (Depo-Provera)
		DTRs	deep tendon reflexes
AST	aspartate transaminase	DUB	dysfunctional uterine bleeding
AV	arteriovenous	DVT	deep venous thrombosis
AZT	analogs—zidovudine	ECG	electrocardiogram
β-hCG	β-human chorionic gonadotropin	EDC	estimated date of confinement
BID	twice a day	EDD	estimated date of delivery
BP	blood pressure	EFW	estimated fetal weight
BPP	biophysical profile	EIF	echogenic intracardiac focus
BUN	blood urea nitrogen	ELISA	enzyme-linked immunosorbent assay
BV	bacterial vaginosis	EMB	endometrial biopsy
CAH	congenital adrenal hyperplasia	EPT	estrogen and progesterone therapy
CBC	complete blood count	ERT	estrogen replacement therapy
CCCT	clomiphene citrate challenge test	ESR	erythrocyte sedimentation rate
CF	cystic fibrosis	ET	estrogen therapy
CHF	congestive heart failure	FAS	fetal alcohol syndrome
CIN	cervical intraepithelial neoplasia	FH	fetal heart
		FHR	fetal heart rate

FIGO	International Federation of Gynecology and Obstetrics	IUFD	intrauterine fetal demise or death
FIRS	fetal immune response syndrome	IUGR	intrauterine growth restricted
FISH	fluorescent in situ hybridization	IUI	intrauterine insemination
FNA	fine-needle aspiration	IUP	intrauterine pregnancy
FSE	fetal scalp electrode	IUPC	intrauterine pressure catheter
FSH	follicle-stimulating hormone	IUT	intrauterine transfusion
FTA-ABS	fluorescent treponemal antibody absorption	IVC	inferior vena cava
		IVF	in vitro fertilization
FTP	failure to progress	IVP	intravenous pyelogram
G	gravidity	KB	Kleihauer–Betke
GA	gestational age	KOH	potassium hydroxide
GBS	group B *streptococcus*	KUB	kidneys/ureter/bladder (X-ray)
GDM	gestational diabetes mellitus	LBW	low birth weight
GFR	glomerular filtration rate	LCHAD	long-chain hydroxyacyl-CoA dehydrogenase
GH	gestational hypertension	LCIS	lobular carcinoma in situ
GI	Gastrointestinal	LDH	lactate dehydrogenase
GLT	glucose loading test	LDL	low-density lipoprotein
GnRH	gonadotropin-releasing hormone	LEEP	loop electrosurgical excision procedure
GTD	gestational trophoblastic disease	LFT	liver function test
GTT	glucose tolerance test	LGA	large for gestational age
GU	genitourinary	LGV	lymphogranuloma venereum
GUSM	genitourinary syndrome of menopause	LH	luteinizing hormone
		LIQ	lower inner quadrant
HAART	highly active antiretroviral therapy	Lletz	large loop excision of the transformation zone
Hb	hemoglobin	LMP	last menstrual period
HbH	hemoglobin H disease	LOQ	lower outer quadrant
hCG	human chorionic gonadotropin	LOT	left occiput transverse
hCS	human chorionic somatomammotropin	LSIL	low-grade squamous intraepithelial lesion
Hct	hematocrit	LTL	laparoscopic tubal ligation
HDL	high-density lipoprotein	MAO	monoamine oxidase
HELLP	hemolysis, elevated liver enzymes, low platelets	MESA	microsurgical epididymal sperm aspiration
HIV	human immunodeficiency virus	MHA-TP	microhemagglutination assay for antibodies to *Treponema pallidum*
hMG	human menopausal gonadotropin	MHT	menopause hormone therapy
HNPCC	hereditary nonpolyposis colorectal cancer syndrome	MI	myocardial infarction
HPL	human placental lactogen	MIF	müllerian inhibiting factor
HPV	human papillomavirus	MLK	myosin light-chain kinase
HRT	hormone replacement therapy	MRI	magnetic resonance imaging
HSG	hysterosalpingogram	MRKH	Mayer–Rokitansky–Küster–Hauser (syndrome)
HSIL	high-grade squamous intraepithelial lesion	MSAFP	maternal serum α-fetoprotein
HSV	herpes simplex virus	MTHFR	methyl tetrahydrofolate reductase
I&D	incision and drainage	NPV	negative predictive value
ICSI	intracytoplasmic sperm injection	NSAID	nonsteroidal anti-inflammatory drug
Ig	immunoglobulin	NST	nonstress test
IM	intramuscular	NT	nuchal translucency
INR	International Normalized Ratio	NTD	neural tube defect
ITP	idiopathic thrombocytopenic purpura		
IUD	intrauterine device		

OA	occiput anterior	SGA	small for gestational age
OCP	oral contraceptive pill	SHBG	sex hormone binding globulin
OCT	oxytocin challenge test	SIDS	sudden infant death syndrome
OI	ovulation induction	SIS	saline infusion sonogram
OP	occiput posterior	SLE	systemic lupus erythematosus
OT	occiput transverse	SNRIs	serotonin and norepinephrine reuptake inhibitors
OTC	over-the-counter		
P	parity	SSRIs	selective serotonin reuptake inhibitors
PALM-COEIN	Polyp, Adenomyosis, Leiomyoma, Malignancy and hyperplasia; Coagulopathy, Ovulatory dysfunction, Endometrial, Iatrogenic and Not yet classified	STD	sexually transmitted disease
		STI	sexually transmitted infection
		SVT	superficial vein thrombophlebitis
		TAC	transabdominal cerclage
		TAHBSO	total abdominal hysterectomy and bilateral salpingo-oophorectomy
PCOS	polycystic ovarian syndrome		
PCR	polymerase chain reaction	TENS	transcutaneous electrical nerve stimulation
PDA	patent ductus arteriosus		
PE	pulmonary embolus	TFTs	thyroid function tests (given in ch 26)
PID	pelvic inflammatory disease	TLC	total lung capacity
PMDD	premenstrual dysphoric disorder	TNM	tumor/node/metastasis
PMOF	premature ovarian failure	TOA	tubo-ovarian abscess
PMS	premenstrual syndrome	TOLAC	trial of labor after cesarean
PO	per os (by mouth)	TOV	transposition of the vessels
POCs	products of conception	TPAL	term, preterm, aborted, living
POI	primary ovarian insufficiency	TRH	thyrotropin-releasing hormone
POP-Q	Pelvic Organ Prolapse Quantification system	TSE	testicular sperm extraction (given in ch 26)
PPCM	peripartum cardiomyopathy	TSH	thyroid-stimulating hormone
PPD	purified protein derivative	TSI	thyroid-stimulating immunoglobulins
PPROM	preterm premature rupture of membranes	TSS	toxic shock syndrome
		TSST	toxic shock syndrome toxin
PPS	postpartum sterilization	TTTS	twin-to-twin transfusion syndrome
PPV	positive predictive value	UAE	uterine artery embolization
PROM	premature rupture of membranes	UG	urogenital
PSTT	placental site trophoblastic tumor	UIQ	upper inner quadrant
PT	prothrombin time	UOQ	upper outer quadrant
PTL	preterm labor	UPI	uteroplacental insufficiency
PTT	partial thromboplastin time	US	ultrasound
PTU	propylthiouracil	UTI	urinary tract infection
PUBS	percutaneous umbilical blood sampling	V/Q	ventilation/perfusion ratio
		VAIN	vaginal intraepithelial neoplasia
QD	each day	VBAC	vaginal birth after cesarean
QID	four times a day	V_D	volume of distribution
RBC	red blood cell	VDRL	Venereal Disease Research Laboratory
RDS	respiratory distress syndrome		
ROM	rupture of membranes	VIN	vulvar intraepithelial neoplasia
ROT	right occiput transverse	VMS	vasomotor symptoms
RPR	rapid plasma reagin	VSD	ventricular septal defect
SAB	spontaneous abortion	VZIG	varicella zoster immune globulin
SCC	squamous cell carcinoma	VZV	varicella zoster virus
SERM	selective estrogen receptor modulator	WBC	white blood cell

PART I OBSTETRICS

1 | Pregnancy and Prenatal Care

PREGNANCY

Pregnancy is the state of having products of conception implanted normally or abnormally in the uterus or occasionally elsewhere. It is terminated by spontaneous or elective abortion or by delivery. Myriad physiologic changes occur in a pregnant woman, affecting every organ system.

DIAGNOSIS

In a patient who has regular menstrual cycles and is sexually active, a period delayed by more than a few days to a week is suggestive of pregnancy. Even at this early stage, patients may exhibit signs and symptoms of pregnancy. On physical examination, a variety of findings indicate pregnancy (Table 1-1).

TABLE 1-1. Signs and Symptoms of Pregnancy

Signs
Bluish discoloration of vagina and cervix (Chadwick sign)
Softening and cyanosis of the cervix at or after 4 wk (Goodell sign)
Softening of the uterus after 6 wk (Ladin sign)
Breast swelling and tenderness
Development of the linea nigra from umbilicus to pubis
Telangiectasias
Palmar erythema
Symptoms
Amenorrhea
Nausea and vomiting
Breast pain
Quickening—fetal movement

Many over-the-counter (OTC) urine pregnancy tests have a high sensitivity and will be positive around the time of the missed menstrual cycle. These urine tests and the hospital laboratory serum assays test for the β subunit of human chorionic gonadotropin (β-hCG). This hormone, produced by the placenta, will rise to a peak of 100,000 mIU/mL by 10 weeks of gestation, decrease throughout the second trimester, and then level off at approximately 20,000 to 30,000 mIU/mL in the third trimester.

A viable pregnancy can be confirmed by ultrasound, which may show the gestational sac as early as 5 weeks on a transvaginal ultrasound or at a β-hCG of 1,500 to 2,000 mIU/mL. Fetal heart (FH) motion may be seen on transvaginal ultrasound as soon as 6 weeks or at a β-hCG of 5,000 to 6,000 mIU/mL.

TERMS AND DEFINITIONS

From the time of fertilization until the pregnancy is 8 weeks along (10 weeks' gestational age [GA]), the conceptus is called an **embryo**. After 8 weeks until the time of birth, it is designated a **fetus**. The term **infant** is used for the period between delivery and 1 year of age. Pregnancy is divided into trimesters. The **first trimester** lasts until 12 weeks but is also defined as up to 14 weeks' GA, the **second trimester** lasts from 12 to 14 until 24 to 28 weeks' GA, and the **third trimester** lasts from 24 to 28 weeks until delivery. An infant delivered prior to 23 to 24 weeks is considered to be **previable**, delivered between 24 and 37 weeks is considered **preterm**, and between 37 and 42 weeks is considered **term**. A pregnancy carried beyond 42 weeks is considered **postterm**.

Gravidity (G) refers to the number of times a woman has been pregnant, and **parity** (P) refers to the number of pregnancies that led to a birth at or beyond 20 weeks' GA or of an infant weighing more than 500 g. For example, a woman who has given birth to one set of twins would be a G1 P1, because a multiple gestation is considered to be just one pregnancy. A more specific designation of pregnancy outcomes divides parity into **term** and **preterm** deliveries and also adds the number of **abortuses** and the number of **living** children. This is known as the TPAL designation. Abortuses include all pregnancy losses prior to 20 weeks, both therapeutic and spontaneous, as well as ectopic pregnancies. For example, a woman who has given birth to one set of preterm twins, one term infant, and had two miscarriages would be a G4 P1-1-2-3.

The prefixes nulli-, primi-, and multi- are used with respect to gravidity and parity to refer to having 0, 1, or more than 1, respectively. For example, a woman who has been pregnant twice, one ectopic pregnancy and one full-term birth, would be multigravid and primiparous. Unfortunately, this terminology often gets misused, with individuals referring to women with a first pregnancy as primiparous, rather than nulliparous. Obstetricians also use the term **grand multip**, which refers to a woman whose parity is greater than or equal to 5.

Dating of Pregnancy

The GA of a fetus is the age in weeks and days measured from the last menstrual period (LMP). **Developmental age** (DA) or conceptional age or embryonic age is the number of weeks and days since fertilization. Because fertilization usually occurs about 14 days after the first day of the prior menstrual period, the GA is usually 2 weeks more than the DA.

Classically, the **Nagele rule** for calculating the **estimated date of confinement** (EDC), or estimated date of delivery (EDD), is to subtract 3 months from the LMP and add 7 days. Thus, a pregnancy with an LMP of January 16, 2017, would have an EDC of October 23, 2017. Exact dating uses an EDC calculated as 280 days after a certain LMP. If the date of ovulation is known, as in assisted reproductive technology, the EDC can be calculated by adding 266 days. Pregnancy dating can be confirmed and should be consistent with the examination of the uterine size at the first prenatal appointment.

With an uncertain LMP, ultrasound is often used to determine the EDC. Ultrasound has a level of uncertainty that increases during the pregnancy, but it is rarely off by more than 7% to 8% at any GA. A safe rule of thumb is that the ultrasound should not differ from LMP dating by more than 1 week in the first trimester, 2 weeks in the second trimester, and 3 weeks in the third trimester. The dating done with crown–rump length in the first half of the first trimester is probably even more accurate, to within 3 to 5 days.

Other measures used to estimate GA include pregnancy landmarks such as auscultation of the FH at 20 weeks by nonelectronic fetoscopy or at 10 weeks by Doppler ultrasound, as well as maternal awareness of fetal movement or "quickening," that usually occurs between 16 and 20 weeks.

Because ultrasound dating of pregnancy decreases in accuracy as the pregnancy progresses, determining and confirming pregnancy dating at the first interaction between a pregnant woman and the health care system is imperative. A woman who presents to the emergency department may not return for prenatal care, so dating should be confirmed at that visit. Pregnancy dating is particularly important because a number of decisions regarding care are based on accurate dating.

One such decision is whether to resuscitate a newborn at the threshold of viability, which may be at 23 or 24 weeks of gestation, depending on the institution. Another is the induction of labor at 41 weeks of gestation. Approximately 5% to 15% of women may be oligo-ovulatory, meaning they ovulate beyond the usual 14th day of the cycle. Thus, their LMP dating may overdiagnose a prolonged (≥41 weeks' gestation) or postterm pregnancy (≥42 weeks' gestation). Luckily, early verification or correction of dating can correct such misdating.

PHYSIOLOGY OF PREGNANCY

Cardiovascular

During pregnancy, **cardiac output** increases by 30% to 50%. Most increases occur during the first trimester, with the maximum being reached between 20 and 24 weeks' gestation and maintained until delivery. The increase in cardiac output is first due to an increase in stroke volume and is then maintained by an increase in heart rate as the stroke volume decreases to near prepregnancy levels by the end of the third trimester. **Systemic vascular resistance** decreases during pregnancy, resulting in a fall in arterial blood pressure. This decrease is most likely due to elevated progesterone, leading to smooth muscle relaxation. There is a decrease in systolic blood pressure of 5 to 10 mm Hg and in diastolic blood pressure of 10 to 15 mm Hg that reaches a nadir at week 24. Between 24 weeks' gestation and term, the blood pressure slowly returns to prepregnancy levels but should never exceed them.

Pulmonary

There is an increase of 30% to 40% in tidal volume (TV) during pregnancy (Fig. 1-1) despite the fact that the total lung capacity (TLC) is decreased by 5% because of the elevation of the diaphragm. This increase in V_T decreases the expiratory reserve volume by about 20%. The increase in V_T with a constant respiratory rate leads to an increase in minute ventilation of 30% to 40%, which in turn leads to an increase in alveolar (PAO_2) and arterial (PaO_2) PO_2 levels and a decrease in $PACO_2$ and $PaCO_2$ levels.

$PaCO_2$ decreases to approximately 30 mm Hg by 20 weeks' gestation from 40 mm Hg during prepregnancy. This change leads to an increased CO_2 gradient between mother and fetus and is likely caused by elevated progesterone levels that either increase the respiratory system's responsiveness to CO_2 or act as a primary stimulant. This gradient facilitates oxygen delivery to the fetus and carbon dioxide removal from the fetus. Dyspnea of pregnancy occurs in 60% to 70% of patients. This is possibly secondary to decreased $PaCO_2$ levels, increased V_T, or decreased TLC.

Gastrointestinal

Nausea and vomiting occur in more than 70% of pregnancies. This has been termed **morning sickness** even though it can occur anytime throughout the day. These symptoms have been attributed to the elevation in estrogen, progesterone, and hCG. They may also be due to hypoglycemia and can be treated with frequent snacking. The nausea and vomiting typically resolve by 14 to 16 weeks' gestation. **Hyperemesis gravidarum** refers to a severe form of morning sickness associated with weight loss (≥5% of prepregnancy weight) and ketosis.

During pregnancy, the stomach has prolonged gastric emptying times, and the gastroesophageal sphincter has decreased tone. Together, these changes lead to reflux and possibly combine with decreased esophageal tone to cause ptyalism, or spitting, during pregnancy. The large bowel also has decreased motility, which leads to increased water absorption and constipation.

Renal

The kidneys increase in size and the ureters dilate during pregnancy, which may lead to increased rates of pyelonephritis. The glomerular filtration rate (GFR) increases by 50% early in pregnancy and is maintained until delivery. As a result of increased GFR, blood urea nitrogen and creatinine decrease by about 25%. An increase in the renin–angiotensin system leads to increased levels of aldosterone, which results in increased sodium resorption. However, plasma levels of sodium do not increase because of the simultaneous increase in GFR.

Hematology

Although the plasma volume increases by 50% in pregnancy, the RBC volume increases by only 20% to 30%, which leads to a decrease in the hematocrit or dilutional anemia. The WBC count increases during pregnancy to a mean of 10.5 million/mL with a range of 6 to 16 million. During labor, stress may cause the WBC count to rise to over 20 million/mL. There is a slight decrease in the concentration of platelets, probably secondary to increased plasma volume and an increase in peripheral destruction. Although in 7% to 8% of patients, the platelet count may be between 100 and 150 million/mL, a drop in the platelet count below 100 million/mL over a short time is not normal and should be investigated promptly.

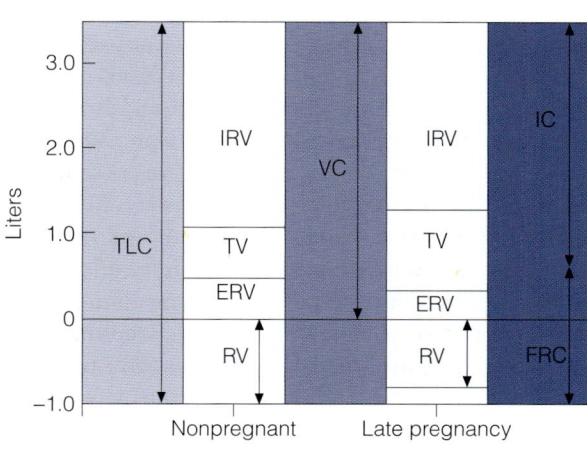

TLC–total lung capacity
VC–vital capacity
IC–inspiratory capacity
FRC–functional residual capacity
IRV–inspiratory reserve volume
TV–tidal volume
ERV–expiratory reserve volume
RV–residual volume

FIGURE 1-1. Lung volumes in nonpregnant and pregnant women.

Pregnancy is considered to be a hypercoagulable state with an increase in the number of thromboembolic events. There are elevations in the levels of fibrinogen and factors VII–X. However, the actual clotting and bleeding times do not change. The increased rate of thromboembolic events in pregnancy may also be secondary to the other elements of Virchow triad, that is, an increase in venous stasis and vessel endothelial damage.

Endocrine

Pregnancy is a hyperestrogenic state. The increased estrogen is produced primarily by the placenta, with the ovaries contributing to a lesser degree. Unlike estrogen production in the ovaries, where estrogen precursors are produced in ovarian theca cells and transferred to the ovarian granulosa cells, estrogen in the placenta is derived from circulating plasma-borne precursors produced by the maternal adrenal glands. Fetal well-being has been correlated with maternal serum estrogen levels, with low estrogen levels being associated with conditions such as fetal death and anencephaly.

The hormone hCG is composed of two dissimilar α and β subunits. The α subunit of hCG is identical to the α subunits of luteinizing hormone (LH), follicle-stimulating hormone (FSH), and thyroid-stimulating hormone (TSH), whereas the β subunits differ. The levels of hCG double approximately every 48 hours during early pregnancy, reaching a peak at approximately 10 to 12 weeks, and thereafter declining to reach a steady state after week 15.

The placenta produces hCG, which acts to maintain the corpus luteum in early pregnancy. The corpus luteum produces progesterone, which maintains the endometrium. Eventually, the placenta takes over progesterone production, and the corpus luteum degrades into the corpus albicans. Progesterone levels increase over the course of pregnancy. Progesterone causes relaxation of smooth muscle, which has multiple effects on the gastrointestinal, cardiovascular, and genitourinary systems. **Human placental lactogen** (hPL) is produced in the placenta and is important for ensuring a constant nutrient supply to the fetus. hPL, also known as human chorionic somatomammotropin (hCS), induces lipolysis with a concomitant increase in circulating free fatty acids. hPL also acts as an insulin antagonist, along with various other placental hormones, thereby having a diabetogenic effect. This leads to increased levels of insulin and protein synthesis. The levels of **prolactin** are markedly increased during pregnancy. These levels decrease after delivery but later increase in response to suckling.

There are two major changes in thyroid hormones during pregnancy. First, estrogen stimulates thyroid binding globulin, leading to an elevation in total T_3 and T_4, but free T_3 and T_4 remain relatively constant. Second, hCG has a weak stimulating effect on the thyroid, likely because its α subgroup is similar to TSH. This leads to a slight increase in T_3 and T_4 and a slight decrease in TSH early in pregnancy. Overall, however, pregnancy is considered a euthyroid state.

Musculoskeletal and Dermatologic

The obvious change in the center of gravity during pregnancy can lead to a shift in posture and lower back strain, which worsens throughout pregnancy, particularly during the third trimester. Numerous changes occur in the skin, including spider angiomata and palmar erythema secondary to increased estrogen levels, and hyperpigmentation of the nipples, umbilicus, abdominal midline (the **linea nigra**), perineum, and face (**melasma** or **chloasma**) secondary to increased levels of the melanocyte-stimulating hormones and the steroid hormones. Pregnancy is also associated with carpal tunnel syndrome, which results from compression of the median nerve. The incidence in pregnancy varies greatly, and symptoms are usually self-limited.

Nutrition

Nutritional requirements increase during pregnancy and breastfeeding. An average woman requires 2,000 to 2,500 kcal/day. The caloric requirement is increased by 300 kcal/day during pregnancy and by 500 kcal/day when breastfeeding. Thus, pregnancy is not the caloric equivalent of eating for two; more accurately, it is approximately eating for 1.15. Most patients should gain between 20 and 30 lb during pregnancy. Overweight women are advised to gain less, between 15 and 25 lb; underweight women are advised to gain more, 28 to 40 lb. Unfortunately, a large proportion of women gain more than the recommended amount, which contributes to a number of complications in pregnancy plus postpartum weight retention and downstream obesity. It is the responsibility of each prenatal care provider to review diet and exercise during pregnancy.

In addition to the increased caloric requirements, there are increased nutritional requirements for protein, iron, folate, calcium, and other vitamins and minerals. The protein requirement increases from 60 to 70 or 75 g/day. Recommended calcium intake is 1.5 g/day. Many patients develop iron deficiency anemia because of the increased demand on hematopoiesis both by the mother and by the fetus. Folate requirements increase from 0.4 to 0.8 mg/day and are important in preventing neural tube defects.

TABLE 1-2. Recommended Daily Dietary Allowances for Nonpregnant, Pregnant, and Lactating Women

	Nonpregnant Women by Age					Pregnant Women	Lactating Women
	11–14 y	15–18 y	19–22 y	23–50 y	51+ y		
Energy (kcal)	2,400	2,100	2,100	2,000	1,800	+300	+500
Protein (g)	44	48	46	46	46	+30	+20
Fat-soluble vitamins	800	800	800	800	800	1,000	1,200
Vitamin A activity (RE) (IU)	4,000	4,000	4,000	4,000	4,000	5,000	6,000
Vitamin D (IU)	400	400	400	–	–	400	400
Vitamin E activity (IU)	12	12	12	12	12	15	15
Water-soluble vitamins							
Ascorbic acid (mg)	45	45	45	45	45	60	80
Folacin (mg)	400	400	400	400	400	800	600
Niacin (mg)	16	14	14	13	12	+2	+4
Riboflavin (mg)	1.3	1.4	1.4	1.2	1.1	+0.3	+0.5
Thiamin (mg)	1.2	1.1	1.1	1	1	+0.3	+0.3
Vitamin B_6 (mg)	1.6	2	2	2	2	2.5	2.5
Vitamin B_{12} (mg)	3	3	3	3	3	4	4
Minerals							
Calcium (mg)	1,200	1,200	800	800	800	1,200	1,200
Iodine (mg)	115	115	100	100	80	125	150
Iron (mg)	18	18	18	18	10	+18	18
Magnesium (mg)	300	300	300	300	300	450	450
Phosphorus (mg)	1,200	1,200	800	800	800	1,200	1,200
Zinc (mg)	15	15	15	15	15	20	25

IU, international unit. (From Gabbe SG, Niebyl JR, Simpson JL. *Obstetrics: Normal and Problem Pregnancies,* 4th ed. New York, NY: Churchill Livingstone; 2002:196.)

All patients are advised to take prenatal vitamins during pregnancy. These are designed to compensate for the increased nutritional demands of pregnancy. Furthermore, any patient whose hematocrit falls during pregnancy is advised to increase iron intake with oral supplementation (Table 1-2).

PRENATAL CARE

Prenatal visits are designed to screen for various complications of pregnancy and to educate the patient. They include a series of outpatient office visits that involve routine physical examinations and various screening tests that occur at different points in the prenatal care. Important issues of prenatal care include initial patient evaluation, routine patient evaluation, safety and housing, nutrition and food security, disease states during the pregnancy, and preparing for the delivery.

INITIAL VISIT

This is often the longest of the prenatal visits because it involves obtaining a complete history and performing a physical examination as well as a battery of initial laboratory tests. It should occur early in the first trimester, between 6 and 10 weeks, although occasionally patients will not present for their initial prenatal visit until later in their pregnancy. At this visit, diet, exercise, and weight gain goals should also be discussed.

History

The patient's history includes the present pregnancy, the LMP, and symptoms during the pregnancy. After this, an obstetric history of prior pregnancies, including date, outcome (e.g., spontaneous abortion [SAB], therapeutic abortion, ectopic pregnancy, and term delivery), mode of delivery, length of time in labor and second stage, birth weight, and any complications, should be obtained. Finally, a complete medical, surgical, family, and social history should be obtained.

Physical Examination

A complete physical examination is performed, paying particular attention to the patient's prior medical and surgical history. The pelvic examination includes a Pap smear according to standard cervical cancer screening guidelines and cultures for gonorrhea and chlamydia. On bimanual examination, the size of the uterus should be consistent with the GA from the LMP. If a woman is unsure of her LMP or if size and dates are not consistent, one should obtain an ultrasound for dating. Accurate dating is crucial for all subsequent obstetric evaluations and interventions.

Diagnostic Evaluation

The panel of tests in the first trimester includes a complete blood count, primarily for hematocrit, blood type, antibody screen, rapid plasma reagin (RPR) or Venereal Disease Research Laboratory (VDRL) screening for syphilis, rubella antibody screen, hepatitis B surface antigen, urinalysis, and urine culture. If a patient has no history of chickenpox, a titer for varicella zoster virus (VZV) antibodies is sent. A purified protein derivative (PPD) is usually placed during the first or second trimester to screen for tuberculosis in high-risk patients. A urine pregnancy test should be sent if the patient is not entirely certain she is pregnant. If there has been any bleeding or cramping, a serum β-hCG level should be obtained. Although there is some debate over the use of routine toxoplasma titers, they are often ordered as well. All patients are counseled about HIV, and testing should be offered routinely (Table 1-3). In addition, first-trimester screening tests for aneuploidy with nuchal translucency (NT) by ultrasound and serum markers are increasingly being obtained in most women via referral to a prenatal diagnosis unit. In addition to this battery of tests, there are a variety of other screens offered to high-risk patients (Table 1-4).

ROUTINE PRENATAL VISITS

Blood pressure, weight, urine dipstick, measurement of the uterus, and auscultation of the FH are performed and assessed on each follow-up prenatal care visit. Maternal blood pressure decreases during the first and second trimesters and slowly returns to baseline during the third trimester; elevation may be a sign of preeclampsia. Maternal weight is followed serially throughout the pregnancy as a proxy for adequate nutrition. Also, large weight gains toward the end of pregnancy can be a sign of fluid retention and preeclampsia. Measurement of the uterine fundal height in centimeters corresponds roughly to the weeks of gestation. If the fundal height is progressively decreasing or is 3 cm less than GA, an ultrasound is

TABLE 1-3. Routine Tests in Prenatal Care

Initial Visit and First Trimester	Second Trimester	Third Trimester
Hematocrit	MSAFP/triple or quad screen	Hematocrit
Blood type and screen	Obstetric ultrasound	RPR/VDRL
RPR/VDRL	Amniocentesis for women interested in prenatal diagnosis	GLT
Rubella antibody screen		Group B streptococcal culture
Hepatitis B surface antigen		
Gonorrhea culture		
Chlamydia culture		
PPD		
Pap smear		
Urinalysis and culture		
VZV titer in patients with no history of exposure		
HIV offered		
Early screening for aneuploidy (NT plus serum markers)		

GLT, glucose loading test; MSAFP, maternal serum alpha fetoprotein; NT, nuchal translucency; PPD, purified protein derivative; RPR, rapid plasma reagin; VZV, varicella zoster virus.

TABLE 1-4. Initial Screens in Specific High-Risk Groups

High-Risk Group	Specific Test
African American, Southeast Asian	Sickle cell prep for African Americans; Hgb electrophoresis for both
Family history of genetic disorder (e.g., hemophilia, sickle cell disease, fragile X syndrome), maternal age 35 or older at time of EDC	Prenatal genetics referral
Prior gestational diabetes, family history of diabetes, Hispanic, Native American, Southeast Asian, obese	Early GLT
Pregestational diabetes, unsure dates, recurrent miscarriages	Dating sonogram at first visit
Hypertension, renal disease, pregestational diabetic, prior preeclampsia, renal transplant, Systemic Lupus Erythematosus	Blood Urea Nitrogen, Cr, uric acid, and 24-h urine collection for protein and creatinine clearance (to establish a baseline)
Pregestational diabetes, prior cardiac disease, hypertension	ECG
Pregestational diabetes	Hgb A1C, ophthalmology for eye examination
Graves disease	Thyroid-stimulating immunoglobulins (can cause fetal disease)
All thyroid disease	TSH, possibly free T_4
PPD+	Chest X-ray after 16 wk's gestation
SLE	AntiRho, antiLa antibodies (can cause fetal complete heart block)

EDC, estimated date of confinement; GLT, glucose loading test; PPD, purified protein derivative; TSH, thyroid-stimulating hormone.

done to more accurately assess fetal growth. After 10 to 14 weeks, Doppler ultrasound is used to auscultate the fetal heart rate (FHR). Urine is routinely dipped for protein, glucose, blood, and leukocyte esterase. The presence of protein may be indicative of preeclampsia, glucose of diabetes, and leukocyte esterase of urinary tract infection (UTI). Pregnant women are at an increased risk for complicated UTIs such as pyelonephritis, given increased urinary stasis from mechanical compression of the ureters and progesterone-mediated smooth muscle relaxation.

At each visit, the patient is asked about symptoms that indicate complications of pregnancy. These symptoms include vaginal bleeding, vaginal discharge or leaking of fluid, and urinary symptoms. In addition, after 20 weeks, patients are asked about contractions and fetal movement. Vaginal bleeding is a sign of possible miscarriage or ectopic pregnancy in the first trimester and of placental abruption or previa as the pregnancy advances. Vaginal discharge may be a sign of infection or cervical change, whereas leaking fluid can indicate ruptured fetal membranes. While irregular (Braxton Hicks) contractions are common throughout the third trimester, regular contractions occurring more frequently than five or six per hour may be a sign of preterm labor and should be assessed. Changes in or the absence of fetal movement should be evaluated by auscultation of the FH in the previable fetus and with further testing such as a nonstress test (NST) or biophysical profile (BPP) in the viable fetus.

First-Trimester Visits

During the first trimester, patients—particularly nulliparous women—need to be familiarized with pregnancy. The symptoms of pregnancy and what will occur at each prenatal visit should be reviewed. At the second prenatal visit, all of the initial laboratory test results should be reviewed with the patient. Those with poor weight gain or decreased caloric intake secondary to nausea and vomiting may be referred to a nutritionist. Patients treated for infections noted at the initial prenatal visit should be cultured for test of cure. Additionally, early screening for aneuploidy, either combined screening with an ultrasound for NT and serum levels of pregnancy-associated plasma protein A and free β-hCG, or with a blood test to assess the relative quantity of fetal DNA (cell-free DNA) for chromosomes 13, 18, and 21, is offered between 11 and 13 weeks of gestation to all women. Of note, the tradeoffs between combined first trimester screening and the new cfDNA screening are evolving and controversial.

Second-Trimester Visits
During the second trimester, much of the screening for genetic and congenital abnormalities is done. This allows a patient to obtain an elective termination if there are abnormalities. Screening for **maternal serum alpha fetoprotein** (MSAFP) is usually performed between 15 and 18 weeks. An elevation in MSAFP is correlated with an increased risk of neural tube defects, and a decrease is seen in some aneuploidies, including Down syndrome. The sensitivity of aneuploidy screening is augmented using β-hCG and estriol along with MSAFP, called the **triple screen**. The addition of inhibin A to this screening test further enhances the ability to detect abnormalities and is known as the **quad screen**. Between 18 and 20 weeks' gestation, most patients are offered a screening ultrasound. This provides the opportunity to screen for common fetal abnormalities. Also noted are the amniotic fluid volume, placental location, and GA.

Historically, these maternal analytes combined with ultrasound were the only options for genetic screening. However, an alternative is now available and is being offered to patients with increasing frequency. Cell Free DNA (cfDNA) is a noninvasive test which identifies cfDNA from the fetal-placental unit which is found in the maternal circulation. This circulating DNA can be detected as early as 5 weeks gestation and increases in relative concentration with advancing gestational age. Prenatal screening for trisomy 21, trisomy 18, trisomy 13 and sex chromosome aneuploidies is now widely available using next-generation sequencing of cfDNA. The cfDNA offers an increased detection rate and a lower false positive rate than the maternal analyte screening though it is important to remember that these remain screening and not diagnostic tests.

The FH is usually first heard during the second trimester, as is the first fetal movement, or "quickening," felt usually between 16 and 20 weeks' GA. Most patients have resolution of their nausea and vomiting by the second trimester, although some continue with these symptoms throughout their pregnancy. Because the risk of SABs decreases after 12 weeks of gestation, childbirth classes and tours of the labor floor are usually offered in the second and third trimesters.

Third-Trimester Visits
During the third trimester, the fetus is viable. Patients will begin to have occasional Braxton Hicks contractions and, if these contractions become regular, the cervix is examined to rule out preterm labor. Prenatal visits increase to every 2 to 3 weeks from 28 to 36 weeks and then to every week after 36 weeks. In addition, patients who are Rh negative should receive RhoGAM at 28 weeks. Beyond 32 to 34 weeks, Leopold maneuvers (see Fig. 3-1) are performed to determine fetal presentation. Either as a routine or if there is any question, an office ultrasound may be used at 35 to 36 weeks to confirm fetal presentation. In the setting of breech presentation, women are offered external cephalic version of the fetus at 37 to 38 weeks of gestation.

Beyond 37 weeks, which is considered term, the cervix is usually examined at each visit. Because a vigorous examination of the cervix, known as "sweeping" or "stripping" the membranes, has been demonstrated to decrease the probability of progressing postterm or requiring an induction of labor, this is commonly offered at all term pregnancy prenatal visits.

Third-Trimester Laboratory Test Results
At 27 to 29 weeks, the third-trimester laboratory test results are ordered. These consist of the hematocrit, RPR/VDRL, and **glucose loading test** (GLT). At this time, the hematocrit is getting close to its nadir. Patients with a hematocrit below 32% to 33% (hemoglobin <11 mg/dL) are usually started on iron supplementation. Because this will cause further constipation, stool softeners are given in conjunction. The GLT is a screening test for gestational diabetes. It consists of giving a 50-g oral glucose loading dose and checking serum glucose 1 hour later. If this value is greater than or equal to 140 mg/dL, a **glucose tolerance test** (GTT) is administered, although some institutions use a lower threshold of 130 or 135 mg/dL.

The GTT is the diagnostic test for gestational diabetes. It consists of a fasting serum glucose measurement and then administration of a 100-g oral glucose loading dose. The serum glucose is then measured at 1, 2, and 3 hours after the oral dose is given. This test is indicative of gestational diabetes if there is an elevation in two or more of the following threshold values: the fasting glucose, 95 mg/dL; 1 hour, 180 mg/dL; 2 hour, 155 mg/dL; or 3 hour, 140 mg/dL.

In high-risk populations, vaginal cultures for gonorrhea and chlamydia are repeated late in the third trimester. These infections are transmitted vertically during birth and should be treated if cultures or DNA tests return positive. In women with latent herpes simplex virus (HSV), antiviral prophylaxis can be initiated at 36 weeks. Active HSV would be an indication for cesarean delivery. At 36 weeks, screening for group B streptococcal infection is also performed. Patients who have a positive culture should be treated with intravenous penicillin when they present in labor to prevent potential neonatal group B streptococcal infection.

ROUTINE PROBLEMS OF PREGNANCY

BACK PAIN

During pregnancy, low back pain is quite common, particularly in the third trimester when the patient's center of gravity has shifted and there is an increased strain on the lower back. Mild exercise—particularly stretching—may release endorphins and reduce the amount of back pain. Gentle massage, heating pads, and Tylenol can be used for mild pain. For patients with severe back pain, muscle relaxants or, occasionally, narcotics can be used. Physical therapy can also be helpful in these patients.

CONSTIPATION

The decreased bowel motility secondary to elevated progesterone levels leads to increased transit time in the large bowel. In turn, there is greater absorption of water from the gastrointestinal tract. This can result in constipation. Increased oral (PO) fluids, particularly water, should be recommended. In addition, stool softeners or bulking agents may help. Laxatives can be used, but are usually avoided in the third trimester because of the theoretical risk of preterm labor.

CONTRACTIONS

Occasional irregular contractions that do not lead to cervical change are considered Braxton Hicks contractions and will occur several times per day up to several times per hour. Patients should be warned about these and assured that they are normal. Dehydration may cause increased contractions, and patients should be advised to drink many (10 to 14) glasses of water per day. Regular contractions, as often as every 10 minutes, should be considered a sign of preterm labor and should be assessed by cervical examination. If a patient has had several days of contractions and no documented cervical change, this is reassuring to both the obstetrician and the patient that delivery is not imminent.

DEHYDRATION

Because of the expanded intravascular space and increased third spacing of fluid, patients have a difficult time maintaining their intravascular volume status. Dietary recommendations should include increased fluids. As mentioned above, dehydration may lead to uterine contractions, possibly secondary to cross-reaction of vasopressin with oxytocin receptors.

EDEMA

Compression of the inferior vena cava (IVC) and pelvic veins by the uterus can lead to increased hydrostatic pressure in the lower extremities and eventually to edema in the feet and ankles. Elevation of the lower extremities above the heart can ease this. Also, patients should be advised to sleep on their sides to decrease compression. Severe edema of the face and hands may be indicative of preeclampsia and merits further evaluation.

GASTROESOPHAGEAL REFLUX DISEASE

Relaxation of the lower esophageal sphincter and increased transit time in the stomach can lead to reflux and nausea. Patients with reflux should be started on antacids, advised to eat multiple small meals per day, and should avoid lying down within an hour of eating. For patients with continued symptoms, H_2 blockers or proton pump inhibitors can be given.

HEMORRHOIDS

Patients will have increased venous stasis and IVC compression, leading to congestion in the venous system. Congestion of the pelvic vessels combined with increased abdominal pressure with bowel movements secondary to constipation can lead to hemorrhoids. Hemorrhoids are treated symptomatically with topical anesthetics and steroids for pain and swelling. Prevention of constipation with increased fluids, increased fiber in the diet, and stool softeners may prevent or decrease the exacerbation of hemorrhoids.

PICA

Rarely, a patient will have cravings for inedible items such as dirt or clay. As long as these substances are nontoxic, the patient is advised to maintain adequate nutrition and encouraged to stop ingesting the inedible items. However, if the patient has been consuming toxic substances, immediate cessation along with a toxicology consult is advised.

ROUND LIGAMENT PAIN

Usually late in the second trimester or early in the third trimester, there may be some pain in the adnexa, lower abdomen, or groin. This pain is likely secondary to the rapid expansion of the uterus and stretching of the ligamentous attachments, such as the round ligaments. This is often self-limited but may be relieved with warm compresses or acetaminophen.

URINARY FREQUENCY

Increased intravascular volumes and elevated GFR can lead to increased urine production during pregnancy. However, the most likely cause of urinary frequency during pregnancy is increasing compression of the bladder by the growing uterus. A UTI may also be present with isolated urinary frequency but is often accompanied by dysuria. A urinalysis and culture should therefore be ordered to rule out infection. If no infection is present, patients can be assured that the increased voiding is normal. Patients should be advised to keep up PO hydration despite urinary frequency.

VARICOSE VEINS

The lower extremities or the vulva may develop varicosities during pregnancy. The relaxation of the venous smooth muscle and increased intravascular pressure, probably both, contribute to the pathogenesis. Elevation of the lower extremities or the use of pressure stockings may help reduce existing varicosities and prevent more from developing. If the problem does not resolve by 6 months postpartum, patients may be referred for surgical therapy.

PRENATAL ASSESSMENT OF THE FETUS

Throughout pregnancy, the fetus is screened and diagnosed by a variety of modalities. Parents can be screened for common diseases such as cystic fibrosis, Tay–Sachs disease, sickle cell disease, and thalassemia. If both parents are carriers of recessive genetic diseases, the fetus can then be diagnosed. Fetal karyotype and genetic screens can be obtained via amniocentesis or chorionic villus sampling (CVS). The fetus can be imaged and many of the congenital anomalies diagnosed via second-trimester ultrasound. First- and second-trimester genetic screening and prenatal diagnosis is discussed further in Chapter 3. Other fetal testing includes fetal blood sampling, fetal lung maturity testing, and assessment of fetal well-being.

ULTRASOUND

Ultrasound can be used to date a pregnancy with an unknown or uncertain LMP and is most accurate in the first trimester. To detect fetal malformations, most patients undergo a routine screening ultrasound at 18 to 20 weeks. Routinely, an attempt is made to identify placental location, amniotic fluid volume, GA, and any obvious malformations. Of note, most patients will think of this ultrasound as the time to find out the fetal sex. Although determination of fetal sex is medically indicated in some settings (e.g., history of fragile X syndrome or other X-linked disorders), it is not necessarily a part of the routine level I obstetric ultrasound. It is useful to clarify this point with patients to establish proper expectations for the ultrasound.

In high-risk patients, careful attention is paid to commonly associated anomalies such as cardiac anomalies in pregestational diabetics. Fetal echocardiography and, rarely, MRI are used to augment assessment of the FH and brain, respectively.

In the third trimester, ultrasound can be used to monitor high-risk pregnancies by obtaining **biophysical profiles** (BPP), fetal growth, and fetal Doppler studies. The BPP looks at the following five categories and gives a score of either 0 or 2 for each: amniotic fluid volume, fetal tone, fetal activity, fetal breathing movements, and the **nonstress test** (NST), which is a test of the FHR. A BPP of 8 to 10 or better is reassuring. Ultrasound with Doppler flow studies can also be used to assess the blood flow in the umbilical cord. A decrease, absence, or reversal of diastolic flow in the umbilical artery is progressively more worrisome for placental insufficiency and resultant fetal compromise.

ANTENATAL TESTING OF FETAL WELL-BEING

Formal antenatal testing includes the NST, the oxytocin challenge test (OCT), and the BPP. The NST is considered formally reactive (a reassuring sign) if there are two accelerations of the FHR in 20 minutes that are at least 15 beats above the baseline heart rate and last for at least 15 seconds. An OCT or contraction stress test (CST) is obtained by getting at least three contractions in 10 minutes and analyzing the FHR tracing during that time. The reactivity criteria are the same as for the NST. In addition, late decelerations with at least half of the contractions constitute a positive test and are worrisome. Commonly, most antenatal testing units use the NST, beginning at 32 to 34 weeks of gestation in high-risk pregnancies and at 40 to 41 weeks for undelivered patients. If the NST is nonreactive, the fetus is assessed via ultrasound. If the FH tracing has any worrisome decelerations or the BPP is not reassuring, an OCT is usually performed or, in more severe cases, consideration is given to delivery.

FETAL BLOOD SAMPLING

Percutaneous umbilical blood sampling (PUBS) is performed by placing a needle transabdominally into the uterus and phlebotomizing the umbilical cord. This procedure may be used when the fetal hematocrit needs to be obtained, particularly in the setting of Rh isoimmunization, other causes of fetal anemia, and hydrops. PUBS is also used for fetal transfusion, karyotype analysis, and assessment of fetal platelet count in alloimmune thrombocytopenia.

FETAL LUNG MATURITY

To test for fetal lung maturity, an amniotic fluid sample obtained through amniocentesis is analyzed. Classically, the lecithin to sphingomyelin (L/S) ratio has been used as a predictor of fetal lung maturity. Type II pneumocytes secrete a surfactant that uses phospholipids in its synthesis. Commonly, lecithin increases as the lungs mature, whereas sphingomyelin decreases beyond about 32 weeks. The L/S ratio should therefore increase as the pregnancy progresses. Repetitive studies have shown that an L/S ratio of greater than 2 is associated with only rare cases of **respiratory distress syndrome** (RDS). Other fetal lung maturity tests include measuring the levels of phosphatidylglycerol, saturated phosphatidyl choline, the presence of lamellar body count, and surfactant to albumin ratio.

KEY POINTS

- A urine pregnancy test will often be positive at the time of the missed menstrual cycle.
- Physiologic changes during pregnancy, mediated by the placental hormones, affect every organ system.
- Cardiovascular changes include a decrease in systemic vascular resistance and blood pressure and an increase in cardiac output.
- The initial prenatal visit is designed to screen for many of the problems that can occur in pregnancy and to verify dating of the pregnancy.
- Much of the screening for genetic and congenital abnormalities is performed in the second trimester.
- Blood pressure, weight gain, fundal height, FHR, and symptoms such as contractions, vaginal bleeding or discharge, and perceived fetal movement are assessed at each prenatal visit.
- Many of the routine problems of pregnancy are related to hormonal effects of the placenta.
- It is important to discuss the side effects of pregnancy in order to best prepare the patient.
- Although pregnancy is often the cause of many somatic complaints, other causes should still be ruled out as in a nonpregnant patient.
- Common screening tests for fetal abnormalities include MSAFP and the triple screen.
- The fetus may be diagnosed for abnormalities, using amniocentesis, CVS, and ultrasound.
- Fetal status can be assessed antepartum with ultrasound, NST, BPP, and OCT.

CLINICAL VIGNETTES

VIGNETTE 1

A 27-year-old woman comes to your practice desiring pregnancy. She has a history of regular, 28-day cycles and has been using oral birth control pills for contraception. She has had two pregnancies in the past, one ending in miscarriage at 9 weeks and one vaginal delivery at 39 weeks. Her last Pap smear was 10 months ago, and she has never had an irregular Pap. She is not taking any medications and has no known medical allergies.

1. On the basis of this woman's obstetric history, find out her TPAL designation.
   a. G3P1011
   b. G3P2001
   c. G2P1011
   d. G2P1101
   e. G1P1001

2. Nutritional supplements she should begin before she gets pregnant include which of the following:
   a. Folate to reduce neural tube defects
   b. Vitamin B_{12} to increase RBC production prior to pregnancy
   c. Vitamin B_1 to reduce beriberi
   d. Vitamin C to reduce scurvy
   e. No supplementation is necessary until pregnancy is confirmed

3. Before leaving your office, she asks how reliable OTC pregnancy tests are and how quickly after conceiving she should expect to test positive. You inform her that:
   a. urine pregnancy tests are notoriously unreliable and that she should come in for blood tests if she thinks she is pregnant

b. OTC tests have high sensitivity for hPL and will be positive around the time of the missed menstrual cycle
   c. OTC tests have high sensitivity for β-hCG and will be positive around the time of the missed period
   d. OTC tests have high specificity, but low sensitivity, so she should repeat the test twice at home to confirm the results
   e. OTC tests are typically positive the day after conception

4. She returns to your office 2 months later pregnant. Her initial prenatal visit should include:
   a. quad screen
   b. abdominal ultrasound
   c. pelvic examination
   d. titer for HSV
   e. Leopold maneuvers

VIGNETTE 2

A 33-year-old G0P0 woman comes to your office for her initial prenatal visit. She tested positive with two home pregnancy tests and has been experiencing breast tenderness and mild nausea for a few weeks. She has a history of regular menstrual periods occurring every 28 to 30 days. This was a planned pregnancy and is the first child for her and for her partner.

1. Your patient was actively tracking her menstrual cycle and is certain that the first day of her LMP was December 2, 2017. Using Nägele rule, estimate her date of delivery.
   a. July 5, 2018
   b. September 2, 2018
   c. September 16, 2018
   d. September 9, 2018
   e. August 26, 2018

2. As her pregnancy continues, you would expect her cardiac output to increase by which of the following mechanisms:
   a. First, an increase in stroke volume, then an increase in heart rate
   b. A decrease in systemic vascular resistance
   c. Cardiac output would not change significantly until the third trimester
   d. An increase in systemic vascular resistance facilitated by elevated progesterone levels
   e. Increased heart rate alone

3. Which of the following is true regarding the physiologic changes she might expect during her pregnancy?
   a. Gastric emptying and large bowel motility are increased in pregnancy
   b. BUN and creatinine will decrease by 25% as a result of an increase in GFR, which will be maintained until delivery
   c. An overall decrease in the number of WBC and platelets
   d. Nausea and vomiting that should be treated aggressively with antiemetics and intravenous hydration
   e. An increase in the tidal volume along with an increase in TLC

4. Which of the following is true regarding hCG in your patient?
   a. The corpus luteum produces hCG throughout pregnancy
   b. It is composed of two dissimilar α and β units
   c. Levels double every 3 to 4 days in early pregnancy
   d. Levels peak after 24 weeks of pregnancy
   e. The α subunits are identical to subunits of prolactin and human growth hormone

5. The major function of hPL is:
   a. To cause a diuretic effect
   b. To cause relaxation of smooth muscle
   c. To maintain the corpus luteum in early pregnancy
   d. To act as an insulin agonist
   e. To induce lipolysis and protein synthesis leading to a constant nutrient supply to the fetus

VIGNETTE 3

A 36-year-old G1P0 is 31 weeks and 5 days by LMP and is sure of her dates. Her pregnancy has been complicated by persistent nausea and vomiting, back pain, and lower extremity swelling. She comes to you for a routine prenatal visit. She had a quad screen at 16 weeks that was normal. She is having a girl.

1. On this visit, her urine is assessed for the presence of protein, glucose, blood, and leukocyte esterase. Which of the following results would be most concerning?
   a. Absent leukocyte esterase
   b. Negative glucose
   c. Trace blood
   d. 4+ protein
   e. Leukocyte esterase positive

2. Her low back pain is no longer relieved with a heating pad, and she finds that she needs pain relief to make it through each work day. Which of the following options would be safest for her?
   a. Ibuprofen
   b. Aspirin
   c. Oxycodone
   d. Flexeril
   e. Tylenol

3. Her nausea and vomiting has extended past the first trimester when most women stop experiencing these symptoms. What would suggest that she has hyperemesis gravidarum?
   a. Less than 5% loss of prepregnancy weight
   b. Jaundice

c. Syncopal episodes
d. Ketonuria
e. Metabolic acidosis

4. She has started experiencing lower abdominal pain and tightening that occurs infrequently (1 to 2 times per hour) and irregularly. This is most likely:
   a. a preterm labor
   b. round ligament pain
   c. Braxton Hicks contractions
   d. an indication of fetal distress
   e. related to constipation

VIGNETTE 4

A G3P2002 woman at 35 weeks is seen in your office for her prenatal visit. She is concerned because she has not felt her baby moving as much as she used to. Her pregnancy has been uncomplicated, and her past two pregnancies ended in full term, normal spontaneous vaginal deliveries.

1. A BPP is done to assess which of the following?
   a. Diastolic flow in the umbilical artery
   b. Lung maturity
   c. Blood flow in the middle cerebral artery
   d. Fetal well-being
   e. Genetic abnormalities

2. An indication for early delivery is identified, but first a test for fetal lung maturity is done. Which of the following is true?
   a. Type I pneumocytes secrete surfactant
   b. A L/S ratio greater than 2 is ideal if an early delivery is indicated
   c. A low L/S ratio is associated with fewer cases of RDS
   d. Typically, lecithin decreases as the lung matures
   e. Sphingomyelin decreases beyond 24 weeks

3. When formal antenatal testing is done, which of the following is most reassuring?
   a. Late decelerations on fetal monitoring
   b. A CST with variable FHR decelerations with contractions, but moderate variability
   c. A NST with two accelerations of the FHR in 20 minutes that are at least 15 beats above baseline and last for at least 15 seconds
   d. An increase in the systolic to diastolic ratio in the umbilical artery blood flow
   e. A score of 6 on a BPP

ANSWERS

VIGNETTE 1 Question 1
1. Answer C:
TPAL designation is written in the following order to reflect the total number of pregnancies: term deliveries, preterm deliveries, abortions including all pregnancy losses prior to 20 weeks, and living children. She has been pregnant twice (G2) and had one term delivery leading to one living child and one spontaneous miscarriage prior to 20 weeks. Although she desires pregnancy, she is not yet pregnant, and so G3 is not correct.

VIGNETTE 1 Question 2
2. Answer A:
Women can reduce the risk of neural tube defects by taking 400 mcg folic acid supplements the month before conception and during the first trimester. The other supplements would not harm, but are not routinely recommended in the time before conception.

VIGNETTE 1 Question 3
3. Answer C:
Many OTC pregnancy tests have improved in recent decades. These are highly sensitive for urine β-hCG and are typically positive around the time of the missed menstrual cycle.

VIGNETTE 1 Question 4
4. Answer C:
A pelvic examination should be conducted, feeling for the size of the uterus, and should include a Pap smear if one has not been done in the past 6 months. Quad screen is done in the second trimester, and Leopold maneuvers are done beyond 32 to 34 weeks to determine fetal presentation. HSV treatment or prophylaxis is initiated on the basis of clinical examination or patient history and not laboratory data. Transvaginal ultrasound is typically used to date the pregnancy in initial, first-trimester visits.

VIGNETTE 2 Question 1
1. Answer D:
Nägele rule gives an EDD by subtracting 3 months and adding 7 days from the LMP.

VIGNETTE 2 Question 2
2. Answer A:
Cardiac output increases by 30% to 50% during pregnancy as a result of an increase in stroke volume and is then maintained by an increase in heart rate. Progesterone levels lead to a decrease in systemic vascular resistance, resulting in a fall in arterial blood pressure.

VIGNETTE 2 Question 3
3. Answer B:
BUN and creatinine will decrease because of a 50% increase in the GFR, which occurs early in pregnancy. Gastric emptying and large bowel motility are decreased as a result of progesterone, leading to reflux and constipation, respectively. WBCs increase in pregnancy, but an increase in plasma volume results in a decrease in the concentration of both platelets and WBCs. Nausea and vomiting is common in early pregnancy and is most often mild. These symptoms should be treated with frequent snacking and oral hydration, although some patients will require more aggressive treatment. Tidal volume increases, but TLC decreases in pregnancy.

VIGNETTE 2 Question 4
4. Answer B:
The placenta produces hCG. Levels double approximately every 48 hours in early pregnancy and peak at 10 to 12 weeks. The α subunits are identical to LH, FSH, and TSH.

VIGNETTE 2 Question 5
5. Answer E:
hPL (also known as hCS) is an insulin antagonist, and its major function is not a diuretic effect. In its role as an insulin antagonist, hCS results in decreased maternal insulin sensitivity and glucose utilization and increases lipolysis with the release of free fatty acids to ensure an adequate fetal supply. In doing so, hCS contributes to the development of gestational diabetes as well. Progesterone causes relaxation of smooth muscle, and hCG maintains the corpus luteum in early pregnancy.

VIGNETTE 3 Question 1
1. Answer D:
Leukocyte esterase and trace blood may be indicative of UTI, which could be complicated by pyelonephritis, but is treatable. Large amounts of blood could be nephrolithiasis, bladder injury, nephrotic syndrome, or even cancer. Absent glucose is normal, whereas the presence of glucose may indicate diabetes. Large amounts of protein are concerning for preeclampsia, which demands a broader assessment. While trace or 1+ protein has only a modest positive predictive value, 3+ or 4+ protein has a very high positive predictive value for significant proteinuria and deserves immediate attention.

VIGNETTE 3 Question 2
2. Answer E:
Ibuprofen and aspirin are contraindicated in pregnancy. Although NSAIDs are occasionally prescribed in the midtrimester for acute pain, in the latter part of the third trimester, they are absolutely contraindicated as they are associated with premature closure of the ductus arteriosus. Narcotics and muscle relaxants are options for patients with severe back pain, but it would be safest to start with Tylenol and gentle massage.

VIGNETTE 3 Question 3
3. Answer D:
Hyperemesis gravidarum is a severe form of morning sickness in which women lose more than 5% of their prepregnancy weight and go into ketosis. With severe vomiting, a metabolic alkalosis would be expected. Syncopal episodes may occur secondary to dehydration but are not a part of the diagnosis. Jaundice is not associated with hyperemesis gravidarum.

VIGNETTE 3 Question 4
4. Answer C:
Occasional irregular contractions that do not lead to cervical change are considered Braxton Hicks contractions and will occur several times per day up to several times per hour. Patients should be warned about these and reassured that they are normal. However, if contractions are more frequent or painful, the patient should be assessed for preterm labor.

VIGNETTE 4 Question 1
1. Answer D:
A BPP is particularly helpful in monitoring high-risk pregnancies. The BPP assesses fetal well-being using amniotic fluid volume, fetal tone, activity, breathing movements, and an NST, receiving either 0 or 2 points for each of the five categories. A score of 8 to 10 is reassuring. A BPP is often done in conjunction with fetal Doppler studies, which assess flow in the umbilical artery. Genetic abnormalities are screened for in the second trimester, using the triple or quad screen. Blood flow in the middle cerebral artery is used when evaluating for fetal anemia in the setting of Rh isoimmunization. Lung maturity is assessed through amniocentesis.

VIGNETTE 4 Question 2
2. Answer B:
An L/S ratio greater than 2 is associated with only rare cases of RDS. Type II pneumocytes secrete surfactant. Lecithin increases as the lung matures and sphingomyelin decreases beyond 32 weeks.

VIGNETTE 4 Question 3
3. Answer C:
This answer describes a formally reactive NST, which is a reassuring sign. On fetal monitoring, late FHR decelerations are concerning for uteroplacental insufficiency. Similarly, on a CST, FHR decelerations with contractions are considered nonreassuring. The fact that the decelerations are variable is a bit less worrisome, but certainly not reassuring. Decreased diastolic flow in the umbilical artery, which leads to an increased systolic to diastolic ratio, is concerning for increased placental resistance. Although a 6/10 on a BPP is not particularly worrisome, it is not formally reassuring and demands a plan for further follow-up.

2 | Early Pregnancy Complications

ECTOPIC PREGNANCY

An **ectopic pregnancy** is one that implants outside the uterine cavity. Implantation occurs in the fallopian tube in 95% to 99% of patients with an ectopic pregnancy (Fig. 2-1). The most common site of implantation in a tubal pregnancy is the ampulla (70%), followed by the isthmus (12%) and fimbriae (11%). Implantation may also occur on the ovary, the cervix, the outside of the fallopian tube, the abdominal wall, or the bowel. The incidence of ectopic pregnancies has been increasing over the past 10 years. Currently, more than 1:100 of all pregnancies are ectopic. This is thought to be secondary to the increase in assisted fertility, sexually transmitted infections(STIs), and pelvic inflammatory disease (PID). Patients who present with vaginal bleeding and/or abdominal pain should always be evaluated for ectopic pregnancy because a ruptured ectopic pregnancy is a true emergency. It can result in rapid hemorrhage, leading to shock and eventually death. Although early diagnosis and treatment of this condition has dramatically decreased the mortality risk, ruptured ectopic pregnancies are still responsible for 6% of all maternal deaths in the United States (*N Eng J Med.* 2009;361:379–387).

RISK FACTORS

Several risk factors predispose patients to extrauterine implantation (Table 2-1). Many of the risk factors commonly affect the fallopian tubes causing either tubal scarring or decreased peristalsis of the tube which may lead to abnormal implantation of a pregnancy. The strongest risk factor is a history of a prior ectopic pregnancy. The risk of a subsequent ectopic pregnancy is 10% after one prior ectopic pregnancy and increases to 25% after more than one prior ectopic pregnancy (*N Eng J Med.* 2009;361:379–387). It has been noted that there is an increased risk (up to 1.8%) of ectopic implantation in pregnancies produced by assisted reproductive technology. Whether this is primarily due to the techniques utilized or the underlying

FIGURE 2-1. Sites of ectopic pregnancies.

TABLE 2-1. Risk Factors for Ectopic Pregnancy
History of STIs or PID
Prior ectopic pregnancy
Previous tubal surgery
Prior pelvic or abdominal surgery resulting in adhesions
Endometriosis
Current use of exogenous hormones including progesterone or estrogen
IVF and other assisted reproduction
DES-exposed patients with congenital abnormalities
Use of an IUD for birth control
Smoking

DES, diethylstilbestrol; IUD, intrauterine device; IVF, in vitro fertilization; PID, pelvic inflammatory disease; STIs, sexually transmitted infections.

tubal disease and pelvic adhesions in such patients is unclear. Although use of an intrauterine device (IUD) for birth control decreases the overall rate of pregnancy, when the contraceptive fails, there is an increased rate of ectopic pregnancy in those women who become pregnant because the IUD prevents normal intrauterine implantation. This risk may be as high as 25% to 50% (*NEJM*. 2009;361:379–387).

DIAGNOSIS

The diagnosis of ectopic pregnancy is made by history, physical examination, laboratory tests, and ultrasound. On history, patients often complain of unilateral pelvic or lower abdominal pain and vaginal bleeding. Physical examination, including speculum and bimanual examination, may reveal an adnexal mass that is often tender, a uterus that is small for gestational age, and bleeding from the cervix. Patients with ruptured ectopic pregnancies may be hypotensive, tachycardic, unresponsive, or show signs of peritoneal irritation secondary to hemoperitoneum. Importantly, however, because many women with ectopic pregnancies are young and otherwise healthy, such signs of intraabdominal hemorrhage may not occur until the patient has lost a large amount of blood.

On laboratory studies, the classic finding is a beta human chorionic gonadotropin (β-hCG) level that is low for gestational age and does not increase at the expected rate. In patients with a normal **intrauterine pregnancy** (IUP), the trophoblastic tissue secretes β-hCG in a predictable manner that should lead to doubling (or at least an increase of two-thirds) approximately every 48 hours. An ectopic pregnancy has a poorly implanted placenta with less blood supply than in the endometrium, and thus levels of β-hCG do not double every 48 hours. The hematocrit may be low or may drop in patients with ruptured ectopic pregnancies.

Ultrasound may reveal an adnexal mass or an extrauterine pregnancy (Fig. 2-2). A gestational sac with a yolk sac seen in the uterus on ultrasound indicates an IUP. However, there is always a small risk of **heterotopic pregnancy**, a multiple gestation with at least one IUP and at least one ectopic pregnancy. This is of particular concern in the setting of in vitro fertilization (IVF) pregnancies when more than one embryo is transferred. At early gestations, neither an IUP nor an adnexal mass can be seen on ultrasound. A hemorrhaging, ruptured ectopic pregnancy may reveal intraabdominal fluid throughout the pelvis and abdomen.

FIGURE 2-2. Endovaginal view of a right adnexal ectopic pregnancy with a gestational sac (*large arrows*) and fetal pole (*small arrow*). The uterus is seen to the right of the image, with a small amount of endometrial fluid (*hollow arrows*).

Patients who cannot be definitively diagnosed with an ectopic versus an IUP are labeled as pregnancy of unknown location. If such patients are stable on examination, they may be followed with serial β-hCG levels every 48 hours. β-hCG levels that do not double (or increase by at least two-thirds) every 48 hours might indicate ectopic pregnancy. As a guideline, an IUP should be seen on transvaginal ultrasonography with β-hCG levels between 1,500 and 2,000 mIU/mL. A fetal heartbeat should be seen with β-hCG level greater than 5,000 mIU/mL.

TREATMENT

If a patient presents with a ruptured ectopic pregnancy and is unstable, the first priority is to stabilize with intravenous fluids, blood products, and vasopressor medications if necessary. The patient should then be taken to the operating room where exploratory laparotomy can be performed to stop the bleeding and remove the ectopic pregnancy. If the patient is stable with a likely ruptured ectopic pregnancy, the procedure of choice at many institutions is an exploratory laparoscopy, which can be performed to evacuate the hemoperitoneum, coagulate any ongoing bleeding, and resect the ectopic pregnancy. Resection can be either through a salpingostomy where the ectopic pregnancy is removed leaving the fallopian tube in place or a salpingectomy where the entire ectopic pregnancy is removed. In the rare case of a cornual (or interstitial) ectopic pregnancy, a cornual resection can be performed.

Patients who present with an unruptured ectopic pregnancy can be treated either surgically (as described above) or medically. At most institutions, clinicians prescribe **methotrexate** in order to treat uncomplicated, nonthreatening, ectopic pregnancies. It is appropriate to use methotrexate for patients who have small ectopic pregnancies (as a general rule, <5 cm, serum β-hCG level <5,000, and without a fetal heartbeat) and for those patients who will be reliable with follow-up. Of note, ectopic pregnancies outside of these parameters have also been treated with methotrexate, but the failure risks are higher, and such patients deserve careful attention and follow-up.

Care of such women involves assessment of baseline transaminases and creatinine, intramuscular methotrexate, and serially following the β-hCG levels. Both single- and multidose methotrexate regimens are available. A single-dose regimen most commonly uses a 50 mg/m^2 dose of intramuscular methotrexate and requires fewer clinic or emergency department visits. However, the success rate is slightly lower with a single- versus a multidose regimen (93% vs. 88%, respectively). Commonly, the β-hCG level will rise the first few days after methotrexate therapy, but should fall by 10% to 15% between days 4 and 7 of the treatment. If β-hCG does not fall to these levels, the patient requires a second dosage of methotrexate. Additionally, these women should be monitored for signs and symptoms of rupture—increased abdominal pain, bleeding, or signs of shock—and advised to come to the emergency department immediately in case of such symptoms.

SPONTANEOUS ABORTION

A **spontaneous abortion** (SAB), or miscarriage, is a pregnancy that ends before 20 weeks' gestation. SABs are estimated to occur in 15% to 25% of all pregnancies. This number may be even higher because losses that occur at 4 to 6 weeks' gestational age are often confused with late menses. The type of SAB is defined by whether any or all of the **products of conception** (POC) have passed and whether or not the cervix is dilated. Definitions are as follows:

- **Abortus**—fetus lost before 20 weeks' gestation or less than 500 g
- **Complete abortion**—complete expulsion of all POC before 20 weeks' gestation (Fig. 2-3).
- **Incomplete abortion**—partial expulsion of some but not all POC before 20 weeks' gestation.

FIGURE 2-3. (**A**) Complete abortion. (**B**) Product of complete abortion. (**C**) Incomplete abortion. (**D**) Product of incomplete abortion.

- **Inevitable abortion**—no expulsion of products, but vaginal bleeding and dilation of the cervix such that a viable pregnancy is unlikely.
- **Threatened abortion**—any vaginal bleeding before 20 weeks, without dilation of the cervix or expulsion of any POC (i.e., a normal pregnancy with bleeding).
- **Missed abortion**—death of the embryo or fetus before 20 weeks with complete retention of all POC.

FIRST-TRIMESTER ABORTIONS

It is estimated that 60% to 80% of all SABs in the first trimester are associated with abnormal chromosomes, of which 95% are due to errors in maternal gametogenesis. In these 95%, autosomal trisomy is the most common chromosomal abnormality. Other factors associated with SABs include infections, maternal anatomic defects, immunologic factors, environmental exposures, and endocrine factors. A large number of first-trimester abortions have no obvious cause.

DIAGNOSIS

Most patients present with bleeding from the vagina (Table 2-2). Other findings include cramping, abdominal pain, and decreased symptoms of pregnancy. The physical examination should include vital signs to rule out shock and febrile illness. A pelvic examination can be performed to look for sources of bleeding other than uterine and for changes in the cervix suggestive of an inevitable abortion. The laboratory tests to be ordered include a quantitative level of β-hCG, complete blood cell count (CBC), blood type, and antibody screen. An ultrasound can assess fetal viability and placentation. As ectopic pregnancies can also present with vaginal bleeding, this must also be considered in the differential diagnosis.

TREATMENT

The treatment plan is based on specific diagnosis and on the decisions made by the patient and her caregivers. Initially, all pregnant and bleeding patients need to be stabilized if hypotensive. A complete abortion can be followed for recurrent bleeding and signs of infection such as elevated temperature. Any tissue that the patient may have passed at home and at the hospital may be sent to pathology, both to assess that POC have passed and for chromosome analysis if applicable.

TABLE 2-2. Differential Diagnosis of First-Trimester Bleeding

SAB
Postcoital bleeding
Ectopic pregnancy
Vaginal or cervical lesions or lacerations
Extrusion of molar pregnancy
Nonpregnancy causes of bleeding

SAB, spontaneous abortion.

An incomplete abortion can be allowed to finish on its own if the patient prefers expectant management, but can also be taken to completion either surgically or medically. The surgical management of a first-trimester abortion requires a dilation and curettage either in the office or operating room. Patients who are hemodynamically unstable generally require urgent surgical management. Medical management includes administration of prostaglandins (e.g., misoprostol) with or without mifepristone to induce cervical dilatation, uterine contractions, and expulsion of the pregnancy. Inevitable abortions and missed abortions are similarly managed.

A patient with a threatened abortion should be followed for continued bleeding and placed on pelvic rest with nothing per vagina. Often, the bleeding will resolve. However, these patients are at increased risk for preterm labor (PTL) and preterm premature rupture of membranes. All Rh-negative pregnant women who experience vaginal bleeding during pregnancy should receive RhoGAM to prevent isoimmunization. Finally, all patients who experience an abortion should be offered contraception if desired.

SECOND-TRIMESTER ABORTIONS

Second-trimester abortions (i.e., abortion at 12 to 20 weeks' gestational age) have multiple etiologies. Infection, maternal uterine or cervical anatomic defects, maternal systemic disease, exposure to fetotoxic agents, and trauma are all associated with late abortions. Abnormal chromosomes are not a frequent cause of late abortions. Late second-trimester abortions and periviable deliveries are also seen with PTL and cervical insufficiency. As in first-trimester abortions, the treatment plan is based on the specific clinical scenario.

Incomplete and missed abortions can be allowed to finish on their own, but are often taken to completion with a D&E (dilation and evacuation). The distinction between a D&C and D&E depends on gestational age at the time of procedure (i.e., first or second trimester). The fetus is larger in the second trimester making the procedure more difficult. Between 16 and 24 weeks, either a D&E may be performed or labor may be induced with high doses of oxytocin or prostaglandins. The advantage of a D&E is that the procedure is self-limited and performed faster than an induction of labor. However, aggressive dilation is necessary prior to the procedure with laminaria (which are small rods of seaweed that are placed in the cervix 1 to 2 days prior to the procedure; these rods then expand as they absorb water, thereby dilating the cervix), and there is a small risk of uterine perforation and cervical lacerations. An induction of labor can take longer, but allows completion of the abortion without the inherent risks of instrumentation. An induction of labor also allows for the possibility of an external genetics examination or autopsy of the POC. Patient preference as well as the capabilities of the facility should be considered when choosing medical or surgical options. With either method, great care should be taken to ensure the complete evacuation of all POC.

In the second trimester, the diagnoses of PTL and cervical insufficiency need to be ruled out. Particularly in the setting of inevitable abortions or threatened abortions, the etiology is likely to be related to the inability of the uterus to maintain the pregnancy. PTL begins with contractions leading to cervical change, whereas cervical insufficiency is characterized by painless dilation of the cervix. In the case of cervical insufficiency, an emergent cerclage may be offered. PTL can potentially be managed with tocolysis.

CERVICAL INSUFFICIENCY

Previously known as cervical incompetence, patients with **cervical insufficiency** present with painless dilation and effacement of the cervix, often in the second trimester of pregnancy. As the cervix dilates, the fetal membranes are exposed to vaginal flora and increased risk of trauma. Thus, infection, vaginal discharge, and rupture of the membranes are common findings in the setting of cervical insufficiency. Patients may also present with short-term cramping or contracting, leading to advancing cervical dilation or pressure in the vagina with the chorionic and amniotic sacs bulging through the cervix. Cervical insufficiency is estimated to cause approximately 15% of all second-trimester losses.

RISK FACTORS

Surgery or other cervical trauma is the most common cause of cervical incompetence (Table 2-3). Causes of cervical trauma might include dilation and curettage, loop electrocautery excisional procedure, or cervical conization. The other possible cause is a congenital abnormality of the cervix that can sometimes be attributed to diethylstilbestrol (DES) exposure in utero. However, many patients who present with cervical incompetence have no known risk factors.

TABLE 2-3. Risk Factors for Cervical Incompetence

History of cervical surgery, such as a cone biopsy or dilation of the cervix
History of cervical lacerations with vaginal delivery
Uterine anomalies
History of DES exposure

DES, diethylstilbestrol

DIAGNOSIS

Patients with cervical insufficiency often present with a dilated cervix noted on routine examination, ultrasound, or in the setting of bleeding, vaginal discharge, or rupture of membranes. Occasionally, patients experience mild cramping or pressure in the lower abdomen or vagina. On examination, the cervix is dilated more than expected with the level of contractions experienced. It is often difficult to differentiate between cervical insufficiency and PTL. However, patients who present with mild cramping and have advancing cervical dilation on serial examinations and/or an amniotic sac bulging through the cervix (Fig. 2-4) are more likely to have cervical insufficiency, with the cramping being instigated by the dilated cervix and exposed membranes rather than the contractions/cramping leading to cervical change as in the case of PTL.

TREATMENT

Individual obstetric issues should be treated accordingly. If the fetus is previable (i.e., <23 to 24 weeks' gestational age), expectant management and elective termination are options. Patients with viable pregnancies are treated with betamethasone

FIGURE 2-4. Hourglass membranes prolapsing through the cervix.

to decrease the risk of prematurity and are managed expectantly with strict bed rest. If there is a component of preterm contractions or PTL, tocolysis may be used during administration of betamethasone with viable pregnancies.

One alternative course of management for cervical insufficiency in a previable pregnancy is the placement of an emergent **cerclage**. The cerclage is a suture placed vaginally around the cervix either at the cervical–vaginal junction (McDonald cerclage) or at the internal os (Shirodkar cerclage). The intent of a cerclage is to close the cervix. Complications include rupture of membranes, PTL, and infection.

If cervical insufficiency was the suspected diagnosis in a previous pregnancy, the patient is usually offered an elective cerclage with subsequent pregnancies (Fig. 2-5). Placement of the elective cerclage is similar to that of the emergent cerclage (with either the McDonald or Shirodkar methods being used), usually at 12 to 14 weeks' gestation. The cerclage is maintained until 36 to 38 weeks of gestation if possible. At that point, it is removed and the patient is followed expectantly until labor ensues. Both types of prophylactic cerclage are associated with 85% to 90% successful pregnancy rate. In patients for whom one or both types of vaginal cerclage have failed, a transabdominal cerclage (TAC) is often the next management offered. This is placed around the cervix at the level of the internal os during a laparotomy. This can be placed electively either prior to the pregnancy or at 12 to 14 weeks. Patients with a TAC need to be delivered via cesarean section. If a patient with cervical insufficiency had a preterm birth (which is usually the case), it is also common to treat her in the subsequent pregnancy with intramuscular (IM) 17-hydroxyprogesterone weekly until 36 weeks' gestation, though this practice is somewhat controversial.

FIGURE 2-5. Cervical cerclage (Shirodkar) for cervical insufficiency in a pregnant patient. (**A**) Placement of the suture. (**B**) Cinching the suture down to tie the knot posteriorly. (**C**) The tightened cerclage almost at the internal os.

RECURRENT PREGNANCY LOSS

A recurrent or habitual aborter is a woman who has had three or more consecutive SABs. Less than 1% of the population is diagnosed with **recurrent pregnancy loss**. The risk of a SAB after one prior SAB is 20% to 25%; after two consecutive SABs, 25% to 30%; and after three consecutive SABs, 30% to 35%.

PATHOGENESIS

The etiologies of recurrent pregnancy loss are generally similar to those of SABs. These include chromosomal abnormalities, maternal systemic disease, maternal anatomic defects, and infection. Fifteen percent of patients with recurrent pregnancy loss have **antiphospholipid antibody** (APA) **syndrome**. Another group of patients are thought to have a **luteal phase defect** and lack an adequate level of progesterone to maintain the pregnancy.

DIAGNOSIS

Patients with recurrent pregnancy loss should be evaluated for the etiology. Patients with only two consecutive SABs are occasionally assessed as well, particularly those with advancing maternal age or for whom continued fertility may be an issue. Patients are often screened in the following manner. First, a karyotype of both parents is obtained, as well as the karyotypes of the POC from each of the SABs if possible. Of note, often obtaining a karyotype from the aborted tissue is impossible; new technology, particularly array complete genome hybridization, can be used to identify chromosomal abnormalities as well with much more success. Second, maternal anatomy should be examined, initially with a hysterosalpingogram (HSG). If the HSG is abnormal or nondiagnostic, a hysteroscopic or laparoscopic exploration may be performed. Third, screening tests for hypothyroidism, diabetes mellitus, APA syndrome, hypercoagulability, and systemic lupus erythematosus should be performed. These tests should include lupus anticoagulant, factor V Leiden deficiency, prothrombin G20210A mutation, ANA, anticardiolipin antibody, Russell viper venom, antithrombin III, protein S, and protein C. Fourth, a level of serum progesterone should be obtained in the luteal phase of the menstrual cycle. Finally, cultures of the cervix, vagina, and endometrium can be taken to rule out infection. An endometrial biopsy can be done during the luteal phase as well to look for proliferative endometrium.

TREATMENT

Treatment of patients with recurrent pregnancy loss depends on the etiology of the SABs. For many (approximately 30% to 50%), no etiology is ever found. For others, the etiology itself needs to be diagnosed (as described above) and can often be treated on an individual basis. For patients with chromosomal abnormalities such as balanced translocations, IVF can be performed using donor sperm or ova. More recently, such patients may undergo preimplantation diagnosis in order to maximize fertilization with their own normal chromosomes. This is where one cell of an embryo harvested through IVF is removed and karyotyped so that abnormal embryos are not implanted. Anatomic abnormalities may or may not be correctable. If cervical insufficiency is suspected, a cerclage may be placed. If a luteal phase defect is suspected, progesterone may be given. Patients with APA syndrome are treated with low-dose aspirin. In the presence of a thrombophilia, SQ heparin (either low molecular weight or unfractionated) may be used. Maternal diseases should be treated with the appropriate therapy (e.g., hypothyroidism with thyroid hormone, infection with antibiotics). However, with some systemic diseases, treatment may not decrease the risk of SAB. Because even patients with three prior consecutive SABs will have a subsequent normal pregnancy two-thirds of the time, it is difficult to estimate whether certain treatments of recurrent abortions are effective.

KEY POINTS

- Approximately 1% of pregnancies are ectopic; that is, implantation of the pregnancy has occurred outside the uterine cavity.
- Initially, when a pregnant woman presents with vaginal bleeding and abdominal pain, an ectopic pregnancy must be ruled out or diagnosed with physical examination, laboratory assessment, and pelvic ultrasound.
- β-hCG levels double approximately every 48 hours in normal intrauterine pregnancies but not in ectopic pregnancies.

(continued)

KEY POINTS (continued)

- Treatment of ectopic pregnancies is often surgical and includes stabilizing the patient and removing the pregnancy. Stable, unruptured ectopic pregnancies can be managed medically with methotrexate therapy.
- The most common cause of first-trimester spontaneous abortions is fetal chromosomal abnormality.
- Incomplete, inevitable, and missed abortions are usually completed with a D&C or medical management with prostaglandins, although expectant management can also be used.
- RhoGAM should be given to all Rh-negative pregnant patients who experience vaginal bleeding.
- Most second-trimester abortions are secondary to uterine or cervical abnormalities, trauma, systemic disease, or infection.
- D&E, prostaglandins, or oxytocic agents can be used for the management of SABs in the second trimester that needs assistance to completion.
- Cervical insufficiency is a painless dilation of the cervix. This dilation may lead to infection, rupture of membranes, or PTL.
- If the fetus is previable, cervical insufficiency is treated with expectant management, elective termination, or emergent cerclage.
- Patients with a history of cervical insufficiency should be offered an elective, prophylactic cerclage at 12 to 14 weeks' gestational age.
- Recurrent pregnancy loss is defined as three or more consecutive SABs.
- Despite extensive evaluation to diagnose the etiology of SABs, the cause of recurrent SABs is undiagnosed in more than one-third of all cases.
- The most common diagnosed causes of recurrent pregnancy loss include APA syndrome and luteal phase defects.
- Treatment is specific to the etiology, but efficacy is difficult to measure because two-thirds of subsequent pregnancies will be normal without therapy.

CLINICAL VIGNETTES

VIGNETTE 1

A 28-year-old P0010 woman presents to the emergency department with abdominal pain since the past day. She reports a 1-week history of nausea with occasional vomiting. She has noticed some breast tenderness as well. She denies dysuria, vaginal bleeding, or any bowel symptoms. She reports that her last period was 4 weeks ago, but was lighter than normal. She has been using condoms for contraception. On arrival, her vital signs include a temperature of 37°C, BP of 117/68, pulse rate of 78 beats per minute, and respiratory rate of 16 breaths per minute. Cardiovascular and respiratory examinations are normal. She notes some suprapubic abdominal discomfort with palpation, but she does not have rebound tenderness or guarding. A speculum examination reveals a closed cervix without bleeding. A pelvic examination is mildly uncomfortable and reveals a normally sized, anteverted uterus, and palpably normal adnexa. A urine pregnancy test is positive.

1. What is the test you should order first?
   a. Type and cross
   b. CBC
   c. Quantitative level of β-hCG
   d. Pelvic ultrasound
   e. Urine gonorrhea and chlamydia testing

2. The quantitative β-hCG level is 1,300 mIU/mL. The patient reveals that this was an unplanned, but desired pregnancy. What follow-up recommendations do you give this patient?
   a. Make an appointment with her primary OB/GYN for an initial prenatal visit
   b. This is likely an ectopic pregnancy and she should proceed with methotrexate therapy
   c. She should undergo urgent laparoscopy for evacuation of an ectopic pregnancy
   d. She should return in 48 hours for a repeat β-hCG
   e. She has likely had a SAB and does not need further follow-up

3. The patient returns 48 hours later per your recommendations. She reports that her abdominal pain is worse and is left-sided. Yesterday, she also had a small amount of vaginal bleeding that has since subsided. She has not been light-headed, short of breath, or had palpitation, and she has been able to tolerate food and drink without difficulty. Her vital signs remain stable. You repeat a β-hCG and the

level is now 1,700 mIU/mL. A pelvic ultrasound reveals a left adnexal mass and nothing in the uterine cavity. What is the most common site of an ectopic pregnancy?
   a. Ampulla
   b. Ovary
   c. Fimbriae
   d. Isthmus
   e. Cervix

4. You explain to the patient that she most likely has an ectopic pregnancy that requires treatment. She would like to avoid surgery. You draw a type and screen, CBC, and complete metabolic panel. Her blood type is O positive, antibody negative. Her hemoglobin is normal as are her liver enzymes. What is your next recommendation?
   a. Her vaginal bleeding suggests an inevitable abortion and she does not need further treatment at this time
   b. Her abdominal pain is concerning and she must undergo urgent laparoscopy for evacuation of the ectopic pregnancy
   c. This is a desired pregnancy; she should return in 48 hours to continue to follow the β-hCG level
   d. She should proceed with methotrexate therapy
   e. She should proceed with mifepristone and misoprostol therapy

5. What additional recommendation would you make at this time?
   a. The patient should receive RhoGAM
   b. She should return in 48 hours for a follow-up test of β-hCG level
   c. She should return in 96 hours for a follow-up test of β-hCG level
   d. She should return in 1 week for a follow-up test of β-hCG level
   e. She should return in 48 hours for a follow-up ultrasound

VIGNETTE 2

A 35-year-old G3P0020 woman presents to the hospital with vaginal bleeding and abdominal pain. She appears pale and states that she feels light-headed when sitting up or standing. She reports that she is currently 9 weeks pregnant. On arrival, her temperature is 37°C, BP is 86/50, pulse rate is 110 beats per minute, and respiratory rate is 18 breaths per minute. Abdominal examination reveals a rigid abdomen with rebound tenderness to palpation. Pelvic examination reveals a small amount of vaginal bleeding, a 6-week-size uterus, and fullness at the right adnexa. A urine β-hCG confirms that she is pregnant. The nurse works to obtain intravenous (IV) access and draw blood for laboratory tests.

1. What is your first step?
   a. Proceed immediately to the operating room for emergency laparotomy
   b. Perform an emergency dilation and suction curettage in the emergency department
   c. Obtain a pelvic ultrasound
   d. Give the patient IM methotrexate
   e. Give the patient oral misoprostol

2. A pelvic ultrasound reveals a right-sided ectopic pregnancy as well as large amounts of fluid, thought to be blood in the abdomen. She now has IV access and a bolus of IV fluids is being given. Her BP is now 78/45 and her pulse rate is 112 beats per minute. Her hematocrit returns as 27.2%. How will you proceed?
   a. Administer IM methotrexate
   b. Transfuse the patient with two units of packed RBCs and transfer her to the intensive care unit (ICU)
   c. Proceed with a laparoscopic salpingectomy
   d. Proceed with emergent laparotomy
   e. Start vasopressors and transfer the patient to the ICU

3. The patient undergoes emergency laparotomy with evacuation of the hemoperitoneum as well as right salpingectomy for removal of the ectopic pregnancy. On postoperative day 1, she explains that this pregnancy was conceived via IVF and was highly desired. What is her risk of having a future ectopic pregnancy?
   a. 1% to 2%
   b. 5%
   c. 10%
   d. 15%
   e. 25%

VIGNETTE 3

A 22-year-old P0 woman presents to the clinic for an annual examination. She reports that her last normal menstrual period was 5 weeks prior. Her menstrual cycles are irregular and she reports that she frequently skips a month between periods. She reports that she is sexually active and uses condoms sporadically for birth control. Pelvic examination reveals a mildly enlarged, anteverted, nontender uterus with palpably normal adnexa bilaterally. The patient consents to a urine pregnancy test that returns as positive. The patient expresses that she is uncertain if this is a desired pregnancy. You perform an in-office transvaginal ultrasound; however, neither an ectopic nor IUP is visualized.

1. What step do you take next?
   a. Obtain a serum quantitative β-hCG level
   b. Explain that the patient likely has a chemical pregnancy that will not develop into a viable pregnancy
   c. Explain to the patient that she likely had a miscarriage

d. Offer the patient IM methotrexate for a presumed ectopic pregnancy
e. Send the patient for an official ultrasound with a high-resolution machine

2. The patient consents to a blood draw before leaving the clinic. Later that day, the patient's β-hCG level returns at 1,300 mIU/mL. You call the patient with the results and she informs you that she would like to continue the pregnancy. What do you recommend next?
   a. You inform her that ultrasound should have detected a pregnancy and she has likely had a miscarriage
   b. She should return in 48 hours for a follow-up β-hCG
   c. She should return in 1 week for a follow-up β-hCG
   d. She should return in 48 hours for a follow-up ultrasound
   e. She should return in 1 week for a follow-up ultrasound

3. Forty-eight hours later, the patient has a repeat β-hCG level that returns at 2,700 mIU/mL. An office ultrasound reveals an intrauterine gestational sac with yolk sac consistent with a 5-week pregnancy. You prescribe a prenatal vitamin and ask the patient to return in 4 weeks for an official prenatal visit. At 8 weeks' gestation, she returns to the clinic with vaginal spotting. A pelvic examination reveals minimal old blood in the vagina and closed cervix. What test or procedure do you perform first?
   a. CBC
   b. Quantitative β-hCG level
   c. Dilation and curettage
   d. Pelvic ultrasound
   e. Gonorrhea and chlamydia testing

4. Fetal heart tones are confirmed with an office ultrasound. What test should you obtain next?
   a. CBC
   b. Gonorrhea and chlamydia
   c. Saline wet mount
   d. Blood type
   e. Quantitative β-hCG level

VIGNETTE 4

A 34-year-old G3P0020 woman presents to the office at 8 weeks' gestation for her first prenatal visit. This is a planned and desired pregnancy. Her obstetric history is significant for one prior elective termination and one SAB. It took her and her partner just over 1 year to conceive this pregnancy. She is afebrile, normotensive with a normal pulse. Pelvic examination reveals a 7- to 8-week-sized uterus with normal adnexa. Her cervix is closed and there is no vaginal bleeding. An office ultrasound is performed and an IUP is seen with a crown–rump length consistent with 7 weeks and 2 days gestation. Unfortunately, no fetal heart beat is seen.

1. What is your diagnosis?
   a. Incomplete abortion
   b. Threatened abortion
   c. Ectopic pregnancy
   d. Missed abortion
   e. Inevitable abortion

2. You offer the patient either medical or surgical management. She opts for medical management and takes mifepristone in the office with the plan to take misoprostol the next day. The following evening, you receive a call that the patient has presented to the emergency department with heavy vaginal bleeding. Her vital signs are as follows: temperature, 37°C; BP, 90/52; pulse rate, 100 beats per minute; respirations, 16 breaths per minute; and 100% oxygen saturation on room air. Pelvic examination reveals active bleeding from an open cervical os. Pelvic ultrasound reveals partial retention of fetal products. What is your new diagnosis?
   a. Incomplete abortion
   b. Threatened abortion
   c. Ectopic pregnancy
   d. Missed abortion
   e. Inevitable abortion

3. The emergency department team obtains IV access and draws blood for a CBC, type and screen and quantitative β-hCG level. An IV fluid bolus is given. Her hematocrit is 30.6%, she is RH positive, and the β-hCG is pending. What is your next step in the management of this patient?
   a. Reassure the patient and send her home
   b. Proceed with dilation and curettage
   c. Administer RhoGAM
   d. Administer vasopressors
   e. Transfer the patient to the ICU

4. The patient stabilizes and is discharged. She follows up in your office 1 week later and wants to know why she had a miscarriage as well as her risk of future miscarriages. Which of the following is not true?
   a. As much as 80% of first-trimester SABs are due to abnormal chromosomes
   b. The most common chromosomal abnormality is autosomal trisomy
   c. Ninety-five percent of the chromosomal abnormalities are due to errors in paternal gametogenesis
   d. Her risk of a third miscarriage is 25% to 30%
   e. Because of her advancing age, she should consider evaluation for recurrent pregnancy loss, starting with parental karyotyping

ANSWERS

VIGNETTE 1 Question 1

1. Answer C:
The next best test is to obtain a quantitative β-hCG level. This will help determine an approximate gestational age for the pregnancy as well as whether you would expect to see anything on ultrasound. Recall that in most institutions, ultrasound should be able to detect an IUP at β-hCG levels between 1,500 and 2,000 mIU/mL. Although a CBC may be ordered to ensure hemodynamic stability, her vital signs are stable and she is not having vaginal bleeding. Similarly, a type and cross is not immediately necessary, as there is no evidence of hemodynamic instability. Given the unremarkable pelvic examination, a pelvic ultrasound may be deferred until you are certain that the β-hCG levels are above the discriminatory zone. Gonorrhea and chlamydia testing is part of routine prenatal care, but is not the best first step.

VIGNETTE 1 Question 2

2. Answer D:
The patient's β-hCG level is below the discriminatory zone and you would not expect to see anything on ultrasound. The patient should return for a repeat β-hCG level in 48 hours so that you can trend the values. With only one β-hCG level, you cannot definitively determine whether this is an intrauterine or ectopic pregnancy. Her abdominal pain is concerning, but not diagnostic for an ectopic pregnancy and it would be premature to recommend methotrexate therapy given that the pregnancy is desired. She is hemodynamically stable and does not need surgery at this point. She has not had any vaginal bleeding to suggest that she has had a SAB. Because you do not know yet if this is an IUP, it would be premature to send the patient for routine prenatal care (a).

VIGNETTE 1 Question 3

3. Answer A:
The most common site of implantation in a tubal pregnancy is the ampulla (70%), followed by the isthmus (12%) and fimbriae (11%). Although an ectopic pregnancy may implant in the cervix or ovary, this is rare.

VIGNETTE 1 Question 4

4. Answer D:
The patient's β-hCG level did not rise by more than two-thirds in 48 hours, which is suggestive of an abnormal pregnancy. This in conjunction with the adnexal mass on ultrasound is highly suggestive of an ectopic pregnancy. She should proceed with treatment. Her β-hCG level is well below the cutoff of 5,000 mIU/mL, that is, at an appropriate level for methotrexate therapy, and this would be the recommended first-line therapy. Vaginal bleeding is a common presenting symptom in an ectopic pregnancy. However, unlike in an IUP, vaginal bleeding does not signify that the pregnancy will pass on its own. Again, the patient's vital signs and CBCs are stable.

She has proven that she is reliable as she returned for her follow-up visit as recommended. She may be offered surgery at this time, but it is not mandatory. Once the diagnosis of ectopic pregnancy is made, the patient should no longer be managed expectantly. Mifepristone and misoprostol therapy is reserved for the treatment of intrauterine pregnancies.

VIGNETTE 1 Question 5

5. Answer C:
The β-hCG level commonly rises in the first few days after methotrexate therapy with a fall of 10% to 15% between days 4 and 7 after administration. Checking β-hCG levels at 48 hours may raise a false concern that the patient needs additional treatment. However, the patient should be seen sooner than 1 week so that additional methotrexate may be administered if necessary. The patient's blood type is Rh positive and RhoGAM is not indicated. Ultrasound is not commonly used to follow the resolution of an ectopic pregnancy.

VIGNETTE 2 Question 1

1. Answer C:
The patient is hemodynamically stable. The first steps should be to obtain IV access with a large-bore IV catheter, bolus the patient with IV fluids, and draw blood for a CBC and a type and screen and/or cross for units of blood. Although the nurse helps with these important steps, it would be prudent to perform an urgent ultrasound to determine if this is an intrauterine versus an ectopic pregnancy, as this will dictate your next steps. The patient will likely need to undergo an urgent procedure, but the type of pregnancy will determine whether a D&C versus abdominal surgery is most appropriate. As the patient is not hemodynamically stable, she is not a candidate for medical therapy at this time.

VIGNETTE 2 Question 2

2. Answer D:
The patient is hemodynamically unstable and has evidence of a ruptured ectopic pregnancy on ultrasound as well as acute blood loss anemia and possible hemoperitoneum. She should be taken for emergent exploratory laparotomy to control the bleeding and remove the ectopic pregnancy. Although a more stable

patient may be offered laparoscopy, it is not the best choice in an unstable patient. The patient may require a blood transfusion, vasopressor support, and ICU care, but not without concurrent surgery to control the bleeding. She is not a candidate for methotrexate because of her hemodynamic instability.

VIGNETTE 2 Question 3
3. Answer C:
The risk of an ectopic pregnancy after IVF has been estimated to be between 1% and 2% and this was likely the patient's baseline risk of ectopic pregnancy. However, after one prior ectopic pregnancy, the risk of a subsequent ectopic pregnancy increases to 10%, which is likely the patient's new risk. The risk of a subsequent ectopic pregnancy after more than one prior ectopic pregnancy increases to 25%.

VIGNETTE 3 Question 1
1. Answer A:
An IUP should be seen on ultrasound with β-hCG levels between 1,500 and 2,000 mIU/mL. Without knowing the patient's β-hCG level, you cannot give any additional advice about the status of the pregnancy.

VIGNETTE 3 Question 2
2. Answer B:
In an IUP, the β-hCG level can be expected to increase by 60% or more every 48 hours. An ectopic pregnancy would be expected to have a slower rate of increase in β-hCG level because of decreased blood supply due to abnormal placentation. Therefore, the next best step would be to ask the patient to return in 48 hours for a repeat β-hCG level. A β-hCG level of 1,300 mIU/mL is not above the discriminatory zone for detection of pregnancy and cannot rule out pregnancy. Repeating an ultrasound in 48 hours may not be necessary if the patient has a normal rise in β-hCG level and is not symptomatic. Returning in 1 week for laboratory tests and/or ultrasound would not be advised prior to determining whether the pregnancy is intrauterine or ectopic.

VIGNETTE 3 Question 3
3. Answer D:
The current diagnosis based on your clinical assessment is a threatened abortion. It is important to confirm the presence or absence of fetal heart tones with ultrasound to appropriately counsel the patient regarding the next steps. She does not have heavy vaginal bleeding and does not need an urgent CBC. At this gestational age, a quantitative β-hCG level will not offer additional information. It would be premature to proceed with dilation and curettage for a desired pregnancy. Cervicitis may cause vaginal spotting, but this is not the initial test of choice.

VIGNETTE 3 Question 4
4. Answer D:
With any bleeding in pregnancy, the patient's Rh status should be obtained. All patients with Rh-negative status should receive RhoGAM to prevent maternal isoimmunization. Again, the patient is not bleeding heavily, so obtaining a CBC would not be the first step. Although gonorrhea, chlamydia, or other vaginal infections may cause spotting, these tests are less urgent than obtaining the patient's blood type. A quantitative β-hCG level does not offer any additional information at this point.

VIGNETTE 4 Question 1
1. Answer D:
Missed abortion is the death of an embryo with complete retention of all POCs. An incomplete abortion is partial expulsion of POCs prior to 20 weeks. This patient has not had any tissue expelled. A threatened abortion does present with vaginal bleeding, but in this type of abortion the patient does not have cervical dilation. This patient has an IUP as confirmed by an intrauterine gestational sac and yolk sac. An inevitable abortion is a pregnancy complicated by vaginal bleeding with a dilated cervix such that the pregnancy is unlikely to be viable.

VIGNETTE 4 Question 2
2. Answer A:
Missed abortion is the death of an embryo with complete retention of all POCs. An incomplete abortion is partial expulsion of POC prior to 20 weeks. This patient has not had any tissue expelled. A threatened abortion does present with vaginal bleeding, but in this type of abortion the patient does not have cervical dilation. This patient has an IUP as confirmed by an intrauterine gestational sac and yolk sac. An inevitable abortion is a pregnancy complicated by vaginal bleeding with a dilated cervix such that the pregnancy is unlikely to be viable.

VIGNETTE 4 Question 3
3. Answer B:
The patient is actively bleeding and controlling this is the first step after stabilizing the patient. Performing a dilation and curettage to remove the remaining fetal tissues will allow the uterus to contract and will likely stop the bleeding. The patient should not be sent home with heavy vaginal bleeding and unstable vital signs. She is Rh positive and does not require RhoGAM. She has not yet become so unstable as to require vasopressors or be transferred to the ICU.

VIGNETTE 4 Question 4
4. Answer C:
Ninety-five percent of the chromosomal abnormalities are due to errors in maternal gametogenesis. All of the other statements are true.

3 | Prenatal Screening, Diagnosis, and Treatment

Prenatal screening, diagnosis, and treatment is a relatively new field within obstetrics. It has been particularly tied to the advent and advancement of real-time ultrasound imaging over the last three decades as well as the new kinds of genetic testing that are being rapidly introduced today. Prenatal genetic diagnoses are and will be increasingly available as the association between specific genes, large chromosomal aberrations, and submicroscopic chromosomal losses and gains, and their phenotypes are discovered. Imperative to understand prenatal diagnosis is the distinction between screening and diagnostic tests. **Screening** allows high-risk individuals to be selected out of a low-risk population at risk for a given diagnosis or complication. The sensitivity and specificity and resulting false-negative and false-positive rates of screening tests are highly important because of both the number of patients missed by a screen and the number of patients who are falsely concerned. The cell-free fetal DNA (cffDNA) test is a recently developed screening tool that may maximize sensitivity and minimize false positives, but is not currently a diagnostic test. **Prenatal diagnosis** is nearly always diagnostic and usually far more specific than screening, but diagnostic procedures such as amniocentesis and chorionic villus sampling (CVS) bear a greater risk of complications, in particular, pregnancy loss.

SCREENING PATIENTS FOR GENETIC DISEASES

Many diseases are passed genetically from parents to their offspring. This is best understood using the principles of Mendelian genetics. **Autosomal dominant** diseases are usually inherited from one parent with the disease via a single gene defect. The risk of disease and recurrence (if the partners choose to have another child) is usually 50%. **Autosomal recessive** (AR) diseases require two affected alleles. Thus, assuming both parents are carriers, the risk to the child is 25%. **X-linked disorders** (e.g., hemophilia and fragile X) are usually carried by the mother who is unaffected (in X-linked recessive) or mildly affected (X-linked dominant) and passed only to her sons. The sons are affected 50% of the time and the daughters are unaffected or mildly affected carriers 50% of the time. **X-linked dominant** disorders can be passed from mothers to their sons and daughters, and theoretically from fathers to their daughters. In some X-linked dominant disorders, the disorder is lethal in males, as in Aicardi syndrome. One important tenet of X-linked inheritance is that there is no male-to-male transmission, which is a key component of the family history. Phenotypes can vary, especially in females, because of X-chromosome lyonization. The first step in determining fetal risk is to screen the mother for the disease, which is usually done in higher risk groups (e.g., by ethnicity or family history). In this section, we review several of the common genetic diseases that have prenatal screening and diagnosis.

CYSTIC FIBROSIS

Cystic fibrosis (CF) is an AR disease resulting from an abnormality in the CF transmembrane conductance regulator (CFTR), which is the gene responsible for chloride channels. Almost all CF patients have chronic lung disease because of recurrent infections, leading eventually to irreversible lung damage and strain on the right ventricle (cor pulmonale). Eighty-five percent of CF patients have pancreatic insufficiency manifested by chronic malabsorption and failure to thrive. Chronic lung disease and its sequelae are the life-limiting factors for most CF patients. Median survival is close to 40 years for CF patients born today in the United States with high phenotypic variability.

In CF, two mutant copies (gene changes) of the CFTR gene are required (homozygosity) for disease, though, for the majority of AR disorders, affected individuals have two different allelic mutations at the same locus (compound heterozygote). For example, ΔF508/G542X are two of the most common mutations in CF. These two specific mutations can be screened for in asymptomatic carrier patients. If the mother has a positive screen, her partner can be screened as well and if he is also positive, then the risk of the fetus being affected is 25%. If desired, amniocentesis or CVS can then be performed to diagnose the fetus. The CF mutations are more common in Caucasians (approximately 1:25 to 29 is a carrier). One challenge in screening for CF is that more than 1,300 disease-causing mutations have been identified in the CFTR gene. Therefore, even with a negative screen of the most common disease-causing mutations, there remains a small probability that a child could be affected. Although the risk of carrier status is less common in other races/ethnicities (e.g., Asian and Hispanic), the relative proportion of disease common mutations is fewer as well, making the screening test less sensitive in these women. One way to improve the sensitivity of screening is to screen for additional mutations, and a number of commercial laboratories offer screening for up to 97 mutations.

SICKLE CELL ANEMIA

Sickle cell anemia is an AR disease caused by a single point mutation in the gene for the β chain in hemoglobin. The resulting hemoglobin (Hb S) forms polymers that when deoxygenated cause the cells to lose their biconcave shape and become "sickled" in appearance. As a result, patients have a hemolytic anemia, shortened life expectancy, and frequent pain crises secondary to vaso-occlusion of small vessels by the dysmorphic erythrocytes. Because this disease is more common among African Americans, all persons of African descent should be screened during pregnancy. Individuals with one abnormal sickle cell allele are known as having sickle cell trait. It is likely that the increased carrier status in those of African ancestry was selected because of **heterozygote advantage**. This is observed because resistance to malaria in individuals heterozygous for sickle cell anemia was greater than those without the gene defect. In these individuals, RBCs function in normal conditions but are inhospitable to *Plasmodium vivax*, the parasitic protozoan responsible for malaria. Interestingly, a recent study demonstrated a lower rate of preterm birth among women with sickle cell trait.

The maternal screen is usually accomplished with a hemoglobin electrophoresis. This test distinguishes Hb S from normal Hb A. If the patient is positive, then her partner can also be screened. If he is also positive, then the fetus carries a 25% chance of being affected, and the couple can choose to undergo invasive fetal diagnosis.

TAY–SACHS DISEASE

Tay–Sachs is an AR disease that is most commonly observed in Eastern European Jews and French Canadians. Approximately 1 in 27 to 31 Ashkenazi Jews is a carrier for an abnormal Tay–Sachs allele, which means that the incidence of Tay–Sachs in this population is approximately 100 times greater than in other populations. This is thought to be due to a **founder effect**, in which the high frequency of a mutant gene in a population is founded by a small ancestral group when one or more individuals are a carrier for the mutation.

Infants with Tay–Sachs disease develop symptoms approximately 3 to 10 months after birth. These symptoms include a loss of alertness and an excessive reaction to noise (hyperacusis). There is a progressive developmental delay and neurologic degeneration in intellectual and neurologic function. Myoclonic and akinetic seizures can present 1 to 3 months later. One physical examination finding is a cherry-red spot seen on funduscopic eye examination, where the prominent red macular fovea centralis is contrasted by the pale retina. These children eventually suffer from paralysis, blindness, and dementia, and typically die by age of 4 years.

Tay–Sachs disease occurs due to the deficiency of hexosaminidase A (hex A), the enzyme responsible for the degradation of GM2 gangliosides. Hex A is a multimeric protein composed of three parts: α and β subunits, which comprise the enzyme, and an activator protein. The activator protein must associate with both the enzyme and the substrate before the enzyme can cleave the ganglioside between the N-acetyl-α-galactosamine and galactose residues. Gangliosides are continually degraded in lysosomes, where multiple degradative enzymes function to sequentially remove terminal sugars from the gangliosides. The impact of Tay–Sachs disease is primarily in the brain, which has the highest concentrations of gangliosides, particularly in the gray matter. The deficiency of hex A results in the accumulation of gangliosides in the lysosomes, which in turn results in enlarged neurons containing lipid-filled lysosomes, cellular dysfunction, and ultimately neuronal death.

Similar to other AR syndromes, Tay–Sachs is screened for particularly among high-risk patients (e.g., Ashkenazi Jews), and their partners if they are positive. Fetal diagnosis can then be performed if both partners are carriers.

THALASSEMIA

The **thalassemias** are a set of hereditary hemolytic anemias that are caused by mutations that result in the reduction in the synthesis of either the α or β chains that make up the hemoglobin molecule. The reduction of a particular chain leads to the imbalance of globin chain synthesis and subsequently a distortion in the α:β ratio. As a result, unpaired globin chains produce insoluble tetramers that precipitate in the cell and cause damage to membranes. The RBCs are susceptible to premature red cell destruction by the reticuloendothelial system in the bone marrow, liver, and spleen.

β-THALASSEMIA

In **β-thalassemia**, there is an impairment of β-chain production that leads to an excess of α chains. These disorders are typically diagnosed several months after birth because the presence of β-chain is important only postnatally when it would normally replace the γ-chain as the major non-α chain. There are multiple mutations that can lead to β-thalassemia. Almost any point mutation that causes a decrease in the synthesis of mRNA and the subsequent protein can cause this disease. β-Thalassemia is essentially an AR disorder seen more commonly among patients of Mediterranean descent as well as Asians and Africans. Because the heterozygotes will have a mild hemolytic anemia and low MCV (<80 fL), they can be screened by getting a complete blood count (CBC). Confirmation can then be made by hemoglobin electrophoresis, which will show an increase in α:β ratio (Hgb A_2).

α-Thalassemia

The α chain is encoded by four alleles on two chromosomes. Additionally, two of the four mutations can occur *cis* or *trans*, with *cis* being on the same chromosome and *trans* being on two different chromosomes. *cis* mutations are seen more commonly among women of Southeast Asian descent, whereas *trans* mutations are seen more commonly among women of African descent. With α-thalassemia, deletions, or alterations of two, three, or four genes cause an increasingly severe phenotype; however, deletion of one allele has no clinical significance. The most severe form of α-thalassemia causes fetal hydrops and is incompatible with life. The infants are delivered premature and are pale, hydropic, severely anemic, and have splenomegaly. A fetal hemoglobin electrophoresis would reveal no HbF, no HbA, and approximately 90% to 100% Hbα4 also referred to as **Hb Bart**. **Hemoglobin H disease** (HbH) is due to the deletion of three α globin genes, resulting in the accumulation of excess β chains in the red cell. β tetramers form, which are unstable and undergo oxidation. Membrane damage results, and these RBCs are susceptible to early clearance and destruction. These infants develop moderate hemolytic anemia, and the initial hemoglobin electrophoresis shows some Hb Bart and some HbH. Within the following few months, Hb Bart disappears and the hemoglobins detected are HbH and HbA. **α-Thalassemia trait** (two deletions) carries a milder phenotype with mainly a microcytic anemia and a normal hemoglobin electrophoresis. Patients with only one gene deletion are silent carriers and usually have an MCV of less than 85 fL. In such a case, diagnosis is confirmed by targeted mutation analysis.

Like β-thalassemia, α-thalassemia is also screened for with a CBC in high-risk groups. Patients can then undergo hemoglobin electrophoresis if they have a microcytic anemia, which is typically normal. Molecular testing is needed to determine the number of genes lost. Sorting out whether patients are *cis* or *trans* is particularly important. When both partners have a *cis* mutation, their child has a 25% chance of getting the most severe variant that usually results in fetal death. If they both have the *trans* mutation, the child will end up with the *trans* mutation, as well, and primarily remain an asymptomatic carrier.

CHROMOSOMAL ABNORMALITIES

In addition to genetic disorders caused by single gene mutations, another family of genetic disorders in the fetus is caused by chromosomal abnormalities. Aneuploidy, that is, extra or missing chromosome(s), is generally the cause of these syndromes. These chromosomal abnormalities are usually accompanied by obvious phenotypic differences and congenital anomalies. However, these may not always be appreciated on prenatal ultrasound. Thus, fetal karyotype remains the only way to achieve a definitive diagnosis of aneuploidy. Screening tests exist for some types of aneuploidy—specifically trisomies 21 and 18. Women may choose to undergo first-trimester screening at

11 to 14 weeks, second-trimester screening, or a combination of the two called sequential screening. The components of first-trimester screening include a nuchal translucency (NT), which is combined with pregnancy-associated plasma protein A (PAPP-A) and β-hCG. The second-trimester portion is called the quadruple (quad) screen and includes maternal serum α-fetoprotein (MSAFP), estriol, β-hCG, and inhibin. Recent advancements have allowed researchers to examine cffDNA in maternal serum to make a "noninvasive prenatal diagnosis." These tests are highly sensitive and specific for specific aneuploidies, but have a number of limitations (e.g., not applicable in twins, chromosomal mosaicism, etc.) and do not currently assess all of the chromosomal aneuploidies as one can do with a karyotype. Although trisomy and monosomy of any of the chromosomes theoretically exist, most result in early miscarriage. In addition, triploidy (i.e., three sets of chromosomes) may also occur and usually results in miscarriage or gestational trophoblastic disease. Despite the high rate of miscarriage, an infant is occasionally born with triploidy and survival for up to 1 year has been described.

DOWN SYNDROME

Trisomy 21, or an extra chromosome 21, is the most common cause of **Down syndrome**. This chromosomal aneuploidy results in higher rates of both miscarriage and stillbirth. However, several thousand infants with Down syndrome are born each year. Because chromosomal abnormalities increase with maternal age, the overall average risk per patient is increasing in the United States as more women delay childbearing. The typical phenotype of Down syndrome is that of a short stature, classic facies, developmental delay, and mental retardation with IQs ranging from 40 to as high as 90. Associated anomalies include cardiac defects, duodenal atresia or stenosis, and short limbs. Some of these anomalies can be seen by ultrasound, but up to 40% to 50% of fetuses with Down syndrome will not have diagnosable anomalies by ultrasound, making this a poor screening tool.

Currently, women undergo screening for Down syndrome using the first-trimester screen (NT with PAPP-A and hCG) and/or the quad screen (MSAFP, hCG, estriol, and inhibin A) between 15 and 20 weeks' gestation. The sensitivity of the first-trimester screen is 82% to 87% for Down syndrome and for the quad screen alone has just more than 80% sensitivity. The combination of these two tests results in a sensitivity of 95% with a screen positive rate of 5%, while the sensitivity of the NT alone is 64% to 70%. When the serum analytes are used alone, free β-hCG and PAPP-A can achieve a 60% sensitivity. First-trimester screening has been studied in several large trials and affords women to have information earlier in gestation to allow decisions on prenatal diagnostic testing as early as 12 weeks. The newer, cell-free DNA (cfDNA) tests originally focused on identifying trisomy 21, and indeed, these tests have the highest sensitivity and specificity at 99.3% and 99.8%, respectively (*N Engl J Med*. 2015;372:1589–1597).

TRISOMY 18

Trisomy 18 (Edward syndrome) is another common trisomy that can also be screened for using the first- and second-trimester screening with a sensitivity approaching 90% in women who choose sequential screening. cfDNA screening has been shown in recent studies to be greater than 97% sensitive at a much lower screen positive rate (0.3%) in high-risk populations. Trisomy 18 is a lethal aneuploidy and nearly all neonates die within the first 2 years of life. This syndrome is associated with multiple congenital anomalies, which are typically seen on ultrasound (in approximately 95% of cases), making this modality a reasonable screening tool. Edward syndrome is classically associated with clenched fists, overlapping digits, and rocker bottom feet. Cardiac defects including ventricular septal defect (VSD) and tetralogy of Fallot, omphalocele, congenital diaphragmatic hernia, neural tube defects (NTDs), and choroid plexus (CP) cysts have also been associated with trisomy 18 (Fig. 3-1). Although trisomy 18 is

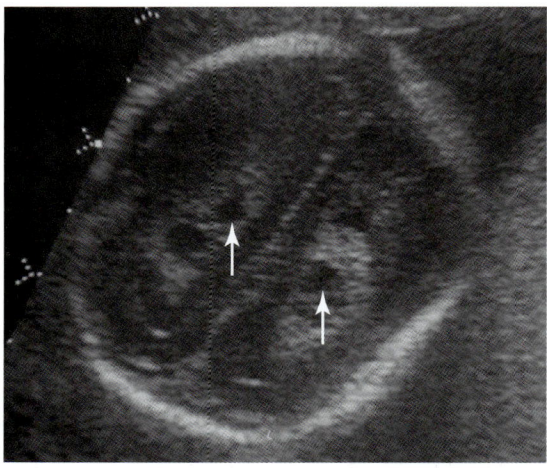

FIGURE 3-1. CP cysts located in the lateral ventricles of the brain. (Image provided by Departments of Radiology and Obstetrics & Gynecology, University of California, San Francisco, CA.)

rarely missed on ultrasound, the advantage of early diagnosis with a screening test is an earlier, safer, termination of pregnancy.

TRISOMY 13

Trisomy 13 (Patau syndrome) has many findings similar to trisomy 18. Eighty-five percent of these newborns will not live past the first year of life. Commonly associated anomalies include holoprosencephaly, cleft lip and palate, cystic hygroma, single nostril or absent nose, omphalocele, cardiac anomalies including hypoplastic left heart, and limb anomalies including clubfoot and clubhand, polydactyly, and overlapping fingers. Unfortunately, the serum analytes of the first trimester and quad screen are variable in these pregnancies, making this a poor screening test, and thus it is typically not reported. Early studies of noninvasive prenatal diagnosis suggest that the detection of trisomy may also be possible. It is very rare that trisomy 13 fetuses would not have anomalies visible on ultrasound, and thus will be commonly diagnosed by routine ultrasound examination. Similar to trisomy 18, the newer, cfDNA screening test can be used to identify trisomy 13 as well, at a sensitivity of 91.6%. Although trisomy 13 is likely missed even less than trisomy 18 on ultrasound, the advantage of early diagnosis with a screening test is an earlier, safer, termination of pregnancy.

SEX CHROMOSOMAL ABNORMALITIES

45,X (**Turner syndrome** or monosomy X) and 47,XXY (**Klinefelter syndrome**) are the most common sex chromosome aneuploidies. This may be because 47,XXX and 47,XYY karyotypes exhibit little variation from standard phenotypes and are not identified as often. Individuals affected by Turner syndrome are phenotypically female and of short stature. They experience primary amenorrhea, sexual infantilism, webbed neck, low-set ears, low posterior hairline, epicanthal folds, wide carrying angle of the arms, shield-like chest, wide-set nipples, short fourth metacarpal, renal anomalies, lymphedema of the extremities at birth, and cardiovascular anomalies, especially coarctation of the aorta. The only anomaly in Turner syndrome commonly seen on ultrasound is cystic hygroma. Currently, it is possible to screen for sex chromosomal abnormalities using noninvasive prenatal testing; however, the use of cffDNA for this purpose has additional challenges. The sensitivity is 91% and the lack of identification of a Y chromosome can identify a female fetus, or inability of the test to pick up the Y chromosome. Thus, patients must be counseled (as discussed previously) that this can only be used as a screening test and is not diagnostic. Additionally, both these and other sex chromosome abnormalities are diagnosed by karyotype when patients undergo amniocentesis or CVS. In patients with Klinefelter syndrome, testicular development is initially normal in these individuals. However, the presence of at least two X chromosomes causes the germ cells to die when they enter meiosis, eventually resulting in small, firm testes and hyalinization of the seminiferous tubules. Other classic findings in Klinefelter syndrome include infertility, gynecomastia, mental retardation, and elevated gonadotropin levels due to the decreased levels of circulating androgens.

FETAL CONGENITAL ANOMALIES

Congenital anomalies can occur in any organ system and may be due to an intrinsic abnormality such as a gene change, aneuploidy, or related to a teratogenic agent. The affected organ system often depends on which time during gestation a teratogenic insult is received by the fetus. These teratogens can include medications ingested by the mother or infections, most commonly a viral infection that the mother contracts and transmits transplacentally, and rarely chemotherapy. Radiation doses resulting in a congenital malformation are considerably higher than any diagnostic radiologic study (>20 rads). In order to better understand how these anomalies occur, a review of organogenesis is useful.

EARLY EMBRYOGENESIS AND ORGANOGENESIS

After fertilization of the ovum by the sperm, the resulting zygote undergoes a series of cell divisions, reaching the 16-cell morula stage by day 4 (Fig. 3-2). After the morula enters the uterine cavity, an influx of fluid separates the morula into the inner and outer cell masses, which forms the blastocyst. This gives rise to the embryo and the trophoblast, respectively. The blastocyst implants into the endometrium by the end of week 1. By the start of week 2, the trophoblast begins to differentiate into the inner cytotrophoblast and the outer syncytiotrophoblast, and together they eventually give rise to the placenta. Meanwhile, the inner cell mass divides into the bilaminar germ disc composed of the epiblast and the hypoblast.

During week 3 of development, the embryo is primarily preoccupied with the process of gastrulation.

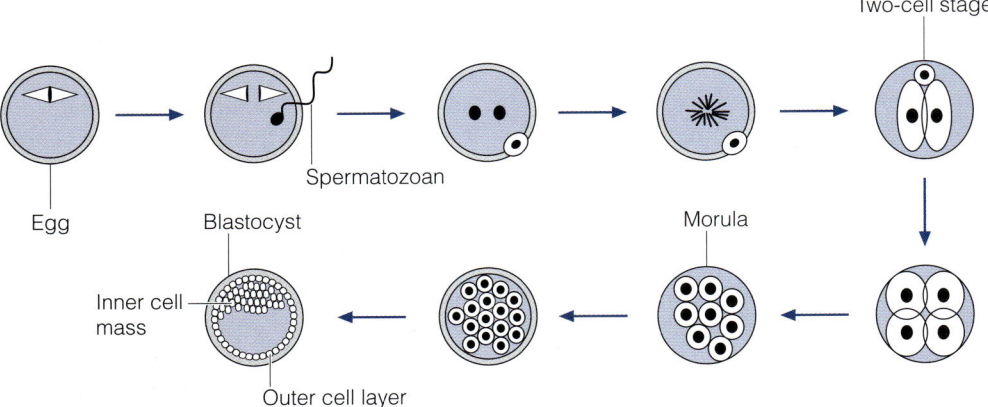

FIGURE 3-2. Progression of the ova through fertilization to the blastula phase.

This is characterized by the formation of the primitive streak on the epiblast, followed by the invagination of epiblast cells to form the three germ layers of the embryo: the inner endoderm, the middle mesoderm, and the outer ectoderm. The endodermal layer eventually gives rise to the gastrointestinal and respiratory systems. The mesoderm forms the cardiovascular, musculoskeletal, and genitourinary systems. The ectoderm layer will differentiate into the nervous system, skin, and many sensory organs (e.g., hair, eyes, nose, and ears). The period of organogenesis primarily lasts from weeks 3 to 8 after conception (i.e., weeks 5 to 10 gestational age [GA]) and is the time when most of the major organ systems are formed.

NEURAL TUBE DEFECTS

The formation of the neural tube begins on days 22 to 23 after conception (week 4) in the region of the fourth and sixth somites. Fusion of the neural folds occurs in cranial and caudal directions. The anterior neuropore (future brain) closes by day 25 and the posterior pore (future spinal cord) closes by day 27. Closure of the neural tube coincides with establishment of its vascular supply. The majority of **neural tube defects** (NTDs) develop as a result of defective closure by week 4 of development (6 weeks' GA by last menstrual period [LMP] dating).

NTDs, including spina bifida and anencephaly, are classic examples of multifactorial inheritance, emphasizing the interactions between environmental and genetic factors. Geographic and ethnic variations may reflect environmental and genetic influences on the incidence of NTDs. Decreased levels of maternal folic acid are associated with the development of NTDs. Supplementation with periconceptional folic acid effectively reduces the incidence as well as recurrence of NTDs. The risk of NTDs is doubled in cases of homozygosity for a common mutation in the gene for methyl tetrahydrofolate reductase (MTHFR), the C677T allelic variant that encodes an enzyme with reduced activity. However, even if the association was causal, this MTHFR variant would account for only a small fraction of NTDs prevented by folic acid. The risk of NTDs seen with certain genotypes may vary depending on maternal factors, such as the blood levels of vitamin B_{12} or folate.

Fetuses with **spina bifida** can be identified on ultrasound, which is accomplished not by visualization of the opening of the spinal canal (Fig. 3-3), but by the associated findings. Spina bifida leads to classic ultrasound findings of the "lemon" sign (concave

FIGURE 3-3. Meningomyelocele—nonclosure of the neural tube at the lower aspect of the spine. (Image provided by Departments of Radiology and Obstetrics & Gynecology, University of California, San Francisco, CA.)

FIGURE 3-4. Cerebral findings of the "lemon" and "banana" signs in spina bifida. (Image provided by Departments of Radiology and Obstetrics & Gynecology, University of California, San Francisco, CA.)

frontal bones), and the "banana" sign (a cerebellum that is pulled caudally and flattened) (Fig. 3-4). Ventriculomegaly and clubfeet are also seen. Prior to the existence of real-time ultrasound, one of the first prenatal screening programs was created using MSAFP to screen for NTDs. An open neural tube leads to elevated amniotic fluid α-fetoprotein (AFP) that crosses into the maternal serum.

Function of the infant and child with spina bifida is entirely dependent on the level of the spinal lesion. If the lesion is quite low in the sacral area, bowel and bladder function may be normal, and ambulation can be achieved with assistance. However, in higher lesions, there may be complete inability to use the lower extremities as well as lack of bowel or bladder control. Currently, there are multiple centers across the United States, which perform intrauterine repair of these lesions on a select subset of patients. Early data suggest that fetuses who undergo surgery have improved outcomes with decreased need for ventricular shunt procedures after delivery, increased ability to walk and improved neurodevelopmental outcomes, however also have increased risk of preterm delivery, oligohydramnios, pulmonary edema, and uterine dehiscence at the surgical scar. Long-term outcomes are continuing to be followed.

CARDIAC DEFECTS

Although the heart is merely a four-chamber pump, there are a number of ways to change the structure that can lead to some interesting pathophysiology. Cardiac development begins during week 3 after conception, when an angiogenic cell cluster forms at the anterior central portion of the embryo. As the embryo folds cephalocaudally, the cardiogenic area also folds into a heart tube. Even at this early stage, the embryonic heart tube is already receiving venous flow from its caudal end and pumping blood through the first aortic arch and into the dorsal aorta. Simultaneously, mesoderm around the endocardial tube forms the three layers of the heart wall composed of an outer epicardium, a muscular wall of myocardium, and the endocardium that is the internal endothelial lining. Between days 23 and 28, the heart tube elongates and bends to create the cardiac loop with a common atrium and a narrow atrioventricular junction connecting it to the primitive ventricle. The bulbus cordis is the caudal section of the heart tube and will eventually form three structures: the proximal third will form the trabeculated part of the right ventricle, the midportion (conus cordis) will form the outflow tracts of the ventricles, and the distal segment (truncus arteriosus) will eventually give rise to the proximal portions of the aorta and pulmonary artery (Fig. 3-5).

Between days 27 and 37, the heart continues to develop through the formation of the major septa. Septum formation is achieved via the formation of tissue, called endocardial cushions, which subdivide the lumen into two cavities. The right and left atria are created by the formation of the septum primum and septum secundum that subdivides the primitive atrium, while allowing for an interatrial opening (foramen ovale) to continue the right-to-left shunting of blood. At the end of week 4, endocardial cushions also appear in the atrioventricular canal to form the right and left canals as well as the mitral and tricuspid valves. During this time, the medial walls of the ventricles gradually fuse together to form the muscular interventricular septum. The conus cordis comprises the middle third of the bulbus cordis, and during week 5 of development, cushions subdivide the conus to form the outflow tract of the right and left ventricle as well as the membranous portion of the interventricular septum. Cushions also appear in the truncus arteriosus (distal third of bulbus cordis) and grow in a spiral pattern to form the aorticopulmonary septum and divide the truncus into the aortic and pulmonary tracts.

Any of these points of development can go awry, leading to disastrous complications. For example, if the ventricular walls fail to fuse, there is a VSD, which, if not repaired, can lead to Eisenmenger physiology, that is, right ventricular hypertrophy, pulmonary hypertension, and a right-to-left shunt. A commonly seen constellation of cardiac findings is tetralogy of Fallot. This is a VSD with an overriding

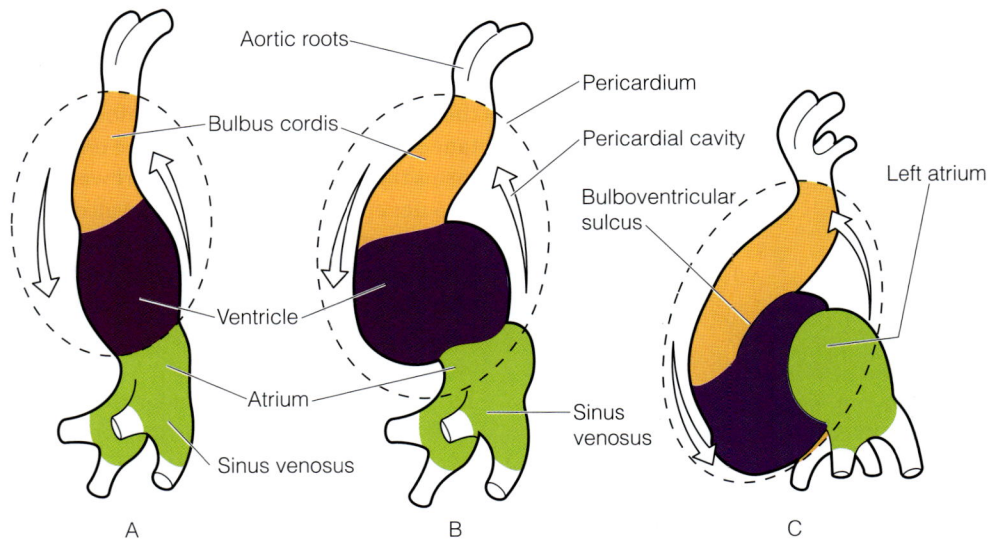

FIGURE 3-5. (**A–C**) Folding of the heart tube into the four-chamber heart.

aorta, pulmonary stenosis (or atresia), and right ventricular hypertrophy. Just as the chambers and valves can be anomalous, so can the great vessels as seen in transposition of the vessels, where the pulmonary artery and the aorta are connected to the wrong ventricles. Other common anomalies of vessels are coarctation of the aorta, an atretic portion prior to the insertion of the ductus arteriosus; and a patent ductus arteriosus, which can also lead to Eisenmenger physiology.

Diagnosis of these anomalies varies widely and depends on the lesion and the quality of the sonographer imaging the fetal heart. Some of the more common lesions will be identified by the standard four-chamber view of the heart, but many—including coarctation of the aorta, small VSDs, and ASD—often will not. Outcomes of these congenital anomalies are quite variable. Most of these may be surgically repaired, although hypoplastic left heart, in particular, can have high mortality at a young age.

POTTER SYNDROME

Potter syndrome results from renal failure leading to anhydramnios, which in turn causes pulmonary hypoplasia and contractures or deformations of the limbs in the fetus. Potter disease is a bilateral renal agenesis. However, a fetus can also develop renal failure if there is distal obstruction of the urinary system as with posterior urethral valves. To better understand the etiology of this system, we should consider its embryology.

The kidneys are formed from intermediate mesoderm. Kidney development begins in week 4 with the formation of the first of three kidney scaffolds that arise and regress sequentially before the permanent kidney develops. This first scaffold is the pronephros, which is nonfunctional. In week 5, the *meso*nephros develops and functions briefly, creating the *meso*nephric duct (Wolffian duct). The ureteric bud is an offshoot of the mesonephric duct that dilates and subdivides to form the urinary collecting system (collecting tubules, calyces, renal pelvis, and ureter) in both males and females. In the presence of testosterone, the mesonephric duct in males also forms the vas deferens, epididymis, ejaculatory duct, and seminal vesicles. In females, it degenerates entirely except for the vestigial Gartner's duct that can form a benign cyst along the broad ligament. The third scaffold—the *meta*nephros—also appears in week 5 of gestation and becomes the functioning kidney by week 9 of gestation. The ureteric bud from the *meso*nephric duct contacts the *meta*nephros and induces it to form nephrons. If this contact does not occur, renal agenesis results. The adjacent dorsal aorta also sends out collaterals into the *meta*nephros that ultimately develop into glomerular tufts.

Before week 7, the cloaca (the proximal portion of the allantois distally connected to the yolk sac) is divided into the urogenital (UG) sinus and the anorectal canal. During this process, the caudal-most portion of the mesonephric duct is absorbed. Thus, the ureteric bud no longer buds off of the mesonephric duct but enters the UG sinus directly. As such, the UG sinus forms the bladder and the ureteric buds form the ureters. The UG sinus forms the bladder and is continuous with the urethra caudally and the allantois cranially. The urachus is the fibrotic cord that remains when the allantois is obliterated and becomes the median umbilical ligament in the adult.

There are many renal anomalies (e.g., horseshoe kidney, ectopic kidney, and double ureter) that go undiagnosed and are without much consequence. Renal agenesis, however, is not one of these. Without kidneys, the fetus can still excrete waste via placental exchange; however, renal agenesis ultimately results in anhydramnios and leads to other potentially lethal issues. Without amniotic fluid, the fetal lungs do not have the constant pressure that would normally cause them to expand and grow. This leads to pulmonary hypoplasia. Without amniotic fluid, the fetus cannot move much and so develops dramatic deformations called contractures of the limbs. There have been attempts to put amniotic fluid into the amniotic cavity via amniocentesis. However, this has been unsuccessful because the fluid is resorbed rapidly. An indwelling catheter has also been considered, but the infectious risks are quite high. At this point in time, there is minimal treatment available for Potter disease. However, in Potter syndrome secondary to bladder outlet obstruction, there have been attempts to place catheters into the bladder or to perform in utero laser ablation of the obstruction. In theory, as long as the fetal kidneys have not been damaged, this idea should work. However, the recent trials indicate that pulmonary function may be improved but renal injury is much more difficult to prevent.

PRENATAL SCREENING

Screening for fetal chromosomal and congenital anomalies is dependent on developing screens that are both sensitive and specific for the condition being screened. Before we move on to discuss these modalities, we should quickly review the terms used with screening tests.

EPIDEMIOLOGY

The classic two-by-two table in epidemiology is divided into cases and controls versus exposed and unexposed. In screening tests, the two dimensions are affected/not affected versus screen positive/screen negative (Table 3-1).

As can be seen in Table 3-1, the sensitivity is the proportion of individuals who are affected and test positive. On the other hand, the specificity is that proportion of individuals who are unaffected and test negative. Sometimes we are more interested in what it means to have a particular test result. In this setting, the positive predictive value (PPV) reports what percentage of patients with a positive screen is affected. The negative predictive value (NPV) is the percentage of people with a negative screen who indeed are not affected. Another set of useful test characteristics is likelihood ratios. The positive likelihood ratio (LR+) tells how much to multiply the prior odds to get the posterior odds; that is, if one knows the odds of some event occurring is 1:100, and runs a test with an LR of 5, then the odds after getting a positive result is 5:100. Similarly, the negative likelihood ratio (LR−) does the same for a negative result.

TABLE 3-1. 2×2 Table

	Screen Positive (Pos)	Screen Negative (Neg)
Affected	a	b
Not affected	c	d

Sensitivity (sens) = a/(a + b); specificity (Spec) = d/(c + d); false negative = b/(a + b); false positive = c/(c + d); PPV = a/(a + c); NPV = d/(b + d); LR+ = sens/(1 − spec) = [a/(a + b)]/[c/(c + d)]; LR− = (1 − sens)/spec = [b/(a + b)]/[d/(c + d)].

FIRST-TRIMESTER SCREENING

First trimester was traditionally the time for the first prenatal visit and to get laboratory tests done. However, first-trimester screening has become a routine part of prenatal care and this has two theoretical benefits. One is to find screening tests that are more sensitive than the current second-trimester tests. The other is that by making the diagnosis sooner, the option of termination is safer. **Nuchal translucency** (NT) appears to be an excellent way to screen for aneuploidy and Down syndrome in particular. NT involves a measurement of the posterior fetal neck taken in profile view (Fig. 3-6). Its sensitivity for Down syndrome has been reported to be between 60% and 90% and is generally assumed to be about 70% or greater.

Several maternal serum analytes have been studied to generate a first-trimester serum screen. Currently, a combination of free or total β-hCG and PAPP-A is being studied alone and in combination with NT. Using a 5% false-positive rate, they appear to have a sensitivity of approximately 60% when used alone, and when combined, the two appear to give an approximate sensitivity of 80%. Commonly, thresholds

FIGURE 3-6. Posterior fetal neck, posterior view.

for these tests are established at a 5% false-positive rate, or where the posterior probability of disease is somewhere between 1:190 and 1:300.

SECOND-TRIMESTER SCREENING

The initial second-trimester serum screen was the MSAFP. This was designed to screen for fetuses with NTDs. When the data from studies were being analyzed, it was noted that the cases of Down syndrome had low MSAFP. This has been combined with low serum estriol and high β-hCG and inhibin as the quadruple screen (Table 3-2). Overall, the quadruple screen has only a 75% to 80% sensitivity for Down syndrome with a 5% false-positive rate. Maternal age is essentially another screening tool because it has been found that the risk of aneuploidy increases exponentially beyond age 35 (Fig. 3-7). At age 35, the overall risk is about 1:190 of aneuploidy. The quad screen is combined with maternal age to generate an overall risk profile of both Down syndrome and trisomy 18. Among women older than age 35, the quadruple (quad) screen has a sensitivity of more than 80%, whereas in women younger than age 35, the sensitivity drops to about 60%. One advantage of the quad screen over the first-trimester screens is that specially trained ultrasound technologists and sonologists are not necessary for performing the test so it is more widely available. Also, because a proportion of the pregnant population does not present for care in the first trimester, the quad screen is the only test available for them. Of importance, the first-trimester screen can be followed by the second-trimester screen called a sequential screen that leads to an even greater sensitivity for Down syndrome of approximately 95%.

Another finding from studies of MSAFP has been in patients whose MSAFP was elevated, but did not have an open NTD. Common reasons for this include inaccurate dating (MSAFP increases with gestation), abdominal wall defects, multiple gestations, placental abnormalities, and fetal demise. Patients whose MSAFP is elevated without an elevated amniotic fluid AFP or these other etiologies have been found to be at greater risk of pregnancy complications

TABLE 3-2. Quadruple Screen Table

	Trisomy 21	Trisomy 18	Trisomy 13
MSAFP	Decreased	Decreased	Depends on defects
Estriol	Decreased	Decreased	Depends on defects
β-hCG	Elevated	Decreased	Depends on defects
Inhibin	Elevated	Decreased	Depends on defects
MSAFP, maternal serum α-fetoprotein.			

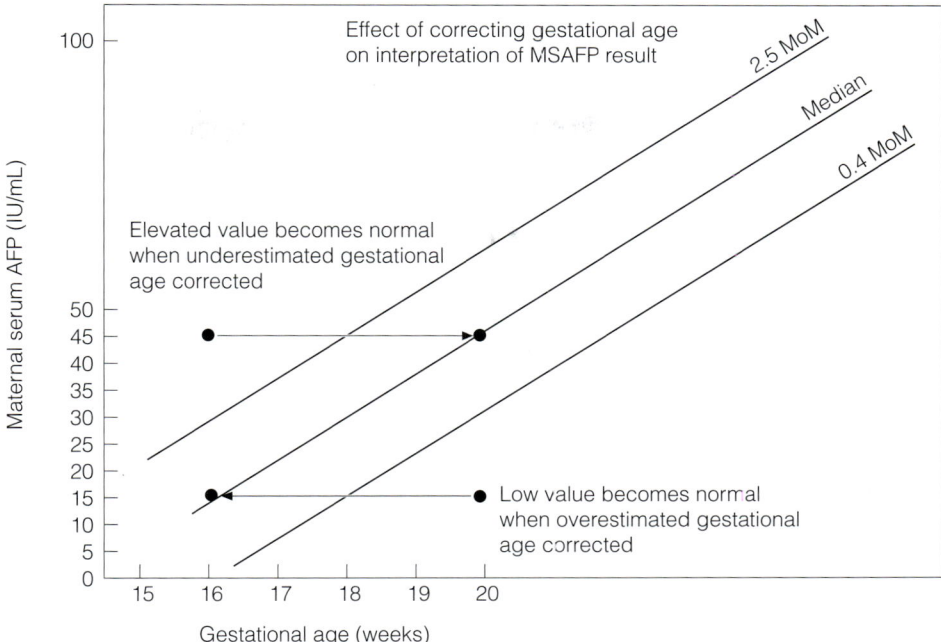

FIGURE 3-7. Median MSAFP levels throughout gestation. Increasing values with increasing GA require accurate dating to interpret low or high MSAFP. GA, gestation age; MSAFP, maternal serum α-fetoprotein.

associated with the placenta: placental abruption, preeclampsia, intrauterine growth restriction, and possibly intrauterine fetal demise. These problems have been associated with elevated β-hCG as well.

Real-time ultrasound is used to document a singleton, viable gestation and a rudimentary anatomy scan in more than 90% of pregnancies in the United States. The level I or screening obstetric ultrasound scan is a fair screening tool, but its sensitivity varies between providers. One study showed that there was a two- to threefold difference in the number of anomalies identified between primary and tertiary medical centers. The level I ultrasound is not designed to be all encompassing and does not look at fetal limbs, identify sex, show the face, or provide extensive views of the heart. These are generally all done in a level II, detailed or targeted ultrasound. A level II ultrasound is used in patients who are at risk for congenital anomalies or who have had an abnormal level I scan. These tests are generally performed by specially trained perinatologists or radiologists.

There are a number of "soft" findings on obstetric ultrasound that have been associated with aneuploidies. Trisomy 18 has been associated with the finding of a CP cyst, and Down syndrome has been associated with many ultrasound findings, most notably the **echogenic intracardiac focus** (EIF). Pathologically, the EIF (Fig. 3-8) is a calcification of the papillary

FIGURE 3-8. Echogenic intracardiac focus. (Image provided by Departments of Radiology and Obstetrics & Gynecology, University of California, San Francisco, CA.)

muscle without any particular pathophysiology. It is seen in 5% of pregnancies and is more common in the fetuses of Asian women. Unfortunately, the LR for this test is 1.5 to 2.0, so it at most double the pretest odds. For example, a young, 25-year-old woman whose Down syndrome risk is 1:1,000 prior to finding the EIF will therefore have an "increased" risk of 1:500 after finding the EIF. Thus, these tests end up needlessly worrying many patients only to identify a few abnormal fetuses.

CELL-FREE DNA SCREENING

Noninvasive prenatal diagnosis has been thought about and discussed for more than 25 years. It is known that both fetal cells and fetal DNA end up in the maternal circulation. Thus, it would be much less invasive to extract this genetic information from a blood draw from the mother than from either the amniotic fluid around the baby (amniocentesis) or a placental biopsy (CVS). Currently, there are several cfDNA tests on the market. These tests are relatively new and therefore should still be considered very good screening tests as opposed to perfectly diagnostic. The currently available tests all rely on the fact that there are free fetal DNA fragments circulating in the maternal plasma. From a maternal blood draw, a technique called massive parallel sequencing, is performed in which millions of small fragments of DNA are sequenced and counted. The relative ratio of fetal chromosome 21 is compared to the maternal 21 (or any other chromosome of interest) based on the proportion of fetal DNA in the maternal circulation. Potential advantages of this test include the high sensitivity (>98%), low false-positive rates (approximately 0.2%), and the ability to obtain samples early in pregnancy (10 weeks). Recent work has been performed looking at these tests in low-risk populations. Although the sensitivity and specificity rates remained about the same, the PPV was lower due to the lower incidence rate, thus resulting in a higher false-positive rate. Disadvantages of this test are that it is not useful in twins or cases of mosaicism, only screens for the most common aneuploidies, does not evaluate risk for structural abnormalities (such as NTD or cardiac defects), and is costly. Although this test's use appears to be increasing, it is controversial and several recent publications suggest that while it has a greater sensitivity and specificity for Down syndrome and other common aneuploidies than other traditional serum screening, it does not screen for more rare aneuploidies that can be identified on sequential screening, for example (*Am J Obstet Gynecol*. 2016;214:727.e1–727.e6). Another important limitation of cfDNA screening is that between 2% and 6% of women will not get results from the test. The risk of "no-results" is higher in obese women and in women with an aneuploidy. Because of this increased risk of aneuploidy, some clinicians have called for such patients to be called screen positive, but this would lead to many more women being offered invasive testing. Thus, this issue also remains controversial.

Patients who are known carriers of a genetic disease, at high risk for aneuploidy based on age, who have a positive screening test, or simply those who wish to have greater certainty about their fetus' risk of aneuploidy may choose to undergo a prenatal diagnostic test. This involves obtaining fetal cells in order to perform a karyotype and possibly DNA tests. There are currently three ways that fetal cells are obtained: amniocentesis, CVS, and percutaneous umbilical blood sampling (PUBS).

AMNIOCENTESIS

An amniocentesis is generally performed beyond 15 weeks to obtain a fetal karyotype, once the chorion and amnion have fused. Early amniocentesis prior to that has been studied and appears to be associated with higher pregnancy loss rates. **Amniocentesis** involves placing a needle transabdominally through the uterus, into the amniotic sac, and withdrawing some of the fluid. The fluid contains sloughed fetal cells that can be cultured. These cultured cells can then be karyotyped and also used in DNA tests.

The cultures take about 5 to 7 days to grow, and additional techniques—**fluorescent in situ hybridization** (FISH)—can be used to identify aneuploidy and give results in 24 to 48 hours. Additionally, chromosomal abnormalities (e.g., deletions) that are below the detection threshold of the traditional karyotype may be detected by FISH or microarray comparative genomic hybridization (CGH). Generally, the risk of complications secondary to amniocentesis is considered to be about 1:200, but more recent studies indicate a lower risk, perhaps 1 in approximately 350 or even less. The common risks are rupture of membranes, preterm labor, and, rarely, fetal injury. This risk of 1:200 is one of the reasons why the threshold risk for offering patients fetal diagnosis is about 1:200, which is roughly equivalent to age 35. Although it is true that the numbers are approximately the same, the outcomes—Down syndrome and miscarriage—are quite different. Thus, there has been a recent push to discard the maternal age 35 threshold in favor of counseling patients regarding their risk and allowing them to make their own decision incorporating risks and benefits of screening and diagnosis. The most recent bulletin on prenatal diagnosis from the American College of Obstetricians and Gynecologists suggests that both prenatal screening and prenatal diagnosis should be made available to all pregnant women.

With the improvement in maternal serum screening tests for aneuploidy, and now the advent of the noninvasive free fetal DNA tests, there is a de-emphasis on invasive prenatal diagnostic testing. Although this is a personal, individual decision for each pregnant woman, obviously, patients can be swayed by the medical culture. One potential issue with screening tests is that they look for trisomy 21, 18, and occasionally 13. There are other common aneuploidies, for example, the sex chromosomal aneuploidies, that some couples would choose to terminate. But, they often do not even know about these anomalies. Another relatively common chromosomal problem is a microdeletion, which is a break or loss of a small piece of chromosome. Small is a relative term; these microdeletions can be missing thousands of base pairs. Similarly, there can be an insertion called a microduplication. The best way to screen for microdeletion/microduplication syndromes is through a complete genome hybridization array (array cGH). This test can identify these microdeletions/microduplications and research studies are being done to determine the clinical utility for these tests. For example, the risk of such syndromes is higher in the setting of fetal abnormalities on an ultrasound, so it is commonly recommended to obtain array cGH in that setting (*N Engl J Med*. 2012;367:2175–2184). Importantly, if a pregnant woman or couple wants such a test, fetal DNA obtained from an invasive prenatal diagnostic test would be necessary.

Thus, while there are improvements in sensitivity and specificity, in the end, one cannot replace the certainty of a diagnostic test. It is important for patients to understand the difference between a screening and diagnostic test when they are being seen for prenatal care. If the primary clinician is not comfortable explaining the tests, referral to a genetic counselor or other expert in prenatal diagnosis is merited.

CHORIONIC VILLUS SAMPLING

Chorionic villus sampling (CVS) can be used to obtain a fetal karyotype sooner than amniocentesis because it can be performed between 9 and 12 weeks. CVS involves placing a catheter into the intrauterine cavity, either transabdominally or transvaginally, and aspirating a small quantity of chorionic villi from the placenta. The risk of complications from CVS is likely higher than the amniocentesis rate of 1:200. Because a greater amount of cells is obtained, CVS results are often faster than those of amniocentesis. However, the cells are from the placenta; therefore, in rare cases of confined placental mosaicism, the cells may be misleading. Complications include preterm labor, premature rupture of membranes, previable delivery, and fetal injury. When performed earlier than 9 weeks of gestation, CVS has been associated with fetal limb anomalies, which is assumed to be secondary to vascular interruption.

FETAL BLOOD SAMPLING

PUBS is performed by placing a needle transabdominally into the uterus and phlebotomizing the umbilical cord. This procedure may be used when a fetal hematocrit or platelet count needs to be obtained, particularly in the setting of Rh alloimmunization and other causes of fetal anemia. PUBS may also be used for rapid karyotype analysis. The PUBS needle can also be used to transfuse the fetus in cases of fetal anemia. Intrauterine transfusion was performed before the advent of real-time ultrasound by placing needles into the fetal peritoneal cavity and performing intraperitoneal transfusions, but transumbilical transfusions are more effective.

FETAL IMAGING

Currently, ultrasound is used most commonly to image a fetus prenatally. As described above, a level I or level II ultrasound is commonly performed between 18 and 22 weeks. The fetal anatomy can be difficult to visualize well prior to 18 weeks of gestation, giving the lower threshold for detection of anomalies. For the upper threshold, if an anomaly is seen, the further workup can take more than a week, giving the patient just a few days prior to 24 weeks of gestation to decide about termination of the pregnancy in the setting of congenital anomalies. A targeted, level II ultrasound can identify cleft lip, polydactyly, clubfoot (Fig. 3-9),

FIGURE 3-9. Clubfoot—the fibula and tibia can be seen with the foot at almost a right angle to them. (Image provided by Departments of Radiology and Obstetrics & Gynecology, University of California, San Francisco, CA.)

fetal sex, NTDs, abdominal wall defects, and renal anomalies. It can usually identify some cardiac and brain anomalies as well, but may not be able to make a specific diagnosis. It is poor at identifying esophageal atresia and tracheoesophageal fistula, in which sometimes the only sign may be a small or nonvisualized stomach in the setting of polyhydramnios.

Fetal echocardiogram is usually used to make specific diagnoses of fetal cardiac anomalies detected on ultrasound. Doppler ultrasound can characterize the blood flow through the chambers of the heart as well as the vessels entering and leaving the heart. Fetal echo is used in some institutions as the first-line diagnostic modality in patients at high risk for cardiac anomalies, in particular, pregestational diabetic patients.

Fetal MRI is one of the newest modalities to image a fetus. It is particularly useful in examining the fetal brain and may recognize changes associated with hypoxic damage sooner than ultrasound. It is also superior in measuring volumes. Another new modality that may be better in measuring volumes is three-dimensional (3-D) ultrasound. Although the image provided by 3-D ultrasound certainly looks more like an actual fetus than the more common 2-D images, it is unclear whether 3-D ultrasound offers increased diagnostic capabilities.

KEY POINTS

- Mothers can be asymptomatic carriers of AR diseases and can often be screened for carrier status. Geographic ancestry is used to provide pretest counseling and inform testing.
- If a mother is a carrier, the father of the baby can be screened as well to determine his carrier status. If the father is negative, there is no risk to the baby; if he is positive, there is a 25% chance of the disease in the fetus.
- The two common ways that AR disorders are introduced and maintained in a population are the founder effect (Tay–Sachs) and heterozygote advantage (sickle cell disease).
- Having an abnormal number of chromosomes usually leads to miscarriage. However, several aneuploidies exist that commonly survive until birth and beyond.
- Of all the autosomal trisomies, Down syndrome is the hardiest. Although they have foreshortened life expectancies, these individuals commonly survive into their 50s.
- The most common aneuploidies are those of the sex chromosomes. These individuals are less severely affected than the autosomal aneuploidies.
- Fetal congenital anomalies primarily arise during embryogenesis. However, they can progress (as seen in Potter syndrome) as development continues.
- NTDs are associated with folate deficiency and can be screened for by noting an elevated MSAFP.
- Cardiac anomalies that are surgically repaired can often result in minimal impairment, although this is highly lesion dependent.
- Organ systems are often interconnected during development, as in the case of the lungs and kidneys in Potter syndrome.
- The sensitivity of a screening test is that percentage of patients who would be identified by the test.
- Common screening tests for fetal abnormalities include first-trimester screening, the quad screen, and level I ultrasound.
- cfDNA testing appears to have great sensitivity and specificity for trisomies 13, 18, and 21 but does not screen for less common aneuploidies and has other limitations.
- Karyotype, array cGH, and specific DNA tests require fetal or trophoblastic cells for analysis.
- Fetal diagnosis in the first trimester is by CVS, which obtains trophoblastic cells.
- In the second trimester, amniocentesis is used to obtain fetal cells in the amniotic fluid.
- Prenatal diagnosis can also be made by imaging studies, most commonly 2-D ultrasound. Fetal echocardiogram, MRI, and 3-D ultrasound are also used.

Chapter 3 / Prenatal Screening, Diagnosis, and Treatment • 41

CLINICAL VIGNETTES

VIGNETTE 1

A 40-year-old G_2P_0 woman at 7 weeks gestational age (GA) by last menstrual period (LMP) presents for her first prenatal visit. She spontaneously conceived after 18 months of trying. She is excited about the pregnancy, but at the same time is concerned about potential risks for herself as well as the baby because of her age. Her husband is 52 years old, healthy, and has fathered two children from a prior marriage. The week prior to the visit, she experienced spotting that lasted 3 days and then resolved. Currently, she has no complaints. She has no past medical or surgical history except for a miscarriage 3 years ago. She has regular periods every 30 days.

1. You offer her which of the following prenatal screening/diagnostic tests?
   a. Chorionic villus sampling (CVS)
   b. Amniocentesis
   c. First-trimester screening
   d. Quad screening
   e. All of the above

2. She undergoes both first- and second-trimester screening. All of the screening tests are relatively reassuring as her risk of Down syndrome is reduced below the screen positive threshold at 1 in 967. She also has a normal screening ultrasound. You explain that these are screening tests and that she still has some risk for aneuploidy. Which of the following aneuploidies would be most common in the setting of otherwise normal screening?
   a. Trisomy 21
   b. Trisomy 18
   c. Trisomy 13
   d. Sex chromosomal aneuploidy
   e. None of the above

3. Because of the lack of certainty, she is considering an amniocentesis. The risks of amniocentesis include which of the following?
   a. Alloimmunization of an Rh-negative woman carrying an Rh-positive fetus
   b. Preeclampsia
   c. Premature rupture of membranes
   d. a, b, and c
   e. a and c only

4. In the end, she decides not to undergo amniocentesis. She goes on to deliver a normal-appearing baby boy at 39 weeks' gestation without complications. The counseling you gave to facilitate her decision-making specifically emphasized which of the following?
   a. Beneficence
   b. Justice
   c. Autonomy
   d. Paternalism
   e. None of the above

VIGNETTE 2

You are providing prenatal care to a 22-year-old G_1P_0 woman at 16 weeks GA by LMP. She has had a relatively smooth pregnancy without complications thus far. At 5,950 and 215 lb she has an obese BMI, otherwise without medical or surgical history. She presented to prenatal care at 14 1/2; weeks, and so missed first-trimester screening. She undergoes the quad screen and has an elevated level of maternal serum α-fetoprotein (MSAFP).

1. Given the elevation in MSAFP, her pregnancy is at increased risk for which of the following?
   a. Gestational diabetes
   b. Gastroschisis
   c. Down syndrome
   d. Klinefelter syndrome
   e. All of the above

2. You discuss the potential meaning of the elevated MSAFP. After a long conversation, the patient decides to undergo her second-trimester ultrasound. Which of the following findings seen on ultrasound would NOT be an explanation for the elevated MSAFP?
   a. Double bubble-duodenal atresia
   b. A membrane-covered mass protruding through the abdominal wall
   c. Fetal bowel floating around in the amniotic fluid
   d. Lack of a fetal skull
   e. A small membrane-covered outpouching in the lower back/spine

3. The ultrasound reveals a myelomeningocele. Which of the following is true and may be used in counseling?
   a. This is generally a lethal anomaly
   b. Delivery must be by cesarean to protect the baby
   c. Fetal surgery includes laser therapy
   d. Fetal surgery has been shown to improve some outcomes
   e. Fetal surgery is experimental and has no known benefits

4. The increased incidence of this finding is associated with which of the following medications when used in pregnancy?
   a. Valproic acid
   b. Lithium

c. Fluoxetine
d. Prednisone
e. Acetaminophen

5. In a subsequent pregnancy, prevention of recurrence would include:
   a. low-dose aspirin
   b. low molecular weight heparin
   c. prenatal vitamins taken twice per day
   d. 4 mg folic acid
   e. increased dietary calcium

VIGNETTE 3

A 25-year-old G2P1 woman presents at 9 weeks' gestation for routine prenatal care. She has a history of a prior term birth 2 years earlier in which she developed preeclampsia and required induction of labor at 38 weeks' gestation. This led a vaginal delivery of a viable baby girl. She is interested in first-trimester screening.

1. Which of the following is true about first-trimester screening?
   a. First-trimester serum screening has an 80% sensitivity for Down syndrome
   b. NT screening alone has a 70% sensitivity for Down syndrome
   c. Combined first-trimester screening has a 90% sensitivity for Down syndrome
   d. Increased NT in the setting of normal karyotype is associated with limb anomalies
   e. First-trimester screening has a sensitivity for Down syndrome that is greater than the sequential screen

2. Her tests come back with a risk for Down syndrome of 1 in 420 at 11 weeks' gestation. What do you report to the patient?
   a. The test is negative
   b. The test is positive
   c. The risk for Down syndrome is 1 in 420
   d. She will need an amniocentesis
   e. She will not need an amniocentesis

3. The patient chooses to delay prenatal diagnosis at this time and plans on obtaining second-trimester screening and an obstetric ultrasound. Which of the following is true about obstetric ultrasound and Down syndrome
   a. Ultrasound has a higher sensitivity for Down syndrome than the first-trimester screening
   b. Ultrasound has higher sensitivity for Down syndrome than the quad screening
   c. A finding of caudal regression syndrome on ultrasound is pathognomonic for Down syndrome
   d. Down syndrome fetuses with normal ultrasound findings have lower IQs than those with major anomalies
   e. Classic findings of Down syndrome on obstetric ultrasound are an AV canal and pyloric stenosis

VIGNETTE 4

A 24-year-old G_1P_0 woman presents for prenatal care at 8 weeks by LMP. She has regular menses every 28 to 30 days and you confirm her GA with an ultrasound today in the office. She has no past medical or surgical history. She and her husband of 6 months planned the pregnancy and they have both been reading about pregnancy and prenatal care. You discuss the prenatal tests for the first visit as well as the plan throughout the rest of the pregnancy.

1. As part of this discussion, you offer her which of the following prenatal screening/diagnostic tests?
   a. CVS
   b. Amniocentesis
   c. First-trimester screening
   d. Quad screening
   e. All of the above

2. The patient opts to undergo first-trimester screening, which returns with a risk for Down syndrome of 1 in 1,214 and risk of trisomy 18 of 1 in 987. At 18 weeks, she gets a quad screen, and her estriol, β-hCG, and α-fetoprotein (AFP) are all low. She has an ultrasound, which shows a fetus consistent with 16 weeks' size, increased amniotic fluid, clubfoot, omphalocele, choroid plexus cyst, and possible heart defect. On the basis of the patient's history and data provided, what is the most likely diagnosis?
   a. Trisomy 21
   b. Trisomy 18
   c. Trisomy 13
   d. Turner syndrome
   e. Klinefelter syndrome

3. The patient and her husband wish to have a definitive diagnosis. Which of the following tests do you offer her?
   a. Amniocentesis
   b. CVS
   c. Array CGH
   d. Quad screen
   e. Noninvasive prenatal diagnosis

4. Because of their anxiety about the diagnosis, the patient and her husband wonder if there is a faster test one could do to obtain a diagnosis more quickly. Which of the following do you offer them?
   a. Array CGH
   b. Fetal MRI
   c. Fluorescent in situ hybridization (FISH)
   d. MCA Doppler
   e. Quad screen

ANSWERS

VIGNETTE 1 Question 1
1. Answer E:
Decision-making about prenatal screening and diagnosis is going to be different for each woman/couple, instead of as with much of medical care where clinicians make strong recommendations. In prenatal diagnosis, the key is to not make specific recommendations, but to educate regarding the options. Because there are some young women who would prefer not to have a child with aneuploidy and are willing to bear the risk of invasive prenatal diagnosis, all pregnant women should be offered invasive prenatal diagnosis alongside options of screening. Conversely, older women who historically were recommended to undergo invasive prenatal diagnosis may wish to have a screening test and will live with the uncertainty of a screening test to avoid the risk of a pregnancy loss from invasive prenatal diagnosis.

VIGNETTE 1 Question 2
2. Answer D:
The sex chromosomal abnormalities include 45 X,O—Turner syndrome, 47 XXY—Klinefelter syndrome, as well as the less commonly diagnosed 47 XXX and 47 XYY. Unfortunately, the serum screens in the first and second trimester do not screen for the sex chromosomal abnormalities, so having a normal screen does not reduce the risk. Turner syndrome will commonly be found on first-trimester NT screen because these patients may have a cystic hygroma. However, this still does not reduce the risk of sex chromosomal abnormality below a screening threshold. Trisomy 21 thresholds are generally 1 in 200 to 1 in 300 varying by states and countries. Trisomies 18 and 13 will also commonly manifest multiple congenital anomalies, so their risk is quite low after a normal ultrasound. The four most common sex chromosomal abnormalities range in risk from approximately 1 in 500 to 1 in 1,000 live births, and the most common, Turner syndrome and Klinefelter syndrome, appear to be due to paternal nondisjunction rather than maternal. Thus, maternal age itself does not appear to be a risk factor.

VIGNETTE 1 Question 3
3. Answer E:
There are risks of amniocentesis that include pregnancy loss, infection (chorioamnionitis), preterm premature rupture of the membranes, risk of fetal injury with the needle, risk of puncturing the umbilical cord leading to loss of fetal blood, exposure to the fetus of maternal infection (e.g., HIV), and exposure to the mother of the fetal cells (e.g., alloimmunization of mother). There is no evidence that the risk of preeclampsia is any higher in the setting of amniocentesis.

VIGNETTE 1 Question 4
4. Answer C:
In many aspects of medical decision-making, it is important to emphasize patient autonomy in the decision-making process. This is because while the patient may not have as much information about the medical issues, she will have the most information about her preferences toward the outcomes. Thus, shared medical decision-making is at its best when the clinician provides information, pros and cons, and the patient incorporates her values and preferences to make the ultimate decision.

VIGNETTE 2 Question 1
1. Answer B:
Elevated MSAFP can be seen in a variety of pregnancy complications. It is primarily used to screen for NTDs such as spina bifida, meningomyelocele, or anencephaly. It is also elevated in pregnancies that are not dated as far along as they should be, have abdominal wall defects such as omphalocele or gastroschisis, and have placental abnormalities like previa or accreta. MSAFP is decreased in Down syndrome and has no relationship with Klinefelter syndrome.

VIGNETTE 2 Question 2
2. Answer A:
Double bubble is seen in the setting of duodenal atresia, which is seen more commonly in Down syndrome and is not associated with an elevated MSAFP. The membrane-covered mass through the abdominal wall is an omphalocele. Along with the bowel floating in the amniotic fluid, gastroschisis, these abdominal wall defects are associated with an increased MSAFP. NTDs such as anencephaly, no skull or cerebral cortex, or spina bifida, a lack of closure of the neural tube at various levels of the spine leads to an increased MSAFP.

VIGNETTE 2 Question 3
3. Answer D:
Myelomeningocele, a common form of spina bifida, is not usually lethal, but leads to long-term morbidity in a large majority of affected children. In order to reduce the morbidity, a recent prospective trial of closure of the defect while the fetus was still in utero was conducted. The study demonstrated improvement in several outcomes including ambulation at 30 months of age. Laser is used for in utero ablation of connecting vessels in the setting of twin-to-twin transfusion

syndrome, not in myelomeningocele repair. Some providers recommend cesarean delivery for fetuses with NTDs. This is not a uniform recommendation and is not accompanied with much evidence in favor of its practice.

VIGNETTE 2 Question 4
4. Answer A:
NTDs are increased in the setting of diabetes and women with seizure disorders. The latter is thought to be associated with the use of several antiepileptic drugs, including carbamazepine and valproic acid. Lithium is associated with Ebstein anomaly, a displacement of the tricuspid valve. Fluoxetine and several other SSRIs have been associated with an increase in fetal cardiac anomalies. Prednisone does not cross the placenta. However, it can lead to hyperglycemia, which may, in turn, cause fetal effects. It is important to have women on prednisone in pregnancy check blood glucose values. Acetaminophen has not been associated with any fetal anomalies.

VIGNETTE 2 Question 5
5. Answer D:
Folic acid supplementation has been shown to decrease the risk of NTDs. Folic acid has been added to grains in the United States, which has led to lower rates of NTDs. There is 0.4 mg of folic acid in standard prenatal vitamins. However, in high-risk patients, the recommendation is currently to take 10 times that dose, or 4 mg/day. Further work delineating the dose response and threshold effect still needs to be done. Low-dose aspirin has been shown to slightly reduce the risk of preeclampsia, and both low-dose aspirin and LMWH have been used in women with known thrombophilias. Low dietary calcium intake has been shown to be associated with preeclampsia, but intervention trials are equivocal on the potential benefits.

VIGNETTE 3 Question 1
1. Answer B:
First-trimester screening for Down syndrome has become the standard of care, though not all women can get access to the testing because of the lack of availability of trained sonologists to provide NT ultrasound and variability in the insurance coverage for first-trimester testing. The serum screen is composed of PAPP-A and free β-hCG and has a 60% sensitivity for Down syndrome alone. NT alone has a 70% sensitivity and when added to the serum screen, the two together have an 80% sensitivity. If the NT is increased and there is no aneuploidy, the fetus is at increased risk, in particular, for cardiac anomalies. The sequential screen is a test that combines the first-trimester and second-trimester tests. This combination gets to a 90% to 95% sensitivity, so it has a greater sensitivity than first-trimester screening alone.

VIGNETTE 3 Question 2
2. Answer C:
The question is not meant as a trick question, but to make the point that across most clinical settings, clinicians think of the Down syndrome screening tests as positive or negative. However, in the setting of Down syndrome screening because patient preferences are so important, the best way to counsel women is to present them with the absolute risks instead of calling a test positive or negative. Now, it is true that most Down syndrome screening thresholds range from 1 in 150 to 1 in 350, so this 1 in 420 would be considered a "negative" test from that standpoint. However, given that this risk is approximately twice her age-related risk should also be mentioned.

VIGNETTE 3 Question 3
3. Answer E:
Down syndrome fetuses will have findings on ultrasound about 60% of the time. This makes obstetric ultrasound a poor screening test for Down syndrome, worse than both first-trimester combined screening and quad screening. There are no good studies that suggest that the function of individuals with Down syndrome varies by ultrasound findings. However, mortality and some morbidity will be greater in those with serious cardiac anomalies. The classic cardiac anomaly in Down syndrome is the AV canal defect. Pyloric stenosis is also common and should raise concern for Down syndrome. Caudal regression is seen in diabetic pregnancies.

VIGNETTE 4 Question 1
1. Answer E:
As explained in Case 1, all prenatal screening and diagnostic options should be offered to all women. Case 1 discussed a 40-year-old woman and this one is about a 24-year-old woman; however, all options should be made available to both women. This is contrary to historic practice and teaching as recently as 5 to 10 years ago when clinicians would recommend invasive prenatal diagnosis to higher risk women and recommend against it to lower risk women. Many clinicians today, because they were trained in this prior era, still practice this way. Thus, in contrast to much of medical care wherein clinicians make strong recommendations, nondirective counseling by clinicians will make decision-making about prenatal screening and diagnosis different for each woman/couple. In prenatal diagnosis, the key is to not make specific recommendations, but to educate regarding the options. Because there are some young women who would prefer not to have a child with aneuploidy and are willing to bear the risk of invasive prenatal diagnosis, all pregnant women should be offered invasive prenatal diagnosis alongside options of screening. Conversely,

older women who historically were recommended to undergo invasive prenatal diagnosis may wish to have a screening test and will live with the uncertainty of a screening test to avoid the risk of a pregnancy loss from invasive prenatal diagnosis.

VIGNETTE 4 Question 2
2. Answer B:
The quad screen with low estriol, β-hCG, and MSAFP is consistent with trisomy 18. So is the finding of the multiple anomalies on ultrasound, including the growth restriction. Trisomy 13 may also have multiple anomalies on ultrasound, though these findings are more consistent with trisomy 18. Trisomy 21, Turner syndrome, and Klinefelter syndrome will all often have a normal ultrasound, though trisomy 21 will have soft findings or anomalies on ultrasound about 60% of the time. One part of the case that may have been confusing was her first-trimester test results, which revealed a risk of approximately 1 per 1,000 of both trisomies 21 and 18. Of note, while a 1 per 1,000 risk of trisomy 21 is roughly the background baseline, the risk of trisomy 18 of 1 per 1,000 is an increase over the background risk, which is 1 per 5,000 to 1 per 10,000. Further, this reminds us that these are simply screening tests, not diagnostic tests.

VIGNETTE 4 Question 3
3. Answer B:
In order to achieve a definitive diagnosis, one must obtain fetal DNA. This is usually done via CVS or amniocentesis. At 18 weeks' gestation, the preferred route is amniocentesis. Array CGH can be performed on the cells from the amniocentesis to look for microdeletions. This is relatively new technology and is not universally covered by insurance, so one would obtain a karyotype first and then order CGH if karyotype was negative. The quad screen was already performed on the patient and is just a screening test. Noninvasive prenatal diagnostic testing using free fetal DNA in the maternal circulation is available for trisomies 21, 18, and 13. However, this is still thought of as a high-order screening test, not a diagnostic test.

VIGNETTE 4 Question 4
4. Answer C:
A karyotype usually takes 5 to 10 business days to return a result. FISH can be used to get quick results in 2 to 3 days for commonly known problems such as trisomies 21, 18, 13, and aneuploidies of X or Y. FISH can also be used to screen for particular aberrations in components of the genome such as the 22q deletion seen in DiGeorge syndrome. Array CGH could also give the results potentially sooner than amniocentesis. However, currently turnaround times are not as fast as FISH and there are still relatively few laboratories performing this test. Fetal MRI can allow better visualization of anomalies, but would not give a genetic diagnosis. MCA Doppler is used to screen for fetal anemia by measuring the peak systolic velocity in the middle cerebral artery. As mentioned previously, the quad screen is a screening test that she has already had. She obtains the FISH testing, which is consistent with trisomy 18 as is the follow-up karyotype.

4 | Normal Labor and Delivery

LABOR AND DELIVERY

When a patient first presents to the labor floor, a quick initial assessment is made using the history of present pregnancy, obstetric history, and the standard medical and social history. Routinely, patients are queried regarding contractions, vaginal bleeding, leakage of fluid, and fetal movement. Beyond the standard physical examination, the obstetric examination includes maternal abdominal examination for contractions and the fetal lie, presentation, and size (**Leopold maneuvers**), cervical examination, fetal heart tones, and a sterile speculum examination if rupture of membranes is suspected. Increasingly, this obstetric examination is augmented with obstetric ultrasound evaluation of the cervical length and fetal presentation.

OBSTETRIC EXAMINATION

The physical examination includes determination of fetal lie, presentation, an estimated fetal weight, and a cervical examination. **Fetal lie**, that is, whether the infant is longitudinal or transverse within the uterus, is relatively easy to determine with Leopold maneuvers (Fig. 4-1). The maneuvers involve palpating first at the fundus of the uterus in the maternal upper abdominal quadrants, then on either side of the uterus (maternal left and right), and, finally, palpation of the presenting part just above the pubic symphysis. Determination of **fetal presentation**, either breech or vertex (cephalic), can be more difficult, and even the most experienced examiner may require ultrasound to confirm presentation, particularly in the obese patient.

RUPTURE OF MEMBRANES

In 10% of pregnancies, the membranes surrounding the fetus rupture prior to the onset of labor; this is called premature rupture of membranes (PROM).

FIGURE 4-1. (**A–D**) Leopold maneuvers used to determine fetal presentation, position, and engagement.

When PROM occurs more than 18 hours before labor, it is considered prolonged PROM and puts both mother and fetus at increased risk for infection. PROM is often confused with PPROM, which is preterm, premature rupture of membranes, with preterm being before 37 weeks of gestation.

Diagnosis

Diagnosis of rupture of membranes (ROM) is suspected with a history of a gush or leaking of fluid from the vagina, although sometimes it is difficult to differentiate between stress incontinence and small leaks of amniotic fluid. Diagnosis can be confirmed by the **pool**, **nitrazine**, and **fern** tests.

Using a sterile speculum to examine the vaginal vault, the pool test is positive if there is a collection of fluid in the vagina. This can be augmented by asking the patient to cough or bear down, potentially allowing one to observe fluid escaping from the cervix. Vaginal secretions are normally acidic, whereas amniotic fluid is alkaline. Thus, when amniotic fluid is placed on nitrazine paper, the paper should immediately turn blue. The estrogens in the amniotic fluid cause crystallization of the salts in the amniotic fluid when it dries. Under low microscopic power, the crystals resemble the blades of a fern, giving the test its name (Fig. 4-2). Caution should be exercised to sample fluid that is not directly from the cervix because cervical mucus also ferns and may result in a false-positive reading. If these tests are equivocal, an ultrasound examination can determine the quantity of fluid around the fetus. If the fluid volume was previously normal and there is no other reason to suspect low fluid, **oligohydramnios** is indicative of ROM. In situations in which an accurate diagnosis is necessary (e.g., PPROM where antibiotic prophylaxis would be indicated),

amniocentesis may be used to inject dilute indigo carmine dye into the amniotic sac to look for leakage of fluid from the cervix onto a tampon (the amnio dye test or tampon test). More recently, a rapid test called Amnisure has been developed. This test uses rapid molecular testing to identify placental α-microglobulin-1 via immunoassay, which appears to have a higher sensitivity and specificity than conventional tests for PROM. The clinical utility and cost-effectiveness of using this test continue to be explored, but the test is used widely in some clinical practices.

CERVICAL EXAMINATION

The cervical examination allows the obstetrician to determine whether a patient is in labor, the phase of labor, and how labor is progressing. The five components of the cervical examination are dilation, effacement, fetal station, cervical position, and consistency of the cervix. These five aspects of the examination make up the **Bishop score** (Table 4-1). A Bishop score greater than 8 is consistent with a cervix favorable for both spontaneous labor and, as it is more commonly used, induced labor.

Dilation is assessed by using either one or two fingers of the examining hand to determine how open the cervix is at the level of the **internal os**. The measurements are in centimeters and range from closed, or 0 cm, to fully dilated, or 10 cm. On average, a 10-cm dilation is necessary to accommodate the term infant's biparietal diameter.

Effacement is also a subjective measurement made by the examiner. It determines how much length is left of the cervix and how effaced (i.e., thinned out) it is (Fig. 4-3). Effacement can commonly be reported by percent or by cervical length. The typical cervix is 3 to 5 cm in length; thus, if the cervix feels like it is about 2 cm from external to internal os, it is 50% effaced. Complete or 100% effacement occurs when the cervix is as thin as the adjoining lower uterine segment.

FIGURE 4-2. Fern test. (From Beckmann CRB, Ling LW, Laube DW, et al. *Obstetrics and Gynecology*. 4th ed. Baltimore, MD: Lippincott Williams & Wilkins; 2002.)

TABLE 4-1. The Bishop Score				
Score	0	1	2	3
Cervical (cm)	Closed	1–2	3–4	<5 dilation
Cervical (%)	0–30	40–50	60–70	<80 effacement
Station	−3	−2	−1, 0	<+1
Cervical consistency	Firm	Medium	Soft	
Cervical position	Posterior	Mid	Anterior	

FIGURE 4-3. (**A**) The absence of cervical effacement prior to labor. (**B**) The cervix is approximately 50% effaced. (**C**) The cervix is as thin as the adjoining lower uterine segment, 100% effaced.

The relation of the fetal head to the ischial spines of the female pelvis is known as **station** (Fig. 4-4). When the most descended aspect of the presenting part is at the level of the ischial spines, it is designated 0 station. Station is negative when the presenting part is above the ischial spines and positive when it is below. There are two systems for measuring the distance of the presenting part in relation to the ischial spines. One divides the distance to the pelvic inlet into thirds, and, thus, station is −3 to 0 and then 0 to +3, which is at the level of the introitus. The other system uses centimeters, which gives stations of −5 to +5. Either system is effective, and both are widely used among different institutions; however the American College of Obstetricians and Gynecologists (ACOG) recommends the usage of the −5 to +5 system in its clinical guidelines.

Cervical **consistency** is self-explanatory. Whether the cervix feels firm, soft, or somewhere in between should be noted. Cervical **position** ranges from posterior to mid to anterior. A posterior cervix is high in the pelvis, located behind the fetal head and often quite difficult to reach, let alone examine. The anterior cervix can usually be felt easily on examination and is often lower down in the vagina. During early labor, the cervix often changes its consistency to soft and advances its position from posterior to mid to anterior.

Although cervical evaluation through a physical examination has been the standard throughout modern obstetrics, cervical evaluation through ultrasound has become increasingly common. There are clinical studies that find greater inter-observer reliability with ultrasound measures of cervical length as opposed to a digital physical examination of the cervix. So, particularly in the evaluation of preterm patients with concern for preterm labor, many clinicians will use ultrasound to measure the cervical length.

FETAL PRESENTATION AND POSITION

The fetal presentation can be **vertex** (head down), **breech** (buttocks down), or **transverse** (neither down). Although presentation may already be known from the Leopold maneuvers, it can be confirmed by examination of the presenting part during cervical examination. Assuming that the cervix is somewhat dilated, the fetal presenting part may be palpated as well during this examination. In the early stages of labor when the cervix is not very dilated, digital examination of the presenting part can be difficult, leading to inaccurate determination of presentation. However, palpation of hair or sutures on the fetal vertex or the gluteal cleft or anus on the breech usually leaves little doubt. A fetus presenting head-first should actually be designated cephalic rather than vertex, unless the head is flexed and the vertex is truly presenting. If the fetus is cephalic with an extended head, it may be presenting with either the face or the brow. If the fetal vertex is presenting along with a fetal extremity such as an arm, this is deemed a compound presentation.

With face presentations, the chin or mentum is the fetal reference point, while with breech presentations, the reference is the fetal sacrum (Fig. 4-5). If fetal presentation cannot be determined by physical examination, ultrasound can confirm presentation. Ultrasound is also useful in determining whether a

FIGURE 4-4. The relationship of the leading edge of the presenting part of the ischial spine determines the station. +1 station is depicted in the frontal view on the left; approximately −2 station is depicted in the lateral view on the right.

breech presentation is frank, complete, or footling. Breech presentations are discussed further in Chapter 6.

Fetal **position** in the vertex presentation is usually based on the relationship of the fetal occiput to the maternal pelvis. An abnormal fetal position such as occiput transverse (OT) or occiput posterior (OP) can lead to prolonged labor and a higher rate of cesarean delivery. Thus, OT or OP position may be suspected with an abnormally long labor. Position is determined by palpation of the sutures and fontanelles. The vault, or roof, of the fetal skull is composed of five bones: two frontal, two parietal, and one occipital. The **anterior fontanelle** is the junction between the two frontal bones and two parietal bones and is larger and diamond-shaped. The **posterior fontanelle** is the junction between the two parietal bones and the occipital bone and is smaller and more triangular. In the setting of extensive molding of the fetal skull or asynclitism, where the sagittal suture is not midline within the maternal pelvis, palpation of the fetal ear can be used to determine position. Ultrasound can also be useful in determining fetal position on labor and delivery and has been noted to be more accurate than vaginal examination.

NORMAL LABOR

Labor is defined as contractions that cause cervical change in either effacement or dilation. **Prodromal labor** or "false labor" is common in the differential diagnosis of labor. These patients usually present with irregular contractions that vary in duration, intensity, and intervals and yield little or no cervical change.

The diagnosis of labor strictly defined is regular uterine contractions that cause cervical change. However, clinicians use many other signs of labor, including patient discomfort, bloody show, nausea and vomiting, and palpability of contractions. These signs and symptoms vary from patient to patient; although they can add to the assessment, clinicians should rely on an objective definition.

INDUCTION AND AUGMENTATION OF LABOR

Induction of labor is the attempt to begin labor in a nonlaboring patient, whereas **augmentation of labor** is intervening to increase the already present contractions. Labor is induced with **prostaglandins**, **oxytocic agents**, mechanical dilation of the cervix, and/or **artificial ROM**. The indications for induction are based on maternal, fetal, or fetoplacental reasons. Common indications for induction of labor include postterm pregnancy, preeclampsia, diabetes mellitus, nonreassuring fetal testing, and intrauterine growth restriction. The patient's desire to end the pregnancy is *not* an indication for induction of labor, and is characterized as an elective induction of labor.

Induction of labor has become increasingly common in the United States with as many as one

50 • **BLUEPRINTS** Obstetrics & Gynecology

FIGURE 4-5. (A–H) Various possible positions of the fetal head in the maternal pelvis.

A Occiput anterior
B ROA
C ROT
D ROP
E Occiput posterior
F LOP
G LOT
H LOA

in five pregnancies ending up with an induction of labor. It has been conjectured that the rise in inductions of labor, particularly those at 35 and 36 weeks of gestation, has contributed to the overall rise in the rate of preterm birth. Elective inductions at 37 and 38 weeks of gestation, while technically at term, have been shown to lead to higher rates of neonatal morbidity and should be avoided. Although elective induction of labor at 39 and 40 weeks of gestation has been demonized as contributing to the overall rise in cesarean delivery, it is unclear whether elective induction is truly associated with an increase in cesareans. The majority of studies compare elective induction to spontaneous labor, but the actual clinical decision is between induction and expectant management. Expectant management can lead to spontaneous labor, but it also leads to a larger fetus, an older placenta, and a proportion of these patients will go on to develop preeclampsia or a postterm pregnancy requiring induction of labor as well. In studies of elective induction of labor at 41 weeks of gestation, there appears to be a decrease in the overall rate of cesarean. In three very small, non-US studies of elective induction of labor prior to 41 weeks of gestation, there appears to be a decrease in the overall rate of cesarean as well. Future studies, particularly ones that will reflect practice in a variety of settings, will be necessary to demonstrate such a potential benefit.

Preparing for Induction

When proper indications for induction exist, the situation should be discussed with the patient and a plan for induction formed. When the indication is more pressing, induction should be started without significant delay. The success of an induction (defined as achieving vaginal delivery) is higher with favorable cervical status as defined by the **Bishop score**. A Bishop score of 5 or less may lead to a failed induction as often as 50% of the time. In these patients, prostaglandin E_2 (PGE_2) gel, PGE_2 pessary (Cervidil), or PGE_1M (misoprostol) is often used to "ripen" the cervix. The use of cervical ripening agents with prostaglandins or a mechanical means to dilate the cervix can reduce the risk of cesarean delivery.

There are both maternal and obstetric contraindications for the use of prostaglandins. Maternal reasons include asthma and glaucoma. Obstetric reasons include having had a prior cesarean delivery and nonreassuring fetal testing. Because PGE_2 gel cannot be turned off with the ease of oxytocin, there is a risk of uterine hyperstimulation and tetanic contractions. In this setting, a mechanical dilator such as a 30mL or 60 mL Foley bulb can be used. The Foley is inserted into the cervix adjacent to the amniotic sac, inflated, and placed on gentle traction. It usually dilates the cervix 2 to 3 cm within 4 to 6 hours, but may stay in for up to 12 hours.

Induction

Labor may begin with the ripening and dilation of the cervix performed with prostaglandins or mechanical means. However, labor induction is usually begun pharmacologically with oxytocin (Pitocin). This is a synthesized, but identical, version of the octapeptide oxytocin normally released from the posterior pituitary that causes uterine contractions. Pitocin is given continuously via IV drip because it is rapidly metabolized.

Labor may also be induced by **amniotomy**. Amniotomy is performed with an amnio hook that is used to puncture the amniotic sac around the fetus and release some of the amniotic fluid. After the amniotomy is performed, a careful examination should be performed to ensure that prolapse of the umbilical cord has not occurred. When performing amniotomy, it is important not to elevate the fetal head from the pelvis to release more of the amniotic fluid because this may lead to prolapse of the umbilical cord beyond the fetal head.

Augmentation

Oxytocin and amniotomy are also used to augment labor. The indications for augmentation of labor include those for induction in addition to inadequate contractions or a prolonged phase of labor. The adequacy of contractions is indirectly assessed by the progress of cervical change. It may also be measured directly using an **intrauterine pressure catheter** (IUPC) that determines the absolute change in pressure during a contraction and thus estimates the strength of contractions. Aggressive augmentation, deemed active management of labor, involves both oxytocin and amniotomy and has been demonstrated to lead to shorter labor courses but no difference in cesarean delivery rates.

MONITORING OF THE FETUS IN LABOR

It is easy to monitor the mother in labor with vital signs and laboratory studies. Monitoring the infant is indirect and thus more difficult than maternal assessment. Determination of the baseline rate and assessment of fetal heart rate variations with contractions can be done by auscultation. The normal range for the fetal heart rate is between 110 and 160 beats per minute. With baselines above 160, fetal distress secondary to infection, hypoxia, or anemia is of concern. Any prolonged fetal heart rate deceleration of greater than 2 minutes' duration with a heart rate less than 90 beats per minute is of concern and requires immediate action.

External Electronic Monitors

Since the advent of electronic fetal monitoring, intermittent auscultation is rarely used in the hospital setting. Continuous fetal heart monitors are standard in most hospitals in the United States because they afford several advantages over auscultation. The information gathered is more subtle and includes variations in heart rate. Arguably, the greatest advantage is that the information is easier to gather and record. This allows more time for analyzing the data and has economic advantages because one nurse can readily monitor multiple patients. In one of the largest studies conducted in Dublin at the National Maternity Hospital and published in 1985, the rate of cesarean was slightly greater in the continuous fetal monitoring group (2.4% vs. 2.2%) and the rate of operative vaginal delivery was higher (8.2% vs. 6.3%). However, there were more fetuses identified with abnormal umbilical cord pH values. Intermittent auscultation has been found to be associated with a higher rate of neonatal seizures, though no difference in cerebral palsy in long-term follow-up. There are very few recent studies examining these two fetal monitoring methods in a modern obstetric population. The decision making surrounding the use of such monitoring varies between different labor and delivery units. Intermittent auscultation is predominantly driven by midwives and pregnant women who desire less intervention.

The external tocometer has a pressure transducer that is placed against the patient's abdomen, usually near the fundus of the uterus. During uterine contractions, the abdomen becomes firmer, and this pressure is transmitted through the transducer to a tocometer that records the contraction. The relative heights of the tracings on different patients or at different locations on the same patient cannot be used to compare strength of contractions. External tocometers are most useful for measuring the frequency of contractions and comparing to the fetal heart rate tracing to determine the type of decelerations occurring.

A fetal heart tracing is evaluated by visual inspection. A fetal heart rate tracing is examined for several characteristics that are considered reassuring. First, the baseline is determined and should be in the normal range (110 to 160 beats per minute). Then the variations from the baseline should be examined. The beat-to-beat variation from the baseline is called fetal heart rate variability. Fetal heart rate variability is interpreted as absent (<3 beats per minute of variation), minimal (3 to 5 beats per minute of variation), moderate (5 to 25 beats per minute of variation), and marked (more than 25 beats per minute of variation). The tracing should be jagged from the beat-to-beat variability of the heart rate. Although a fetal heart rate tracing with minimal variability is not reassuring, this may also occur while the fetus is asleep or inactive. A flat tracing with absent variability is more worrisome and demands that another test to determine fetal well-being be conducted. There should also be at least three to five cycles per minute of the heart rate around the baseline. Finally, a tracing can be considered formally reactive (Fig. 4-6), if there are at least two accelerations of at least 15 beats per minute over the baseline that last for at least 15 seconds within 20 minutes.

Decelerations of the Fetal Heart Rate

The fetal heart rate tracing should also be used to examine decelerations and can be used along with the tocometer to determine the type and severity. There are three types of decelerations: early, variable, and late. **Early decelerations** begin and end approximately at the same time as contractions (Fig. 4-7A). They are a result of increased vagal tone secondary to head compression during a contraction. **Variable decelerations** can occur at any time and tend to drop more precipitously than either early or late decelerations (Fig. 4-7C). They are a result of umbilical cord compression. Repetitive variables with contractions can be seen when the cord is entrapped either under a fetal shoulder or around the neck and is compressed with each contraction. **Late decelerations** begin at the peak of a contraction and slowly return to baseline after the contraction has finished (Fig. 4-7B). These decelerations are a result of uteroplacental insufficiency and are the most worrisome type. They may degrade into bradycardias as labor progresses, particularly with stronger contractions.

Fetal Scalp Electrode

In the case of repetitive decelerations or in fetuses that are difficult to trace externally with Doppler, a **fetal scalp electrode** (FSE) is often used. A small electrode is attached to the fetal scalp that senses the potential differences created by the depolarization of the fetal heart. The information obtained from the scalp electrode is more sensitive in terms of the beat-to-beat variability and is in no danger of being lost during contractions as the fetal position changes. Contraindications include a history of maternal hepatitis or HIV or fetal thrombocytopenia.

Fetal Heart Rate Evaluation

Although fetal heart rate monitoring has been used widely since the 1970s and 1980s, consistent algorithms to evaluate the tracing have not been

FIGURE 4-6. (**A**) Normal short- and long-term beat-to-beat variability. (**B**) Reduced variability. This may occur during fetal sleep, following maternal intake of drugs, or with reduced fetal CNS function, as in asphyxia.

developed and adopted. Thus, the fetal heart rate abnormalities that were thought to contribute to the rapid rise in cesarean deliveries three decades ago are still poorly understood. This lack of understanding and consensus led to a National Institutes of Health (NIH) conference in 2008. This conference arrived at a three-tier categorization of the fetal heart rate:

Category I—This is a normal fetal heart rate tracing characterized by a normal baseline, moderate variability, and no variable or late decelerations.
Category II—This is an indeterminate fetal heart tracing and includes a variety of fetal heart tracings, including those with variable and late decelerations, bradycardia and tachycardia, minimal variability, marked variability, and even absent variability without decelerations. The best way to remember Category II is that it is not Category I and not Category III, but every other fetal heart tracing.
Category III—This is an abnormal fetal heart rate tracing. Category III tracings consist of those with absent fetal heart variability and recurrent late or variable decelerations or bradycardia. The other fetal heart rate tracing that also is Category III is the sinusoidal pattern consistent with fetal anemia.

Although these categories are a step in the right direction to provide a consistent approach to fetal heart rate monitoring, they should not be perceived as the final word on fetal heart rate monitoring. In particular, there has been criticism of the three-tiered system as not being granular enough and having too broad a range of tracings in Category II. Ongoing work will hopefully shed light on this incredibly important topic to allow us to better identify those fetuses at risk for injury and also maintain or even decrease the cesarean delivery rate.

Intrauterine Pressure Catheter

The external tocometer records the onset and end of contractions. The absolute values of the readings mean little and are entirely position dependent. Further, on some patients—particularly those who are obese—the tocometer does not show much in the way of fluctuation from the baseline. If it is particularly important to determine the timing or strength of contractions, an intrauterine pressure catheter (IUPC) may be used (Fig. 4-8). This catheter is threaded past the fetal presenting part into the uterine cavity to measure the pressure changes during contractions. The baseline intrauterine pressure is usually between 10 and 15 mm Hg. Contractions during labor will increase by 20 to 30 mm Hg in early labor and by 40 to 60 mm Hg as labor progresses. The most commonly used measurement of uterine contractions is the **Montevideo unit**, which is an average of the variation of the intrauterine pressure from the baseline multiplied by the number of contractions in a 10-minute period. Some institutions use the Alexandria unit, which multiplies the Montevideo units by the length of each contraction as well.

Fetal Scalp pH, Pulse Oximetry, and ST-Analysis

If a fetal heart rate tracing is nonreassuring, the fetal scalp pH may be obtained to directly assess fetal hypoxia and acidemia (Fig. 4-9). Fetal blood is obtained by making a small nick in the fetal scalp and drawing up a small amount of fetal blood into capillary tubes. The results are reassuring when the scalp pH is greater than 7.25, indeterminant when it is between 7.20 and 7.25, and nonreassuring when it is less than 7.20. Care must be taken to avoid contamination of the blood sample with amniotic fluid, which is basic and will elevate the results falsely. Although this tool is used less frequently now that technology has improved fetal monitoring,

FIGURE 4-7. (**A**) An early deceleration pattern is depicted in this FHR tracing. Note that each deceleration returns to baseline before the completion of the contraction. The remainder of the FHR tracing is reassuring. (**B**) Repetitive late decelerations in conjunction with decreased variability. (**C**) Variable decelerations are the most common periodic change of the FHR during labor. Repetitive mild to moderate variable decelerations are present. The baseline is normal.

FIGURE 4-8. Technique for continuous electronic monitoring of FHR and uterine contractions.

FIGURE 4-9. Technique for fetal scalp blood sampling via an amnioscope. After making a small stab incision in the fetal scalp, the blood is drawn off through a capillary tube.

it can still provide additional information on fetal well-being. Interestingly, it is almost never used in the United States any longer, but still used in 5% or more of fetuses in the United Kingdom.

Another modality for assessing fetal status that is still experimental at this point is fetal pulse oximetry. Using technology similar to the monitors placed on ears, fingers, and toes, the fetal pulse oximeter is placed intrauterine along the fetal cheek and measures fetal oxygen saturation. A normal fetal pulse oximeter reading is above 30%. Because fetal variability and decelerations have a poor predictive value of fetal hypoxemia and acidemia, it is theorized that the fetal pulse oximeter would be useful in such patients. A large, multicenter trial demonstrated that many of these fetuses with nonreassuring tracings do have normal pulse oximeter readings. However, the use of the pulse oximeter did not have an effect on either the cesarean delivery rate or fetal outcomes. Thus, the FDA did not approve fetal pulse oximetry, and it is unclear whether this technology has the potential for future use. Recently, STAN (ST-Analysis of the fetal electrocardiogram) has been examined in a variety of settings. Although initial studies were promising, with lower cesarean rates and lower rates of neonatal acidemia, a recent, large trial in the United States showed no benefit of either reducing cesareans or reducing neonatal acidemia at delivery.

THE PROGRESSION OF LABOR

Labor is assessed by the progress of cervical effacement, cervical dilation, and descent of the fetal presenting part. To assess the progress of labor, it is important to understand the cardinal movements or mechanisms of labor.

Cardinal Movements of Labor

The cardinal movements are engagement, descent, flexion, internal rotation, extension, and external rotation (also called restitution or resolution) (Fig. 4-10). When the fetal presenting part enters the pelvis, it is

FIGURE 4-10. (A–H) Cardinal movements of labor.

said to have undergone **engagement**. The head will then undergo **descent** into the pelvis, followed by **flexion**, which allows the smallest diameter to present to the pelvis. With descent into the midpelvis, the fetal vertex undergoes **internal rotation** from an OT position so that the sagittal suture is parallel to the anteroposterior diameter of the pelvis, commonly to the occiput anterior (OA) position. Disruption of the internal rotation or improper rotation can lead to a fetus maintained in OT position or malrotated to the OP position. As the vertex passes beneath and beyond the pubic symphysis, it will **extend** to deliver. Once the head delivers, **external rotation** occurs and the shoulders may be delivered.

Stages of Labor
Labor and delivery are divided into three stages. Each stage involves different concerns and considerations.

Stage 1 begins with the onset of labor and lasts until dilation and effacement of the cervix are completed. Stage 2 is from the time of full dilation until delivery of the infant. Stage 3 begins after delivery of the infant and ends with delivery of the placenta.

Stage 1

The first stage of labor ranges from the onset of labor until complete dilation of the cervix has occurred. An average first stage of labor lasts approximately 10 to 12 hours in a nulliparous patient and 6 to 8 hours in a multiparous patient. The range of what is considered within normal limits is quite wide, from 6 to 20 hours in a nulliparous patient and from 2 to 12 hours in a multiparous patient. The first stage is further divided into the latent and active phases (Fig. 4-11).

The **latent phase** generally ranges from the onset of labor until 6 cm of dilation and is characterized by slow cervical change. The **active phase** follows the latent phase and extends until complete dilation, and is defined by the period of time when the slope of cervical change against time is at its maximum. A third phase has been delegated just prior to complete dilation called deceleration or transition phase.

Historically, the values of the length of the first stage were primarily derived from studies of labor by Dr. Emmanuel Friedman in the 1950s and 1960s. These studies found that during the active phase, at least 1.0 cm/hour of dilation could be expected in a nulliparous woman and 1.2 cm/hour in a multiparous woman. This minimal expectation was approximately the fifth percentile of women undergoing labor, and the median rates of dilation range from 2.0 to 3.0 cm/hour during the active phase as designated by the Friedman curve. Further, the Friedman studies suggested that the active phase began at 3 to 4 cm of cervical dilation as seen in Fig 4-11. However, studies over the last decade reveal longer first and second stages of labor and variation by maternal race/ethnicity, age, and body habitus; thus, longer norms have been created and the new threshold for active labor is 6 cm of dilation.

The three "Ps"—power, passenger, and pelvis—can all affect the transit time during the active phase of labor. The "power" is determined by the strength and frequency of uterine contractions. The size and position of the infant affect the duration of the active phase, as do the size and shape of the maternal pelvis. If the "passenger" is too large for the "pelvis," **cephalopelvic disproportion** (CPD) results. If the rate of change of cervical dilation falls below the fifth percentile (1.0 cm/hour), these three Ps should be assessed to determine whether a vaginal delivery can be expected. Strength of uterine contractions can be measured with an IUPC and is considered adequate with greater than 200 Montevideo units. Signs of CPD include development of fetal caput and extensive molding of the fetal skull with palpable overlapping sutures.

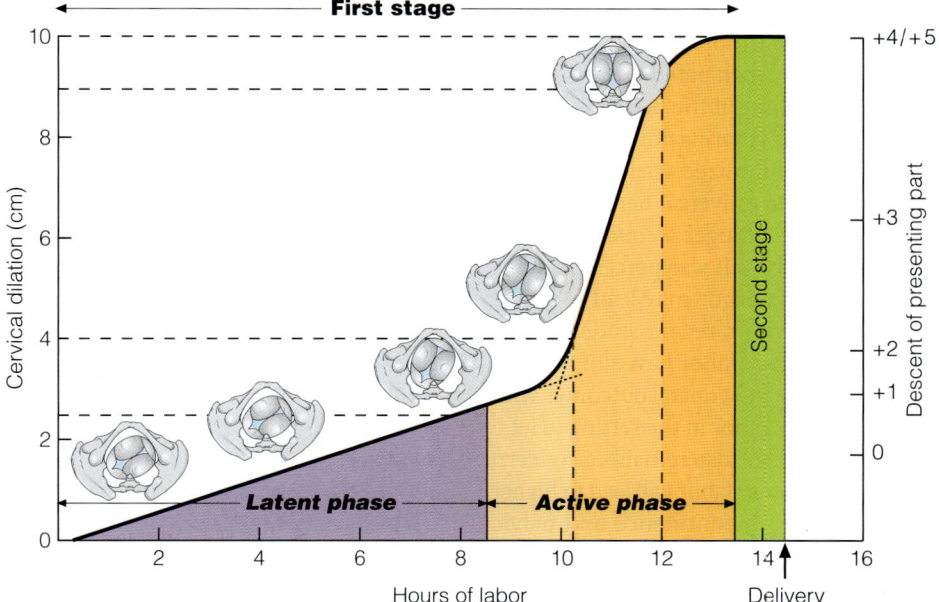

FIGURE 4-11. The progress of rotation of OA presentation in the successive stages of labor.

If there is no change in either cervical dilation or station for 2 hours in the setting of adequate Montevideo units during the active phase of labor, this is deemed active phase arrest and is an extremely common indication for cesarean. However, in the past decade, several studies have indicated that if clinicians exhibited more patience in this setting by waiting up to 4 or more hours to make this diagnosis, then more than half of these women will go on to deliver vaginally. Although the issue deserves more research, in a setting with continuous fetal monitoring and no worrisome signs from either the mother or the fetus, it appears reasonable to manage such pregnancies expectantly to allow for the possibility of vaginal birth.

Stage 2

When the cervix has completely dilated, stage 2 has begun. Stage 2 is completed with delivery of the infant. Stage 2 is considered prolonged if its duration is longer than 3 hours in a nulliparous patient, although at least an extra hour is allowed in patients who have epidurals. In multiparous women, stage 2 is prolonged if its duration is longer than 2 hours without an epidural and at least 3 hours with an epidural. In multiparous women without an epidural, it is rare for stage 2 to last longer than 60 minutes unless there is fetal macrosomia, persistent occiput posterior or transverse position, compound presentation, or asynclitism. However, epidurals can have a profound effect on the length of the second stage in both nulliparous and multiparous women.

One reason for the effect on the second stage is that often women will have little urge to push, little sensation, and even a strong motor block and so have less ability to push. Often, such patients are given an hour or two without pushing at the beginning of the second stage; this is called "laboring down" or "passive descent." Prospective randomized trials of laboring down do not demonstrate universal benefit, and all find that women will have a longer second stage with laboring down. Traditionally, it was perceived that a prolonged second stage of labor may lead to worse neonatal outcomes. However, recent studies of the length of the second stage of labor have not actually demonstrated a difference in neonatal outcomes with prolonged second stage of labor in the setting of fetal heart rate monitoring. There also remains a concern that prolonged second stage of labor will lead to higher rates of maternal urinary incontinence and pelvic relaxation, but to date, no large, prospective studies have been performed. Thus, management of the second stage of labor remains somewhat controversial.

Monitoring Repetitive early and variable decelerations are common during the second stage. The clinician can be reassured if these decelerations resolve quickly after each contraction and there is no loss of variability in the tracing. Repetitive late decelerations, bradycardias, and loss of variability are all signs of nonreassuring fetal status. With these tracings, the patient should be placed on face mask O_2, turned onto her left side to decrease inferior vena cava (IVC) compression and increase uterine perfusion; if it is being used, the oxytocin should be immediately discontinued until the tracing resumes a reassuring pattern. If a prolonged deceleration is felt to be the result of uterine **hypertonus** (a single contraction lasting 2 minutes or longer) or **tachysystole** (greater than five contractions in a 10-minute period), which can be diagnosed by palpation or examination of the tocometer, the patient can be given a dose of terbutaline to help relax the uterus. If a nonreassuring pattern does not resolve with these interventions, the fetal position and station should be assessed to determine whether an operative vaginal delivery can be performed. If fetal station is above 0 station (though many clinicians will require the fetus to be +2 station or lower) or the position cannot be determined, cesarean delivery is the mode of choice.

More recently, it has been recognized that uterine tachysystole, even in the setting of no fetal heart rate decelerations, can lead to higher rates of complications. Thus, with uterine tachysystole and a Category I tracing, if an agent is being used to induce or augment the labor, either that medication will be decreased or an IUPC will be used to more accurately estimate the Montevideo units being generated by the uterine contractions. If uterine tachysystole with a Category I tracing occurs spontaneously, it deserves close follow-up. If a Category II or III tracing occurs in this setting, terbutaline can be given to reduce the frequency of contractions.

Vaginal Delivery As the fetus begins crowning, the delivering clinician should be dressed with eye protection, sterile gown, and sterile gloves (for self-protection as much as for prevention of maternal/fetal infection) and have two clamps, scissors, and suction bulb. Historically, when meconium was suspected or confirmed many units used a DeLee suction trap to aspirate meconium from the neonatal airway after the head is delivered and prior to delivery of the rest of the body before breaths can be taken. However, after a large, prospective, randomized trial was conducted and demonstrated no benefit from

FIGURE 4-12. Near completion of the delivery of the fetal head by the modified Ritgen maneuver. Moderate upward pressure is applied to the fetal chin by the posterior hand covered with a sterile towel while the suboccipital region of the fetal head is held against the symphysis.

such suctioning, the routine use of the DeLee for meconium is no longer recommended.

Various approaches can be taken to vaginal delivery, but most clinicians would agree that a smooth, controlled delivery leads to less perineal trauma. Thus, one hand is commonly used to support or massage the perineum, while the other hand is used to flex the head to keep it from extending too quickly and causing periurethral or labial lacerations. The fingers on the hand controlling the fetal head can also be used to massage the labia over the head during delivery. When a delivery needs to be expedited, a modified Ritgen maneuver (Fig. 4-12) using the heel of the delivering hand to exert pressure on the perineum and the fingers below the woman's anus to extend the fetal head to hasten delivery and maintain station between contractions may be performed. This procedure tends to lead to greater perineal lacerations, but is effective during a prolonged deceleration to effect delivery.

Once the head of the infant is delivered, the mouth and upper airway are bulb suctioned. After suctioning is complete, the infant's neck is checked for a wrapped umbilical cord. If such a nuchal cord exists, an attempt is made to reduce the cord over the infant's head. If it is too tight, two options exist: If the clinician is extremely confident that delivery will be accomplished shortly, the cord is clamped and cut at this point. If a shoulder dystocia is suspected, an attempt is made to deliver the infant with the nuchal cord intact.

Delivery of the rest of the infant follows first with delivery of the anterior shoulder by exerting direct downward pressure on the infant's head. Once the anterior shoulder is visualized, a direct upward pressure is exerted to deliver the posterior shoulder (Fig. 4-13). After this, exertion of gentle traction will deliver the torso and the rest of the infant. At this point, the cord is clamped and cut and the infant passed either to the labor nurse and mother or to the waiting pediatricians.

Episiotomy An **episiotomy** is an incision made in the perineum to facilitate delivery. Indications for episiotomy include need to hasten delivery and

FIGURE 4-13. (**A**) Delivery of the anterior shoulder. (**B**) Delivery of posterior shoulder.

impending or ongoing shoulder dystocia. A relative contraindication for episiotomy is the assessment that there will be a large perineal laceration, because episiotomies have been associated with higher risk of severe perineal lacerations. Once the episiotomy is done, great care should be taken to support the perineum around the episiotomy to avoid extension into the rectal sphincter or rectum itself. In the past, episiotomies were used routinely in the setting of spontaneous and operative vaginal deliveries. However, evidence suggests that the rate of third- and fourth-degree lacerations increases with the use of routine midline episiotomy.

There are two common types of episiotomies: median (or midline) and mediolateral (Fig. 4-14). The median episiotomy, the most common type used in the United States, uses a vertical midline incision from the posterior fourchette into the perineal body. The mediolateral episiotomy is an oblique incision made from the 5- or 7-o'clock position on the perineum and cut laterally. Historically, it has been used less frequently and reportedly causes more pain and wound infections. However, mediolateral episiotomies are thought to lead to fewer third- and fourth-degree extensions, particularly in patients with short perineums or with operative deliveries.

▮ **Operative Vaginal Delivery** In the case of a prolonged second stage, maternal exhaustion, or the need to hasten delivery, an operative vaginal delivery may be indicated. The two possibilities are forceps delivery or vacuum-assisted delivery. Both are effective methods to facilitate vaginal delivery and have similar indications. The choice of method depends on the clinician's preference and experience, though they carry slightly different risks of maternal and neonatal complications.

▮ **Forceps Delivery** **Forceps** (Fig. 4-15) have blades that are placed around the fetal head and are shaped with a cephalic curve to accommodate the head. In addition, most have a pelvic curve that conforms to the maternal pelvis. The blade of each forceps is at the end of a shank that is connected to a handle. The two forceps are connected at the lock between the shank and the handle. Once the forceps are placed around the fetal head, the operator uses varying vector forces on the handles to aid maternal expulsive efforts and guide the fetal head through the curvature of the pelvis (Table 4-2).

The conditions necessary for safe application of forceps include full dilation of the cervix, ruptured membranes, engaged head and at least +2 station, absolute knowledge of fetal position, no evidence of CPD, adequate anesthesia, empty bladder, and—most important—an experienced operator. In some institutions, midforceps applications (fetal station between 0 and +2) and rotational forceps (fetal head more than 45 degrees from either direct OA or OP position) are also used. An experienced operator is, again, the most important component of these deliveries. Using high forceps with the fetal vertex above 0 station is no longer considered a safe obstetric procedure. Complications from forceps application include bruising on the face and head, lacerations to the fetal head, cervix, vagina, and perineum, facial nerve palsy, and, rarely, skull fracture and/or intracranial damage.

▮ **Vacuum Extraction** The **vacuum extractor** consists of a vacuum cup that is placed on the fetal scalp and a suction device that is connected to the cup to create the vacuum. Conditions for the safe use of the vacuum extractor are identical to that of forceps. Vacuum should never be chosen when position is unknown or the station is too high. Exertion on the cup and consequently on the fetal scalp is made parallel to the axis of the maternal pelvis concomitant with maternal bearing-down efforts and uterine contractions. The most common complications of use of the vacuum are scalp laceration and cephalohematoma. However, a rare complication from the vacuum extractor is the subgaleal hemorrhage, which can be a neonatal emergency.

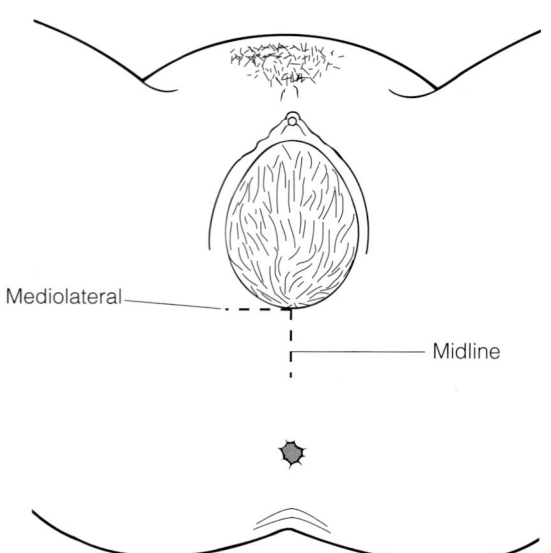

FIGURE 4-14. Placement of mediolateral and midline episiotomy.

FIGURE 4-15. Forceps.

TABLE 4-2.	Classification of Forceps Delivery According to Station and Rotation
Type of Procedure	**Classification**
Outlet forceps	1. Scalp is visible at the introitus without separating the labia 2. Fetal skull has reached pelvic floor 3. Sagittal suture is in anteroposterior diameter or right or left occiput anterior or posterior position 4. Fetal head is at or on perineum 5. Rotation does not exceed 45 degrees
Low forceps	Leading point of fetal skull is at station 2 or greater, but not on the pelvic floor
	Rotation <45 degrees (left or right occiput anterior to occiput anterior, or left or right occiput posterior to occiput posterior)
	Rotation >45 degrees
Midforceps	Station above +2 cm but head engaged
High forceps	Not included in classification

From Cunningham FG, Gant NF, Leveno KJ, et al. *Williams Obstetrics*, 19th ed. Norwalk, CT: Appleton & Lange; 1993:557.

Forceps vs. Vacuum A subject of great debate between clinicians is which of these forms of operative delivery is safer. In several studies that compare the two modes of operative vaginal delivery, the rates of severe neonatal complications such as intracranial hemorrhage are not statistically different. However, vacuums are associated with a higher rate of cephalohematomas and shoulder dystocias, whereas forceps are associated with a higher rate of facial nerve palsies. With respect to maternal complications, forceps are associated with higher rates of third- and fourth-degree perineal lacerations. Some of the differences between these instruments are related to design. The forceps are applied around the fetal head, and the tips of the blades lie on the fetal cheek and are thus more likely to cause compression of the facial nerve. The vacuum exerts its entire force on the fetal scalp; thus, fetal cephalohematomas are a common complication. Because of the higher placement and their rigidity, forceps can be used to generate greater downward force on both the fetus and concomitantly the maternal anatomy. This may lead to a lower rate of shoulder dystocia, but higher rates of maternal lacerations. In the end, the most important factor in the use of these instruments is operator experience. Because either of these instruments may be the tool of choice in different given situations, it is important for obstetricians to be trained in the use of both.

Stage 3

Stage 3 begins once the infant has been delivered and is completed with the delivery of the placenta. Placental separation usually occurs within 5 to 10 minutes of delivery of the infant; however, up to 30 minutes is usually considered within normal limits. With the abrupt decrease in intrauterine cavity size after the delivery of the fetus, the placenta is mechanically sheared from the uterine wall with contractions. Classically, the use of oxytocin was contraindicated during stage 3. However, this was established prior to the use of ultrasound out of concern for causing abruption in the case of an undiagnosed twin. If there is no doubt about completion of stage 2, oxytocin can be used during stage 3 to strengthen uterine contractions to decrease both placental delivery time and blood loss.

The three signs of placental separation include cord lengthening, a gush of blood, and uterine fundal rebound as the placenta detaches from the uterine wall. No attempt to deliver the placenta should be made until all these signs are noted. The placenta is delivered by gentle traction on the cord. It is important not to use too much traction because the cord may avulse or uterine inversion may occur. When the patient begins bearing down for delivery of the placenta, it is imperative that one of the examiner's hands is applying suprapubic pressure to keep the uterus from inverting or prolapsing (Fig. 4-16). When the placenta is evident at the introitus, the delivery should be controlled to avoid both further perineal trauma and tearing of any of the membranes that often trail the placenta at delivery.

Retained Placenta

The diagnosis of retained placenta is made when the placenta does not deliver within 30 minutes after the infant. Retained placenta is common in preterm deliveries, particularly previable deliveries. However, it is also a sign of placenta accreta, where the placenta has invaded into or beyond the endometrial stroma. The retained placenta may be removed by manual extraction. A hand is placed in the intrauterine cavity and the fingers used to shear the placenta from the surface of the uterus (Fig. 4-17). If the placenta cannot be completely extracted manually, curettage is performed to ensure no products of conception (POC) are retained.

Laceration Repair

Lacerations are usually repaired after placental delivery. A thorough examination of the perineum, labia, periurethral area, vagina, anus, and cervix is performed to assess lacerations. The most common lacerations are perineal lacerations, which are described by the depth of tissues they involve (Fig. 4-18). A first-degree laceration involves the mucosa or skin. Second-degree lacerations extend into the perineal body but do not involve the anal sphincter. Third-degree lacerations extend into or completely through the anal sphincter. A fourth-degree tear occurs if the anal mucosa itself is entered. A rectal examination should always be performed because occasionally a "buttonhole" fourth-degree laceration will be noted. This is a laceration through the rectal mucosa into the vagina, but with the sphincter still intact.

Repair of any superficial lacerations, including first-degree perineal tears, is usually accomplished with interrupted sutures. A second-degree laceration is repaired in layers. The apex of the laceration, which often lies beyond the hymenal ring, is located and a suture is anchored at the apex. This suture is then run down to the level of the hymenal ring, bringing

FIGURE 4-16. Delivery of the placenta with traction on the cord and suprapubic pressure on the uterus to prevent uterine inversion.

FIGURE 4-17. Manual removal of placenta. The fingers are alternately abducted, adducted, and advanced until the placenta is completely detached.

together the vaginal tissue. This suture is then passed beyond the hymenal ring and used to bring together the perineal body. Sometimes, a separate suture is used to place a "crown stitch," which brings together the perineal body. Finally, the skin of the perineum is closed with a subcuticular closure (Fig. 4-19).

Third-degree lacerations require repair of the anal sphincter with several interrupted sutures, and then the rest of the repair is completed as in a second-degree repair. Fourth-degree repairs are begun with the repairing of the anal mucosa. Mucosal repair is performed meticulously to prevent fistula formation. Once the rectum is repaired, a fourth-degree laceration is completed just as a third-degree repair.

Cesarean Delivery Cesarean delivery or cesarean section has been used effectively throughout the twentieth century and is one of the most common operations performed today. The cesarean rate in the United States in 2009 had increased to 32.9%, which represented a 50% rise over the previous 15 years. However, in 2014, the cesarean rate had declined slightly to 32.2%, perhaps in response to nationwide efforts from ACOG and other organizations. It is not entirely clear why the cesarean delivery rate rose so rapidly in the 1990s and 2000s, but it is likely multifactorial, including (1) biologic reasons such as higher rates of multiple gestations, an older population with more medical disorders, and higher rates of overweight and obesity; (2) patient preferences toward elective cesarean, also known as cesarean delivery on maternal request (CDMR); and (3) clinician preferences related to the escalating medical–legal environment and inadequate economic incentives to encourage clinician patience. Although maternal mortality from cesarean section is low, approximately 0.01% to 0.02%, it is still higher than from vaginal delivery. Further, the morbidity from infections, thrombotic events, wound dehiscence, and recovery time is greater than that of vaginal delivery. In addition, the risk in subsequent pregnancies from having a

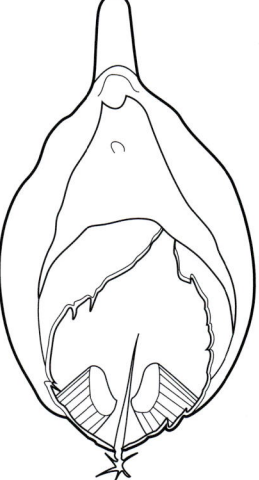

First-degree tear (Superficial)   Second-degree tear (Into the body of the perineum)   Third-degree tear (Into the anal sphincter)   Fourth-degree tear (Into the rectum)

FIGURE 4-18. Perineal tears.

A B C

FIGURE 4-19. Repair of a second-degree laceration. (**A**) The vaginal mucosa is repaired down to the level of the hymenal ring. (**B**) The subcutaneous tissue of the perineum is then brought together. (**C**) Finally, the skin of the perineum is reapproximated in a subcuticular fashion.

prior cesarean delivery is an important aspect to consider when performing the first cesarean. These include the need for future cesareans and the risk of future placenta previa and accreta.

The most common indication for primary cesarean delivery is that of failure to progress in labor. Failure to progress can be caused by problems with any of the three Ps. If the pelvis is too small or the fetus too large (depending on the viewpoint taken), the diagnosis is CPD, which leads to failure to progress. If the uterus simply does not generate enough pressure during contractions, labor can stall and lead to failure to progress. If labor seems to be stalling, there are a number of measures that can be taken to augment it, such as oxytocin or ROM. Commonly, 2 hours without cervical change in the setting of adequate uterine contractions in the active phase of labor is deemed failure to progress or active phase arrest, often leading to cesarean delivery. However, a recent study suggests that it is reasonable to wait at least 4 hours for cervical stage in the active phase of labor, leading to a vaginal delivery in the majority of these patients.

Other common indications for primary cesarean section (Table 4-3) are breech presentation, transverse lie, shoulder presentation, placenta previa, placental abruption, fetal intolerance of labor, nonreassuring fetal status, cord prolapse, prolonged second stage, failed operative vaginal delivery, or active herpes lesions. Overall, the most common indication for cesarean section is a previous cesarean section.

TABLE 4-3. Indications for Cesarean Section

Type	Indication
Maternal/fetal	Cephalopelvic disproportion Failed induction of labor

Maternal	Maternal diseases
	   Active genital herpes
	   Untreated HIV (elevated viral load)
	   Cervical cancer
	Prior uterine surgery
	   Classical cesarean section
	   Full-thickness myomectomy
	Prior uterine rupture
	Obstruction to the birth canal
	   Fibroids
	   Ovarian tumors

Fetal	Nonreassuring fetal testing
	   Bradycardia
	   Absence of FHR variability
	   Scalp pH <7.20
	Cord prolapse
	Fetal malpresentations
	   Breech, transverse lie, brow
	Multiple gestations
	   Nonvertex first twin
	   Higher-order multiples
	Fetal anomalies
	   Hydrocephalus
	   Osteogenesis imperfecta

Placental	Placenta previa Vasa previa Abruptio placentae

Vaginal Birth after Cesarean

Vaginal birth after cesarean (VBAC) can be attempted if the proper setting exists. This includes an in-house obstetrician, anesthesiologist, surgical team, and informed patient consent. The prior hysterotomy needs to be either a Kerr (low transverse incision) or Kronig (low vertical incision) without any extensions into the cervix or upper uterine segment. The greatest risk during a trial of labor after cesarean (TOLAC) is that of rupture of the prior uterine scar, which occurs approximately 0.5% to 1.0% of the time. Prior classical hysterotomies, or vertical incisions through the thick upper segment of the uterine corpus, are at a higher risk for uterine rupture in labor, and women who have had this type of cesarean are not usually allowed to attempt a trial of labor. Similarly, multiple prior cesarean deliveries increase the risk of uterine rupture and are a relative contraindication. Unfortunately, induction of labor in the setting of prior cesarean delivery has been associated with higher rates of uterine rupture, though induction of labor is not an absolute contraindication. Women with a medical indication for delivery prior to the onset of labor should be counseled about the relative risks of induction of labor and repeat cesarean delivery and informed consent should be obtained. Other factors associated with success or failure of a TOLAC and with uterine rupture are listed in Table 4-4. Common signs of rupture include abdominal pain, FHR decelerations or bradycardia, sudden decrease in pressure on an IUPC, and maternal sensation of a "pop." Therefore, the patient needs to be monitored closely in labor and delivered emergently if uterine rupture is suspected. Over the last decade, the rate of VBAC in the United States has plummeted from as high as 40% to 50% in some populations to below 10%. Because of medical–legal issues, many hospitals no longer sanction TOLAC. These trends have contributed to the overall rising cesarean delivery rate. Because of lack of access to in-hospital TOLAC, some patients have opted to attempt VBAC at home.

OBSTETRIC ANALGESIA AND ANESTHESIA
Natural Childbirth

Certainly, a component of the discomfort during labor comes from the anticipation of pain and the apprehension that accompanies this event. The concept behind natural childbirth is to educate patients regarding the experiences of labor and delivery in order to prepare them for the event. In addition, a variety of relaxation techniques, showers, and massages are used to help patients cope with the pain from uterine contractions. These practices have been formalized in a variety of characterized techniques, such as the Lamaze method, which involves a series of classes that teach both the patient and a birthing coach relaxation and breathing techniques.

Systemic Pharmacologic Intervention

Either narcotics or sedatives can be useful in the first stage of labor to relax patients and decrease pain. These commonly include fentanyl, Nubain, and Stadol. Early in labor, IM morphine sulfate is commonly used to achieve patient pain relief and rest. Sedating medications should not be used close to the time of expected delivery because they cross the placenta and may result in a depressed infant. Other complications of these medications are maternal respiratory depression and increased risk of aspiration.

Pudendal Block

The pudendal nerve travels just posterior to the ischial spine at its juncture with the sacrospinous ligament. With the pudendal block, anesthetic is injected at that site, bilaterally, to give perineal anesthesia. A pudendal block is commonly used in the case of operative vaginal delivery with either forceps or vacuum. It may be combined with local infiltration of the perineum to ensure perineal anesthesia (Fig. 4-20).

TABLE 4-4. Risk Factors for Uterine Rupture and Success or Failure in a TOLAC

Increased Success of TOLAC	Increased Risk of Uterine Rupture
Prior vaginal birth	More than one prior cesarean delivery
Prior VBAC	Prior classical cesarean
Nonrecurring indication for prior C/S (herpes, previa, breech)	Induction of labor Use of prostaglandins Use of high amounts of oxytocin
Presentation in labor at: >3 cm dilated >75% effaced	Time from last cesarean <18 mo
	Uterine infection at time of last cesarean
Decreased Success of TOLAC	**Decreased Risk of Uterine Rupture**
Prior C/S for cephalopelvic disproportion	Prior vaginal birth
Induction of labor	

TOLAC, trial of labor after cesarean; VBAC, Vaginal birth after cesarean.

FIGURE 4-20. Technique for transvaginal pudendal block.

Local Anesthesia

In patients without anesthesia who are going to require an episiotomy, local infiltration with an anesthetic is used. Local anesthetic is also used before repair of vaginal, perineal, and periurethral lacerations.

Epidural and Spinal Anesthesia

Epidurals are commonly administered to patients who wish to have anesthesia throughout the active phase and delivery of the infant. Many patients worry about nerve damage and the pain of the epidural itself. An early consult with an anesthesiologist to help answer questions about the epidural can be reassuring. The epidural catheter is placed in the L3–L4 interspace when the patient requires analgesia, although usually not until labor is deemed to be in the active phase. Once the catheter is placed, an initial bolus of anesthetic is given and a continuous infusion is started. Again, the epidural does not commonly remove all sensation and can actually be detrimental to the ability to push during the second stage if it does so. However, if the patient requires cesarean delivery, a bolus of epidural can be given, and this usually provides adequate anesthesia.

Spinal anesthesia provides anesthesia over a region similar to that of an epidural, but differs in that it is given in a one-time dose directly into the spinal canal, leading to more rapid onset of anesthesia. It is used more commonly for cesarean section than for vaginal delivery. A common complication of both forms of anesthesia is maternal hypotension secondary to decreased systemic vascular resistance, which can lead to decreased placental perfusion and fetal bradycardia. A more serious complication can be maternal respiratory depression if the anesthetic reaches a level high enough to affect diaphragmatic innervation. A spinal headache due to the loss of cerebrospinal fluid is a postpartum complication seen in less than 1% of patients.

General Anesthesia

Although general anesthesia is rarely used for vaginal delivery, it may be used for cesarean delivery, particularly in the emergent setting. For less urgent cesarean sections, epidural or spinal anesthesia is usually preferred. The two principal concerns of general anesthesia are the risk of maternal aspiration and the risk of hypoxia to mother and fetus during induction. Thus, when choosing the route of anesthesia for a cesarean section, the urgency of the delivery must be assessed. Common reasons for an emergent cesarean section are abruption, fetal bradycardia, umbilical cord prolapse, uterine rupture, or hemorrhage from a placenta previa.

KEY POINTS

- The physical examination of a pregnant woman in labor and delivery often includes Leopold maneuvers, a sterile speculum examination, and a cervical examination.
- It is important to determine both the presentation of the fetus and the status of the cervix. The cervical examination includes dilation, effacement, station, consistency, and position.
- Labor can be induced or augmented with prostaglandins, oxytocin, laminaria, Foley bulb, and artificial ROM.
- The fetus can be monitored in labor with external fetal monitoring, fetal scalp electrode, ultrasound, and fetal scalp pH.
- Labor is divided into three stages: the first stage extends until complete cervical dilation, the second stage extends until delivery of the infant, and the third stage extends until delivery of the placenta.
- Forceps delivery and vacuum extraction are two forms of operative vaginal delivery that are used to expedite vaginal delivery.
- Cesarean delivery has multiple indications and is the most common operation performed in the United States.
- Because the most common indication for cesarean delivery is a prior cesarean delivery, attempts should be made to achieve vaginal delivery in the first pregnancy.
- Obstetric anesthesia allows for more patient comfort throughout labor.
- Epidurals are commonly used during labor, whereas spinals are used more often for cesarean section.
- Epidural anesthesia leads to a longer second stage of labor, but offers better control during crowning.
- Occasionally, general anesthesia is used in the emergent setting.

CLINICAL VIGNETTES

VIGNETTE 1

A 31-year-old G1P0 woman at 39 weeks and 4 days presents to the labor and delivery unit, with regular contractions occurring every 3 to 5 minutes. Her contractions last 30 to 90 seconds. She is not sure if she has been leaking any fluid from her vagina. You take her history and conduct a physical examination.

1. ROM would be supported by which of the following?
   a. Nitrazine paper remaining orange when exposed to fluid in the vagina
   b. A negative fern test
   c. An ultrasound with a normal AFI
   d. A negative tampon test
   e. Speculum examination with evidence of pooling in the vagina

2. You determine her membranes have ruptured and admit her for active management of labor. The first stage of labor:
   a. includes an active and latent phase
   b. begins when the cervix has completely dilated
   c. is considered prolonged if its duration is longer than 2 hours in a nulliparous woman
   d. begins with the onset of Braxton Hicks contractions
   e. is commonly associated with repetitive early and variable decelerations

3. On examination, you attempt to determine the presentation of the fetus. Which of the following presentations and positions would be most favorable to achieve a vaginal delivery?
   a. Breech
   b. Transverse
   c. Vertex with occiput posterior
   d. Vertex with occiput anterior
   e. Vertex with occiput transverse

4. The patient dilates without difficulty to 10 cm, and the second stage of labor begins. She is pushing effectively, but during contractions you notice decelerations on fetal heart tracings. Which of the following would be most concerning?
   a. Isolated early decelerations
   b. Repetitive variable decelerations that resolve quickly after each contraction
   c. Repetitive early decelerations and variable decelerations

d. Repetitive late decelerations and loss of variability between contractions
e. Absence of decelerations

5. She pushes the head to the perineum, and you deliver the head and shoulders without complication. The cord is clamped and the placenta delivered. You examine her for lacerations. A second-degree laceration:
   a. involves the anal mucosa
   b. is commonly associated with buttonhole lacerations
   c. involves the mucosa or the skin only
   d. will heal well without repair
   e. extends into the perineal body, but does not involve the anal sphincter

VIGNETTE 2

A 26-year-old G2P2001 woman at 40 weeks and 2 days is seen in clinic for prenatal care. She is experiencing occasional contractions and has a sense of pressure in her vagina, but does not feel like she is in labor (as she experienced in her first delivery). Her first child was born at 41 weeks following an induction, resulting in a normal spontaneous vaginal delivery. She is interested in an induction for this pregnancy as well. You perform a cervical examination and discuss options with her.

1. Which of the following cervical examinations is the most favorable for induction of labor?
   a. Cervix closed, posterior, firm with 0% effacement
   b. Cervix soft, midposition, 3 cm dilated, 50% effaced with −2 station
   c. Cervix soft, anterior, 4 cm dilated, 80% effaced with −1 station
   d. Cervix medium, posterior, consistent, 2 cm dilated, 30% effaced
   e. Cervix soft, midposition, 3 cm dilated, 50% effaced with −3 station

2. For women undergoing induction of labor with a Bishop score of 5 or less, which of the following is a commonly used first step?
   a. Nonstress test
   b. Oxytocin drip
   c. Cervical application of prostaglandin E^2
   d. Cesarean section
   e. Attempts at induction should be avoided at a Bishop score of less than 5

3. Which of the following is not a contraindication to use of prostaglandins in labor induction?
   a. Maternal asthma
   b. Nonreassuring fetal testing
   c. A prior cesarean section
   d. Maternal glaucoma
   e. Maternal SLE

4. Once the patient is in active labor and 6 cm dilated, you notice that on two subsequent examinations she is failing to make progress. Which of the following would be appropriate for evaluating the adequacy of contractions?
   a. Fetal scalp electrode
   b. Intrauterine pressure catheter
   c. Abdominal ultrasound
   d. Speculum examination
   e. Serum oxytocin levels

VIGNETTE 3

A 34-year-old G3P2002 woman at 38 weeks and 6 days was admitted to the labor and delivery unit for active management of labor after it was determined that her membranes had ruptured and she was dilated to 3 cm. Her cervix has been steadily dilating, and now she is at 6 cm. She is very uncomfortable and finds her contractions very painful. Her partner is also very concerned that she needs pain relief.

1. You advise your patient that:
   a. narcotics are available, but should be reserved for closer to the time of delivery when her pain will be greatest
   b. if she continues with natural childbirth and eventually needs a cesarean section, she will require general anesthesia
   c. spinal anesthesia is her best option because it gives a constant infusion of medicine over a long period of time
   d. she cannot have an epidural yet because she is not yet in the active phase of labor
   e. a variety of relaxation techniques can be incorporated into her labor in addition to pain medication

2. With adequate pain control she dilates to 10 cm, and the second stage begins. Which of the following is the correct order of the cardinal movements of labor?
   a. Internal rotation, engagement, descent, flexion, extension, external rotation
   b. Engagement, descent, extension, internal rotation, flexion, external rotation
   c. Internal rotation, descent, engagement, flexion, extension, external rotation
   d. Engagement, descent, flexion, internal rotation, extension, external rotation
   e. Engagement, descent, internal rotation, extension, flexion, external rotation

3. An uncomplicated vaginal delivery typically includes which maneuver?
   a. Perineal support to decrease perineal trauma
   b. An episiotomy to hasten delivery
   c. Vacuum extraction if the fetal station is low

d. Forceps to aid maternal efforts
   e. The McRoberts maneuver
4. Stage 3 begins following the delivery of the infant and typically involves which of the following?
   a. Placental separation
   b. Stopping oxytocin drips if they were used during stage 2
   c. An abrupt increase in the size of the intrauterine cavity
   d. Uterine prolapse
   e. A delay of 60 minutes before the placenta is delivered

VIGNETTE 4

A 24-year-old G2P1001 woman at 39 weeks and 3 days is seen in clinic. She has been experiencing more frequent contractions and thinks she might be in labor. Her last pregnancy ended with a cesarean delivery after a stage 1 arrest. There was no evidence of cephalopelvic disproportion. Earlier in the course of her current pregnancy, she had desired a scheduled repeat cesarean, but now that she might be in labor she would like to try and deliver vaginally.

1. What would be a contraindication to a trial of labor after cesarean (TOLAC)?
   a. Prior classical hysterotomy
   b. Prior Kerr hysterotomy
   c. Small-for-gestational-age (SGA) fetus
   d. Oligohydramnios
   e. GBS + mother
2. After counseling and consent, the patient agrees to a trial of labor and after dilating to 10 cm, she begins to push. After 1 hour of pushing, the fetal heart tracing has absent variability and a baseline that has risen to the 180 beats per minute. The baby's station is low enough to consider using either forceps or vacuum. Which of the following is not required for forceps delivery?
   a. Adequate anesthesia
   b. Evidence of cephalopelvic disproportion
   c. Full dilation of the cervix
   d. At least two station and engaged head
   e. Knowledge of fetal position
3. You decide to attempt vacuum extraction. Which of the following is the most common complication of vacuum extraction?
   a. Fetal facial nerve palsy
   b. Maternal perineal laceration
   c. Cephalohematoma
   d. Fetal skull fracture
   e. Prolonged stage 3

ANSWERS

VIGNETTE 1 Question 1
1. Answer E:
Diagnosis of ROM is suspected with a history of a gush or leaking of fluid from the vagina. It can be confirmed by the pool, nitrazine, and fern tests. If tests are equivocal, an ultrasound examination can evaluate the amount of fluid around the fetus. The tampon test is used in situations where accurate diagnosis is necessary and involves using amniocentesis to inject dilute indigo carmine dye and looking for leaking of the blue fluid from the cervix onto a tampon.

VIGNETTE 1 Question 2
2. Answer A:
The first stage of labor includes an active and latent phase. Braxton Hicks are irregular contractions that do not result in cervical change, which is common in the third trimester of pregnancy. The other answer choices are associated with the second stage of labor.

VIGNETTE 1 Question 3
3. Answer D:
Fetal position in the vertex position depends on the relationship of the fetal occiput to the maternal pelvis. Occiput transverse and occiput posterior can lead to a prolonged labor and a higher rate of cesarean delivery. Breech and transverse presentations are also associated with prolonged labor, and, when identified, are treated either by external cephalic version or, if that fails, by cesarean delivery in most labor wards in the United States. Breech vaginal delivery is still offered at some labor units, but even in that setting, the risk of cesarean delivery is still higher than in vertex presentations.

VIGNETTE 1 Question 4
4. Answer D:
Repetitive early and variable decelerations that resolve quickly between contractions are common in the second stage. Repetitive late decelerations, bradycardias, and loss of variability are all signs of nonreassuring fetal status.

VIGNETTE 1 Question 5

5. Answer E:
Second-degree lacerations extend into the perineal body, but do not involve the anal sphincter, whereas first-degree lacerations involve only the mucosa or skin, and fourth-degree lacerations can occasionally be buttonhole, wherein the rectal mucosa is torn but the sphincter is intact. All but shallow first-degree lacerations are typically repaired after placental delivery.

VIGNETTE 2 Question 1

1. Answer C:
The Bishop score is a method of evaluating the cervix and associated points for fetal station and for cervical dilation, effacement, consistency, and position. The higher the Bishop score, the greater the likelihood of successful vaginal delivery following induction of labor. Soft is the best consistency, anterior the best position, and greater dilation and effacement are more favorable.

VIGNETTE 2 Question 2

2. Answer C:
A Bishop score of 5 or less may lead to a failed induction as often as 50% of the time. In these patients, prostaglandin E^2 (PGE^2) gel, PGE2 pessary (Cervidil), or PGE1M (misoprostol) is often used to "ripen" the cervix. Oxytocin is used to induce labor with a Bishop score greater than 5.

VIGNETTE 2 Question 3

3. Answer E:
There are both maternal and obstetric contraindications for the use of prostaglandins. Maternal reasons include asthma and glaucoma, whereas obstetric reasons include having had a prior cesarean section and nonreassuring fetal testing. All of these are relative contraindications that allow individual clinicians to decide, depending on the specific clinical situation. Because PGE2 gel cannot be turned off with the ease of oxytocin, there is a risk of uterine hyperstimulation and tetanic contractions.

VIGNETTE 2 Question 4

4. Answer B:
The intrauterine pressure catheter (IUPC) is inserted into the uterine cavity to directly measure the pressure changes during contractions and can evaluate the adequacy of contractions. A fetal scalp electrode can directly monitor fetal heart rate and variability. Abdominal ultrasound and speculum examinations are not used to assess adequacy of contractions. Serum oxytocin levels are not routinely measured.

VIGNETTE 3 Question 1

1. Answer E:
A variety of relaxation techniques, including the Lamaze method, have been developed to ease the pain of labor. She is in active labor now that she has dilated past 4 cm and is therefore eligible for an epidural. Spinal anesthesia is given as a one-time bolus. Narcotics should not be used close to the time of delivery, as they may lead to decreased respiratory drive in the infant. General anesthesia is only rarely used in emergent situations for cesarean deliveries.

VIGNETTE 3 Question 2

2. Answer D:
The correct order of the cardinal movements of labor is engagement, descent, flexion, internal rotation, extension, and external rotation.

VIGNETTE 3 Question 3

3. Answer A:
Perineal support is usually provided with the fingers of the deliverer's hand, keeping pressure on the perineum to prevent a sudden, uncontrolled delivery to minimize the extent and depth of the perineal laceration. Episiotomy is used to hasten delivery, particularly in the case of impending or ongoing shoulder dystocia. Forceps and vacuum extractors are both forms of operative delivery used commonly in the case of prolonged second stage or to hasten delivery. The McRoberts maneuver is used in the setting of shoulder dystocia.

VIGNETTE 3 Question 4

4. Answer A:
Placental separation occurs secondary to mechanical shearing due to an abrupt decrease in intrauterine cavity size after delivery of the fetus. This is perceived by the provider as a gush of blood, cord lengthening, and uterine fundal rebound. Uterine prolapse can be a serious complication, and so the provider should apply suprapubic pressure when the patient begins bearing down for placental delivery. Oxytocin is used in the third stage to decrease placental delivery time and blood loss.

VIGNETTE 4 Question 1

1. Answer A:
A prior classical hysterotomy or other vertical uterine incision is an absolute contraindication to TOLAC given the increased risk of uterine rupture. Prior Kerr (low horizontal) or Kronig (low vertical) incisions are required for TOLAC. GBS + mothers should receive prophylactic antibiotics during labor, but may proceed with TOLAC. Oligohydramnios and SGA fetus are not contraindications to TOLAC.

VIGNETTE 4 Question 2
2. Answer B:
Adequate anesthesia, full dilation of the cervix, station 2 or lower with an engaged head, and knowledge of the fetal position are all required for forceps delivery. Evidence of cephalopelvic disproportion is a contraindication to forceps.

VIGNETTE 4 Question 3
3. Answer C:
Facial nerve palsy, maternal laceration, and skull fracture are associated with forceps delivery. Prolonged stage 3 is commonly seen in preterm deliveries and in placenta accreta and is not associated with mode of delivery. Cephalohematoma and scalp lacerations are the most common complications of vacuum extraction.

5 | Antepartum Hemorrhage

Obstetric hemorrhage is a leading cause of maternal death in the United States and one of the leading causes of perinatal morbidity and mortality. In 2012, hemorrhage was the fourth leading cause of maternal deaths due to obstetric factors in the United States. Bleeding during pregnancy has different etiologies depending on the trimester. As discussed in Chapter 2, first-trimester bleeding is associated with spontaneous abortion, ectopic pregnancy, and even normal pregnancies. Third-trimester vaginal bleeding occurs in 4% to 5% of pregnancies and may be obstetric or nonobstetric (Table 5-1). Hemorrhage can occur antepartum or postpartum (Chapter 12), with the major causes of antepartum hemorrhage including placenta previa (20%) and placental abruption (30%).

TABLE 5-1.	**Differential Diagnosis of Antepartum Bleeding**
Obstetric causes	
Placental	Placenta previa, placental abruption, vasa previa
Maternal	Uterine rupture
Fetal	Fetal vessel rupture
Nonobstetric causes	
Cervical	Severe cervicitis, polyps, cervical dysplasia/cancer
Vaginal/vulvar	Lacerations, varices, cancer
Other	Hemorrhoids, congenital bleeding disorder, abdominal or pelvic trauma, hematuria

Adapted from Hacker N, Moore JG. *Essentials of Obstetrics and Gynecology*. Philadelphia, PA: WB Saunders; 1992:155.

PLACENTA PREVIA

PATHOGENESIS

Placenta previa is defined as abnormal implantation of the placenta over the internal cervical os (Fig. 5-1). **Complete previa** occurs when the placenta completely covers the internal os. **Partial previa** occurs when the placenta covers a portion of the internal os. **Marginal previa** occurs when the edge of the placenta reaches the margin of the os. A **low-lying placenta** is implanted in the lower uterine segment in close proximity but not extending to the internal os. Rarely, a fetal vessel may lie over the cervix; this is known as a **vasa previa** (discussed later in this chapter).

It is unclear why some placentas implant in the lower uterine segment rather than in the fundus. Uterine scarring may predispose to placental implantation in the lower uterine segment. Up to 6% of pregnant women display sonographic evidence of placenta previa on early ultrasound. With the progression of pregnancy, more than 90% of these low-lying placentas identified early in pregnancy will appear to move away from the cervix and out of the lower uterine segment. Although the term **placental migration** has been used, most experts do not believe the placenta actually moves. The apparent movement of the placenta is most likely due to the development of the lower uterine segment. Additionally, it may be that the placenta grows preferentially toward a better vascularized fundus (trophotropism), whereas the placenta overlying the less well-vascularized cervix may undergo atrophy. In some cases, this atrophy leaves vessels running through the membranes, unsupported by placental tissue or umbilical cord. If this occurs over the cervix, it is termed a **vasa previa**. In cases where the atrophy is incomplete, leaving a

FIGURE 5-1. Classifications of placenta previa.

placental lobe discrete from the rest of the placenta, it is termed a **succenturiate lobe**.

The bleeding associated with placenta previa results from small disruptions in the placental attachment during normal development and thinning of the lower uterine segment during the third trimester. Blood acts as an irritant to the uterus, stimulating uterine contractions, which in turn stimulates further placental separation and bleeding. Although they may be a reason for hospitalization, these initial bleeds are rarely a major problem. In labor, as the cervix dilates and effaces, there is usually placental separation and unavoidable bleeding. As a result, profuse hemorrhage and shock can occur, leading to significant maternal and fetal morbidity and mortality. Maternal mortality is estimated to occur in 0.03% of cases of placenta previa in the United States. Although the maternal and perinatal mortality from placenta

TABLE 5-2.	Fetal Complications Associated with Placenta Previa
Preterm delivery and its complications	
PPROM	
IUGR	
Malpresentation	
Congenital abnormalities	

IUGR, intrauterine growth restriction; PPROM, preterm premature rupture of membrane.
Adapted from Hacker N, Moore JG. *Essentials of Obstetrics and Gynecology*. Philadelphia, PA: WB Saunders; 1992:155.

previa has dropped rapidly in the United States over the last few decades, the perinatal mortality rate is still 10 times higher than in the general population. Most of this morbidity and mortality is associated with preterm delivery, which is responsible for 60% of perinatal deaths. Other fetal risks associated with placenta previa are listed in Table 5-2.

Placenta previa may also be complicated by an associated placenta accreta (placenta previa accreta). **Placenta accreta** is a condition in which the placenta invades into and is inseparable from the uterine wall. When the invasion extends into the myometrium, this is termed a **placenta increta**. When the invasion is through the myometrium and the serosa, this is termed a **placenta percreta**. In some cases of placenta percreta, the invasion may involve other organs such as the bladder anteriorly or the rectum posteriorly.

Placenta accreta causes an inability of the placenta to properly separate from the uterine wall after the delivery of the fetus. This can result in profuse hemorrhage and shock with substantial maternal morbidity and mortality, such as need for hysterectomy, surgical injury to the ureters, bladder, and other viscera, adult respiratory distress syndrome, renal failure, coagulopathy, and death. The average blood loss at delivery in women with placenta accreta is 3,000 to 5,000 mL. Historically, the most frequent indication for a peripartum hysterectomy has been uterine atony. Recent literature suggests that this may be shifting, as abnormal placentation is increasingly becoming a more common reason for peripartum hysterectomy. With the increasing cesarean section rate, as well as a decrease in vaginal birth after cesarean (VBAC) section, this number is likely to further increase in the future. Indeed, in several centers, placenta accreta has become the leading reason for cesarean hysterectomy.

Two-thirds of women with both a placenta previa and an associated accreta require a hysterectomy at the time of delivery (**peripartum hysterectomy**). Rarely, placenta accreta may lead to spontaneous uterine rupture in the second or third trimester, resulting in intraperitoneal hemorrhage, a life-threatening emergency. Minor degrees of placenta accreta may occur, which may lead to slightly heavier postpartum bleeding, but may not require the aggressive management that is often employed with more extensive placenta accreta. Table 5-3 summarizes the abnormalities of placentation.

TABLE 5-3.	Abnormalities of Placentation
Circumvallate placenta	Occurs when the membranes double back over the edge of the placenta, forming a dense ring around the periphery of the placenta. Often considered a variant of placental abruption, it is a major cause of second-trimester hemorrhage
Placenta previa	Occurs when the placenta develops over the internal cervical os Types include complete, partial, and marginal
Placenta accreta	Abnormal adherence of part or all of the placenta to the uterine wall May be associated with a placenta in normal locations, but incidence increases in placenta previa
Placenta increta	Abnormal placentation in which the placenta invades the myometrium
Placenta percreta	Abnormal placentation in which the placenta invades through the myometrium to the uterine serosa Occasionally, placentas may invade into adjacent organs such as the bladder or rectum
Vasa previa	Occurs when a velamentous cord insertion causes the fetal vessels to pass over the internal cervical os Also seen with velamentous and succenturiate placentas
Velamentous placenta	Occurs when blood vessels insert between the amnion and the chorion, away from the margin of the placenta, leaving the vessels largely unprotected and vulnerable to compression or injury
Succenturiate placenta	An extra lobe of the placenta that is implanted at some distance away from the rest of the placenta Fetal vessels may course between the two lobes, possibly over the cervix, leaving these blood vessels unprotected and at risk for rupture

EPIDEMIOLOGY

Placenta previa occurs in approximately 3.5 to 5 per 1,000 births and accounts for nearly 20% of all antepartum hemorrhage. Previa occurs in as many as 1% to 5% of women with a prior cesarean section. Because a bleeding previa often results in delivery, which may occur preterm, it is a common indication for preterm delivery. Placenta previa can also be complicated by an associated placenta accreta (placenta previa accreta) in approximately 5% of cases. The risk of placenta accreta is increased in women with placenta previa in the setting of prior cesarean delivery. In the setting of a placenta previa, the risk of concurrent placenta accreta is approximately 3%, 11%, 40%, 61%, and 67% for one, two, three, four, and five prior cesarean sections, respectively.

Abnormalities in placentation are the result of events that prevent normal migration of the placenta during normal progressive development of the lower uterine segment during pregnancy (Table 5-4). Previous placental implantations and prior uterine scars are thought to contribute to abnormal placentation in subsequent pregnancies. Thus, the risk of placenta previa is increased in patients with prior uterine surgeries such as myomectomy or uterine septum resection. Other risk factors include uterine anomalies, multiple gestations, multiparity, advanced maternal age, smoking, and previous placenta previa. The likelihood of placenta previa increases significantly with each additional cesarean delivery, putting those women with repeat cesarean section at significant risk with each additional pregnancy. Of note, because many patients receive a routine obstetric ultrasound, marginal previa or low-lying placenta is commonly diagnosed in the second trimester. This is diagnosed when the placental edge is <2 cm from, but not covering, the internal os. Most resolve on repeat ultrasound by "moving" up and away from the cervix during the third trimester as the lower uterine segment develops. The later in pregnancy that placenta previa is diagnosed, the higher the likelihood of persistence to delivery. Women who at 20 weeks have a low-lying placenta that does not overlie the internal os will not have a placenta previa at term and need no further sonographic examinations for placental location. However, the presence of a low-lying placenta in the second trimester is a risk factor for developing a vasa previa, and therefore, in these cases, an ultrasound should be performed later in pregnancy to exclude that condition.

CLINICAL MANIFESTATIONS

History

Patients with placenta previa classically present with sudden and profuse **painless vaginal bleeding**. The first episode of bleeding—the "sentinel" bleed—usually occurs after 28 weeks of gestation. During this time, the lower uterine segment develops and thins, disrupting the placental attachment resulting in bleeding. Placenta accreta (and increta) is usually asymptomatic. On rare occasions, however, a patient with a percreta into the bladder or rectum may present with hematuria or rectal bleeding.

Physical Examination

Vaginal examination is contraindicated in placenta previa because the digital examination can cause further separation of the placenta and trigger catastrophic hemorrhage. Because many women have an ultrasound examination that can diagnose placenta previa, diagnosis by digital examination of the placenta previa is uncommon today. However, in the rare patient that is undiagnosed, the cervical examination may reveal soft, spongy tissue just inside the cervix. Because of the increased vascularity, there may be notable varices in the lower uterine segment or cervix, which can be visualized on speculum examination or palpated. A marginal previa can be palpated at the edge of, or quite near, the internal os.

DIAGNOSTIC EVALUATION

The diagnosis of placenta previa can be made via ultrasonography with a sensitivity of greater than 95% (Fig. 5-2). If made before the third trimester in pregnancy, a follow-up ultrasound is often obtained in the third trimester to determine if the previa has resolved. Although transabdominal sonography is frequently used for placental location, this technique lacks some precision in diagnosing placenta previa. Numerous studies have demonstrated the accuracy and superiority of transvaginal sonography for the diagnosis of placenta previa. One study of 131 women believed to have a placenta previa by transabdominal sonography found that anatomic landmarks crucial for the accurate diagnosis were poorly recognized

TABLE 5-4. Predisposing Factors for Placenta Previa
Prior cesarean section and uterine surgery (e.g., myomectomy)
Multiparity
Multiple gestation
Erythroblastosis
Smoking
History of placenta previa
Increasing maternal age

FIGURE 5-2. Complete placenta previa. *p*, placenta; *c*, cervix; *b*, bladder.

in 50% of cases. In 26% of the cases of suspected placenta previa, the initial diagnosis was changed after transvaginal sonography demonstrated the diagnosis to be incorrect.

The superiority of transvaginal sonography over transabdominal sonography can be attributed to several factors:

1. If a transabdominal ultrasound is performed with a full maternal bladder, placenta previa may be overdiagnosed. Compression of the anterior and posterior walls of the lower uterine segment with bladder filling can result in the perception of a longer cervix. Consequently, a normally situated placenta may falsely appear to be a previa. Therefore, it is important to have the bladder entirely emptied before this portion of the ultrasound is performed if a previa is a possibility.
2. Vaginal probes are closer to the region of interest, and typically of higher frequency, and therefore obtain higher resolution images than transabdominal probes.
3. The internal cervical os and the lower placental edge frequently cannot be imaged adequately by the transabdominal approach. The position of the internal os is assumed rather than actually seen.
4. The fetal head may obscure views of the lower placental edge when using the transabdominal approach, and a posterior placenta previa may not be adequately imaged.

The improved accuracy of transvaginal sonography over transabdominal sonography means that fewer false-positive diagnoses are made. Thus, the rate of placenta previa is significantly lower when using transvaginal sonography as compared to using transabdominal sonography. One study found that the incidence of placenta previa is considerably lower (1.1%) when routine transvaginal sonography is performed at 15 to 20 weeks versus the previously reported incidence (15% to 20%) in the second trimester when using transabdominal sonography.

Numerous studies have demonstrated the safety of transvaginal sonography for the diagnosis of placenta previa. Importantly, this imaging technique does not lead to an increase in bleeding. The two main reasons for this are (1) the vaginal probe is introduced at an angle that places it against the anterior fornix and anterior lip of the cervix and (2) the optimal distance for visualization of the cervix is 2 to 3 cm away from the cervix, so the probe is generally not advanced sufficiently to make contact with the placenta. Nonetheless, the examination should be performed by personnel experienced in transvaginal sonography, and the transvaginal probe should always be inserted carefully, with the examiner looking at the monitor to avoid putting the probe in the cervix.

Translabial sonography has been suggested as an alternative to transvaginal sonography, and it has been shown to be superior to transabdominal sonography for placental location. However, because transvaginal sonography appears to be accurate, safe, and well tolerated, it should be the imaging modality of choice.

Of note, placenta accreta can also be diagnosed by ultrasound with a sensitivity of 77% to 87% (*Ultrasound Obstet Gynecol*. 2011;37:324–327). Findings on ultrasound suggestive of a placenta accreta include irregular shaped placental lacunae, thinning of the myometrium over the placenta, loss of the retroplacental space, protrusion of the placenta into the bladder, increased vascularity of the uterine serosa–bladder interface, and turbulent blood flow through the lacunae on ultrasound. This diagnosis is important to make prenatally because this allows effective multidisciplinary planning and management to minimize morbidity. This diagnosis can also be made with MRI, but given its cost and questionably superior diagnostic capabilities, it is more commonly used as an adjunct modality instead of a first line diagnostic tool. Placenta accreta should be suspected in women who have both a placenta previa and a history of cesarean delivery or other uterine surgery. Close surveillance is particularly indicated when the placenta is anterior and overlies the cesarean scar.

TREATMENT

Management of patients with placenta previa varies between providers. Although there is minimal data to support the efficacy of avoidance of intercourse and excessive activity, antepartum patients with a placenta previa are commonly managed with strict pelvic rest (i.e., no intercourse) after 20 weeks, earlier if they have experienced bleeding, and decreased physical activity. However, some clinicians will not institute this conservative management until the patient presents with a sentinel bleed.

In asymptomatic women without bleeding outpatient management until their scheduled cesarean is preferred. Following a sentinel bleed, inpatient versus outpatient management remains an area of controversy. In symptomatic women, the decision for inpatient management usually depends on the frequency and severity of the bleeding episode or episodes. In one of the few prospective randomized studies dealing with placenta previa, 53 women with placenta previa at gestational ages between 24 and 36 weeks, who had been initially stabilized in hospital after a bleeding event, were randomized to inpatient or outpatient management. The investigators found no significant difference in clinical outcomes between the two groups. Thus, women who are stable and asymptomatic, and who are reliable and have quick access to the hospital, may be considered for outpatient management.

Unstoppable labor, fetal distress, and life-threatening hemorrhage are all indications for immediate cesarean delivery regardless of gestational age. There is consensus that patients with complete or partial placenta previa require delivery by cesarean. In patients with a low-lying placenta or marginal previa (<2 cm from the internal os), some authors suggest that patients should have a transvaginal ultrasound in the late third trimester to evaluate the distance of the placental edge from the os and that those with a placental edge less than 1 to 2 cm should be delivered by cesarean given the risk of antepartum hemorrhage. A study demonstrated, however, that in patients where the distance between the placental edge and internal os is >1 cm, the risk of antepartum hemorrhage is 3% and the majority will deliver vaginally with minimal morbidity and therefore may generally be allowed to have a trial of labor as long as there is no evidence of fetal distress or excessive hemorrhage. Of note, there is potential for postpartum hemorrhage in women with a placenta that extends into the noncontractile lower uterine segment. In case of preterm pregnancy, if the bleeding is not profuse, fetal survival can be enhanced by aggressive expectant management. However, 70% of patients with placenta previa have a recurring bleeding episode and will require delivery before week 36. For patients who make it to week 36, typical management involves delivery by cesarean section between 36 and 37 weeks. Evaluation of fetal lung maturity prior to delivery is no longer recommended, the rationale being that the risks associated with continuing the pregnancy (hemorrhage, emergency delivery) outweigh the risks of prematurity at this gestation.

Advanced planning and interdisciplinary collaboration are fundamental because as gestational age increases, so does the risk of emergent bleeding. The following should be the course of action in the case of vaginal bleeding and suspected placenta previa and/or placenta accreta:

1. **Stabilize the patient**. Every patient with vaginal bleeding and a known or suspected previa should be hospitalized, placed on continuous fetal monitoring, and have IV access established. If the patient presents with a particularly large bleed, two large-bore IV catheters will commonly be placed. Laboratory evaluation includes hematocrit, type and cross, and, if considerable bleeding or coagulopathy is suspected, fibrinogen level, activated partial thromboplastin time (aPTT), and prothrombin time (PT). For an Rh-negative woman, a Kleihauer–Betke test should be performed to determine the extent of any fetomaternal transfusion so that the appropriate amount of RhoGAM can be administered to prevent alloimmunization.

2. **Prepare for catastrophic hemorrhage**. Expectant management in the stabilized patient includes hospitalization, limited activity, hematocrit monitoring, and consideration of limiting any oral intake. Two or more units of blood should be typed, cross-matched, and made available. Transfusions are usually given to maintain a hematocrit of 25% or greater.

3. **Prepare for preterm delivery**. Generally, at the time of admission, women between 24 and 36 weeks of gestation with vaginal bleeding should be given steroids to promote fetal lung maturity. Magnesium sulfate should be given for neuroprotection in patients between 24 and 32 weeks if delivery is occurring within 24 hours. The patient and her family should

have a neonatology consultation so that the management of the infant after birth may be discussed. In women who have a history of cesarean delivery or uterine surgery, detailed ultrasonography should be performed to exclude placenta accreta. Because prematurity is the main cause of perinatal mortality associated with placenta previa, it is desirable to prolong the pregnancy as long as safely possible. Therefore, before 32 weeks of gestation, moderate to severe bleeding without maternal or fetal compromise may be managed aggressively with blood transfusions, rather than moving toward delivery. Cautious use of tocolytics in women with placenta previa who are having contractions appears reasonable to assist in prolonging the pregnancy up to 34 weeks of gestation, as long as both mother and fetus are stable. Indomethacin should be avoided, however, given its inhibitory effect on platelets.

Following are additional considerations for suspected placenta accreta/increta/percreta:

1. **Plan for total abdominal hysterectomy at the time of cesarean section** as this is the accepted management plan for patients with a placenta accreta. In addition, there is almost universal consensus that the placenta should be left in place; attempts to detach the placenta frequently result in massive hemorrhage. However, the physician should be aware that focal placenta accreta may exist, which may not require such aggressive therapy.
2. **Schedule delivery at approximately 34 weeks of gestation**. A study comparing emergency with elective peripartum hysterectomy found that women in the emergency hysterectomy group had greater intraoperative blood loss, were more likely to have intraoperative hypotension, and were more likely to receive blood transfusions than women who had elective obstetric hysterectomies.
3. **Plan ahead and have back-up available**. The patient should be counseled regarding hysterectomy and blood transfusion. The patient should be type and crossed for blood products and these should be readily available at the time of cesarean section. Urology, urogynecology, and/or gynecologic oncology should be aware of the patient in the event of percreta or catastrophic blood loss.

PLACENTAL ABRUPTION

PATHOGENESIS

Placental abruption (abruptio placentae) is the premature separation of the normally implanted placenta from the uterine wall, resulting in hemorrhage between the uterine wall and the placenta. Fifty percent of abruptions occur before labor and after 30 weeks of gestation, 15% occur during labor, and 30% are identified only on placental inspection after delivery. Large placental separations may result in premature delivery, uterine tetany, disseminated intravascular coagulation (DIC), hypovolemic shock, and even perinatal death.

The primary cause of placental abruption is unknown, although it is associated with a variety of

TABLE 5-5. Predisposing and Precipitating Factors for Placental Abruption

Predisposing factors
Hypertension
Previous placental abruption
Advanced maternal age
Multiparity
Uterine distension
Multiple pregnancy
Polyhydramnios
Vascular deficiency
Diabetes mellitus
Collagen vascular disease
Cocaine use
Methamphetamine use
Cigarette smoking
Alcohol use (>14 drinks/wk)
Circumvallate placenta
Short umbilical cord
Precipitating factors
Trauma
External/internal version
Motor vehicle accident
Abdominal trauma
Sudden uterine volume loss
Delivery of first twin
Rupture of membranes with polyhydramnios
PPROM

PPROM, preterm premature rupture of membrane.

predisposing and precipitating factors (Table 5-5). These factors include maternal hypertension, prior history of placental abruption, maternal cocaine use, tobacco use, external maternal trauma, and rapid decompression of the overdistended uterus. Abnormal placental vasculature, thrombosis, and reduced placental perfusion are some of the mechanisms that have been proposed to explain the pathogenesis of placental separation and that these anomalies might have some genetic basis.

At the initial point of separation, nonclotted blood courses from the injury site. The enlarging collection of blood may cause further separation of the placenta. In 20% of placental separations, bleeding is confined within the uterine cavity and is referred to as a **concealed hemorrhage** (Fig. 5-3). In the remaining 80% of placental separations, the blood dissects downward toward the cervix, resulting in a **revealed** or **external hemorrhage**. Because there is an egress for the blood, revealed hemorrhages are less likely to result in larger retroplacental clots, which are associated with fetal demise. The result of hemorrhage from torn placental vessels can vary from maternal anemia in mild cases to shock, acute renal failure, and maternal death in severe cases.

Global maternal mortality from placental abruption varies from 0.5% to 5.0%. Most deaths are due to hemorrhage, cardiac failure, or renal failure. Population-based studies estimate the perinatal mortality rate associated with abruption to be about 12% with rates as high as 35% for clinically relevant antepartum placental abruptions and 50% to 80% in cases of severe placental abruption. The cause of fetal demise is usually due to hypoxia resulting from decreased placental surface area and maternal hemorrhage.

EPIDEMIOLOGY

Placental abruption occurs in about 0.2% to 1% of pregnancies and is responsible for 30% of cases of third-trimester bleeding and 12% of perinatal mortality. Abruption occurs in about 0.7% to 1.0% of singleton births and in twins the incidence ranges from 1% to 2%. Although relatively uncommon, placental abruption is a major cause of fetal and neonatal mortality. The high mortality associated with abruptio placentae has been demonstrated to be due to its strong association with preterm birth. Abruption is implicated as the cause of approximately 10% of all preterm deliveries and perinatal death related to preterm delivery in this cohort occurs in at least 30% of cases. While the incidence of placental abruption increases with the number of gestations (triplets > twins > singletons), perinatal mortality is greatest among singletons, followed by twins, and surprisingly least among triplets. The predisposing and precipitating factors for placental abruption are listed in Table 5-5. The strongest factor associated with increased incidence of abruption is history of previous abruption, carrying an 8- to 12-fold increase in risk. The risk of abruption in future pregnancy is 10% after one abruption and 25% after two prior abruptions. This is followed closely by hypertension that carries a fivefold increase in risk, whether it is chronic, the result of preeclampsia, or maternal ingestion of cocaine or methamphetamine. In cases of abruptions that are severe enough to cause fetal death, 50% are due to hypertension: 25% of these are from chronic hypertension and 25% are from preeclampsia.

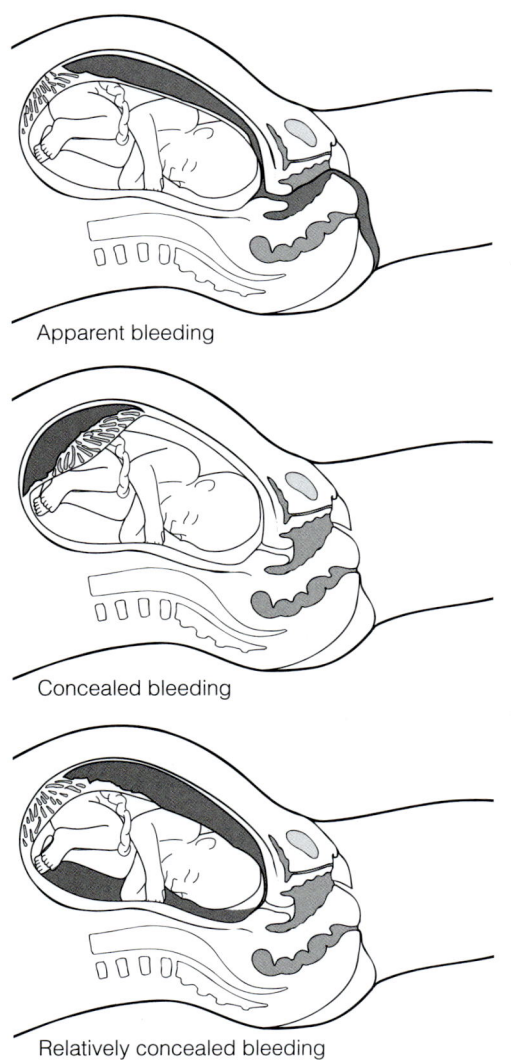

FIGURE 5-3. Types of placental separation.

CLINICAL MANIFESTATIONS

History
The classic presentation of placental abruption is third-trimester vaginal bleeding associated with severe abdominal pain and/or frequent, strong contractions. However, about 30% of placental separations are small with few or no symptoms and are identified only after inspection of the placenta at delivery. It has historically been taught that **painful** uterine bleeding signifies placental abruption, whereas **painless** uterine bleeding is indicative of placenta previa. The differential diagnosis is usually not this straightforward, and labor accompanying previa may cause pain suggestive of placental abruption. Alternatively, pain from abruption may mimic normal labor, or it may be painless, especially with a posterior placenta. At times, the cause of vaginal bleeding remains obscure even after delivery. The symptoms of abruption and their rate of occurrence are listed in Table 5-6.

Physical Examination
On physical examination, a patient with placental abruption will often have vaginal bleeding and a firm, tender uterus. On tocometer, small frequent contractions are usually seen along with tetanic contractions. On fetal monitoring, nonreassuring fetal heart tracing is frequently seen secondary to hypoxia. A classic sign of placental abruption that can only be seen at the time of cesarean delivery is the Couvelaire uterus, which is a life-threatening condition and occurs when there is enough blood from the abruption that markedly infiltrates the myometrium to reach the serosa, especially at the cornua, that it gives the myometrium a bluish purple tone that can be seen on the surface of the uterus.

DIAGNOSTIC EVALUATION
The diagnosis of placental abruption is primarily clinical. Only 2% to 25% of abruptions are diagnosed by ultrasound (evidenced by a retroplacental clot). However, because abruption can present clinically in a similar fashion to placenta previa with vaginal bleeding, ultrasonography is routinely performed to rule out previa in cases of suspected abruption. Importantly, negative findings on ultrasound examination do **NOT** exclude placental abruption. The diagnosis of abruption may be confirmed by inspection of the placenta at delivery. The presence of a retroplacental clot with overlying placental destruction confirms the diagnosis.

ADDITIONAL CLINICAL FINDINGS

Hypovolemic Shock
One study showed that in women with abruption severe enough to kill the fetus, the cumulative blood loss often amounted to at least half of the pregnant blood volume. Due to the overall healthy state of pregnant women, tachycardia and hypotension may not occur, even with extreme concealed hemorrhage, until they have already lost 1 to 1.5 L of blood. Oliguria from inadequate renal perfusion that is observed in these circumstances is responsive to vigorous IV fluid and blood infusion.

Consumptive Coagulopathy
Placental abruption is one of the most common causes of clinically significant consumptive coagulopathy in obstetrics. In approximately one-third of women with an abruption severe enough to kill the fetus, there are measurable changes in coagulation factors; specifically, clinically significant hypofibrinogenemia (i.e., plasma levels <150 mg/dL). In 10% to 20% of cases acute DIC also occurs, where significant hypofibrinogenemia is coupled with increased fibrinolysis (elevated levels of fibrin degradation products and/or D-dimers). Other coagulation factors are also variably decreased. Consumptive coagulopathy is more likely with a concealed abruption. In cases where the fetus survives, severe coagulation defects are seen less commonly. In general, if serious coagulopathy develops, it is usually evident by the time abruption symptoms appear.

The major mechanism of consumptive coagulopathy in the setting of abruption is activation of intravascular coagulation with varying degrees of defibrination. Procoagulants are also consumed in the retroplacental clots, although the amounts recovered are insufficient to account for all of the missing fibrinogen. An important consequence of intravascular coagulation is the activation of plasminogen to plasmin, which lyses fibrin microemboli

TABLE 5-6. Presentation of Abruptio Placentae

Symptom	Occurrence (%)
Vaginal bleeding	80
Uterine tenderness/abdominal or back pain	67
Abnormal contractions/increased uterine tone	34
Fetal distress	50
Fetal demise	15

to maintain microcirculatory patency. With placental abruption severe enough to kill the fetus, there are always pathological levels of fibrinogen–fibrin degradation products and/or D-dimers in maternal serum. Overt thrombocytopenia may or may not accompany severe hypofibrinogenemia initially, but commonly becomes evident after repeated blood transfusions.

TREATMENT

The potential for rapid deterioration (e.g., hemorrhage, DIC, fetal hypoxia) necessitates delivery in some cases of placental abruption. However, most abruptions are small and noncatastrophic, and do not therefore necessitate immediate delivery. Treatment of placental abruption varies depending on gestational age and the status of the mother and fetus. Emergency cesarean delivery is chosen by most clinicians if vaginal delivery is not imminent and the fetus is of viable gestational age. With massive external bleeding, intensive resuscitation with blood products, crystalloid fluids, and prompt delivery to control hemorrhage are lifesaving for the mother and, hopefully, for the fetus. If the diagnosis is uncertain and the fetus is alive but without evidence of compromise, then close observation can be practiced in facilities capable of immediate intervention.

The following should be done in case of suspected placental abruption:

1. **Stabilize the patient**. When placental abruption is known or suspected, the patient should be hospitalized with continuous fetal monitoring and IV access gained (ideal to have two large-bore IV catheters). Laboratory evaluation should include complete blood count (CBC), type and cross, PT/PTT, fibrinogen, and D-dimer or fibrin split products. For an Rh-negative woman, RhoGAM should be administered to prevent alloimmunization. The anesthesiologist should be notified of the patient's condition in case emergent cesarean delivery is indicated.

2. **Prepare for the possibility of future hemorrhage**. Standard antishock measures should be taken, including placement of large-bore IV catheters, infusion of lactated Ringer's solution, and preparation of units of cross-matched blood (whole or packed red blood cells [RBCs]). Blood loss due to placental abruption is commonly grossly underestimated because of concealed bleeding. If cross-matched blood is not available, O-negative blood may be given in an emergency to help prevent massive blood loss and development of a consumptive coagulopathy/DIC. Additionally, patients should also be transfused fresh frozen plasma and occasionally cryoprecipitate as well as platelets in similar ratios as RBCs. This 1:1:1 transfusion is usually described in massive transfusion protocols for trauma (i.e., 1 unit of packed RBCs:1unit FFP:1 unit of platelets) and has been widely adopted in order to improve maternal outcomes.

3. **Prepare for preterm delivery**. In the preterm pregnancy, betamethasone may be given to promote fetal lung maturity and some providers tocolyze to assist in prolonging the pregnancy to week 36 for pregnancies complicated by suspected abruption with no evidence of fetal compromise. Others view abruption as a contraindication to tocolysis. Similarly, magnesium sulfate should be administered for neuroprotection in fetuses less than 32 weeks.

4. **Deliver if bleeding is life threatening or fetal testing is nonreassuring**. Delivery should be performed in patients with a life-threatening hemorrhage. This is a clinical determination, but any patient whose vital signs are unstable or have a coagulopathy should be delivered regardless of gestational age and steroid administration. Vaginal delivery is preferred as long as bleeding is controlled and there are no signs of fetal distress. Vaginal delivery is also preferred in the case of intrauterine fetal demise in the setting of severe placental abruption. Because the uterus is typically hyperactive and persistently hypertonic in patients with an abruption, a rapid labor and delivery (L&D) should be expected. If the fetal heart rate (FHR) tracing is nonreassuring, delivery should occur for fetal indications.

UTERINE RUPTURE

PATHOGENESIS

Uterine rupture represents a potential obstetric catastrophe and can lead to both maternal and fetal death. Most complete uterine ruptures occur during the course of labor. More than 90% of all uterine ruptures are associated with a prior uterine scar either from cesarean section or other uterine surgery. Uterine ruptures without a prior uterine scar may be related to an abdominal trauma (e.g., auto accidents, external or internal version procedures), associated with labor or delivery (e.g., improper oxytocin use or excessive fundal pressure), or spontaneously initiated (e.g., placenta percreta, multiple gestation, grand multiparity, invasive mole, or choriocarcinoma).

The primary maternal complications from a ruptured uterus include hemorrhage and hypovolemic shock. The overall maternal mortality for uterine rupture is less than 1%, but if rupture occurs in the antepartum patient at home, it is likely to be higher. The perinatal mortality for uterine rupture ranges from 5% to 6%, again depending on where the patient is when the uterine rupture occurs.

EPIDEMIOLOGY

Uterine rupture is rare, occurring in an estimated 1 in 15,000 to 20,000 deliveries of patients with no prior uterine surgery. In women with a prior low-transverse cesarean delivery, it is estimated to occur in 0.5% to 0.1% of deliveries. However, in women with a prior classical cesarean delivery (vertical uterine incision), the incidence of uterine dehiscence or rupture is estimated to be 6% to 12%. Risk factors for uterine rupture are conditions that predispose to a weakened uterine wall, including uterine scars, overdistension, inappropriate and aggressive use of uterotonic agents, maternal congenital uterine anomalies, and abnormal placentation (Table 5-7).

CLINICAL MANIFESTATIONS

The presentation of uterine rupture is highly variable. Typically, it is characterized by the sudden onset of intense abdominal pain. Vaginal bleeding, if present, may vary from spotting to severe hemorrhage. Nonreassuring fetal testing, abnormal abdominal contour, cessation of uterine contractions, disappearance of fetal heart tones, and regression of the presenting fetal part are other signs of uterine rupture.

TABLE 5-7. Risk Factors for Uterine Rupture

Prior uterine surgery/uterine scar
Injudicious use of oxytocin
Grand multiparity
Marked uterine distension
Abnormal fetal lie
Large fetus
External version
Trauma

TREATMENT

Management of uterine rupture requires immediate laparotomy and delivery of the fetus. If feasible, the rupture site should be repaired and hemostasis obtained. In cases of large rupture extensions, repair may not be feasible and the patient may require a hysterectomy. Patients are usually discouraged to attempt future pregnancies given the high risk of recurrent rupture. Trial of labor would be avoided in any subsequent pregnancy, and the patient would commonly be delivered via repeat cesarean section between 36 and 37 weeks.

FETAL VESSEL RUPTURE

PATHOGENESIS

Most pregnancies complicated by rupture of a fetal vessel are due to **velamentous cord insertion** where the blood vessels insert between the amnion and chorion away from the placenta instead of inserting directly into the chorionic plate (Table 5-3). Because the vessels course unprotected through the membranes before inserting on the placental margin, they are vulnerable to rupture, shearing, or laceration. In addition, these unprotected vessels may cross over the internal cervical os (**vasa previa**), making them vulnerable to compression by the presenting fetal part or to being torn when the membranes are ruptured. Although vasa previa is rare, perinatal mortality is high (approximately 40% to 60%) and increases if the membranes are also ruptured. The condition is important because, when the membranes rupture, spontaneously or artificially, the fetal vessels running through the membranes have a high risk of concomitant rupture, frequently resulting in fetal exsanguination and death. Because the fetal blood volume is only about 80 to 100 mL/kg, loss of even small amounts of blood could prove disastrous to the fetus. Additionally, pressure on the unprotected vessels by the presenting fetal part could lead to fetal asphyxia and death.

Unprotected fetal vessels and vasa previa may occur with a **succenturiate lobe** of the placenta. In this case, the bulk of the placenta is implanted in one portion of the uterine wall, but a small lobe of the placenta is implanted in another location. The vessels that connect these two portions of the placenta are unprotected and may course over the cervix and present as a vasa previa.

EPIDEMIOLOGY

Only 0.1% to 0.8% of pregnancies are complicated by the rupture of a fetal vessel. The incidence of vasa previa is approximately 1:2,500 pregnancies. Risk factors for fetal vessel rupture include abnormal placentation leading to a succenturiate lobe as well as multiple gestations that increase the risk of velamentous insertion. Although the rate of velamentous insertion is only 1% in singleton gestations, it increases up to as high as 4% to 12% for twin gestations (4% to 7% for dichorionic twins and 10% to 12% for monochorionic twins), and 28% to 50% for triplet gestations. There is an increased incidence of both velamentous cord insertion and vasa previa in pregnancies that result from in vitro fertilization (IVF), particularly in twin pregnancies.

CLINICAL MANIFESTATIONS

In fortunate cases of unknown vasa previa, the fetal vessels are palpated and recognized through the dilated cervix. More commonly, the presentation of a fetal vessel rupture is vaginal bleeding associated with a sinusoidal variation of the FHR indicative of fetal anemia. Whenever bleeding accompanies rupture of the membranes in labor, especially if there are associated FHR decelerations, fetal bradycardia, or a sinusoidal FHR pattern, the obstetrician should have a high index of suspicion for a ruptured vasa previa.

DIAGNOSIS

Unfortunately, diagnosis is often made after a large bleed and fetal compromise have already occurred. With advancing capabilities of ultrasound, velamentous insertion of the umbilical cord and succenturiate placental lobes can be diagnosed in the antepartum period. Further, with the use of color Doppler, vasa previa may also be diagnosed antepartum, but the sensitivity ranges widely in studies from 53% to 100% and is likely related to the experience of the sonographer and/or sonologist and ultrasound equipment available. Several small prospective studies have demonstrated that the majority of cases of vasa previa in asymptomatic women can be diagnosed prenatally through a policy of routinely evaluating the placental cord insertion when an ultrasound examination is performed, and considering vaginal sonography with color Doppler if the placental cord insertion cannot be identified, or if there is a low-lying placenta or a suspected succenturiate placental lobe. These studies found that sonographic identification of placental cord insertion was accurate, sensitive, and added little or no extra time to the duration of the obstetric sonographic examination. In the prenatally diagnosed cases, the neonatal survival of infants without congenital malformations was approximately 97%. This is dramatic when compared to the 45% neonatal survival rate when the diagnosis was not made prenatally.

Diagnosis at the time of vaginal bleeding can be accomplished by the **Apt test** or examination of the blood for nucleated (fetal) RBCs. The Apt test involves diluting the blood with water, collecting the supernatant, and combining it with 1% NaOH. If the resulting mixture is pink, it indicates fetal blood; a yellow-brown color is seen with maternal blood. However, when acute bleeding occurs from a ruptured vasa previa, emergent delivery is frequently indicated, and there is usually no time to test for fetal blood cells.

TREATMENT

Given the high risk of fetal exsanguination and death (the vascular volume of the term fetus is <250 mL), the treatment of a ruptured fetal vessel is emergent cesarean delivery. Even when the neonate has lost considerable blood, immediate transfusion may be lifesaving. Now that vasa previa can occasionally be diagnosed antepartum, these patients are often given the option of elective cesarean delivery, although there are few data as to the fetal risk with expectant management. One study suggests that women with prenatally diagnosed vasa previa be offered elective delivery by cesarean at about 35 weeks of gestation. This is earlier than the 39 weeks that is generally recommended for elective cesarean delivery. The mean age of delivery for the cases *not* diagnosed prenatally in this series was approximately 38 weeks. In these cases, perinatal mortality was 56%. The risks associated with prematurity at 35 weeks of gestation must be weighed against the risk of a dismal outcome should the membranes rupture, especially because approximately 8% of women at term will have ruptured membranes before the onset of labor. Unfortunately, membrane rupture, even in a hospital, often results in infants with low Apgar scores and who require transfusions, suggesting significant morbidity. If patients with known vasa previa elect to undergo a trial of labor, artificial rupture of membranes is contraindicated.

NONOBSTETRIC CAUSES OF ANTEPARTUM HEMORRHAGE

Nonobstetric causes of antepartum hemorrhage are listed in Table 5-1. Patients with these conditions usually present with spotting rather than frank bleeding. Typically, there are no uterine contractions or abdominal pain. The diagnosis is usually made by speculum examination, Papanicolaou test, cultures, or colposcopy as indicated. Other than advanced maternal neoplasia, which is associated with poor maternal outcome, most nonobstetric causes of antepartum hemorrhage require relatively simple management and have good outcomes. Vaginal lacerations and varices can be located and repaired. Infections may be treated with appropriate agents, cervical polyps can be removed, and benign neoplasms usually require simple treatment.

KEY POINTS

- Placenta previa accounts for 20% of antepartum hemorrhage and is associated with placenta accreta in up to 5% of cases without prior cesareans and in 3% to 67% of cases with prior cesarean deliveries.
- Previa occurs more often in patients with prior placenta previa, uterine scars, or multiple gestations.
- The classic presentation of placenta previa is **painless** vaginal bleeding in the third trimester and it is usually diagnosed via ultrasound.
- Placenta previa is associated with antepartum hemorrhage, preterm delivery, preterm premature rupture of membranes (PPROM), intrauterine growth restriction (IUGR), and increases the risk of puerperal hysterectomy.
- Patients with placenta previa are delivered by cesarean section in the case of unstoppable preterm labor, large hemorrhage, nonreassuring fetal testing, or at 36 weeks.
- Placenta accreta is the abnormal attachment of the placenta to the uterus. When the placenta invades into the myometrium, it is known as placenta increta, whereas when it invades through the myometrium and to the serosa, it is known as placenta percreta.
- Placental abruption accounts for 30% of all third-trimester hemorrhages and is seen more often in women with chronic hypertension, with preeclampsia, using cocaine or methamphetamines, using tobacco, or with a history of abruption.
- Women with placental abruption usually present with vaginal bleeding, painful contractions, and a firm, tender uterus; 20% of patients present with no bleeding (concealed hemorrhages).
- Placental abruption can be complicated by hypovolemic shock, DIC, and preterm delivery. Women can be delivered vaginally if they are stable; cesarean delivery is necessary in the unstable patient or when fetal testing is nonreassuring.
- Uterine rupture is a rare obstetric catastrophe, but is seen in 325 per 100,000 laboring women with a prior cesarean delivery.
- Maternal and fetal morbidity and mortality are increased in the setting of uterine rupture.
- Uterine rupture requires immediate laparotomy, delivery of the fetus, and either repair of the rupture site or hysterectomy.
- Fetal vessel rupture is a rare obstetric complication and is usually associated with multiple gestation and/or a velamentous cord insertion.
- Fetal vessel rupture is associated with a perinatal mortality of up to 60% of cases.
- Patients may present with vaginal bleeding and a sinusoidal FHR pattern, which requires emergent cesarean delivery.
- Nonobstetric causes of antepartum hemorrhage include cervical and vaginal lacerations, hemorrhoids, infections, and neoplasms.
- Nonobstetric causes of antepartum hemorrhage generally require simple management and have good outcomes.

CLINICAL VIGNETTES

VIGNETTE 1

A 30-year-old G3P2002 Asian woman at 28 weeks 0 days by last menstrual period (LMP) consistent with a 7-week ultrasound presents for her follow-up ultrasound. At 20 weeks' gestation, she had a complete previa on ultrasound. No concerns today. No vaginal bleeding, no leakage of fluid, no discharge, just starting to feel fetal movement. No significant past medical history (PMH). Past surgical history was significant for two prior low-transverse cesarean sections at term, first cesarean section for breech at 39 weeks secondary to failed external cephalic version in 2007 and second for repeat cesarean section at 39 weeks in 2009. On ultrasound, the fetus is noted to have normal anatomy, normal amniotic fluid index, and an anterior placenta that is noted to be completely covering the internal os of the cervix. Transvaginal ultrasound confirms complete anterior placenta previa.

1. What is this patient most at risk for given her history and ultrasound findings?
   a. Preterm labor
   b. Placenta abruption
   c. Intrauterine fetal demise
   d. Placenta accreta
   e. Preeclampsia

2. What care precautions should be given to this patient?
   a. Complete bed rest for the remainder of the pregnancy or until previa resolves
   b. Complete pelvic rest for the remainder of the pregnancy or until previa resolves
   c. No special precautions necessary
   d. Bed rest and pelvic rest for the remainder of the pregnancy or until previa resolves
   e. Limited activity but pelvic rest is unnecessary

3. What further imaging, if any, might be helpful in the diagnosis of placenta accreta in this patient?
   a. No further imaging would be helpful
   b. Noncontrast CT of the abdomen/pelvis
   c. Noncontrast MRI of the abdomen/pelvis
   d. Cystoscopy by urologist
   e. Continue with serial ultrasound but no additional imaging

4. What is the most appropriate management plan if this patient continues to labor?
   a. Attempt to tocolyze the patient and give a steroid course for fetal lung maturity
   b. Cesarean section with manual extraction of the placenta, followed by hysterectomy
   c. Cesarean section, leaving the placenta in situ, followed by hysterectomy
   d. Expectant management and spontaneous vaginal delivery if she continues to labor

VIGNETTE 2

A 32-year-old G1P0 Caucasian woman presents for her anatomy ultrasound at 18 weeks by IVF dating. On ultrasound, the fetus is noted to have an anterior placenta with a posterior succenturiate lobe. She has no concerns. Her pregnancy is otherwise uncomplicated at this time.

1. What does the finding of an anterior placenta with a posterior succenturiate lobe on ultrasound put this patient at risk for?
   a. Placenta previa
   b. Placental abruption
   c. Cervical incompetence
   d. Vasa previa
   e. Preterm labor

2. What is the preferred mode of delivery in patients with this finding?
   a. Emergent cesarean delivery
   b. Scheduled cesarean delivery
   c. Induction of labor, including artificial rupture of membranes
   d. Spontaneous vaginal delivery, including spontaneous rupture of membranes
   e. None of the above

3. What does the sinusoidal pattern on the fetal monitoring strip suggest?
   a. Fetal anemia
   b. Uteroplacental insufficiency
   c. Cord compression
   d. Head compression
   e. Normal tracing for twin gestation

VIGNETTE 3

A 24-year-old G2P1001 Hispanic woman at 38 weeks by LMP consistent with 10-week ultrasound presents to L&D triage, complaining of painful uterine contractions every 4 to 5 minutes. She has no significant PMH. Her obstetric history is significant for one prior low-transverse cesarean section for breech at 39 weeks' gestation. On sterile vaginal examination, the patient is initially found to be 2 cm dilated, 50% effaced, and −3 station. The patient strongly desires to have a vaginal delivery if at all possible.

1. What is the best initial management for this patient?
   a. Close observation in triage with continuous fetal monitoring and repeat sterile vaginal exam in 2 to 4 hours
   b. Discharge home and follow-up in 1 week at clinic
   c. Admission to L&D triage and repeat cesarean delivery without a trial of labor
   d. Admission to L&D triage, continuous fetal monitoring, and start oxytocin augmentation

2. What is next best step?
   a. Admission to L&D triage, continuous fetal monitoring, counsel patient regarding trial of labor after cesarean (TOLAC), proceed with expectant management of labor if she desires to proceed with TOLAC
   b. Discharge home and follow-up in 1 week at clinic
   c. Admission to L&D triage and repeat cesarean delivery without a trial of labor
   d. Admission to L&D triage, continuous fetal monitoring, counsel patient regarding TOLAC, and start oxytocin augmentation if she desires to proceed with TOLAC

3. What is the best explanation for these findings?
   a. Placental abruption
   b. Fetal head compression
   c. Umbilical cord compression
   d. Uterine rupture
   e. None of the above

4. What is the most appropriate next step?
   a. Stop the oxytocin and observe expectantly
   b. Place an intrauterine pressure catheter and start an amnioinfusion
   c. Administer tocolysis to stop the uterine contractions
   d. Proceed to the operating room for emergent cesarean delivery
   e. None of the above

VIGNETTE 4

A 22-year-old G1P0 African-American woman at 36 weeks by LMP consistent with 12-week ultrasound with limited prenatal care presents via ambulance to the L&D triage unit complaining of severe abdominal pain and profuse vaginal bleeding. The patient is unstable and unable to communicate coherently. The emergency medical technician (EMT) reports that initially her BP was 180/100 mm Hg and pulse rate was 110 beats per minute, but she has lost at least 500 mL blood en route. On examination, her BP is 90/50 mm Hg, pulse rate is 120 beats per minute, she appears to be in significant pain, is unable to answer questions, and her abdomen feels rigid.

1. What is the most likely diagnosis in this patient?
   a. Placenta previa
   b. Normal labor
   c. Vasa previa
   d. Cervical tear after intercourse
   e. Placental abruption

2. What is the best next step?
   a. Sterile speculum examination, followed by sterile vaginal examination
   b. Abdominal ultrasound
   c. Stabilize the patient, obtain two large-bore IV catheters, and start IV fluid bolus while checking for fetal heart tones
   d. Emergent cesarean section
   e. Transvaginal ultrasound

3. The nurse attempts to find fetal heart tones (FHTs) and they seem to be about 70 beats per minute but the nurse is unsure. You quickly do a bedside ultrasound and confirm that FHTs are 70 beats per minute. What is the best next step?
   a. Proceed immediately to the operating room (OR) for emergent cesarean delivery
   b. Sterile vaginal examination to see if the patient is in labor
   c. Transfuse two units of packed RBCs while continuously monitoring the fetus
   d. Expectant management
   e. None of the above

4. What is the most important laboratory test to order for this patient emergently?
   a. Type and cross
   b. CBC
   c. Urine drug screen
   d. Chemistry
   e. PT, PTT, international normalized ratio (INR)

5. What does this patient now have as a result of her abruption and significant blood loss?
   a. Anemia
   b. Thrombocytopenia
   c. Hypovolemia
   d. Consumptive coagulopathy
   e. All of the above

ANSWERS

VIGNETTE 1 Question 1
1. Answer D:
If the patient's placenta previa persists into the third trimester, then she is most at risk for placenta accreta in the presence of an anterior placenta previa and a history of two previous cesarean sections. With the progression of pregnancy, more than 90% of low-lying placentas identified early in pregnancy will appear to move away from the cervix and out of the lower uterine segment. However, placenta previa occurs in as many as 1% to 4% of women with a prior cesarean section. If placenta previa persists, it can be complicated by an associated placenta accreta (placenta previa accreta) in approximately 5% of cases. The risk of placenta accreta is increased in women with placenta previa in the setting of one or more prior cesarean deliveries: approximately 3%, 11%, 40%, 61%, and 67% for one, two, three, four, and five prior cesarean sections, respectively. While Asian women are at a higher risk for having a placenta previa than are Caucasian women, there is no known association between placenta accreta and race. The patient is at increased risk of preterm labor and preterm delivery if she has an antepartum hemorrhage as a result of her placenta previa but her risk of placenta accreta is likely higher given her two prior cesarean deliveries. She does not have any other risk factors for preterm labor/preterm delivery. This patient is not at increased risk from the general population for placental abruption or preeclampsia. She does not have any significant risk factors for intrauterine fetal demise.

VIGNETTE 1 Question 2
2. Answer B:
It is recommended for patients with a complete or partial previa to have complete pelvic rest, meaning no intercourse, in order to prevent significant vaginal bleeding. If significant bleeding occurs, it can lead to both maternal and fetal anemia and potentially preterm labor. There is no evidence that complete bed rest will help prevent vaginal bleeding or preterm labor in patients with complete or partial placenta previa. The special precautions regarding placenta previa are complete pelvic rest and close observation. Although it is reasonable to limit the patient's activity, particularly if they experience preterm contractions or bleeding, it is more important for them to observe pelvic rest.

VIGNETTE 1 Question 3
3. Answer C:
Because this patient has had two prior cesarean sections, has an anterior placenta previa, and because the sonographer cannot distinguish the placenta from the bladder, it might be helpful to get further imaging to rule out a placenta accreta, increta, or percreta. MRI is the imaging modality of choice to evaluate for the myometrial and/or bladder invasion of the placenta, particularly when it is not clear on ultrasound. Further imaging to rule out placenta accreta (or increta/percreta) can be helpful in cases such as this, where the diagnosis is unclear on ultrasound. CT is not the modality of choice in this case as MRI is far superior to evaluate the muscular planes of the uterine wall and bladder. Although it may be necessary for the patient to have cystoscopy by an urologist or urogynecologist at some point, it is more helpful to get an MRI of the abdomen and pelvis first. Cystoscopy is often indicated if there is evidence of accreta/increta/percreta on ultrasound or MRI, or if the patient develops significant hematuria. Although it is important to continue performing serial ultrasounds of the fetus and placenta in order to evaluate fetal growth and fluid, cervical length, and the placenta, additional imaging with MRI can be helpful and should be considered.

Further imaging reveals complete anterior previa with evidence of placental invasion into the bladder. Four weeks later, at 32 weeks' gestation, the patient presents to L&D triage complaining of passing two large blood clots with continued spotting. She denies contractions but on the tocometer is noted to have contractions every 2 to 4 minutes. A sterile speculum examination is performed and her cervix is dilated to approximately 2 cm. The patient also reports noting blood in her urine over the last few days. Of note, she does not desire future fertility and would like a tubal ligation after delivery, if possible.

VIGNETTE 1 Question 4
4. Answer A:
The most appropriate management plan if the patient continues to labor would be to tocolyze her so as to prolong the pregnancy long enough to administer a steroid course to improve fetal lung maturity in the event that she continues to labor. It is reasonable to attempt to tocolyze at this early gestation as long as the patient remains hemodynamically stable with minimal vaginal bleeding. However, if the patient bleeds significantly, she may need to be delivered prior to completion of the steroid course. Although in some cases it is reasonable to allow a patient to have a trial of labor after two cesarean sections, it is not appropriate in a patient with a complete placenta previa, as it would result in significant hemorrhage and likely both maternal and fetal compromise. Because the patient has had

two prior cesarean sections, has complete placenta previa, and is now experiencing hematuria, this is concerning for a placenta percreta with invasion into the bladder. If she indeed has a percreta documented by cystoscopy or MRI, the mode of delivery would be a cesarean section, often followed by hysterectomy. A hysterectomy outright without removal of the placenta will minimize hemorrhage. However, because of the challenges of making certain diagnoses, if the patient desires future fertility, then some clinicians will attempt placental removal in an attempt to avoid hysterectomy. If she does have complete previa and placenta percreta, the most common delivery plan is to proceed with a cesarean section (often a high vertical or transverse hysterotomy to avoid the placenta), deliver the fetus, leave the placenta in situ (rather than extraction), and to proceed with hysterectomy. By leaving the placenta in situ, closing the hysterotomy, and proceeding with hysterectomy, the surgeon avoids the significant bleeding that can occur from the placental bed after manual extraction of the placenta. In this patient's case, because she does not desire future fertility and was planning on a tubal ligation, the more appropriate choice would be to leave the placenta in situ so as to minimize blood loss during the procedure.

VIGNETTE 2 Question 1
1. Answer D:
There is an increased incidence of vasa previa when there is a succenturiate lobe, particularly when this lobe is noted to be some distance from the rest of the placenta. A succenturiate lobe is an accessory placental lobe. In this case, the bulk of the placenta is implanted in one portion of the uterine wall, but a small lobe of the placenta is implanted in another location. The vessels that connect these two portions of the placenta are unprotected and may course over the cervix and present as a vasa previa. When a vasa previa is present in the case of a succenturiate lobe, these unprotected vessels may cross over the internal cervical os, making them vulnerable to compression by the presenting fetal part or to being torn when the membranes are ruptured. In this case, the bulk of the placenta is anterior and the succenturiate lobe is posterior so it is possible that the vessels connecting the two lobes could course over the internal os of the cervix resulting in a vasa previa. There is no significant increase in the incidence of placenta previa, placental abruption, cervical incompetence, or preterm labor as a result of a succenturiate posterior lobe of the placenta.

On transvaginal ultrasound, color Doppler demonstrates that there are vessels from the anterior placental lobe coursing over the internal os to connect to the posterior succenturiate placental lobe. The fetus is noted to be in the vertex presentation. Otherwise, the pregnancy continues to be uncomplicated.

VIGNETTE 2 Question 2
2. Answer B:
In patients with a known vasa previa diagnosed on ultrasound, generally a cesarean delivery is the preferred mode of delivery so as to decrease the risk of rupture of the fetal vessels. There are very few studies on this; however, because a ruptured fetal vessel leads to catastrophic neonatal outcomes of cognitive injury and death, when a vasa previa is diagnosed, most clinicians recommend a cesarean delivery. There is a significantly higher neonatal survival rate in those infants who have a vasa previa diagnosed prenatally, most likely because when it is not diagnosed prenatally, the diagnosis is usually made at the time of fetal vessel rupture, which in turn leads to significant fetal anemia and often death. Ideally, cesarean delivery should be scheduled before the patient goes into labor and/or spontaneously ruptures in order to prevent fetal vessel rupture at the time of the rupture of membranes. This is commonly done at 36 weeks' gestation, though some clinicians have even recommended earlier. Although not preferable, if the patient does desire to have a vaginal delivery and there is evidence of fetal anemia on continuous fetal monitoring, emergent cesarean delivery would then be necessary. Also, if the patient does choose to undergo a vaginal delivery (induction or spontaneous), artificial rupture of membranes is contraindicated, as the risk of fetal vessel rupture is higher than with spontaneous rupture of membranes.

The patient presents to L&D triage at 34 weeks and complains of leakage of fluid, vaginal bleeding, and contractions. On sterile speculum examination, the patient appears to have PPROM and to be 4 cm dilated. There appears to be a sinusoidal pattern on the continuous fetal monitoring tracing strip.

VIGNETTE 2 Question 3
3. Answer A:
A sinusoidal pattern on continuous FHR monitoring indicates fetal anemia. Although this can sometimes be confused with a pseudosinusoidal pattern, when there is a true sinusoidal pattern, it is considered to be nonreassuring because it indicates fetal anemia. Given the small fetal blood volume, a sinusoidal pattern should prompt an emergent delivery (as fast as possible) by the obstetrician. Fetal anemia in this case was most likely caused by rupture of the fetal vessels (vasa previa) upon rupture of the membranes. Uteroplacental insufficiency is not associated with a sinusoidal FHR tracing. Late decelerations are the typical fetal tracing finding when uteroplacental insufficiency occurs. These can be subtle or overt but if they are recurrent with every contraction for more than three contractions, the obstetrician should undertake immediate intervention. Cord compression causes variable decelerations, rather than a sinusoidal pattern. This can usually be

resolved with an intraamniotic infusion using an intrauterine pressure catheter. By instilling the uterus with fluid, the cord has more protection from compression during uterine contractions. Head compression during labor is usually associated with early decelerations that start before a contraction and recover by the end of the contraction. A true sinusoidal tracing is never normal and is indicative of nonreassuring fetal status.

VIGNETTE 3 Question 1
1. Answer A:
Because the patient is 2 cm dilated, 50% effaced, and −3 station, with painful contractions every 4 to 5 minutes, and has a known uterine scar (from her previous cesarean delivery), the most appropriate initial course of action is to continue close observation with continuous fetal monitoring, and reevaluate in 2 to 4 hours (or earlier if clinically necessary). Although the patient does not seem to be in active labor and is only 2 cm dilated, the patient is painfully contracting and is at risk of uterine rupture so she needs to be adequately ruled out for active labor before being sent home. It is not appropriate to proceed immediately to repeat cesarean delivery at this stage, as it is not clear that she is laboring and there is no other indication for cesarean section at this time. A prospective, randomized, controlled trial showed that in the setting of latent labor admission and augmentation led to a higher risk of uterine rupture. Therefore, admission to L&D triage for labor augmentation is not indicated. In general, in the setting of TOLAC, the patient is at increased risk of uterine rupture with oxytocin augmentation and so oxytocin should not be started unless it is necessary.

The patient is expectantly managed in L&D triage for 2 hours. On repeat vaginal examination, she is found to have changed to 6 cm dilated, 75% effaced, and −1 station. She is now contracting painfully every 1 to 2 minutes. The FHR tracing is reactive with no decelerations.

VIGNETTE 3 Question 2
2. Answer A:
The next best step now that the patient has changed from 2 to 6 cm, that is, active labor, is to admit her to L&D triage, to continue with fetal monitoring, and to counsel her regarding the risks, benefits, alternatives, and indications for TOLAC versus repeat cesarean delivery. If after counseling the patient considers the risks of TOLAC and desires to have a vaginal delivery (VBAC), then most physicians would expectantly manage her active labor. Because oxytocin augmentation has been shown to double the risk of uterine rupture, it is more appropriate to follow expectant management than to immediately start oxytocin augmentation on admission to L&D triage. It is better to wait to start oxytocin until it is clear she is not continuing to change her cervix or contract regularly after 4 hours (provider dependent). It is not appropriate to send an actively laboring patient with a prior cesarean section, and who is dilated to 6 cm, home with follow-up. Given the risk of uterine rupture, at the very least the patient needs to be expectantly managed with continuous fetal monitoring. It is an option to proceed immediately to repeat cesarean delivery if there is concern for uterine rupture, fetal distress, or if the patient desires a repeat cesarean after being counseled regarding the risks, benefits, alternatives, and indications for TOLAC and repeat cesarean delivery.

The patient labors spontaneously without an epidural but after 4 hours her cervical examination is unchanged. The FHR tracing continues to be reactive with no late decelerations noted. Oxytocin augmentation is started. Two hours later the patient is found to be 8 cm dilated, 90% effaced, and 0 station. Approximately 1 hour later, the nurse calls you to the room because the patient is complaining of severe abdominal pain with and without contractions. On sterile vaginal exam (SVE), the patient is now noted to be 8 cm dilated, 90% effaced, but station has changed from 0 to −3. You note that there had been several recurrent deep variable decelerations with each contraction on the FHR tracing that now shows fetal bradycardia.

VIGNETTE 3 Question 3
3. Answer D:
The most likely explanation for these findings in this clinical scenario is uterine rupture of the prior cesarean scar. The rupture of the scar disrupts uterine blood flow to the placenta, resulting in uteroplacental insufficiency, which in turns causes late decelerations. Additionally, the umbilical cord or fetal parts can be extruded into the patient's abdomen leading to cord compression and severe variable decelerations or frank bradycardia. Severe abdominal pains with loss of station of the fetal head on vaginal examination are classic findings in a uterine rupture, especially when associated with a nonreassuring fetal status on the continuous fetal monitoring. While placental abruption can result in recurrent late decelerations as a result of uteroplacental insufficiency and can occur with a uterine rupture, it is unlikely in this situation as there is minimal bleeding noted. Additionally, loss of station is not generally found on a placental abruption unless it occurs concurrently with uterine rupture. Fetal head compression causes early decelerations, not late decelerations, and does not result in the loss of station on vaginal examination. Umbilical cord compression is not generally associated with pain worse than usual with contractions, causes variable decelerations, and does not cause loss of station of the fetal head.

VIGNETTE 3 Question 4

4. Answer D:
Uterine rupture is an obstetric emergency. It can result in placental abruption, or if the fetus is delivered through the uterine dehiscence into the abdomen, it can result in significant fetal hypoxic injury because of complete cord compression. Additionally, there is risk for significant maternal blood loss; thus, immediate delivery via cesarean section is imperative. Once the neonate is delivered, the surgeon should then assess the uterine rupture site for the feasibility of repair and to obtain hemostasis. If it cannot be repaired or hemostasis cannot be obtained, peripartum hysterectomy is indicated. While intuitively it is important to stop the oxytocin augmentation when one suspects uterine rupture, expectant management would not be appropriate. An amnioinfusion is not appropriate in this clinical situation, as there is no evidence of cord compression. While there may be uterine tetany as a result of excess oxytocin, once the uterus has dehisced, tocolysis is neither appropriate nor helpful in this situation.

VIGNETTE 4 Question 1

1. Answer E:
Given the patient's hemodynamic instability, significant vaginal bleeding resulting in profound blood loss, and rigid abdomen, along with severe abdominal pain, the most likely clinical diagnosis is placental abruption. Normal labor does not cause significant blood loss with cervical change except in the instance of placenta previa. While patients who labor with a placenta previa can have pain from the contractions and profuse vaginal bleeding, they are not usually hemodynamically unstable nor are they usually in severe pain with a rigid abdomen. Also, the initial elevated BP of 180/100 mm Hg suggests preeclampsia or superimposed preeclampsia, which is a known risk factor for placental abruption. Vasa previa can lead to profuse vaginal bleeding if a patient ruptures her membranes and the fetal vessels also rupture, but it does not result in maternal hemodynamic instability. A cervical tear from intercourse can cause significant pain and vaginal bleeding but does not fit with this clinical scenario.

VIGNETTE 4 Question 2

2. Answer C:
Typically, when a patient in this scenario presents to the emergency department or obstetrics triage unit, multiple steps are undertaken at the same time. However, the best next step is to start stabilizing the patient and to assess the fetal status. Given the patient's hemodynamic instability (hypotension, tachycardia, and profuse bleeding), two large-bore IV catheters should be placed, a bolus of IV fluids (normal saline or lactated Ringer's) should be given, while another nurse or clinician is attempting to assess the fetal status. This is important to do immediately, as it determines the speed with which the team must mobilize the patient to the OR for an emergent cesarean section. If the fetus is dead, the team's sole focus can be placed on the mother's status before addressing the fetus and delivery planning. If the fetal status cannot be determined with external fetal monitoring quickly, an abdominal ultrasound is the next step but should not supersede gaining IV access and fetal Doppler. Often in these cases, the FHTs are difficult to determine as they are usually bradycardic (and/or similar to maternal heart rate). Ultrasound becomes critical to determine the fetal status, as it can be used to visualize the FHR, particularly in the setting of terminal bradycardia as is often found in these cases. Ultrasound is also important to determine the location of the placenta if there is any concern for a placenta previa. Given this patient's limited prenatal care and profuse vaginal bleeding, ultrasound is important in this situation but, again, should not supersede obtaining maternal IV access and starting her stabilization. Sterile vaginal examination and speculum examination are important steps in the evaluation process but should not come before IV access or assessing the fetal status and location of the placenta. Often it is not necessary at all in the setting of placental abruption as most proceed to emergent cesarean delivery if the fetus has a documented heart rate. Emergent cesarean delivery should follow shortly after obtaining maternal vital signs, IV access, fetal assessment, and ultrasound if placental abruption is strongly suspected and there is fetal bradycardia or nonreassuring fetal status on external fetal monitoring. Transvaginal ultrasound should come later if the patient stabilizes and needs further assessment of placental location because placenta previa is suspected.

VIGNETTE 4 Question 3

3. Answer A:
In the setting of suspected placental abruption, once the fetus is determined to have a heart rate and to be in distress, emergent cesarean delivery is indicated. Unless the patient appears to be laboring with delivery imminent, when FHTs are about 50 beats per minute, it is best to proceed with emergent cesarean delivery. Often there is time in the OR to do a vaginal examination to assess cervical dilation. If delivery is imminent, then the patient can begin pushing, but otherwise one should proceed with emergent cesarean section. While the patient should be transfused two units of packed RBCs during the cesarean delivery, it is not appropriate to wait for the blood transfusion to proceed to the OR for cesarean delivery in the setting of terminal fetal bradycardia. Expectant management is similarly not appropriate.

VIGNETTE 4 Question 4

4. Answer A:

While all the above laboratory tests are important and should be ordered as soon as possible, the most important laboratory test to send immediately is a type and cross because it will allow you to start preparing blood and FFP to transfuse to the patient. While the patient can be given O-negative blood in this type of emergency, in the case of placental abruption, the patient will likely need multiple units of packed RBCs, platelets, FFP, and cryoprecipitate as patients frequently lose more than 2 L of blood and can develop consumptive coagulopathy. A CBC is important to assess the patient's baseline Hgb/Hct and platelet count. A urine drug screen is important because placental abruption frequently occurs in the setting of cocaine abuse and this patient in particular is at high risk for cocaine abuse. A chemistry and coagulation laboratory test results (PT/PTT, INR) are also important to establish the patient's baseline renal function and clotting ability, particularly if the patient develops a consumptive coagulopathy.

The patient undergoes delivery with Apgar scores of 1 and 5, at 5 and 10 minutes, respectively. The placenta is removed easily and 500 mL clot follows the delivery of the placenta. Total estimated blood loss (EBL) from cesarean section is 1,500 mL (2,500 mL EBL including blood lost in the field). Intraoperative hematocrit is 20%, platelet count 70,000, fibrinogen level 50, INR value 3, and creatinine level 1.5.

VIGNETTE 4 Question 5

5. Answer E:

In addition to patient's obvious anemia, thrombocytopenia, hypofibrinogenemia, elevated INR, hypovolemia, and acute renal failure, the patient appears to have consumptive coagulopathy caused by the massive hemorrhage from the placental abruption. Consumptive coagulopathy is commonly associated with placental abruption, particularly in the setting of preeclampsia. It can be fatal if adequate resuscitation is not administered in a timely fashion. It is important to anticipate profound blood loss and coagulopathy with placental abruption. Consumptive coagulopathy often occurs when the patient's blood loss is underestimated and she is under-resuscitated, particularly if she is given packed RBCs without FFP in a ratio of at least 4:1. Recent literature suggests that these patients should be managed more like a trauma patient and transfused with a ratio of 1:1:1 (packed red blood cells [PRBC] to FFP to platelets). It is also important to follow fibrinogen and to transfuse cryoprecipitate as needed. Acute renal failure as a result of acute tubular necrosis is common in this scenario and usually resolves with adequate resuscitation.

6 Complications of Labor and Delivery

PRETERM LABOR

Labor that occurs before week 37 is called **preterm labor** (PTL). Many patients present with preterm contractions, but only those who have cervical change as measured on cervical examination are diagnosed as having PTL. It differs from **cervical insufficiency**, which is a silent, painless dilation, and effacement of the cervix. Both can result in preterm delivery, which is the leading cause of fetal morbidity and mortality in the United States. The incidence of preterm delivery in the United States reached a peak in 2005 to more than 12% of all births but since then has been steadily declining and as of 2014 was 9.6%. Unfortunately, the reason for the rise was predominantly from iatrogenic deliveries, and thus the recent decline has more to do with policy interventions to avoid unindicated, iatrogenic preterm delivery as opposed to medical interventions that have decreased preterm births. Despite this recent decline, large racial and ethnic disparities in preterm birth still exist; for example, as of 2014, African American infants were 50% more likely to be born preterm compared with their Caucasian counterparts.

PRETERM DELIVERY

Infants born before 37 weeks' gestation are termed **preterm**. There are three subcategories of preterm birth based on gestational age at the time of delivery: extremely preterm (<28 weeks), very preterm (28 to <32 weeks), and moderate to late preterm (32 to <37 weeks). Infants can also be classified by **birth weight**, again subgrouped into three categories: low birth weight (LBW), <2,500 g; very LBW, <1,500 g; and extremely LBW, <1,000 g. Infants who have not grown appropriately for their gestational age have **intrauterine growth restriction** (IUGR) or are **small for gestational age**. Thus, an IUGR infant can be born after week 37 but still be LBW, and similarly, a preterm LBW infant may still be appropriate size for their gestational age. Morbidity and mortality of preterm infants are dramatically affected by gestational age and birth weight. Prematurity immediately puts infants at increased risk of respiratory distress syndrome (RDS), intraventricular hemorrhage, sepsis, and necrotizing enterocolitis. Infants born on the cusp of viability at 23 weeks' gestation have a greater than 50% mortality rate, whereas infants born after week 34 have a mortality rate that is only slightly higher than that of full-term neonates. Long-term complications of prematurity include bronchopulmonary dysplasia and asthma; neurologic disorders, including cerebral palsy, behavioral problems, and learning disabilities; retinopathy of prematurity; and hearing loss.

ETIOLOGY AND RISK FACTORS

The defining physiologic mechanism that causes the onset of labor is unknown. However, various risk factors have been associated with PTL. These include but are not limited to preterm rupture of membranes (ROM); chorioamnionitis; multiple gestations; uterine anomalies, such as a bicornuate uterus; previous preterm delivery; maternal prepregnancy weight less than 50 kg; placental abruption; maternal disease, including preeclampsia, infections, intra-abdominal disease or surgery; substance abuse; and low socioeconomic status.

TOCOLYSIS

Tocolysis is the attempt to prevent contractions and the progression of labor. Many tocolytics are used in the United States, but only ritodrine—a β-mimetic agent—is FDA approved for this purpose. It is difficult to conduct placebo-controlled studies of new tocolytics because most patients and clinicians are unwilling to allow contractions to proceed without some tocolytic therapy. Thus, many of the current trials compare currently used tocolytics with other tocolytics. Because the evidence for which of the tocolytic agents may be the most effective is unclear, institutions and practitioners vary widely in practice.

The principal goal of tocolytic therapy is to delay delivery by at least 48 hours. This is because the principal benefit is to allow treatment with steroids to enhance fetal lung maturity and reduce the risk of complications associated with preterm delivery. **Betamethasone**, a glucocorticoid, has been shown to reduce the incidence of RDS and other complications from preterm delivery. Prior to 34 weeks of gestation, the advantages of treating with steroids need to be weighed against the risks of prolonging the pregnancy. From 34 to 36 weeks and 6 days, betamethasone has now been shown to be beneficial but is not used with concomitant tocolysis (*N Engl J Med*. 2016;374:1311–1320). There are many situations in which PTL should be allowed to progress. Chorioamnionitis, nonreassuring fetal testing, and significant placental abruption are absolute indications to allow labor to progress and often to hasten delivery. Many other issues, such as maternal disease—particularly preeclampsia or poor placental perfusion—an assessment of the severity of the situation, the precipitous nature of the complication, and the risks from prematurity, contribute to the decision of whether or not to tocolyze.

TOCOLYTICS

The goal of a tocolytic is to decrease or halt the cervical change resulting from contractions. In the case of preterm contractions without cervical change, hydration can often decrease the number and strength of the contractions. This operates along the principle that a dehydrated patient has increased levels of vasopressin or **antidiuretic hormone** (ADH), the octapeptide synthesized in the hypothalamus along with oxytocin. Because ADH differs from oxytocin by only one amino acid, it may bind with oxytocin receptors and lead to contractions. Thus, hydration, which decreases the level of ADH, may also decrease the number of contractions. For patients who do not respond to hydration or whose cervices are actively changing, a variety of tocolytics may be used. Currently, in the United States, the most commonly used tocolytics are nifedipine and indomethacin.

Calcium Channel Blockers

Calcium channel blockers decrease the influx of calcium into smooth muscle cells, thereby diminishing uterine contractions. In vitro, they have been shown to decrease myometrial contractions. In clinical trials, **nifedipine** has been the principal drug studied and has been shown to reduce the risk of delivery within 48 hours compared with placebo/no treatment but was not statistically different when compared with other classes of tocolytics. Because nifedipine is a peripheral vasodilator, its main side effects include headaches, flushing, and dizziness. Nifedipine is given orally and, as with other tocolytics, should be loaded. Typically, a 10-mg dose Q 15 minutes is given for the first hour or until contractions have ceased. This is followed by a maintenance dosage of 10 to 30 mg Q 4 to 6 hours as tolerated according to the patient's BP (up to 180 mg/day). The optimal dosing of nifedipine, however, has not been established, and so loading and maintenance doses may vary between providers. Nifedipine is contraindicated in women with preload-dependent cardiac lesions and hypotension and should be used with caution in women with left ventricular dysfunction. Also, the concomitant use of nifedipine and magnesium sulfate necessitates caution given their potential synergistic effect that results in respiratory depression.

Prostaglandin Inhibitors

Prostaglandins increase the intracellular levels of calcium and enhance myometrial gap junction function, thereby increasing myometrial contractions. Thus, they are commonly used to induce labor and to heighten contractions in postpartum patients with uterine atony. Conversely, antiprostaglandin agents are used to inhibit contractions and possibly halt labor. **Indomethacin**—a nonsteroidal anti-inflammatory drug (NSAID) that blocks the enzyme cyclooxygenase and decreases the level of prostaglandins—is used as a tocolytic. In clinical trials, it has been shown to effectively decrease contractions and forestall labor with minimal maternal side effects. However, it has been associated with a variety of fetal complications, including premature constriction of the ductus arteriosus, pulmonary hypertension, and oligohydramnios secondary to reduced fetal urine output as a result of enhanced vasopressin action and reduced renal blood flow. Furthermore, one study showed an increased risk of necrotizing enterocolitis and intraventricular hemorrhage in extremely premature fetuses that had been exposed to indomethacin within 48 hours of delivery. Currently, indomethacin is most commonly used before 32 weeks' gestation and generally only for 48 to 72 hours. If indomethacin is used, the amniotic fluid index should be checked before initiating the drug and again after 48 hours, to monitor for development of oligohydramnios. Indomethacin should be stopped promptly if amniotic fluid is decreased. Maternal contraindications to indomethacin include platelet dysfunction, hepatic dysfunction, gastrointestinal ulcerative disease, renal dysfunction, and asthma. Indomethacin is given orally as a 50-mg loading dose followed by 25 mg every 6 hours for 48 hours.

Magnesium Sulfate

Magnesium decreases uterine tone and contractions by acting as a calcium antagonist and a membrane stabilizer. Although magnesium can stop contractions, in small placebo-controlled trials, it has not been shown to change gestational age of delivery. In larger trials, the efficacy of magnesium did not vary significantly from that of β-mimetics. Side effects such as flushing, headaches, fatigue, and diplopia are seen. At toxic levels of magnesium (>10 mg/dL), respiratory depression, hypoxia, and cardiac arrest have been seen. Deep tendon reflexes (DTRs) are depressed at magnesium levels of 6 to 10 mg/dL. Therefore, a reliable and quick assessment for magnesium toxicity can be achieved with serial DTR exams. Pulmonary edema has also been seen in women treated with magnesium sulfate, although it may be secondary to the concomitant IV fluid given to patients in PTL. Generally, magnesium sulfate should be loaded as a 6-g bolus over 20 minutes, and then maintained at a 2 g/hour continuous infusion. A slower infusion should be used in the case of renal insufficiency because magnesium is cleared via the kidneys.

β-Mimetics

Uterine myometrium is composed of smooth muscle fibers. The contraction of these fibers is regulated by myosin light-chain kinase (MLK), which is activated by calcium ions through their interaction with calmodulin (Fig. 6-1). By increasing the level of cAMP, calcium is sequestered in the sarcoplasmic reticulum, causing a decrease in the level of free calcium ions and a decrease in uterine contractions. Conversion of ATP to cAMP is increased by β-agonists that bind and activate $β_2$ receptors on myometrial cells.

The two **β-mimetics** historically used for PTL were **ritodrine** and **terbutaline**. Although both are certainly effective in halting preterm contractions, randomized controlled studies in which patients were truly in PTL showed that β-agonists increased gestation an average of only 24 to 48 hours further over hydration and bed rest alone. Side effects of these drugs include tachycardia, headaches, and anxiety. More seriously, pulmonary edema may occur and, in rare cases, maternal death. Ritodrine was given as continuous IV therapy, whereas terbutaline was usually given as 0.25 mg SC, loaded Q 20 minutes three times dosages, and then Q 3 to 4 hours maintenance. Because terbutaline may cause maternal death and cardiac events, including tachycardia, transient hyperglycemia, hypokalemia, cardiac arrhythmias, pulmonary edema, and myocardial ischemia, the FDA has now added a black box warning to the use of terbutaline IV beyond 24 to 48 hours. Similarly, ritodrine was pulled from the U.S. market. Subcutaneous terbutaline is still used to acutely stop contractions in the setting of uterine hypertonicity leading to an abnormal fetal heart tracing.

Oxytocin Antagonists

Oxytocin antagonists (e.g., atosiban) are selective oxytocin–vasopressin receptor antagonists that, in theory, seem to be an obvious choice for an effective tocolytic and should have minimal side effects. They are commonly used in Europe but are not available in the United States. Although they have shown to decrease uterine myometrial contractions, clinical studies have been small and have not demonstrated an improvement in outcomes. Current use has been limited to experimental trials that have shown no clinical difference from the other commonly used tocolytics, and the FDA had concerns about the drug's safety when used in pregnancies less than 28 weeks (higher rate of fetal and infant death in patients taking atosiban).

PRETERM AND PREMATURE RUPTURE OF MEMBRANES

ROM occurring before week 37 is considered **preterm rupture of the membranes**, whereas ROM occurring before the onset of labor is termed **premature rupture of the membranes** (PROM). If the two occur together, it is termed **preterm premature rupture of the membranes** (PPROM). Anytime ROM lasts longer than 18 hours before delivery, it is described as **prolonged rupture of membranes**.

PRETERM ROM

Spontaneous rupture of the fetal membranes before week 37 is a common cause of PTL, preterm delivery, and chorioamnionitis. Without intervention, approximately 50% of patients who have ROM will go into labor within 24 hours, and up to 75% will do so within 48 hours. These rates are inversely correlated with

FIGURE 6-1. Control of myometrial contractility: myosin light-chain kinase (MLK) is the key enzyme. (**A**) Activation of myosin light chain kinase (MLK) by calcium bound to calmodulin. (**B**) Increased cytoplasmic calcium concentration results from calcium release from storage sites (Sarcoplasmic reticulum and mitochondria) and extracellular influx through voltage operated and receptor mediated channels. (**C**) Activation of adenylate cyclase by β-agonists and subsequent formation of cAMP results in deactivation of MLK and uterine relaxation.

gestational age at ROM; thus, patients with ROM before 26 weeks are more likely to gain an additional week when compared with those at greater than 30 weeks. Although maintaining the pregnancy to gain further fetal maturity would seem beneficial, prolonged PPROM has been associated with increased risk of chorioamnionitis, abruption, and cord prolapse.

Diagnosis

Commonly, a patient complains of a gush of fluid from the vagina. However, any increased vaginal discharge or complaints of stress incontinence should be evaluated to rule out ROM. The diagnosis is made by obtaining a history of leaking vaginal fluid, pooling on speculum examination, and positive nitrazine and fern tests. If these tests are equivocal, an ultrasound can be performed to examine the level of amniotic fluid. Some providers and hospitals will use the Amnisure test (discussed in Chapter 4). If the diagnosis is still unconfirmed, an amniocentesis dye test can be performed by injecting a dye via amniocentesis and observing whether or not the dye leaks into the vagina. This is also known as the **tampon test** because the dye is usually identified by its absorption into a tampon. If there is concern for chorioamnionitis, maternal temperature, WBC count, uterine tenderness, and the fetal heart tracing should all be checked for signs of infection.

Treatment

The management of PROM varies depending on the gestational age of the fetus. The rationale for the management of PPROM is that at some gestational age, usually somewhere between 32 and 36 weeks, the risk from prematurity is equal to the risk of infection. Up to this point, the risk of prematurity drives management, whereas after this point, the risk of infection motivates delivery. The exact gestational age at which the risk of infection is greater is debatable. Some practitioners prefer to wait until week 36, but the most common practice across the country is delivery at 34 weeks' gestation. With that said, in the setting of intrauterine infection, acute placental abruption, or nonreassuring fetal testing, expeditious delivery regardless of gestational age is appropriate. PPROM presenting >34 weeks generally should be managed with induction or augmentation of labor.

For those pregnancies presenting with PPROM <34 weeks, there is strong evidence that the use of antibiotics leads to a longer latency period before the onset of labor. Thus, ampicillin with erythromycin (48 hours IV followed by 5 days of oral erythromycin and amoxicillin) or azithromycin (oral) once and 48 hours of IV ampicillin and 5 days of oral amoxicillin is recommended in the setting of PPROM. The use of tocolysis in the setting of PPROM is the subject of debate. Tocolysis seems to add little, if any, benefit in PPROM and may even be harmful in the setting of chorioamnionitis. However, at many institutions, tocolysis is used for 48 hours, particularly at earlier gestational ages, in order to gain time to administer a course of corticosteroids. Currently, the recommendation is to use corticosteroids in the setting of PPROM up to 36 weeks because of the fetal benefits, despite any concern regarding immunosuppression.

PREMATURE RUPTURE OF THE MEMBRANES

PROM at term complicates 8% of pregnancies. The most significant risk of PROM is the development of chorioamnionitis. The risk of chorioamnionitis increases with the length of ROM. Antibiotics are recommended for women with prolonged ROM and women with unknown group B streptococcus (GBS) status. Commonly, labor is induced/augmented if ROM occurs anytime after 34 weeks. Studies have demonstrated that induction of labor in the setting of PROM reduces time to delivery and decreases rates of chorioamnionitis, endometritis, and NICU admission without increasing rates of cesarean delivery when compared with expectant management. Some patients may elect to bear the risk of increased infection to await the onset of spontaneous labor. This may be acceptable in patients with no clinical evidence of infection at the time of presentation and reassuring fetal status so long as they have been counseled regarding the risks of prolonged PROM (infection, prolonged labor, etc.). One large, randomized, controlled trial demonstrated that there was no difference in length of labor or mode of delivery with immediate induction/augmentation of PROM, but the rate of chorioamnionitis was higher among those with expectant management.

OBSTRUCTION, MALPRESENTATION, AND MALPOSITION

Although the most common form of delivery is the spontaneous vertex vaginal delivery, other presentations and deliveries also occur. Many of the malpresentations lead to cesarean delivery.

CEPHALOPELVIC DISPROPORTION

One of the most common indications for cesarean section is failure to progress (FTP) in labor, most often caused by **cephalopelvic disproportion** (CPD). The three "Ps"—pelvis, passenger, and power—are primarily responsible for a vaginal delivery. If the pelvis is too small, the fetal presenting part is too large, or the contractions are inadequate, there will be FTP. The strength of uterine contractions can be measured with an intrauterine pressure catheter and augmented with oxytocin, but little can be done about the other two factors that contribute to CPD.

Diagnosis

The maternal pelvis is described as one of four dominant types: **gynecoid**, **android**, **anthropoid**, and **platypelloid** (Fig. 6-2). Many pelvises have characteristics from more than one of these types. Common measurements of the pelvis include those of the pelvic inlet, the midpelvis, and the pelvic outlet. The **obstetric conjugate** is the distance between the sacral promontory and the midpoint of the symphysis pubis, and the shortest anteroposterior (AP) diameter of the pelvic inlet. The AP diameter of the pelvic outlet is the distance from the tip of the sacrum to the inferior margin of the pubic symphysis and usually ranges from 9.5 to 11.5 cm. These measurements are performed with both clinical and X-ray pelvimetry, but it is rare to assume CPD based on measurements alone.

The fetal skull is composed of the face, the base, and the vault. The face and base are composed of fused bones that do not change during labor; however, the bones of the vault are not fused and can undergo

FIGURE 6-2. Characteristics of four types of pelvises.

molding to conform to the maternal pelvis. The vault is composed of five bones: two frontal, two parietal, and one occipital. The spaces between the bones are known as sutures; the two places where the sutures intersect are the **anterior** and **posterior fontanelles**. How the fetal head presents to the maternal pelvis is important in accomplishing a vaginal delivery. There is great variation in the diameter of the skull at various levels and with various inclinations. When the fetal skull is properly flexed, the suboccipitobregmatic diameter presenting to the pelvis averages 9.5 cm in a term infant. When the sagittal suture is not located midline in the pelvis (asynclitism), the diameter of the skull being accommodated is effectively increased. Given our poor ability to predict the course and outcome of labor, even in the setting of suspected CPD, it is worthwhile to attempt a trial of labor. True CPD usually presents as arrest of labor in stage 1 or stage 2, necessitating a cesarean delivery.

BREECH PRESENTATION

Breech presentation occurs in 3% to 4% of all singleton deliveries. Factors associated with breech presentation include previous breech delivery, uterine anomalies, polyhydramnios, oligohydramnios, multiple gestation, PPROM, hydrocephaly, and anencephaly. Persistent breech presentation is also associated with placenta previa and fetal anomalies. Complications of a vaginal breech delivery include prolapsed cord and entrapment of the head.

Types of Breech
There are three categories of the breech presentation (Fig. 6-3): **frank**, **complete**, and **incomplete** or **footling**. The frank breech has flexed hips and extended knees, and thus the feet are near the fetal head. The complete breech has flexed hips, but one or both knees are flexed as well, with at least one foot near the breech. The incomplete or footling breech has one or both of the hips not flexed so that the foot or knee lies below the breech in the birth canal.

Diagnosis
The breech presentation may be diagnosed in several ways. With abdominal examination using the Leopold maneuvers, the fetal head can be palpated near the fundus while the breech is palpated in the pelvis. With vaginal examination, the breech can be palpated using common landmarks such as the gluteal cleft and the anus or, in the case of an incomplete breech, the fetal lower extremity. Diagnosis is often made or confirmed with ultrasound. On ultrasound, it is easy to confirm breech and then to determine the type of breech. With bedside Doppler, the fetal heartbeat is often heard in the upper part of the uterus.

FIGURE 6-3. Types of breech presentations.

Treatment

Breech presentation is typically managed with external cephalic version of the breech or elective cesarean delivery. Because of a single, large, randomized trial that found a higher risk of asphyxia and traumatic injury during vaginal delivery of a breech fetus, cesarean delivery has become the preferred mode of delivery in this setting. Because of specific criticisms of this trial and that the long-term outcomes did not differ, there are still a minority of providers who will offer a trial of labor in the setting of breech presentation. External version consists of manipulation of the breech infant into a vertex presentation. It is rarely performed before 36 to 37 weeks' gestation because of the potential for spontaneous version before this point and the risk of delivery after version secondary to abruption or ROM. External version is usually attempted without anesthesia, and if successful, the patient can continue the pregnancy with a 5% to 10% risk of the fetus reverting to breech presentation. If the version is not successful, a second attempt is often made under spinal anesthesia at 39 weeks of gestation at the time of scheduled cesarean. If successful, then either labor can be induced or the patient can continue the pregnancy. If the second attempt fails, often the patient will proceed with a cesarean delivery.

Trial of breech vaginal delivery can be attempted in the proper setting but is becoming increasingly rare in the United States. Complications of breech deliveries include cord prolapse, entrapment of the fetal head, and fetal neurologic injury. A favorable pelvis (by clinical examination, pelvic radiograph, MRI, or CT pelvimetry), a flexed head, estimated fetal weight between 2,000 and 3,800 g, and frank or complete breech are common criteria used for trial of labor of breech presentation. Relative contraindications include nulliparity, estimated fetal weight greater than 3,800 g, and incomplete breech presentation. Patients with these contraindications are usually recommended to undergo cesarean delivery. However, if a patient wishes to attempt vaginal delivery, careful monitoring of the fetus and progress of labor are imperative and should be conducted only with an experienced provider available for delivery.

OTHER MALPRESENTATION

Malpresentation can occur even in the setting of a cephalic or vertex presentation. The face, brow, or a compound presentation with a fetal upper extremity can complicate the cephalic presentation. Additionally, the shoulder can present in the setting of a transverse lie.

Face

The diagnosis of face presentation (Fig. 6-4) can be made with vaginal examination and palpation of the nose, mouth, eyes, or chin (mentum). Mentum anterior is the only face presentation that will allow for a vaginal delivery. With mentum posterior or

Face presentation

FIGURE 6-4. (A) Mechanisms of labor for right mentum posterior position with subsequent rotation of mentum anterior and delivery. **(B)** Face presentation with fetal head well engaged in the mentolateral position.

transverse, the fetus must rotate to mentum anterior to deliver vaginally; otherwise, a cesarean delivery is necessary. Augmentation is used only sparingly with a face presentation because the pressure on the face leads to edema. Of note, many anencephalic fetuses have a face presentation.

Brow

Brow presentation (Fig. 6-5) occurs when the portion of the fetal skull just above the orbital ridge presents. With the brow presenting, a larger diameter must pass through the pelvis. Therefore, unless the fetal head is particularly small (e.g., preterm) or the pelvis is particularly large, the brow presentation must convert to vertex or face to deliver.

Compound Presentation

A fetal extremity presenting alongside the vertex or breech is considered a compound presentation (Fig. 6-6). This occurs in less than 1 in 1,000 pregnancies. The rate increases with prematurity, multiple gestations, polyhydramnios, and CPD. A

Brow presentation

FIGURE 6-5. Brow presentation with mentovertex diameter presenting.

common complication of compound presentation is umbilical cord prolapse. The diagnosis is often made with vaginal examination when the fetal extremity is palpated alongside the presenting part. At this point, it should be determined whether the prolapsed fetal part is a hand or foot. Ultrasound may be used to determine the type of extremity presenting.

FIGURE 6-6. Compound presentation with the left hand lying in front of the vertex. With further labor, the hand and arm may retract from the birth canal, and the head may then descend normally.

Often, if an upper extremity is presenting alongside the vertex, the part may be gently reduced. However, prolapse of a lower extremity in vertex presentation is far less likely to deliver vaginally. Compound presentation of a lower extremity with a breech is considered a footling or incomplete breech presentation and calls for cesarean delivery. In all cases of compound presentation, the risk of umbilical cord prolapse should be remembered, and careful monitoring with continuous fetal heart tracings should be performed.

Shoulder

If the fetus is in a transverse lie, often the shoulder is presenting to the pelvic inlet. Diagnosis of this malpresentation can be made with abdominal or vaginal examination and ultrasound confirmation. Unless there is spontaneous conversion to vertex, shoulder presentations are delivered via cesarean section because of the increased risk of cord prolapse, increased risk for uterine rupture, and the difficulty of vaginal delivery.

MALPOSITION

The fetal position that optimizes the probability of the fetal head passing through the maternal pelvis is occiput anterior (OA). Left OA (LOA) and right OA (ROA) are also normal and commonly complete internal rotation to OA by the late first stage or second stage of labor. However, if the fetus is occiput transverse (OT) or occiput posterior (OP), it is called malposition, particularly in active first or second stage of labor. Fetal malposition has an association with a higher rate of cesarean delivery. Interestingly, it is seen more commonly with epidural use. The epidural itself does not cause the fetus to become OP or OT, but rather for those fetuses in OP or OT position at the time of epidural placement, they are more likely to stay OP or OT than in pregnancies where an epidural was not obtained.

Persistent Occiput Transverse and Posterior Position

The most common position of the fetus at the onset of labor is either left OT (LOT) or right OT (ROT). From the transverse position, the cardinal movement of internal rotation usually converts the fetus to the OA position. However, it is not uncommon for the fetus to stay in the OT position or rotate to the OP position. If this occurs, the progress of labor may be arrested. Diagnosis is made by palpation of the fetal sutures and fontanelles and following the progress of labor.

A persistent OT position leading to arrest of labor is more common in women with a platypelloid pelvis. If the cervix is not fully dilated, a minority of clinicians will make an attempt at manual rotation to the OA position. However, if the cervix is fully dilated, rotation to the OA position can be attempted manually or with forceps. Additionally, in the setting of full dilation, an attempt at vacuum delivery may be effective as the traction on the fetal scalp may lead to autorotation to the OA position.

During descent, OP positions may rotate to OA, although this does not always occur and can slow progress in labor. The management is similar to that for OA position: patiently watch and wait. However, spontaneous vaginal delivery occurs less often. In the setting of OP or OT position and active phase arrest, manual rotation prior to complete cervical dilation has been described, although it may be associated with injury to the cervix. If the second stage of labor is prolonged, the options include delivery of the fetus with forceps or vacuum in the OP position, rotation with forceps, or manual rotation. In either the OT or OP position, if the attempt at rotation or operative vaginal delivery fails, cesarean delivery is commonly required. Whereas OP-position fetuses deliver vaginally in about 50% of cases, OT-position fetuses rarely deliver vaginally in the OT position and must rotate to either OA or OP to deliver vaginally.

OBSTETRIC EMERGENCIES

FETAL BRADYCARDIA

A most common event in labor and delivery that leads to anxiety among both the practitioners and the patients is fetal heart rate (FHR) bradycardia. Anytime the FHR is below 100 to 110 beats per minute for longer than 2 minutes, it is called a **prolonged deceleration**. Longer than 10 minutes is termed **bradycardia**. Older terminology deemed a deceleration lasting longer than 2 minutes a bradycardia, and so this term is commonly used in labor and delivery in the setting of prolonged decelerations. Either way, these FHR decelerations are associated with a number of complications such as placental abruption, cord prolapse, uterine tetanic contraction, uterine rupture, pulmonary embolus (PE), amniotic fluid embolism (AFE), and seizure. They have also been associated with poor fetal outcome.

The etiology of prolonged FHR decelerations can be considered to be preuterine, uteroplacental, or postplacental. Preuterine issues would be any event leading to maternal hypotension or hypoxia. These would include seizure, AFE, PE, Myocardial Infarction (MI), respiratory failure, or recent epidural or spinal placement leading to hypotension. Uteroplacental issues include placental abruption, infarction, and hemorrhaging previa, as well as uterine hyperstimulation. Postplacental etiologies include cord prolapse, cord compression, and rupture of a fetal vessel such as vasa previa.

Diagnosis

FHR decelerations are usually not subtle. However, the FHR can easily be confused with the maternal heart rate, which is commonly between 60 and 100 beats per minute, and therefore, these should be differentiated. This can be done by placing a fetal scalp electrode on the fetal scalp and concomitantly an O_2 saturation monitor on the mother. In facilities without access to these tools, palpation of the maternal pulse while listening to the FHR can usually help differentiate between the two.

Diagnosis of the etiology of the bradycardia is often more important than the diagnosis of bradycardia, which is relatively straightforward in the era of continuous fetal monitoring. A simple algorithm to diagnose the etiology of bradycardia is as follows:

1. Look at the mother for signs of respiratory compromise or change in mental status. This should commonly diagnose seizures, PE, and AFE.
2. While putting on a glove for a cervical examination, assess the maternal BP and heart rate. This will diagnose maternal hypotension, which is commonly seen after epidural placement and is a potential cause of FHR decelerations. This will also aid in determining whether the FHR being recorded could be maternal.
3. Immediately before the examination, assess for vaginal bleeding. With increased vaginal bleeding, placental abruption and uterine rupture should be considered. If placentation is unknown, placenta previa is also a possibility. Rarely, vaginal bleeding is secondary to rupture of a fetal vessel, as in vasa previa.
4. Examine the patient with one hand on the maternal abdomen and the other hand vaginally feeling for cervical dilation, fetal station, and prolapsed umbilical cord. The abdominal hand should feel for uterine hyperstimulation and fetal parts outside the uterus. If the fetal station is dramatically lower than expected, then the prolonged FHR deceleration may be because of rapid descent and vagal stimulation. If the fetal station is much higher than expected, uterine rupture should be suspected. If the cervix is fully dilated and the fetus is in the pelvis, operative vaginal delivery can be performed if the FHR decelerations do not resolve in a timely fashion.

Treatment

In the setting of prolonged FHR deceleration, the initial management is standardized. The patient is moved to the left or right lateral decubitus position to resolve a FHR deceleration secondary to compression of the inferior vena cava, leading to decreased preload or, more commonly, a compressed umbilical cord by the fetus. Oxygen by face mask is commonly administered to the mother in case hypoxia is an issue. The examination is performed as described earlier, and the individual etiologies are diagnosed and treated appropriately. In the setting of maternal hypotension, the patient can be given aggressive IV hydration and ephedrine. The management of seizure, AFE, and uterine rupture is discussed later in this chapter, and the management of PE is discussed in Chapter 11. Tetanic uterine contraction is treated with nitroglycerin, usually administered via a sublingual spray, and/or terbutaline (a β-agonist tocolytic). If umbilical cord prolapse is identified, there have been case reports of replacement into the uterus; but most commonly, this requires an emergent cesarean delivery, performed with the examining clinician lifting the fetal head to avoid compression of the prolapsed cord. In the setting of previa, cesarean delivery should be expedited. If abruption is suspected, and the patient is remote from delivery, cesarean section may be necessary. In all of these settings with a fetal bradycardia, an emergent cesarean delivery, one that is done as fast as is safely possible, should be performed.

It is imperative that the timing of these events is followed very closely. Clinicians need to know the capabilities of their labor and delivery units and the rapidity of response of the anesthesiologists and other members of the OR team. Commonly, a patient is moved from the labor room to the OR after 4 to 5 minutes of FHR deceleration. If the FHR is checked in the OR (at this time, usually 8 minutes) and the bradycardia persists, plans for emergent cesarean delivery should proceed. The rapidity of this delivery may not allow all of the most common sterile techniques typically employed because delivery of the fetus within the next 2 to 4 minutes is the goal.

SHOULDER DYSTOCIA

Once the head of the fetus is delivered, if there is difficulty in delivering the shoulders, particularly because of impaction of the anterior shoulder behind the pubic symphysis, this is termed **shoulder dystocia**. Risk factors for shoulder dystocia include fetal macrosomia (weight greater than 4,000 g), preconceptional and gestational diabetes, previous shoulder dystocia, maternal obesity, postterm pregnancy, prolonged second stage of labor, and operative vaginal delivery. The incidence of shoulder dystocia has been reported to be between 0.2% and 3% of all vaginal deliveries. Increased morbidity and mortality are associated with shoulder dystocia. Fetal complications include fractures of the humerus and clavicle, brachial plexus nerve injuries (Erb palsy), phrenic nerve palsy, hypoxic brain injury, and death.

Diagnosis

The actual diagnosis of a shoulder dystocia is made when routine obstetric maneuvers fail to deliver the fetus. When antepartum risk factors are present, shoulder dystocia can be predicted, prepared for, and possibly even prevented. Preparation for a shoulder dystocia includes placing the patient in the dorsal lithotomy position, having adequate anesthesia, and having several experienced clinicians present at the birth. At the time of delivery, suspicion is increased with prolonged crowning of the head and then with the "turtle" sign of either incomplete delivery of the head or the chin tucking up against the maternal perineum. Because of the concern for shoulder dystocia, when a fetus is suspected to weigh greater than 5,000 g in women without diabetes and greater than 4,500 g in women with diabetes, elective cesarean delivery should be offered.

Treatment

As with any obstetric emergency, it is important to have all members of the health care team effectively working together. Once a shoulder dystocia is identified, the labor and delivery alert should be sounded, and the pediatric team should be called. Similar to a code, someone needs to be running the shoulder dystocia emergency; in a teaching hospital, this is usually the attending or chief resident, and in a private hospital, this is usually the delivering obstetrician. Someone should be assigned to keep track of time, because a shoulder dystocia can lead to entrapment and complete compression of the umbilical cord, and thus delivery in less than 5 minutes is imperative. Two individuals should be assigned to hold the patient's legs, and one person to give suprapubic pressure.

The specific series of maneuvers for delivering an infant with a shoulder dystocia are as follows:

- **McRoberts maneuver**—Hyperflexion of the maternal hips towards the maternal abdomen flattens the lumbar spine and ventrally rotates the maternal pelvis and symphysis increasing the

FIGURE 6-7. Sharp flexion of both maternal hips (McRoberts maneuver) brings the pelvic inlet and outlet into a more vertical alignment, facilitating delivery of the fetal shoulders.

space of the posterior outlet and allowing for easier disimpaction of the anterior shoulder (Fig. 6-7).
- **Suprapubic pressure**—pressure applied just above the maternal pubic symphysis at an oblique angle to dislodge the anterior shoulder from behind the pubic symphysis (Fig. 6-8).
- **Rubin maneuver**—pressure on either accessible shoulder toward the anterior chest wall of the fetus to decrease the bisacromial diameter and free the impacted shoulder (Fig. 6-9).
- **Wood corkscrew maneuver**—pressure behind the posterior shoulder to rotate the infant and dislodge the anterior shoulder.
- **Delivery of the posterior arm/shoulder**—delivery of the posterior arm by sweeping the posterior arm across the chest to allow the bisacromial diameter to rotate to an oblique diameter of the pelvis and the anterior shoulder to be freed.

If these maneuvers are unsuccessful, they may be performed again. If the infant is still undelivered, there are several other maneuvers that can be performed. If delivery of the posterior arm or other maneuvers cannot be accomplished because of a tight perineum, a generous episiotomy may provide more room. Placement of the patient on

FIGURE 6-8. Moderate suprapubic pressure is often the only additional maneuver necessary to free the anterior fetal shoulder.

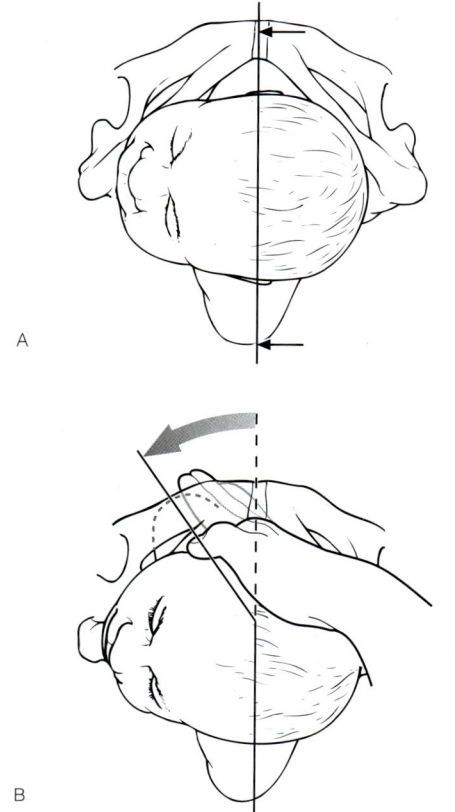

FIGURE 6-9. Rubin maneuver. (**A**) The shoulder-to-shoulder diameter is shown as the distance between the two small arrows. (**B**) The most easily accessible fetal shoulder (the anterior is shown here) is pushed toward the anterior chest wall of the fetus. Most often, this results in abduction of both shoulders, reducing the shoulder-to-shoulder diameter, and freeing the impacted anterior shoulder.

hands and knees, the so-called Gaskin maneuver, has been successful as well. It has been described to fracture or cut the fetal clavicle in order to disimpact the anterior shoulder. If these maneuvers fail, the **Zavanelli** maneuver, which involves placing the infant's head back into the pelvis and performing cesarean delivery, can be attempted as well. Additionally, symphysiotomy, cutting the maternal pubic symphysis, will often release the infant; however, this is a morbid procedure often complicated by infection, healing difficulties, and chronic pain. Thus, it should be reserved for the true emergency, and in the United States, most clinicians would simply do a cesarean and attempt to facilitate delivery abdominally before performing a symphysiotomy.

UTERINE RUPTURE

Uterine rupture of an unscarred uterus is estimated to occur in 1 in 5,700 to 20,000 deliveries. Associated complications in these patients include uterine fibroids, uterine malformations, obstructed labor, and the use of uterotonic agents, such as oxytocin and prostaglandins. In patients who have had a prior uterine scar from myomectomy or cesarean delivery, the risk of uterine rupture is theoretically 0.5% to 1.0%. The risk is increased in patients who have more than one cesarean scar, have a "classical" or high vertical scar, undergo labor induction, and/or are treated with uterotonic agents.

Uterine rupture is suspected in the setting of FHR decelerations in patients with prior scars on their uterus. Patients may feel a "popping" sensation or experience sudden abdominal pain. On physical examination, the fetus may be palpable in the extrauterine space, there may be vaginal bleeding, and commonly, the fetal presenting part is suddenly at a much higher station than previously. If a uterine rupture is strongly suspected, the patient should be taken to the OR for immediate cesarean delivery and exploratory laparotomy.

MATERNAL HYPOTENSION

Pregnant women commonly have a BP as low as 90/50 mm Hg. However, BPs much lower than the 80/40 mm Hg range are unusual and can lead to poor maternal and uterine perfusion. Common etiologies of maternal hypotension include vasovagal events, regional anesthesia, overtreatment with antihypertensive drugs, hemorrhage, anaphylaxis, and AFE. Most of these events can be differentiated quickly by the clinical scenario.

Treatment of maternal hypotension may vary depending on the etiology, but the mainstays are aggressive IV hydration and adrenergic medications to constrict peripheral vessels and increase both the preload and the afterload. If the event occurs in close proximity to medication administration, Benadryl and epinephrine should be considered for a possible anaphylactic reaction. If the patient has an AFE, the mortality rate is quite high. The definitive diagnosis of AFE is the finding of fetal cells in the pulmonary vasculature at autopsy.

SEIZURE

Seizures on labor and delivery are usually quite startling and can be dangerous. In patients with a history of a seizure disorder as well as those with preeclampsia, careful observation for particular seizure precursors is maintained. However, many patients who have seizure on labor and delivery have no history and may be normotensive.

Many vasovagal events are misdiagnosed as a seizure because the patient may have several tonic–clonic movements. One of the key ways to differentiate between the two is the presence of a postictal period after the event. To help sort out the etiology, patients should have a full preeclamptic workup, toxicology panel, chemistry panel, and, when it is safe for the patient to leave the unit, obtain a head CT. A neurology consult is also indicated. Acutely, the patients should be managed with the ABCs of resuscitation and with antiseizure medications (Table 6-1). In pregnancy, magnesium sulfate is the antiseizure medication of choice.

TABLE 6-1. Management of a Pregnant Patient with Seizures or in Status Epilepticus

Assess and establish airway and vital signs, including oxygenation
Assess FHR or fetal status
Bolus magnesium sulfate, or give 10 g IM
Bolus with lorazepam 0.1 mg/kg, 5.0–10.0 mg at no more than 2.0 mg/min
Load phenytoin 20 mg/kg, usually 1–2 g at no more than 50 mg/min
If not successful, load phenobarbital 20 mg/kg, usually 1–2 g at no more than 100 mg/min
Laboratory tests include CBC, metabolic panel, Antiepileptic Drug (AED) levels, and toxicology screen
If fetal testing is not reassuring, move to emergent delivery

CBC, Complete blood count; FHR, fetal heart rate.

KEY POINTS

- Preterm delivery occurs in roughly 10% of all pregnancies.
- PTL is treated with tocolytic therapy such as nifedipine (calcium channel blocker) and indomethacin (NSAIDs).
- Current tocolytics are only marginally effective but may buy time for a course of betamethasone to accelerate fetal lung maturity.
- Preterm ROM is ROM that occurs before 37 weeks of gestation; PROM is ROM that occurs before the onset of labor.
- The latency period before the onset of labor is inversely correlated with gestational age in PPROM.
- Once ROM is confirmed, the therapeutic course depends on gestational age, risk of infection, and fetal lung maturity; any patient who shows signs of infection or fetal distress needs delivery.
- If the fetal head is too large to pass through the maternal pelvis, it is deemed CPD.
- Unless ultrasound and CT have been used to document a fetal head larger than the maternal pelvis, in the case of suspected CPD, a trial of labor should be attempted.
- There are three types of breech: frank, complete, and incomplete or footling.
- Breech presentations may be managed by external version to vertex, cesarean delivery, and, less frequently, a trial of labor. The complications of labor and delivery of breech presentation include cord prolapse and entrapment of the fetal head.
- Vertex malpresentations include face, brow, compound, and persistent OP. These presentations will often deliver vaginally but need closer monitoring and sometimes require different maneuvers.
- Prolonged FHR decelerations may have a variety of etiologies and can be thought of as preuterine, uteroplacental, and postplacental.
- A quick examination and verification of vital signs will often determine the etiology of a prolonged deceleration.
- If there is no sign of resolution of the FHR deceleration in 4 to 5 minutes, the patient should either be delivered vaginally or moved to the OR for cesarean delivery.
- Shoulder dystocia can result in fetal fractures, nerve damage, and hypoxia.

(continued)

KEY POINTS (continued)

- Risk factors for shoulder dystocia include fetal macrosomia, diabetes, previous dystocia, maternal obesity, postterm deliveries, and prolonged stage 2 of labor.
- The maneuvers to reduce a shoulder dystocia include McRoberts maneuver, suprapubic pressure, Rubin maneuver, Wood corkscrew maneuver, delivery of posterior arm, episiotomy, and, rarely, the fracture or cutting of the clavicle or pubic symphysis, or the Zavanelli maneuver.
- Uterine rupture is uncommon in patients with no prior uterine scar; it is seen in 0.5% to 1.0% of patients who labor with a prior cesarean delivery.
- Maternal hypotension may have a variety of etiologies, such as regional anesthesia, hemorrhage, vasovagal events, AFE, and anaphylaxis.
- The first-line treatment of patients with seizures in pregnancy is IV or IM magnesium sulfate.

CLINICAL VIGNETTES

VIGNETTE 1

A 29-year-old G3P1102 woman at 29 weeks 3 days presents to labor and delivery triage for evaluation of abdominal pain. Her pain started 2 hours ago and comes and goes every 5 minutes. She denies any leaking fluid, change in vaginal discharge, or vaginal bleeding. Her baby has been active. Her pregnancy is complicated by a history of a urinary tract infection at 10 weeks with group B streptococcus (GBS) and a history of preterm birth at 31 weeks with her last child. She is currently taking progesterone injections weekly and a prenatal vitamin. On vaginal examination, her cervix is closed, 25% effaced, and −3 station. Uterine contractions are noted every 4 to 5 minutes with a category 1 tracing. A fetal fibronectin test returns positive. Repeat examination after 1 hour shows dilation of 1 cm, 50% effacement, and −2 station. The team decides to start her on magnesium sulfate for tocolysis and administers the first dose of betamethasone.

1. Which of the following is the mechanism of action of magnesium sulfate on cellular calcium?
   a. Increases conversion of ATP to cAMP, which results in decreased levels of free calcium ions through sequestration in the sarcoplasmic reticulum
   b. Antagonizes calcium and stabilizes cell membranes
   c. Decreases influx of calcium into cells
   d. Blocks cyclooxygenase and decreases levels of prostaglandins

2. What side effects or complications should you counsel your patient that she might experience from magnesium sulfate?
   a. Flushing, diplopia, headache
   b. Headache, tachycardia, anxiety
   c. Headache, flushing, dizziness
   d. Constriction of the ductus arteriosus in the neonate

3. Magnesium sulfate has a potential for serious complications such as respiratory depression, hypoxia, cardiac arrest, and even death. Which of the following clinical tests is most useful to monitor patients who are receiving magnesium sulfate infusions?
   a. Serum magnesium levels every 4 hours
   b. Serum magnesium levels every 2 hours
   c. Serial BP measurements
   d. Serial deep tendon reflex (DTR) examination
   e. Serial pulmonary examination

4. What is the next best step in clinical management of this patient?
   a. NICU consult
   b. Penicillin G 5 million units loading dose, followed by 2.5 million units every 4 hours
   c. Fetal ultrasound for growth
   d. Complete blood count (CBC), type and screen, urine dip

5. What is the next best step in management?
   a. Recommend cesarean section for placental abruption remote from delivery
   b. Continue expectant management, bleeding is likely from the cervix
   c. Send a CBC, type and screen, Kleihauer–Betke test, and place a second IV
   d. Consent the patient for transfusion of packed red blood cells (PRBCs)
   e. Place fetal scalp electrode (FSE) and intrauterine pressure catheter (IUPC) to better monitor fetus and contractions

VIGNETTE 2

A 35-year-old G2P1001 woman at 40 weeks 6 days presents to labor and delivery triage with a 5-hour history of painful contractions. Monitoring reveals contractions every 3 minutes, and cervical examination on arrival is 3 cm dilated, 50% effaced, and −2 station. Her pregnancy has been complicated by A1 gestational diabetes and 45 lb weight gain in pregnancy (BMI, 24). In her first pregnancy, she presented at 2 cm dilation and 90% effacement. Her labor progressed slowly with dilation of 1 cm every 3 hours until labor arrested at 7 cm. A healthy baby girl weighing 4,200 g was delivered by cesarean section after arrest at 7 cm for 4 hours. Today, your patient requests a trial of labor after cesarean section. You recheck her cervix 2 hours later and find that it is 4 cm dilated, 90% effaced, and −1 station. The estimated fetal weight by Leopold maneuvers is 9 lb. A recent ultrasound performed at 38 weeks estimated the fetal weight at 3,900 g. You admit the patient to labor and delivery for expectant management.

1. Which of the following factors was least likely to result in her prior failure to progress (FTP)?
    a. Obstetric conjugate diameter of the pelvis greater than 11.5 cm
    b. Inadequate strength of uterine contractions
    c. Fetal size or position
    d. Maternal pelvis shape

2. Which of the following factors places the patient at greatest risk for shoulder dystocia?
    a. Gestational diabetes
    b. Prior FTP
    c. 45 lb weight gain in pregnancy
    d. Suspected fetal macrosomia
    e. Prior fetus weighing 4,200 g

3. What is the name of the maneuver used to relieve the shoulder dystocia?
    a. McRoberts maneuver
    b. Wood corkscrew maneuver
    c. Rubin maneuver
    d. Zavanelli maneuver

4. What is the most common fetal complication of shoulder dystocia?
    a. No complication
    b. Erb palsy
    c. Humerus fracture
    d. Hypoxic brain injury
    e. Clavicle fracture

VIGNETTE 3

A 32-year-old G3P2002 woman presents for routine prenatal care at 37 weeks. Her pregnancy is complicated by Rh-negative status, depression, and a history of low-grade Squamous Intraepithelial Lesion (LSIL) Pap smear with normal colposcopy in the first trimester. Today, she reports good fetal movement and denies leaking fluid or contractions. During your examination, you measure the fundal height at an appropriate 37 cm and find fetal heart tones located in the upper aspect of the uterus. A bedside ultrasound reveals frank breech presentation.

1. Which of the following is the next best step in management of this patient?
    a. Schedule a cesarean delivery for 39 weeks
    b. Return visit in 1 week to reassess fetal position
    c. Schedule an external cephalic version
    d. Offer a trial of vaginal breech delivery

2. Prior to discharging the patient from labor and delivery triage after her successful external cephalic version, which of the following should you do first?
    a. Schedule induction for 39 weeks
    b. Place abdominal binder to help hold fetus in cephalic presentation
    c. Prescribe tocolytic
    d. Give RhoGAM
    e. Check fetal position with ultrasound

3. Which of the following findings would deter you from offering this patient a trial of breech delivery?
    a. Frank breech presentation
    b. Fetal weight of 3,200 g
    c. Complete breech presentation
    d. Fetal weight of 4,100 g

4. Which of the following is not associated with increased risk for breech presentation?
    a. Fetal anencephaly
    b. Uterine anomalies
    c. Polyhydramnios
    d. Chorioamnionitis

VIGNETTE 4

You are working in the emergency department when an 18-year-old Caucasian woman arrives via ambulance. EMS reports that she was found seizing in a local drug store approximately 10 minutes ago. She appears to be 7 to 8 months pregnant. She had no family or friends with her, but police have contacted family who are on the way to the emergency department. Her vital signs on arrival are as follows: BP, 180/116 mm Hg; heart rate, 76 beats per minute; respiratory rate, 16 beats per minute; oxygen saturation, 98%. Her pants are soiled, and she is not responding to questions at this time. Bedside ultrasound demonstrates fetal cardiac activity in the 130s. Quick bedside biometry estimates gestation age to be 32 weeks 1 day.

1. What is the best first step in managing this patient?
    a. Obtain formal fetal ultrasound for gestational age
    b. Obtain complete blood count (CBC), metabolic panel, serum toxicology screening
    c. Order CT head

    d. Emergent cesarean section
    e. Begin empiric magnesium sulfate therapy

2. What is the most appropriate next step in management?
    a. Intubation to protect airway
    b. IV labetalol
    c. Head CT
    d. Lumbar puncture to rule out infection
    e. Delivery

3. What do you recommend next?
    a. Load phenytoin for seizure control
    b. Begin induction of labor
    c. Give betamethasone for fetal lung maturity
    d. Lumbar puncture to rule out meningitis and encephalitis
    e. Cesarean section

4. At what stage of pregnancy is eclampsia most likely to occur?
    a. First trimester
    b. Second trimester
    c. Third trimester
    d. Immediately postpartum within 48 hours of delivery
    e. Postpartum period between 48 hours and 4 weeks

ANSWERS

VIGNETTE 1 Question 1

1. Answer B:
Uterine myometrium is composed of smooth muscle fibers whose contraction is regulated by MLK, which is activated by calcium ions. Magnesium decreases uterine tone and contractions by acting as a calcium antagonist and a membrane stabilizer. Terbutaline acts by increasing conversion of ATP to cAMP, which decreases free calcium ions through sequestration in the sarcoplasmic reticulum. Calcium channel blockers decrease intracellular calcium, which reduces uterine contractility. Indomethacin blocks the enzyme cyclooxygenase and decreases the level of prostaglandins, which decreases intracellular levels of calcium and therefore decreases myometrial contractions.

VIGNETTE 1 Question 2

2. Answer A:
Flushing, diplopia, and headache are common side effects of magnesium sulfate. Women taking terbutaline often note headache, tachycardia, and anxiety. Calcium channel blockers such as nifedipine can cause headache, flushing, and dizziness. Lastly, indomethacin has been associated with the premature closure of the ductus arteriosus in the neonate.

VIGNETTE 1 Question 3

3. Answer D:
The most effective test to monitor patients for magnesium toxicity is through serial DTR examination. DTRs are diminished and then lost with magnesium serum levels between 6 and 10 mg/dL. Toxic levels of magnesium (>10 mg/dL) result in respiratory depression, hypoxia, and cardiac arrest. Serial DTR examination is therefore a cost-effective screening test for magnesium toxicity. Serum levels are not necessary unless there is concern for absent DTRs or patients show symptoms of respiratory depression. Serial pulmonary examination and BP monitoring are useful tests when monitoring patients with preeclampsia who are being treated with magnesium sulfate to prevent eclampsia, but are not the most effective monitoring method.

VIGNETTE 1 Question 4

4. Answer B:
Early in pregnancy, this patient had a urinary tract infection, which demonstrated GBS bacteriuria. Patients with GBS bacteriuria are colonized and should be treated with penicillin if in labor or threatened PTL. As a result, it is important to treat this patient with GBS prophylaxis as long as labor is threatened. The goals of GBS prophylaxis are to have antibiotics in the mother 4 hours prior to ruptured membranes or delivery. Antibiotics are discontinued when labor is no longer threatened. In a patient without a history of GBS bacteriuria, a GBS culture swab is collected on presentation and diagnosis of PTL, and antibiotics are continued until the results either return negative for GBS or labor is no longer threatened. A NICU consult should be obtained for the family so they can gather information on the risks of delivery of a preterm fetus. Fetal ultrasound, if not performed in the previous 4 weeks, can provide additional information on the well-being of the fetus. Routine CBC, type and screen, and urine dip should also be collected but are not as important as starting GBS prophylaxis.

The nurse calls you to the patient's room to evaluate her vaginal bleeding. You look at the tocometer and see that uterine contractions are every 2 minutes. The fetal heart tracing shows a baseline of 135 beats per minute with moderate variability and accelerations. There are occasional early decelerations. You examine the cervix and find 5 cm dilation, 100% effacement, and −1 station. There is a moderate amount of bright red blood on your glove.

VIGNETTE 1 Question 5
5. Answer C:
This scenario describes the development of placental abruption. The description of the fetal monitoring and maternal status tells us that the situation is not emergent and that trial of vaginal delivery can continue. However, it is important to be prepared for worsening vaginal bleeding or need for emergent delivery should the fetal status or maternal status deteriorate. Therefore, you should check the maternal blood counts, prepare for transfusion, evaluate for fetal–maternal exposure of blood, and place a second IV in case blood products or fluids need to be administered for resuscitation. Cesarean delivery is not necessary at this time. You could discuss blood transfusion at this time, but it is not the best answer choice. Lastly, the question does not suggest that fetal or contraction monitoring is difficult, and, therefore, FSE or internal contraction monitoring with an IUPC is not indicated.

VIGNETTE 2 Question 1
1. Answer A:
FTP is commonly associated with the three Ps—power, passenger, and pelvis. Power refers to the strength of uterine contractions. Contraction strength is most commonly measured by the Montevideo unit, and data are collected from an IUPC. Montevideo units are a measure of average uterine strength of contractions in millimeters of mercury multiplied by the number of contractions in 10 minutes, and 200 to 250 Montevideo units define adequate labor in the active phase of labor. Optimal uterine contractions are believed to be necessary for vaginal birth and are also measured by cervical dilation and effacement. The second P, the passenger or fetus, can be too large to deliver or be malpositioned for delivery. Lastly, the pelvic outlet may not be the right shape or size, in combination with the fetal position, to allow delivery. Generally, an obstetric conjugate of 11.5 cm should be adequate to deliver a cephalic fetus because the suboccipitobregmatic diameter presenting to the pelvis averages 9.5 cm.

VIGNETTE 2 Question 2
2. Answer D:
Shoulder dystocia is reported to occur in 0.2% to 3% of all vaginal deliveries. Traditionally, shoulder dystocia is associated with fetal macrosomia, but up to one-half of shoulder dystocia events occur in neonates weighing less than 4,000 g. However, an 11-fold increased relative probability of shoulder dystocia has been found in pregnancies where the neonate weighed greater than 4,000 g. Approximately 7% of neonates will weigh greater than 4,000 g and 2% will weigh greater than 4,500 g. In those deliveries where neonates weighed greater than 4,500 g, the relative probability of shoulder dystocia during delivery was 22-fold. With fetal macrosomia, the trunk and chest grow larger relative to the fetal head. Macrosomia is more common in gestational diabetes but also occurs in prolonged pregnancies. Maternal obesity, previous fetus weighing greater than 4,000 g, prolonged second stage of labor, prolonged deceleration phase (8 to 10 cm), and prior shoulder dystocia all appear to be related to fetal macrosomia. Some studies have shown increased maternal age and excess maternal weight gain in pregnancy to be associated with shoulder dystocia.

Over the course of the next 6 hours, the patient progresses to 8 cm dilation. Her progress slows, and she does not make any change over the next 2 hours. You place an IUPC, and Montevideo units are 160. Pitocin is started. Three hours later, she is completely dilated, 100% effaced, and 0 station. She has a strong urge to push, so you begin pushing. Two hours into pushing, she is at +2 station. An hour later, the fetus is crowning and you see the turtle sign. You immediately announce, "I have a shoulder dystocia," and call for additional help from nursing, anesthesia, and neonatology. You ask the patient to stop pushing. The time of the shoulder dystocia is noted. You ask to have the patient's hips flexed and ask another nurse to apply pressure just above the maternal pubic symphysis directed obliquely. The anterior fetal shoulder remains trapped. Next you place your hand inside the vagina and attempt to put pressure on the posterior shoulder to decrease the biacromial diameter and facilitate the anterior shoulder's delivery. The maneuver works, and the fetus delivers and is handed to the awaiting neonatology team. The shoulder dystocia lasted 65 seconds.

VIGNETTE 2 Question 3
3. Answer C:
Rubin maneuver. This maneuver involves pressure on either fetal shoulder to diminish the biacromial diameter in an effort to free the anterior shoulder and allow delivery of the fetus. In this scenario, McRoberts maneuver is described first and involves flexing the maternal hips, which results in ventral rotation of the maternal pelvis and an increase in the size of the pelvic outlet. It is the least invasive of maneuvers. Next, suprapubic pressure is applied by directing force just above the pubic symphysis in an oblique direction.

The goal of this maneuver is to disimpact the anterior shoulder. It is very important that pressure be applied obliquely to free the shoulder, because downward pressure will not change the biacromial diameter. Wood cork maneuver involves placing a hand behind either the anterior or posterior fetal shoulder and rotating the fetus 180 degrees to lead to descent and delivery of the shoulders. Lastly, if all other attempts are unsuccessful and approximately 4 to 5 minutes has passed, consideration should be given to Zavanelli maneuver and emergent cesarean section. Zavanelli involves replacement of the fetal head by reversing the cardinal movements of labor.

VIGNETTE 2 Question 4
4. Answer A:
In 90% to 95% cases of shoulder dystocia, there are no long-term sequelae. Depending on the type of maneuver used to deliver the baby, clavicle or humerus fracture may be more likely. This is true for delivery of the posterior arm. Erb palsy results from brachial plexus injury. This injury is due to traction on the anterior shoulder, because it is trapped behind the pubic symphysis. It is important that the mother does not push while the shoulder is impacted, because this can worsen risk for injury. Brachial plexus injuries can occur without shoulder dystocia and are thought to be due to uterine forces on the fetus while delivering. Hypoxic brain injury occurs when a shoulder dystocia is prolonged. This risk increases after 3 minutes but is highly variable and depends on the reserve of the fetus prior to the shoulder dystocia. This is the rarest of complications from shoulder dystocia and the most severe apart from fetal demise.

VIGNETTE 3 Question 1
1. Answer C:
Given her gestational age prior to 39 weeks, it would be best to try an external cephalic version. If unsuccessful, a second trial of version at 39 weeks with epidural or spinal anesthesia should be offered. If the version is successful prior to 39 weeks, the patient is followed expectantly with routine prenatal care. If the version is accomplished after 39 weeks, she may be induced at that time. If the version is unsuccessful on second attempt with anesthesia, delivery by cesarean section is recommended. External cephalic versions carry the risk of cord compression and placental abruption. It is critically important to monitor the fetus for a period of time after the procedure. Occasionally, an emergent delivery is indicated by cesarean following a trial of version due to nonreassuring fetal testing. If the patient declines a trial of version, she should be scheduled for an elective cesarean section after 39 weeks' gestation. In a select population, trial of vaginal breech delivery can be attempted but requires stringent criteria be met.

VIGNETTE 3 Question 2
2. Answer D:
Because the patient is Rh negative, she should receive a dose of RhoGAM prior to discharge. External cephalic version carries the risk of placental abruption and also the possibility of maternal exposure to fetal blood through disruption in the placental interface. In Rh-negative mothers, this could lead to formation of antibodies against Rh factor if the fetus is Rh positive. In future pregnancy with an Rh-positive fetus, maternal antibodies can cross the placenta and destroy fetal blood cells, resulting in anemia and fetal hydrops. A dose of RhoGAM can prevent this problem. Other risk factors of external cephalic version include fetal distress, failed rotation, and need for urgent cesarean section. Induction is generally scheduled at 39 to 40 weeks, and abdominal binders are commonly used to prevent the fetus from returning to breech presentation, but these are not the best answers. There is no role for use of tocolytics at this stage of pregnancy. Lastly, rechecking the fetal position is possible and reasonable, especially if the mother describes a large fetal movement, but it is not necessary or the best answer choice.

VIGNETTE 3 Question 3
3. Answer D:
Fetal weight of 4,100 g is a relative contraindication to offering a trial of breech delivery. The criteria recommended to offer a trial of breech labor include an adequate pelvis as determined by pelvimetry and imaging (generally X-ray, CT, or MRI), frank or complete breech, a flexed fetal head, and estimated fetal weight of 2,500 to 3,800 g. Relative contraindications to offering a vaginal breech trial of labor include weight greater than 3,800 g, nulliparity, and incomplete breech, such as footling breech presentation.

VIGNETTE 3 Question 4
4. Answer D:
Breech presentation is associated with fetal anomalies such as anencephaly and hydrocephaly as well as uterine anomalies. Both oligohydramnios and polyhydramnios are also associated with risk of breech presentation. Prior breech delivery, multifetal gestation, and PPROM are also associated risk factors. Chorioamnionitis is not a direct cause of breech presentation but can occur as a result of PPROM or be the cause of PPROM.

VIGNETTE 4 Question 1
1. Answer E:
Any pregnant woman with a seizure is presumed to have eclampsia until proven otherwise. Treatment begins with a 6-g bolus of magnesium given over 15 to 20 minutes, followed by 2 g/hour. The goal of treatment with magnesium sulfate in eclampsia is

to prevent recurrent convulsions. However, approximately 10% of women with eclampsia will have a second convulsion after treatment with magnesium, and a second bolus of 2 g can be given over 3 to 5 minutes. Other antiepileptic medications can be given as well, such as lorazepam, phenytoin, and phenobarbital in status epilepticus. Fetal age is important, but you already have an estimate, and fetal age will not change management of eclampsia at this time. CBC, metabolic panel, and serum toxicology should be obtained but are not as important as preventing future convulsions. If focal deficits are suspected, CT head may be warranted, but, again, this is not as critical as starting magnesium sulfate. Delivery is ultimately the treatment of eclampsia but not the first step in management.

VIGNETTE 4 Question 2
2. Answer B:
On arrival, BP is reported to be elevated at 180/116 mm Hg. The second step in the management of eclampsia is to control severe hypertension. The goal of treating severe hypertension in eclampsia is to avoid loss of cerebral autoregulation and prevent congestive heart failure without compromising cerebral or placental perfusion, which can be reduced in women with eclampsia. Treatment is usually given IV, and labetalol or hydralazine is an appropriate agent. Target BP is between 140 and 160 mm Hg systolic and 90 and 110 mm Hg diastolic. Because she has normal oxygen saturation and is therefore protecting her airway, intubation is not warranted at this time. Again, unless focal deficits are noted on examination, CT head is not as important as controlling BP. Although infection is a common cause of seizure in the general population, it is less likely the etiology in a pregnant woman. Delivery is reasonable but not the best answer. Ultimately, delivery is the treatment of eclampsia but will not improve her condition as acutely as BP control.

Family arrives and informs you of the patient's due date, making her 33 weeks 2 days. They also reveal that the patient has been feeling unwell for the past 2 days. She has had a severe frontal headache associated with visual changes, which she described as blurry vision. She has also been nauseated and had worsening swelling in her legs. She missed her last doctor's appointment and has not been seen in over 5 weeks. Her medical history is significant only for asthma, and this is her first pregnancy. It has been 20 minutes since her first seizure. The patient develops a glazed look on her face and twitching. She then begins having another tonic–clonic seizure. A repeat bolus of 2 g magnesium sulfate is given, and the seizure subsides within 2 minutes.

VIGNETTE 4 Question 3
3. Answer E:
At this point in management, cesarean delivery is indicated. The patient is remote from delivery, and the definitive treatment of eclampsia is delivery. There is no time to begin induction of labor or wait to give betamethasone for fetal lung maturity. Treatment with phenytoin to prevent additional seizures is reasonable but not the best answer. Lastly, an LP is not the best answer because all signs and symptoms point to eclampsia as the etiology of her seizures.

VIGNETTE 4 Question 4
4. Answer C:
Eclampsia can occur antepartum, intrapartum, or postpartum. Antepartum eclampsia occurs in 38% to 53%, whereas postpartum eclampsia ranges from 11% to 44%, and most cases occur in the immediate postpartum period within 48 hours. Late postpartum eclampsia after 48 hours is rare but does occur. Reviewing the intrapartum history will often reveal that these women had preeclampsia and were treated with magnesium sulfate. Almost all cases of eclampsia occur in the third trimester (91%), 7.5% of cases will occur in the second trimester, and approximately 1.5% cases in the first trimester. Eclampsia in the first trimester is often associated with a molar or hydropic degeneration of the placenta.

7 Fetal Complications of Pregnancy

DISORDERS OF FETAL GROWTH

Newborns with birth weight less than the 10th percentile or greater than the 90th percentile are easily identified. However, the accuracy of antepartum estimates of fetal weight can vary. Ultrasound is the most commonly used modality to estimate fetal weight. Fetuses whose estimated fetal weight (EFW) is less than the 10th percentile are termed **small for gestational age** (SGA). Fetuses whose EFW is greater than the 90th percentile are termed **large for gestational age** (LGA). SGA fetuses are further described as either symmetric or asymmetric. *Symmetric* implies that the fetus is proportionally small. *Asymmetric* implies that certain organs of the fetus are disproportionately small. Classically, an asymmetric infant will have wasting of the torso and extremities while preserving the brain. Thus, the fetal head will be at a greater percentile than the rest of the body. Screening for disorders of fetal growth is done during routine prenatal care. Once the fetus is at or greater than 20 weeks' gestational age, the uterine fundal height (in centimeters) should be approximately equal to the gestational age (in weeks). Fetal growth can therefore be followed by serial examinations of the fundal height. Before making the diagnosis of either SGA or LGA, it is imperative that accurate dating of the pregnancy is ascertained. If the fundal height varies by more than 3 cm from the gestational age, ultrasound is usually obtained. Of note, although birth percentiles are useful in identifying small neonates, they fail to distinguish between infants who reached their growth potential and those with disproportionate growth. For example, a small infant may have normally grown because of his/her genetic potential, whereas another may be small because of genetic disease.

FETAL GROWTH REGULATION

Regulation of fetal growth begins early in the first trimester when the placental cytotrophoblast villi anchor to the uterine decidua. Because vascular connections form between the maternal circulation and the intervillous spaces, endocrine and paracrine signaling promotes adaptation of the maternal circulation, which provides both oxygen and nutrients to the developing fetus. Placental growth is supported by increased substrate delivery and perfusion, which is critical to its intricate function. As the site of maternal–fetal exchange, the placenta provides active transport to glucose, amino acids, and free fatty acids, which is facilitated by its low-resistance and high-capacitance vascular network. By term, 600 mL/min of maternal cardiac output will pass through the placental exchange network, which has an area of up to 12 m^2. The ultimate growth potential of the fetus is felt to be predetermined genetically. When the expected regulatory processes occur in the fetus, mother, and placenta, normal growth ensues. However, fetal growth regulation can be impacted both positively and negatively depending on genetic potential, maternal diet, pathophysiology, and placental function.

SMALL FOR GESTATIONAL AGE

SGA refers to a neonate with signs of fetal growth disruption but in whom the causative factor for small size is unknown. Intrauterine growth restriction (IUGR) generally refers to a fetus whose growth has been interfered with in some pathologic fashion, but IUGR and SGA are not uncommonly used interchangeably. SGA infants are associated with higher rates of mortality and morbidity for their gestational age. Even within the SGA category, infants with birth weight less than the 5th percentile or even less than the 3rd percentile have even worse outcomes. However, SGA infants do better than infants with the same weight delivered at earlier gestational ages. For example, an SGA neonate born at 34 weeks that weighs the same as a 28-week neonate will have lower morbidity and mortality rates. Factors that can result in infants being SGA can be divided into those that lead to **decreased growth potential** and those that lead to **intrauterine growth restriction** (**IUGR**) (Table 7-1).

Decreased Growth Potential

Congenital abnormalities account for approximately 10% to 15% of SGA infants. Trisomy 21 (Down syndrome), trisomy 18 (Edward syndrome), and trisomy 13 (Patau syndrome) all lead to SGA babies. Turner syndrome (45,XO) leads to a decrease in birth weight. Infants with osteogenesis imperfecta, achondroplasia, neural tube defects, anencephaly, and a variety of autosomal recessive syndromes may all be SGA.

Many intrauterine infections—particularly **cytomegalovirus** (CMV) and **rubella**—lead to SGA infants. These probably account for 10% to 15% of all SGA babies. Exposure to **teratogens**, most chemotherapeutic agents, and other drugs during pregnancy can also lead to decreased growth potential. The two most common teratogens causing SGA are alcohol and cigarettes. Up to 10% of SGA fetuses are constitutionally small based purely on parental stature or their genetic potential, and this appears to vary by race/ethnicity.

Intrauterine Growth Restriction

As noted earlier, IUGR is generally considered to be a pathologic interference with fetal growth, and yet another term, fetal growth restriction, is also utilized. Fetal growth can be divided into two phases: prior to 20 weeks of gestation, growth is primarily hyperplastic (increasing number of cells), and after 20 weeks, it is primarily hypertrophic (increasing cell size). As a consequence of this, an insult occurring prior to 20 weeks will most likely result in symmetric growth restriction, whereas an insult occurring after 20 weeks, in a prolonged fashion, will most likely result in asymmetric growth. Asymmetric growth is presumably caused by decreased nutrition and oxygen being transmitted across the placenta, which is then shunted to the fetal brain. Two thirds of the time growth restriction is asymmetric and can be identified by increased head-to-abdominal measurements.

Maternal risk factors include baseline hypertension, anemia, chronic renal disease, antiphospholipid antibody syndrome, systemic lupus erythematosus, and severe malnutrition. Severe diabetes with extensive vascular disease may also lead to IUGR. Placental factors leading to diminished placental blood flow may lead to IUGR. These factors include placenta previa, velamentous and marginal cord insertion, and placental thrombosis with or without infarction. Multiple gestations often lead to lower birth weights because of earlier delivery and SGA infants.

Diagnosis

The risk of having an SGA neonate increases in mothers with a previous SGA neonate or with any of the above etiologies. The intrauterine growth of these fetuses should be followed carefully. Fundal height is measured at each prenatal visit. Oligohydramnios and SGA fetuses tend to have fundal heights less than expected. Anytime a fundal height is 3 cm less than expected, fetal growth should be estimated via ultrasound. Of note, the use of fundal height as a screening tool for either SGA or LGA is quite poor with sensitivities much less than 50% and positive predictive values less than 50% as well. Thus, with concern in the setting of the risk factors listed previously, ultrasound to evaluate fetal growth is common even without abnormal fundal height measurements.

If SGA is suspected, the accuracy of the pregnancy's dating should be verified. Any infant at risk for IUGR

TABLE 7-1. Risk Factors for SGA Infants

Decreased growth potential
Genetic and chromosomal abnormalities
Intrauterine infections
Teratogenic exposure
Substance abuse
Radiation exposure
Small maternal stature
Pregnancy at high altitudes
Female fetus
Intrauterine growth restricted
Maternal factors, including hypertension, anemia, chronic renal disease, malnutrition, and severe diabetes
Placental factors, including placenta previa, chronic abruption, placental infarction, and multiple gestations

SGA, small for gestational age.

or being SGA is followed with serial ultrasound scans for growth every 2 to 3 weeks. A fetus with decreased growth potential will usually start small and stay small, whereas one with IUGR will progressively fall off the growth curve. Another test to differentiate IUGR fetuses is Doppler investigation of the umbilical artery. Normal flow through the umbilical artery is higher during systole and decreases only 50% to 80% during diastole (Fig. 7-1). The flow during diastole should never be absent or reversed (Fig. 7-2). However, in the setting of increased placental resistance, which can be seen with a thrombosed or calcified placenta, diastolic flow decreases or even becomes absent or reversed. Reversed diastolic flow is particularly concerning and is associated with a high risk of intrauterine fetal demise. Thus, an SGA fetus with normal Doppler values is often expectantly managed to term, whereas those with abnormal Doppler values are often delivered early.

Treatment
For patients with a history of SGA infants, the underlying etiology should be explored. If malnutrition or drugs like alcohol or cigarettes were issues in a prior pregnancy, these should be dealt with at each prenatal visit. Patients with a history of placental insufficiency, preeclampsia, collagen vascular disorders, or vascular disease are often treated with low-dose aspirin. Patients with prior placental thrombosis, thrombophilias, or antiphospholipid antibody syndrome have been treated with heparin and corticosteroids as well, with mixed results.

There is no indication to expedite delivery in SGA fetuses that have consistently been small throughout the pregnancy. However, the neonatal risk of delivery is likely to be lower than that of remaining in the intrauterine environment for some SGA fetuses in the late preterm and early term period who have fallen off the growth curve. This risk is assessed with fetal testing, such as a nonstress test (NST), oxytocin challenge test (OCT), biophysical profile (BPP), and umbilical Doppler velocimetry. With increasing placental resistance due to calcifications or thromboses, the umbilical arterial diastolic flow will decrease, halt, and occasionally reverse. Doppler investigation of the fetal umbilical cord is particularly useful because

FIGURE 7-1. Normal umbilical artery Doppler. Note that the ratio between systolic peak and diastolic trough is 3.29:1.

FIGURE 7-2. Reversed diastolic flow on umbilical artery Doppler in the setting of IUGR.

of the high predictive value of poor outcomes in the setting of absent or reversed end-diastolic flow. If fetal testing is nonreassuring, the fetus should be delivered. The decision of whether to deliver SGA fetuses remote from term is based on how the infant will do in a neonatal intensive care unit versus how it will be maintained in the intrauterine environment. For those left undelivered, frequent antenatal testing with NSTs, OCTs, and BPPs; frequent (every 2 to 3 weeks) ultrasounds for fetal growth; antenatal corticosteroids to accelerate fetal lung maturity; and, possibly, admission to the hospital for continuous monitoring may be indicated.

LARGE FOR GESTATIONAL AGE AND FETAL MACROSOMIA

An LGA fetus is defined as having an EFW greater than the 90th percentile. Although LGA identifies neonates with increased growth at a particular gestational age, it is considered less important than the diagnosis of fetal macrosomia, which is better correlated with identifying fetuses at higher risk for birth trauma or cesarean delivery. Although definitions of macrosomia vary, the American College of Obstetricians and Gynecologists (ACOG) uses **a birth weight greater than 4,500 g**. Birth weights of greater than 4,000 or 4,200 g are also used by many clinicians and researchers to define macrosomia. Macrosomic fetuses have a higher risk of shoulder dystocia and birth trauma with resultant brachial plexus injuries with vaginal deliveries. Other neonatal risks include low Apgar scores, hypoglycemia, polycythemia, hypocalcemia, and jaundice. LGA infants are at a higher risk for childhood leukemia, Wilms tumor, and osteosarcoma.

Mothers with LGA or macrosomic fetuses are at increased risk for cesarean delivery, perineal trauma, and postpartum hemorrhage. There is a higher rate of cesarean delivery in women with macrosomic infants because of failure to progress in labor. In addition, some women with suspected fetal macrosomia elect to have a cesarean delivery out of concern for increased risk of shoulder dystocia and the possibility of neonatal injury. Clinicians are generally obligated to offer such elective cesareans with an EFW of 5,000 g or greater in women without gestational diabetes and 4,500 g or greater in women with gestational diabetes.

Etiology

The most classically associated risk factor for fetal macrosomia is preexisting or gestational diabetes mellitus. **Maternal obesity**, with a BMI greater than 30 or weight greater than 90 kg, is also strongly associated with an increased risk for fetal macrosomia, as is increased maternal weight gain in pregnancy. This association is seemingly independent of maternal stature and gestational diabetes. Any woman who has previously delivered an LGA infant is at increased risk in ensuing pregnancies for fetal macrosomia. **Postterm pregnancies** have an increased rate of macrosomic infants. **Multiparity** and **advanced maternal age** are also risk factors (Table 7-2), but these are mostly secondary to the increased prevalence of diabetes and obesity.

Diagnosis

In the course of routine prenatal care, patients with macrosomic infants will more often be of a size greater than dates on measurement of the fundal height, and by the late third trimester, Leopold examination may reveal a fetus that seems large. Patients whose fundal heights are greater than dates by more than 3 cm are referred to ultrasound for EFW. Again, as noted under the SGA section, fundal height screening has a relatively poor sensitivity and specificity for fetal growth disorders. Unfortunately, ultrasound is not particularly accurate for the identification of LGA fetuses either. Ultrasound uses the biparietal diameter, femur length, and abdominal circumference to estimate fetal weight. These estimates are usually accurate to within 10% to 15%; however, with estimates beyond the 90th percentile, the positive predictive value of the weight being greater than or equal to that predicted is less than 50%. As with SGA fetuses, pregnancy date should be verified. In many institutions, any patient with diabetes or a previous LGA infant merits an EFW by ultrasound in the late third trimester.

Treatment

Management of LGA and macrosomic infants includes prevention, surveillance, and, in some cases, induction of labor before the attainment of macrosomia. The key to prevention of LGA in the broad obstetric population is counseling women about the goals for gestational weight gain, including specific counseling about diet and exercise in pregnancy. Women with type 1 and 2 pregestational diabetes or gestational diabetes are at increased risk of LGA fetuses and will benefit from tight control of blood glucose level during pregnancy. Well-controlled blood glucose level has been shown to decrease the incidence of macrosomic infants in this population. Specifically, studies of gestational diabetes have demonstrated a decrease in birth weight when women maintained good control of blood glucose level.

Maternal obesity is an independent risk factor for LGA infants. With the epidemic of obesity in the United States, approximately one third of pregnant women are obese and another third are overweight. Preconception counseling should be incorporated into the annual well-women examination of all reproductive age women, whether they receive care from an obstetrician/gynecologist or another primary care provider. Obese patients must be encouraged to lose weight before conception and offered specific programs to help them do so. Once pregnant, these patients should be advised to gain less weight (but never to lose weight) than the average patient, and they should be referred to a nutritionist for assistance in maintaining adequate nutrition, with some control of caloric intake.

Given the risk for birth trauma and failure to progress in labor secondary to cephalopelvic disproportion, LGA pregnancies are often induced before the fetus can attain macrosomic status. The risks of this course of action are thought to be an increased rate of cesarean section for failed induction and potentially neonatal complications of prematurity in a poorly dated pregnancy. Thus, induction should be used primarily when there is either excellent dating or lung maturity as assessed via amniocentesis. For

TABLE 7-2. Risk Factors for Macrosomic Infants
Diabetes
Maternal obesity
Postterm pregnancy
Previous LGA or macrosomic infant
Maternal stature
Multiparity
Advanced maternal age
Male infant
Beckwith–Wiedemann syndrome (pancreatic islet cell hyperplasia)

LGA, large for gestational age.

induction in the setting of an unfavorable cervix, prostaglandins and mechanical means should be used to achieve cervical ripening, and this can often take several days to accomplish. Interestingly, prospective studies of the practice of induction for impending macrosomia have not demonstrated an increase in cesarean delivery rates but do appear to lead to lower rates of macrosomia. Most recently, a large, randomized trial of this question demonstrated a decreased risk of neonatal birth injury as well. Vaginal delivery of the suspected macrosomic infant involves preparing for a shoulder dystocia and counseling patients on the risks and treatment options. Operative vaginal delivery with forceps or vacuum is generally not advised in the setting of known macrosomia because of the increased risk of shoulder dystocia; however, this decision is one to be made in a setting of shared decision making with the patient.

DISORDERS OF AMNIOTIC FLUID

The amniotic fluid reaches its maximum volume of about 800 mL at approximately 28 weeks. This volume is maintained until close to term when it begins to fall to about 500 mL at week 40. The balance of fluid is maintained by production of the fetal kidneys and lungs, resorption by fetal swallowing, and the interface between the membranes and the placenta. A disturbance in any of these functions may lead to a pathologic change in amniotic fluid volume.

Ultrasound can be used to evaluate the amniotic fluid volume. The classic measure of amniotic fluid is the **amniotic fluid index** (AFI). The AFI is calculated by dividing the maternal abdomen into quadrants, measuring the largest vertical pocket of fluid in each quadrant in centimeters, and summing them. An AFI of less than 5 is considered **oligohydramnios**. An AFI greater than 20 or 25 is used to diagnose **polyhydramnios**, depending on gestational age. More recently, a single deepest vertical pocket (DVP) to identify amniotic fluid disorders has been proposed, but both approaches are still utilized.

OLIGOHYDRAMNIOS

Oligohydramnios in the absence of rupture of membranes (ROM) is associated with a 40-fold increase in perinatal mortality. This is partially because without the amniotic fluid to cushion it, the umbilical cord is more susceptible to compression, thus leading to fetal asphyxiation. It is also associated with congenital anomalies, particularly of the genitourinary system, and growth restriction. In labor, nonreactive NSTs, fetal heart rate (FHR) decelerations, meconium, and cesarean delivery due to nonreassuring fetal testing are all associated with an AFI of less than 5.

Etiology

The cause of oligohydramnios can be thought of as either decreased production or increased withdrawal. Amniotic fluid is produced by the fetal kidneys and lungs. It can be resorbed by the placenta, swallowed by the fetus, or leaked out into the vagina. Chronic uteroplacental insufficiency (UPI) can lead to oligohydramnios because the fetus likely does not have the nutrients or blood volume to maintain an adequate glomerular filtration rate. UPI is commonly associated with growth-restricted infants.

Congenital abnormalities of the genitourinary tract can lead to decreased urine production. These malformations include renal agenesis (Potter syndrome), polycystic kidney disease, or obstruction of the genitourinary system. The most common cause of oligohydramnios is ROM. Even without a history of leaking fluid, the patient should be examined to rule out this possibility.

Diagnosis

Oligohydramnios is diagnosed when AFI is less than 5 as measured by ultrasound. Some centers use the DVP of amniotic fluid less than 2 cm as diagnostic for oligohydramnios. Patients screened for oligohydramnios include those measuring size less than dates, with a history of ruptured membranes, with suspicion of IUGR, and who have a postterm pregnancy. Once the diagnosis of oligohydramnios is made, the etiology needs to be determined before creating a management plan.

Treatment

Management of oligohydramnios depends entirely on the underlying etiology. In pregnancies that are IUGR, a host of other data should be considered, including the rest of the BPP, umbilical artery Doppler flow, gestational age, and the cause of the IUGR. Labor is usually induced in the case of a pregnancy at term or postdate. In the case of a fetus with congenital abnormalities, the patient should be referred to maternal–fetal medicine care for genetic counseling and prenatal diagnosis. A plan for delivery should be made in coordination with the pediatricians and, if necessary, pediatric surgeons. Severely preterm patients with no other etiology are usually managed expectantly with frequent antenatal fetal testing.

Labor is induced in patients with ROM at term if they are not already in labor. If there is meconium or frequent variable decelerations in the FHR, an amnioinfusion may be performed to increase the AFI. Traditionally, amnioinfusion has been performed to dilute any meconium present in the amniotic fluid, and therefore decrease the risk of meconium aspiration syndrome. However, in a large, multinational, randomized trial, amnioinfusion in the setting of meconium did not improve neonatal outcomes, and it is decreasingly used for this indication. In the setting of recurrent variable decelerations, there is evidence to suggest that amnioinfusion does decrease the number of variable decelerations caused by cord compression, and it is still used commonly for this indication, despite less clear evidence for neonatal benefit. Preterm premature ROM has already been discussed in Chapter 6.

POLYHYDRAMNIOS

Polyhydramnios, defined by an AFI greater than 20 or 25, is present in 2% to 3% of pregnancies. Fetal structural and chromosomal abnormalities are more common in polyhydramnios. It is associated with maternal diabetes and malformations such as neural tube defects, obstruction of the fetal alimentary canal, and fetal hydrops; however, the majority of cases of polyhydramnios have no associated diagnosis or cause.

Etiology

Polyhydramnios is not as ominous a sign as oligohydramnios. However, it is associated with an increase in congenital anomalies. It is also more common in pregnancies complicated by diabetes, hydrops, and multiple gestation. An obstruction of the gastrointestinal tract (e.g., tracheoesophageal fistula, duodenal atresia) may render the fetus unable to swallow the amniotic fluid, leading to polyhydramnios. Just as in other diabetic patients, the increased levels of circulating glucose can act as an osmotic diuretic in the fetus, leading to polyhydramnios. Hydrops secondary to high-output cardiac failure is generally associated with polyhydramnios. Monozygotic multiple gestations can lead to twin-to-twin transfusion syndrome with polyhydramnios around one fetus and oligohydramnios around the other. Polyhydramnios has also been associated with stillbirth and with preeclampsia.

Diagnosis

Polyhydramnios is diagnosed by ultrasound in patients being scanned for size greater than dates, routine screening of diabetic or multiple-gestation pregnancies, or as an unsuspected finding on an ultrasound performed for other reasons. Polyhydramnios is further classified as mild (AFI 25–30 cm or DVP 8–12 cm), moderate (AFI 30–35 cm or DVP 12–16 cm), or severe (AFI >35 cm or DVP >16 cm).

Treatment

As in oligohydramnios, the particular setting of polyhydramnios dictates the management of the pregnancy. Although polyhydramnios has been associated with an increased risk of stillbirth, there is no consensus on whether routine antenatal testing or early induction should routinely be done in cases of idiopathic polyhydramnios. Patients with polyhydramnios are at risk for malpresentation and should be carefully evaluated during labor. There is an increased risk of cord prolapse with polyhydramnios. Thus, ROM should be performed in a controlled setting if possible and only if the head is truly engaged in the pelvis. Upon spontaneous ROM, a sterile vaginal examination should be performed to verify fetal presentation and rule out cord prolapse.

RH INCOMPATIBILITY AND ALLOIMMUNIZATION

If a woman is Rh negative and her fetus is Rh positive either in a prior or current pregnancy, she may become sensitized to the Rh antigen. An individual may also become sensitized from a prior blood transfusion and develop anti-Rh antibodies. These IgG antibodies cross the placenta and cause hemolysis of fetal RBCs in a fetus that is Rh positive. The incidence of Rh negativity varies among race (Table 7-3), with the highest incidence of 30% seen among individuals in the Basque region of Spain. In the United States, the incidence of sensitization is decreasing because of both careful management of transfusions and the use of Rh immunoglobulin (RhoGAM) in pregnancy. Interestingly, because

TABLE 7-3. Prevalence of Rh Negativity by Race and Ethnicity

Race and Ethnicity	Percent Rh Negative
Caucasian	15
African American	8
African	4
Native American	1
Asian	<1

the risk of sensitization during pregnancy is due to transplacental passage of fetal cells that then present the Rh antigen, ABO incompatibility actually decreases the risk of Rh sensitization as a result of destruction of these fetal cells by anti-A or anti-B antibodies.

In sensitized patients with Rh-positive fetuses, the antibodies cross the placenta and cause hemolysis, leading to disastrous complications in the fetus. The anemia caused by hemolysis leads to increased extramedullary production of fetal red cells. **Erythroblastosis fetalis**, or fetal hydrops (Fig. 7-3): The anemia can lead to a syndrome that includes a hyperdynamic state, high-output heart failure, diffuse edema (Fig. 7-4), ascites (Fig. 7-5), pleural effusion, and pericardial effusion. Fetal hydrops is specifically defined as accumulation of fluid in the extracellular space in at least two body compartments. Bilirubin, a breakdown product of RBCs, is cleared by the placenta before birth but can lead to jaundice and neurotoxic effects in the neonate.

FIGURE 7-4. Scalp edema (e).

FIGURE 7-3. Fetal hydrops caused by the accumulation of fluid in fetal tissues. (From Sadler TW. *Langman's Medical Embryology*, 10th ed. Philadelphia, PA: Lippincott Williams & Wilkins; 2006.)

FIGURE 7-5. Note the large ascites (a) and pleural effusion (e) in this fetus with hydrops.

THE UNSENSITIZED RH-NEGATIVE PATIENT

If a patient is Rh negative but has a negative antibody screen, the goal during pregnancy is to keep her from becoming sensitized. Anytime during the pregnancy, if there is a possibility that a patient may be exposed to fetal blood (in the form of intact cells or free DNA), such as during amniocentesis, miscarriage, vaginal bleeding, abruption, and delivery, she should be given RhoGAM, an anti-D immunoglobulin (Rh

IgG). An antibody screen is performed at the initial visit to detect prior sensitization. RhoGAM should be administered at 28 weeks and postpartum if the neonate is Rh positive.

A standard dose of RhoGAM, 0.3 mg of Rh IgG, will eradicate 15 mL of fetal RBCs (30 mL of fetal blood with a hematocrit of 50%). This dose is adequate for a routine pregnancy. However, in the setting of placental abruption or any antepartum bleeding, a Kleihauer–Betke test for the amount of fetal RBCs in the maternal circulation can be done. If the amount of fetal RBCs is more than what can be eliminated by the single RhoGAM dose, additional dosages can be given.

THE SENSITIZED RH-NEGATIVE PATIENT

If the antibody screen for Rh comes back positive during the initial prenatal visit, the titer is checked as well. Antibody titers of 1:16 and greater have been associated with fetal hydrops. If paternity is not in question, blood type can be performed on the father of the baby to determine whether the fetus is at risk. However, because approximately 5% of all pregnancies have unknown or incorrect paternity, the safest course is to treat all pregnancies as if the fetus is at risk.

Throughout pregnancy, the antibody titer is followed approximately every 4 weeks. As long as it remains less than 1:16, the pregnancy can be managed expectantly. However, if it becomes 1:16 or greater, serial amniocentesis is begun as early as 16 to 20 weeks. At the first amniocentesis, fetal cells can be collected and analyzed for the Rh antigen to determine fetal Rh status. If negative, the pregnancy can be followed expectantly. However, if the fetus is Rh positive, fetal anemia is screened for using fetal middle cerebral artery (MCA) Doppler measurements. It was demonstrated more than a decade ago that in anemic fetuses, there is greater blood flow to the brain, and thus the MCA Doppler measures peak systolic velocity (PSV). In fetuses with greater PSV measurements, concern for fetal anemia merits more invasive testing and, potentially, treatment.

Historically, prior to the use of MCA Doppler measurements, the evaluation of Rh-positive fetus in a Rh-negative woman with positive titers 1:16 or greater was done with serial amniocenteses to assess the amniotic fluid by a spectrophotometer. Because the breakdown products of hemoglobin include bilirubin, which discolors the amniotic fluid, the light absorption (ΔOD_{450}) by bilirubin will increase, as it is concentrated in the amniotic fluid with increasing fetal hemolysis. These measurements are plotted on the Liley curve (Fig. 7-6), which predicts the severity of disease. The curve is divided into three zones.

Zone 1 is suggestive of a mildly affected fetus, and follow-up amniocentesis can be performed approximately every 2 to 3 weeks. Zone 2 is suggestive of a moderately affected fetus, and amniocentesis should be repeated every 1 to 2 weeks. The severely affected fetus will fall into zone 3. Once in zone 3, it is likely that the fetus has anemia.

Because most centers currently screen for fetal anemia with MCA Doppler measurements of blood flow, amniocentesis has been reserved for those with questionable results or in the setting of a positive MCA Doppler screen prior to intervention. A potentially enormously beneficial procedure, percutaneous umbilical blood sampling (PUBS) and intrauterine transfusion (IUT) are the treatments for fetal anemia. PUBS can be used to obtain a fetal hematocrit to verify fetal anemia and to perform an IUT. If a PUBS or IUT cannot be performed, fetal intraperitoneal transfusion may be performed. Although the risk of immediate delivery may be as high as 3%, this risk is preferred to worsening fetal anemia, hydrops, and likely fetal death.

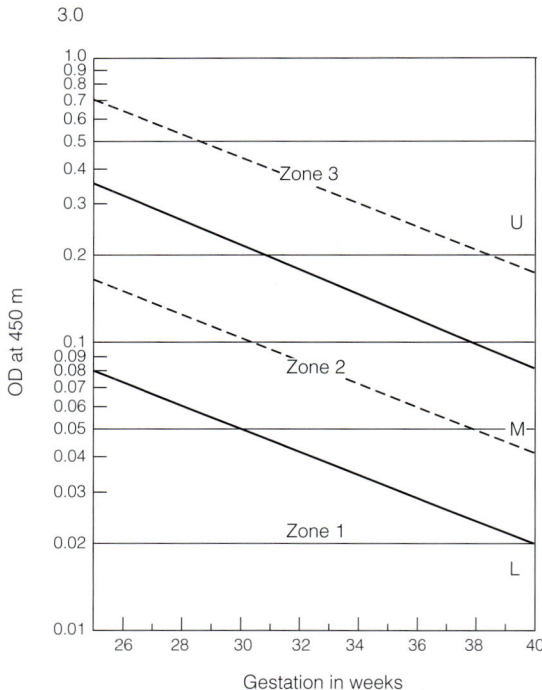

FIGURE 7-6. Liley curve used to predict severity of fetal hemolysis with red-cell isoimmunization.

OTHER CAUSES OF IMMUNE HYDROPS

There are a variety of other RBC antigens, including the **ABO** blood type, antigens **CDE** in which D is the Rh antigen, **Kell**, **Duffy**, and **Lewis**. Some may cause fetal hydrops (e.g., Kell and Duffy), whereas others may lead to a mild hemolysis but not severe immune hydrops (e.g., ABO, Lewis). With the advent of treatment with RhoGAM, the incidence of Rh alloimmunization has decreased, and the other causes of immune-related fetal hydrops now account for a greater percentage of cases. Sensitized patients are managed similar to Rh-negative patients with antibody titers, MCA Doppler measurements, PUBS, and transfusions. Although most of the RBC antigens lead to a hemolytic anemia alone, anti-Kell antibodies lead also to suppression of the marrow and decreased RBC production. Thus, the advent of MCA Doppler screening has made an enormous difference in the management of such patients.

FETAL DEMISE

Intrauterine fetal demise (IUFD) or stillbirth is a rare but disastrous occurrence, occurring in approximately 0.5% to 1% of pregnancies overall and approximately 1:1,000 term births. The risk of IUFD increases with a variety of medical and obstetric complications of pregnancy, including abruption, congenital abnormalities, infection, and postterm pregnancy. Chronic placental insufficiency secondary to rheumatologic, vascular, or hypertensive disease may lead to IUGR and eventually IUFD. When there is no explanation for a fetal demise, it is usually attributed to a "cord accident." A retained IUFD greater than 3 to 4 weeks can lead to hypofibrinogenemia secondary to the release of thromboplastic substances from the decomposing fetus. In some cases, full-blown disseminated intravascular coagulation (DIC) can result.

DIAGNOSIS

Early in pregnancy, before 20 weeks, the diagnosis of fetal death (missed abortion) is suspected by lack of uterine growth or cessation of symptoms of pregnancy. Diagnosis is confirmed with serially falling human chorionic gonadotropin (hCG) and ultrasound documentation. After week 20, fetal death is suspected with absence of fetal movement noted by the mother or absence of uterine growth. Diagnosis can be confirmed by ultrasound. Given the importance of making an appropriate, accurate diagnosis, the absence of fetal heart motion is usually verified by two clinicians.

TREATMENT

Because of the risk of DIC with retained IUFD, the best treatment is delivery. Early gestations can be evacuated from the uterus by dilation and evacuation or with mifepristone and misoprostol in some cases. After 20 weeks, the pregnancy is usually terminated by induction of labor with prostaglandins or high-dose oxytocin. Helping patients understand what may have caused the fetal death is imperative to helping them cope with the situation. Tests for causes of fetal death include screening for collagen vascular disease or hypercoagulable state, fetal karyotype, and often TORCH titers (i.e., toxoplasmosis, rapid plasma reagin [RPR], CMV, and Herpes Simplex virus [HSV]). Because the cells of an IUFD will often not grow to obtain karyotype, recent studies have examined performing microarray studies of the fetal or placental genome to look for both aneuploidy and other genetic abnormalities, such as copy number variants. It is also extremely important to get an autopsy on the fetus, which can contribute valuable information. Despite this extensive battery of tests, the etiology of fetal demise will likely remain unknown in the majority of cases.

POSTTERM PREGNANCY

A postterm pregnancy is defined as one that goes beyond 42 weeks' gestational age or greater than 294 days past the last menstrual period (LMP). As many women are induced at 41 weeks of gestation, this gestation is occasionally labeled as "postdates," but this term is not consistently used. The categories of term pregnancies recognized by ACOG are early term (37 0/7 to 38 6/7), full term (39 0/7 to 40 6/7), and late term (41 0/7 to 41 6/7), with 42 weeks and beyond continuing to be how we define postterm pregnancy. It is estimated that 3% to 10% of all pregnancies will go postterm. This is an important obstetric issue because of the increased risk of macrosomic infants, oligohydramnios, meconium aspiration, intrauterine fetal death, and dysmaturity syndrome. There is also greater risk to the mother because of a greater rate of cesarean delivery (approximately doubled) and delivery of large infants. With improved dating, there are an increasing number of studies that show these complications of pregnancy may increase after 40 or 41 weeks of gestation and may benefit from delivery prior to 42 weeks of gestation.

ETIOLOGY

The most common reason for the diagnosis of postterm pregnancy is inaccurate dating; therefore, accurate dating is imperative. Postterm pregnancy appears to be more common in overweight and obese women as well. Because the physiologic basis for the onset of labor is poorly understood, the mechanisms for preterm or postterm labor are also unclear. There are a few rare conditions of the fetus associated with postterm pregnancy. These include anencephaly, fetal adrenal hypoplasia, and absent fetal pituitary. All are notable for diminished levels of circulating estrogens.

DIAGNOSIS

Again, the diagnosis is made by accurate dating. Because ultrasound can be off by as much as 3 weeks near term, this cannot be used to confirm dating. Accurate dating is made by a certain LMP consistent with a first- or second-trimester ultrasound. Dating by a third-trimester ultrasound or unsure LMP is more suspect.

TREATMENT

The varying approaches to the postterm pregnancy generally involve more frequent visits, increased fetal testing, and plans for eventual induction. A typical plan for following a postterm pregnancy is outlined as follows:

Patients whose pregnancies go past 40 weeks of gestation usually receive an NST during the 41st week of pregnancy. Induction is indicated with nonreassuring fetal testing. During the 42nd week (between 41 and 42 weeks of gestation), the patient should be seen twice for antenatal testing. Alternatively, many practitioners use the modified BPP (an NST and AFI) for fetal testing at each visit past the due date. Because oligohydramnios is a marker for worsening placental function and would likely be seen prior to an abnormal NST, the advantage of this test is that it may improve the sensitivity for fetuses at risk for IUFD. Induction is indicated with nonreassuring fetal testing or electively with an inducible cervix (Bishop score >6). After 42 weeks of gestation, the patient is offered induction of labor regardless of cervical examination.

In most practices, patients are offered induction of labor at 41 weeks of gestation, as a result of improved dating by ultrasound, patient demand, as well as the risk-averse environment of obstetrics. Several randomized trials have demonstrated that induction of labor at 41 weeks of gestation when compared with expectant management leads to lower rates of cesarean delivery (even with an unfavorable cervix) as well as lower rates of meconium aspiration syndrome in the neonate. The lower rate of cesarean delivery with induction of labor is counterintuitive to most clinicians and patients. However, this makes sense when one considers that the common indications for cesarean delivery (a fetus that is too big for the maternal pelvis or a nonreassuring fetal tracing) increase with increasing gestational age at term. The key is to allow active labor to ensue in an induction of labor, which can take longer than in spontaneous labor. Because of this evidence regarding induction of labor at 41 weeks' gestation, ACOG supported routine induction of labor at 41 weeks as a component of the approach to reduce cesarean deliveries.

MULTIPLE GESTATIONS

If a fertilized ovum divides into two separate ova, monozygotic, or "identical," twins result. If ovulation produces two ova and both are fertilized, dizygotic twins result. Without assisted fertility, the rate of twinning is approximately 1:80 pregnancies, with 30% of those monozygotic. The rate of dizygotic twinning varies between races and is influenced by maternal age and parity. By race/ethnicity, the frequency of dizygotic twins is lowest in Asians, intermediate in Caucasians, and higher in African Americans. The rate of naturally occurring triplets is approximately 1:7,000 to 8,000 pregnancies. However, with ovulation-enhancing drugs and in vitro fertilization (IVF), the incidence of multiple gestations has increased dramatically.

COMPLICATIONS OF MULTIPLE GESTATIONS

Multiple gestations result in an increase in a variety of obstetric complications, including preterm labor, placenta previa, cord prolapse, postpartum hemorrhage, cervical incompetence, gestational diabetes, and preeclampsia. The fetuses are at increased risk for preterm delivery, congenital abnormalities, SGA, and malpresentation. The average gestational age of delivery for twins is between 36 and 37 weeks; for triplets it is between 33 and 34 weeks, and for quadruplets it is between 28 and 29 weeks. Neonates delivered from multiple gestations weigh less than their singleton counterparts and have a greater overall mortality rate as a result of prematurity and low birth weight. Monochorionic (one placenta), diamniotic (two amniotic sacs) twins, also referred to as Mo-Di twins, often have placental vascular communications and can develop **twin-to-twin transfusion syndrome** (TTTS). Monochorionic, monoamniotic (Mo-Mo) twins have an extremely high mortality rate (reported as high as 40% to 60%) secondary to cord accidents from entanglement.

Pathogenesis

Monozygotic twinning results from division of the fertilized ovum or cells in the embryonic disk. If separation occurs before the differentiation of the trophoblast, two chorions and two amnions (Di-Di) result (Fig. 7-7). After trophoblast differentiation and before amnion formation (days 3 to 8), separation leads to a single placenta, one chorion, and two amnions (Mo-Di). Division after amnion formation leads to a single placenta, one chorion, and one amnion (Mo-Mo) (days 8 to 13) and, rarely, conjoined or "Siamese" twins (days 13 to 15). Division of cells beyond day 15 or 16 will result in a singleton fetus. Monozygotic twinning does not follow any inheritable pattern. Risk factors include assisted reproductive techniques (as high as 5% rate of monozygotic twinning) and a slight increased rate with advancing maternal age.

Dizygotic twins result primarily from fertilization of two ova by two sperm. There are varying risk factors associated with dizygotic twinning. Dizygotic twins tend to run in families and are more common in people of African descent. Globally, the rate of dizygotic twins ranges from 1:1,000 in Japan to 1:20 in several Nigerian tribes. The rate of all multiple gestations has increased sharply since the onset of medical treatment of infertility. Clomiphene citrate, a fertility-enhancing drug, increases the rate of dizygotic twinning up to 8%. The use of multiple embryos in IVF to improve the pregnancy rates also leads to increased rates of twinning and higher order multiple gestations. Although the rate of higher order multiple gestations has decreased over the past decade, many infertility practices have a rate of twin gestations of 30% to 40% or greater.

Diagnosis

Multiple gestations are usually diagnosed by ultrasound. Multiple gestations are indicated by rapid uterine growth, excessive maternal weight gain, or palpation of three or more fetal large parts (cranium and breech) on Leopold examination. Family history and use of reproductive technology also raise suspicion for multiples. The levels of β-hCG, human placental lactogen, and maternal serum α-fetoprotein are all elevated for gestational age. Rarely, diagnosis will be made after delivery of the first fetus with palpation of the aftercoming fetus(es). Differentiation

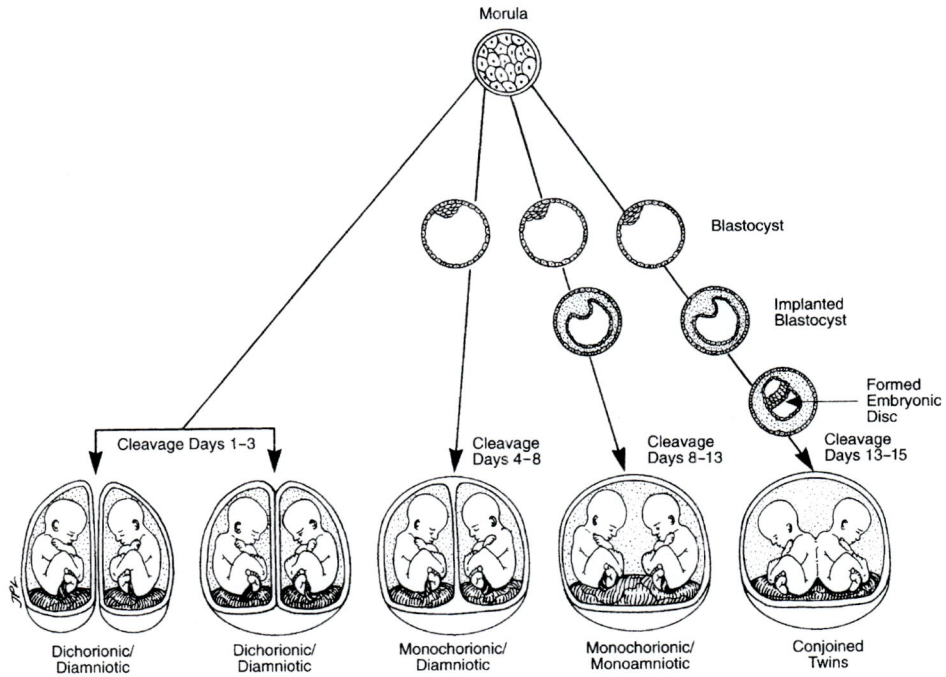

FIGURE 7-7. The relationship between the timing of cleavage and the resulting amnionicity/chorionicity in monozygotic twinning. (From LifeART image copyright © 2006 Lippincott Williams & Wilkins. All rights reserved.)

FIGURE 7-8. Monochorionic–diamniotic (Mo-Di) twins. Note the single chorion but two developing amniotic sacs.

between Di-Di and Mo-Di twins is easier the earlier the ultrasound is performed. For example, quite early in pregnancy, one can see a single chorion and two amniotic sacs (Fig. 7-8) indicative of Mo-Di twins. Later in pregnancy, sonologists rely on the thickness of the membrane and the "twin peak" sign (Fig. 7-9), which is formed by the two placentae fusing together in the setting of Di-Di twins. Mo-Mo twins are usually the easiest because they have no intertwin membrane.

Treatment

Given the increased risk of complications, multiple-gestation pregnancies are managed as high-risk pregnancies, usually in conjunction with a perinatologist. Aside from the antenatal management of the complications, the principal issue in twin gestations is mode of delivery. With higher order multiple gestations, triplets and above, selective reduction down to twins or even a singleton is commonly recommended. Although there is a chance of losing the entire pregnancy in the setting of selective reduction, if successful, the chances of delivering a severely premature infant are also dramatically reduced. However, the question of the risks and benefits of selective reduction from twins to a singleton gestation is unanswered at this time.

TWIN-TO-TWIN TRANSFUSION SYNDROME

Polyhydramnios–oligohydramnios (poly–oli) sequence or TTTS has been described for several centuries and results in a small, anemic twin and a large, plethoric, polycythemic, and occasionally hydropic twin. The etiology of TTTS appears to be secondary to unequal flow within vascular communications between the twins in their shared placenta, leading to one twin becoming a donor and the other a recipient of this unequal blood flow. In particular, an abundance of unidirectional arteriovenous connections without adequate bidirectional arterio-arterial or venovenous connections to rescue this shunting appears to predispose to a higher risk of TTTS. This can result in one fetus with hypervolemia, cardiomegaly, glomerulotubal hypertrophy, edema, and ascites, and the other with hypovolemia, growth restriction, and oligohydramnios. Given the risk of this syndrome in Mo-Di twins, serial ultrasounds examining the amniotic fluid and fetal growth should be obtained every 2 weeks after diagnosis. The syndrome can present at any gestational age; however, earlier diagnosis is associated with worse outcomes.

TTTS has historically been managed with serial amnioreduction, which can reduce preterm contractions secondary to uterine distension and maternal symptoms, but only occasionally actually cures the fetal syndrome. More recently, as these vascular connections have been identified as the etiology of the syndrome, coagulating these vessels has been proposed as the treatment of choice in more severe

FIGURE 7-9. The fused chorionic and amniotic membranes lead to the "twin peak" sign in the middle of image in Di-Di twins.

cases. This is accomplished by fetal surgeons using a fetoscopically placed laser to coagulate the vessels. Risks of the procedure include maternal risks, loss of the pregnancy entirely, and eventual preterm delivery. Because TTTS leads to an extremely high rate of poor pregnancy outcomes, the procedure appears to be beneficial to these patients. However, because of the potential risks, pregnancy termination should always be offered as an option as well.

MO-MO TWINS

Given the risk of cord entanglement and IUFD, Mo-Mo twins are often managed with frequent antenatal testing and early delivery. Unfortunately, frequent antenatal testing has not, in and of itself, appeared to make a difference in the rate of IUFD in these cases. As a result, some patients are offered admission to the hospital and continuous electronic fetal monitoring from weeks 28 to 34, during which time delivery is performed via cesarean section. Mo-Mo and conjoined twins are almost always delivered via cesarean section.

DELIVERY OF TWINS

There are four possibilities for twin presentation: both vertex (40%), both breech, vertex then breech (40%), and breech then vertex. When deciding mode of delivery, all breech-presenting twins (20%) are considered together. Patients should be thoroughly counseled on all possible presentations and delivery options.

Vertex/vertex twins should undergo a trial of labor, with cesarean section reserved for the usual indications. Vertex/nonvertex twins can also undergo a trial of labor if the twins are concordant or the presenting twin is larger. Generally, the twins should be between 1,500 and 3,500 g, although there are scant data that breech extraction between 500 and 1,500 g leads to any worse outcomes. Breech extraction for delivery of the second twin has advantages over a vertex second twin because the second twin's lower extremity can be grasped and delivery expedited quickly. In the setting of a vertex second twin, occasionally, placental abruption occurs, necessitating a rapid delivery. However, if the cervix is no longer fully dilated or the fetal vertex is above 0 station, a cesarean delivery may be necessary. External cephalic version and internal podalic version have also been used for delivery of the second twin, but small studies have found lower Apgar scores than with breech extraction. Furthermore, the chances of failure of such maneuvers are higher. Nonvertex presenting twins are usually delivered via cesarean section.

DELIVERY OF TRIPLETS

Most triplet gestations are delivered via cesarean section. Rarely, triplets will be concordant, with vertex presenting, all greater than 1,500 to 2,000 g, and a vaginal delivery can be attempted. Multiple gestations beyond triplets are all delivered via cesarean section.

KEY POINTS

- Fetuses whose EFW is less than the 10th percentile are considered SGA, although the rate of poor neonatal outcomes rises significantly below the 5th and 3rd percentiles.
- Common causes of decreased growth potential include congenital abnormalities, drugs, infections, radiation, and small maternal stature.
- IUGR infants are commonly born to women with systemic diseases, leading to poor placental blood flow.
- An LGA fetus has an EFW greater than the 90th percentile at any particular gestational age.
- Both 4,000 and 4,500 g have been used as the threshold for defining fetal macrosomia.
- LGA and macrosomic fetuses are at greater risk for birth trauma, hypoglycemia, jaundice, lower Apgar scores, and childhood tumors.
- Increased size in the fetus is seen with maternal diabetes, maternal obesity, increased maternal height, postterm pregnancies, multiparity, advanced maternal age, and male sex.
- Oligohydramnios is defined by an AFI of less than 5 cm and can be caused by decreased placental perfusion, decreased fluid production by the fetus, and ROM.
- Pregnancies at term complicated by oligohydramnios should be delivered.

(continued)

KEY POINTS (continued)

- Polyhydramnios is diagnosed by an AFI greater than 20 cm on ultrasound and is associated with diabetes, multiple gestations, hydrops, and congenital abnormalities.
- Obstetric management of polyhydramnios should include careful verification of presentation and close observation for cord prolapse.
- Rh-sensitized women with Rh-positive fetuses have antibodies that cross the placenta, leading to hemolysis and anemia in the fetuses. If the anemia is severe enough, hydrops develops with edema, ascites, and heart failure.
- Rh-negative patients who are not sensitized should be treated with antepartum RhoGAM to prevent sensitization. Postpartum, they should receive another dose of RhoGAM if the fetus is Rh positive.
- Rh-negative patients undergoing miscarriage, abruption, amniocentesis, ectopic pregnancy, and vaginal bleeding should also be given RhoGAM.
- Rh-negative patients who are sensitized are followed closely with serial MCA Doppler velocities and ultrasound. If fetal anemia is suspected, PUBS and IUT can be performed.
- Although IUFD is more common with disorders of the placenta, the actual cause of most IUFDs is usually unknown and is often attributed to cord accidents.
- Retained IUFD can lead to DIC; thus, delivery soon after diagnosis is indicated.
- Postterm pregnancy is defined as greater than 42 weeks' gestational age.
- Postterm pregnancies are at increased risk for fetal demise, macrosomia, meconium aspiration, and oligohydramnios.
- Increased fetal surveillance and labor induction are the most common management options for postterm pregnancies.
- Monozygotic twins carry identical genetic material, whereas dizygotic twins are from separate ova and sperm.
- Multiple gestations are at increased risk for preterm labor and delivery, placenta previa, postpartum hemorrhage, preeclampsia, cord prolapse, malpresentation, and congenital abnormalities.
- There is a genetic predisposition for dizygotic twinning, whereas the rate of monozygotic twinning is the same throughout all races and families.
- Monozygotic twins are at risk for TTTS and should have frequent ultrasound examinations to diagnose this early.
- Vaginal delivery of vertex/vertex presenting twins is preferred and is possible with vertex/nonvertex twins under the right circumstances. Nonvertex presenting twins are delivered by cesarean section.was

CLINICAL VIGNETTES

VIGNETTE 1

A 23-year-old G1P0 woman at 30 weeks 3 days presents to clinic for routine prenatal care. Her pregnancy is dated by last menstrual period (LMP) consistent with a 10-week ultrasound. She has had three prenatal visits, and her pregnancy has been complicated by vaginal bleeding in the first trimester and the development of heartburn at 25 weeks. She has no complaints today. She continues to smoke half a pack of cigarettes daily, which has decreased from one pack per day at the beginning of her pregnancy. Her medical history is significant for asthma. Ultrasound at 20 weeks' gestation showed no evidence of fetal abnormality, posterior placenta, Amniotic fluid index (AFI) of 10.6 cm, and fetal growth in the 20th percentile. Her current weight is 130 lbs, and her height is 5 ft 6 in. She has gained 10 lbs so far in pregnancy. Urine dip is negative for protein, glucose, ketones, and leukocytes. BP is 112/64 mm Hg and heart rate is 80 beats per minute. Fetal heart tones are in the 130s. Fundal height measures 25 weeks. Of note, during her last visit at 25 weeks, fundal height measured 23 weeks, and she had a normal glucose tolerance test and complete blood count.

1. Which of the following is the next best step in managing this patient's pregnancy?
   a. Nonstress test (NST)
   b. Fetal ultrasound
   c. Group B streptococcus culture

d. TORCH titers
   e. Amniocentesis

2. Which of the following is the most likely risk factor for this patient's small for gestational age (SGA) fetus?
   a. Congenital anomaly such as cardiac anomaly
   b. Congenital cytomegalovirus (CMV) infection
   c. Tobacco abuse
   d. History of chemotherapy exposure as a child
   e. Genetic potential

3. Ultrasound demonstrates that the fetus measures less than the 10th percentile for head circumference, femur length, and abdominal circumference. Doppler velocimetry of the fetal umbilical artery was normal. Amniotic fluid index (AFI) was 11.2 cm. Which of the following is the most appropriate component of the treatment strategy at this time?
   a. Induction of labor
   b. Continue routine prenatal care
   c. Fetal ultrasound every 2 to 3 weeks
   d. Admission to the hospital for daily NST and biophysical profile (BPP)
   e. Daily Doppler velocimetry

4. The patient has a repeat ultrasound performed at 33 weeks of gestation. Fetal growth is noted to be at the 4th percentile with intermittently elevated umbilical cord Dopplers and an AFI of 8.4 cm. What do you recommend at this time?
   a. Repeat growth ultrasound in 4 to 6 weeks
   b. Amniocentesis for fetal lung maturity and delivery if mature
   c. Admission to hospital for continuous fetal monitoring until delivery
   d. Induction of labor
   e. Betamethasone administration

5. The patient is admitted to the antepartum service for inpatient monitoring. Repeat ultrasound on hospital day 5 is notable for AFI of 4.3 cm, and umbilical Doppler is elevated with absent end-diastolic flow. NST is nonreactive and a BPP is 6 out of 8. The decision is made to induce labor. Bishop score is 2, and a Foley bulb is placed for cervical ripening. Which of the following is not a complication commonly associated with oligohydramnios in labor?
   a. Meconium amniotic fluid
   b. Cesarean delivery
   c. Fetal heart rate (FHR) decelerations
   d. Cord prolapse
   e. Nonreactive fetal tracing

VIGNETTE 2

A 38-year-old G3P2002 woman presents at 40 weeks 3 days with contractions to labor and delivery triage. Contractions started 1 hour ago and are very painful. The patient denies leaking fluid but did notice blood and mucus on her underwear. The baby has not been particularly active since contractions started. Her pregnancy has been complicated by gestational diabetes for which she was treated with insulin. Fasting blood glucose levels are usually between 80 and 90 mg/dL with 1-hour postprandial values between 120 and 140 mg/dL. Her prepregnancy weight was 130 lb, and she is 5 ft 5 in (BMI 21.6). She has gained 30 lb this pregnancy (BMI, 26.6). Hemoglobin A1C is 6.0%. Fetal ultrasound at 20 weeks demonstrated normal fetal anatomy. Repeat ultrasound for growth at 38 weeks demonstrated fetus with weight in the 90th percentile and an EFW of 4,350 g. Her last pregnancy was complicated by A1GDM, and she delivered a 4,200-g infant without complications. Initial cervical examination reveals dilation of 6 cm, 50% effacement, and −1 station. Two hours later, the nurse calls you to the room after the patient's water breaks. Examination shows complete dilation and effacement, and fetus at +1 station. The patient has a strong urge to push and begins pushing.

The delivery is complicated by a second degree perineal laceration and a postpartum hemorrhage of 600 mL. Fetal weight is 4,560 g, and the Apgar scores are 6, 8.

1. What neonatal outcomes are most commonly present in macrosomic fetuses?
   1. Jaundice
   2. Hypoglycemia
   3. Hyperglycemia
   4. Birth trauma
   5. Asthma
   6. Hypocalcemia
      a. 1, 2, 4, 6
      b. 1, 3, 4, 5
      c. 3, 4, 5
      d. 1, 3, 5, 6
      e. 2, 4, 5, 6

2. Which of the following is most likely the cause of fetal macrosomia in this case?
   a. Maternal weight gain in pregnancy
   b. Gestational diabetes
   c. Poor glycemic control
   d. Advanced maternal age
   e. Postterm pregnancy

3. The patient returns to your clinic for her 6-week postpartum visit. You ask her about contraception, and she states that she would like to have one more child in the near future. She is breastfeeding, and it is going well. What do you also recommend as part of her postpartum care in this setting?
   a. Immediate weight loss to 20% under prepregnancy weight
   b. RPR
   c. Continue insulin regimen postpartum

- d. Start metformin
- e. Perform a 2-hour glucose tolerance test

4. The patient returns 2 years later to your office. She is now 8 weeks 3 days pregnant by certain LMP. She weighs 160 lb (BMI, 26.6). She has been very nauseated this pregnancy and is eating frequent small snacks. She has not seen a physician since her last postpartum visit with you during her last pregnancy. What test, in particular, do you recommend performing, in addition to routine prenatal laboratory studies?
   - a. Preeclampsia panel (creatinine, AST, BUN, platelets, uric acid)
   - b. 24-hour urine protein collection
   - c. Referral for eye examination to evaluate for retinopathy
   - d. Glucose tolerance test
   - e. Hemoglobin A1C

VIGNETTE 3

A 35-year-old woman with a history of primary infertility presents with her partner for initial prenatal visit. They had been attempting pregnancy for the past 3 years and have now conceived through IVF. She had one embryo transferred 7 weeks ago. The patient's medical history is significant for rheumatoid arthritis and polycystic ovarian syndrome. She is overweight. In reviewing their family history, she tells you that her grandmother was a twin and there is no family history of congenital abnormalities or known genetic disorders in their family. Today, she reports nausea and vomiting, which is worse in the morning. She has not had any vaginal bleeding or cramping. You perform a transvaginal ultrasound and notice not one but two embryos. There appears to be a thin dividing membrane between the two. Heart rate for each embryo is around 150 beats per minute.

1. At what stage of division in the embryonic disk does monochorionic–diamniotic twining occur?
   - a. Before the differentiation of the trophoblast
   - b. After trophoblast differentiation and before amnion formation
   - c. After amnion formation
   - d. Not until after day 15 of development

2. During your visit with the couple, you explain to them that you will be monitoring fetal growth of their twins closely because they are at risk for SGA and twin-to-twin transfusion syndrome. You also explain that multiple gestations are at risk for preterm labor, preterm birth, placental abnormalities, cesarean section due to malpresentation, preeclampsia, and gestational diabetes. In twin-to-twin transfusion syndrome, the recipient twin may suffer from which of the following complications?
   - a. Fetal hydrops
   - b. Anemia
   - c. Growth restriction
   - d. Oligohydramnios
   - e. Hypovolemia

3. The couple returns for routine prenatal care at 30 weeks. The patient has been feeling well. She reports mild low back pain and fatigue. The babies are very active. The last ultrasound showed only 12% discordance in fetal weights, with baby A estimated to be 200 g larger than baby B. Baby A is currently cephalic and baby B is frank breech. The couple would like a trial of labor. You begin counseling them on the risks and benefits of vaginal birth with twins, including breech extraction, and cesarean section. In which of the following pairs would trial of labor not be recommended?
   - a. Twin A 2,800 g cephalic; twin B 2,650 g cephalic
   - b. Twin A 2,850 g cephalic; twin B 3,775 g breech
   - c. Twin A 3,150 g cephalic; twin B 3,010 g frank breech
   - d. Twin A 3,440 g cephalic; twin B 3,220 g footling breech
   - e. Twin A 1,645 g cephalic; twin B 1,550 g cephalic

VIGNETTE 4

A 33-year-old G8P5116 woman with a fundal height of 39 cm presents for initial prenatal visit in your clinic. She is currently an inmate at a local jail. She is imprisoned on charges of marijuana possession. She has had no prenatal care. She is unsure of her last period but reports that she started feeling the baby move approximately 5 months ago. She denies vaginal bleeding, leaking fluid, or contractions during the pregnancy. She reports using marijuana nearly daily throughout the pregnancy. She has not been taking any medications in pregnancy and has had no other exposures. The father of the baby is not involved. She does not have custody of her other children and has an open DHS case. She hopes to regain custody and is interested in drug rehabilitation. Ultrasound performed in your clinic shows gestational age to be approximately 40 weeks 3 days.

1. What is the most common cause of a diagnosis of postterm pregnancy?
   - a. Inaccurate dating
   - b. Fetal anomaly
   - c. Delayed presentation to prenatal care
   - d. Advanced maternal age
   - e. Multiparity

2. In a routine pregnancy, NST should be started during which week of pregnancy to monitor for fetal well-being?
   - a. 38
   - b. 39
   - c. 40

d. 41
e. 42

3. Postterm pregnancy is associated with all the following except
   a. Transient tachypnea of the newborn
   b. Oligohydramnios
   c. Macrosomia
   d. Meconium aspiration
   e. Intrauterine fetal demise

4. You receive a call from the infirmary nurse at the jail at 4:30 PM. Your patient reports decreased fetal movement for the past 2 days. She is now 41 weeks 2 days. She had monitoring 3 days ago, and fetal testing was reassuring. The nurse reports that the patient denies any contractions, leaking fluid, or vaginal bleeding. She last felt the baby move once this morning and felt the baby move only twice yesterday. What do you recommend to the nurse?
   a. Perform kick counts and phone back if less than 10 movements in 2 hours
   b. Schedule NST with BPP for first thing tomorrow morning
   c. Schedule induction of labor tomorrow morning
   d. Evaluation on labor and delivery triage as soon as possible
   e. Schedule patient for evaluation in clinic first thing tomorrow morning

ANSWERS

VIGNETTE 1 Question 1
1. Answer B:
Fetal ultrasound to evaluate growth is the next best step in management. At each routine prenatal visit after 20 weeks of gestation, the fundal height is measured to evaluate fetal growth. For each week of gestation over 20 weeks, the corresponding fundal height should match in centimeters. For example, at 28 weeks this patient's fundal height should be close to 28 cm. When the fundal height and gestational age are discordant by 3 or more centimeters, a fetal ultrasound is indicated to better assess fetal growth. It is also very important to reevaluate the patient's dating criteria to ensure that the growth discrepancy is not related to dating error. Fetal NSTs can be used to evaluate fetal well-being but not to determine fetal growth, which is most concerning at this time. Group B streptococcus cultures are collected around 35 to 36 weeks of gestation or sooner if preterm birth is suspected. Intrauterine infection can lead to SGA fetuses. TORCH titers are commonly collected in the evaluation of the SGA fetus: "To" stands for toxoplasmosis, "R" for Rubella, "C" for CMV, and "H" for herpes. Toxoplasmosis is acquired either by consuming infected undercooked meat or through contact with infected cat feces. One third of women have antibodies to toxoplasmosis, indicating previous exposure. The frequency of seroconversion during pregnancy is approximately 5%. In women who are exposed to toxoplasmosis for the first time in pregnancy, rates of fetal infection are 10% to 15% in the first trimester, 25% in the second trimester, and 60% in the third trimester. Although increasing gestational age is associated with increased risk of infection, the severity diminishes. Fifty-five percent to 85% of infants will develop sequelae to infection with toxoplasmosis, which includes IUGR, microcephaly, chorioretinitis, intracranial calcifications, hearing loss, mental retardation, hepatosplenomegaly, ascites, periventricular calcifications, ventriculomegaly, and seizures. Fetal rubella infection depends on gestational age and is worse if acquired in early gestation. Fetal growth retardation is the most common effect, followed by sensorineural hearing loss, cardiac lesions, and eye defects. These findings are generally seen only in fetuses infected in the first 12 weeks of gestation. Primary maternal infection with CMV complicates 0.7% to 4% of pregnancies and results in mental retardation, microcephaly, chorioretinitis, and cerebral calcifications. It is the most common congenital infection in pregnancy. Congenital herpes virus is rare and is associated with growth restriction, eye disease, microcephaly, or hydranencephaly. Amniocentesis can be performed to evaluate for fetal chromosomal abnormalities or intrauterine infection. It is not indicated at this point in the evaluation for SGA.

VIGNETTE 1 Question 2
2. Answer C:
Tobacco abuse causes IUGR by directly affecting fetal growth. Tobacco use reduces uterine blood flow to the placenta and impairs fetal oxygenation. It is a major cause of growth restriction in women who are tobacco smokers. It is imperative to counsel women who smoke on the risks of IUGR and provide support for smoking cessation in pregnancy. Congenital anomalies are a cause of IUGR but are unlikely to be a major source of IUGR in this patient, who had a normal ultrasound at 20 weeks. Congenital CMV infection is less likely to be the cause of IUGR in this case. Seroconversion in the mother is more common in day care workers, individuals of lower socioeconomic status, as well as those with increased parity, abnormal Pap smear

history, and multiple sexual partners. Chemotherapy exposure during pregnancy is a known risk for IUGR. Prior history of chemotherapy should not directly impact a pregnancy. Genetic potential refers to the fetus's inherent growth potential. In this mother, we know that she is of average height and weight. Poor nutritional status can contribute to IUGR. There is not enough information to gather what the fetus's growth potential may be otherwise, and therefore, this is not the best answer.

VIGNETTE 1 Question 3
3. Answer C:
Although no one answer is perfect, the best answer is fetal ultrasound every 2 to 3 weeks. It is important to monitor the fetus for interval growth and ensure that fetal growth continues. Ultrasound is usually combined with fetal testing such as NST or BPP with AFI on a weekly or twice weekly basis. At 30 weeks of gestation, NST is not a great modality because it may be more commonly false negative (falsely nonreassuring), but it is commonly used in this setting. Induction of labor is not yet indicated at this time. Delivery is warranted when the benefits of the intrauterine environment are outweighed by the risks to the fetus. Fetal testing done with NST or BPP suggests a compromised intrauterine environment when testing indicates acidemia. A reactive NST displaying two accelerations in 20 minutes reassures the provider that the fetus is not acidotic. Similarly, an abnormal BPP can help predict the pH in an IUGR fetus. Before induction of labor of a 30-week fetus, the mother should receive betamethasone to improve fetal outcomes after birth. Given the fetus' poor growth, this patient's care is no longer routine and will require additional testing and monitoring. Admission to the hospital for daily NST and BPP is not the best answer. Although this may be an option for management, it is more common to start with twice weekly testing with NST and once weekly BPP and Doppler testing. If abnormal testing develops, it may become appropriate to admit the patient to the hospital for more frequent monitoring such as daily NST, twice weekly BPP, AFI, and Doppler testing. Doppler velocimetry is a valuable tool to try to predict placental dysfunction. Decreased oxygen delivery to the fetus can trigger changes in the vascular smooth muscle tone of the fetus. Changes in the flow resistance through the umbilical artery can be measured and used to predict fetal well-being and placental dysfunction. Late signs of dysfunction such as reversed end-diastolic flow suggest fetal acidemia, and delivery is warranted. Frequent Doppler testing is only performed when abnormalities have been identified on prior testing. In that scenario, repeat testing is done to help guide delivery planning.

VIGNETTE 1 Question 4
4. Answer E:
This scenario describes IUGR. Elevated Doppler of the umbilical artery and declining weight raise the concern for fetal well-being. It is possible that this patient may require premature delivery if fetal condition deteriorates further. To improve outcomes in the neonate, betamethasone should be administered at this time. Ultrasound should be repeated in 2 to 3 weeks to assess growth. Even with fetal lung maturity documented, one would not deliver on this basis alone. The decision to deliver in this setting would be based on nonreassuring fetal testing, for example, a worsening Doppler ultrasound of the umbilical artery or a nonreassuring BPP. If fetal status changes, such as absent or reversed Doppler flow, delivery will be indicated regardless of fetal lung maturity.

VIGNETTE 1 Question 5
5. Answer D:
Cord prolapse is not a direct consequence of oligohydramnios, nor is it strongly associated with oligohydramnios. It is seen more commonly in women with polyhydramnios. Meconium, cesarean section, FHR decelerations, and nonreactive fetal tracing are all associated with oligohydramnios in labor.

VIGNETTE 2 Question 1
1. Answer A:
Macrosomic neonates are most at risk for neonatal jaundice, hypoglycemia, birth trauma, hypocalcemia, and childhood cancers such as leukemia, osteosarcoma, or Wilms tumor. Asthma has not been shown to be associated with fetal macrosomia. Hypoglycemia is thought to be due to maternal hyperglycemia resulting in fetal hyperglycemia and hyperinsulinemia. Beta-cell hyperplasia also occurs, and immediately after birth when the umbilical cord is clamped, the neonate experiences a sudden drop in blood glucose level likely because of an exaggerated insulin release after delivery. In macrosomic infants, as many as 50% can experience hypoglycemia, and this rate is lowered to 5% to 15% when tight glucose control is achieved in the latter half of pregnancy as well as during the labor process. Neonatal jaundice occurs in approximately 25% to 50% of pregnancies complicated by GDM. The pathogenesis is unclear but may be related to polycythemia. Birth trauma is directly related to the risk of shoulder dystocia in mothers with diabetes and macrosomic infants. Birth injury can be a transient palsy to permanent neurologic deficits or even death.

VIGNETTE 2 Question 2
2. Answer B:
This mother has gestational diabetes. Fetal macrosomia complicates as many as 50% of pregnancies in women

with gestational diabetes, including women treated with intensive glycemic control. The Pedersen hypothesis proposes that maternal hyperglycemia results in fetal hyperglycemia and hyperinsulinemia, which in turn results in excessive fetal growth. Although the patient gained 35 lb, it is still within the recommended weight gain guidelines of 25 to 35 lb for a woman with a normal prepregnancy BMI. She actually achieved good glucose control during the pregnancy. Target fasting levels are less than 90; 1-hour postprandial values should be less than 140, and 2-hour postprandial values less than 120. However, even with reasonable control, women with GDM are at increased risk of having a fetus with macrosomia. Advanced maternal age has been found to be associated with macrosomia but may be related because of an increased rate of diabetes in older women. Postterm pregnancies are at increased risk for fetal macrosomia because of the additional time in utero that the fetus has to grow. However, postterm is beyond 42 weeks' gestation.

VIGNETTE 2 Question 3

3. Answer E:
Perform a 2-hour glucose tolerance test. Women who develop GDM are at increased risk of developing type 2 diabetes later in life. All women with GDM should have a 2-hour glucose challenge test at or around their 6-week postpartum visit. It is best to actually give the patient the laboratory slip to obtain the test prior to the 6-week follow-up visit so that the results can be discussed at the visit. This test helps to identify those women who either have type 2 diabetes or who remain at high risk because of insulin insensitivity. Education, diet, and exercise are mainstay treatments to improve insulin sensitivity. Although this patient should eventually lose weight down to and even slightly below her prepregnancy weight, this does not need to occur immediately. She does not need to lose 20% of her body weight, which would potentially make her underweight. Weight loss can be challenging after childbirth, and breastfeeding is a very effective way for women to return toward their prepregnancy weight in the postpartum period. The RPR is often obtained twice during pregnancy, but not needed postpartum. Once the placenta is delivered, the patient's insulin demands decline dramatically. For type 1 and type 2 diabetic patients, prepregnancy doses of insulin are resumed. For patients with gestational diabetes, all medications are stopped. It is not standard of care to continue GDM patients on antihyperglycemic medications unless there is a suspicion for type 2 diabetes or they have a diagnostic 2-hour glucose tolerance test.

VIGNETTE 2 Question 4

4. Answer D:
In patients with a history of gestational diabetes, it is valuable to perform an early glucose tolerance test to evaluate for type 2 diabetes. Because she has not had any routine health care in the past 2 years, she has not been screened for development of diabetes. Early diagnosis improves outcomes because patients can be educated on diet and started on insulin-lowering medications if indicated. If the patient has elevated blood glucose values that suggest type 2 diabetes, then answer options a, b, c, and e should be performed for the patient at that time. In patients with type 2 diabetes, eye examination is recommended to evaluate for retinopathy, which can worsen in pregnancy.

VIGNETTE 3 Question 1

1. Answer B:
Monochorionic–diamniotic twinning results from cleavage between 3 and 8 days and occurs after placental differentiation has occurred but prior to amnion formation. This leads to the formation of a single placenta but two amnions. Dichorionic–diamniotic twins result from cleavage of the fertilized ovum during the first 2 to 3 days. Cleavage at this stage occurs before cells are differentiated to form the trophoblast. As a result, two placentas (chorions) and two amnions develop. Embryo cleavage between days 8 and 13 again occurs after differentiation of the trophoblast but also after formation of the amnion. This results in a monochorionic and monoamniotic gestation. After day 15 of development, only a singleton pregnancy will result.

VIGNETTE 3 Question 2

2. Answer A:
Twin-to-twin transfusion syndrome (TTTS) is characterized by one twin who is the donor and the other who is the recipient. The placenta has shared vascular connections between monochorionic twins, and in some gestations, these connections are markedly unequal and result in one twin receiving more blood flow than the other. The donor twin is typically smaller, anemic, and has less amniotic fluid, which can lead to hypovolemia, growth restriction, and oligohydramnios. The recipient twin is generally larger, polycythemic, and occasionally hydropic as the result of hypervolemia. Cardiomegaly and glomerulotubal hypertrophy, edema, and ascites result. Monitoring for development of TTTS is recommended early in the gestation, and ultrasounds to assess fetal growth should occur every 2 weeks, starting around 16 weeks. About 15% of monochorionic twins will develop TTTS. The earlier it is diagnosed, the poorer the prognosis. The mainstay of treatment of severe cases of TTTS today is laser ablation of placental anastomoses with perinatal survival rates between 53% and 69%. Other treatments include serial reduction amniocentesis and amniotic septostomy. Anemia, growth restriction, oligohydramnios, and hypovolemia are all findings in the donor twin.

VIGNETTE 3 Question 3

3. Answer B:
In this answer, twin A is 925 g smaller than twin B, so more than 20% discordant (925/3,775). For twins, if both are cephalic, vaginal delivery is usually reasonable to attempt. However, with vertex/breech twins, the second twin should not be more than 20% discordant; if the second twin is significantly larger than the first, then there can be head entrapment during the breech extraction. In fact, some clinicians are uncomfortable with offering breech extraction of the second twin if it is even slightly larger than the first. In all cases, counseling and informed consent should include discussion of the possible need for an emergent cesarean delivery of the second twin should cord prolapse, fetal distress, or placental abruption occur and delivery not be imminent. Answer options a, c, d, and e are appropriate scenarios for a trial of labor.

VIGNETTE 4 Question 1

1. Answer A:
The most common reason for postterm pregnancy is inaccurate dating. It is very common for a woman to be uncertain of the first date of her LMP. As a result, we must rely on ultrasound for dating the pregnancy, and ultrasound is not without errors. Ultrasound dating is best when performed in the first trimester and may have up to a 1 week error in either direction of the proposed due date. For pregnancies dated during the second trimester, the error may be as great at 2 weeks, and in the third trimester, as much as 3 weeks. Fetal anomaly is occasionally a cause of postterm pregnancy but is not the most common cause. Delayed presentation to prenatal care is a problem that contributes to delay and inaccurate dating but is not the most specific answer in this case. Advanced maternal age (AMA) and multiparity do not contribute to postterm pregnancy.

VIGNETTE 4 Question 2

2. Answer D:
NSTs are generally not indicated in a routine pregnancy until the pregnancy goes into the 41st week. Therefore, in a routine pregnancy, a patient is usually scheduled for an NST during the 41st week, which is between the 40 0/7 and 41 0/7 weeks of gestation. If the pregnancy continues into the 42nd week, in other words between 41 and 42 weeks, the patient should receive an NST twice during that week as well as a BPP on one of the visits. If nonreassuring testing is identified, induction of labor is initiated.

VIGNETTE 4 Question 3

3. Answer A:
Postterm pregnancy is not associated with transient tachypnea of the newborn, which is seen more commonly in cesarean deliveries and in early term births at 37 and 38 weeks of gestation. Oligohydramnios, macrosomia, meconium aspiration, and intrauterine fetal demise are all risks associated with postterm pregnancy.

VIGNETTE 4 Question 4

4. Answer D:
The patient should be seen on labor and delivery triage as soon as possible. Given her gestational age and risk for adverse pregnancy outcome, it is best to perform monitoring this evening. Delayed care could have disastrous consequences. In patients less than 40 weeks of gestation, it may be acceptable to have them perform kick counts at home prior to presentation. Kick counts involve the women resting in a quiet room and counting fetal movements over time. In general, 6 movements in the first hour or 10 movements in 2 hours suggest reassuring fetal status. However, although widely used, there is no strong evidence to support the use of kick counts in predicting fetal well-being. Answer options b, c, and e all delay presentation and evaluation of fetal well-being and are therefore not the best answer choices. At 41 2/7 weeks, even if the fetal testing were reassuring, it would be reasonable to recommend induction of labor in this setting.

8 | Hypertension and Pregnancy

One of the physiologic changes that occur during pregnancy is a decrease in blood pressure (BP). This occurs as a result of decreased systemic vascular resistance starting in the latter half of the first trimester and reaching its nadir in the midsecond trimester. During the third trimester, BP will slowly increase back to baseline, but should not become higher than a patient's prepregnancy BP. Abnormal BP during pregnancy is classified into categories based on preexisting hypertension (chronic hypertension) and gestational hypertension (GH). Chronic hypertension is seen increasingly in pregnancy and is associated with increased risk of maternal and neonatal morbidity. Alternatively, hypertension may be caused by the pregnancy, as with GH, preeclampsia, and eclampsia (Table 8-1). Liver injury is seen in a small percentage of patients with preeclampsia and is associated with two diseases in pregnancy with high morbidity and mortality: HELLP (hemolysis, elevated liver enzymes, and low platelet count) syndrome and acute fatty liver of pregnancy (AFLP). Complications from these disorders are consistently among the leading causes of maternal death in both developed and developing countries. Because treatment is delivery, these disorders are also the leading causes of premature delivery.

PREECLAMPSIA

PATHOGENESIS

Although no definitive cause for preeclampsia has been determined, it is well accepted that the underlying pathophysiology involves both maternal and fetal factors resulting in abnormal development of placental vasculature and maternal systemic endothelial dysfunction. The downstream effect of abnormal placental vascular development is placental underperfusion resulting in possible growth restriction and hypoxia. From a maternal standpoint, the endothelial dysfunction is thought to be primarily related to circulating antiangiogenic factors. This results in increased vascular permeability, activation of the coagulation cascade, microangiopathic hemolysis, and vasoconstriction manifesting clinically as hypertension, proteinuria, and other clinical manifestations of the disease.

As outlined in Table 8-2, major fetal complications of preeclampsia are caused by prematurity. Also, the generalized vasoconstriction of preeclampsia can result in decreased blood flow to the placenta. This may manifest as acute uteroplacental insufficiency, resulting in abruption or fetal hypoxia. The uteroplacental insufficiency may also be chronic in nature and result in an intrauterine growth restricted (IUGR) fetus.

Maternal complications associated with preeclampsia (Table 8-3) are related to the generalized arteriolar vasoconstriction that affects the brain (seizure and stroke), kidneys (oliguria and renal failure), lungs (pulmonary edema), liver (edema and subcapsular hematoma), and small blood vessels (thrombocytopenia and disseminated intravascular coagulation [DIC]). Studies now indicate that the complications of preeclampsia extend past the peripartum period, with preeclamptic women being at increased risk of developing cardiovascular disease later in life.

In 2013, the American College of Obstetricians and Gynecologists (ACOG) published a report from the Task Force on Hypertension in Pregnancy that created new category names for preeclampsia. Historically, preeclampsia had been described as mild or severe, but the Task Force delineated these two as preeclampsia without severe features and preeclampsia with severe features. About 10% of patients with preeclampsia with severe features develop HELLP syndrome. HELLP syndrome is a further

TABLE 8-1. Hypertensive States of Pregnancy
GH (or pregnancy-induced hypertension)
Preeclampsia without severe features
Preeclampsia with severe features
Chronic hypertension
Chronic hypertension w/superimposed preeclampsia (with or without severe features)
HELLP syndrome
AFLP
AFLP, acute fatty liver of pregnancy; GH, gestational hypertension; HELLP, hemolysis, elevated liver enzymes, and low platelet count.

subcategory of preeclampsia in which the patient presents with HEmolysis, Elevated Liver enzymes, and Low Platelets. Hypertension and proteinuria may be minimal or even absent in these patients. HELLP syndrome is uncommon, but patients who experience it decline rapidly, resulting in poor maternal and fetal outcomes. Despite careful management, HELLP syndrome results in a high rate of stillbirth (10% to 15%) and neonatal death (20% to 25%).

EPIDEMIOLOGY

Preeclampsia occurs in 5% to 6% of all live births and can develop anytime after the 20th week, but is most commonly seen in the third trimester near term. When hypertension is seen early in the second trimester (14 to 20 weeks), a hydatidiform mole or previously undiagnosed chronic hypertension should be considered. Unlike other preeclamptic patients, the patient with HELLP syndrome is more likely to be less than 36 weeks' gestation at the time of presentation. Although 80% of patients develop HELLP syndrome after being diagnosed with preeclampsia (30% with preeclampsia without severe features and 50% with

TABLE 8-2. Fetal Complications of Preeclampsia
Complications related to prematurity (if early delivery is necessary)

Acute uteroplacental insufficiency
    Placental infarct and/or abruption
    Intrapartum fetal distress
    Stillbirth (in severe cases)

Chronic uteroplacental insufficiency
    Asymmetric and symmetric SGA fetuses
    IUGR

Oligohydramnios
SGA, small for gestational age; IUGR, intrauterine growth restricted.

TABLE 8-3. Maternal Complications of Preeclampsia
Medical manifestations
Seizure
Cerebral hemorrhage
DIC and thrombocytopenia
Renal failure
Hepatic rupture or failure
Pulmonary edema
Obstetric complications
Uteroplacental insufficiency
Placental abruption
Increased premature deliveries
Increased cesarean section deliveries
DIC, disseminated intravascular coagulation.

preeclampsia with severe features), 20% of patients with HELLP syndrome have no previous history of hypertension before their diagnosis and will present merely with the symptom of right upper quadrant (RUQ) pain. Thus, any patient who presents with RUQ pain, epigastric pain, or nausea and vomiting in the third trimester should be seen immediately to rule out HELLP syndrome.

RISK FACTORS

Risk factors for preeclampsia fall essentially into two categories: those related to the manifestations of the disease (like chronic hypertension or renal disease) and those related to the immunogenic nature of preeclampsia (Table 8-4). African American race

TABLE 8-4. Risk Factors for Preeclampsia
Primarily disease related
Chronic hypertension
Chronic renal disease
Antiphospholipid antibody syndrome (APLS)
Collagen vascular disease (e.g., SLE)
Pregestational diabetes
African American
Maternal age (<20 or >35)
Primarily immunogenic related
Nulliparity
Previous preeclampsia
Multiple gestation
Abnormal placentation
New paternity
Family history
Female relatives of parturient
Mother-in-law
Cohabitation <1 y
SLE, systemic lupus erythematosus.

has been put into the disease manifestations category, because these women are more likely to have chronic hypertension, obesity, and type 2 diabetes, all of which are underdiagnosed and associated with preeclampsia. The risk factors posited to be immunogenic are particularly interesting. For example, it has been shown that in addition to a family history in the parturient, if the mother of the father of her baby (mother-in-law) had preeclampsia, the patient is at greater risk of developing preeclampsia. Further, it has been demonstrated that parental ethnic discordance slightly increases the risk of developing preeclampsia. Although multiparous women who have not had preeclampsia in the past have a decreased risk, if a woman conceives with a new father of her baby, her risk increases back to that of a nulliparous woman. A tolerance effect is seen in women who cohabitate with the father of the baby longer than 1 year prior to conceiving in comparison to women who conceive sooner. These risk factors support a theory that preeclampsia has an alloimmunogenic pathophysiology. Interestingly, smoking appears to be associated with a decreased risk of preeclampsia, a phenomenon that has not been explained.

CLINICAL MANIFESTATIONS, DIAGNOSES, AND TREATMENT

Gestational Hypertension

The diagnosis of GH is reserved for patients with elevated systolic BP of above 140 and/or diastolic BP above 90 mm Hg on two occasions at least 4 to 6 hours apart. BP should be evaluated while the patient is in a seated position because when patients lie in the supine position on their side, it lowers their BP; therefore, BP should always be taken in the seated position to obtain the most accurate reading. In all women with elevated BP, it is important to rule out preeclampsia (discussed below). Patients diagnosed with GH should be delivered at 37 weeks' gestation. Because GH is believed to be part of a continuum of hypertensive diseases in pregnancy, which includes preeclampsia, patients diagnosed prior to 37 weeks should be monitored closely for the development of preeclampsia, with twice weekly BP checks and weekly laboratory testing and antenatal fetal testing.

Preeclampsia without Severe Features

As shown in Table 8-5, preeclampsia without severe features is classically defined as a third-trimester BP greater than or equal to 140 mm Hg systolic and/or 90 mm Hg diastolic on two occasions, at least 6 hours apart, accompanied by proteinuria greater than 300 mg/24 hours or a protein to creatinine ratio of greater than or equal to 0.3. Of note, women with a protein to creatinine ratio less than 0.3 can still have greater than 300 mg on a 24-hour urine protein collection. Thus, to rule out preeclampsia, it is common to still obtain the 24-hour protein collection with a protein to creatinine ratio less than 0.3. Some investigators have proposed 0.15 as an absolute screening threshold, with those women who have a ratio less than 0.15 extremely unlikely to have 300 mg or greater of protein on a 24-hour urine collection.

Although not included in the diagnostic criteria, peripheral edema, especially of the face, hands, and feet, is commonly seen in preeclampsia. Women diagnosed with preeclampsia without severe features should be delivered at 37 weeks. Changes in recent ACOG guidelines no longer recommend administration of magnesium sulfate ($MgSO_4$) for seizure prophylaxis in this patient population. Again, given the continuum of hypertensive diseases in pregnancy and high risk of patients with preeclampsia developing severe features, these women, if diagnosed prior to 37 weeks, are commonly managed as inpatients with very close monitoring of BP, laboratory values, and fetal testing. However, in women with no other pregnancy comorbidities diagnosed prior to 37 weeks, it is possible to manage them as outpatients, provided careful patient selection and practitioner preference are ensured.

Preeclampsia with Severe Features

Criteria for preeclampsia with severe features (Table 8-5) include: BP greater than or equal to 160 mm Hg systolic and/or 110 mm Hg diastolic minutes apart in addition to proteinuria (24-hour urine protein greater than or equal to 300 mg or a protein to creatinine ratio greater than or equal to 0.3) or a BP greater than or equal to 140 mm Hg systolic and/or 90 mm Hg diastolic on two occasions in addition to one of the following: thrombocytopenia (platelets less than 100,000 μL^{-1}), renal insufficiency (creatinine greater than 1.1 mg/dL or double baseline serum creatinine), impaired liver function (liver transaminases twice normal), pulmonary edema, or cerebral or visual disturbances. Many clinical manifestations of preeclampsia are explained by vasospasm leading to necrosis and hemorrhage of organs. Patients diagnosed with preeclampsia with severe features should be delivered at 34 weeks. They should be treated with $MgSO_4$ (usually a 4 to 6 g loading dose followed by 1 to 2 g/hour through

TABLE 8-5. Criteria for Diagnosis of GH and Preeclampsia	
Gestational Hypertension	
BP	• SBP ≥ 140 mm Hg and/or DBP ≥ 90 mm Hg on two occasions at least 4 h apart after 20 wks' gestation in women with previously normal BP
Preeclampsia without severe features	
BP	• SBP ≥ 140 mm Hg and/or DBP ≥ 90 mm Hg on two occasions at least 4 h apart after 20 wks' gestation in women with previously normal BP
and	
Proteinuria	• ≥300 mg/24 h or protein/creatinine ratio ≥0.3 or dipstick reading of +1 (used only if other quantitative methods are unavailable)
Preeclampsia with severe features	
BP	• SBP ≥ 140 mm Hg and/or DBP ≥ 90 mm Hg on two occasions at least 4 h apart after 20 wk gestation in women with previously normal BP • SBP ≥ 160 mm Hg and/or DBP ≥ 110 mm Hg confirmed within a short interval (minutes) to facilitate antihypertensive therapy
and	
Proteinuria	• ≥300 mg/24 h or protein/creatinine ratio ≥0.3 or dipstick reading of +1 (used only if other quantitative methods are unavailable)
Or in the absence of proteinuria and severe range blood pressures, new onset hypertension with the new onset of any of the following:	
Thrombocytopenia	• Platelet count less than 100,000 μL^{-1}
Renal insufficiency	• Serum creatinine concentrations greater than 1.1 mg/dL or a doubling of the serum baseline creatinine concentration in the absence of other renal disease
Impaired liver function	• Elevated blood concentrations of liver transaminases to twice normal concentration
Pulmonary edema	
Cerebral or visual symptoms	

SBP, systolic blood pressure; DBP, diastolic blood pressure.

24 hours postpartum) for seizure prophylaxis. Women with BPs greater than or equal to 160 mm Hg/110 mm Hg should be quickly managed with antihypertensive therapies (usually IV labetalol, IV hydralazine, or PO nifedipine) to bring BPs out of the severe range given risk of stroke. In the event that preeclampsia with severe features is diagnosed prior to 34 weeks and maternal and fetal conditions are stable, it is recommended that women be managed expectantly until 34 weeks. Patients should receive betamethasone for fetal lung maturity through 36 weeks. Preeclampsia with severe features is not an indication for cesarean delivery, and if delivery is needed, induction of labor in appropriate patients is recommended.

Even though delivery is the cure for preeclampsia, patients can have lingering effects for up to several weeks. In fact, some women will worsen acutely in the immediate postpartum period, possibly because of the increased placental antigen exposure during labor and delivery. Because of this, seizure prophylaxis is usually continued 24 hours postpartum or until the patient improves markedly. In the setting of chronically elevated BPs, antihypertensive medications (most commonly labetalol and nifedipine) should be initiated, and, in some cases, patients may need to continue medications for several weeks after release to home.

HELLP Syndrome

As noted above, HELLP syndrome stands for hemolysis, elevated liver enzymes, and low platelets. As the name suggests, this disorder is characterized by rapidly deteriorating liver function, evidence of hemolysis, and thrombocytopenia. In addition, a number of patients will develop DIC. The criteria for diagnosis and relevant laboratory tests are outlined in Table 8-6. Liver

TABLE 8-6. Diagnosis of HELLP Syndrome

Hemolytic anemia

Schistocytes on peripheral blood smear
Elevated lactate dehydrogenase
Elevated total bilirubin

Elevated liver enzymes

Increase in aspartate aminotransferase
Increase in alanine aminotransferase

Low platelets

Thrombocytopenia

HELLP, hemolysis, elevated liver enzymes, and low platelet count.

capsule distension can produce epigastric pain, often with progressive nausea and vomiting, and can lead to hepatic rupture. Patients with HELLP syndrome who present with frank hepatic failure should be screened for AFLP. Women with HELLP syndrome diagnosed after 34 0/7 weeks should be delivered soon after maternal stabilization. Those diagnosed prior to 34 weeks should be delivered 24 to 48 hours after administration of betamethasone for fetal lung maturity if maternal and fetal conditions remain stable. These women should also be given $MgSO_4$ for seizure prophylaxis through 24 hours postpartum.

Acute Fatty Liver of Pregnancy

It is unclear whether AFLP is truly in the spectrum of preeclamptic syndromes or an entirely separate entity with similar signs and symptoms. More than 50% of patients with AFLP will also have hypertension and proteinuria. It presents in approximately 1 in 10,000 pregnancies and has a high mortality rate. Interestingly, it has been found that a number of AFLP patients will have fetuses with long-chain hydroxyacyl-CoA dehydrogenase deficiency or medium-chain hydroxyacyl-CoA dehydrogenase deficiency. AFLP can be difficult to distinguish from HELLP syndrome, but typically women with AFLP exhibit evidence of liver failure, including an elevated ammonia level, blood glucose less than 50 mg/dL, and markedly reduced fibrinogen and antithrombin III levels. Management of such patients involves maternal stabilization and prompt delivery of the fetus regardless of gestational age. AFLP is associated with significant morbidity, including the need for liver transplant and high maternal mortality rates.

Follow-Up

Women who develop preeclampsia during their first pregnancy will have a 25% to 33% recurrence rate in subsequent pregnancies. In patients with both chronic hypertension and preeclampsia, the risk of recurrence is 70%. It is now recommended that women with a history of preeclampsia, multiple gestations, chronic hypertension, diabetes, renal disease, or autoimmune disease receive low-dose aspirin after 12 weeks to help reduce the risk of preeclampsia. Calcium supplementation has also been associated with decreased rates of subsequent preeclampsia, but one large randomized controlled trial found no difference between calcium and placebo.

ECLAMPSIA

Eclampsia is the occurrence of grand mal seizures in the preeclamptic patient that cannot be attributed to other causes. A seizure in a pregnant woman should be assumed to be eclampsia until proven otherwise. It occurs in 2% to 3% of women with severe features of preeclampsia but can also occur in women with preeclampsia without severe features. The overall incidence of eclampsia is roughly 2 to 10 per 10,000. The cause of eclampsia is poorly understood but is thought to result from a breakdown in the autoregulatory system of cerebral circulation due to hyperperfusion, endothelial dysfunction, and brain edema. Complications of eclampsia include cerebral hemorrhage, aspiration pneumonia, hypoxic encephalopathy, and thromboembolic events.

CLINICAL MANIFESTATIONS

Seizures in the eclamptic patient are tonic–clonic in nature and may or may not be preceded by an aura. These seizures may develop before labor (59%), during labor (20%), or after delivery (21%). Most postpartum seizures occur within the first 48 hours after delivery, but will occasionally occur as late as several weeks after delivery. Fetal bradycardia can also occur during and after an eclamptic seizure. In general, the fetal tracing improves with supportive maternal care, fetal resuscitative measures, and seizure resolution.

TREATMENT

Eclampsia is a clinical diagnosis and should be treated promptly upon recognition. Treatment strategies for eclamptic patients include seizure management, BP control, and prophylaxis against further convulsions. Seizure management should always start with the ABCs (airway, breathing, circulation), although the majority of seizures are unwitnessed by clinicians and will resolve spontaneously without major morbidity. Hypertension management can usually be achieved using hydralazine or labetalol

TABLE 8-7. Clinical Response to Serum MgSO$_4$ Concentrations

Serum Concentration MgSO$_4$ (mg/mL)	Clinical Response
4.8–8.4	Therapeutic seizure prophylaxis
8	CNS depression
10	Loss of deep tendon reflexes
15	Respiratory depression/paralysis
17	Coma
20–25	Cardiac arrest

MgSO$_4$, magnesium sulfate; CNS, central nervous system.

to lower the BP to less than 160/110 mm Hg. For seizure control and prophylaxis, eclamptic patients are treated with MgSO$_4$ to decrease hyperreflexia and prevent further seizures by raising the seizure threshold. In prospective, randomized studies, magnesium has been found to be as good as or better than phenytoin, carbamazepine, and phenobarbital in the prevention of recurrent seizures in eclamptic patients. In eclampsia, MgSO$_4$ therapy is initiated at the time of diagnosis and continued for 12 to 24 hours after delivery. The goal of MgSO$_4$ therapy is to reach a therapeutic level, although avoiding toxicity through careful clinical monitoring (Table 8-7). In the case of overdose, 10 mL 10% calcium chloride or calcium gluconate should be rapidly administered intravenously for cardiac protection.

Delivery should be initiated only after the eclamptic patient has been stabilized and convulsions have been controlled. It is common for prolonged fetal heart rate (FHR) decelerations to occur in the setting of an eclamptic seizure. The most appropriate way to treat the fetus is to stabilize the mother by establishing adequate maternal oxygenation and cardiac output. Occasionally, the FHR abnormalities will not resolve, and emergent cesarean delivery will be necessary. Otherwise, cesarean delivery should be reserved for obstetric indications, and such patients can undergo an induction of labor after they are stabilized.

CHRONIC HYPERTENSION

PATHOGENESIS

Chronic hypertension is defined as hypertension present before conception, before 20 weeks' gestation, or persisting more than 6 weeks postpartum. For women who present without prenatal care prior to 20 weeks of gestation, this can be difficult to differentiate from GH. Approximately one-third of patients with chronic hypertension in pregnancy will develop superimposed preeclampsia. Because of poor vascular development, the fetus may suffer from IUGR, and the mother is at increased risk for superimposed preeclampsia, premature delivery, and abruptio placentae.

TREATMENT

Treatment of mild chronic hypertension is controversial. However, patients with controlled BPs tend to have fewer complications in pregnancy. Patients with chronic hypertension whose BPs in early pregnancy are consistently 140/90 mm Hg or less can be managed expectantly. Antihypertensives are used in patients with persistently elevated BPs or in those who were already on medications prior to pregnancy. The two most common medications used are labetalol (a beta-blocker with concomitant alpha blockade) and nifedipine (a peripheral calcium channel blocker). In retrospective studies, beta-blocker use has been associated with decreased birth weight. However, these studies are likely biased by the severity of disease. Because these patients are at risk for other complications of chronic hypertension, baseline labs (complete blood count, complete metabolic panel [CMP]) and a baseline 24-hour urine collection for creatinine clearance and protein should be obtained. This will also help differentiate superimposed preeclampsia from chronic renal disease later in pregnancy. It is also important to get a baseline ECG in patients with chronic hypertension to ensure that there is no current cardiac compromise requiring further evaluation. Low-dose aspirin should be initiated after 12 weeks to reduce the risk of developing superimposed preeclampsia.

CHRONIC HYPERTENSION WITH SUPERIMPOSED PREECLAMPSIA

One-third or more of patients with chronic hypertension will develop superimposed preeclampsia. Because the hypertension is longstanding, complications such as IUGR and placental abruption are more common. The diagnosis can sometimes be difficult to make because many of these patients will have concomitant renal disease at baseline. The diagnosis of superimposed preeclampsia can be made in patients with increasingly elevated BPs and new or worsening proteinuria. Patients meet criteria for superimposed preeclampsia with severe features if they exhibit evidence of end-organ damage (Table 8-5). Historically, an increase in the systolic blood pressure (SBP) of 30 mm Hg or in the SBP of 15 mm Hg over prepregnancy BP was also indicative of superimposed preeclampsia, but experts disagree on how to use BP changes in the diagnosis of superimposed preeclampsia. If a 24-hour urine protein becomes elevated and is greater than 300 mg/24 hours, the diagnosis is clearly superimposed preeclampsia; if not, then the BP can be managed with increasing dosages of medications. In patients who have baseline renal disease as well, an elevated uric acid above 6.0 to 6.5 is sometimes used to differentiate preeclampsia from exacerbation of hypertension. Of course, if any of the severe preeclampsia signs and symptoms are present, this points to a diagnosis of severe superimposed preeclampsia.

KEY POINTS

- Preeclampsia without severe features is the presence of hypertension (≥140/90 mm Hg) and proteinuria (protein to creatinine ratio ≥0.3 or ≥300 mg/24 hours).
- Preeclampsia has an incidence of 5% to 6% of all live births and occurs most commonly in nulliparous women in their third trimester.
- Preeclampsia is characterized by generalized multiorgan endothelial dysfunction and vasospasm that can lead to seizure, stroke, renal failure, liver damage, DIC, or fetal demise.
- Risk factors for preeclampsia include nulliparity, multiple gestation, and chronic hypertension.
- Preeclampsia is ultimately treated with delivery, but seizures can be prevented with magnesium sulfate, and BPs can be controlled with antihypertensive medications.
- Eclampsia is the occurrence of grand mal seizures in the preeclamptic patient that cannot be attributed to other causes.
- Patients present with eclamptic seizures occurring before labor (59%), during labor (20%), or after delivery (21%).
- Eclampsia is treated with seizure management and prophylaxis with magnesium sulfate, hypertension management with hydralazine, and delivery only after the patient has been stabilized.
- Chronic hypertension is defined as hypertension occurring before conception, before 20 weeks' gestation, or persisting more than 6 weeks postpartum.
- Chronic hypertension leads to superimposed preeclampsia in one-third of patients.
- Chronic hypertension is generally treated with antihypertensives, commonly nifedipine or labetalol.
- Baseline laboratory values (CBC, AST, ALT, and Cr), an ECG, and a 24-hour urine collection for protein and creatinine should be performed in patients with chronic hypertension.

CLINICAL VIGNETTES

VIGNETTE 1

A 36-year-old G2P1001 woman at 12 weeks' gestation presents to clinic for a routine prenatal visit. She reports that her nausea has resolved and denies vaginal bleeding. Her pregnancy has been uncomplicated. Her prior pregnancy 2 years ago was complicated by the diagnosis of GH that led to an induction of labor and cesarean delivery. She has no other medical history. On examination, her BP is 138/84 mm Hg, her body mass index (BMI) is 36 kg/m, and a urine dip shows trace protein.

1. Given her history of gestational hypertension (GH) and the BP today, what diagnosis is most likely?
    a. Gestational diabetes
    b. GH
    c. Preeclampsia
    d. Chronic hypertension
    e. HELLP syndrome

2. Which of the following laboratory tests should be ordered today?
   a. Quad screen
   b. 24-hour urine protein collection
   c. HgbA1c
   d. Low-density lipoprotein (LDL)
   e. Herpes simplex virus (HSV) titer

3. Which of the following pregnancy complications is not associated with chronic hypertension?
   a. Superimposed preeclampsia
   b. Placental abruption
   c. Placenta previa
   d. Preterm delivery
   e. Intrauterine growth restriction

4. The patient's 24-hour urine shows 100 mg of protein. You counsel the patient on the pregnancy complications associated with chronic hypertension as well as management. What is the next best step in her management?
   a. Expectant management with close observation for early signs of preeclampsia and fetal growth restriction
   b. Start antihypertensive therapy
   c. Hospitalization for further maternal and fetal testing
   d. Bed rest
   e. Recommend termination of pregnancy

VIGNETTE 2

A 17-year-old G1P0 woman presents at 25 weeks' gestation complaining of headache for the past 36 hours. She has had regular prenatal visits going back to her first prenatal visit at 8 weeks' gestation. A 20-week ultrasound redated her pregnancy by 2 weeks because it was 15 days earlier than her last menstrual period dating. She has a BP of 155/104 mm Hg.

1. Which of the following is the most important question to ask on history?
   a. Do you have heartburn?
   b. Do you have low back pain?
   c. Are you constipated?
   d. Do you have pain in your right upper abdomen?
   e. Do you have urinary frequency?

2. Which of the following would NOT help to determine her diagnosis?
   a. Baseline or prepregnancy BP
   b. Bilirubin levels
   c. Urine dip for protein
   d. Complete blood count (CBC)
   e. AST and ALT

3. You review her medical record and determine that she does not have chronic hypertension. The patient denies having right upper quadrant (RUQ) pain, but because of your high suspicion of preeclampsia with severe features, you order a CBC, liver enzymes, renal function test, and a urine protein to creatinine (P/C) ratio. Her laboratory test results reveal a normal platelet count and liver enzymes but a slightly elevated P/C ratio of 0.5. Her headache has resolved after a dose of acetaminophen. What is the next best step in her management?
   a. Give her a prescription for labetalol and have her follow-up in clinic in 2 weeks
   b. (a) plus bed rest
   c. Hospitalization for further evaluation and treatment
   d. Immediate delivery
   e. Begin induction of labor

4. Over the next 12 hours, her systolic blood pressures (SBPs) rise above 160 mm Hg on several occasions, most notably to 174/102 mm Hg 2 hours after admission and to 168/96 mm Hg 9 hours after admission. Her headache does not return, and she has no RUQ pain or visual symptoms. A set of repeat laboratory test results is unchanged, and by increasing her labetalol dose to 400 mg TID, her BPs decrease to 140s to 150s/70 to 90 mm Hg. She is also started on magnesium sulfate ($MgSO_4$). What change in physical or laboratory examination do you observe that would indicate delivery?
   a. Another BP of 174/102 mm Hg
   b. Headache returning
   c. Double vision
   d. Platelets of 108
   e. AST of 265

5. Forty-eight hours later, she has completed the course of betamethasone, her $MgSO_4$ is stopped, and her laboratory test results have been stable, and she has had no further headaches. Your next plan of care is:
   a. Discharge home for expectant management
   b. Discharge home on bed rest
   c. Continue to expectantly manage in hospital with close monitoring
   d. Remain in hospital for 48 more hours and then consider discharge home on bed rest
   e. Continue to expectantly manage in hospital for 48 more hours and then move toward delivery

VIGNETTE 3

A 26-year-old G1P0 woman presents for a prenatal visit at 34 weeks' gestation. She complains of some mild nausea and vomiting over the past 3 days. She has no headache and no visual changes. Her BP is 142/83 mm Hg. On examination, she has +1 lower extremity pitting edema, and +3 reflexes bilaterally with four beats of clonus. A urinalysis dip has +1 protein.

1. Which of the following questions would be helpful?
   a. Do you have double vision?
   b. Do you have pain radiating down your legs?
   c. Are you constipated?
   d. Do you have pain in your right upper abdomen?
   e. Do you have ringing in your ears?

2. Which of the following laboratory tests would NOT be helpful at this point?
   a. Platelets
   b. WBC
   c. Liver function tests (LFTs)
   d. Lactate dehydrogenase (LDH)
   e. Obstetric ultrasound

3. The laboratory test results come back with elevated LFTs, low platelets, a normal hematocrit (Hct), and an elevated LDH. What is her diagnosis?
   a. Preeclampsia
   b. Eclampsia
   c. Chronic hypertension
   d. HELLP syndrome
   e. GH

4. The next step in her management is:
   a. Schedule a follow-up appointment in 1 week
   b. Start oral nifedipine
   c. IV hydralazine
   d. induction of labor
   e. immediate cesarean delivery

VIGNETTE 4

A 17-year-old G1P0 woman presents to labor and delivery complaining of contractions at 38 weeks' gestation. Her BP at the beginning of pregnancy was 90/60 mm Hg. She has gained 46 lb throughout pregnancy (10 lb in the past 4 weeks). Her BP on presentation was 145/80 mm Hg. A urine dip is +1 protein. On examination, her cervix is 3 cm dilated, 90% effaced, 1 station.

1. What is the next step in her management?
   a. $MgSO_4$
   b. Betamethasone
   c. Send laboratory tests
   d. Artificial rupture of the membranes
   e. Send home until in active labor

2. While you are writing a note, the patient's nurse calls out of the room that the patient is having a seizure. As you run to the patient's room, you plan your next step, which is:
   a. IV $MgSO_4$
   b. IV midazolam
   c. IV phenytoin
   d. Check the fetal heart rate (FHR)
   e. Assess the patient's airway

3. The patient's seizure is self-limited, and she is in a postictal state. Her BP is 145/96 mm Hg, O_2 saturation 96%, FHR 160s, minimal variability after a 4-minute prolonged deceleration. The IV is in and you begin a bolus of $MgSO_4$. All of the labor rooms are full, so she remains in triage. Thirty minutes later, you evaluate the fetal heart tracing. There are contractions every minute, accompanied by late decelerations with most of the contractions. The fetal heart tracing demonstrates another 6-minute prolonged late deceleration down to the 60 beats per minute, and you:
   a. wait an additional 4 to 5 minutes doing fetal resuscitative measures
   b. move immediately to the operating room
   c. perform an emergency cesarean in triage
   d. rebolus the $MgSO_4$
   e. look up her laboratory test results

ANSWERS

VIGNETTE 1 Question 1

1. Answer D:
This patient's age, BMI, history of GH, and BP indicate that the patient most likely has a diagnosis of chronic hypertension. Chronic hypertension complicates up to 5% of pregnancies in the United States. Its prevalence varies depending on the woman's age, race, and BMI. With the increasing prevalence of advanced maternal age mothers and obesity in the United States, there has been an increase in chronic hypertension during pregnancy. In pregnant women, chronic hypertension is defined as hypertension that is present before pregnancy, sustained hypertension before 20 weeks' gestation, or hypertension persisting for more than 6 weeks postpartum. As is the case with this patient, the diagnosis may be difficult in women with previously undiagnosed chronic hypertension because of the physiologic decrease in BP that usually begins in the latter half of the first trimester. This decrease may result in normal BP readings (systolic <140 mm Hg and diastolic <90 mm Hg), which will eventually increase in the third trimester. Subsequently, these women are more likely to be misdiagnosed with GH. Gestational diabetes is impairment in glucose metabolism that first presents during pregnancy. Although the patient is obese, she has no other risk factors for or history to suggest that she

has gestational diabetes. GH is defined as elevated BPs (≥140/90 mm Hg) after 20 weeks' gestation. Although GH is on the differential, this patient's elevated BPs in the first trimester make chronic hypertension more likely. Although the patient could have superimposed preeclampsia and/or HELLP syndrome, in addition to chronic hypertension, again these diagnoses are made after 20 weeks' gestation, and we need more laboratory data to make those diagnoses.

VIGNETTE 1 Question 2
2. Answer B:
The initial evaluation of women with chronic hypertension includes assessing for the presence of other medical complications and target end-organ damage associated with chronic hypertension. A baseline 24-hour urine collection should be done to assess protein and creatinine clearance. In addition to establishing a baseline, this will help to differentiate between chronic renal disease and superimposed preeclampsia later in the pregnancy. A baseline ECG is important to obtain in order to determine the patient's baseline cardiac status. A quad screen is a maternal blood screening test that looks at the levels of alpha fetoprotein, β-human chorionic gonadotropin, estradiol, and inhibin A to assess the probability of potential genetic abnormalities. Quad screens are usually performed in the second trimester between 15 and 18 weeks, assuming the patient desires genetic testing. Hemoglobin A1c, LDL, and HSV titers are not evaluated unless there is an indication. Women with pregestational diabetes may have their HgbA1c measured to assess their glucose control. LDL levels are not routinely tested because they tend to increase in pregnancy and then return to normal after delivery. HSV titers may be checked to differentiate between a primary and secondary infection if a woman has an outbreak during pregnancy. On the basis of the information given, there are no indications to test her HgbA1c, LDL, or HSV titer.

VIGNETTE 1 Question 3
3. Answer C:
Pregnant women with chronic hypertension do not have an increased risk of placenta previa. However, they are at increased risk of superimposed preeclampsia, placental abruption, preterm delivery, and small-for-gestational age infants. Depending on the severity of disease, one-third or more of pregnant women with chronic hypertension will develop superimposed preeclampsia. The diagnosis is made by worsening BPs and the presence of new onset or worsening proteinuria or evidence of end-organ damage after 20 weeks' gestation. In addition to pregnancy complications, these women are also at increased risk of maternal complications such as pulmonary edema, cerebral hemorrhage, and acute renal failure.

VIGNETTE 1 Question 4
4. Answer A:
Although treatment of mild chronic hypertension is controversial, women who are early in pregnancy with mild chronic hypertension without superimposed preeclampsia are usually managed expectantly. Although most are not treated with antihypertensives, these women are still monitored closely for signs of superimposed preeclampsia and fetal growth restriction by scheduled ultrasounds and regular laboratory tests. Those who develop severe hypertension (BPs ≥ 160/110 mm Hg) may be hospitalized for further maternal and fetal testing and then started on antihypertensive medications such as labetalol or nifedipine. Women who develop severe persistent hypertension and/or superimposed preeclampsia may be hospitalized and managed expectantly with antihypertensives until 34 weeks' gestation, when delivery is indicated. Although this patient is at increased risk of pregnancy complications, there would be no reason to recommend termination of pregnancy.

VIGNETTE 2 Question 1
1. Answer D:
This patient's BP and headache are concerning for severe preeclampsia. Although her BP may not meet severe criteria (SBP ≥160 mm Hg or diastolic blood pressure ≥ 110 mm Hg), severe preeclampsia can also be diagnosed in patients who develop other associated conditions. These include thrombocytopenia (less than 100,000 μL^{-1}), serum creatinine ≥ 1.1 mg/dL or double the baseline creatinine, transaminitis of double normal, headache or visual disturbances, and pulmonary edema. It is important to evaluate for these conditions when preeclampsia with severe features is suspected. It is thought that the pathophysiology of preeclampsia involves endothelial dysfunction, vasospasm, hemoconcentration, and capillary leakage, resulting in ischemia and hemorrhage of maternal organs such as a hepatic subscapular hematoma leading to RUQ pain. Heartburn, low back pain, constipation, and urinary frequency are common complaints associated with routine problems of pregnancy. Although it is important to address these issues, the concern for severe preeclampsia takes precedence because of the increased risk of maternal and fetal mortality.

VIGNETTE 2 Question 2
2. Answer B:
Bilirubin levels are not part of the criteria for diagnosing preeclampsia with severe features. Prepregnancy BP is important in differentiating preeclampsia with severe features from superimposed preeclampsia in a woman who has chronic hypertension, because the two diseases are managed differently and they have different prognoses. The diagnosis of preeclampsia with severe features is outlined in Table 8-5.

VIGNETTE 2 Question 3
3. Answer C:
Although the patient does not yet meet criteria for preeclampsia with severe features at this point, because her BPs are not severe and her head has resolved, her clinical picture at 25 weeks is very concerning for impending preeclampsia with severe features. Because this patient is at significant risk of developing preeclampsia with severe features at such an early gestational age, she should be hospitalized for close observation and monitoring. Management in this situation includes antihypertensive medications as indicated to keep BPs ≤ 160/110 mm Hg using oral agents such as labetalol or nifedipine, ultrasound to assess fetal growth, daily nonstress tests, and at least daily preeclampsia laboratory tests (CBC, liver enzymes, basic metabolic panel, LDH, and uric acid). Additionally, betamethasone should be given to facilitate fetal maturation, particularly the pulmonary system in women less than 36 weeks.

VIGNETTE 2 Question 4
4. Answer E:
At this gestational age, there are few clinical scenarios that force one's hand to deliver at 25 weeks' gestational age. Rapidly worsening HELLP syndrome is one of those situations. An AST of 265 is markedly elevated, far above the reference range. Elevated BPs are expected and can be managed by maxing out the first antihypertensive agent and then adding a second agent. If the headache returns, it may be due to the high BPs, so it may resolve with better BP control. Further, her previous dose of acetaminophen was several hours ago, and she can be given another dose. Double vision is common with $MgSO_4$, and although double vision is not concerning, if the patient develops scotomata in the setting of HELLP syndrome, that is concerning for worsening end-organ damage and vasospasm. Platelets of 108 are not normal but are still greater than 100,000 and so are not an indication for a 25-week delivery.

VIGNETTE 2 Question 5
5. Answer C:
Because of her elevated BPs, this patient carries a diagnosis of preeclampsia with severe features. Preeclampsia with severe features is managed in the hospital because of the need for close monitoring and treatment with antihypertensives. Thus, she should not be discharged. Rather, she should be managed expectantly with at least daily fetal and laboratory testing. Further, because she is still quite early in gestation, she should be managed expectantly until she reaches 34 weeks' gestation if maternal and fetal status allows.

VIGNETTE 3 Question 1
1. Answer D:
Although one might ask any of the questions on review of systems, the question about RUQ pain is important when evaluating a patient whose signs/symptoms are concerning for preeclampsia. In a pregnant patient with nausea and vomiting in the third trimester, it is important to know about RUQ pain because it can be related to preeclampsia with severe features and/or HELLP syndrome. Of note, another cause of nausea, vomiting, and RUQ pain common in pregnancy is cholelithiasis. Women in pregnancy can occasionally get gall bladder symptoms, even without stones, from gall bladder sludge in the setting of a fatty meal.

VIGNETTE 3 Question 2
2. Answer B:
Although one frequently orders a WBC as part of a CBC, it is not particularly useful in the setting of preeclampsia. Platelets, LFTs, LDH, Cr, Hct, and uric acid are all useful in determining whether the patient has preeclampsia. An obstetric ultrasound would be useful to assess fetal growth. If the ultrasound were to demonstrate fetal growth restriction, then assessment of umbilical artery Dopplers would also be indicated.

VIGNETTE 3 Question 3
3. Answer D:
HELLP syndrome is hemolysis, elevated liver enzymes, and low platelets. This is a severe form of preeclampsia that is typically not managed expectantly. Before 28 to 32 weeks' gestation, expectant management of HELLP syndrome has been employed in order to administer a course of betamethasone to improve fetal lung maturity followed by prompt delivery. In order to manage this disease expectantly, the patient needs to be fully informed because expectant management is more dangerous to the mother than the fetus. When expectant management of HELLP syndrome is employed, if the patient develops severe symptoms, has worsening of the laboratory test results, or when the patient completes the betamethasone course, the patient should then be delivered.

VIGNETTE 3 Question 4
4. Answer D:
HELLP syndrome is a subtype of preeclampsia with severe features. Patients with HELLP syndrome should be delivered promptly. As maternal and fetal status allow, one can defer delivery in patients with HELLP syndrome for 24 to 48 hours to administer betamethasone. In contrast, patients with preeclampsia with severe features can be expectantly managed until 34 weeks. Although some clinicians opt for delivery via cesarean in the setting of preeclampsia with severe features or HELLP syndrome, there are few data to

suggest that cesarean delivery is necessary or better than attempting induction and a trial of labor as long as the fetal status remains reassuring. The patient's BPs are not severely elevated, so she does not need IV hydralazine or oral nifedipine.

VIGNETTE 4 Question 1
1. Answer C:
This patient does not have a diagnosis of preeclampsia. However, because her BP at the beginning of pregnancy was 90/60 mm Hg, this new acute elevation is likely a sign of underlying GH or preeclampsia and should cause the astute clinician to be concerned. In order to fully evaluate this patient, serial BPs, particularly between contractions when she is in less pain, would be helpful. In addition, a set of preeclamptic laboratory tests and a urine P/C ratio should be ordered.

VIGNETTE 4 Question 2
2. Answer E:
With seizures, ABCs are first—airway, breathing, circulation. The vast majority of eclamptic seizures are self-limited, and thus there will be no need for emergent antiseizure medications. However, this is not always true, and so a basic understanding of an antiseizure algorithm is always good to have. With eclampsia, $MgSO_4$ should be given IV or IM. In this patient who is unlikely to have an IV as of yet, 10 g of IM $MgSO_4$ (two separate 5 g IM doses) is the ideal way to load the patient to prevent future seizures. However, her initial seizure does not stop, and often the fastest way to break her seizure is do with an IV benzodiazepine such as midazolam. Once the patient has been stabilized, it is important to determine the FHR. It is common for the FHR to have a deceleration during the seizure and to return to baseline after the seizure activity has resolved. If it does not, an emergent cesarean delivery may be indicated, and thus the operating room should be notified and all other key staff notified of a potential emergent cesarean delivery.

VIGNETTE 4 Question 3
3. Answer B:
First, it is not appropriate to leave a patient with presumed eclampsia in triage. They should be placed in a labor room with 1:1 nursing if at all possible. Given the frequent contractions, it is likely that she is having a placental abruption, and thus this late deceleration may be a prolonged bradycardia, necessitating an emergent delivery. By moving her to the operating room, you are better prepared to perform an emergent cesarean delivery if necessary. It is inappropriate in this setting to wait 4 to 5 minutes to see if the fetal bradycardia resolves. It is important to remember that it typically takes at least 5 minutes to move a patient to the operating room and assemble the necessary staff to start an emergent cesarean. It will take time to consent the patient in the postictal state, for the anesthesiologist to evaluate the patient, and to get the patient prepped for a cesarean. Thus, moving her to the operating room should be your top priority in this situation. Another option would have been to perform a cervical examination. If she was complete, one could perform an emergent forceps delivery. She could also have had a cord prolapse or a tetanic uterine contraction, both of which can be diagnosed by cervical examination. This should happen as one prepares to move the patient to the operating room. She is not having another seizure; there is no need for rebolusing the $MgSO_4$. Her laboratory test results are of interest, and if the anesthesiologist is planning to attempt to perform regional anesthesia, her platelet count is important to know. However, this is all secondary to moving the patient immediately to the operating room.

9 Diabetes During Pregnancy

Diabetes during pregnancy encompasses a range of disease entities that includes gestational diabetes and overt diabetes mellitus (Table 9-1). In the nonpregnant state, diabetic patients are subgrouped into two types based on the pathophysiology of their disease, whereas during pregnancy, diabetes is usually characterized as pregestational or gestational. Patients with pregestational diabetes include all those diagnosed with type 1 and type 2 diabetes mellitus prior to pregnancy. Patients with gestational diabetes are those diagnosed with carbohydrate intolerance during pregnancy. Because of a lack of routine screening for diabetes in many nonpregnant women, this latter group may occasionally include women with undiagnosed pregestational diabetes mellitus.

GESTATIONAL DIABETES MELLITUS

True **gestational diabetes mellitus** (GDM) is an impairment in carbohydrate metabolism that first manifests during pregnancy. These patients may have borderline carbohydrate metabolism impairment at baseline or be entirely normal in the nonpregnant state. However, during pregnancy, human chorionic somatomammotropin (a.k.a. human placental lactogen) and other hormones produced by the placenta act as anti-insulin agents leading to increased insulin resistance and generalized carbohydrate intolerance. This increased insulin resistance occurs in all pregnant women, but those in whom the balance between insulin function and resistance is tipped beyond a usual carbohydrate metabolism state will have elevated postprandial and occasionally fasting glucose. Because this balance between insulin production and insulin sensitivity appears to be important, it has also been hypothesized that beta cell function in the pancreas may also play a part. In particular, in animal models, it appears that there is beta cell hypertrophy that occurs in the first half of pregnancy that enables enough insulin production to overcome the increased insulin resistance produced by the placental hormones.

Because these placental hormones increase in volume with the size and function of the placenta, the carbohydrate metabolism abnormalities usually are not apparent until the late second trimester or early third trimester. Thus, women with GDM generally are not at increased risk for congenital anomalies like women with pregestational diabetes. They do, however, carry an increased risk of fetal macrosomia and birth injuries as well as neonatal hypoglycemia, hypocalcemia, hyperbilirubinemia, and polycythemia like those with pregestational diabetes. Further, these women have a 4- to 10-fold increased risk of developing type 2 diabetes mellitus (T2DM) during their lifetime.

EPIDEMIOLOGY

The incidence of GDM ranges from 1% to 12% of pregnant women depending on the population and on the screening or diagnostic test utilized. In the United States, it often has been reported to range between 5% and 8%. Higher rates of GDM are seen in women of Hispanic/Latina, Asian/Pacific Islander, and Native American descent. There is also evidence to suggest that paternal race/ethnicity in these three groups is associated with GDM. Initial studies found higher rates of GDM among African-American women. However, subsequent studies controlling for maternal BMI have found little difference in incidence between African Americans and Caucasians. Other risk factors include increasing maternal age, obesity, family history of diabetes, history of a previous infant weighing more than 4,000 g, and previous stillborn infant.

TABLE 9-1. White Classification for Diabetes During Pregnancy

Classification	Description
Class A₁	Gestational diabetes; diet controlled
Class A₂	Gestational diabetes; insulin controlled
Class B	Onset: age 20 or older Duration: <10 y
Class C	Onset: age 10–19 Duration: 10–19 y
Class D	Onset: before age 10 Duration: >20 y
Class F	Diabetic nephropathy
Class R	Proliferative retinopathy
Class RF	Retinopathy and nephropathy
Class H	Ischemic heart disease
Class T	Prior renal transplantation

DIAGNOSTIC EVALUATION

The best time to screen for diabetes during pregnancy is at the end of the second trimester between 24 and 28 weeks of gestation in women with low risk for GDM. However, to identify women with preexisting T2DM, patients with one or more risk factors for developing GDM should be screened at their first prenatal visit as part of initial prenatal laboratory tests. If such testing is negative, patients are screened for GDM in the early third trimester (24 to 28 weeks of gestation).

There are a variety of proposed methods of screening for diabetes during pregnancy (Table 9-2). In the United States, the most common laboratory screening test consists of giving a 50-g glucose load and then measuring the plasma glucose 1 hour later. If the 1-hour glucose level is greater than 140 mg/dL, then the test is considered positive, and a glucose tolerance test (GTT), which often consists of a 100-g glucose load, is indicated. Screening thresholds of 130 or 135 mg/dL have been proposed; this would increase the sensitivity of the test but at a cost of a larger proportion of women who will screen positive and thus need subsequent confirmatory testing. Thus, the optimal screen-positive threshold that maximizes sensitivity and costs is still under intense research and requires further elucidation.

Women with a positive screening test are diagnosed with a 100-g, 3-hour oral GTT to evaluate their carbohydrate metabolism (Table 9-3). To conduct the GTT, the patient is given 100 g of oral glucose after an 8-hour overnight fast preceded by a 3-day special carbohydrate diet. Glucose levels are measured immediately before glucose administration (fasting) and again at 1, 2, and 3 hours after the load. If two or more of the four values are elevated, a diagnosis of GDM is made. The values shown in Table 9-3 reflect recently lowered values that will increase the number of women diagnosed with GDM.

More recently, the American Diabetes Association (ADA), the World Health Organization, and the International Association of Diabetes in Pregnancy Study Group have recommended that women in pregnancy are screened and diagnosed with a single test similar to that for nonpregnant individuals. The test would be a fasting blood glucose followed by a 75-g load and then a 1-hour and a 2-hour blood glucose assessments. The diagnosis of GDM would be made with one out of the three values being elevated. These recommendations are in part based on the findings from the Hyperglycemia and Pregnancy Outcomes (HAPO) study. In the HAPO study, women with either an elevated fasting blood glucose, 1-hour postprandial glucose, or 2-hour postprandial glucose all had higher risks of a wide range of neonatal complications. Thus, those

TABLE 9-2. Glucose Screening Tests During Pregnancy

	Normal Glucose Test Level (mg/dL)
Fasting	<105
1 h after a 50-g glucose load	<140

TABLE 9-3. Three-Hour GTT: Venous and Plasma Criteria for GDM[a]

Timing of Glucose Measurement	Normal Venous Blood Glucose (mg/dL)	Normal Whole Plasma Glucose (mg/dL)
Fasting	90	105
1 h	165	190
2 h	145	165
3 h	125	145

[a]Results reflect upper limits of normal. Diagnosis of gestational diabetes is made if fasting value or any two values are exceeded. GTT, glucose tolerance test; GDM, gestational diabetes mellitus.

groups recommending the lower threshold, single test justify the change because of this prior work. Of note, a benefit in treating these patients has not, specifically, been demonstrated. The downside of this change in care would be an estimated 17% of the pregnant population being diagnosed with GDM and how to care for them all.

TREATMENT

Once the diagnosis of GDM is made, the patient is usually started on a diet recommended for patients with diabetes. The ADA diet plan of 2,200 calories per day is recommended for all patients with diabetes during pregnancy, although the total carbohydrate intake is more important. The recommended intake is approximately 200 to 220 g of carbohydrates per day. In addition, both the timing and the content of meals are important; therefore, a meal plan based on intake of 30 to 35 kcal/kg of ideal body weight is suggested. Patients are taught to count carbohydrates, and meals are designed to contain between 30 and 45 g of carbohydrates at breakfast, 45 and 60 g of carbohydrates for lunch and dinner, and 15 g of carbohydrates for snacks. Although on this diet, the patient also monitors her blood glucose levels four times per day, which includes a fasting and three postprandial values. In addition to diet, mild exercise, usually postprandial walking, is encouraged as well. The best way for walking to enhance postprandial blood glucose control is to have the woman walk for 15 minutes about 30 to 40 minutes after the meal.

If the recommended diet plus exercise controls the blood glucose levels within the target range (fasting values <90 mg/dL and 1-hour postprandial values <140 mg/dL or 2-hour postprandial values <120 mg/dL), then this management is continued throughout the pregnancy. These patients are classified as Class A_1 or diet-controlled gestational diabetic patients in the **White classification of GDM**. This classification is used as a prognostic tool to determine the likely severity of a woman's diabetes and its interaction with pregnancy; it was originally designed to predict perinatal survival. However, if more than 25% to 30% of a patient's blood glucose values are elevated, medication—usually insulin or an oral hypoglycemic agent—is indicated. These individuals are then considered Class A_2 or medication-controlled gestational diabetic patients.

In true gestational diabetic patients, fasting values are commonly normal, although postprandial values are elevated. This is because the pathophysiology is related to metabolism of large carbohydrate boluses rather than carbohydrate intolerance at baseline. These patients can be started on short-acting insulin in combination with an intermediate-acting insulin in the morning (to cover breakfast and lunch) and a short-acting insulin at dinner. Commonly, the short-acting insulin is Humalog (lispro) or NovoLog, and the intermediate-acting insulin is NPH. Regular insulin had long been the mainstay of diabetic management; however, it has been replaced by Humalog because of the latter's faster onset of action and shorter length of action. Humalog's profile better represents normal physiology and leads to better control of postprandial blood glucose with less hypoglycemia.

Historically, the oral hypoglycemic agents were not used in pregnancy owing to concerns regarding fetal hypoglycemia. However, recent studies indicate that in some patients, adequate blood glucose control can be achieved without particular harm to the fetus. Because of the ease of patient administration and possibly improved compliance, oral agents such as glyburide or metformin are now being used by some clinicians. With respect to glyburide, there have been only three relatively small, randomized prospective trials, and these were not adequately powered to examine all important neonatal outcomes, and long-term results are not yet available. Recent meta-analyses of glyburide versus insulin demonstrate that short-term outcomes are worse in glyburide-treated pregnancies. Thus, glyburide should not be a first-line treatment of GDM. A recent randomized trial comparing metformin and insulin demonstrated no differences in outcomes. However, because the oral agents cross the placenta and long-term outcomes have not been adequately assessed, metformin should be used as a second-line agent only in those women who will not take insulin. The American College of Obstetricians and Gynecologists still considers the use of oral hypoglycemic agents during pregnancy to be experimental, although they are used in clinical practice widely.

FETAL MONITORING

In A_2 GDM patients who are started on insulin or an oral hypoglycemic agent, fetal monitoring via nonstress test (NST) or modified biophysical profile (BPP) is typically begun between 32 and 36 weeks of gestation and continued until delivery on a weekly or biweekly basis. Because of the increased risk of macrosomia, these patients commonly receive an obstetric ultrasound for an estimated fetal weight (EFW) between 34 and 37 weeks. It is not common to offer fetal monitoring to A_1 GDM patients who are well controlled on diet alone. The decision to offer these patients an ultrasound for EFW varies among practitioners.

DELIVERY MANAGEMENT

The intrapartum management of diet-controlled gestational diabetic patients does not differ from that of nondiabetic women, provided that a random glucose check on admission does not reveal significant hyperglycemia that requires correction to avoid neonatal hypoglycemia. It is unclear whether well-controlled gestational diabetic patients have any particular increased risk for peripartum complications other than the theoretical risk of macrosomia. A closer evaluation of fetal weight at term may be prudent in patients whose pregnancy extends beyond their due date.

Scheduled delivery (typically via induction of labor) at 39 weeks of gestation is common in patients on insulin or a hypoglycemic agent (Class A_2 GDM). One concern about allowing their pregnancies to proceed is that there may be an increased risk of hypoglycemia because their placental function decreases toward the end of pregnancy. These patients are commonly brought in to labor and delivery at 39 weeks for induction, where their long-acting hypoglycemic agents are discontinued and blood glucose monitored every hour. Dextrose and insulin drips are used if necessary to maintain blood glucose within reference limits (<120 mg/dL). Patients with poor glycemic control are offered delivery between weeks 37 and 39. Patients who have an EFW above 4,000 g have increased risks of shoulder dystocia, and their labor curves should be followed closely. Some clinicians offer these patients an elective cesarean birth, but, more commonly, elective cesarean delivery is offered to those with an EFW greater than 4,500 g.

At the time of delivery, forceps and vacuum are generally not used if macrosomia is suspected because of the increased risk of shoulder dystocia, except in the case of true outlet forceps for nonreassuring fetal monitoring. To prepare for a possible shoulder dystocia, there should be at least one experienced obstetrician in the delivery room and usually several extra nurses/assistants. This allows one individual to perform suprapubic pressure, two others to perform McRoberts maneuver, although another can be available to time events and function as an assistant.

FOLLOW-UP

Among patients with GDM, over 50% will experience GDM in subsequent pregnancies, and 25% to 35% will go on to develop overt diabetes within 5 years.

Women with GDM should be screened for T2DM at the postpartum visit, and every year thereafter, most commonly with a fasting serum blood glucose or a 75 g, 2-hour GTT. The infants of patients with GDM have an increased incidence of childhood obesity and T2DM during early adulthood and later in life. Unfortunately, only a minority of patients actually obtain the recommended GTT follow-up test postpartum. However, there are several small intervention studies that find that scheduling such follow-up testing or sending reminders by a nurse improves test completion rates.

PREGESTATIONAL DIABETES

Diabetes during pregnancy can have devastating effects on both the mother (Table 9-4) and the fetus (Table 9-5). Women with diabetes are four times more likely to develop preeclampsia or eclampsia than women without diabetes. They are also twice as likely to have a spontaneous abortion. In addition, the risks of infection, polyhydramnios, postpartum hemorrhage, and cesarean delivery are all increased for diabetic mothers. Similarly, diabetes can have an adverse effect on the fetus, including a fivefold increase in perinatal death and a two- to threefold increase in the risk of congenital malformations, depending on glycemic control.

TABLE 9-4. Maternal Complications of Diabetes During Pregnancy

Obstetric complications
Polyhydramnios
Preeclampsia
Miscarriage
Infection
Postpartum hemorrhage
Increased cesarean section
Diabetic emergencies
Hypoglycemia
Ketoacidosis
Diabetic coma
Vascular and end organ involvement
Cardiac
Renal
Ophthalmic
Peripheral vascular
Neurologic
Peripheral neuropathy
Gastrointestinal disturbance

TABLE 9-5. Fetal Complications of Diabetes Mellitus

Macrosomia
Traumatic delivery
Shoulder dystocia
Erb palsy

Delayed organ maturity
Pulmonary
Hepatic
Neurologic
Pituitary–thyroid axis

Congenital malformations
Cardiovascular defects
Neural tube defects
Caudal regression syndrome
Situs inversus
Duplex renal ureter

IUGR
Intrauterine death

IUGR, intrauterine growth restriction.

Control of maternal glucose levels in overtly diabetic women is a particularly important factor in determining fetal outcome. In older studies, with minimal glycemic management in gravid diabetic women, the perinatal mortality was as high as 30%. However, with careful management by specialists, this risk can be reduced to less than 1%. The fetuses of diabetic mothers are more likely to develop congenital anomalies, including both cardiac anomalies and neural tube defects, and most dramatically, caudal regression syndrome. The fetus is also at risk for fetal growth abnormalities and sudden intrauterine fetal demise.

EPIDEMIOLOGY

Less than 1% of pregnant women have pregestational diabetes. However, with improved management of type 1 diabetes mellitus (T1DM) and increased rates of T2DM in the setting of the obesity epidemic, the number of women with pregestational diabetes who become pregnant is increasing.

RISK FACTORS

The White classification system was originally designed to prognosticate perinatal survival; with changing management of diabetes as a chronic disease, it has, however, become less applicable. The length of illness used to differentiate classes B, C, and D has little predictive value at this point because there are likely some Class B patients with poor control and many Class D patients with excellent control, and thus less likely to be at risk of perinatal complications. However, the severity of illness as reflected by classes R (retinopathy), F (nephropathy), and H (heart disease) is certainly predictive of worsened perinatal outcomes in these patients. Along with the White classification, other prognostic factors include hypertension, pyelonephritis, ketoacidosis, and poor glycemic control. Glycemic control is often measured by $HgbA_1c$, which gives an estimate of the average blood glucose control over the prior 8 to 12 weeks. Patients with an $HgbA_1c$ less than 6.5% generally have good outcomes, whereas patients with an $HgbA_1c$ greater than or equal to 12% are estimated to have a 25% rate of congenital anomalies.

TREATMENT

The goals of managing the diabetic patient include thorough patient education, control of maternal glucose, as well as careful maternal and fetal monitoring and testing. To achieve these goals, tight glycemic control should be maintained prior to conception and throughout pregnancy. Studies now show that stricter control of serum glucose levels during pregnancy can decrease the rate of maternal and neonatal complications. To achieve euglycemia, diet, insulin, and exercise must all be regulated.

Diabetic patients have become increasingly aware of the differences that tight control can make as well as the importance of this management during pregnancy. Ideally, these patients should be seen prior to conception to discuss the risks and benefits of pregnancy. In these visits, a diabetic woman can be counseled regarding the risks to her health, particularly in the setting of chronic renal disease that has been shown to worsen during pregnancy. The patient can also be counseled about the risk of congenital anomalies in the fetus based on her $HgbA_1c$. If she is not in optimal control, this can be tightened to prepare for pregnancy. Because these patients are at higher risk of neural tube defects, they are also placed on 4 mg of folate daily.

It has been standard for patients to follow the ADA diet plan of 2,200 calories per day. More recently, however, the focus on diabetic diet management has shifted to total carbohydrate intake rather than caloric intake. Generally, patients keep their carbohydrate intake at 30 to 45 g for breakfast, and at 45 to 60 g for lunch and dinner, and at 15 g for snacks. Patients can increase or decrease protein and fat depending on whether they need more or fewer calories to gain or maintain weight. These carbohydrate-focused diets should be maintained during pregnancy, although the total caloric intake is usually about 300 kcal higher than for nonpregnant patients.

TYPE 1 DIABETES MELLITUS

Historically, patients with T1DM had extremely poor maternal and perinatal outcomes, many of which can be attributed to long-standing disease and difficulty in maintaining euglycemia. Nowadays, many T1DM patients are checking their blood glucose seven or more times per day, doing carbohydrate counting, and maintaining their HgbA$_1$c below 6.0% to 6.5%. When patients are able to maintain tight control prior to and during their pregnancies, the risks of microvascular disease, renal disease, and hypertension are significantly decreased. These lower rates of baseline disease lead to fewer complications during pregnancy.

Because of the correlation of outcome with prepregnant disease, patients are extensively screened at their first visit (if not preconceptionally). Routinely, patients should obtain an ECG, particularly those with long-standing disease, hypertension, advanced maternal age, or renal disease. A 24-hour urine collection for creatinine clearance and protein should be sent to assess baseline renal function. An HgbA$_1$c is ordered to assess baseline glucose management as well as thyroid function tests (thyroid-stimulating hormone and free T4) because these patients are at risk for other autoimmune endocrinopathies. In addition, a referral to an ophthalmologist should be made to check for baseline retinopathy.

Because patients with T1DM require insulin, they are usually very experienced at managing their disease. However, this experience may not be applicable during pregnancy, when glycemic control can be dramatically different. During the first half of pregnancy, the patient's prior dosing regimen is usually increased slightly, but can increase substantially during the latter half of pregnancy as insulin resistance increases. If patients have been managed on an insulin pump, this practice should be continued. In fact, because an insulin pump can help maintain patients in tight control, it is often begun either preconception for patients planning to conceive or after the first trimester in patients who are becoming increasingly difficult to manage with NPH and Humalog insulin shots. Some patients will have excellent control prepregnant with Lantus (glargine insulin). This insulin is a slow-release insulin that gives a very flat steady-state level of insulin for 24 hours. Unfortunately, the experience in pregnancy is minimal. Although generally not recommended during pregnancy at this time, it is being used increasingly by clinicians who care for preconceptional diabetic patients during pregnancy.

TABLE 9-6. Glucose Monitoring and Insulin Dosing During Pregnancy

Insulin Type and Dose Time	Time Impact Seen	Target Glucose Level (mg/dL)
Evening NPH	Fasting	70–90
Morning Humalog	Postbreakfast	100–139
Morning NPH	Postlunch	100–139
Evening Humalog	Postdinner	100–139

Table 9-6 demonstrates the relationship among the time of insulin dose, the time of glucose testing, and the target blood glucose levels. When adjusting a patient's dosing schedule, it is important to consider other factors that may alter insulin requirements, such as diet, exercise, stress, and infection. When insulin changes become necessary, there are a few simple rules that aid in the process (Table 9-7). In addition to the schedules given in Tables 9-6 and 9-7, patients on insulin pumps should also check premeal glucose values throughout the day to get a sense of how well blood glucose levels are being managed at baseline.

Because the level of physical activity affects the plasma glucose level, consistent levels of physical activity are suggested. Keep in mind that a hospitalized patient who achieves euglycemia in the context of relatively low activity may encounter bouts of hypoglycemia when discharged home on the same insulin regime because her physical activity level increases at home, thus lowering the need for insulin. Physical activity can also be used to help manage blood glucose. If a patient consistently has an elevated postmeal blood glucose, the premeal insulin or postmeal activity can be increased. It is also important to consider differences between weekday and weekend activity.

TABLE 9-7. Instructions for Adjusting Insulin Dosage

1. Establish a fasting glucose level between 70 and 90 mg/dL
2. Adjust only one dosing level at a time
3. Do not change any dosage by more than 20% per day
4. Wait 24 h between dosage changes to evaluate the response

Some patients will require entirely different insulin regimens on the weekends.

TYPE 2 DIABETES MELLITUS

The pathophysiology of T2DM differs from T1DM. Patients with T1DM have had autoimmune destruction of their pancreatic islet cells, resulting in diminished or absent insulin production, whereas patients with T2DM have peripheral insulin resistance. Many type 2 diabetic patients are managed prior to pregnancy with oral hypoglycemic agents or diet alone. However, in pregnancy, most will require insulin. Oral hypoglycemic agents have not generally been used during pregnancy because of concerns regarding fetal hypoglycemia or potential teratogenicity, but recent studies have not demonstrated any particular association with congenital anomalies, and patients are often initially maintained on these medications during pregnancy. However, eventually, most of these patients will be hyperglycemic even on the maximum doses of the oral agents and need to be switched to insulin.

When oral hypoglycemic agents do not adequately maintain glucose control during pregnancy, insulin can be substituted or supplemented. In general, insulin is started as neutral protamine Hagedorn (NPH) at bedtime to control fasting blood glucose and in the morning to provide a longer acting substrate throughout the day. A short-acting insulin, usually Humalog or lispro, is used at meals to control immediate carbohydrate intake. Once patients are started on insulin, management is very similar to that of type 1 diabetic patients, although the doses are often higher depending on the patient's degree of insulin resistance. Again, although regular insulin has been used traditionally, it is a poor substitute for the newer fast-acting insulins for postprandial blood glucose control.

Fetal Testing and Delivery

In the patient with pregestational diabetes, antenatal testing to evaluate the growth and well-being of the fetus usually begins at 32 weeks. Earlier testing is recommended in the setting of poor glycemic control. Testing regimens vary, but may resemble the following: antenatal fetal assessment consisting of weekly NSTs until 36 weeks, during which time biweekly testing is implemented, including weekly NST alternating with weekly modified BPP to assess amniotic fluid measurement as well. In addition to the weekly testing, an ultrasound to assess fetal growth is usually obtained between 32 and 36 weeks of gestation.

In general, well-controlled pregestational insulin-dependent diabetic patients with no complications are offered induction of labor at 39 weeks of gestation. This is a change from older management plans that delivered such patients at 37 or 38 weeks of gestation who were given a reassuring amniocentesis for fetal lung maturity. Thus, expectant management beyond 37 weeks is acceptable, but the clinician needs to follow the patient closely beyond that point. Indications for earlier delivery include nonreassuring fetal testing, poor glycemic control, worsening or uncontrolled hypertension, worsening renal disease, or poor fetal growth.

Blood glucose levels can be extremely difficult to manage in the laboring diabetic woman. The physical effort of labor and delivery decreases the overall insulin requirements. Patients are usually begun on dextrose and insulin drips to maintain blood glucose between 100 and 120 mg/dL. If the blood glucose level increases above 120 mg/dL, the insulin can be increased. Conversely, if the blood glucose level drops to between 80 and 100 mg/dL, an infusion of dextrose can be started or increased.

After delivery, maternal insulin requirements decrease significantly because of the removal of the placenta, which contains many insulin antagonists. In fact, insulin requirements may go below prepregnant levels during the puerperium, particularly in breastfeeding women. Type 2 diabetic patients may require no insulin during this period. However, type 1 diabetic patients should always be maintained on at least a small amount of insulin because they do not produce any endogenously.

Follow-Up

In the puerperal period, pregestational diabetic patients should resume their prepregnancy regimens. Patients, who were on oral hypoglycemic agents, however, are often not advised to resume their use of breastfeeding because of concerns regarding neonatal hypoglycemia. This complication is more theoretical because it has not been documented in any large case series or cohort studies. In patients with preexisting renal disease, a 24-hour urine collection for creatinine clearance and protein is usually done at 6 weeks postpartum to assess worsening of disease. In addition, an ophthalmologic appointment is usually scheduled 12 to 14 weeks postpartum. After 6 to 8 weeks postpartum, management of the patient's diabetes should be transferred back to her primary provider or endocrinologist.

KEY POINTS

- GDM occurs in 1% to 12% of pregnant women.
- Risk factors for GDM include Hispanic, Asian American, and Native American ethnicity, obesity, family history of diabetes, and prior pregnancy complicated by GDM, macrosomia, shoulder dystocia, or fetal death.
- All pregnant women should be screened for diabetes between weeks 24 and 28. High-risk women should also be screened at their first prenatal visit.
- Fetal complications of GDM include macrosomia, shoulder dystocia, and neonatal hypoglycemia.
- Pregnancy management should include frequent health care visits, thorough patient education, ADA diet plan, glucose monitoring, fetal monitoring, and insulin or an oral hypoglycemic agent as indicated.
- Patients with good glycemic control should generally be induced between 39 and 40 weeks of gestation. Intrapartum insulin and dextrose are used to maintain tight control during delivery. Cesarean section is offered if fetal weight is over 4,500 g.
- Maternal complications of diabetes during pregnancy include hyperglycemia, hypoglycemia, urinary tract infection, worsening renal disease, hypertension, and retinopathy.
- Fetal complications of diabetes during pregnancy include spontaneous abortion, congenital anomalies, macrosomia, intrauterine growth restriction, neonatal hypoglycemia, respiratory distress syndrome, and perinatal death.
- Pregnancy management is optimized by a preconception visit, early prenatal care, thorough patient education, tight glucose monitoring and management with insulin, fetal monitoring, and thoughtful plan for delivery.
- Motivated type 1 diabetic patients can usually maintain tighter control on an insulin pump. Management in labor and delivery usually requires an insulin drip; however, insulin requirements decrease dramatically postpartum.

CLINICAL VIGNETTES

VIGNETTE 1

A 32-year-old G0 woman with type 1 diabetes mellitus (T1DM) presents for a preconception visit. She was diagnosed with T1DM at age 4, and other than some challenges with glucose control during her teenage years, she generally has good control per her report. She uses a subcutaneous insulin pump. She has no history of retinopathy, renal disease, heart disease, proteinuria, peripheral neuropathy, or any other medical conditions. On examination, she is 60″ tall and weighs 122 lb. Her blood pressure is 128/76 mm Hg.

1. During your counseling, which of the following do you NOT mention that she or her fetus is at increased risk for during pregnancy?
   a. Preeclampsia
   b. Congenital abnormalities
   c. Breech presentation
   d. Cesarean delivery
   e. Fetal macrosomia

2. You order a laboratory test and her HgbA$_1$c returns at 11. You advise her which of the following?
   a. She should go ahead and start trying to get pregnant
   b. She should aggressively try to lower her HgbA$_1$c to less than 9 to reduce the risk of preterm birth
   c. She should aggressively lower her HgbA$_1$c to less than 5 in order to reduce her risk of preeclampsia
   d. She should aggressively lower her HgbA$_1$c to less than 7 to reduce her risk of congenital anomalies
   e. She should go ahead and start trying to get pregnant, but also slowly reduce her blood glucoses with a HgbA$_1$c target of less than 9

3. In addition to the above, what other tests/recommendations do you make?
   a. Perform a 24-hour urine collection for protein and creatinine clearance
   b. Obtain a baseline ECG
   c. Obtain a baseline ophthalmology examination
   d. Check a thyroid test—thyroid-stimulating hormone (TSH)
   e. All of the above

4. She returns 6 months later with a positive pregnancy test and a last menstrual period (LMP) that was 6 weeks ago. You check that her HgbA$_1$c is now 8.6. Given her baseline medical history, what is her White classification?
   a. Class A
   b. Class B
   c. Class C
   d. Class D
   e. Class F

5. You review her blood glucose levels with her. Her fasting blood glucose levels range from 102 to 188 mg/dL; preprandial values range from 102 to 168 mg/dL, and postprandial values range from 120 to 179 mg/dL. Given these values and her current HgbA$_1$c of 8.6, what management do you recommend?
   a. Add glyburide to the medical management
   b. Add metformin to the medical management
   c. Increase her basal insulin throughout the day and night
   d. Increase her insulin boluses at mealtimes
   e. No changes at this time to avoid hypoglycemia

VIGNETTE 2

A 29-year-old G2P1 woman with obesity, a history of gestational diabetes mellitus (GDM) in the prior pregnancy, and a strong family history for type 2 diabetes mellitus (T2DM) presents at 7 weeks of gestation by LMP. In her previous pregnancy, she required insulin therapy. She delivered at 39 weeks and her baby boy weighed 4,300 g (or approximately 9 1/2 lb).

1. In addition to the routine prenatal laboratory tests, what other testing do you also obtain at this point?
   a. A glucose challenge test with fasting blood glucose
   b. An ultrasound to estimate fetal weight
   c. Anti-insulin antibodies
   d. No testing at this point; we would get a glucose challenge test at 24 weeks' gestation
   e. No other testing needed; we assume she has GDM

2. Laboratory test results return, and her fasting blood glucose is 145 mg/dL. An ultrasound reveals the pregnancy to be 7 weeks and 2 days, consistent with LMP, and anti-insulin antibodies are negative. Her diagnosis is:
   a. A$_1$ GDM
   b. A$_2$ GDM
   c. T1DM
   d. T2DM
   e. no diabetes in pregnancy

3. In order to reduce her risk of congenital anomalies, you start her on:
   a. glyburide
   b. metformin
   c. Humalog insulin with meals only
   d. NPH insulin and Humalog insulin
   e. Lantus insulin only

4. Her pregnancy progresses without complication. At 34 weeks of gestation, she begins antenatal testing with nonstress tests (NSTs) and amniotic fluid indices twice weekly. This is done in order to:
   a. prevent preterm birth
   b. prevent preeclampsia
   c. prevent macrosomia
   d. prevent shoulder dystocia
   e. prevent stillbirth

VIGNETTE 3

A 36-year-old Hispanic G1P0 woman presents for consultation after undergoing a 50 g glucose loading test, which returned with a value of 168 mg/dL. She carries a diagnosis of asthma, but her pregnancy has been otherwise uncomplicated with routine first and second prenatal laboratory tests. She is 5'2" and weighs 150 lb. Her mother has T2DM.

1. What is the next step in management?
   a. Begin dietary management of GDM
   b. Begin insulin treatment
   c. Further glucose testing
   d. No need for further management—routine prenatal care
   e. Begin treatment with glyburide

2. What in her history does not increase her risk for GDM?
   a. Maternal weight
   b. Maternal age
   c. Maternal race/ethnicity
   d. Family history of diabetes
   e. History of asthma

3. Once she is diagnosed with GDM, the next step in management is to:
   a. begin low-fat diet
   b. exercise three times per week
   c. have blood glucose checks on the glucometer four times per day
   d. begin insulin
   e. begin glyburide

VIGNETTE 4

A 28-year-old G1P0 woman presents to the diabetes clinic at 28 weeks with a recent diagnosis of GDM. On the 3-hour test, she had two elevated values. Her pregnancy has otherwise been uncomplicated. She undergoes counseling with a nutritionist who discusses carbohydrate counting and the need for between-meal snacks. She is also given a glucometer to check some blood glucose values.

1. As part of her routine counseling, you mention that she is at increased risk of all of the following except:
   a. preeclampsia
   b. fetal macrosomia
   c. her baby having jaundice
   d. her baby having a shoulder dystocia
   e. her baby having a cardiac defect

2. She returns in 1 week with blood glucose values ranging from 75 to 85 mg/dL fasting (threshold goal <90 mg/dL), postbreakfast values ranging from 120 to 142 mg/dL (threshold goal values <140 mg/dL), postlunch values ranging from 128 to 148 mg/dL (threshold goal values <140 mg/dL), and postdinner values ranging from 124 to 152 mg/dL (threshold goal values <140 mg/dL). Your next step in management is to:
   a. continue checking blood glucose values
   b. discuss exercise plan, including walking after each meal
   c. begin insulin
   d. begin glyburide
   e. begin metformin

3. By 37 weeks of gestation, she has been started on medical treatment with insulin before each meal. The insulin dosing has increased until 36 weeks when her glycemic control was excellent with all values below threshold. You schedule her for induction of labor at:
   a. 37 weeks
   b. 38 weeks
   c. 39 weeks
   d. 40 weeks
   e. 41 weeks

ANSWERS

VIGNETTE 1 Question 1
1. Answer C:
Women with preexisting diabetes mellitus, both type 1 and type 2, are at increased risk for a number of complications in pregnancy. First, because of elevated blood glucose during the first trimester, there is increased risk of congenital anomalies including cardiac and a pathognomonic finding of caudal regression sequence. Throughout the rest of the pregnancy, there is an increased risk of preterm birth, preeclampsia, induction of labor, cesarean delivery, and hyperglycemia, which can lead to fetal macrosomia and predispose to a shoulder dystocia at vaginal delivery. Neonates delivered from women with pregestational diabetes are at increased risk of hyperbilirubinemia, respiratory distress syndrome, and hypoglycemia, but are not particularly at increased risk for malpresentation.

VIGNETTE 1 Question 2
2. Answer D:
In pregnancy, the goal is to get the $HgbA_1c$ as low as possible, within reason. Commonly, less than 7 or less than 6 may be used as targets. With an $HgbA_1c$ of 11, her risk of a congenital anomaly is in the 20% to 30% range, which would be reduced to less than 5% with $HgbA_1c$ less than 7. Thus, it is worth delaying attempting to get pregnant for a few months in order to improve glycemic control. Although getting the $HgbA_1c$ even lower to less than 6 may further improve outcomes, being too aggressive to get $HgbA_1c$ less than 5 may lead to too many hypoglycemic events and is not encouraged. Further, it does not appear that lowering $HgbA_1c$ levels necessarily reduces the risk of either preterm birth or preeclampsia.

VIGNETTE 1 Question 3
3. Answer E:
Yes, all of these are things one would get on a preconceptional diabetic patient. Some clinicians would obtain only an ECG on women 35 years or older, but in this woman who has had diabetes for more than 30 years, it seems like a good idea. The 24-hour urine collection is to establish baseline renal function, and the baseline ophthalmology examination is to look for diabetic retinopathy. Because women with T1DM are more likely to have autoimmune thyroid disease, a TSH screening test is always good to obtain. One would also start this patient on folate supplementation to lower the risk of neural tube defects, and make tight glycemic control recommendations.

VIGNETTE 1 Question 4
4. Answer D:
The White classification of diabetes in pregnancy relies on the number of years an individual has had diabetes and the number of medical complications of diabetes she has. Class A is gestational diabetes (A_1, diet controlled; A_2, medically controlled). Classes B, C, and D are all related to either the amount of time the patient has had diabetes or her age of onset of

diabetes, whichever leads to the higher class. By years of disease, less than 10 years is Class B, 10 to 20 years is Class C, and 20 years or greater is Class D. By age of onset, older than 20 years is Class B, age 10 to 20 years is Class C, and age younger than 10 years is Class D. Because she was diagnosed at age 4, it makes her Class D, and because she has had the disease for 28 years, it makes her D as well. Class F is for nephropathy, Class R is for retinopathy, and Class H is for heart disease.

VIGNETTE 1 Question 5
5. Answer C:
She has increased basal and preprandial blood glucose levels. Thus, she needs greater amounts of basal insulin overnight and throughout the day. Although her postprandial blood glucose levels are also elevated, the reference range for the mealtime glucose excursion is about 20 to 40 mg/dL, and her excursions seem reasonable. Thus, if we lower her preprandial blood glucose levels, her postprandial glucose levels should improve as well. Women with true T1DM do not take glyburide or metformin. Glyburide stimulates the beta cells in the pancreas to release more insulin, but a T1DM patient with the disease for 28 years would not have any beta cell function. Metformin decreases insulin resistance, but most T1DM patients will have minimal insulin resistance because they do not get exposed to chronic hyperglycemic diets like T2DM patients do.

VIGNETTE 2 Question 1
1. Answer A:
A patient such as this with obesity, prior history of GDM, and a family history of T2DM is at relatively high risk of having T2DM. Thus, one would obtain testing at the very first prenatal visit. Such a test could simply be the standard 75-g load with fasting and a 2-hour blood glucose that is done to diagnose T2DM. For others, clinicians go for the pregnancy 50-g load and 1-hour blood glucose check; in such a case, it is advisable to obtain a fasting blood glucose as well. Anti-insulin antibodies can be seen in women with T1DM, which seems less likely in this setting. Despite her being a high-risk patient, most clinicians will still do GDM testing in such a patient because as many as one-third will not have GDM in a subsequent pregnancy.

VIGNETTE 2 Question 2
2. Answer D:
Until recently, women with elevated blood glucose values in pregnancy were not given a formal diagnosis of T2DM during pregnancy. They had to wait until 6 weeks postpartum to do a no-pregnant glucose challenge test with the 75-g load to receive a diagnosis. Recently, this was changed, as it was realized that, particularly early on, there should only be mild elevations in blood glucose values so that women who exceeded the standards commonly used, greater than 125 mg/dL on a fasting blood glucose or greater than 200 mg/dL 2 hours after a 75-g load, should be diagnosed with T2DM. If this woman had GDM, we would not know whether it was A_1 or A_2 until we followed some blood glucose levels.

VIGNETTE 2 Question 3
3. Answer D:
In this patient with T2DM, some clinicians will manage with either glyburide or metformin. It is likely that either of those medications will not adequately control a patient with T2DM in pregnancy and she will eventually require insulin. However, in this setting, in particular with a need to rapidly control her blood glucose to reduce the risk of congenital anomalies, a combination of long- and short-acting insulin is indicated. Often, in this setting, such a patient will be admitted to the hospital and placed on an insulin drip for 24 hours to assess the potential total need for insulin. However, with a reliable patient, it is reasonable to give a dose of 0.7 units/kg split between long- and short-acting insulin and frequently revise the dosages based on the glucometer values. We would recommend doing so every 1 to 2 days for the first week in order to rapidly titrate the dosing.

VIGNETTE 2 Question 4
4. Answer E:
Women with pregestational diabetes are at increased risk of having an intrauterine fetal demise or stillbirth. This is thought to be due to the elevated blood glucose values, the wide swings in glucose values, or the effect of diabetes on placental function. Antenatal testing including NSTs and BPPs is performed to identify any fetal complications before they occur, in particular to decrease the risk of stillbirth. It would not do any of the other four options given. Treatment of diabetes in pregnancy by controlling blood glucose does seem to lower the risk of complications such as preterm birth, preeclampsia, macrosomia, and shoulder dystocia.

VIGNETTE 3 Question 1
1. Answer C:
This patient has an elevated GLT. Thresholds for the GLT that have been used include 140, 135, or 130 mg/dL. This patient has a positive screen by any measure. However, the GLT is just a screening test, and a follow-up diagnostic test is indicated. There are some clinicians who will not do any further testing for GLT values greater than 200 mg/dL, but will instead consider such values diagnostic of GDM and start blood glucose monitoring at that point. This patient with a value of 168 mg/dL on GLT should undergo the 3-hour, 100-g load test to confirm the diagnosis of

GDM. Once she is diagnosed, we could move forward with answer option a or b.

VIGNETTE 3 Question 2
2. Answer E:
There are a number of risk factors for developing GDM. These include maternal risk factors such as an elevated BMI, increased maternal age, family history of T2DM, or maternal race ethnicity including Asian/PI, Hispanic, or Native American. African-American race has also been noted to be a risk factor in some studies. Maternal history of a macrosomic baby or a history of GDM also increases the risk of GDM. Asthma is not known as a risk factor for GDM. However, an asthma patient who is on chronic systemic steroids can, occasionally, be diagnosed and needs to be treated for GDM.

VIGNETTE 3 Question 3
3. Answer C:
Once diagnosed with GDM, the next step in the care is to check the patient's blood glucose values four times per day. At the same time, she should begin a carbohydrate-controlled diet with 30 g of carbohydrates in the morning, 45 g for lunch and dinner, and 15 g for snacks between meals. Daily exercise, particularly exercise after each meal, can help to control blood glucose values. Although three times per week exercise (or more) is a great part of a baseline of healthy exercise, it is the frequent, postprandial activity that makes a larger difference on blood glucose control.

VIGNETTE 4 Question 1
1. Answer E:
Although all of these complications can be seen in pregestational diabetic patients, women with GDM do not have an appreciable increased risk in congenital anomalies.

VIGNETTE 4 Question 2
2. Answer B:
In this patient with only slight postprandial elevations, walking after each meal is likely to reduce her blood glucose values into the reference range. Given that conservative management has only been tried for 1 week, reviewing dietary plan and reinforcing exercise, particularly after meals, is important with follow-up in another week. It is not yet time to begin medical therapy with hypoglycemic agents.

VIGNETTE 4 Question 3
3. Answer C:
Women with well-controlled pregestational diabetes and A_2 GDM are usually induced at 39 weeks of gestation. This allows enough time for the fetus to reach full maturity and minimize fetal metabolic complications, but prevents stillbirth and overgrowth that would occur in subsequent weeks of gestation. A_1 GDM patients are usually managed expectantly until 40/41 weeks of gestation. Finally, pregestational or A_2 GDM patients who have poor glycemic control are commonly delivered earlier, typically 36 to 38 weeks of gestation.

10 Infectious Diseases in Pregnancy

In pregnancy, the immune system is altered, so that the mother does not immunologically reject the fetus. As such, infections pose important challenges to the pregnant patients and affect maternal, fetal, and pregnancy outcomes. In this chapter, we discuss common infections that increase or whose complications increase in pregnancy, infections specific to pregnancy, and infections that can affect the fetus (Table 10-1). The infectious complications that are common to the puerperium (postpartum period), such as endomyometritis and wound infections, are discussed in Chapter 12.

URINARY TRACT INFECTIONS

Urinary tract infection (UTI) is one of the most common medical complications of pregnancy. A UTI consists of infection anywhere along the urinary tract and includes cystitis and pyelonephritis. UTIs occur in up to 20% of pregnancies and account for as many as 10% of antepartum hospitalizations. The incidence of UTIs increases during pregnancy, and moreover, asymptomatic bacterial colonization of the urinary tract is relevant. Asymptomatic bacteriuria (ASB) is screened for as a part of routine pregnant care and is associated with significant risk in pregnancy.

The prevalence of ASB (i.e., >100,000 colonies on culture) in pregnant women ranges from 2% to 11%, with the majority of studies reporting 4% to 7%. An increased prevalence of bacteriuria in women has been associated with lower socioeconomic status, diminished availability of medical care, and increased parity. Although this prevalence is similar to that in the nonpregnant population, women with ASB in early pregnancy are at a 20- to 30-fold increased risk of developing acute pyelonephritis during pregnancy when compared with pregnant women without

TABLE 10-1. Infectious Diseases in Pregnancy

Infections whose complications increase during pregnancy
UTIs
Bacterial vaginosis
Surgical wound
Group B streptococcal
Infections more common in pregnancy and the puerperium
Pyelonephritis
Endomyometritis
Mastitis
Toxic shock syndrome (TSS)
Infections specific to pregnancy
Chorioamnionitis
Septic pelvic thrombophlebitis
Episiotomy or perineal lacerations
Infections that affect the fetus
Neonatal sepsis (e.g., Group B *Streptococcus*, *Escherichia coli*)
HSV
VZV
Parvovirus B19
CMV
Rubella
HIV
Hepatitis B and C
Gonorrhea
Chlamydia
Syphilis
Toxoplasmosis
Zika virus

CMV, cytomegalovirus; HSV, herpes simplex virus; UTIs, urinary tract infections; VZV, Varicella zoster virus.

bacteriuria. ASB in pregnancy is further associated with preterm birth and low–birth-weight infants.

UTI and ASB in pregnancy present risks to the pregnancy and fetus. A recent meta-analysis demonstrated a significant association between bacteriuria and preterm delivery. This also demonstrated a statistically significant reduction in the incidence of low–birth-weight infants among women with bacteriuria who were treated in eight placebo-controlled treatment trials. Untreated ASB will progress to cystitis or pyelonephritis in 25% to 40% of pregnant patients. Before the advent of universal screening for ASB in early pregnancy, the reported rate of acute pyelonephritis in pregnancy was 3% to 4%; afterward, it was 1% to 2%. Of the cases of pyelonephritis, up to 15% may be complicated by bacteremia, sepsis, or adult acute respiratory distress syndrome (ARDS). In pregnant women with sickle-cell disease, the rate of ASB doubles to 10%, although it has been shown that there is no increased risk in sickle-cell trait carriers.

PATHOGENESIS

Women are 14 times more likely to develop UTIs compared with men. Presumably, this women predominance is the result of several factors, including (1) a shorter urethra in women, (2) continuous exposure of the external one-third of the urethra by pathogenic bacteria from the vagina and rectum, (3) a greater incidence of incomplete emptying during voiding, and (4) movement of bacteria into the female bladder during sexual intercourse.

Additionally, pregnant women have a higher incidence of UTI for several reasons, including hormonal, mechanical, and immunologic changes that predispose to infection. During pregnancy, the smooth muscle relaxation effects of progesterone decrease bladder tone and cause ureteral and renal pelvis dilation, as well as decrease ureteral peristalsis. This results in urinary stasis throughout the urinary tract that can be seen radiologically as physiologic hydronephrosis of pregnancy. In addition, mechanical compression from the enlarged uterus can cause obstruction of the ureters, leading to additional stasis. In pregnancy, there is an increased capacity and an incomplete emptying of the bladder, all of which predispose pregnant women to vesicoureteral reflux. Hypotonia of the vesicle musculature and the vesicoureteral reflux and dilation of the ureters and renal pelves result in static columns of urine in the ureters, facilitating the ascending migration of bacteria to the upper urinary tract after bladder infection is established. Moreover, the altered immune response in pregnancy has been demonstrated to be involved in a predisposition to UTI. TLR4 response is inhibited during pregnancy, and this has a major role in responding to uropathogenic *Escherichia coli*. The combination of hormonal influences on smooth muscle, mechanical pressures, and predisposition to reflux with altered immune response provides an environment where pathogenic bacteria can be quite virulent.

DIAGNOSIS

UTIs are diagnosed with clinical signs and symptoms of dysuria, urinary frequency, and urinary urgency in conjunction with a positive urine culture. The gold standard for diagnosing a UTI has been a quantitative culture containing at least 100,000 CFU/mL. Because urine cultures may take 3 to 4 days to become positive, a urinalysis is often used as a proxy during initial evaluation. The urinalysis may be positive for leukocyte esterase, nitrates, or hematuria, and the urine sediment will have elevated WBCs and bacteria. Nitrates are sensitive and specific to gram-negative bacteria. Because ASB has been shown to be higher in the first trimester, commonly, a routine urine culture is used to screen for ASB between 12 and 16 weeks of gestation.

UTIs are distinguished into cystitis or lower UTI and pyelonephritis or upper UTI. Acute cystitis is a distinct syndrome characterized by urinary urgency, frequency, dysuria, and suprapubic discomfort (tenderness on palpation) in the absence of systemic symptoms, such as high fever and costovertebral angle tenderness. Gross hematuria may be present; the urine culture is invariably positive for bacterial growth. Pyelonephritis is diagnosed with signs of systemic symptoms and is discussed below.

TREATMENT

E. coli accounts for greater than 80% of all ASB and UTIs, and the remaining is caused by gram-negative enterobacteria (e.g., *Klebsiella*, *Proteus* species) and gram-positive bacteria, such as coagulase-negative staphylococci, group B-streptococci (GBS), and enterococci. Because most UTIs are caused by *E. coli*, initial treatment of ASB is usually with amoxicillin, nitrofurantoin (Macrodantin), trimethoprim/sulfamethoxazole (Bactrim), or cephalexin. In the first trimester, penicillins and cephalosporins are considered first-line treatment. Some authorities advise caution when using nitrofurantoin or trimethoprim/sulfamethoxazole in the third trimester because it may cause kernicterus in fetuses/neonates with G6PD deficiency. Treatment duration for

ASB consists of a 3- to 7-day course of antibiotics, although many authorities prefer 7-day treatment course for pregnant women. Single-dose therapy is not recommended. Cystitis is recommended to be treated with 7-to 10-day course of identical antibiotics, with adjustment of medication depending on culture-sensitivity results. Because ASB may persist, a test-of-cure culture should be obtained 2 weeks after completion of therapy. If the test of cure is positive, a different regimen should be initiated, and this should be continued for 14 days. Continuous nightly antibiotic prophylaxis is recommended for women who have two or more UTIs during pregnancy. Either nitrofurantoin or trimethoprim/sulfamethoxazole can be used for prophylaxis. In addition to treating the infection, in patients with dysuria or bladder pain, phenazopyridine (Pyridium), which is concentrated in the urine and acts as a local anesthetic to reduce the pain, is commonly used for symptomatic relief. Of note, patients should be counseled that Pyridium will cause the urine to turn bright orange.

PYELONEPHRITIS

The most common complication of a lower UTI is an ascending infection to the kidneys, or **pyelonephritis**. Pyelonephritis is estimated to complicate as many as 1% to 2.5% of pregnancies despite universal screening for ASB. Recurrence during the same pregnancy is frequent, occurring in 10% to 18% of cases. The major risk factors for developing pyelonephritis are previous pyelonephritis, history of vesicoureteral reflux, and ASB. Among pregnant women not receiving antibiotic prophylaxis to prevent acute pyelonephritis in pregnancy, recurrence has been noted to be up to 60%; conversely, in pregnant women on suppressive therapy, recurrence is less than 10%. Although ASB is not more frequent in pregnant women, pyelonephritis is a much more frequent complication. The most common organisms associated with acute antepartum pyelonephritis are similar to those in ASB and acute cystitis: *E. coli* (70%), *Klebsiella/Enterobacter sp.* (3%), *Proteus sp.* (2%), and gram-positive bacteria, including GBS (10%).

DIAGNOSIS

Acute pyelonephritis is characterized by fever, chills, flank pain, dysuria, urgency, and frequency. It is sometimes associated with nausea and vomiting. On physical examination, fever and costovertebral angle tenderness are often present. Pyelonephritis is a clinical diagnosis that is confirmed by laboratory testing. Laboratory abnormalities include pyuria, bacteriuria, and elevated WBC count. WBC casts are highly associated with pyelonephritis. Onset of symptoms is often abrupt, and fever is universally present.

Pyelonephritis is not only a risk factor for preterm labor but also has particularly serious associated maternal complications, including septic shock and ARDS. Up to 20% of pregnant women with acute pyelonephritis develop multiorgan system involvement secondary to endotoxemia, resulting in sepsis. Endotoxin release results in increased capillary permeability and decreased perfusion of vital organs. Fulminant sepsis can develop quickly and can be fatal. ARDS, the most severe complication of severe sepsis, develops in 2% to 8% of pregnant women with acute pyelonephritis. ARDS should be suspected in patients who present with hypoxemia, dyspnea, tachypnea, and radiographic evidence of pulmonary edema.

TREATMENT

Because of the associated risks, pyelonephritis during pregnancy is usually treated aggressively with hospital admission, intravenous (IV) hydration, and IV antibiotics—often cephalosporins for broad-spectrum activity (cefazolin, cefotetan, or ceftriaxone) or ampicillin and gentamicin—until the patient is afebrile and asymptomatic for 24 to 48 hours. Aggressive IV hydration is imperative because there is often transient renal dysfunction in patients with pyelonephritis. The patient is then transitioned to an oral antibiotic regimen for 10 to 14 days. Given the high incidence of resistance by *E. coli* to ampicillin and first-generation cephalosporins (cephalexin or cefazolin), these agents are not recommended. Women with signs of ARDS should have an ICU consult and consideration of transfer, and women in the third trimester should be monitored for preterm delivery. Of note, small trials have examined the possibility of treating these patients with a single dose of IV or IM antibiotics, such as ceftriaxone, followed by outpatient oral antibiotic regimen. Although these treatments seem to be effective in certain groups, consideration of appropriate patient criteria, including absence of signs of sepsis, compliance, ability to tolerate oral medications, and gestational age (GA), is imperative. If the patient is not improving on IV antibiotics, a renal ultrasound should be performed to evaluate for a perinephric or renal abscess. Pregnant women with one episode of pyelonephritis or two or more episodes of ASB and/or cystitis are generally placed on antimicrobial prophylaxis for the remainder of the duration of the pregnancy.

INFLUENZA

Influenza is caused by influenza A or influenza B virus. The influenza epidemics that occur annually can be particularly important for pregnant women. It is currently recommended that all pregnant women are vaccinated for influenza with the inactivated influenza vaccine. This vaccine has been well studied in pregnancy and is thought to be safe and without association with miscarriage or congenital anomalies. All pregnant women should be counseled on the importance of this vaccine and recommended to receive the vaccine during fall months. The vaccine offered is different each year and is based on the predictions on the variations in antigenic properties of the predicted seasonal virus. Influenza viruses (particularly influenza A) are notable for their mutation rate and ability to change antigenic glycoproteins to evade the immune system. As such, it is important to note that the vaccine may or may not be effective against the epidemic strain, depending on the success of predicting the antigenic variation and formulation of the vaccine. Studies have found that women who receive the influenza vaccine have a lower risk of preterm birth and a lower chance of neonates with influenza.

Influenza during pregnancy is associated with increased morbidity and mortality. This may be associated with the physiologic decreased lung capacity and changes in cell-mediated immunity. Studies have shown that pregnancy confers an increased risk of pneumonia, sepsis, ICU admission, and ARDS. In particular, this was highlighted in the 2009 H1N1 influenza pandemic where the mortality from influenza approached 5%. During the pandemic, of women hospitalized with influenza, 20% to 40% required ICU admission, and a higher rate of maternal mortality was seen. The fetal effects of influenza in pregnancy are not well defined, but some studies have demonstrated a risk of preterm labor and delivery. Women with influenza should be closely monitored, and those with hypoxia, tachycardia, and fetal tachycardia should be assessed and hospitalization strongly considered.

A high index of suspicion is warranted to test for influenza in pregnancy in women with a cough and fever, because treatment with neuraminidase inhibitors may decrease the length of time of symptoms and the complication rate. This has not been well studied in pregnancy, but in nonpregnant patients, treatment has been shown to be beneficial. Oseltamivir is the preferred medication in pregnancy, and ideally, treatment is indicated for women who are within 24 hours of symptom onset. Some have recommended that all women are treated regardless of time of onset because the complications during pregnancy can be so severe.

BACTERIAL VAGINOSIS IN PREGNANCY

Several large studies have demonstrated that **bacterial vaginosis** (BV) increases the risk for preterm premature rupture of membranes (PPROM), preterm delivery, and puerperal infections, including chorioamnionitis and endometritis. Because of this, it has been proposed that patients with BV should be treated and followed up with a test of cure to decrease their risk of preterm delivery. Several studies have also demonstrated a reduction of preterm births when high-risk asymptomatic pregnant women (those with prior preterm delivery or PPROM) were treated for BV with an oral agent. However, the largest, prospective randomized trial of screening and treating asymptomatic women did not demonstrate benefit. Therefore, screening for BV in asymptomatic women is not routinely recommended. Treatment of symptomatic women who are diagnosed in pregnancy is recommended.

DIAGNOSIS AND TREATMENT

Diagnosis of BV is made on the combination of symptoms and laboratory findings. Common symptoms of BV include malodorous, copious discharge, or vaginal irritation. Diagnosis can be made with three of the four following findings (Amsel criteria): (1) presence of thin, white or gray, homogeneous discharge coating the vaginal walls; (2) an amine (or "fishy") odor noted with addition of 10% KOH ("whiff" test); (3) pH of greater than 4.5; (4) presence of more than 20% of the epithelial cells as "clue cells" (squamous epithelial cells so heavily stippled with bacteria that their borders are obscured) on microscopic examination. There are generally few leukocytes and less lactobacilli than usual on wet mount. Gram stain with examination of bacteria in the vaginal discharge is considered the gold standard for BV diagnosis. Common BV organisms include *Gardnerella vaginalis*, *Bacteroides*, and *Mycoplasma hominis*. Oral metronidazole (Flagyl) for 1 week is recommended for treatment of BV in pregnancy.

Clindamycin (as oral dose) for 1 week may also be used. Because a majority of studies have demonstrated adverse perinatal events when intravaginal forms of clindamycin were used for treatment of BV, an oral form is preferred for pregnant women. In pregnancy, because of high rates of asymptomatic infection and because treatment of high-risk patients may prevent adverse perinatal outcomes, a test of cure may be considered 1 month after treatment completion.

GROUP B STREPTOCOCCUS

GBS refers to the β-hemolytic gram-positive bacteria *Streptococcus agalactiae* and is commonly responsible for UTIs, chorioamnionitis, and endomyometritis during pregnancy. It is also a major pathogen in neonatal sepsis, which has severe implications. Although early-onset neonatal sepsis occurs in 2 to 3 per 1,000 live births, the mortality rate with GBS sepsis ranges from 2% to 50%, depending on GA at the time of delivery. One recent study showed an overall mortality rate of 4%, 2% in term infants and 16% in preterm infants. GBS is a commensal organism that colonizes the gastrointestinal (GI) and genitourinary (GU) tracts. Various studies have demonstrated a wide range of asymptomatic colonization in pregnant women, from 10% to 35%. To protect infants from GBS infections, widespread screening programs have been implemented utilizing a rectovaginal culture for GBS colonization between 35 and 37 weeks. Large prospective studies have demonstrated that these screening programs decrease the rate of neonatal sepsis from GBS. Of note, there are concerns that the increase in prophylactic antibiotics given to these patients will increase widespread antibiotic resistance. Another concern is that by focusing clinical attention on GBS, the incidence of *E. coli* sepsis, which has an even higher mortality rate, will increase.

DIAGNOSIS AND TREATMENT

GBS screening is performed by a culture from a swab of the vagina and rectum between 35 and 37 weeks of gestation. Women with positive GBS cultures are subsequently treated with IV penicillin G at the time of labor or rupture of membranes (ROM). Women with an unknown GBS status who are in labor and meet certain risk-based criteria are also treated. Risk-based criteria include experiencing labor before 37 weeks of gestation, ROM greater than 18 hours, and temperature >100.4°F. Women with a history of GBS UTI or a history of a previous infant with GBS disease should be treated independent of screening.

Of note, GBS results are only good for 5 weeks, such that if a woman is screened at 35 weeks of gestation and is negative, she should have repeat screening done at 40 weeks of gestation. For cesarean delivery before ROM and labor, GBS prophylaxis is not indicated. Because of the difficulty of obtaining the correct dosage of penicillin G, ampicillin is commonly used instead. However, ampicillin is a broader-spectrum antibiotic than penicillin, and some authorities feel that its use should be discouraged because of the risk of developing resistance of other bacteria. For GBS-colonized women with an allergy to penicillin but low risk for anaphylaxis (i.e., rash allergy), cefazolin (Ancef) is used for prophylaxis during labor. In women with a significant penicillin allergy (i.e., high risk for anaphylaxis), clindamycin is the drug of choice, but it can be used only if the GBS susceptibilities are known. In patients with a severe penicillin allergy where GBS is resistant to clindamycin or of unknown susceptibility, vancomycin is the drug of choice for GBS prophylaxis.

CHORIOAMNIONITIS

Chorioamnionitis is an infection of the membranes and amniotic fluid surrounding the fetus. It is frequently associated with preterm and prolonged ROM but can also occur without ROM. Clinical chorioamnionitis occurs in 0.5% to 10% of pregnancies, whereas histologic chorioamnionitis is present in up to 20% of term deliveries and more than 50% of preterm deliveries. Clinical chorioamnionitis has been recently reviewed and suggested to be renamed as intrauterine inflammation, infection or both (Triple I) and is the most common precursor of neonatal sepsis, which has a high rate of neonatal mortality. Triple I has elevated risk of neonatal respiratory distress, pneumonia, meningitis, periventricular leukomalacia, and cerebral palsy. Additionally, it has maternal sequelae of uterine atony, postpartum hemorrhage, need for cesarean delivery, endomyometritis, and, in some cases, septic shock.

DIAGNOSIS

The diagnosis of Triple I requires a high index of suspicion. Diagnosis is made by the combination of fever ≥39°C or 102.2°F based on oral maternal temperature with another clinical sign, including elevated maternal WBC count (>15,000/mL), purulent fluid from cervical os or fetal tachycardia (>160 beats per minute), or evidence from an amniocentesis that is consistent with microbial invasion. Of note, a temperature ≥38°C but <39°C does not by itself meet diagnosis for fever for Triple I according to updated guidelines. In this case, the temperature should be repeated after 30 minutes, and if both are ≥38°C and there is a presence of an additional clinical factor, it would lead to a diagnosis of Triple I.

Because Triple I is significant and necessitates delivery, other physiologic events that may have similar signs and symptoms should be excluded. Other loci of maternal infection may cause maternal fever, elevated WBC count, as well as fetal tachycardia. Elevations in maternal temperature have been seen in patients undergoing labor induction with prostaglandins as well as in those patients with epidurals. Fetal tachycardia may be congenital. Thus, a prior baseline fetal heart rate can be useful. Fetal tachycardia can also be caused by medications administered to the mother, such as β-agonist tocolytic agents and promethazine. The maternal WBC count is elevated in pregnancy and further elevated with the onset of labor. The WBC count is also increased when corticosteroids are given.

In patients at term, if the constellation of the above signs exists without any other etiology, the diagnosis of Triple I should be presumed and treatment started. In preterm patients whose fetuses would benefit from remaining in utero for more time, a more aggressive means to reach the diagnosis can be taken if there is any doubt. The gold standard for diagnosis of chorioamnionitis is a culture of the amniotic fluid, which can be obtained via amniocentesis. At the same time, the amniotic fluid can be sent for the following tests: glucose, WBC count, protein, and Gram stain. Unfortunately, these tests have a sensitivity that ranges from 40% to 70%. The lack of a single sensitive and specific test has led to the proposal for a clinical diagnosis of Triple I as described above.

TREATMENT

When acute chorioamnionitis is strongly suspected, most experts agree that prompt initiation of IV antibiotics and delivery of the fetus are required. Commonly, the causative organisms are polymicrobial and include those that colonize the vagina and rectum. Thus, broad-spectrum coverage should be used, most commonly, a second- or third-generation cephalosporin or ampicillin and gentamicin. Multiple studies have shown that there are decreased rates of neonatal sepsis and maternal morbidity if antibiotics are begun intrapartum, rather than immediate postpartum. In addition to antibiotics, delivery should be hastened with induction and augmentation by vaginal delivery or, in the case of a nonreassuring fetal tracing, by cesarean delivery. In the case of delivery by cesarean section, anaerobic organism coverage is recommended using either these specific drugs (metronidazole or clindamycin) or a broad-spectrum antibiotic, which covers anaerobes. Additionally, it is commonly recommended that antibiotics are continued after cesarean section for 12 to 24 hours.

INFECTIONS THAT AFFECT THE FETUS

HERPES SIMPLEX VIRUS

The frequency of neonatal herpes ranges from 8 to 60 per 100,000 live births. The majority of these infections occur from exposure to herpes simplex virus (HSV) from the genital tract during delivery. Neonatal herpes is a serious infection with significantly associated morbidity and mortality.

Genital herpes is caused by **herpes simplex virus**, a DNA virus transmitted through skin contact. There are two types based on peripheral glycoproteins: HSV-1 and HSV-2. HSV-2 classically causes genital herpes, but the rates of genital HSV-1 have been increasing in young women and, recently, have been reported to cause as much genital HSV-1 herpes as HSV-2. Infection with HSV is chronic and divided into primary infection and latent infection. Primary infections are asymptomatic in 50% of patients and are responsible for approximately 90% of neonatal herpes. The risk of transmission to the neonate with a primary outbreak is 20% to 50%. In comparison, the risk of transmission with recurrent herpes with active lesions is approximately 1%. Latent infection occurs after a primary infection. In this infection, the virus resides in the dorsal root ganglion, and the peripheral nerves can shed virus symptomatically or asymptomatically. A symptomatic outbreak after a primary outbreak is also referred to as recurrent herpes.

Routine serologic screening for all pregnant women is not recommended. It is important to ask if women are at risk by asking if their partner has genital HSV, or if they have a history of genital lesions. Approximately 10% of seronegative women have positive partners and are at risk for infection. Some have suggested that these women abstain from intercourse during the third trimester. Any patient with vesicular lesions should be tested for HSV because clinical diagnosis alone has a sensitivity of 40% and a specificity of 99% and a false-positive rate of 20%. Diagnosis of HSV is based on the presence of both (1) viral tests and (2) serologic tests. A symptomatic, suspected infection should be tested with both a viral test and a serologic test to help distinguish if the outbreak is primary or a recurrence. The ideal method of testing for genital herpes is through scraping of the lesions and sending for viral detection through Polymerase Chain Reaction (PCR). Viral culture is less sensitive than PCR, and additional assays are less specific. Because viral shedding is intermittent, a negative result does not rule out the presence of an infection. The antibody detection techniques include the use of serologic tests to detect the presence of antibodies to either HSV-1 or HSV-2. A positive viral detection result and negative serologic test indicate a primary infection. A positive serologic test indicates a latent infection or recurrence. There is not thought to be a role for IgM in serologic testing for herpes. Importantly, in a woman with no history of lesions who is asymptomatic, a positive serologic test could indicate oral herpes, rather than genital herpes.

HSV-2 can be detected at term in asymptomatic individuals by culture (approximately 2%) or PCR (approximately 8% to 15%) in genital secretions, but neonatal herpes occurs in less than 1% of those with detectable viral shedding, because the majority of transmission is through a primary infection, much of which is asymptomatic. The risk of vertical transmission to the neonate when a primary outbreak occurs at the time of delivery is approximately 30% to 60% and most often occurs through delivery and cervical viral shedding but also can be transplacental. Several factors are thought to contribute to the increased risk of transmission. First, with a primary infection, there is a reduced transplacental passage of protective HSV antibodies. As such, higher titers of neutralizing antibodies in the neonate have been associated with a reduced risk of neonatal infection. Second, neonatal exposure to the amount of virus in the genital tract may be increased. The genital viral shedding in women with primary infection is of higher concentration and longer duration than shedding that occurs with recurrent episodes. Cervical shedding has been detected by viral culture in 90% of women with primary infection. In contrast to a primary outbreak, the presence of protective antibodies and a lower concentration of viral shedding are thought to lead to significantly decreased rates of transmission in recurrent outbreaks.

Patients with a history of herpes should have a thorough examination for genital lesions when presenting in labor because of the risk of vertical transmission of HSV to the fetus during vaginal delivery. The vulva, vagina, and cervix should be inspected, and any suspicious lesions should be swabbed and sent for viral testing. If lesions are present, cesarean delivery is recommended for prevention of vertical transmission. The risk reduction of vertical transmission with cesarean delivery is not well characterized, but a large study showed reduction of transmission from 8% to 1%. Of note, cesarean delivery does not completely prevent vertical transmission to the neonate because transmission has been shown to occur transplacentally.

Antiviral medications are used to treat primary and recurrent outbreaks as well as prevent recurrent outbreaks. Acyclovir, valacyclovir, and famciclovir are category B in pregnancy and are overall well tolerated. Primary outbreaks at any time in pregnancy are recommended to be treated both to reduce the duration and severity of the symptoms and to reduce the duration of viral shedding. In patients who have severe disease, oral treatment can be extended for more than 10 days if lesions are incompletely healed at that time. Acyclovir may be administered intravenously to pregnant women with severe genital HSV infection or with disseminated herpetic infections. Case reports have associated significant improvement in expected survival with acyclovir treatment in cases of pregnant women with disseminated HSV, herpes pneumonitis, herpes hepatitis, and herpes encephalitis.

Patients with an HSV genital outbreak during their pregnancies are also offered acyclovir prophylaxis from week 36 until delivery to prevent recurrent lesions. Acyclovir has been shown to decrease both viral shedding and cesarean section at term. Treatment has not been clearly shown to decrease neonatal infections. Women with a history of genital HSV, but without an outbreak in pregnancy, are more controversial, although the majority of clinicians also recommend acyclovir prophylaxis beyond 36 weeks of gestation. Asymptomatic shedding during the antepartum period does not predict asymptomatic shedding at delivery, and viral shedding is associated with a 300-fold risk of neonatal transmission.

As noted above, HSV can cause severe infections in the neonate. Neonatal herpes usually is acquired during the intrapartum period through exposure to the virus in the genital tract, although rarely in utero and postnatal infections can also occur. Primary infection acquired near the time of labor is associated with the highest risk of transmission to the neonate during delivery. Primary infection in the first trimester has been associated with congenital HSV infection and associated chorioretinitis, microcephaly, and

FIGURE 10-1. Newborn with disseminated herpes simplex virus (HSV) infection. Note the healing ulcerations on the abdomen of the infant. (From Sweet R, Gibbs R. *Atlas of Infectious Diseases of the Female Genital Tract*, Philadelphia, PA: Lippincott Williams & Wilkins; 2005.)

hydrocephalus. More commonly, neonatal infection from exposure to the genital tract presents after delivery and is classified as disseminated disease (25%); CNS disease (30%); and disease limited to the skin, eyes, or mouth (45%) (Fig. 10-1). The infection in the neonate can progress to a viral sepsis, pneumonia, and herpes encephalitis, which can lead to neurologic devastation and death. Infected infants are treated with IV acyclovir as soon as infection is suspected, but even in the setting of adequate treatment, cognitive difficulties and developmental delay can persist. Mortality has decreased substantially over the past two decades, decreasing to 30% for disseminated disease and 4% for CNS disease. Approximately 20% of the survivors of neonatal herpes have long-term neurologic sequelae, and relapses of CNS infections can occur.

VARICELLA ZOSTER VIRUS

Varicella zoster virus (VZV) is a highly contagious DNA herpes virus that is transmitted by respiratory droplets or close contact and causes the disease chicken pox. It can later reactivate to cause herpes zoster or shingles. The attack rate among susceptible contacts is 60% to 90% after exposure. The virus enters the mucus membranes and establishes a viremia. This leads to prodromal symptoms, including headache, malaise, and fever. The prodromal symptoms are followed by a diffuse maculopapular rash that becomes vesicular. The incubation period after infection is 10 to 20 days, with a mean of 14 days. The period of infectivity begins 48 hours before the rash appears and lasts until the vesicles crust over. After the primary infection, VZV remains dormant in sensory ganglia and can be reactivated to cause a vesicular erythematous skin rash known as herpes zoster (or shingles). The antibody to VZV develops within a few days after the onset of infection, and prior infection with VZV confers lifelong immunity. VZV causes several syndromes relevant to pregnancy, including maternal varicella pneumonia, congenital varicella syndrome, and neonatal varicella infection.

Because it is primarily a disease of childhood, more than 90% of adults are immune to VZV infection in the United States. Severe complications, such as encephalitis and pneumonia, are more common in adults than in children. VZV pneumonia in pregnancy is a risk factor for maternal mortality. Likewise, pregnancy carries additional risk, and maternal varicella pneumonia has significant maternal morbidity and mortality; as many as 40% will require mechanical ventilation, and mortality is 3% to 14%. The incidence of maternal varicella pneumonia with primary infection has been reported with case series 10% to 40%, and more recent population-based studies have shown an incidence of 2% to 3%. Varicella infection is uncommon in pregnancy (occurring in 0.4 to 3 per 1,000 patients) because of the high prevalence of natural immunity, and thus, studies are limited due to small case numbers.

Pregnancy complicated by maternal varicella infection is also associated with fetal and neonatal effects. Vertical transmission occurs transplacentally. More recent, large studies do not demonstrate an increased risk of spontaneous abortion during maternal VZV infection in the first trimester. Investigations have shown that the frequency of fetal anomalies was less than 1% when maternal infection occurred in weeks 1 through 12 of pregnancy and 2% or less when infection occurred in weeks 13 through 20. However, VZV is associated with congenital malformations characterized as congenital varicella syndrome (Fig. 10-2) in approximately 0.5% to 2% of cases, resulting predominantly when mothers are infected between 8 and 20 weeks of gestation. Congenital varicella syndrome is characterized by skin scarring, limb hypoplasia, chorioretinitis, and microcephaly. It is associated with 30% mortality in the first month of life. The mechanism of congenital varicella syndrome is thought to be reactivation of VZV in utero (similar to herpes zoster). With maternal infection in the late third trimester, the virus can cross the placenta, and the infant has insufficient cell-mediated immunity to prevent hematogenous dissemination of virus and cause neonatal varicella. Neonatal VZV infection is associated with a high

FIGURE 10-2. Congenital varicella syndrome characterized by long-bone defects, chorioretinitis, and cerebral cortical atrophy. (From Sweet R, Gibbs R. *Atlas of Infectious Diseases of the Female Genital Tract*, Philadelphia, PA: Lippincott Williams & Wilkins; 2005.)

neonatal death rate. In this setting, maternal disease develops between 5 days before delivery and up to 48 hours postpartum, and as a result of the relative immaturity of the neonatal immune system and the lack of protective maternal antibody, the infants have a disseminated infection. Neonatal varicella with postnatal infection may range from a benign course (like chicken pox) to a fulminant disseminated infection, leading to death. In the absence of timely antiviral chemotherapy, up to 30% of infected infants die of complications of neonatal varicella. Other infants may show no signs of infection at birth; however, they will develop shingles (recurrent herpes zoster outbreaks) at some point later in childhood. Infants of mothers who develop varicella disease within 5 days before delivery or 2 days after should also receive Varicella Zoster Immunoglobulin (VZIG) and/or treatment with antiviral agents, such as acyclovir or valacyclovir. Of note, maternal herpes zoster, recurrent VZV outbreaks, is not associated with congenital anomalies or neonatal varicella.

Varicella titers may be evaluated during pregnancy for those patients who are unsure about exposure history. Women who present preconceptionally can be screened for VZV titers and, if negative, be immunized prior to conceiving. The varicella vaccine (Varivax) is a live virus vaccine that is highly immunogenic and, therefore, contraindicated in pregnancy to avoid transmission to the fetus. The Centers for Disease Control (CDC) guidelines indicate that the vaccine may be considered in breastfeeding mothers, although there is little information about whether the vaccine virus is excreted in breast milk. Vaccine recipients pose minimal risk of transmitting infection to susceptible contacts if no rash develops after the vaccination. If a rash does develop, there is a very small risk of transmission to susceptible contacts.

If a susceptible pregnant patient is exposed to someone with varicella, she should be treated within 72 to 96 hours with one of two agents to prevent active infection. Varicella zoster immune globulin preparation (VariZIG) is recommended for postexposure prophylaxis, and any woman who has exposure without a history of chicken pox or history of vaccination should be treated. This recommendation has been extended for up to 10 days after exposure. The efficacy of this in preventing maternal and neonatal complications is not well characterized, but preliminary studies have suggested a decrease in maternal complications. An alternative method of prophylaxis is to administer oral acyclovir (800 mg, five times daily for 7 days) or oral valacyclovir (1,000 mg, three times daily for 7 days). Pregnant women who develop varicella despite immunoprophylaxis should be treated with oral acyclovir or valacyclovir in the same dose as outlined for prophylaxis. Patients who have evidence of pneumonia, encephalitis, or disseminated infection and those who are immunosuppressed should be hospitalized and treated with IV acyclovir. Of note, women who are treated with postexposure prophylaxis should be vaccinated after delivery.

PARVOVIRUS

Parvovirus B19 is a DNA virus that causes erythema infectiosum (fifth disease), a common childhood illness. The virus is transmitted primarily by respiratory droplets and infected blood products. In pregnancy, the virus is transmitted transplacentally in about 35% of infected women. Immunity to parvovirus increases progressively throughout childhood and young adult life. Approximately 50% to 60% of women of reproductive age have evidence of prior infection, and immunity is long-lasting. Parvovirus B19 infects rapidly dividing cells and is cytotoxic for erythroid progenitor cells. Erythema infectiosum is usually manifested by a low-grade fever, malaise, myalgias, arthralgias, and a red macular "slapped cheek" facial rash. An erythematous, lace-like rash also may extend to the torso and upper extremities. In children, parvovirus infection can also cause transient aplastic crisis. This same disorder may occur in adults who have an underlying hemoglobinopathy.

Erythema infectiosum usually resolves with minimal intervention. In pregnancy, vertical transmission of the virus is associated with severe sequelae and fetal death. First-trimester infections have been associated with miscarriage, whereas midtrimester and later infections are associated with fetal hydrops. The risk of hydrops is directly related to the GA at which maternal infection occurs. If infection develops during the first 12 weeks of gestation, the risk of hydrops is 5% to 10%. If infection occurs during weeks 13 through 20, the risk of infection decreases to 5% or less. If infection occurs beyond the 20th week of gestation, the risk of fetal hydrops is <1%.

Vertical transmission occurs 1 to 3 weeks after maternal infection during the peak viral load. The virus can cross the placenta and infects and lyses RBC progenitors in the fetal bone marrow. This suppresses erythropoiesis, thereby resulting in severe anemia and high-output congestive heart failure. This same antigen is also present in fetal myocardial cells, and, in some fetuses, the viral infection causes a cardiomyopathy that further contributes to heart failure (i.e., hydrops). The heart failure manifests as fluid overload and nonimmune hydrops fetalis. The hydrops can lead to rapid fetal death or can resolve spontaneously. Additional manifestations include nervous system damage, thrombocytopenia, hyperechoic bowel, and non-hydrops–associated fetal death.

If parvovirus exposure is suspected in the mother, acute infection can be diagnosed by checking parvovirus IgM and IgG levels. If IgM is negative and IgG is positive, then the patient has prior immunity and is protected against a second infection. If IgM and IgG are both negative, then the patient does not have an acute infection but is susceptible to future infections. In patients with a strong exposure history and negative IgG and IgM, serum viral PCR should be considered because an IgM response takes 10 days. If studies indicate an acute parvovirus infection (positive IgM and positive or negative IgG) beyond 20 weeks of gestation, then the fetus should undergo serial ultrasounds for 12 and up to 20 weeks after maternal infection is suspected to have occurred. However, by the time sonographic evidence of hydrops is present, the fetal hematocrit is likely to be less than 20%. Therefore, a more precise way to detect evolving fetal anemia is to use Doppler velocimetry to examine the peak systolic velocity of the middle cerebral artery (MCA). Increases in peak systolic velocity are associated with fetal anemia. If velocimetry indicates fetal anemia, a cordocentesis should be performed to determine the fetal hematocrit. If anemia is confirmed, an intrauterine blood transfusion should be performed. Management of parvovirus infection with intrauterine blood transfusion can correct fetal anemia and may reduce the mortality of parvovirus infection significantly. Although this intervention has not been studied in large populations, there are several studies that have shown that timely intrauterine blood transfusion in cases of severe hydrops in patients who are infected prior to 20 weeks of gestation decreases the risk of stillbirth. A few cases of spontaneous resolution of hydrops caused by parvovirus infection have been described. Most clinicians choose to proceed with transfusion when the fetal blood sample shows anemia, even if there is already an evidence of recovery of erythropoiesis by a high reticulocyte count. Because of the rarity of the disease and ethical considerations, a randomized trial to find the best policy is unlikely ever to be performed.

During outbreaks, pregnant child-care workers and school workers who are susceptible for infection can consider avoiding the workplace. Vaccine studies have been limited by side effects, and a vaccine is not available.

CYTOMEGALOVIRUS

Cytomegalovirus (CMV) is the most common cause of a congenital viral infection. CMV is a DNA virus in the herpes virus family. CMV is not highly contagious; close personal contact is required for infection to occur. Horizontal transmission may result from infected blood, sexual contact, or contact with contaminated saliva or urine. Vertical transmission may occur as a result of transplacental infection, exposure to contaminated genital tract secretions during delivery, or breastfeeding. The incubation period of CMV ranges from 28 to 60 days. CMV infections in the mother usually cause either a subclinical or mild viral illness. Only rarely will it lead to hepatitis or a mononucleosis-like syndrome. Thus, maternal infections are rarely diagnosed. After the initial infection, CMV remains latent in host cells; recurrent infection can occur following reactivation of latent virus. In rare cases, recurrent CMV infection can occur by infection with a new strain of virus. Approximately 50% to 80% of adult women in the United States have serologic evidence of past CMV infection. Maternal antibodies do not prevent reactivation of latent virus or reinfection with a new strain and are not perfectly protective against vertical transmission of infection from mother to fetus. Therefore, pregnant women with either recurrent or primary infection pose a risk to their fetus.

Diagnosis of CMV infection in adults is usually confirmed by serologic testing. Serum samples collected 3 to 4 weeks apart, tested in parallel for anti-CMV IgG, are essential for the diagnosis of primary infection. Seroconversion from negative to positive or a significant increase (greater than fourfold, e.g., from 1:4 to 1:16) in anti-CMV IgG titers is an evidence of infection. When there is a question of acute infection, IgG avidity testing can be performed. If high-avidity CMV is detected, a recent infection can be ruled out. In contrast, the presence of CMV-specific IgM is a useful but not completely reliable indication of a primary infection. IgM titers may not be positive during an acute infection, or they may persist for months after the primary infection.

Congenital CMV may be suspected prenatally after a documented maternal primary infection or, more typically, after detection of ultrasound findings suggestive of infection. The most sensitive and specific test for diagnosing congenital CMV infection is the identification of CMV in amniotic fluid by either culture or PCR. Identification of the virus in amniotic fluid by culture or PCR does not necessarily indicate the severity of fetal injury. The principal sonographic findings suggestive of serious fetal injury are microcephaly, ventriculomegaly, intercerebral calcification, fetal hydrops, growth restriction, and oligohydramnios. Less common findings include fetal heart block, echogenic bowel, meconium peritonitis, renal dysplasia, ascites, and pleural effusions. Fetuses that demonstrate abnormalities, particularly if they involve the CNS, generally have a much poorer prognosis.

CMV is the most common congenital infection, occurring in approximately 1% to 2% of all neonates, and is the leading cause of congenital hearing loss. Vertical transmission may occur at any stage of pregnancy, with the overall risk of infection greatest when the infection occurs during the third trimester. However, more serious fetal sequelae occur after maternal CMV infection during the first trimester. With primary maternal CMV infection, the risk of transmission to the fetus is 30% to 40%. Approximately 5% to 15% of infants who develop congenital CMV infection as a result of primary maternal infection are symptomatic at birth. The incidence of severe fetal infection is much lower after recurrent maternal infection than after primary infection. Vertical transmission after a recurrent infection is 0.15% to 2%. Infants infected after maternal CMV reactivation generally are asymptomatic at birth. Congenital hearing loss is the most common severe sequela of secondary infection, and congenital infection following recurrent infection is unlikely to produce multiple sequelae. CMV infection acquired as a result of exposure to infected cervical secretions or breast milk is typically asymptomatic and is not associated with severe neonatal sequelae. Infants who are symptomatic can develop cytomegalic inclusion disease manifested by a constellation of findings, including hepatomegaly, splenomegaly, thrombocytopenia, jaundice, cerebral calcifications, chorioretinitis, and interstitial pneumonitis (Fig. 10-3). The most

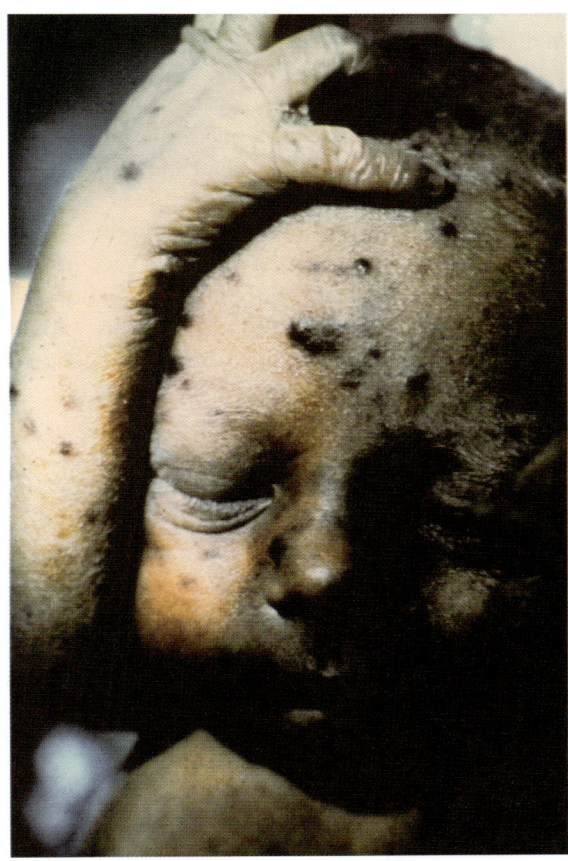

FIGURE 10-3. Congenital cytomegalovirus (CMV) "blueberry muffin" baby with jaundice and thrombocytopenia purpura. (From Sweet R, Gibbs R. *Atlas of Infectious Diseases of the Female Genital Tract*, Philadelphia, PA: Lippincott Williams & Wilkins; 2005.)

common clinical manifestations of severe neonatal infection are hepatosplenomegaly, intracranial calcifications, jaundice, growth restriction, microcephaly, chorioretinitis, hearing loss, thrombocytopenia, hyperbilirubinemia, and hepatitis. Approximately 30% of severely infected infants die, and 80% of survivors have severe neurologic morbidity, such as mental retardation, sensorineural hearing loss, and neuromuscular disorders. Among the 85% to 90% of infants with congenital CMV infection who are asymptomatic at birth, 10% to 15% subsequently develop hearing loss, chorioretinitis, or dental defects within the first 2 years of life, whereas 85% will have no sequelae of the infection.

Currently, there is no treatment or prophylaxis for the disease. Studies reporting use of IV hyperimmune globulin and antiviral medications have been published, and these treatments are supported by some clinicians. In particular, the use of IVIG demonstrated improvement in outcomes, but large randomized trials demonstrating decrease in fetal infection are still lacking. A vaccine for the prevention of disease in the mother is also being investigated.

RUBELLA VIRUS

Rubella (also called "German measles") is caused by an RNA virus. With licensure of an effective vaccine in 1969, the frequency of rubella declined markedly. Such that rubella is no longer endemic in the United States. Yet in other regions of the world vaccination is not optimal, and persistence of this infection appears to be caused by failure to vaccinate susceptible individuals, rather than by a lack of immunogenicity of the vaccine. Rubella infection in adults leads to a mild illness with a widely disseminated, nonpruritic, erythematous maculopapular rash; arthritis; arthralgias; and a diffuse lymphadenopathy that lasts 3 to 5 days. Postauricular adenopathy and mild conjunctivitis also are common. The infection can be transmitted to the fetus and cause congenital rubella infection, which may lead to **congenital rubella syndrome**. Rubella virus crosses the placenta by hematogenous dissemination, and the frequency of congenital infection critically depends on the time of exposure to the virus. The fetus is not at risk from infection before the time of conception. However, approximately 50% to 80% of infants exposed to the virus within 12 weeks after conception will manifest signs of congenital infection. The rate of congenital infection declines sharply with advancing GA, so that very few fetuses are affected if infection occurs after 18 weeks of gestation. The maternal–fetal transmission rate is highest during the first trimester, as are the rates of congenital abnormalities. However, transmission may occur at any time during pregnancy.

The four most common anomalies associated with congenital rubella syndrome (CRS) are deafness (affecting 60% to 75% of fetuses); eye defects, such as cataracts or retinopathy (10% to 30%); CNS defects (10% to 25%); and cardiac malformations (10% to 20%). The most common cardiac abnormality is patent ductus arteriosus, although supravalvular pulmonic stenosis is perhaps the most pathognomonic. Other possible abnormalities include microcephaly, mental retardation, pneumonia, fetal growth restriction, hepatosplenomegaly, hemolytic anemia, and thrombocytopenia. Specifically, if maternal rubella infection occurs during the period of organogenesis, any fetal organ system may be affected. There are a variety of latent sequelae, including the delayed onset of diabetes, thyroid disease, deafness, ocular disease, and growth hormone deficiency. The prognosis for infants with CRS is guarded. Approximately 50% of affected individuals have to attend schools for the hearing-impaired. An additional 25% require at least some special schooling because of hearing impairment, and only 25% are able to attend mainstream schools.

The diagnosis of maternal rubella infection is made with serology studies. IgM titers will result from primary infection and reinfection with rubella. Because IgM does not cross the placenta, IgM titers in the infant are indicative of infection. IgG titers that are elevated over time support the diagnosis of CRS in an infant as well. Fetal blood, obtained by cordocentesis, can be used to determine the total and viral-specific IgM concentration. However, cordocentesis technically is difficult before 20 weeks of gestation, and fetal immunoglobulins usually cannot be detected before 22 to 24 weeks of gestation. Chorionic villi, fetal blood, and amniotic fluid samples all can be tested via PCR for rubella antigen. Because of its lower complication rate, amniocentesis is the procedure of choice. Although these tests can demonstrate that rubella virus is present in the fetal compartment, they do not indicate the degree of fetal injury. Furthermore, the possibility of false-positive test results cannot be excluded. Accordingly, detailed ultrasound examination is the best test to determine whether serious fetal injury has occurred as a result of maternal rubella infection. Possible anomalies detected by ultrasound include growth restriction, microcephaly, CNS abnormalities, and cardiac malformations.

Currently, there is no treatment for rubella. The incidence of CRS in the United States has declined dramatically. Fewer than 10 cases of congenital rubella occur each year. However, approximately 10% to 20% of women in the United States remain susceptible to rubella, and their fetuses are at risk for serious injury if infection occurs during pregnancy. Ideally, women of reproductive age should have a preconception appointment when they are contemplating pregnancy. At that time, they should be evaluated for immunity to rubella. If serologic testing demonstrates that they are susceptible, they should be vaccinated with rubella vaccine before conception occurs. If preconception counseling is not possible, patients should have a test for rubella at the time of their first prenatal appointment. Women who are susceptible to rubella should be counseled to avoid exposure to other individuals who may have viral exanthems. If a susceptible woman subsequently is exposed to rubella, serologic tests should be obtained to determine whether acute infection has occurred. If acute infection is documented by identification of IgM antibody, the patient should be counseled about the risk of CRS. The diagnostic tests for detection of congenital infection should be reviewed, and the patient should be offered the option of pregnancy termination, depending on the assessed risk of serious fetal injury. In pregnancy, the rubella titer is checked during the first trimester. Because of theoretic risk of transmission of the live virus in the vaccine, patients do not receive the measles, mumps, and rubella vaccine until postpartum, and patients are advised to avoid pregnancy for 1 month following vaccination.

HUMAN IMMUNODEFICIENCY VIRUS

Globally, the cumulative rate of vertical HIV transmission (in utero, intrapartum, and postpartum) is 35% to 40% without intervention. The rate of transmission correlates with viral load, although transmission can occur even with undetectable viral load. With implementation of current recommendations (discussed below), the rates of perinatal HIV transmission have decreased to less than 1%. In 2014, there were 174 pediatric cases of HIV in the United States, and 88% were perinatally acquired. The rate of transmission is associated with a marked racial disparity. In the majority of cases of perinatal transmission, there are limitations in health-care delivery and uptake. It is important to identify and monitor these barriers of care to prevent perinatal transmission. For this reason, women who are found to be HIV positive should have additional counseling to identify barriers for treatment with combination antiretroviral therapy (cART) (homelessness, drug use, domestic violence, etc.) and interventions focused on reducing barriers to access to treatment should be implemented.

Interventions that have been effective and are recommended for decreasing perinatal HIV transmission can be divided into several areas: (1) screening all patients, (2) initiating treatment with cART during antepartum course, (3) interventions during intrapartum care to minimize body fluid exposure, and (4) postpartum prophylaxis of infants. Additional focus on serodiscordant couples has recommended treatment of the infected partner, use of donor sperm, and use of sperm preparation techniques to lower the exposure to genital fluid for conception.

It is recommended that HIV screening be offered to all pregnant women at their first prenatal visit or preconception visit on an informed "opt-out" basis and again in the third trimester if the woman has specified risk factors for HIV infection (i.e., other sexually transmitted infections diagnosed during pregnancy, IV drug use, discordant couples). HIV screening is performed with either HIV1/2 antigen or antibody test with an enzyme immunoassay, and if positive, the result is confirmed through western blot or immunofluorescent antibody. Of note, if at any time during pregnancy, the woman is within the window of seroconversion and has a suspected acute HIV infection, then a plasma HIV PCR should also be used and repeated in 2 weeks.

Testing should also be performed in the intrapartum and/or neonatal periods if serostatus has not been previously determined. Despite the increasingly simple and straightforward approach recommended for prenatal testing, because approximately 15% of HIV-infected women receive no or minimal care and 20% do not initiate care until the third trimester, a number of women will still arrive in labor and delivery suites with unknown serostatus. Because intrapartum and early neonatal prophylaxis, even in the absence of antepartum therapy, can reduce the risk of mother-to-child transmission, efforts should be made during labor to rapidly discern the serostatus of those women whose results were not previously known. Expedited serum HIV tests are recommended with a fourth generation antigen/antibody test, and if positive, treatment should be initiated while a confirmatory test is pending.

Antepartum care for an HIV-infected woman includes cART with the goal to maintain an undetectable viral load. The importance of adherence should be discussed, and identifying barriers to adherence is an important part of prenatal care. CD4 measurements, viral load measurements, baseline blood counts, liver and renal function tests, and drug resistance should be tested at the initial visit, and it is recommended that these tests are repeated every 3 months during pregnancy. HIV-positive pregnant women should receive indicated vaccines if they have not previously vaccinated, including hepatitis A, hepatitis B, and pneumococcal vaccinations. Transplacental passage of antiretrovirals is thought to be an important part of infant pre-exposure prophylaxis, and a medication with high placental transfer is recommended as part of cART. Antiviral use is associated with an increased risk of preterm delivery, small for GA infants, and hypertensive disorders, but these associations are controversial, and cART should not be withheld due to these concerns.

Intrapartum care for HIV-infected women is based on viral load; in women on cART with a viral load less than 1,000 copies/mL near delivery, a vaginal delivery can be considered. During labor, every precaution should be taken to minimize contact between the infant's skin and mucous membranes and contaminated maternal blood and genital tract secretions. Specifically, amniotomy, scalp monitoring, scalp pH assessment, episiotomy, and instrumental delivery should be avoided if at all possible. In women with a viral load >1,000 copies/mL, intravenous zidovudine (ZDV) is recommended 3 hours prior to delivery (regardless of cART use), and cesarean delivery is recommended at 38 weeks. Cesarean delivery has been shown to lower transmission rates by 80% compared with vaginal delivery in patients without onset of labor or ROM or in the setting of high viral load.

Regardless of maternal viral load, all babies born to HIV-infected women should be bathed immediately and within 12 hours should receive a course of ZDV therapy, which should be continued for 4 to 6 weeks. Of note, combination therapy has been shown to be superior than monotherapy in infants of women infected with HIV with no antepartum prophylaxis, and a two-drug (ZDV plus nevirapine) or three-drug regimen (ZDV plus nelfinavir and lamivudine) results in reducing rates of HIV transmission.

Furthermore, in resource-rich nations where safe bottle-feeding alternatives are available, breastfeeding is contraindicated in HIV-infected woman, because virus is found in breast milk and can lead to HIV transmission to the infant. Postnatal HIV transmission from breast milk at 2 years may be as high as 25%. Furthermore, studies are lacking regarding the efficacy of maternal antiretroviral therapy for prevention of transmission of HIV through breast milk and the toxicity of antiretroviral exposure of the infant via breast milk. Conversely, randomized controlled trials of breast- versus bottle-feeding in Africa have shown that the advantage of bottle-feeding in reducing neonatal deaths from AIDS is counterbalanced by increases in neonatal deaths from other illnesses, malnutrition, and dehydration.

Neisseria Gonorrhoeae

Gonococcal infections are associated with pelvic inflammatory disease in early pregnancy, as well as preterm delivery, PPROM, and puerperal infections throughout pregnancy duration. Studies have shown an association between untreated maternal endocervical gonorrhea and perinatal complications, including premature rupture of the membranes (PROM), preterm delivery, chorioamnionitis, neonatal sepsis, and maternal postpartum sepsis. The amniotic infection syndrome is an additional manifestation of gonococcal infection in pregnancy. This condition is characterized by placental, fetal membrane, and umbilical cord inflammation that occurs after PROM and is associated with infected oral and gastric aspirate, leukocytosis, neonatal infection, and maternal fever. Preterm delivery is common, and perinatal morbidity may be significant. The prevalence of gonorrhea in pregnancy ranges from 0% to 10% with marked variations according to risk status and geographic locale. The infection is transmitted during passage of the neonate through the birth canal. Neonatal infection most commonly affects the eye as ophthalmia neonatorum. Infection causes ulceration, scarring, and visual impairment that is irreversible and manifests 5 to 10 days after birth. Because of the severity of disease, neonatal prophylaxis with erythromycin ointment is universally recommended. *Neisseria gonorrhoeae* can also infect the oropharynx, external ear, and anorectal mucosa. These infections can furthermore become disseminated, causing arthritis and meningitis.

Screening for gonorrhea should be performed for pregnant women with risk factors in the first prenatal visit and again in the third trimester. Screening for gonorrhea during pregnancy is clearly cost-effective if the prevalence exceeds 1%. Therefore, the CDC recommends that all pregnant women at risk for gonorrhea, as well as those living in an area where the prevalence of *N. gonorrhoeae* is high, be tested for *N. gonorrhoeae* at their first prenatal visit. The CDC and the American College of Obstetricians and Gynecologists (ACOG) recommend that at-risk women be rescreened for *N. gonorrhoeae* during the third trimester. A recent study demonstrated the value of a repeat screen in the third trimester for *N. gonorrhoeae* among at-risk women who had an initial negative early pregnancy screen. In this study, approximately one-third of at-risk women tested positive for *N. gonorrhoeae* only on the repeat third-trimester screen. The diagnosis is made by nucleic acid amplification tests (NAATs) or culture. Treatment is with IM ceftriaxone and oral azithromycin in directly observed fashion. Combination therapy is recommended due to rising resistant profiles of *N. gonorrhoeae*. A test of cure is recommended 3 months after treatment.

Chlamydia Trachomatis

Chlamydial infection during pregnancy is associated with several adverse maternal outcomes, including preterm delivery, premature rupture of the membranes, low birth weight, and neonatal death. Untreated *Chlamydia trachomatis* infection also may result in neonatal conjunctivitis or pneumonia or both. The infection is transmitted during delivery from the genital tract to the infant. Infants born to women with a chlamydial infection of the cervix are at a 60% to 70% risk of acquiring the infection during passage through the birth canal. Approximately 25% to 50% of exposed infants acquire conjunctivitis in the first 2 weeks of life, and 10% to 20% develop pneumonia within 3 or 4 months.

Asymptomatic infection is common. The prevalence of *C. trachomatis* infection among pregnant women is about 2% to 3% but may be higher in certain high-risk populations. In the Preterm Prediction Study of the National Institute of Child Health and Human Development Maternal–Fetal Medicine Units Network, the overall prevalence of *C. trachomatis* among pregnant women was found to be 11%. Therefore, many authorities recommend that all pregnant women should be screened in the first prenatal visit and, if deemed as high risk, again in the third trimester. The treatment of choice for chlamydial infection in pregnancy is azithromycin, amoxicillin, or erythromycin. In 2006, azithromycin, as a single 1-g dose, was added to the list of recommended regimens for treatment of chlamydial infection during pregnancy. Single-dose therapy with azithromycin definitely improves patient compliance. Repeat testing (preferably by NAATs) 3 weeks after completion of therapy is recommended for all pregnant women to ensure cure, in light of the sequelae that can occur in the mother and newborn infant if chlamydial infection persists. Sex partners should be referred for evaluation, testing, and treatment.

HEPATITIS B

Viral hepatitis caused by the **hepatitis B** DNA virus can be acquired from sexual contact, exposure to blood products, and transplacentally. The clinical manifestations of the disease range from mild hepatic dysfunction to fulminant liver failure and death (<1%). It can be diagnosed using a variety of antibody and antigenic markers. Acute hepatitis B occurs in 1 or 2 of every 1,000 pregnancies in the United States. The chronic carrier state is more frequent, occurring in 6 to 10 of 1,000 pregnancies (approximately 10% of those infected). Worldwide, more than 400 million individuals are chronically infected with hepatitis B virus. In the United States alone, approximately 1.25 million people are chronically infected.

During the prenatal period, all patients are screened for hepatitis B surface antigen (HBsAg). Those with a positive HBsAg test are likely to have chronic disease and are at risk for transmission to the fetus. In order to confirm an active hepatitis B infection, hepatitis B core antibody and hepatitis B surface antibody IgM and IgG should also be checked. Patients with acute hepatitis B are positive for the HBsAg and positive for IgM antibody to the core antigen. Patients with chronic hepatitis B are positive for the surface antigen and positive for IgG antibody to the core antigen. Acutely or chronically infected patients may or may not be positive for the hepatitis B e antigen. If this latter antigen is present, it denotes active viral replication and a high level of infectivity. In the absence of intervention, approximately 20% of mothers who are seropositive for hepatitis B surface antigen will transmit infection to their neonates. Approximately 90% of mothers who are positive for both the surface antigen and the e antigen transmit infection. Fortunately, excellent immunoprophylaxis for prevention of perinatal transmission of hepatitis B infection is now available. Neonates delivered to seropositive mothers should receive hepatitis B immune globulin within 12 hours after birth. Before their discharge from the hospital, these infants also should begin the hepatitis B vaccination series. The CDC now recommends universal vaccination of all infants for hepatitis B. In addition, the vaccine should be offered to all women of reproductive age.

SYPHILIS

Syphilis is caused by infection with the spirochete *Treponema pallidum* and is transmitted via sexual contact or transplacentally to the fetus. Primary syphilis is characterized by a painless chancre. Secondary syphilis is characterized by a systemic rash, mucosal sores, fatigue, and myalgias. Tertiary or latent syphilis is characterized by a long dormant phase followed by systemic organ dysfunction, including paralysis, blindness, and dementia. Vertical transmission can occur at any time during pregnancy, and while *T. pallidum* can cross the placenta and infect the fetus as early as 6 weeks of gestation, clinical manifestations are not apparent until after 16 weeks of gestation when fetal immunocompetence develops. Transmission may also occur intrapartum via contact with active genital lesions in the mother. Women with primary or secondary syphilis are more likely to transmit infection to their offspring than are women with latent disease. Maternal primary syphilis and secondary syphilis are associated with a 50% probability of congenital syphilis and a 50% rate of perinatal death; early latent syphilis, with a 40% risk of congenital syphilis and a 20% mortality rate; and late latent syphilis, with a 10% risk of congenital syphilis. More than 70% of infants born to mothers with untreated syphilis will be infected (with a 40% perinatal death rate and 40% developing congenital syphilis), compared with 1% to 2% of infants born to women who received adequate treatment during pregnancy. Despite prenatal screening and readily available treatment, there are still several hundred cases of congenital syphilis annually in the United States, and this has been on the rise nationally since 2011.

Syphilis during pregnancy that results in vertical transmission may lead to a late abortion, intrauterine fetal demise, hydrops, preterm delivery, neonatal death, early congenital syphilis, and the classic stigmata of late congenital syphilis. The most severe adverse pregnancy outcomes occur with primary or secondary syphilis. Pregnant women diagnosed with syphilis are usually diagnosed during secondary syphilis. Consequently, about two-thirds of infants with early congenital syphilis are asymptomatic at birth and do not develop evidence of active disease for 3 to 8 weeks. Chancres do not occur unless the disease is acquired at the time of passage through the birth canal. Neonates with early congenital syphilis (onset at younger than 2 years of age) present with a systemic illness accompanied by a maculopapular rash, snuffles (a flu-like syndrome associated with a nasal discharge), hepatomegaly, splenomegaly, hemolysis, lymphadenopathy, jaundice, pseudoparalysis of Parrot caused by osteochondritis, chorioretinitis, and iritis. Diagnosis of congenital syphilis can be made by identification of IgM antitreponemal antibodies, which do not cross the placenta. If early congenital syphilis is untreated, manifestations of late congenital syphilis can develop, including saber shins, mulberry molars (Fig. 10-4), Hutchinson teeth, saddle nose, and neurologic manifestations (eighth nerve deafness, mental retardation, hydrocephalus, optic nerve atrophy, and Clutton joints).

All pregnant women should be screened at the initial prenatal visit using nonspecific antibody tests, including either the Venereal Disease Research Laboratory (VDRL) test or the rapid plasma reagin (RPR) test. If the test is positive, a titer is sent. Treponema-specific tests are employed for confirming the diagnosis of syphilis in patients who have reactive VDRL or RPR results. All positive results must then be confirmed with fluorescent treponemal antibody absorption (FTA-ABS), because there are false positives with both RPR and VDRL. There are several conditions that can cause false-positive RPR, including systemic lupus erythematosus and antiphospholipid antibody syndrome. Confirmatory tests include the FTA-ABS test and the *T. pallidum* particle agglutination test. Once reactive, specific treponemal tests usually remain positive for life. In pregnancy, it is best to consider all seropositive women as infected unless an adequate treatment history is documented and sequential serologic antibody titers have declined. High-risk patients should be rescreened at 28 weeks of gestation. In areas with high rates of congenital syphilis, rescreening at admission in labor is also recommended.

Penicillin remains the only treatment with sufficient evidence demonstrating efficacy for treating maternal infection, preventing maternal syphilis transmission to

FIGURE 10-4. Congenital syphilis—mulberry molar. (From Sweet R, Gibbs R. *Atlas of Infectious Diseases of the Female Genital Tract*, Philadelphia, PA: Lippincott Williams & Wilkins; 2005.)

the fetus, and for treating fetal infection. Therefore, if a pregnant patient diagnosed with syphilis is penicillin allergic, she must undergo desensitization and then be treated with penicillin. A high-maternal VDRL titer at the time of diagnosis, unknown duration of infection, treatment within 4 weeks of delivery, and ultrasound signs of fetal syphilis (e.g., hepatomegaly, fetal hydrops, placentomegaly) are associated with failure to prevent congenital syphilis. It is important to distinguish whether a patient has primary, secondary, latent, or tertiary syphilis in order to determine the length of treatment. If the patient has primary syphilis, one dose of 2.4 million units benzathine penicillin G is sufficient. However, if the patient has secondary or latent syphilis, the patient will require weekly treatments of 2.4 million units of benzathine penicillin G for 3 consecutive weeks. Syphilis can involve the CNS during any stage of disease. Therefore, any patient with syphilis who demonstrates clinical evidence of neurologic involvement should have a lumbar puncture to assess the cerebrospinal fluid for evidence of neurosyphilis. Patients with neurosyphilis should be treated with high doses of aqueous penicillin G. For primary and secondary syphilis, patients should be reexamined clinically and serologically at 6 and 12 months after treatment. A two-dilution (fourfold) decline in the nontreponemal titer at 1 year after treatment is used to define response.

TOXOPLASMOSIS

Toxoplasma gondii is a common protozoan parasite that can be found in humans and domestic animals. *T. gondii* has three distinct life forms: trophozoite, cyst, and oocyst. The life cycle of this organism depends on wild and domestic cats, which are the only known host for the oocyst. The oocyst is formed in the intestine of the cat and subsequently is excreted in feces. Mammals, such as cows, ingest the oocyst, which is disrupted in the animal's intestine, releasing the invasive trophozoite. The trophozoite then is disseminated throughout the body, ultimately forming cysts in brain and muscle. Human infection occurs when infected meat is ingested or oocysts are ingested via contamination by cat feces. Infection rates are highest in areas of poor sanitation and crowded living conditions. Stray cats and domestic cats that eat raw meat are most likely to carry the parasite but any mammal that eats the oocyst can become infected. The cyst is completely destroyed by heating.

Approximately half of all adults in the United States have antibodies to this organism and have lifelong immunity. The exception for this is in the case of immunosuppression where reinfection can occur. The prevalence of antibody is highest in lower socioeconomic classes. The frequency of seroconversion during pregnancy is approximately 5%, and about 3 in 1,000 infants show evidence of congenital infection. Clinically significant infection occurs in only 1 in 8,000 pregnancies. Immunity to this infection is mediated primarily through T lymphocytes. The infections in immunocompetent hosts are often subclinical. Occasionally, a patient will develop fevers, malaise, lymphadenopathy, and a rash as with most viral infections. A pregnant woman who is infected can transmit the disease transplacentally to the fetus. Approximately 40% of neonates born to mothers with acute toxoplasmosis have evidence of infection. Transmission is more common when the disease is acquired in the third trimester, although neonatal manifestations are usually mild or subclinical. Infections acquired in the first trimester are transmitted less commonly; however, the infection has far more serious consequences in the fetus.

Severe congenital infection can involve fevers, seizures, chorioretinitis, hydro- or microcephaly, hepatosplenomegaly, and jaundice (Fig. 10-5). The usual clinical manifestations of congenital toxoplasmosis include a disseminated purpuric rash, enlargement of the spleen and liver, ascites, chorioretinitis, uveitis, periventricular calcifications, ventriculomegaly, seizures, and mental retardation. Chronic or latent infection in the mother is unlikely to be associated with serious fetal injury. Thus, the differential diagnosis for this infection includes nearly all other commonly acquired intrauterine infections.

Because women with previous *Toxoplasma* exposure are likely to be protected from further infections, high-risk patients can be screened with titers for IgG to ascertain whether or not they are at risk for infection. Pregnant women are advised to avoid contact with cat litter boxes and significant gardening without glove and mask protection during pregnancy, because the organism is found in cat feces and soil that may be contaminated with animal feces. Toxoplasmosis in pregnancy can be diagnosed with maternal IgM and IgG titers. Because IgM may persist for years, the presence of IgM antibody cannot confirm an acute infection. Given the wide variability of IgM assays, diagnosis of an acute infection should be confirmed by a reference laboratory. If maternal diagnosis is made or suspected early in pregnancy, evaluation of amniotic fluid with DNA PCR for *T. gondii* via amniocentesis at least 4 weeks after maternal infection is the recommended procedure for evaluation of fetal infection. Fetal blood evaluation via percutaneous umbilical blood

FIGURE 10-5. Congenital toxoplasmosis with hepatosplenomegaly, jaundice, and thrombocytopenia purpura. (From Sweet R, Gibbs R. *Atlas of Infectious Diseases of the Female Genital Tract*, Philadelphia, PA: Lippincott Williams & Wilkins; 2005.)

sampling is discouraged given the low sensitivity, because absence of fetal IgM does not completely rule out fetal infection and, in turn, has the potential of transplacental fetal infection. Once amniocentesis has confirmed toxoplasmic infection, targeted ultrasound examination is indicated to look for specific findings suggestive of severe fetal injury. Diagnosis may influence the decision of whether to terminate a pregnancy in the first two trimesters. When acute toxoplasmosis occurs during pregnancy, treatment is indicated because maternal therapy reduces the risk of congenital infection and decreases the late sequelae of infection. Maternal disease without evidence of fetal disease can be treated with spiramycin. Spiramycin is preferable in pregnant women because no teratogenic effects are known. However, because spiramycin does not cross the placenta, it is not effective in treatment of fetal infection. Therefore, pyrimethamine and sulfadiazine are recommended for treatment of documented fetal infection. Pyrimethamine is not recommended for use during the first trimester of pregnancy because of possible teratogenicity. Folic acid is concurrently administered due to the bone marrow suppression effects of pyrimethamine and sulfadiazine, given their folate antagonist effects. Aggressive early treatment of infants with congenital toxoplasmosis is indicated and consists of combination therapy with pyrimethamine, sulfadiazine, and leucovorin for 1 year. Early treatment reduces, but does not eliminate, the late sequelae of toxoplasmosis, such as chorioretinitis. Early treatment of the neonate appears to be comparable in effectiveness with in utero therapy.

ZIKA VIRUS

Zika virus is a DNA flavivirus that is similar to dengue virus. There are three viral subtypes, and the Asian subtype has recently been noted to cause large epidemics in French Polynesia and Brazil. The virus is transmitted by *Aedes aegypti* mosquito bite and through sexual transmission. Zika virus causes systemic symptoms of fever, arthralgia, conjunctivitis, and a maculopapular rash. It is asymptomatic in approximately 40% of infected women. Zika virus has been associated with miscarriage and pregnancy loss in the first and second trimesters, and studies have shown Zika is present in pregnancy tissues and amniotic fluid. Additionally, Zika virus has been shown to demonstrate a distinct neurotropism. It has been found in the brains and spinal cords of infants at much higher concentration than other body compartments. As such, Zika virus is associated with microcephaly, intracerebral calcifications, and ocular damage. The incidence of microcephaly in infected women is estimated at 20% in one population-based retrospective study of Brazil. Testing for Zika virus is recommended for any woman with recent travel to a Zika-endemic location. Testing is through Enzyme-linked Immunosorbent assay (ELISA), which must be confirmed by PCR because the EIA also cross reacts with dengue virus and yellow fever, which have a similar geographic distribution. Patients are recommended to be followed by serial ultrasounds every 3 to 4 weeks. Of note, this is an area of rapidly expanding research and changing guidelines.

KEY POINTS

- Five percent of pregnant women have ASB and are at increased risk for cystitis and pyelonephritis.
- Lower UTIs can be treated with oral antibiotics, whereas pyelonephritis in pregnancy is usually treated initially with IV antibiotics, with change to oral regimen once afebrile for 24 to 48 hours.
- Pyelonephritis may be complicated by septic shock and ARDS.
- Symptomatic BV is associated with preterm delivery.
- BV treatment in pregnancy consists of oral metronidazole for 7 days.
- GBS has traditionally been a leading cause of neonatal sepsis.
- Screening for GBS and using prophylactic antibiotics in labor have been shown to decrease GBS neonatal sepsis.
- GBS screening is performed between 35 and 37 weeks of gestation.
- Chorioamnionitis/Triple I is diagnosed by maternal fever with uterine tenderness, elevated maternal WBC count, and fetal tachycardia.
- Although the infection is often polymicrobial, GBS colonization has a high correlation with both chorioamnionitis and neonatal sepsis.
- Chorioamnionitis/Triple I is treated by IV antibiotics and delivery.
- It is important to differentiate between infections that are transmitted transplacentally and those that are acquired from passage through the birth canal.
- Infections during the first trimester, during organogenesis, are more likely to cause congenital abnormalities and spontaneous abortions.
- Congenital infections can lead to serious infections in the neonatal period, often with severe long-term sequelae, including mental retardation, blindness, and deafness.
- CMV is the most common congenital infection and cause of congenital deafness.
- All patients who are HIV positive should be started on cART.
- HIV, gonorrhea, and *Chlamydia* are screened for in pregnancy.

CLINICAL VIGNETTES

VIGNETTE 1

A 27-year-old G1P0 woman at 9 weeks' gestational age (GA) presents to your office to initiate prenatal care. She has no significant medical or surgical history. She has mild nausea throughout the day, but on review of systems, has no other concerns. You explain to her recommendations for prenatal screening tests at the first visit.

1. Which of the following are not recommended as part of routine prenatal laboratory test screening?
   a. Urine culture
   b. Herpes simplex antibody screen
   c. *Chlamydia* PCR
   d. HIV antibody screen
   e. Rubella immune status

2. The screening urine culture returns with 100,000 colony forming units of *E. coli*. Which of the following are not complications of asymptomatic bacteriuria (ASB) in pregnancy?
   a. Pyelonephritis
   b. Preterm labor
   c. Low–birth-weight infants
   d. Urinary tract infection (UTI)
   e. Oligohydramnios

3. You prescribe a 7-day course of Macrodantin. Two days later, the sensitivities return, and the *E. coli* is resistant to Macrodantin and sensitive to ciprofloxacin, amoxicillin, and cephalexin. Of these antibiotics, which would you avoid in the first trimester?
   a. Ciprofloxacin
   b. Amoxicillin
   c. Cephalexin
   d. None

4. You prescribe a 7-day course of amoxicillin to treat the *E. coli* bacteriuria. She does not fill the amoxicillin and continues to take the Macrodantin. She presents to the emergency department 1 week later with fever, urinary frequency, and right flank

pain. She is mildly tachycardic and has a fever of 38.4°C. Her examination is significant for right-sided costovertebral angle tenderness. A urinalysis shows moderate leukocyte esterase, large nitrites, and many WBCs. In addition to hospital admission, what is the best initial treatment for this patient?
   a. Direct admission to the ICU and aggressive intravenous (IV) fluid hydration
   b. IV vancomycin
   c. IV ceftriaxone
   d. Oral amoxicillin
   e. Oral Keflex

5. What is the most concerning complications of pyelonephritis during pregnancy?
   a. Nephrolithiasis
   b. Pneumonia
   c. Acute respiratory distress syndrome (ARDS)
   d. Chorioamnionitis
   e. Oligohydramnios

VIGNETTE 2

A 28-year-old G2P1001 woman at 39 and 4/7 weeks' GA presents to labor and delivery. Her contractions started 10 hours ago and now have increased in frequency to every 5 minutes. She reports a spontaneous gush of fluid, which was clear, just before the contractions started. She has continued to leak clear fluid and denies any vaginal bleeding. Her vital signs are significant for maternal heart rate of 110 beats per minute. You put her on the monitor and note the fetal heart rate to be in the 170s and reactive. You perform a sterile speculum examination and confirm rupture of membranes (ROM) and note the fluid is cloudy with a foul odor. An abdominal examination confirms cephalic presentation but is notable for mild uterine tenderness.

1. What additional information would help you confirm the diagnosis?
   a. Maternal fever greater than 39°C
   b. Decreased maternal WBC
   c. Decreased amniotic fluid
   d. Blood cultures
   e. Urine culture

2. You diagnose her with chorioamnionitis/Triple I and admit her for IV antibiotics and augmentation of her labor. What is the most common causative organism(s)?
   a. *Listeria monocytogenes*
   b. *Gardnerella vaginosis*
   c. Polymicrobial infection of rectovaginal organisms
   d. Group B streptococcus (GBS)
   e. *Enterococcus*

3. Which of the following is one of the recommended antibiotic regimens?
   a. IV penicillin
   b. IV vancomycin
   c. IV ceftriaxone
   d. IV ampicillin and gentamicin
   e. IV clindamycin

4. Which of the following is not a complication of chorioamnionitis/Triple I?
   a. Endomyometritis
   b. Maternal sepsis
   c. Postpartum hemorrhage
   d. Neonatal pneumonia
   e. Pyelonephritis

VIGNETTE 3

A 28-year-old G1P0 woman at 28 weeks' GA comes to your office for a routine prenatal visit. She works as a kindergarten teacher, and one of her students was recently sent home with a rash and fever. She states that the child had a rash on both cheeks, and the pediatrician said it was a viral infection called fifth disease. She relates the baby is moving well and denies any vaginal bleeding, abnormal vaginal discharge, or contractions. She wonders if she needs any more testing to see if she has been affected.

1. What is the most likely causative organism of the child's infection?
   a. Parvovirus
   b. Varicella
   c. Cytomegalovirus (CMV)
   d. Toxoplasmosis
   e. Listeriosis

2. You send serologies for the agent above, and they come back showing the patient has a positive IgM and negative IgG consistent with an acute infection. What is the most common fetal/neonatal complication of this infection during pregnancy?
   a. Fetal anemia
   b. Preterm labor
   c. Premature preterm ROM
   d. Fetal anomalies
   e. Oligohydramnios

3. You perform an ultrasound of the fetus to evaluate for fetal anemia and hydrops. The ultrasound shows elevated middle cerebral artery (MCA) Doppler peak systolic velocity measurements consistent with fetal anemia. There is no evidence of fetal hydrops. What is the mechanism by which parvovirus infection causes fetal anemia?
   a. Hemolysis
   b. Bone marrow suppression
   c. Sequestration of RBCs in the spleen
   d. Fetal intracranial hemorrhage
   e. Fetomaternal hemorrhage

VIGNETTE 4

A 24-year-old G2P0010 woman at 8 weeks' GA presents for an initial prenatal visit. Her pregnancy is complicated by a history of IV drug use as a teenager and HIV. She had never been on cART medication prior to this pregnancy. You order a viral load, and it returns at 10,000. Her CD4 count is normal (>500). She is otherwise healthy and has no other significant medial history.

1. When would you recommend her to start cART?
   a. At this visit
   b. At 37 weeks in preparation for delivery
   c. At the beginning of the second trimester
   d. Immediately after delivery
   e. Only if it is medically indicated for maternal health

2. She returns at 14 weeks and you start her on a three-drug cART regimen of ZDV, lamivudine, and lopinavir/ritonavir, which she tolerates well for the remainder of her pregnancy. Her viral load in the second trimester decreases to 5,000, and you consult an infection disease specialist to consider adjusting her medications. A repeat viral load at 37 weeks has decreased to 1,250. At 38 weeks, she is admitted to labor and delivery in active labor. What would you recommend to her in order to further decrease neonatal transmission?
   a. Early artificial ROM for labor augmentation
   b. Placement of a fetal scalp electrode to monitor for signs of fetal distress
   c. Assisted vaginal delivery with vacuum or forceps
   d. Stopping all antiviral therapy to decrease risk of neonatal resistance
   e. Cesarean delivery and IV zidovudine (ZDV)

3. The patient has an uncomplicated delivery of a vigorous female infant. Mother and baby are transferred to the postpartum ward. Which of the following activities would increase the risk of transmission to her baby?
   a. Breastfeeding
   b. Treatment of the infant on ZDV prophylaxis
   c. Treatment of the infant with ZDV plus nevirapine
   d. Continuation of maternal cART
   e. Encouraging good hand washing and standard precautions at home

ANSWERS

VIGNETTE 1 Question 1
1. Answer B:
Herpes simplex antibody screening is not recommended for routine prenatal screening in the first visit. It is not recommended to screen for this infection, because there has been no demonstrated benefit in decreasing rates of vertical transmission to neonates.

It is recommended to screen for ASB with a urine culture at the initial prenatal visit given the risk of progression to a UTI or pyelonephritis. ASB is also associated with preterm birth and low–birth-weight infants. Screening is used to provide early treatment to decrease these risks.

Asymptomatic infection with *Chlamydia* is common, and therefore, the CDC recommends that all pregnant women be screened at the beginning of pregnancy.

Given the proven benefit of antiretroviral therapy to decrease vertical transmission of HIV to 1% to 2%, it is recommended that all women be screened at the onset of pregnancy in order to diagnose those that would benefit from this intervention.

Rubella infection during pregnancy can lead to significant congenital malformations. Screening at the beginning of pregnancy is recommended in order to counsel women to avoid possible exposures. In addition, it is recommended that women who are rubella nonimmune receive vaccination postpartum.

VIGNETTE 1 Question 2
2. Answer E:
Oligohydramnios is unrelated to maternal UTIs. Some factors that may lead to oligohydramnios include chromosomal abnormalities, uteroplacental insufficiency, hypertension, postterm pregnancy, and twin–twin transfusion syndrome.

There is a risk of approximately 25% to 40% that ASB will progress to cystitis or pyelonephritis. Treatment should be initiated shortly after confirming the diagnosis, and a test of cure should be performed to prove adequate treatment. Bacteriuria has also been associated with preterm birth and low–birth-weight infants.

VIGNETTE 1 Question 3
3. Answer A:
Ciprofloxacin has been associated with renal anomalies in the fetus, particularly in the first-trimester exposure. Because some fetal complications have been associated with ciprofloxacin even in later exposure, this medication is generally not given in pregnancy. Amoxicillin and Keflex are thought to be safe in pregnancy; both are category B, which means there were no adverse outcomes in animal reproduction studies.

VIGNETTE 1 Question 4
4. Answer C:
Pyelonephritis is estimated to complicate as many as 1% to 2% of pregnancies and has particularly serious associated complications, including septic shock and ARDS. Because of these risks, pyelonephritis during pregnancy is usually treated aggressively with hospital admission, IV hydration, and IV antibiotics—often cephalosporins (cefazolin, cefotetan, or ceftriaxone) or ampicillin and gentamicin—until the patient is afebrile and asymptomatic for 24 to 48 hours. The patient is then transitioned to an oral antibiotic regimen. Small trials have examined the possibility of treating these patients with a single dose of IV or IM antibiotics, such as ceftriaxone, followed by outpatient oral antibiotic regimen. Although these treatments seem to be effective in certain groups, consideration of appropriate patient criteria, including absence of signs of sepsis, compliance, ability to tolerate oral medications, and GA, is imperative. Treatment duration for pyelonephritis consists of a total of 10 to 14 days of combined IV and oral antibiotics.

VIGNETTE 1 Question 5
5. Answer C:
Pyelonephritis has significant morbidity during pregnancy and is associated with high rates of ICU admission and ARDS. Because of this, it is recommended that pregnant women be admitted to the hospital for observation and treatment. IV fluids should be used judiciously, given the risk of pulmonary edema and ARDS. Pregnant women are also at increased risk for urosepsis and septic shock. Initial antibiotic choice is usually ceftriaxone. Women should improve after 24 to 48 hours of therapy and once afebrile for 48 hours can be transitioned to oral therapy based on sensitivities. Oral antibiotics should be continued for total course of 10 to 14 days. For the remainder of the pregnancy, it is recommended the patient takes prophylactic antibiotics, usually 100 mg Macrobid daily.

Pyelonephritis has not been shown to cause nephrolithiasis. However, UTIs with *Proteus mirabilis* and other urea-splitting bacteria are commonly associated with struvite kidney stones. These stones are usually found in patients who are predisposed to UTIs, such as those with spinal cord injury or neurogenic bladder syndromes.

Pneumonia is not a common complication of pyelonephritis. However, pyelonephritis can lead to pulmonary edema from the release of endotoxin that causes increased vascular and alveolar capillary permeability.

Pyelonephritis may lead to urosepsis, but the placenta serves as a barrier, and there is no increased risk of intra-amniotic infection. In addition, placental function is unchanged, and as a result, there is no increased risk of oligohydramnios.

VIGNETTE 2 Question 1
1. Answer A:
Chorioamnionitis/Triple I is a clinical diagnosis that complicates 2% to 4% of term pregnancies. Diagnostic criteria require a maternal fever of greater than 39°C and at least one of the following signs: elevated maternal WBC count, maternal tachycardia, uterine tenderness, fetal tachycardia, and foul-smelling amniotic fluid. The gold standard for diagnosis of chorioamnionitis is a culture of the amniotic fluid, which can be obtained via amniocentesis. At the same time, the amniotic fluid can be sent for the following tests: glucose, WBC count, protein, and Gram stain. Amniocentesis is most commonly used in preterm patients whose fetuses would benefit from remaining in utero for more time and where a more aggressive means to reach the diagnosis can be taken if there is any doubt.

VIGNETTE 2 Question 2
2. Answer C:
Chorioamnionitis/Triple I at term is most commonly caused by polymicrobial infections of bacteria from the vagina and rectum. In some studies, almost 60% had more than one organism present from amniotic fluid culture. The most common organisms regardless of GA are genital *Mycoplasma* species (*Ureaplasma* and *Mycoplasma*). Other common organisms include *G. vaginosis*, *E. coli*, *Enterococcus*, *Bacteroides* species, and GBS.

VIGNETTE 2 Question 3
3. Answer D:
When chorioamnionitis/Triple I is suspected, the patient should be admitted and IV antibiotics started. Because chorioamnionitis is a polymicrobial infection caused by organisms that colonize the vagina and rectum, broad-spectrum coverage should be used. Most commonly, treatment is with cefoxitin (or other second- or third-generation cephalosporin) or ampicillin and gentamicin. In addition to antibiotics, delivery should be hastened with induction and augmentation by vaginal delivery, or, in the case of a nonreassuring fetal tracing, by cesarean delivery.

The patient's initial cervical examination was 7-cm dilation, 100% effacement, and 0 station. After starting IV fluids, ampicillin and gentamicin, and giving Tylenol, the maternal fever resolves and the fetal tachycardia improves. You start oxytocin for augmentation, and the fetal heart tracing remains reassuring. She progresses to complete dilation and delivers a vigorous infant. The neonatal resuscitation team is in attendance, and due to the risk of neonatal sepsis, they recommend that the baby be admitted to the NICU for blood cultures and IV antibiotics.

VIGNETTE 2 Question 4
4. Answer E:
Chorioamnionitis/Triple I is the most common precursor of neonatal sepsis, which has a high rate of fetal mortality. Other neonatal complications include pneumonia and meningitis. Neonatal morbidity and mortality appear to be increased for infants and earlier GAs. The most common maternal complications include dysfunctional labor and need for cesarean section, uterine atony, and postpartum hemorrhage. Other maternal complications include endomyometritis, bacteremia, adult ARDS, and septic shock. With early initiation of IV antibiotics, the more severe complications of ARDS and sepsis are quite rare.

VIGNETTE 3 Question 1
1. Answer A:
Parvovirus B19 causes erythema infectiosum (fifth disease). Classically, this mild infection presents with a low-grade fever and a red macular rash giving the "slapped cheek" appearance and usually resolves with minimal intervention. Approximately one-third to one-half of pregnant women have IgG to the virus and are immune from a prior infection. Among pregnant women who do not have immunity, the incidence of acute parvovirus infection during pregnancy is around 3%. If parvovirus exposure is suspected in the mother, acute infection can be diagnosed by checking parvovirus IgM and IgG levels.

VIGNETTE 3 Question 2
2. Answer A:
Acute parvovirus infections during pregnancy may be transmitted through the placenta to the fetus. First-trimester infections have been associated with miscarriage, but midtrimester and later infections are associated with fetal anemia and hydrops. If studies indicate an acute parvovirus infection (positive IgM and positive or negative IgG) beyond 20 weeks of gestation, then the fetus should undergo serial ultrasounds, up to 8 to 10 weeks after maternal infection. Currently, Doppler ultrasound to examine the peak systolic velocity of the MCA is frequently used to identify fetal anemia. Small studies have shown a benefit of fetal transfusion for fetal anemia leading to hydrops; however, these studies also reported fetal deaths from complications related to transfusion, so this procedure is likely to be reserved for the most severe cases.

VIGNETTE 3 Question 3
3. Answer B:
Parvovirus B19 causes fetal anemia by bone marrow suppression. The virus is cytotoxic to RBC precursors, leading to decreased production. Severe anemia can lead to high-output cardiac failure, hydrops, and fetal death. Parvovirus can also lead to pancytopenia in the fetus, and this has important clinical implications because fetal thrombocytopenia can increase the risk of exsanguination and fetal death during attempts at intrauterine transfusion. It is also important to note that this mechanism for fetal anemia is different from that of Rh alloimmunization, which leads to fetal anemia via hemolysis.

VIGNETTE 4 Question 1
1. Answer A:
Antiretroviral therapy is recommended for all HIV positive pregnant women regardless of viral load or CD4 level. Currently, antiretroviral therapy in pregnancy includes a three-drug regimen generally started preconception or at time of HIV diagnosis. With improved antiretroviral treatment during pregnancy, rates of perinatal transmission have decreased from 1,650 in 1991 to less than 200 per year in 2014 (CDC). Transmission occurs in utero (one-third), generally late in pregnancy or during labor and delivery (two-third). In 1994, Pediatric AIDS Clinical Trials Group (PACTG) protocol 076 demonstrated that a three-part regimen of ZDV administered during pregnancy and labor and to the newborn could reduce the risk of perinatal transmission by two-thirds. Additionally, with the use of cART to further decrease viral load with potent regimens, the rate of transmission can be further decreased to less than 1% to 2% with an undetectable viral load. Increased transmission can be seen with higher viral burden or advanced disease in the mother, rupture of the membranes, and invasive procedures during labor and delivery that increase neonatal exposure to maternal blood.

VIGNETTE 4 Question 2
2. Answer E:
Cesarean delivery has been shown to lower transmission rates by roughly two-thirds compared with vaginal delivery in patients on no therapy and particularly without onset of labor or ROM or in the setting of high viral load. However, in women with viral loads of less than 1,000 copies/mL, there is no additional benefit of cesarean delivery versus vaginal delivery in HIV perinatal transmission. Therefore, cesarean delivery should be considered in HIV-infected pregnant women with viral loads greater than 1,000 copies/mL and without long-standing onset of labor or ROM.

VIGNETTE 4 Question 3
3. Answer A:
In resource-rich nations where safe bottle-feeding alternatives are available, breastfeeding is contraindicated in HIV-infected women because virus is found in breast milk and responsible for HIV transmission to the infant. Postnatal HIV transmission from breast milk at 2 years may be as high as 15%. Furthermore, studies are lacking regarding the efficacy of maternal

antiretroviral therapy for prevention of transmission of HIV through breast milk and the toxicity of antiretroviral exposure of the infant via breast milk. In resource-poor nations, breastfeeding is encouraged because of increased risk of neonatal mortality from diarrheal diseases, pneumonia, and other infectious diseases. In resource-rich nations, infants are placed on a 6-week course cART to reduce risk of transmission. Standard precautions and good hand washing behavior should always be encouraged because they may not lower the risk of transmission but would not increase the risk either.

11 | Other Medical Complications of Pregnancy

The previous three chapters discussed about hypertension, diabetes, and infectious diseases in the context of the pregnant patient. In this chapter, a variety of the other common medical complications of pregnancy are discussed. Pregnancy affects every physiologic system in the body as well as many disease states. Disease management in pregnancy requires consideration of any potential fetal effects of treatment or imaging modalities.

HYPEREMESIS GRAVIDARUM

Nausea and vomiting in pregnancy, or "morning sickness," are common. Seen in 88% of pregnancies, morning sickness usually resolves by week 16. Various etiologies have been proposed, including elevated levels of human chorionic gonadotropin (HCG), thyroid hormone, or the intrinsic hormones of the gut. Additionally, progesterone decreases gastric motility and relaxes the esophageal sphincter that can contribute to nausea and vomiting in pregnancy. Despite nausea and vomiting in early pregnancy, patients are usually able to maintain adequate nutrition. However, some women can become significantly dehydrated and potentially develop electrolyte abnormalities. The diagnosis of **hyperemesis gravidarum** is made when a woman has persistent vomiting, weight loss of greater than 5% of prepregnancy body weight, and ketonuria. In particular, hyperemesis is common in the setting of molar pregnancies (likely because HCG levels can be very high), and a viable intrauterine pregnancy should always be documented in patients with hyperemesis.

TREATMENT AND PROGNOSIS

For patients with hyperemesis gravidarum, symptoms may persist into the third trimester and, rarely, until term. The goal of therapy is to maintain adequate nutrition. Treatment consists of antiemetics and supplements and hydration. Persistent nausea and vomiting during pregnancy can be treated with vitamin B_6 and doxylamine (Unisom). Ginger and supplementation with vitamin B_{12} have been shown to be effective and can be used as adjuncts to antiemetic therapy. First-line antiemetic therapy is usually with promethazine, followed by the addition of metoclopromide, prochlorperazine, and Tigan. If these fail, droperidol and ondansetron can also be used safely in pregnancy. If symptoms persist to dehydration, patients should be rehydrated and electrolyte abnormalities corrected. Because a hypochloremic alkalosis often results from extensive vomiting, normal saline with 5% dextrose is commonly used for IV hydration. In the acute setting, antiemetics should be given intravenously, intramuscularly, or as suppositories because oral medications may be vomited prior to systemic absorption.

Long-term management of hyperemesis includes maintaining hydration, adequate nutrition, and symptomatic relief from the nausea and vomiting. Many patients respond to antiemetics and IV hydration. Once they are rehydrated, they can use the antiemetic to control nausea so that they are able to maintain oral intake. In addition, because hypoglycemia may contribute to nausea, frequent small meals can help to maintain more stable blood glucose and decrease nausea.

Rarely, patients will not respond to antiemetics and recurrent rehydration. In these cases, treatment with corticosteroids has been shown to decrease symptoms. Other alternative treatments shown to decrease nausea include acupuncture, acupressure, hypnotherapy, and nerve stimulation. A small percentage of patients for whom the treatment fails will require feeding tubes or even parenteral nutrition for the course of the pregnancy. As long as hydration and adequate nutrition are maintained, pregnancy outcomes are usually good.

SEIZURE DISORDERS

Approximately 20,000 women with seizure disorders give birth each year. Seizures have implications for fetal and maternal health, and concerns during these pregnancies include risk of fetal malformations, miscarriage, perinatal death, and increased seizure frequency. Maternal mortality in women with epilepsy is increased by approximately 10-fold. Women with a seizure disorder are encouraged to continue on their antiepileptic drugs (AEDs) with the goal to optimize maternal and fetal outcomes. Yet, AEDs are not without risk. Women with epilepsy appear to have a greater baseline risk of fetal malformations that is further increased with the use of AEDs. When managing these women in pregnancy, the risks of increased seizures versus the use of AEDs need to be weighed carefully.

SEIZURE FREQUENCY

In pregnancy, there is an increase in seizures that is not completely understood and is likely multifactorial. Concerns regarding fetal effects lead to decreased compliance with AEDs. Additionally, normal physiologic changes of pregnancy include increased volume of distribution (V_D) and increased hepatic metabolism of AEDs. The combination of these factors is thought to contribute to increased seizure frequency in 17% to 33% of pregnancies. There are a variety of possible etiologies proposed for the increase in seizure frequency seen in some pregnancies. Increased levels of circulating estrogen during pregnancy in turn increase the function of the P_{450} enzymes, which leads to more rapid hepatic metabolism of AEDs. In addition, renal function increases during pregnancy with a 50% rise in creatinine clearance that affects the metabolism of carbamazepine, primidone, and the benzodiazepines. The increase in total blood volume and concomitant rise in the V_D leads to decreased levels of circulating AEDs. Hormonal changes, added stress, and decreased sleep during pregnancy likely lower seizure threshold and have been shown to increase seizure frequency in nonpregnant patients. Finally, many women may have decreased compliance with AEDs because of concerns regarding fetal effects.

Increased levels of estrogen and progesterone may both have direct effects on seizure activity during pregnancy. Estrogen has been shown to be epileptogenic, decreasing seizure threshold. Thus, rising estrogen levels in pregnancy that peak in the third trimester may have some impact on the observed increase in seizure frequency. Conversely, progesterone seems to have an antiepileptic effect. It has been observed that women with seizure disorders have fewer seizures during the luteal phase of the menstrual cycle. Sleep deprivation and stress may also play a role in increased seizures in pregnancy. The best predictor of seizure frequency in pregnancy appears to be the amount of seizures in the year prior to pregnancy. Ideally, plasma AED concentrations are individualized based on seizure history and prepregnancy therapeutic concentrations.

FETAL CONGENITAL ABNORMALITIES AND ADVERSE OUTCOMES

The earliest reports of congenital malformations associated with AEDs occurred in the 1960s. Since then, unique malformations and syndromes have been ascribed to phenytoin, phenobarbital, primidone, valproate, carbamazepine, and trimethadione. However, there are similarities between most of the congenital abnormalities caused by the AEDs (Table 11-1). There is evidence that epileptic women have an increased risk of fetal malformations even without AED use. Although some studies suggest that monotherapy does not increase that baseline risk, there are other studies that do show evidence of an increase in fetal malformations with AED polytherapy. Ideally, a patient is started on or transitioned to a single medication with the lowest risk of malformation (lamotrigine, levetiracetam, and oxacarbemazepine) preconception.

Specific increases in congenital abnormalities seen in infants born to epileptic mothers include a fourfold increase in cleft lip and palate, and a three- to fourfold increase in cardiac anomalies. There is also an increase in the rate of neural tube defects (NTDs) seen in the offspring of epileptic patients who are using carbamazepine or valproic acid. Long-term studies on neurodevelopment show higher rates of abnormal electroencephalogram (EEG) findings, higher rates of developmentally delayed children, and lower IQ scores. Specific neurodevelopmental outcomes have been attributed to particular AEDs, and valproic acid, topiramate, and phenobarbital have been reported as having the greatest risk at 6% to 9%, 4% to 7%, and 5.5%, respectively. Lamotrigine has the lowest risk at 0% to 2%, and baseline risk of women with epilepsy is 1% to 3%.

TABLE 11-1. Fetal Anomalies Associated with AEDs

Fetal Anomaly	Phenytoin	Phenobarbital	Primidone	Valproate	Carbamazepine	Trimethadione
NTD				X	X	
IUGR	X					X
Microcephaly					X	X
Low IQ	X		X			
Distal digital hypoplasia	X	X	X			
Low-set ears	X	X				X
Epicanthal fold	X	X		X	X	X
Short nose	X	X		X	X	
Long philtrum			X		X	
Lip abnormalities	X	X	X	X		
Hypertelorism	X	X				
Developmental delay		X			X	X
Other	Ptosis	Ptosis	Hirsutism of forehead		Hypoplastic nails	Cardiac anomalies

AEDs, antiepileptic drugs; NTD, neural tube defect; IUGR, intrauterine growth restriction.

MECHANISMS OF TERATOGENICITY

The mechanisms of teratogenicity of AEDs have not been fully characterized. Phenobarbital, primidone, and phenytoin act as folate antagonists. Certainly, it appears that folate deficiency can lead to an increase in congenital malformations, particularly NTDs. Folate prior to conception has therefore been recommended for prophylaxis. Because all AEDs have a similar central mechanism to control seizures, there may be a common pathway—disrupted during embryogenesis—that leads to the similarities in the syndromes described. This may explain why there is an additive effect in polytherapy.

Recent studies in teratogenesis—particularly in the fetal hydantoin syndrome—point to a genetic predilection for the generation of epoxides. Specifically, children whose enzyme activity of epoxide hydrolase is one-third less than normal have an increased rate of fetal hydantoin syndrome. Anomalies have also been observed in children exposed to carbamazepine with low epoxide hydrolase activity.

CLINICAL MANAGEMENT

Because exposure to multiple AEDs seems to be more teratogenic than monotherapeutic, patients are advised to switch to a single AED prior to conception and taper down to the lowest possible dose. Patients who have been seizure-free for 2 to 5 years may wish to attempt complete withdrawal from AEDs prior to conception. Because there is particular evidence that high peak plasma levels of valproic acid may be more teratogenic than constant steady-state levels, it should be dosed three to four times per day rather than the standard twice per day dosing. However, epileptic patients should be counseled that they are still at a greater risk (4% to 6% vs. 2% to 3%) for fetal anomalies than the baseline population. Folate supplementation has been shown to decrease NTDs in patients without epilepsy. Therefore, patients should be advised to take supplemental folate prior to conception, particularly those using either valproic acid or carbamazepine.

Because of the increased risk of anomalies, a targeted ultrasound at 19 to 20 weeks of gestation should be performed with careful attention to the face, central nervous system (CNS), and heart (Table 11-2). Because of the increased risk of NTDs, a maternal serum α-fetoprotein (MSAFP) screening test should be offered. The decision to perform an amniocentesis routinely for α-fetoprotein and acetylcholinesterase is controversial. Because the sensitivity of amniocentesis is higher than either MSAFP or ultrasound for NTDs, many practitioners recommend amniocentesis in the setting of a family history of NTDs or with the use of valproic acid or carbamazepine.

Recent studies of seizure frequency show less of an increase than older studies, which suggests that

TABLE 11-2. Management of Women with Epilepsy During Pregnancy
Check total and free levels of AEDs on a monthly basis
Consider early genetic counseling
Check MSAFP
Level II ultrasound for fetal survey at 19–20 wks' gestation
Consider amniocentesis for α-fetoprotein and acetylcholinesterase
Supplement with oral vitamin K 20 mg daily (QD) starting at 37 wks until delivery (optional)
AEDs, antiepileptic drugs; MSAFP, maternal serum α-fetoprotein.

the practice of closer monitoring of AED dosing and levels may have some effect on the number of seizures during pregnancy. A recent study shows that 38% of pregnant patients with epilepsy require changes in their AED dosing to achieve seizure control. Assuming that monotherapy with one of the AEDs has been achieved preconceptionally, total and free serum levels of the AED should be obtained on a monthly basis (see Table 11-2).

LABOR AND DELIVERY

Management of the epileptic patient on labor and delivery should involve preparation and close monitoring. All care providers—obstetricians, neurology, nursing, anesthesia, and pediatrics—should be informed about an epileptic patient in labor and delivery. AED levels should be checked upon admission. If the level is low, patients may be given extra dosing or switched to IV benzodiazepines or phenytoin, bearing in mind that benzodiazepines can cause respiratory depression in both the mother and the newborn. Because trauma and hypoxia from a seizure can put both the mother and the fetus at risk, treatment of seizures should be discussed a priori with the group of practitioners caring for the patient. Management of seizures on labor and delivery is discussed in Chapter 6. One difference is that the drug of choice in patients with a known seizure disorder is usually phenytoin compared with magnesium used in preeclamptic patients.

There have been reports of increased risk of spontaneous hemorrhage in newborns because of the inhibition of vitamin K-dependent clotting factors (i.e., II, VII, IX, and X) secondary to increased vitamin K metabolism and inhibition of placental transport of vitamin K by AEDs. Although the risk is small, conservative management is to overcome this theoretical vitamin K deficiency by aggressive supplementation with vitamin K toward the end of pregnancy. This has not been conclusively shown to demonstrate benefit of supplementation. Upon delivery, clotting studies can be performed on the cord blood and vitamin K administered to the infant. If the cord blood is deficient in clotting factors, fresh frozen plasma may be required to protect the newborn.

MATERNAL CARDIAC DISEASE

Recent studies demonstrate that cardiac disease is leading to an increasing proportion of maternal mortality in the United States. The cardiovascular system undergoes a number of dramatic changes in pregnancy with a 50% increase in blood volume, decrease in systemic vascular resistance, increase in cardiac stroke volume, and actual remodeling of the myocardium to accommodate some of these changes. When caring for patients with cardiac disease preconceptionally or during pregnancy, these changes are paramount when counseling them regarding their options and managing their disease. In particular, patients with primary pulmonary hypertension (PH), Eisenmenger physiology, severe mitral or aortic stenosis, and Marfan syndrome are at a high risk of maternal mortality in pregnancy (reportedly ranging from 15% to 70% in small case series). In patients with cardiac disease and an increased risk of maternal mortality, the option to terminate the pregnancy should always be offered and discussed at length with the patient. Unfortunately, as such women often may not be able to adopt because of their illness, they may think of their own pregnancy as the only way to have children.

PRINCIPLES OF MANAGEMENT

Cardiac diseases vary widely but the principles of management are similar. Many of the diseases are stable prior to pregnancy with medical management, but during pregnancy they can become quite unstable in response to the physiologic changes. Additionally, medications used during pregnancy may be different from those used outside of pregnancy. In particular, many of the newest antihypertensives and antiarrhythmics have been sparsely studied in pregnant women, and are thus commonly avoided. Of the more common agents, angiotensin-converting enzyme inhibitors, diuretics, and warfarin (Coumadin) have all been associated with congenital anomalies and other fetal effects and are usually discontinued in pregnancy. The 2007 American Heart Association Guidelines state that routine vaginal delivery or cesarean section are not indications for subacute bacterial endocarditis (SBE) prophylaxis. However, SBE prophylaxis may be considered for women with high-risk lesions (mechanical or prosthetic valves, unrepaired cyanotic lesions, etc.), and an infection that could cause bacteremia (chorioamnionitis or pyelonephritis).

Patients who would benefit from surgical repair of a lesion as in mitral or aortic stenosis should undergo surgical repair a year or more before becoming pregnant. Because of high maternal risk, those who become pregnant before surgical repair should be offered termination of the pregnancy as the first line of management. It is important that patients and their families are aware of the risks of disabling morbidity and mortality if they decide to continue the pregnancy. Management and early intervention during labor and delivery can help to reduce risk for cardiac patients. Early epidural analgesia to control pain can minimize the cardiac stress of labor and delivery. Likewise, an assisted vaginal delivery (using forceps or vacuum) can diminish the potential detrimental cardiac effect of Valsalva with pushing. In addition, careful fluid monitoring should be maintained, possibly with a central venous pressure monitor and arterial line. After delivery, massive fluid shifts make the immediate postpartum period a particularly dangerous transition for women with congenital heart disease. These fluid shifts have two main sources. First, postpartum women have increased venous return because they no longer have an enlarged uterus compressing the vena cava. Second, the uterus clamps down after placental expulsion and demands less circulation, leading to an effective autotransfusion of its blood supply (approximately 500 cc).

CARDIOVASCULAR DISEASE

Rising average maternal age in pregnancy means that there will be an increasing number of patients with a history of a myocardial infarction who become pregnant. Small case series show that, if optimally managed, these patients do relatively well in pregnancy. A baseline ECG and adjustment of medications, if necessary, should be performed at the initial visit. Throughout pregnancy and during labor and delivery, it is important to minimize increased demand on the heart.

EISENMENGER SYNDROME AND PULMONARY HYPERTENSION

Patients with right-to-left shunts and PH are among the sickest pregnant women, with mortality rates estimated at 50% and higher. The most common right-to-left shunts are patent ductus arteriosus and ventricular septal defect, which have reversed as a result of Eisenmenger syndrome. In Eisenmenger syndrome, an initial left-to-right shunt overfills the right heart. This, in turn, leads to increased flow through the pulmonary vasculature, pulmonary capillary damage, and the formation of scar tissue. As a result, patients develop right ventricular hypertrophy and PH and eventually a right-to-left shunt.

These patients are chronically hypoxic secondary to the mixing of deoxygenated blood and are encouraged to terminate their pregnancies. Patients who elect to continue their pregnancies are followed with serial echocardiograms to measure the pulmonary pressures and cardiac function. Some have been managed with inhaled nitric oxide, but this has not been shown to significantly improve the measured clinical indicators of disease or the outcomes. These women often decompensate in the third trimester of pregnancy. Labor and assisted vaginal delivery are preferable to elective cesarean delivery. Perhaps the greatest concentrated risk of morbidity and mortality is in the postpartum period for approximately 2 to 4 weeks after delivery. It has been hypothesized that this risk is secondary to the sudden changes in hormones. Unfortunately, attempts to counter these changes with progesterone and estrogen supplementation have had little success.

VALVULAR DISEASE

Although the manifestations of the different valvular diseases vary, they are similar in that surgical treatment or repair prior to becoming pregnant is preferred for moderate or severe disease carrying increased risk of maternal mortality. Patients with aortic stenosis and aortic insufficiency require a decreased afterload to maintain cardiac output, and thus initially may have diminished symptoms in response to the decreased systemic vascular resistance seen in pregnancy. Patients with mitral stenosis may be unable to meet the increased demands of pregnancy and experience a backup into the pulmonary system leading to congestive heart failure. Patients with pulmonary stenosis who elect to continue their pregnancy may actually undergo valvuloplasty during the pregnancy if they have severe disease.

MARFAN SYNDROME

Patients with Marfan syndrome have a deficiency in their elastin that can lead to a number of valvular cardiac complications as well as dilation of the aortic root. During pregnancy, the hyperdynamic state can increase the risk of aortic dissection and/or rupture, particularly in those patients with an aortic root diameter greater than 4 cm. In order to decrease some of the pressure on the aorta, women are advised to maintain a sedentary lifestyle and are often placed on beta-blockers to decrease cardiac output.

PERIPARTUM CARDIOMYOPATHY

A small percentage of patients will be found to have heart failure secondary to a dilated cardiomyopathy immediately before, during, or after delivery. Some of these patients likely have a baseline mild cardiomyopathy, whereas others have a postinfectious dilated cardiomyopathy. However, the epidemiology supports the idea that, at least in some cases, **peripartum cardiomyopathy** (PPCM) is specifically caused by pregnancy. Patients present with classic signs and symptoms of heart failure and on echocardiogram have a dilated heart with an ejection fraction far below normal in the 20% to 40% range.

Patients with PPCM should be managed according to the gestational age (GA) of the fetus. Beyond 34 weeks of GA, the risks to the mother of remaining pregnant are usually greater than those of premature delivery of the fetus. At earlier GAs, however, betamethasone should be administered to promote fetal lung maturity, and the patient delivered accordingly. The patient's heart failure is managed similar to other patients with heart failure using diuretics, digoxin, and vasodilators. Well over half of the patients with PPCM have excellent return to baseline of their cardiac activity within several months of delivery.

MATERNAL RENAL DISEASE

Pregnancy can affect kidney function in patients with chronic renal disease by causing a permanent decline in kidney function. The risk of permanent declining function is based on the severity of underlying renal disease. Chronic renal disease can be divided into mild (Cr < 1.5), moderate (Cr from 1.5 to 2.8), and severe (Cr > 2.8), although other thresholds have been used. Renal blood flow and creatinine clearance increase during pregnancy in patients without renal disease, and this is also true initially in patients with renal disease. In fact, patients with mild renal disease will usually experience improvement in renal function throughout much of pregnancy. Only 10% of patients with mild disease will have permanent changes in glomerular filtration rate. Moderate and severe patients, however, may experience decreasing renal function in the latter half of pregnancy that may persist postpartum in as many as half of pregnancies. Because of this, it is important to counsel these patients preconceptionally regarding the risks to them from pregnancy—in particular, the increased risk of requiring dialysis and its concomitant morbidities.

Patients with chronic renal disease have increased risk of preeclampsia, preterm delivery, gestational diabetes, and intrauterine growth restriction (IUGR) in addition to worsening renal disease, and therefore, they should be screened at least once per trimester with a 24-hour urine for creatinine clearance and protein. Patients who present in early pregnancy should be counseled regarding these risks and offered termination of pregnancy, particularly for the mother's health. Because of the risk to the fetus, antenatal fetal testing usually begins at 32 to 34 weeks of gestation. For patients who have baseline proteinuria and hypertension, the diagnosis of preeclampsia can be difficult to make. In these patients, a baseline uric acid is assessed and, if normal at baseline, can be used in the setting of worsening blood pressures (BPs) to help diagnose preeclampsia. Additionally, monitoring platelets and liver function tests can be helpful in delineating preeclampsia from worsening renal disease. An increase in BP of 30/15 mm Hg above prepregnancy BPs can also be used, although experts disagree on its utility.

An interesting subgroup of women is those who are status postrenal transplant. It seems that such women will have outcomes similar to women with similar creatinine clearance. These women need to be closely monitored for adverse maternal outcomes because declining renal function in a transplant patient has grave consequences. As such, the rates of successful pregnancy are decreased in transplant patient, and the average GA of delivery is 30 weeks. In addition to closely watching renal function, monitoring the transplant is also important. Commonly, these women will be on immunosuppressants such as cyclosporine, tacrolimus, prednisone, and Imuran. Because of increased metabolism and V_D, dosages of these medications may need to be adjusted during pregnancy. If this is not done, the risk of acute rejection increases due to under treatment. Similarly, because women may be concerned about the effects of these medications on the developing fetus, they may stop taking the medications and be at increased risk for rejection. Medication levels, creatinine, and creatinine clearance are commonly checked monthly in such women.

COAGULATION DISORDERS

Pregnancy is generally considered a "hypercoagulable" state. The pathogenesis of this state has not been elucidated, but several mechanisms have been proposed, including increased coagulation factors, endothelial damage, and venous stasis (Virchow triad). The risk for superficial vein thrombosis (SVT), deep vein thrombosis (DVT), and pulmonary embolus (PE) is further increased postpartum, and PE remains one of the leading causes of maternal mortality. Additionally, women with a preexisting thrombophilia may get pregnant. These women, in particular, are at high risk for developing DVT or PE.

PATHOGENESIS

No single cause of the hypercoagulability of pregnancy has been found, but there are several possible mechanisms hypothesized. The first is that there is an intrinsic increase in coagulability of the serum itself. In pregnancy, the production of all clotting factors is increased except for II, V, and IX. Turnover time for fibrinogen is also decreased during pregnancy, and there are increased levels of fibrinopeptide A, which is cleaved from fibrinogen to make fibrin. Additionally, there are increased levels of circulating fibrin monomer complexes. These levels increase further at the time of delivery and immediately postpartum. Finally, it has been hypothesized that the placenta synthesizes a factor that decreases fibrinolysis, but there is minimal evidence for this.

Another proposed source of hypercoagulability is increased exposure to subendothelial collagen as a result of increased endothelial damage during pregnancy, although no mechanism has been proposed. It has also been hypothesized that endothelial damage in the venous system during parturition increases the amount of thrombogenesis postpartum. This seems feasible, particularly as the etiology of pelvic vein thrombosis, but it does not account for the hypercoagulability throughout pregnancy.

Venous stasis may also account for some of the increase in venous thromboses during and after pregnancy. There are two principal causes for venous stasis in pregnancy. The first is decreased venous tone during pregnancy, which may be related to the smooth muscle relaxant properties of this high progesterone state. Second, the uterus, as it enlarges, compresses the inferior vena cava, the iliac, and pelvic veins. This compression, in particular, likely contributes to the increase in pelvic vein thromboses.

Finally, the increased estrogen in pregnancy and the initial postpartum state also likely contribute to hypercoagulability. Estrogen and progestogens have been associated with DVT and stroke outside of pregnancy, and the exact pathophysiology of this is yet to be elucidated. Nevertheless, these hormonal factors likely contribute to the thrombotic state of pregnancy and early postpartum.

SUPERFICIAL VEIN THROMBOSIS

Although **superficial vein thrombosis** (SVT) is a painful complication of hypercoagulability, it is believed to be unlikely to lead to emboli. The diagnosis is usually obvious with a palpable, usually visible, venous cord that is quite tender, with local erythema and edema. Because of the low risk of emboli from SVT, it is not routinely treated other than symptomatically with warm compresses and analgesics. However, the patient should be informed of the signs and symptoms of DVTs and PEs because she may be at an increased risk for either.

DEEP VEIN THROMBOSIS

Diagnosis of **deep vein thrombosis** (DVT) is often made clinically with confirmation by Doppler studies or venography. The typical patient presents with unilateral lower extremity pain and swelling. It is important to note that the majority (over 90%) of patients with a DVT in pregnancy will have it in the left leg. On examination, patients will often have edema, local erythema, tenderness, venous distension, and a palpable cord underlying the region of pain and tenderness. When clinical suspicion is high, the patient is usually sent for noninvasive lower extremity studies with the Doppler ultrasound for confirmation of a venous obstruction. Rarely, venography, the gold standard, will be used.

Treatment of DVT during pregnancy involves the use of adjusted dose low-molecular-weight heparin (enoxaparin 1 mg/kg twice daily [BID]) or unfractionated heparin (goal activated partial thromboplastin time (aPTT) of 1.5 to 2.5 times normal). Low-molecular-weight heparin has become the preferred option because levels do not need to be checked, and it is also thought to be safer due to a lower risk of heparin-induced thrombocytopenia. When using unfractionated heparin, the initial treatment is with IV heparin, which is later transitioned to subcutaneous heparin throughout the remainder of the pregnancy and postpartum. Warfarin therapy is contraindicated in pregnancy because it is teratogenic. When given in the first trimester, it causes warfarin embryopathy, a combination of nasal hypoplasia and skeletal abnormalities. In addition, warfarin appears to cause diffuse CNS abnormalities, including optic atrophy, when given during pregnancy.

PULMONARY EMBOLUS

Pulmonary embolus (PE) results when emboli from DVTs travel to the right side of the heart and then lodge in the pulmonary arterial system, leading to **pulmonary hypertension**, **hypoxia**, and, depending on the extent of the emboli, **right-sided heart failure** and **death**. Clinical suspicion of PE is raised whenever a patient presents with acute onset of shortness of breath, simultaneous onset of pleuritic chest pain, hemoptysis or tachycardia, and/or concomitant signs of DVT.

The diagnosis of PE usually depends on the clinical picture correlated with a variety of diagnostic tests. A chest X-ray may be entirely normal. However, when abnormal, two common signs on chest X-ray are the abrupt termination of a vessel because it is traced distally and an area of radiolucency in the region of lung beyond the PE. An ECG may also be entirely normal or simply shows sinus tachycardia. On occasion, however, it will show signs of right-heart strain with right-axis deviation, nonspecific ST changes, and peaked T-waves. Spiral CT scan is the most common diagnostic tool for PE in both the pregnant and nonpregnant patient. The risk of radiation exposure must be weighed against the suspected risk of a PE and the dangers that a PE poses to a pregnant woman's health. As with other life-threatening medical conditions, the woman's health should be the primary consideration and she should receive the same standard of care as that of a nonpregnant patient. Previously more common, ventilation/perfusion (V/Q) scanning is now used less frequently. The V/Q scan is a radionuclide scan that first allows visualization of lung perfusion by detecting a radioisotope in the pulmonary circulation (Fig. 11-1). An entirely normal perfusion scan rules out PE. However, if there is a defect in perfusion, a ventilation scan is performed. Mismatched defects in the ventilation and perfusion scans are suggestive of PE. Pulmonary angiography is the gold standard for diagnosis of PE. The pulmonary artery is catheterized, and a radiopaque dye is injected. Diagnosis is made by the presence of intraluminal filling defects, or if sharp vessel cutoffs are seen (Fig. 11-2).

Treatment of mild PE is similar to the treatment of DVT, with low-molecular-weight heparin (enoxaparin) being the preferred choice in hemodynamically stable patients. In the hypotensive or unstable patient, IV heparin is the recommended option. Massive PE leading to an unstable hypoxic patient is often treated with streptokinase for thrombolysis in addition to supportive measures. Enoxaparin has a long half-life and is thus sometimes switched for unfractionated heparin at 36 weeks of gestation. This allows women the option of regional anesthesia (e.g., epidural) without an increased risk for epidural hematoma.

FIGURE 11-1. In these posterior views, the perfusion lung scan (left) reveals segmental defects that are not matched in the normal ventilation scan (right). This is consistent with a high probability of pulmonary embolism. (Reproduced with permission from Clark SL, Cotton DB, Hankins GDV, Engel EL. *Critical Care Obstetrics*, 2nd ed. Cambridge: Blackwell Science; 1991:162.)

FIGURE 11-2. Arteriogram of the left pulmonary artery showing filling defects, and an unperfused segment of lung as demonstrated by the absence of contrast dye. (Reproduced with permission from Clark SL, Cotton DB, Hankins GDV, Engel EL. *Critical Care Obstetrics*, 2nd ed. Cambridge: Blackwell Science; 1991:162.)

In the postpartum period, warfarin can be used as well, although some women choose to remain on enoxaparin because of the need for serial blood draws to check prothrombin time (PT)/PTT and international normalized ratio (INR) on warfarin. Patients are usually treated for a minimum of 6 months.

Of note, the newer direct oral anticoagulants (antithrombin and factor Xa inhibitors) are not well studied in pregnancy and in general are not used.

MATERNAL THYROID DISEASE IN PREGNANCY

Management of thyroid disease changes in pregnancy because of the V_D, increased circulating thyroid binding globulin, and sex hormone binding globulin (SHBG), which also binds thyroid hormone. Each of these leads to decreased availability of thyroid hormone. Additionally, because metabolic demands increase in pregnancy, thyroid-stimulating hormone (TSH) and FT4 levels are commonly followed every 6 to 8 weeks.

HYPERTHYROIDISM

The most common cause of hyperthyroidism is **Graves disease**. Patients with medically managed Graves disease can continue their **propylthiouracil** (PTU) or methimazole, which decrease the production of the T4 moiety, and in the case of PTU, block its peripheral conversion to T3. Because Graves disease is the result of thyroid-stimulating immunoglobulins (TSIs), TSI levels are checked at the initial visit. If levels are elevated, the fetus is at risk of developing a fetal goiter and should undergo a fetal survey at 18 to 20 weeks of gestation as well as an ultrasound in the third trimester to look for fetal goiter. Antenatal testing with serial nonstress tests is also recommended given the risk of fetal hyperthyroidism, which can be diagnosed with fetal tachycardia. Finally, PTU and methimazole can cross the placenta and can lead to fetal goiter as well. Thus, during pregnancy, it is best to use the minimum dosage possible. Occasionally, patients with Graves disease can be tapered off of their medications.

Given these issues, it is important to follow both symptoms of hyperthyroidism and the thyroid function laboratory test results closely. Although in the general population, TSH should be kept between 0.5 and 2.5, in pregnancy, it should be kept closer to 0.5 than 2.5 if possible.

HYPOTHYROIDISM

The most common etiology for hypothyroidism is **Hashimoto** thyroiditis, and the second is ablation or removal of the thyroid after Graves disease or cancer. Several physiologic changes in pregnancy increase demand for thyroid hormone including increased V_D, increased binding globulin (in particular, SHBG), increased clearance, and increased basal metabolic rate. These changes occur throughout pregnancy and as a result, all women on levothyroxine (Synthroid) supplementation should have their dose increased from 25% to 30%, and TSH levels should be checked each trimester. TSH levels should be kept low normal by increasing levothyroxine supplementation throughout pregnancy and following the TSH level. In women with a history of thyroid cancer, TSH levels should be kept below the reference range of TSH to prevent recurrence of disease.

SYSTEMIC LUPUS ERYTHEMATOSUS

Systemic lupus erythematosus (SLE) and other associated collagen vascular disorders such as Sjögren syndrome, scleroderma, and antiphospholipid antibody syndrome confer increased risk for serious complications during pregnancy. Lupus confers a 20-fold increase in risk for maternal mortality and elevated risk of thrombosis, infection, transfusion, cesarean section, preterm labor, and preeclampsia. There is particular concern in patients with concomitant hypertension or renal disease because these patients bear an even greater risk of developing preeclampsia, IUGR, and having preterm deliveries than women with SLE without these manifestations. The natural history of SLE in pregnancy follows the one-third rule; that is, one-third improve, one-third worsen, and one-third remain unchanged. In general, it also seems that patients who are without flares immediately prior to pregnancy have a better course. Medications such as aspirin and corticosteroids are continued in pregnancy, whereas cyclophosphamide and methotrexate are not.

EARLY PREGNANCY COMPLICATIONS

Patients with SLE and, in particular, antiphospholipid antibody syndrome have a high risk of early pregnancy loss in both the first and second trimesters. The pathophysiology of these losses is placental thrombosis. The high rate of second-trimester losses is a hallmark of these diseases, and they will often show symmetric IUGR by 18 to 20 weeks of gestation. Treatment and prophylaxis with low-dose aspirin, heparin, and corticosteroids have been tried with some improvement in prognosis.

LATER PREGNANCY COMPLICATIONS

Just as in the early pregnancy losses, the placenta can become thrombosed in the third trimester as well, leading to IUGR and intrauterine fetal demise (IUFD). Because of this risk, frequent antenatal testing is performed, usually starting at week 32. Subcutaneous (SQ) heparin or Lovenox prophylaxis and low-dose aspirin have also been used, each exhibiting some improvement in prognosis. However, even on these agents, the risks are still higher than those of the baseline population. Patients are also at increased risk of developing preeclampsia.

LUPUS FLARES VERSUS PREECLAMPSIA

One of the most difficult differential diagnoses to sort out is that of a lupus flare versus preeclampsia in the pregnant lupus patient. Both diseases are likely mediated by circulating antigen–antibody complexes or tissue-specific antibodies that cause a vasculitis. The similarity between the two diseases is remarkable (Table 11-3). One method of differentiating between the two is checking complement levels. Patients having a lupus flare will have reduced C3 and C4, whereas patients with preeclampsia should have normal levels. In addition, lupus flares are often accompanied by active urine sediment, whereas preeclampsia is not. Differentiating between the two conditions is important because the management for each is distinct. A lupus flare is managed with high-dose corticosteroids and, if unresponsive, cyclophosphamide. Worsening preeclampsia, in contrast, is managed by delivery.

NEONATAL LUPUS

As with other maternal diseases, lupus can affect the fetus and neonate. In addition to increased rates of IUGR, still birth, and preterm birth, there are two specific complications of interest. The first is a lupus syndrome related to maternal antigen–antibody complexes that have crossed the placenta and cause lupus in the neonate. These flares can be quite severe and cause skin lesions, hepatosplenomegaly, and low blood counts. The other complication seen is that of irreversible congenital heart block. Lupus patients (and more commonly Sjögren syndrome patients) can produce antibodies called anti-Ro (SSA) and anti-La (SSB) that are tissue specific to the fetal cardiac conduction system. Because these antibodies damage the AV node in particular, congenital heart block is seen in 5% of patients. Of these antibodies, anti-Ro

TABLE 11-3. Lupus Flare versus Severe Preeclampsia

Organ System	Lupus Complication	Severe Preeclampsia
Neuro	Lupus cerebritis, seizures	Seizures, visual changes
cardiovascular (CV)	Hypertension	Hypertension
Pulmonary	Pulmonary edema	Pulmonary edema
Renal	Worsening renal disease	Significant proteinuria, oliguria, renal failure
gastrointestinal (GI)	Hepatitis	Liver dysfunction, ↑ transaminases, hepatic edema
Heme	Thrombocytopenia	Thrombocytopenia, hemolytic anemia
	Hemolytic anemia	DIC

DIC, disseminated intravascular coagulation.

is more likely than anti-La to cause heart block. Patients are screened for these antibodies at the first prenatal visit, and treatments include corticosteroids, plasmapheresis, and intravenous immunoglobulin (IVIG). It is unclear whether any of these interventions improves outcomes, and because these treatments have complications and are quite expensive, many clinicians use serial screening for the fetuses at risk of heart block. Such screening includes serial fetal monitoring and serial fetal echocardiogram to identify cases of potential heart block early in the process.

SUBSTANCE ABUSE IN PREGNANCY

Substance abuse in pregnancy contributes to maternal and fetal morbidity and mortality in both the antepartum and postpartum periods. The most commonly used substances are alcohol and cigarettes, both of which contribute to poor outcomes of pregnancy. The most common illicit drugs used in pregnancy are tetrahydrocannabinol (THC), opiates, methamphetamines, and cocaine, each of which has associated problems for the infant. Finally, even when infants are born with minimal effects from the intrapartum insult, substance abuse is an indicator for other social problems that may contribute to a poor environment for child rearing.

ALCOHOL

A constellation of abnormalities in the infants born to women who abuse alcohol during pregnancy have been included in the diagnosis of **fetal alcohol syndrome** (FAS). The syndrome has a spectrum of increasing severity in children of women who drink more heavily (two to five drinks per day) during pregnancy. However, there is no safe amount of alcohol in pregnancy that confers no risk. FAS, which includes growth retardation, CNS effects, and abnormal facies, is estimated to occur in approximately 1 in 2,000 live births. Many milder cases may go unrecognized. Diagnosis is made by a history of alcohol abuse in the mother combined with the constellation of infant abnormalities. Other teratogenic effects of alcohol include almost every organ system. Cardiac defects are particularly associated with alcohol abuse.

Treatment
Several studies show that aggressive counseling programs for expectant mothers have led to a significant decrease in alcohol intake in greater than 50% of participants. For patients who are at risk for alcohol withdrawal, barbiturates are often used for withdrawal symptoms because of the potential teratogenicity of benzodiazepines. Because alcoholics are at higher risk for nutritional deficiencies, special care should be taken to ensure adequate nutrition during pregnancy.

CAFFEINE

Caffeine is found in coffee (30 to 170 mg/cup), tea (10 to 100 mg/cup), and caffeinated soft drinks (30 to 60 mg/12 oz). It is the most commonly used drug during pregnancy, with almost 80% of all pregnant women being exposed in the first trimester. Studies on rats show teratogenicity at high levels of caffeine exposure. However, the studies in humans are inconsistent.

CIGARETTES

Cigarette smoking in pregnancy has been correlated with increased risk of spontaneous abortions, preterm births, abruptio placentae, and decreased birth weight. Further, infants exposed to cigarette smoking in the womb are at an increased risk for sudden infant death syndrome and respiratory illnesses of childhood. A dose–response effect has been noted for many of these outcomes. In the Ontario Perinatal Mortality Study, smokers were divided into those having less than one pack per day (PPD) and those having more than one PPD. A 20% increase in the risk of fetal death was found in those pregnancies in which patients smoked less than one PPD, whereas a 35% increase was found in the more than one PPD group.

Treatment
There is no demonstrated safe amount of smoking. But because of the demonstrated dose–response effect of smoking, patients should be counseled on the increased risks for the fetus and advised, at minimum, to decrease cigarette use. Several studies show that smoking cessation programs targeting pregnant patients are more effective than those for nonpregnant patients. Further, primary care providers of women of childbearing age should begin this counseling prior to pregnancy.

MARIJUANA

Marijuana is the most common illicit substance used in pregnancy. Owing to increased legality of recreational marijuana, the use in pregnancy is on the rise. Studies have demonstrated that 40% to 60% of women who use marijuana prior to pregnancy continue to use during pregnancy and that many women feel that it is relatively safe. In pharmacokinetic studies, chemical products from marijuana can be transferred across the placenta and into breast milk, and some animal studies show that THC can be concentrated particularly after repeated exposure. Studies of marijuana use in pregnancy are limited due to multiple confounding factors and likely under reporting but have demonstrated an association with low birth weight, preterm birth, and stillbirth. Marijuana smoke contains many of the carcinogens and toxins found in tobacco smoke, and cannabinoids are thought to affect neurodevelopment.

Treatment
Women who smoke or use marijuana should ideally be identified preconception, and current guidelines recommend counseling for cessation. In particular, women who use marijuana for nausea and vomiting in pregnancy should be counseled on safer, better studied medications.

COCAINE AND METHAMPHETAMINES
Cocaine use in pregnancy is associated with abruptio placentae, IUGR, and an increased risk for preterm labor and delivery. The adverse events related to cocaine use during pregnancy are consistent with the physiologic effects of cocaine, which include vasoconstriction and hypertension. Cocaine crosses the placenta and the blood–brain barrier. Mounting evidence shows that children who were exposed to cocaine in utero are also at increased risk for CNS complications, including developmental delay. Cocaine toxicity may mimic preeclampsia and cause hypertension and end organ hypoxic damage.

Methamphetamine use in pregnancy is also associated with adverse pregnancy outcomes. Geographically methamphetamine use is associated with the west coast but has spread across the United States. The use in pregnancy is less studied than opiates or cocaine use, but is associated with low birth weight infants, IUFD, preeclampsia, and neurodevelopmental sequelae in children. Additionally, methamphetamines can induce hypertension, cardiomyopathy, and cardiac arrhythmias. Long-term users can display paranoia and psychosis.

Treatment
Patients who admit to cocaine and methamphetamine use should be advised of its risks to both the mother and the fetus. Social services should be involved in prenatal care, and patients who continue to abuse the drug should be encouraged to enter a detoxification center. Cocaine toxicity is managed with hydralazine, and β-blockade is contraindicated.

OPIATES
The most common narcotics used in pregnancy are oxycodone, heroin, and methadone. The use of opiates in the United States and in pregnancy has garnered national attention during the current epidemic. There are no known teratogenic effects of narcotics. In fact, there is some evidence that opioid withdrawal may pose a greater risk to the fetus than the chronic narcotic use. The risks of opioid withdrawal include miscarriage, preterm delivery, and fetal death. Patients using narcotics in pregnancy should therefore be enrolled in maintenance programs rather than advised to quit outright. Women undergoing withdrawal from opiates should be encouraged to present to an inpatient setting for start and titration of an opiate maintenance program. A new medication for opiate maintenance, buprenorphine (Subutex), is increasingly common for managing opiate withdrawal in pregnancy. Methadone can also be used. Once infants are delivered they are at risk for neonatal abstinence syndrome (NAS). Neonates with NAS require careful monitoring and slow withdrawal from their narcotic addiction using opiates.

KEY POINTS

- Nausea and vomiting in pregnancy are common; however, patients with hyperemesis gravidarum will not be able to maintain adequate hydration and nutrition.
- Acute management of hyperemesis gravidarum involves IV hydration, electrolyte repletion, and antiemetics; chronic management includes antiemetics and occasionally tube feeding or parenteral nutrition.
- The increase in seizure frequency may be related to increased metabolism of AEDs, decreased patient compliance, lower seizure threshold, and/or hormonal changes in pregnancy; patients should be followed frequently in pregnancy with monthly AED level.
- Although patients with seizure disorders have an increased baseline risk for congenital anomalies, this risk is likely increased with the use

- of AEDs, particularly in cases of polytherapy. Because of the risk for congenital anomalies, all patients should have a targeted ultrasound/fetal survey.
- The changes in cardiac physiology during pregnancy can have an enormous impact on cardiac disease. Common aspects of management include offering termination of pregnancy, medical stabilization, surgical or valvuloplasty repair if necessary, and consideration of the changes of pregnancy.
- On labor and delivery, cardiac patients are commonly given an early epidural, careful fluid monitoring, and an assisted vaginal delivery to minimize maternal stress and strain. The most risky period of time for cardiac patients is during labor, delivery, and the puerperium.
- Patients with mild renal disease suffer minimal effects, but may carry an increased risk of preeclampsia and IUGR, which is associated with the underlying diagnosis.
- Patients with moderate or severe renal disease are at risk for preeclampsia and IUGR, as well as worsening renal disease during and after the pregnancy. Careful monitoring of the patient's renal function and of fetal status is an hallmark of the management of these patients during pregnancy.
- Pregnancy is a hypercoagulable state with increased clotting factors, endothelial damage, and venous stasis.
- PE is the leading cause of maternal death. DVT and PE may be treated with enoxaparin or unfractionated heparin. Thrombolysis may be necessary for the unstable patient.
- In pregnancy, there are particular changes to the thyroid system including increased V_D and metabolism.
- In hyperthyroidism, TSIs should be screened for and, if elevated, fetal surveillance initiated to screen for fetal goiter and IUGR.
- In hypothyroidism, increased Synthroid requirements are common.
- Patients with SLE are at risk of developing complications throughout pregnancy. Prophylaxis against pregnancy loss, preeclampsia, and IUGR has been tried with low-dose aspirin, heparin, and corticosteroids, all of which have some possible benefit.
- Lupus flares and preeclampsia can be differentiated on the basis of complement levels.
- Mothers with anti-Ro and anti-La antibodies are at risk of having a fetus with congenital heart block.
- Alcohol abuse in pregnancy is correlated with FAS, which includes a constellation of growth restriction, CNS effects, and abnormal facies. Alcohol has also been correlated with other teratogenic effects, particularly cardiac defects.
- Caffeine use greater than 150 mg/day has been correlated with an increased risk of spontaneous abortions.
- Cigarette use during pregnancy has been correlated with growth restriction, abruptions, preterm delivery, and fetal death. Patients should be strongly encouraged to forgo its use during pregnancy.
- Cocaine use has been correlated with abruptio placentae and CNS effects in children. Patients should be advised to quit outright.
- Narcotic abusers should be enrolled in methadone or Subutex programs because the acute withdrawal effects of narcotics are more dangerous to the fetus than the chronic use.

CLINICAL VIGNETTES

VIGNETTE 1

A 28-year-old G2P1001 woman who is 18 weeks pregnant presents to the ED with increasing left lower extremity swelling, redness, and pain. She first noticed these symptoms 2 days ago and has tried elevation and warm compresses, which have not helped. She has no personal or family history of blood clots. She is otherwise healthy, and her only medication is a prenatal vitamin. In the ED, her vital signs are normal. Physical examination is significant for left lower extremity edema, calf tenderness, and erythema. You suspect that she has a lower extremity DVT, and you plan to start her on anticoagulation therapy.

1. Which of the following is the most important test to confirm your diagnosis?
   a. Venography
   b. D-dimer
   c. Left lower extremity venous Doppler ultrasound
   d. MRI of the left lower extremity
   e. No further testing is indicated

2. The lower extremity Doppler studies show a filling defect in the left popliteal vein. What is the best initial treatment for this patient?
   a. Coumadin
   b. IV heparin
   c. Subcutaneous low-molecular-weight heparin
   d. Placement of an inferior vena cava filter
   e. Thrombolytic therapy

3. You start her on 1 mg/kg Lovenox therapy twice daily and discharge her to follow-up with you next week. She returns to the emergency department later that evening with increasing shortness of breath, chest pain, and a small amount of blood when she coughs. Her examination is significant for sinus tachycardia and the left lower extremity edema and erythema. You are concerned that she has developed a PE. Which of the following tests would be most likely to confirm the diagnosis?
   a. Chest X-ray
   b. Pulse oximetry
   c. Echocardiogram
   d. Ventilation/perfusion (V/Q) study
   e. Spiral chest CT

4. The spiral CT shows evidence of a large filling defect in the left pulmonary artery. You admit her for observation and continued treatment. On admission to the medical ward, her heart rate is 105, BP is 80/54 mm Hg, her SaO_2 is 89%, and she is becoming increasingly short of breath. You decide to transfer to the ICU. What is the best treatment at this time for the PE?
   a. Continue subcutaneous Lovenox 1 mg/kg BID
   b. Start IV heparin
   c. Start Coumadin
   d. Start subcutaneous unfractionated heparin
   e. Embolectomy

5. The patient improved in the ICU on IV heparin and is transferred back to the general medical ward on hospital day number 2. She is transitioned back to subcutaneous Lovenox and discharged home on hospital day number 5. You see her for follow-up a few days later, and she asks why you think she had the DVT. Which of the following is not a risk factor for venous thromboembolism during pregnancy?
   a. Increased serum clotting factors
   b. Decreased levels of circulating fibrin
   c. Uterine compression of the IVC
   d. Progesterone-induced decreased venous tone
   e. None of the above

VIGNETTE 2

A 27-year-old G2P0010 woman at 8 weeks of gestational age (GA) comes to your clinic for an initial prenatal visit. A medical history reveals a diagnosis of lupus 2 years ago. She was initially well-controlled with aspirin and cyclophosphamide. When she started trying to conceive, the cyclophosphamide was discontinued, and she has continued the daily aspirin. She has had no lupus flares for over a year. The remainder of her medical history is normal. A physical examination is normal. Her BP today in clinic is 110/60 mm Hg, and she has trace proteinuria. You draw her basic prenatal laboratory tests and perform a Pap smear and GC/CT test. You also order a complete metabolic panel, baseline preeclampsia laboratory tests, complement levels, and anti–double-stranded DNA antibodies.

1. What additional test should you order to determine appropriate management during pregnancy?
   a. Anti-Ro (SSA) and anti-La (SSB)
   b. Chest X-ray
   c. 1-hour GTT
   d. Thrombophilia testing (factor V Leiden, prothrombin, etc.)
   e. Coagulation panel

2. You recommend that she continue the daily aspirin and prenatal vitamin. You counsel her regarding healthy diet and exercise in pregnancy, normal weight gain, and when to call the clinic. You also counsel her regarding the increased risk of complications during this pregnancy due to lupus. Which of the following is not a maternal complication of this condition during pregnancy?
   a. Recurrent miscarriage
   b. Intrauterine growth restriction (IUGR)
   c. Preeclampsia
   d. Stillbirth
   e. Placental abruption

3. Her laboratory test results are notable for an initial creatinine of 1.0, a 24-hour urine protein total of 190 mg, positive anti-Ro (SSA), and negative anti-La (SSB) antibodies. Complement levels were normal. She does well through the first and second trimesters. She had a normal ultrasound and fetal echocardiogram. At 32 weeks, you started twice weekly nonstress tests (NSTs), which have been reactive. At 36 weeks, you see her in the office, and she has 2+ proteinuria and a BP of 165/88 mm Hg. You admit her to labor and delivery triage unit for further evaluation. What finding can help you diagnose her with preeclampsia and not a lupus flare?
   a. Elevated uric acid
   b. BP greater than 140/90 mm Hg
   c. Thrombocytopenia
   d. Increasing urine protein
   e. Normal C3 and C4 levels

4. You diagnose her with severe preeclampsia based on persistently elevated BPs in the severe range and normal complement levels. You start her on IV magnesium for seizure prophylaxis and misoprostol for cervical ripening. Her labor is uncomplicated, and she has a successful spontaneous vaginal delivery (SVD) of a vigorous male infant. Mother and baby do well and are transferred to the postpartum ward. What is the most significant neonatal complication of maternal lupus?
   a. Congenital abnormalities
   b. Neonatal heart block
   c. Neonatal thrombosis
   d. Acute respiratory distress syndrome
   e. Feeding difficulties

VIGNETTE 3

A 26-year-old G3P2002 woman at 9 weeks of GA comes to clinic for an initial prenatal care visit. She has a history of thyroid cancer and had a total thyroidectomy 5 years ago. She has no evidence of recurrent disease. She has been maintained on 50 mcg of Synthroid for the last 3 years and has no symptoms of hypothyroidism. Her other pregnancies occurred prior to the diagnosis of her thyroid cancer, so she is concerned about how this pregnancy might be managed differently.

1. How would you manage her dose of Synthroid at this initial visit?
   a. Increase Synthroid dose by 25%
   b. Triple her Synthroid dose
   c. Decrease Synthroid dose to 25 mcg
   d. Stop Synthroid
   e. No changes

2. You increase her Synthroid dose to 62.5 mcg daily. What is your goal thyroid-stimulating hormone (TSH)?
   a. TSH < 0.5
   b. TSH 1.0
   c. TSH 3.0
   d. TSH 5.0
   e. TSH > 5.0

3. You see another patient in your office who had a thyroidectomy from Graves disease. She is now hypothyroid and on Synthroid replacement. You monitor her TSH and keep it between 0.5 and 2.5. You increase her Synthroid each trimester, and her TSH remains around 2.0 during the entire pregnancy. In addition to monitoring her TSH, what other additional testing should you perform during her pregnancy?
   a. Amniocentesis to determine if the fetus is affected by Graves disease
   b. A detailed fetal ultrasound at 18 to 20 weeks and again in the third trimester should be performed given the increased risk of fetal goiter
   c. Fetal echocardiogram to evaluate for cardiac abnormalities
   d. Umbilical Dopplers to monitor for placental dysfunction
   e. MCA Dopplers to monitor for fetal anemia

VIGNETTE 4

You see a patient for preconception counseling. She is a 24-year-old G3P0020 woman, and her medical history is significant for IgA glomerulonephritis and a recent creatinine of 2.0. She is otherwise healthy.

1. What can you tell her to expect regarding her kidney function if she were to get pregnant?
   a. It will improve
   b. It will stay the same
   c. It will get worse
   d. It is unlikely she will need dialysis by the end of pregnancy
   e. She will need kidney transplant in order to have a successful pregnancy

2. She returns 6 months later and is 8 weeks pregnant. Her creatinine at this time is 1.8. Her baseline 24-hour urine protein is 1,200 mg, and she has a mildly impaired creatinine clearance. You again counsel that this is a high-risk pregnancy and will need close monitoring. Which of the following is she not at risk for during this pregnancy?
   a. Preeclampsia
   b. Preterm delivery
   c. IUGR
   d. Fetal cardiac malformations
   e. Worsening renal disease

3. She decides to continue the pregnancy. She has an uncomplicated course during the first and second trimester. She has baseline proteinuria and dips 3 to 41 proteins on most clinic visits. In the third trimester, her kidney function worsens, and her creatinine rises to 2.8. A screening 24-hour urine protein at 32 weeks is significant for an increased value of 5,000 mg. She does not require dialysis. You see her in your clinic at 35 weeks, and she has a new onset increase in her BP. She has been mildly hypertensive during most of the pregnancy with values ranging between 130/90s and 140/90s mm Hg. Today, her BP is 170/110 mm Hg, and you send her to labor and delivery triage unit for further evaluation. What clinical data are most likely to help you make the diagnosis of preeclampsia?
   a. Proteinuria of 5,000 mg at 32 weeks
   b. An increase in BP of 30/15 mm Hg above prepregnancy values
   c. Elevated uric acid
   d. Increased creatinine to 3.0
   e. Proteinuria of 7,000 mg at 35 weeks

ANSWERS

VIGNETTE 1 Question 1
1. Answer C:
Diagnosis of DVT is often made clinically with confirmation by compression Doppler studies of the suspected extremity. The diagnosis is made by the following ultrasound findings: abnormal compressibility of the vein, abnormal color Doppler flow, the presence of an echogenic band, and abnormal change in diameter of the vessel. Venography, the gold standard, is rarely used because of the invasive nature of test and questionable improved sensitivity. D-dimer levels are elevated during pregnancy and so are not helpful to diagnose DVT in this population. MRI of the left lower extremity is thought to be as accurate as venography to diagnose DVT; however, because of the high cost of MRI, it is unlikely at this time to replace Doppler ultrasound.

VIGNETTE 1 Question 2
2. Answer C:
Treatment of DVT during pregnancy involves the use of adjusted dose low-molecular-weight heparin (enoxaparin 1 mg/kg BID) or unfractionated heparin (goal aPTT of 1.5 to 2.5 times normal). Low-molecular-weight heparin has become the preferred option because you do not need to check levels, and it is also thought to be safer due to a lower risk of heparin-induced thrombocytopenia. IV heparin is difficult to administer and requires hospitalization and frequent blood draws to confirm adequate treatment levels. It is also associated with increased risk of bleeding complications and would not be first-line therapy in this scenario. Warfarin (Coumadin) therapy is contraindicated in pregnancy secondary to evidence of fetal abnormalities caused by warfarin. When given in the first trimester, it causes warfarin embryopathy, which causes nasal hypoplasia and skeletal abnormalities. In addition, warfarin appears to cause diffuse central nervous system abnormalities, including optic atrophy, when given during pregnancy. Placement of an inferior vena cava filter is an invasive procedure that is generally used in situations, where the patient has a contraindication to anticoagulation. The use of thrombolytic therapy for DVT is controversial and not recommended as first-line treatment at this time.

VIGNETTE 1 Question 3
3. Answer E:
The diagnosis of PE usually involves the clinical picture correlated with a variety of diagnostic tests. Spiral CT scan has become the first-line diagnostic tool for PE in both the pregnant and the nonpregnant patients. The risk of radiation exposure must be weighed against the suspected risk of a PE, and the dangers that this poses to a pregnant woman's health. As with other life-threatening medical conditions, the woman's health should be considered first and foremost, and she should be evaluated and treated just as any nonpregnant patient would be in a similar condition. A chest X-ray may be entirely normal and is not likely to confirm the diagnosis. If abnormal, two common signs are the abrupt termination of a vessel, because it is traced distally, and an area of radiolucency in the area of the lung beyond the PE. Hypoxemia on pulse oximetry can raise clinical suspicion for PE, but is not diagnostic. An ECG may also be entirely normal or simply show sinus tachycardia. V/Q studies are recommended as the first-line diagnostic test only in institutions that have limited experience with spiral CT.

VIGNETTE 1 Question 4
4. Answer B:
In the hypotensive or unstable patient, IV heparin is the recommended option. It is also the recommended option if you are concerned about subcutaneous absorption or considering thrombolytics.

Low-molecular-weight heparin (enoxaparin) is the preferred choice in hemodynamically stable patients. Subcutaneous unfractionated heparin is also an option, but is associated with increased risk of heparin-induced thrombocytopenia and bleeding complications. Coumadin is contraindicated in pregnancy (see previous question). Embolectomy is reserved only for severe cases, where thrombolytics are indicated but are either not effective or contraindicated.

VIGNETTE 1 Question 5
5. Answer B:
Actually, the levels of circulating fibrin monomer complexes are increased in pregnancy and thought to be a contributing factor in the hypercoagulability of pregnancy. These levels increase further at the time of delivery and immediately postpartum.

The etiology of the hypercoagulability of pregnancy is thought to be multifactorial. In pregnancy, the production of all clotting factors is increased except for II, V, and IX. Also noted in pregnancy is that the turnover time for fibrinogen is decreased and that there are increased levels of fibrinopeptide A, which is cleaved from fibrinogen to make fibrin. It has also been hypothesized that the placenta synthesizes a factor that decreases fibrinolysis, but there is minimal evidence for this. Another proposed source of hypercoagulability is increased exposure to subendothelial collagen secondary to increased endothelial damage during pregnancy, although no mechanism has been proposed. Venous stasis may also account for some of the increase in venous thromboses during and after pregnancy. There are two principal causes for venous stasis in pregnancy. The first is decreased venous tone during pregnancy, which may be related to the smooth muscle relaxant properties of this high progesterone state. Second, the uterus, because it enlarges, compresses the inferior vena cava, the iliac, and pelvic veins. This compression, in particular, likely contributes to the increase in pelvic vein thromboses.

VIGNETTE 2 Question 1
1. Answer A:
Systemic lupus erythematosus (SLE) patients (and more commonly Sjögren syndrome patients) can produce antibodies called anti-Ro (SSA) and anti-La (SSB) that are tissue specific to the fetal cardiac conduction system. Because these antibodies damage the AV node in particular, congenital heart block is seen in 5% of patients. Of these antibodies, anti-Ro is more likely than anti-La to cause heart block. Patients are screened for these antibodies at the first prenatal visit, and treatments include corticosteroids, plasmapheresis, and IVIG. It is unclear whether any of these interventions improve outcomes, and because these treatments have complications and are quite expensive, many clinicians use serial screening for the fetuses at risk of heart block. Such screening includes serial fetal monitoring and serial fetal echocardiogram to identify cases of potential heart block early in the process.

Chest X-ray, early diabetes screening, thrombophilia, and a coagulation panel are not routine screening tests for lupus.

VIGNETTE 2 Question 2
2. Answer E:
Placental abruption has not been found to be associated with lupus. Patients with SLE and, in particular, antiphospholipid antibody syndrome have a high risk of early pregnancy loss in both the first and second trimesters. The pathophysiology of these losses is placental thrombosis. The high rate of second-trimester losses is a hallmark of these diseases, and they will often show symmetric IUGR by 18 to 20 weeks of gestation.

Just as in the early pregnancy losses, the placenta can become thrombosed in the third trimester as well, leading to IUGR and intrauterine fetal demise (stillbirth). Because of this risk, frequent antenatal testing is performed, usually starting at week 32. SQ heparin, Lovenox prophylaxis, or low-dose aspirin have also been used, each exhibiting some improvement in prognosis. However, even on these agents, the risks are still much higher than those of the baseline population. Patients are also at increased risk of developing preeclampsia.

VIGNETTE 2 Question 3
3. Answer E:
One of the most difficult differential diagnoses to sort out is that of a lupus flare versus preeclampsia in the pregnant lupus patient. Both diseases are likely mediated by circulating antigen–antibody complexes or tissue-specific antibodies that cause a vasculitis. One method of differentiating between the two is checking complement levels. Patients having a lupus flare will have reduced C3 and C4, whereas patients with preeclampsia should have normal levels. Differentiating between the two conditions is important because the management for each highly differs. A lupus flare is managed with high-dose corticosteroids and, if unresponsive, cyclophosphamide. Worsening preeclampsia, on the other hand, is managed by delivery.

Elevated uric acid, hypertension, thrombocytopenia, and increasing urine protein can be present in both preeclampsia and lupus flares.

VIGNETTE 2 Question 4
4. Answer B:
One of the most significant neonatal complications is that of irreversible congenital heart block. SLE patients (and more commonly Sjögren disease patients) can produce antibodies, called anti-Ro (SSA) and anti-La (SSB), that are tissue specific to the fetal cardiac conduction system and can cause fetal/neonatal heart block. These neonates may need to have a pacemaker placed and will usually require a pacemaker for life.

Maternal lupus can also cause a neonatal lupus syndrome related to maternal antigen–antibody complexes that have crossed the placenta and cause lupus in the neonate. These flares can be quite severe. Maternal lupus has not been associated with congenital abnormalities, neonatal thrombosis, ARDS, or feeding difficulties.

VIGNETTE 3 Question 1
1. Answer A:
Because the demands on thyroid hormone are going to increase in pregnancy owing to increased V_D, increased binding globulin (in particular, SHBG), increased clearance, and increased basal metabolic rate, all women on levothyroxine (Synthroid) supplementation should have their dosage increased 25% to 30% at the beginning of the pregnancy.

Tripling the dose is more likely to cause side effects of hyperthyroidism such as agitation, anxiety, and palpitations. Decreasing or stopping the Synthroid dose may lead to subacute hypothyroidism, which is associated with abnormal neuropsychological development. Subacute hypothyroidism may also be caused by not making changes to her dose at this initial visit.

VIGNETTE 3 Question 2
2. Answer B:
The levels of TSH should be kept low normal (0.5 to 2.5) by increasing levothyroxine supplementation throughout pregnancy and following the TSH level each trimester. For women with a history of thyroid cancer, like this patient, TSH levels should be kept below the reference range of TSH (closer to 1.0) to prevent recurrence of disease.

VIGNETTE 3 Question 3
3. Answer B:
Fetal goiter is a complication of maternal hyperthyroidism from Graves disease and placental transfer of thyroid-stimulating immunoglobulin (TSI) to the fetal circulation, not maternal hypothyroidism. Fetal goiter is a serious complication and, if severe, can lead to compression of the fetal trachea and difficulty with respiration at the time of birth. If present, consultation with a pediatric ENT physician is warranted prior to delivery to determine if intubation or an EXIT procedure is needed at the time of birth. In addition to ultrasound, weekly NSTs should be performed later in pregnancy to monitor for fetal tachycardia, which could be evidence of placental transfer of TSI to the fetal circulation.

Maternal Graves disease is not associated with fetal congenital abnormalities, placental dysfunction, or fetal anemia. Amniocentesis is not indicated because there is no associated test that can determine if the fetus is affected by Graves disease.

VIGNETTE 4 Question 1
1. Answer C:
Chronic renal disease can be divided into mild (Cr < 1.5), moderate (Cr from 1.5 to 2.8), and severe (Cr > 2.8), although other thresholds have been used. Renal blood flow and creatinine clearance increase during pregnancy in patients without renal disease, and this is also true initially in patients with renal disease. Patients with mild renal disease will usually experience improvement in renal function throughout much of pregnancy. Moderate and severe patients, however, may experience decreasing renal function in the latter half of pregnancy that may persist postpartum in as many as half of pregnancies. It is not uncommon for patients with moderate to severe renal dysfunction to require dialysis at some point during the pregnancy or postpartum period.

VIGNETTE 4 Question 2
2. Answer D:
Patients with chronic renal disease have increased risk of preeclampsia, preterm delivery, and IUGR in addition to worsening renal disease. There is no data that suggest an increased risk of fetal malformations, including cardiac abnormalities. Because of the above risks, these patients should be screened at least once per trimester with a 24-hour urine for creatinine clearance and protein. Patients who present in early pregnancy should be counseled regarding these risks and offered termination of pregnancy, particularly for the mother's health. Because of the risk to the fetus, antenatal fetal testing usually begins at 32 to 34 weeks of gestation.

VIGNETTE 4 Question 3
3. Answer B:
For patients who have baseline proteinuria and hypertension, the diagnosis of preeclampsia can be difficult to make. An increase in BP of 30/15 mm Hg above prepregnancy BPs can be used, although some experts disagree on its utility. In this situation, your patient has a significant increase in her BP from baseline, and this is most likely due to preeclampsia.

Increasing proteinuria is expected, and a value of 5,000 mg at 32 weeks with other evidence of preeclampsia is not diagnostic. In addition, a value of 7,000 at 35 weeks would raise your suspicion for preeclampsia but is not diagnostic. An elevated uric acid is not specifically associated with preeclampsia and may be present with worsening kidney function. In addition, her kidney function is expected to worsen, and a creatinine of 3.0 is not unexpected. In isolation, each of the other answers is not diagnostic of preeclampsia.

12 | Postpartum Care and Complications

ROUTINE POSTPARTUM CARE

The puerperium, or postpartum period, is defined as the first 6 weeks after delivery. Although still in the hospital, the patient often needs instruction about care of the neonate, breastfeeding, and her limitations during the ensuing weeks. The patient needs emotional support during the period of adjustment to the new member of the family and to her own physiologic changes. Given that the risk of postpartum complications can extend past the average patient's hospital stay, partners and family should be included in any maternal- or child-care counseling as available.

VAGINAL DELIVERY

Common issues following a vaginal delivery include pain control and perineal care. Usually, pain can be reduced with nonsteroidal anti-inflammatory drugs (NSAIDs) or acetaminophen. Low-dose opioids are occasionally required for adequate patient comfort, particularly at the hour of sleep. For patients with vaginal deliveries that involved either episiotomies or lacerations, perineal care is particularly important. Ice packs around the clock for the first 24 hours can be beneficial for both pain and edema in the perineum and labia. When inspecting the perineum of a postpartum patient, it is important to ensure that the perineal repair is intact, and that no hematomas have developed. These patients should also be on a bowel regimen while their laceration heals; avoiding constipation and bulky stool is an important factor in preventing wound breakdown. It is also important to note whether the patient has hemorrhoids, which are common in pregnancy and postpartum, particularly after a long second stage of labor. These should resolve with time, but patients' symptoms may be ameliorated with over-the-counter medications for hemorrhoids, stool softeners, and ice packs.

CESAREAN DELIVERY

Because more than 30% of deliveries are now by cesarean, wound care and pain management in these women are common components of postpartum care. Local wound care and observation for signs of wound infection or separation are part of routine care. Wound infections include cellulitis or a wound abscess. Wound separations can be at the level of the skin or subcutaneous tissue or deeper at the level of the rectus fascia, also known as a *wound dehiscence*. Postoperative pain is usually managed with opioids, but this can contribute to a postoperative ileus or constipation. Patients on opioids should, therefore, be prescribed stool softeners and, occasionally, laxatives. NSAIDs should be used concomitantly for the cramping pain caused by uterine involution. Patients have usually received a first- or second-generation cephalosporin during the cesarean section as prophylaxis against infection. Although it is routine in many institutions to give additional dosages, this has never been shown to further decrease the risk of infection.

BREASTFEEDING AND BREAST CARE

Although there are rare contraindications, such as infections that may lead to an increase in vertical transmission to the infant or in the case of mothers on medications or using recreational drugs that could be dangerous to a newborn, the vast majority of new mothers should be encouraged to breastfeed. There are various beliefs and racial/cultural differences regarding the practice of breastfeeding, but regardless, the health benefits to babies and mothers are being increasingly identified. Oxytocin release from the pituitary gland with breastfeeding stimulates postpartum uterine contractions, thereby increasing uterine tone and decreasing the risk of bleeding. Numerous studies have demonstrated a decrease in childhood infectious diseases in newborns, and infants of breastfeeding mothers are attributed to the passive immunity transmitted via immunoglobulins in the breast milk. Women who breastfeed are more likely to lose the weight they have gained during pregnancy. Furthermore, women who have breastfed appear to have a lower long-term risk of developing breast and ovarian cancer, osteoporosis, cardiovascular disease, and type 2 diabetes.

Despite all of these benefits, breastfeeding is challenging, particularly for a first-time mother. Historically, women would have likely learned about breastfeeding from female relatives and family, but in today's society in the United States, many women have not had such experiences. Thus, although they may be interested in breastfeeding, many women do not recognize the inherent difficulties and discomforts. A number of barriers to breastfeeding, both iatrogenic and natural, can be introduced in the birthing process and initial postpartum period. In a variety of complicated births, such as a preterm birth, emergency birth, or simply a cesarean delivery, the initial skin-to-skin contact that has been shown to initiate breastfeeding in the neonate is interrupted. Furthermore, although breastfeeding is natural, it is often not instinctive or intuitive to many women. Because they have expectations that breastfeeding should be easier, any delay or drawback can be interpreted as a failure. This misalignment of expectations and reality coupled with concerns about providing adequate nutrition to the neonate leads many women to give up breastfeeding for formula feeding only a few days postpartum. Reassurance that breastfeeding can be challenging and uncomfortable (even painful), but it should become easier and less uncomfortable, can help women to get through the initial weeks of breastfeeding.

All postpartum patients need breast care, regardless of whether or not they are breastfeeding. Patients usually experience the onset of lactation, engorgement or "letdown," approximately 24 to 72 hours postpartum. When this occurs, the breasts usually become uniformly warmer, firmer, and tender. Patients often complain of pain or warmth in the breasts and may experience fever. For patients not breastfeeding, ice packs, a tight bra, analgesics, and anti-inflammatory medications are all useful. Patients who are breastfeeding obtain relief from the breastfeeding itself, although this can lead to its own difficulties, such as tenderness and erosions around the nipple. Although protective creams and barriers can help symptomatically for sore nipples/breasts, providers should also assess breastfeeding positions and the infant's latch onto the breast. If the provider does not have this expertise, referral to a lactation consult is recommended.

POSTPARTUM PREVENTATIVE MEDICATIONS

Previously, it was thought that those who were exposed to pertussis or were vaccinated as children received lifelong immunity. However, recent findings suggest that immunity may only last up to 20 years. Consequently, many women in their childbearing years run the risk of contracting pertussis in the postpartum period and transmitting the disease to their infants prior to their scheduled immunizations at 2 months of age. With a general rise in the incidence of pertussis, routine postpartum immunization of women with Tdap is essential if they have not received the vaccine within the 10 years previous to pregnancy. Caregivers and partners who will be in close contact to the infant should also be vaccinated to create an immunologic cocoon. Mothers found to have low Rubella antibody titers in their prenatal laboratory test results should receive a measles, mumps, and rubella vaccine postpartum as well. The vaccine is a mixture of three attenuated live viruses that cannot be given during pregnancy.

If a woman is found to be Rh negative at the time of her prenatal laboratory tests or a type and screen, it is necessary that she receive an intramuscular injection of Rhogam within 72 hours postpartum. Rhogam contains antibodies to the Rh D factor, such that any Rh-positive fetal cells that mix with maternal blood during the time of delivery will be removed from the circulation, prior to sensitizing the mother's own immune system. Maternal sensitization can lead to the creation of maternal antibodies that, in a subsequent Rh-positive pregnancy, pass into fetal circulation, resulting in hemolytic disease of the newborn. Newborns routinely have their blood typed and screened at birth; only if the infant is found to be Rh negative, will the mother not need to receive Rhogam.

POSTPARTUM CONTRACEPTION

Most patients are advised to have pelvic rest until the 6-week follow-up visit. However, many women resume sexual activity prior to this time. Thus, contraception is an important issue to begin addressing during the prenatal period and continue while patients are still in the hospital postpartum. Because most states require women to consent to a postpartum tubal ligation (PPTL) at least 30 days prior to their estimated date of delivery (EDD), this should be brought up early in the third trimester. For women who desire permanent sterilization, PPTL is an extremely effective form of sterilization. Poor surgical candidates who desire sterilization may consider sterilization of the male partner by means of vasectomy, with equally effective results.

For those women who have not undergone or do not desire PPTL, counseling regarding other options is important. First-line contraception is long-acting reversible contraception (LARC) usually of an intrauterine device (IUD) or an implantable progestin. Uptake of the progesterone-eluting IUD (Mirena) has steadily increased over the past decade. Prior concerns about infections from IUDs in the 1970s or the increased volume and length of menses from the copper IUD are alleviated by the Mirena. Because of the low release of local progesterone, the use of the Mirena can actually lead to lighter, shorter menses and even amenorrhea in 15% to 20% of users. However, the IUD has a higher rate of expulsion in the immediate postpartum period because of the dilated cervix. Thus, in the majority of women, IUD placement is usually done at the 6-week postpartum appointment. In women who are less likely to follow up or for whom contraception is paramount, IUD placement postpartum with several follow-up visits to verify that it is still in situ is increasing in use. The most common implantable progestin used for birth control in the postpartum period is the Nexplanon. This progestin-only device is the size of a matchstick and is implanted superficially in the bicipital groove of the nondominant arm. It is effective for 3 years, and like the Mirena IUD, it is not only an effective and safe form of birth control but also reduces overall menstrual bleeding in one-third of users. Because of the ease of placement in the postpartum period, it is an excellent option for patients with difficulty following up or who are at high risk of short interval unintended pregnancy.

For women who decline LARC, who are interested in hormonal modes of contraception, and who are breastfeeding, the progesterone-only minipill or Depo-Provera is the usual recommended options. Combination estrogen–progesterone oral contraceptive pills (OCPs) in some studies have been shown to decrease milk production, so they are usually recommended only to those women who are not interested in breastfeeding or have excellent milk production (not usually known during the first week postpartum). Although there is a theoretical concern that progestin-based contraception may decrease milk supply, several studies have demonstrated that early administration of progesterone-only contraceptives do not impair lactation and may actually increase quality and duration of lactation. They are, therefore, preferable to combination OCPs for patients who are dedicated to breastfeeding and interested in hormonal forms of birth control.

Women interested in using combination OCPs should wait at least 4 weeks after delivery in order to establish an adequate milk supply given the potential effects of combination OCPs on milk production. If their milk production is adequate after initiation, they can then continue on this form of contraception. Women should also wait 3 weeks after delivery to initiate combined hormonal contraception given the high risk of venous thromboembolism (VTE) in the postpartum period. In women with no other risk factors for VTE, combination OCPs may be initiated after 3 weeks postpartum. However, in women with risk factors for VTE, such as age ≥35 years, previous VTE, thrombophilia, immobility, transfusion at delivery, BMI ≥ 30, postpartum hemorrhage (PPH), post-cesarean delivery, preeclampsia, or active smoking, initiation of combination OCPs should wait until after 6 weeks postpartum.

For patients interested in nonhormonal methods, condoms are particularly good because of the prevention against sexually transmitted infections. The other barrier methods—the diaphragm and cervical cap—should be avoided until 6 weeks postpartum when the cervix has returned to its normal shape and size.

DISCHARGE INSTRUCTIONS

Hospital stays after delivery are short, and although insurance companies have been mandated to cover up to 2 days after a vaginal delivery and 4 days after a cesarean delivery, many hospitals still discharge patients after 1 and 3 days, respectively. After a vaginal delivery, the above issues of perineal care, contraception, and breast care are discussed with the patient. Furthermore, a discussion regarding how common the postpartum "blues" and postpartum depression can be is paramount. Letting patients know that professionals are available to talk the patient through any problems as she transitions to home can be of help. Patients who have a cesarean delivery should be counseled regarding wound care and activity in addition to the above. With Pfannenstiel incisions that were stapled closed, the staples can be removed prior to discharge. Patients are often advised to avoid heavy lifting ("nothing heavier than your baby") and vigorous activities, including driving for 4 to 6 weeks after surgery. Before patients drive, it is recommended that they try to slam on the brakes as an experiment to be sure that they are comfortable enough to drive.

POSTPARTUM COMPLICATIONS

The primary complications that arise postpartum include PPH, endometritis, wound infections and separations, mastitis, and postpartum depression (Table 12-1). PPH usually occurs during the first 24 hours, while the patient is still in the hospital. However, it can also occur in patients with retained products of conception (POCs) for up to several weeks postpartum. Endometritis and wound complications typically occur in the first week to 10 days postpartum, and mastitis typically occurs 1 to 2 weeks after delivery but may present anytime during breastfeeding. Postpartum depression can occur at any time during the puerperium and beyond and is probably grossly underdiagnosed.

POSTPARTUM HEMORRHAGE

PPH occurs in roughly 1% to 5% of all deliveries and is defined as blood loss exceeding 500 mL in a vaginal delivery and greater than 1,000 mL in a cesarean section. If the hemorrhage occurs within the first 24 hours, it is deemed early PPH; after 24 hours, it is considered late or delayed PPH. Common causes of postpartum bleeding include uterine atony, retained POCs, placenta accreta, cervical lacerations, and vaginal lacerations (Tables 12-2 and 12-3). Although the cause of the hemorrhage is being investigated, the patient is simultaneously started on fluid resuscitation, and preparations are made for blood transfusions. With blood loss greater than 2 to 3 L, patients may develop a consumptive coagulopathy and require coagulation factors and platelets. In rare cases, if patients become hypovolemic and hypotensive, Sheehan syndrome, or pituitary infarction, may occur. Sheehan syndrome may manifest with the absence of lactation secondary to the lack of prolactin or failure to restart menstruation secondary to the absence of gonadotropins. Each of the etiologies of PPH is discussed sequentially; the obstetrician often has to consider and/or attempt to treat several etiologies simultaneously.

Vaginal Lacerations and Hematomas

Vaginal lacerations with uncontrolled bleeding should be considered in the case of PPH. Initially after a delivery, the perineum, labia, periurethral area, and deeper aspects of the vagina are examined for lacerations. These should be repaired at that time. However, deep sulcal tears or vaginal lacerations behind the cervix may be quite difficult to visualize without careful retraction. Occasionally, these lacerations will involve arteries and arterioles and lead to a significant PPH. Adequate anesthesia, an experienced obstetrician, and assistance with retraction are all necessary to perform an adequate exploration and repair of these lacerations.

Occasionally, the trauma of delivery will injure a blood vessel without disrupting the epithelium above it. This leads to the development of a hematoma. If a patient has a larger than expected drop in hematocrit, an examination should be performed to rule out a vaginal wall hematoma. A hematoma can be managed expectantly unless it is tense or

TABLE 12-1. Complications of Vaginal and Cesarean Deliveries

	Vaginal Delivery	Cesarean Delivery
Common complications	Postpartum hemorrhage	Postpartum hemorrhage
	Vaginal hematoma	Surgical blood loss
	Cervical laceration	Wound infection
	Retained POCs	Endometritis
	Mastitis	Mastitis
	Postpartum depression	Postpartum depression
Rare complications	Endometritis	Wound separation
	Episiotomy infections	Wound dehiscence
	Episiotomy breakdown	

POCs, products of conception.

TABLE 12-2. Risk Factors for Postpartum Hemorrhage

Prior postpartum hemorrhage

Abnormal placentation
    Placenta previa
    Placenta accreta
    Hydatidiform mole

Trauma during labor and delivery
    Episiotomy
    Complicated vaginal delivery
    Low- or midforceps delivery
    Sulcal or sidewall laceration
    Uterine rupture
    Cesarean delivery or hysterectomy
    Cervical laceration

Uterine atony
    Uterine inversion
    Overdistended uterus
        Macrosomic fetus
        Multiple gestation
        Polyhydramnios
    Exhausted myometrium
        Rapid labor
        Prolonged labor
        Oxytocin or prostaglandin stimulation
        Chorioamnionitis

Coagulation defects—intensify other causes
    Placental abruption
    Prolonged retention of demised fetus
    Amniotic fluid embolism
    Severe intravascular hemolysis
    Severe preeclampsia and eclampsia
    Congenital coagulopathies
    Anticoagulant treatment

TABLE 12-3. Etiology of Postpartum Hemorrhage in Vaginal and Cesarean Deliveries

Vaginal Delivery	Cesarean Delivery
Vaginal lacerations	Uterine atony
Cervical lacerations	Surgical blood loss
Uterine atony	Placenta accreta
Placenta accreta	Uterine rupture
Vaginal hematoma	
Retained POCs	
Uterine inversion	
Uterine rupture	

POCs, products of conception.

---

expanding, in which case it should be opened, the bleeding vessel ligated, and the vaginal wall closed. Rarely, a patient will develop a retroperitoneal hematoma that can lead to a large blood loss into this space. Patients usually complain of low back or rectal pain, and there will be a large drop in hematocrit. Diagnosis is made via ultrasound or CT. If the patient is stable without a falling hematocrit, expectant management may be followed. However, if the patient demonstrates continued bleeding with evidence of expansion of the hematoma or a further drop in hematocrit, interventional radiology can use embolization techniques in order to treat such bleeding. Because these clinicians are not in house at all institutions, early notification of the potential for such an intervention is necessary. If the patient becomes unstable, surgical exploration and ligation of the disrupted vessels may be required.

Cervical Lacerations

Cervical lacerations can cause a brisk PPH. Commonly, they are a result of rapid dilation of the cervix during the stage 1 of labor or maternal expulsive efforts prior to complete dilation of the cervix. If a patient is bleeding at the level of the cervix or above, a careful exploration of the cervix should be performed. The patient should have adequate anesthesia via epidural, spinal, or pudendal block. The walls of the vagina are retracted, so the cervix can be well visualized. When the anterior lip of the cervix is seen, it is grasped with a ring forcep. Then another ring forcep can be used to grasp beyond the first, and in this fashion, the cervix should be "walked" around its entirety, so that no lacerations, particularly on the posterior aspect, are missed. If any lacerations are seen, they are usually repaired with either interrupted or running absorbable sutures.

Uterine Atony

Uterine atony is the leading cause of PPH. Patients are at a higher risk for uterine atony if they have chorioamnionitis, exposure to magnesium sulfate, multiple gestations, a macrosomic fetus, polyhydramnios, prolonged labor, a history of atony with any prior pregnancies, or if they are multiparous, particularly a grand multipara (more than five deliveries). Uterine abnormalities or fibroids may also interfere with uterine contractions leading to and increasing bleeding. The diagnosis of atony is made by palpation of the uterus, which is soft, enlarged, and boggy. Occasionally, the uterine fundus is well contracted, but the lower uterine segment, which has less contractile tissue, will be less so.

Atony is initially treated with IV oxytocin (Pitocin), which is usually given prophylactically after delivery of the infant. Although the oxytocin is being administered, strong uterine massage should be performed to assist the uterus in contracting. If atony continues, the next step is methylergonovine (Methergine), which is contraindicated in hypertensive patients. If the uterus is still atonic, the next step is to give Hemabate (also known as Carboprost or Prostaglandin F2α, PGE-F2α [PGF2]), which is contraindicated in asthma patients. The prostaglandin is thought to be more effective if injected directly into the uterine musculature, either transabdominally or transcervically, although this has not been demonstrated in studies. Misoprostol, a Prostaglandin E1 (PGE1) analog traditionally used for the treatment of gastric ulcers, may also be used off-label for its uterotonic properties. Administered sublingually or rectally, misoprostol is an effective method for decreasing blood loss associated with atony when patients are without IV access. Its shelf-stability makes it suitable for settings that lack electricity, because Pitocin, Hemabate, and methylergonovine all require refrigeration.

If atony continues despite maximal medical management, the patient is brought to the operating room (OR) for a **dilation and curettage** (D&C) to rule out possible retained POCs. Patients with uterine atony unresponsive to these conservative measures, but bleeding at a rate that can tolerate some watchful waiting, may benefit from uterine packing with an inflatable tamponade (Bakri balloon) or occlusion of pelvic vessels (uterine artery embolization) by interventional radiology to prevent the necessity of a hysterectomy. If this is unsuccessful, exploratory laparotomy with ligation of pelvic vessels and possible hysterectomy are required.

Retained Products of Conception

Careful inspection of the placenta should always be performed. However, with vaginal delivery, it can often be difficult to determine whether a small piece of the placenta has been left behind in the uterus. Usually, the retained fetal membranes or placental tissue pass in the lochia. However, they occasionally lead to endometritis and PPH. If suspicion is high for retained POCs, the uterus should be explored either manually if the cervix has not contracted down or by ultrasound. If there is an evidence of a normal uterine stripe, the probability of retained products is much lower. However, if clinical suspicion is high, a D&C would be next for both diagnostic and therapeutic measures. If hemorrhage continues even after ascertaining that there are no further POCs via exploration, placenta accreta should be suspected.

Placenta Accreta

Placenta accreta, increta, and percreta are discussed briefly in Chapter 5 with antepartum hemorrhage. These conditions are the result of abnormal attachment of placental tissue to the uterus that may invade into or beyond the uterine myometrium, leading to incomplete separation of the placenta postpartum and PPH. Risk factors for developing placenta accreta include placenta previa and prior uterine surgery, including cesarean delivery and myomectomy. Often the third stage will have been longer than usual, and the placenta may have delivered in fragments. Accreta involves bleeding that is unresponsive to uterine massage and contractile agents, such as oxytocin, ergonovines, and prostaglandins. Patients with accreta are taken to the OR for surgical management via exploratory laparotomy.

Uterine Rupture

Uterine rupture is estimated to occur in 0.5% to 1.0% of patients with prior uterine scars and in about 1 in 5,700 to 20,000 women with an unscarred uterus. It is an intrapartum complication but may lead to postpartum bleeding. It is rare for rupture to occur in a nulliparous patient. Risk factors include previous uterine surgery, breech extraction, obstructed labor, and high parity. Symptoms usually include abdominal pain and a popping sensation intra-abdominally. Treatment involves laparotomy and repair of the ruptured uterus. If hemorrhage cannot be controlled, hysterectomy may be indicated.

Uterine Inversion

Uterine inversion occurs when the uterine fundus turns partially or completely inside out. Although rare, this is a life-threatening obstetrical emergency. Uterine inversion is estimated to occur in 1 in 2,500 deliveries. Risk factors include fundal implantation of the placenta, uterine atony, placenta accreta, and excessive traction on the cord during the third stage. Diagnosis is made by witnessing the fundus of the uterus attached to the placenta on placental delivery; this usually looks like a round mass protruding from the cervix or vagina accompanied by significant vaginal bleeding. Additionally, patients often experience an intense vasovagal response from the inversion and may require stabilization with the aid of an anesthesiologist before manual replacement of the uterus can be attempted, which should be the first

FIGURE 12-1. Manual replacement of an inverted uterus. To manage a uterine inversion the provider pushes their fist cephalad to replace the uterus with a firm steady force towards the fundus.

step in treatment (Fig. 12-1). Uterine relaxants, such as nitroglycerin, or general anesthesia with halogenated agents may be given to aid uterine relaxation and replacement. If this is unsuccessful, laparotomy is required to surgically replace the uterus. After successful replacement of the uterine fundus, physicians should be prepared to manage the PPH that frequently occurs afterward owing to the use uterine relaxants.

Operative Management of Postpartum Hemorrhage

In the case of vaginal delivery, the management of PPH is as described above. A differential diagnosis is created, and a rapid physical examination is performed to establish the likely etiology. If vaginal and cervical lacerations have been ruled out and the patient is unresponsive to uterotonic agents and massage, the patient should be moved to an OR and a D&C performed. If this fails to stop the bleeding, placement of an inflatable balloon in the uterine cavity may limit further hemorrhage; if these measures fail, a laparotomy is performed.

On entering the abdomen, the surgeon should note whether there is blood in the abdomen, which would indicate a uterine rupture. Unless the patient is unstable and coagulopathic secondary to excessive blood loss, the first surgical procedure is usually bilateral O'Leary sutures to tie off the uterine arteries.

The second is ligation of the hypogastric, or internal iliac, arteries, which requires considerable skill and experience. If uterine atony is the cause of hemorrhage, B-Lynch sutures can be placed in an attempt to compress the uterus and achieve hemostasis. A large Mayo needle with chromic suture is used to enter and exit the uterine cavity laterally across the lower uterine segment. This suture is then looped around the uterus and reenters the uterine cavity laterally on the posterior wall. It is again looped back over anteriorly, and the free ends are pulled tight like suspenders because the uterus is rolled over itself, resulting in uterine compression. If these measures fail to provide hemostasis, often the patient requires a puerperal hysterectomy (known as cesarean hysterectomy if that has been the mode of delivery).

If the patient has been delivered via cesarean section and there is no evidence of placenta accreta, the first step is to close the hysterotomy because this will usually improve uterine atony. If this is unsuccessful, O'Leary sutures can be placed next with the uterus to ligate the uterine arteries, decreasing blood flow to the uterus. Compressive sutures like the B-Lynch described above can also be performed. If these fail, one may consider hypogastric artery ligation; however, this procedure is performed infrequently and should be done by an experienced physician with knowledge and experience in operating the retroperitoneal space. In the event that all of these measures fail, hysterectomy is the definitive procedure.

If a patient has been delivered via cesarean section and there is evidence of accreta, proceeding with a cesarean hysterectomy is appropriate because conservative management of placenta accreta is rarely effective, and the risks associated with delaying hysterectomy, including hemorrhage, coagulopathy, and organ system damage, can be catastrophic.

If a patient is not bleeding too briskly, with either vaginal or cesarean delivery, packing the uterus and obtaining an interventional radiology consult for uterine artery embolization are possible. This is reserved for those patients who are truly stable and desire future fertility.

ENDOMETRITIS

Endometritis is a polymicrobial infection of the uterine lining that often invades the underlying muscle wall. It is most common after cesarean section but may occur after vaginal deliveries as well, particularly in cases of manual extraction of the placenta. Risk factors include meconium, chorioamnionitis, and prolonged rupture of membranes.

The diagnosis is clinical and made in the setting of fever, elevated WBC count, and uterine tenderness, with a higher suspicion after cesarean. Endometritis commonly occurs 5 to 10 days after delivery but may be suspected when all other sources of infection have been ruled out for several weeks after delivery. Because retained POCs can be the etiology of infection, an ultrasound is often obtained to examine the intrauterine contents.

Endometritis is usually treated with broad-spectrum IV antibiotics, or triple antibiotics, although in some institutions a second-generation cephalosporin is used. If retained POCs are identified on ultrasound, a D&C is performed. Because the postpartum uterus is at greater risk for perforation, great care should be taken during dilation, using blunt rather than sharp curettage and ultrasound guidance to limit complications. Antibiotics are continued until the patient is afebrile for 48 hours; uterine pain and tenderness are absent; and the WBC count normalizes.

WOUND COMPLICATIONS
Wound Infections
Wound infections include cellulitis and abscess. Although such infections of the cesarean skin incision are seen in 1% to 5% of cases, these can also be seen in the perineal laceration or episiotomy site. Cellulitis is suspected with local erythema around the surgical site. If the erythema is tender and particularly warm, the level of suspicion is usually high enough to diagnose cellulitis. If these two symptoms are not present, often a line is drawn around the erythema, and if it expands more than 12 to 24 hours, this also makes a diagnosis of cellulitis. Cellulitis can be treated with broad-spectrum antibiotics with a focus on covering skin flora. In the case of a cellulitis not responding to antibiotics and with increasing fever, evidence of pus from the wound, or a palpable collection within the incision, an abscess should be suspected. Wound abscesses need to be treated surgically with incision and drainage (I&D), wound cleaning, and packing. Often, antibiotics are continued until 48 hours afebrile. Anytime a wound abscess is suspected, it should either be ruled out with an imaging study or definitively by opening the wound. Delay in treating a wound abscess may lead to necrotizing fasciitis. One hallmark sign of necrotizing fasciitis is the loss of initial pain from cellulitis caused by nerve injury without change in the visual appearance of the cellulitis. Necrotizing fasciitis requires surgical resection of the necrotic tissue and often repair of the fascia with grafts.

Perineal cellulitis or abscesses are treated similar to abdominal wound infections. However, the diagnosis is often more difficult to make, because the area can be more difficult to readily inspect and women can confuse the infection with normal postpartum perineal pain. Similar treatment with broad-spectrum antibiotics for cellulitis and opening the wound in the setting of an abscess are performed. If such an abscess occurs in the setting of third- or fourth-degree perineal laceration, usually the infection is treated, and a long-delayed closure by a specialist, for example, a urogynecologist or rectal surgeon, is performed. Of note, perineal infections in the setting of third- and fourth-degree lacerations may be decreased by the use of prophylactic antibiotics.

Wound Separations
Even in the absence of an infection, wounds may not heal by primary intention after their first closure. Fluid collections of either serum (seroma) or blood (hematoma) can increase the chances of wound separation by preventing tissue apposition. Thus, continued leaking of either fluid or blood from a wound can signal a seroma or hematoma. Usually, the skin of a transverse incision has adequately healed to remove staples on postoperative day 3 and for a vertical incision by postoperative day 6 or 7. If, when the staples are removed, the skin separates, this is considered a wound separation. In this setting, it is important to make sure it is just a superficial separation, and the wound should be probed to verify that the fascia is still intact. If the fascia is also separated, this is termed as a *wound dehiscence*.

With a superficial wound separation, there are two options. The first is to simply let the wound heal by secondary intention. The wound may be packed with moistened gauze and changed once to two to three times per day. More recently, wounds have been treated with a wound vacuum. By applying negative pressure to the wound, serous fluid is removed, local blood supply to the area improved, and wound edges mechanically reapproximated, and thus decreasing wound healing time. Another alternative is that if the wound is not infected, it can be simply closed by primary intention again.

Because many post-cesarean wounds are complicated by seromas from the surrounding tissue edema, these reattempts at primary closure will often be unsuccessful. For a complete wound dehiscence, the patient requires a trip back to the OR where the fascia is closed, and the skin incision is treated in either fashion detailed above.

MASTITIS

Mastitis is a regional infection of the breast, commonly caused by the patient's skin flora or the oral flora of breastfeeding infants. The organisms enter an erosion or cracked nipple and proliferate, leading to infection. Lactating women will often have bilaterally warm, diffusely tender, and firm breasts, particularly at the time of engorgement or milk letdown. This should be differentiated from focal tenderness, erythema, and differences in temperature from one region of the breast to another, which are all classic signs of mastitis. The diagnosis can be made with physical examination, fever, and an elevated WBC count. Mastitis can be complicated by formation of an abscess, which then requires treatment by I&D.

Mastitis can be treated with oral antibiotics; dicloxacillin is the treatment of choice. In addition, patients should be encouraged to continue breastfeeding, which prevents intraductal accumulation of infected material. Those who are not breastfeeding should be encouraged to use a breast pump in the acute phase of the infection. Women who are unresponsive to oral antibiotics are admitted for IV antibiotics until afebrile for 48 hours. If there is no response to IV antibiotics, a breast abscess should be suspected, and an imaging study obtained.

POSTPARTUM DEPRESSION

More than half of all women will experience postpartum changes in their mood. Many patients experience postpartum blues, often described as rapid mood swings from elation to sorrow, and changes in appetite, concentration, and sleep. These postpartum changes generally occur within 2 to 3 days after delivery, peaking at the fifth day and resolving within 2 weeks. Symptoms of sadness and disinterest that persist may point toward a diagnosis of true postpartum depression, which complicates more than 5% of pregnancies. The pathophysiology of postpartum depression is poorly understood but may be due to the rapid changes in estrogen, progesterone, and prolactin in postpartum patients. It may also be related to the lack of sleep in the postpartum period as well as the psychosocial stress of caring for a newborn. Although all women experience hormonal fluctuation after delivery, some may be more sensitive to these changes, and thereby predisposed to the development of postpartum depression. Such patients include those with a personal history of or family history of depression or other mental illness, depressive symptoms in pregnancy, mood changes with hormonal contraceptive use, as well as those with poor social support networks.

Diagnosis

Most patients have normal changes in appetite, energy level, and sleep patterns in the initial postpartum period that do not necessarily indicate frank depression. However, patients who experience low energy level, anhedonia, anorexia, apathy, sleep disturbances, extreme sadness, and other depressive symptoms for greater than a few weeks may have postpartum depression. These patients often feel incapable of caring for their infants. Occasionally, depressed patients have suicidal or homicidal ideation, which is a much clearer marker for depression and merits close observation. Patients with a history of bipolar disorder should specifically be observed for the development of postpartum psychosis.

Therapy and Prognosis

In patients with postpartum blues, symptoms are usually self-limited with support and encouragement. However, these symptoms can occasionally progress to a more severe postpartum depression or even psychosis. In these situations, the caregiver needs to determine whether the patient is having suicidal or homicidal ideation. A social worker and professional counselor should be involved, as should the immediate family and any other individuals who are close to the patient and can provide support. Although an episode of postpartum blues may resolve quite readily, depression and psychosis should be treated with medications. Selective Serotonin Reuptake Inhibitors (SSRIs) have been used for postpartum depression with good efficacy and compatibility with breastfeeding. Most patients without a history of depression or other mental illness improve, usually to their prepregnant state.

KEY POINTS

- Two central issues in the immediate postpartum period, regardless of the mode of delivery, are pain management and wound care.
- Condoms can be used by anyone postpartum.
- Diaphragms and cervical caps need to be refitted at 6 weeks. IUDs are best placed at 6 weeks as well.
- Depo-Provera, Nexplanon, the progesterone-releasing IUD, and the progesterone-only minipill are the hormonal contraceptives of choice in the puerperium, because they are less likely to decrease milk production in breastfeeding patients and affect risk of venous thromboembolism.
- Discharge instructions should include discussion of medical issues, such as contraception and wound care. Instructions to both patient and partner on social issues, such as the transition to home with the newborn, how to deal with some of the changes related to the delivery, and care of the baby, are also needed.
- Causes of PPH include uterine atony, uterine rupture, uterine inversion, retained POCs, placenta accreta, and cervical or vaginal lacerations.
- Treatment of PPH may require use of blood products, including fresh frozen plasma, cryoprecipitate, and platelets in patients who develop a consumptive coagulopathy.
- Surgical management of PPH ranges from D&C to exploratory laparotomy, uterine artery ligation, hypogastric artery ligation, and, if these fail, hysterectomy.
- In PPH patients who are hemodynamically stable, an alternative to exploratory laparotomy is uterine artery embolization by interventional radiology.
- Endometritis is more common in patients with cesarean section than vaginal delivery, although patients with manual removal of the placenta are also at increased risk.
- Diagnosis of endometritis is clinical with fever, elevated WBC count, and uterine tenderness; treatment is with broad-spectrum antibiotics and D&C for retained POCs.
- Cesarean incisions may be complicated by cellulitis, wound abscess, wound separation, or frank dehiscence. Wound healing is improved by blood glucose level control and smoking cessation.
- Mastitis is differentiated from engorgement by focal tenderness, erythema, and edema, and treatment is usually with oral antibiotics. Breastfeeding/pumping is compatible and encouraged in patients with mastitis.
- Changes in appetite, sleep patterns, and energy level are common in the first few weeks postpartum.
- Postpartum depression is common and probably underdiagnosed. In most patients, the depressive symptoms resolve on their own, but occasionally, antidepressants are required.

CLINICAL VIGNETTES

VIGNETTE 1

You are seeing a 20-year-old single G1P1 woman who is postpartum day 2 after a normal spontaneous vaginal delivery of a healthy female infant. Her pregnancy and delivery were uncomplicated. She is notable for being teary and anxious when you begin providing her discharge instructions. She explains that she has been unable to get any sleep between her baby crying, breastfeeding every 3 hours, and her constant worries about whether she will be able to handle a baby at home by herself. She is particularly bothered by pervasive thoughts that her daughter could roll onto her stomach and be unable to breathe or that she could choke while breastfeeding without her mother recognizing it because of her inexperience and sleep deprivation. She is concerned about the overwhelming responsibility of raising a baby by herself, and that she may never be able to go back to school; she expresses that "this may all have been a bad idea." She denies any history of depression.

1. Which of the following is the most important next step in evaluating the patient?

a. Reassure the patient that she is likely experiencing a common condition called "the baby blues"
b. Contact the father of the baby to ensure that the patient will have an alternative source of childcare when she needs to care for herself
c. Offer a prescription sleep aid to help the patient get a full night's rest
d. Prescribe the patient an SSRI for a new diagnosis of postpartum depression
e. Tell the patient that she likely has postpartum depression and should be seen by a counselor while in the hospital

2. The patient sees you again 6 weeks later for her postpartum appointment and still reports difficulty coping with her new baby. She is still having difficulty with sleep but is now unable to stay asleep even when the baby has been sound asleep. She has been avoiding phone calls from her friends because she does not want them to see her in this state. She has a limited appetite, decreased interest in her normal sources of entertainment, and she reports just generally being sad since the baby was born. Although she has taken her baby to the pediatrician as needed and notes interval weight gain, she reports having ignored her crying baby on more than one occasion over the last few weeks. Which of the following is the most important next step in evaluating the patient?
a. Tell the patient that she likely has postpartum depression and should be seen by a counselor as soon as can be arranged
b. Prescribe the patient an SSRI for a new diagnosis of postpartum depression
c. Provide careful reassurance and arrange for follow-up appointment in 2 weeks to assess for resolution of symptoms
d. Contact the Department of Human Services for your concerns regarding child neglect
e. Assess the patient for any current or historical thoughts of harming herself or her baby

3. After extensive counseling, the patient agrees to pharmacologic therapy for her postpartum depression. In which of the following cases would an SSRI not be recommended for her?
a. The patient is currently breastfeeding
b. She reports a family history of bipolar disease
c. The patient is unlikely to be compliant with a daily medication
d. She desires to become pregnant again in the near future
e. She reports having a glass of wine every other day

VIGNETTE 2

A 36-year-old G7P50015 woman has just delivered a 4,500 g female infant at 39 weeks gestation. She underwent induction of labor with oxytocin for severe preeclampsia diagnosed with systolic BPs elevated to 160 mm Hg. Her pregnancy was complicated by uncontrolled gestational diabetes and resultant polyhydramnios. She was placed on magnesium throughout her induction for seizure prophylaxis. She had an epidural placed during the first stage of labor and remained on a normal labor curve throughout. Her second stage of labor lasted 3 1/2 hours; she was, however, able to deliver vaginally with preemptive McRoberts maneuvers and steady traction. The third stage of labor lasted 10 minutes, and the placenta was delivered intact. Immediately after the third stage, her bleeding was significant with the expulsion of blood clots and a fundus that was notable for bogginess.

1. Which of the following are not risk factors for postpartum hemorrhage (PPH)?
a. Advanced maternal age
b. Grand multiparity
c. Prolonged use of oxytocin during labor
d. Polyhydramnios
e. Prolonged exposure to magnesium during labor

2. Which of the following medications would be contraindicated in the treatment of uterine atony in this patient?
a. Methylergonovine (Methergine)
b. Carboprost (Hemabate, PGF$_2$-α)
c. Intramuscular pitocin
d. Misoprostol (PGE1)
e. Calcium gluconate

3. Prompt use of a 250-mcg IM injection of carboprost manages to increase the tone of her uterus and stop the bleeding; however, you continue to notice a steady stream of blood descending from the vagina. What is the most appropriate next step in the evaluation of this patient's bleeding?
a. Perform a bedside ultrasound for retained products of conception (POCs)
b. Perform a bedside ultrasound to look for blood in the abdomen significant for uterine rupture
c. Perform a manual exploration of the uterine fundus and exploration for retained clots or products
d. Examine the perineum and vaginal sulci for tears sustained during delivery
e. Consult interventional radiology for uterine artery embolization

4. The patient was noted to have a third-degree perineal laceration (affected the external anal sphincter) that was repaired in normal standard fashion. Which of the following considerations in

the treatment and counseling of these patients are false?
a. You should provide a rectal examination to ensure that the mucosa is intact
b. She should be on regular stool softeners throughout the postpartum period
c. She should be given narcotic medications for pain control on a PRN basis
d. She should be counseled about her risk of anal sphincter defect and incontinence
e. She should undergo anal endosonography and/or anal manometry in 1 year to evaluate for sphincter defects

5. You are examining the patient's postpartum hematocrit and note a drop in her antepartum measurement from 33% to 24%. Her estimated blood loss from her vaginal delivery and perineal laceration repair was 400 mL. The nurse reports that the patient has had minimal vaginal bleeding overnight. What is the next best step in her evaluation/treatment?
a. Reassurance and offer iron supplementation postpartum
b. Offer a blood transfusion for palliation of symptoms of anemia
c. Request a procedure room for dilation and curettage (D&C) of the uterus
d. Request an abdominal ultrasound for blood in the uterine or abdominal cavity
e. Examine the site of her laceration repair for hematoma

VIGNETTE 3

A 22-year-old G3P1021 woman recently delivered and is now attempting to breastfeed her baby. Her pregnancy and delivery were uncomplicated. She denies any medical history or social history significant for drug use. She is frustrated by her lack of volume, worried that her son will not gain weight, and is now requesting a bottle and prepared formula.

1. Which of the following statements about the benefits of breastfeeding is false?
a. Breastfed children are more resistant to disease and infection early in life than formula-fed children
b. Breastfeeding women have a lower risk of breast, uterine, and ovarian cancer if they have breastfed for at least 2 years cumulatively
c. Children who are breastfed are significantly less likely to become obese later in childhood
d. Oxytocin released during breastfeeding causes the uterus to return to its normal size more quickly
e. None. All of the above are true statements

2. Your patient is convinced of the benefits of breastfeeding and continues to try, successfully breastfeeding by the end of postpartum day 1. The following morning, however, she develops a low-grade fever of 38.0°C, for which your nurse alerts you. She complains about the pain associated with the engorgement of her breasts bilaterally and very sharp, recurrent pelvic pains. Her vital signs are otherwise normal. What is the most likely explanation for these findings?
a. Lactation fever
b. Mastitis
c. Breast abscess
d. Endometritis
e. Chorioamnionitis

3. Which of the following would be an appropriate form of contraception for this breastfeeding patient?
a. Progesterone-eluting intrauterine device (IUD)
b. Combined oral contraceptive pills
c. Contraceptive vaginal rings
d. Contraceptive patch
e. None of the above

4. Your patient is admitted to the hospital 2 weeks later with rigors and chills and complaint of a swollen and reddened right breast. She has been breastfeeding throughout the last 2 weeks. Her vitals are significant for a fever up to 38.4°C and tachycardia with pulse of 112; all other vital signs are normal. Her physical examination is significant for cracked nipples and engorged breasts bilaterally; her right breast is particularly tense, notable for erythema and increased temperature compared with the left breast without masses. What is the appropriate therapy for the above condition?
a. Dicloxacillin 3, 10 to 14 days
b. Dicloxacillin until afebrile for 48 hours
c. Reassurance, ice, breast support, and breast pumping
d. Protective nipple shields and soothing ointments
e. Ultrasound-guided localization of abscess and aspiration

VIGNETTE 4

A 28-year-old G1P1 woman is being discharged from the hospital on postoperative day 4 after having received a primary low transverse cesarean section for breech presentation, with an estimated blood loss of 700 mL. Her pregnancy was otherwise uncomplicated, and her hospital course was also uncomplicated.

1. Which of the following discharge considerations is accurate?
a. She should have her staples removed as an outpatient at 7 to 10 days postpartum
b. She should avoid vaginal intercourse and tub bathing for 1 to 2 weeks
c. She should not lift anything weighing more than 10 lb or the weight of her baby until her postpartum appointment

d. She should be on strict bed rest for the first week following her cesarean section

2. One week after hospital discharge, the patient ends up in the emergency department complaining of severe abdominal pain. Her vitals are significant for a fever of 39°C and tachycardia. Her physical examination reveals acute fundal tenderness beneath a low transverse skin incision that is well-healed, clean, dry, and intact. She received preoperative antibiotics prior to her procedure. Her staples were removed prior to discharge. She endorses residual vaginal bleeding with a slight odor that is confirmed by speculum examination. What is the most appropriate next step in your treatment of this patient?
   a. Wound exploration
   b. Abdominal and pelvic ultrasound
   c. D&C
   d. Outpatient antibiotics
   e. Inpatient antibiotics

3. Two weeks after her cesarean section, the patient presents to you with a chief complaint of serous drainage from a 1-cm area of skin separation. The borders of the skin are mildly painful, but nonerythematous. Which of the following would be the best approach for the described condition?
   a. The patient's skin separation is a result of infection, requiring immediate administration of antibiotics
   b. She is at risk for necrotizing fasciitis. She should be admitted to the hospital and undergo wound debridement and reapproximation
   c. Skin separation at the incision with serous drainage is normal and needs only be managed by application of a bandage
   d. Skin separation should be evaluated further with a probe to examine whether the fascial layer below it is intact
   e. Skin separation should be closed tightly with suture to prevent recurrence

4. The patient sees you at her 6 week postpartum visit and thanks you for your careful attention to her health; however, she is now thinking about the future and worries about her risk of uterine rupture with subsequent pregnancy. What is this patient's risk of uterine rupture with subsequent trial of labor?
   a. 1%
   b. 5%
   c. 10%
   d. 20%
   e. 50%

ANSWERS

VIGNETTE 1 Question 1

1. Answer A:
More than 75% of new mothers experience some degree of emotional disturbance after delivering their babies. Their feelings do not always meet their expectations of how they would feel while pregnant, with many feeling sad, tired, fragile, anxious, isolated, or even regretful. These feelings may sometimes also be manifested as agitation and anger toward their baby or their caregivers. These feelings, however, are normal and are called the postpartum blues, a period of emotional and hormonal lability following childbirth. They begin approximately 2 to 3 days after birth and resolve within 2 weeks without treatment. Postpartum blues can be alleviated through a team approach where family and friends continue to support and reassure the patient once outside the hospital; however, contacting the father of the baby may not be the correct approach without any further information about their relationship or a history of domestic violence or sexual abuse. Although it may seem like most of the patient's concerns may stem from her tiredness, a pharmacologic sleep aid would not ease her anxieties about motherhood.

VIGNETTE 1 Question 2

2. Answer E:
This patient has developed postpartum depression with symptoms persisting and worsening for more than 2 weeks after childbirth. Although she has no history of depression, postpartum depression can and should be treated like a major depressive episode with a combination of psychotherapy and antidepressant medications. There is no consistent evidence that any one class of antidepressant is superior; patients with a history of depression and treatment should be placed back on the medications that they had responded to previously. Prior to treatment, however, it is more important to assess the severity of her current state; any mention of suicide or infanticide needs to be taken seriously and counseled appropriately, with scheduling of close follow-up. Although it is concerning that the patient has ignored her baby, we can be reassured that the baby has been taken to the pediatrician and has good interval weight gain, indicating that the neglect may not be pervasive and persistent.

VIGNETTE 1 Question 3
3. Answer B:
A number of studies have shown benefit with the use of SSRIs to treat postpartum depression, including sertraline, paroxetine, venlafaxine, and fluvoxamine. SSRIs are generally well tolerated and have a low side-effect profile compared with other antidepressants available. Sertraline is most often recommended for breastfeeding mothers. Although psychotropic medications pass through the breast milk, studies have shown that they are not subsequently detected in infant serum at appreciable levels. Paroxetine should not be prescribed if a woman is planning on becoming pregnant again, because it has been associated with congenital heart defects and persistent pulmonary hypertension. Other SSRIs, however, have been found to be safe in pregnancy and can be prescribed as needed. Monoamine Oxidase Inhibitors (MAOIs) should not be taken while drinking alcohol because of the risk of serotonin syndrome; this, however, does not apply to SSRIs. As family history is one of the strongest predictors of bipolar disorder, it is possible that the use of an antidepressant could trigger mania in a yet undiagnosed, underlying bipolar disorder. In these cases, a mood stabilizer would be the best treatment.

VIGNETTE 2 Question 1
1. Answer A:
PPH in the context of vaginal delivery is defined as an estimated blood loss greater than 500 mL. Most of all PPHs results from uterine atony, the failure of uterine muscles to contract normally after the second and third stages of labor. Without muscular contraction, severed vessels of the placental bed will continue to bleed. Any factor that might cause uterine muscle exhaustion or distend and distort the muscle can cause atony. These factors allow prediction of PPH and preparation of uterotonic medications prior to delivery. Advanced maternal age is not associated with PPH, although it can be associated with multiparity and the development of preeclampsia requiring magnesium.

VIGNETTE 2 Question 2
2. Answer A:
Methylergonovine should **not** be used to treat her atony, because it works by causing systemic vasoconstriction, which would increase her BP even further than it may already be elevated by her preeclampsia. Carboprost, Pitocin, and misoprostol would be suitable options. Carboprost is contraindicated in patients with asthma because the prostaglandin is a bronchoconstrictor. Calcium gluconate may be able to reverse the effects of magnesium, thereby allowing the uterus to better contract; however, it is indicated only in life-threatening cases of hypermagnesemia and, in the setting of preeclampsia, would leave the patient without any seizure prophylaxis.

VIGNETTE 2 Question 3
3. Answer D:
The second most common cause of PPH is genital tract laceration or trauma. Lacerations of the cervix or vagina are common in precipitous deliveries and in deliveries assisted with the vacuum or forceps. Shoulder dystocia can also cause lacerations. In this case, a thorough examination of the vagina should be performed, and if no source is found, a subsequent examination of the cervix would be the correct procedure to evaluate the source of bleeding. Retained POCs or clots would prevent full contraction of the uterus and present as atony. Uterine rupture is rare, especially in women without a history of cesarean. Uterine artery embolization is used infrequently, reserved as a last resort after attempting to stop bleeding by conventional procedures, such as D&C and intrauterine balloon tamponade.

VIGNETTE 2 Question 4
4. Answer E:
Although anal incontinence is one of the reported consequences of vaginal deliveries affected by a third- or fourth-degree laceration and repair, it occurs in women who report having never had a laceration as well. The likelihood of these disorders can depend on the provider's ability to provide a reinforcing repair and the patient's ability to prevent further disruption of the repair with good bowel habits, and such patients are put on round-the-clock stool softeners for 2 to 3 weeks to prevent constipation. Postpartum pain control is important, and nonsteroidal anti-inflammatory drugs (NSAIDs) are first-line treatment option, with opioids being used PRN to prevent associated constipation as well. Routine anal endosonography and manometry are not currently the standard of care for all women affected by deep lacerations.

VIGNETTE 2 Question 5
5. Answer E:
An examination should be performed to rule out either a hematoma from her wound site or an occult hematoma from any blood vessels injured beneath the vaginal mucosa during delivery. Hematomas can often be managed expectantly but should be observed for their enlargement or any increase in tension of the wall of the hematoma. In such cases, the hematoma should be opened, the bleeding vessel ligated, and the vaginal wall closed. A hemogram should be repeated for further drop in hematocrit. Retained products often present with continued vaginal bleeding. Although a blood transfusion may be a part of this patient's ultimate management, it would not be indicated until a source of bleeding has been identified. Reassurance as well should not be given until a source of bleeding has been identified.

VIGNETTE 3 Question 1

1. Answer E:
All of the above responses are reasons to endorse breastfeeding. Breast milk, especially during its initial production (colostrums), is enriched with immunoglobulins that help to protect the infant from disease, such as gastroenteritis, otitis media, and lower respiratory tract infection. Children who are breastfed have a lower likelihood of obesity and even developing type 1 diabetes. In cases of exclusive breastfeeding, women are able to suppress ovulation, believed to thereby decrease the risk of ovarian cancer. The reduction of endogenous estrogen exposure and cycling also contributes to the decreased risk of both breast and endometrial cancers.

VIGNETTE 3 Question 2

2. Answer A:
For the first 24 hours after the initiation of lactation, it is not uncommon for the breasts to become firm, distended, and associated with a rise in temperature. Fevers can be as high as 39°C but rarely do they last for more than 24 hours. They often self-resolve with breastfeeding and pumping and can be treated with a supportive bra, the application of ice, and anti-inflammatory medications. Mastitis and abscesses tend to present unilaterally. The pelvic pain she is having is associated with the release of oxytocin with breastfeeding, causing the uterus to contract. This is normal; nevertheless, infection must always be excluded prior to giving a diagnosis of lactation fever.

VIGNETTE 3 Question 3

3. Answer A:
Any estrogen-containing form of contraception would be contraindicated in a woman attempting to establish breastfeeding. Estrogens have been known to reduce the quantity and quality of breast milk. Estrogen-containing methods may also increase the risk of venous thromboembolism during the first 6 weeks postpartum. Progesterone-only methods, such as the IUD, implant, intramuscular Depo, and progesterone-only contraceptive pills, would be better options. Although the IUD is often not recommended for insertion until after the uterus involutes at 6 weeks postpartum, it can be used in contraceptive-needing patients whose follow-up cannot be guaranteed.

VIGNETTE 3 Question 4

4. Answer A:
The patient has a diagnosis of mastitis, which is caused by infection of the breast most commonly by *Staphylococcus aureus* entering the broken skin sometimes caused by the infant's suckling. Abscess should not be suspected unless an isolated mass is felt in the affected breast that does not resolve with pumping and in cases where the fever is refractory to at least 48 to 72 hours of antibiotics. Treatment is with dicloxacillin to complete a full 10- to 14-day course, even though symptoms may dramatically resolve within 48 hours. Patients should be encouraged to breastfeed through the infection, with counseling on how to improve their baby's latch and avoid further trauma to the nipple.

VIGNETTE 4 Question 1

1. Answer C:
Women who have had a cesarean section will have their staples removed in the hospital, before discharge on postoperative day 3 or 4 as long as they have had a low transverse skin incision. Women who have had a vertical incision will often have to wait to have their staples removed on days 7 to 10. The incision is considered water tight at 48 hours, at which point the patient can shower. Full immersion in a bath should wait, however, until 4 to 6 weeks. Sex should also be delayed for 6 weeks to prevent the introduction of infection from an open cervix and/or continued uterine bleeding. Women who have had a cesarean section are encouraged to walk as soon as possible to decrease their risk of deep vein thrombosis.

VIGNETTE 4 Question 2

2. Answer B:
The patient's presentation is most likely significant for endometritis. Her wound is well-healed and nonerythematous, making a cellulitis unlikely. Were that patient's symptoms to be observed in the hospital during the immediate postoperative period, a simple endometritis could be suspected and treated with antibiotics, with the expectation that involution of the uterus would be sufficient to expel any residual intrauterine contents. In this case, however, the patient continues to have a malodorous discharge that may be significant for retained products that should be evaluated by ultrasound. Failing to perform an ultrasound and performing a D&C without an understanding of expected findings may lead to more vigorous curettage that results in uterine perforation, especially in the setting of a fragile, infected uterine wall. Patients will receive antibiotics after evacuation of uterine contents, which will continue until 48 hours after their last fever.

VIGNETTE 4 Question 3

3. Answer D:
Any skin separation may look innocuous superficially but should be evaluated by a physician to ensure that the fascial layer below it is intact. Any fascial dehiscence could leave the patient prone to the development of a hernia later in life. Skin separation likely stems from the pressurized accumulation of serous fluid in the subcutaneous tissue that ultimately prevents healing. Although the inclination might be to resuture the skin

tightly, doing so would prevent a collection of serous fluid from exiting the wound, thereby leaving a nidus for infection. Given that the patient is not showing any signs of skin erythema, it is unlikely that she has a cellulitis. No prophylactic antibiotics are given for cases of skin separation.

VIGNETTE 4 Question 4
4. Answer A:
Uterine rupture is estimated to occur in 0.5% to 1.0% of patients with prior uterine scars and about 1 in 5,700 to 20,000 women with an unscarred uterus. This risk varies based on a variety of risk factors. For example, the risk appears to be 0.5% or lower in women in spontaneous labor but 1% to 2% in those who are induced. Women with more than one prior cesarean section have an increased risk of subsequent uterine rupture when compared with those with only one. Women with a prior vaginal delivery have a lower risk of uterine rupture when compared with those with no prior vaginal delivery. Additionally, it appears that a two-layered uterine closure is at decreased risk of uterine rupture when compared with a one-layer closure.

PART II GYNECOLOGY

13 | Benign Disorders of the Lower Genital Tract

BENIGN LESIONS OF THE VULVA, VAGINA, AND CERVIX

This chapter encompasses an overview of the many congenital anomalies, epithelial disorders, and benign cysts and tumors of the vulva, vagina, and cervix. Infections of these structures are covered in Chapter 16, and premalignant and malignant lesions are covered in Chapter 27 (vulva and vagina) and Chapter 28 (cervix).

CONGENITAL ANOMALIES OF THE VULVA AND VAGINA

A variety of congenital defects occur in the external genitalia, vagina, and cervix including but not limited to labial fusion, imperforate hymen, transverse vaginal septum, longitudinal vaginal septum, vaginal atresia, and vaginal agenesis. Congenital anomalies of the female genital tract are associated with concomitant anomalies in the upper reproductive tract as well as **anomalies in the genital urinary tract** such as unilateral renal agenesis, pelvic or horseshoe kidneys, or irregularities in the collecting system.

LABIAL FUSION

Labial fusion is associated with **excess androgens**. Most commonly, the etiology is the result of exogenous androgen exposure but may also be due to an enzymatic error leading to increased androgen production. The most common form of enzymatic deficiency is **21-hydroxylase deficiency** (Chapter 23) leading to **congenital adrenal hyperplasia**. This may be phenotypically demonstrated in the neonate with ambiguous genitalia, hyperandrogenism with salt wasting, hypotension, hyperkalemia, and hypoglycemia. The neonates often present in adrenal crisis with salt wasting seen approximately 75% of the time. This autosomal recessive trait occurs in roughly 1 in 40,000 to 50,000 pregnancies. The diagnosis is made by elevated **17α-hydroxyprogesterone** or urine 17-ketosteroid with decreased serum cortisol.

Because cortisol is not being made in the adrenal cortex, the treatment for this disorder is **exogenous cortisol**. The exogenous cortisol then negatively feeds back on the pituitary to decrease the release of adrenocorticotropic hormone, thus inhibiting the stimulation of the adrenal gland that is shunting all steroid precursors into androgens. If salt wasting is documented, a mineralocorticoid (usually fludrocortisone acetate) is also given. Labial fusion and other forms of ambiguous genitalia often require **reconstructive surgery**.

IMPERFORATE HYMEN

The hymen is at the junction between the urogenital sinus and the sinovaginal bulbs (Fig. 13-1). Before birth, the epithelial cells in the central portion of the hymenal membrane degenerate, leaving a thin rim of mucous membrane at the vaginal introitus. This is known as the **hymenal ring**. When this degeneration fails to occur, the hymen remains intact. This is known as an **imperforate hymen**. It occurs in 1 in 1,000 female births. Other congenital abnormalities of the hymen are shown in Figure 13-2. These can result from incomplete degeneration of the central portion of hymen.

An imperforate hymen results in an obstruction to the outflow tract of the reproductive system. This can lead to a buildup of secretions in the vagina behind the hymen (hydrocolpos or mucocolpos) similar to that seen with a transverse vaginal septum (Fig. 13-3). If not identified at birth, an imperforate hymen is often diagnosed at puberty in adolescents who present with **primary amenorrhea** and **cyclic pelvic pain**. These symptoms are due to the accumulation

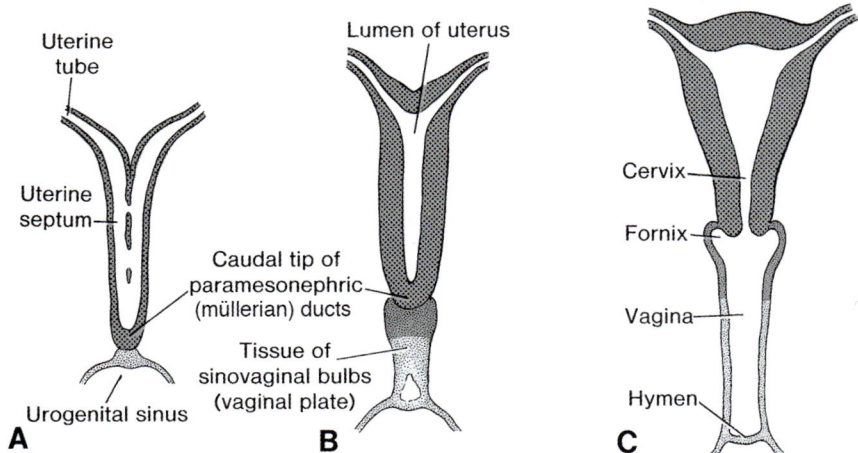

FIGURE 13-1. Embryonic formation of the uterus and vagina. **(A)** 9 weeks. Note the disappearance of the uterine septum. **(B)** At the end of the third month. Note the tissue of the sinovaginal bulbs. **(C)** Newborn. The fornices and the upper portion of the vagina are formed by the vacuolization of the paramesonephric tissue, and the lower portion of the vagina is formed by the vacuolization of the sinovaginal bulbs. (From Sadler T. *Langman's Medical Embryology,* 9th ed. Baltimore, MD: Lippincott Williams & Wilkins; 2003.)

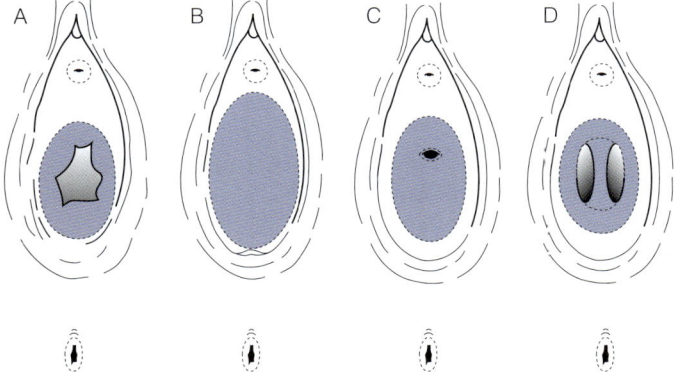

FIGURE 13-2. Congenital abnormalities of the hymen. **(A)** Normal. **(B)** Imperforate. **(C)** Microperforate. **(D)** Septate.

FIGURE 13-3. Transverse vaginal septum.

of menstrual flow behind the hymen in the vagina (hematocolpos) and uterus (hematometra). In these patients, the physical examination may be notable for the absence of an identifiable vaginal lumen, a tense bulging hymen, and possibly increasing lower abdominal girth. Treatment of imperforate hymen and other hymenal abnormalities is with **surgery to excise the extra tissue**, evacuate any obstructed material, and create a normal-sized vaginal opening (Fig. 13-4).

TRANSVERSE VAGINAL SEPTUM

The **upper vagina** is formed as the paramesonephric (Müllerian) ducts elongate and meet in the midline. The internal portion of each duct is canalized and the remaining septum between them dissolves

Chapter 13 / Benign Disorders of the Lower Genital Tract • 217

The vagina is formed as the Müllerian system from above joins the sinovaginal bulb-derived system from below. This takes place at the Müllerian tubercle (Fig. 13-1B). The Müllerian tubercle must be canalized for a normal vagina to form. If this does not occur, the tissue may be left as a **transverse vaginal septum**. These septa often lie near the junction between the lower two-thirds and upper one-third of the vagina (Fig. 13-3) but can be found at various levels in the vagina. This occurs in approximately 1 in 30,000 to 1 in 80,000 women. Similar to the imperforate hymen, diagnosis is usually made at the time of puberty in adolescents who present with **primary amenorrhea** and **cyclic pelvic pain** accompanied by menstrual symptoms. On physical examination, patients typically have normal external female genitalia, and a short vagina that appears to end in a blind pouch. The transverse vaginal septa are usually less than 1 cm thick and may have a central perforation. **Ultrasound and MRI** can be used to characterize the thickness and location of the septum and to confirm the presence of other parts of the reproductive tract. **Surgical correction** is the only form of treatment.

VAGINAL ATRESIA

Vaginal atresia (also known as agenesis of the lower vagina) is often confused with imperforate hymen or transverse vaginal septum. It occurs when the **lower vagina fails to develop** and is replaced by fibrous tissue. The ovaries, uterus, cervix, and upper vagina are all normal. Developmentally, vaginal atresia results when the urogenital sinus fails to contribute the lower portion of the vagina (Fig. 13-1). It presents during adolescence with **primary amenorrhea** and **cyclic pelvic pain**. Physical examination reveals the absence of an introitus and the presence of a **vaginal dimple**. Pelvic imaging with ultrasound and/or MRI may show a large **hematocolpos** and confirm the presence of a normal upper reproductive tract. **Surgical correction** can be achieved by incising the fibrous tissue, and dissecting it until the normal upper vagina is identified. Any accumulated blood or materials can be evacuated, and the normal upper vaginal mucosa is then brought down to the introitus and sutured to the hymenal ring. This is known as a vaginal pull-through procedure.

VAGINAL AGENESIS

Vaginal agenesis, also known as **Mayer–Rokitansky–Küster–Hauser syndrome**, occurs in 1 to 2.5 per 10,000 female births. It is characterized by the congenital **absence of the vagina** (Fig. 13-5) and the

FIGURE 13-4. Imperforate hymen. Note bulging hymen (**A**) and subsequent drainage of obstructed material once the hymenal tissue is excised (**B**). (From Rock J, Johns H. *TeLinde's Operative Gynecology,* 9th ed. Philadelphia, PA: Lippincott Williams & Wilkins; 2003.)

(Fig. 13-1A). The caudal portion of the Müllerian ducts develops into the uterus and upper vagina (Fig. 13-1B and C). The **lower vagina** is formed as the urogenital sinus evaginates to form the sinovaginal bulbs (Fig. 13-1B). These then proliferate to form the vaginal plate. The lumen of the lower vagina is then formed as the central portion of this solid vaginal plate degenerate (Fig. 13-1C). This process is known as canalization or vacuolization.

FIGURE 13-5. Vaginal agenesis is also known as Mayer–Rokitansky–Küster–Hauser syndrome. Notable for congenital absence of the vagina with variable uterine development. (From Emans J, Laufer M, Goldstein DP. *Pediatric & Adolescent Gynecology*, 5th ed. Philadelphia, PA: Lippincott Williams & Wilkins; 2005.)

FIGURE 13-6. McIndoe procedure to make a neovagina. The skin graft is sewn around a mold. (Image from Emans J. *Pediatric & Adolescent Gynecology*, 5th ed. Philadelphia, PA: Lippincott Williams & Wilkins; 2004.)

absence or hypoplasia of all or part of the cervix, uterus, and fallopian tubes. These patients typically have normal external genitalia, normal secondary sexual characteristics (breast development, axillary, and pubic hair), and normal ovarian function. MRKH patients are phenotypically and genotypically female with normal **46,XX karyotypes**. These patients typically present in adolescence with primary amenorrhea. Pelvic imaging with **ultrasound and MRI** can be used to assess the vagina, uterus, ovaries, and kidneys because patients with MRKH will often have **associated urologic and skeletal anomalies**.

Treatment for patients with vaginal agenesis involves a combination of psychosocial support, counseling, nonsurgical, and surgical correction individualized to the patient. In motivated patients, a vagina can be created using **serial vaginal dilators** pressed into the perineal body (Frank and Ingram procedures). This can take 4 months to several years depending on the patient. If this nonsurgical approach fails, a variety of vaginal, laparoscopic, and abdominal procedures are available to create a neovagina. The most commonly used is the **McIndoe procedure**. In this procedure, a split-thickness skin graft is taken from the buttocks and is placed over a silicone mold to create a tube with one closed end (Fig. 13-6). A transverse incision is then made at the vaginal dimple and the fibrous tissue in the location of the normal vagina. The tissue is then dissected to the level of the peritoneum. The mold and graft are inserted into the neovagina. Once the mold is removed, dilators must still be used for several months to maintain vaginal patency. Although normal sexual intercourse is possible after these surgical and nonsurgical procedures, the patient will be unable to carry a pregnancy. She can, however, have her eggs harvested for use with a gestational surrogate.

VULVAR AND VAGINAL DERMATOSES

The nonneoplastic epithelial disorders of the vulva, including lichen sclerosus (LS), lichen planus (LS), lichen simplex chronicus (LSC; eczema and atopic dermatitis), and vulvar psoriasis, were formerly known as the vulvar dystrophies. "Dystrophy" is no longer an acceptable term; in 2006 the International Society for the Study of Vulvovaginal Disease (ISVVD) developed a new nomenclature and classification system for vulvar dermatoses based on the most common histologic patterns seen in these disorders. This classification system allows gynecologists, dermatologists, and pathologists to use a shared terminology for these disorders. These lesions often require **histologic examination** (Table 13-1) to identify and treat the disorder and to differentiate the lesion from vulvar and vaginal intraepithelial neoplasia and cancer (Chapter 27).

Lichen Sclerosus (LS) is an inflammatory dermatosis that can be found on the vulva of women of all age groups, but has major significance in **postmenopausal women**, where it is associated with a 3% to 5% risk of vulvar squamous cell cancer. The etiology is unknown, but it may be autoimmune related with secondary genetic and

TABLE 13-1. Vulvar and Vaginal Dermatoses

	Physical Findings	Symptoms	Treatment Options
Lichen Sclerosus (LS)	White, thinned skin on labia, perineum, and perianal region; resorption of the labia minora into the labia majora, clitoral phimosis, narrowed introitus. Not found in the vagina. Can scar	Often asymptomatic; May report itching, pain, dysuria, dyspareunia; Chronic waxing and waning course	High-potency topical steroid ointment (clobetasol or halobetasol 0.05%) 1–2×/d for 6–12 wk, then a maintenance dosing vs. episodic flare treatment with topical steroid. SQ triamcinolone if refractory. Pelvic floor PT for vaginal dilator therapy.
Lichen Planus (LP)	Bright red erosions with white borders (Wickham's striae) of the inner labia minora and vestibule. Can have narrowed introitus with inflamed vagina from erosions; may have vaginal adhesions or occlusion. LP can be found on vulva, vagina and oral mucous membranes. Can scar	Pruritus with mild inflammation to severe erosions. Can have itching, burning, irritation, painful intercourse	High-potency topical steroids (clobetasol or halobetasol 0.05%) 1–2×/d for 6–12 wk, then maintenance dosing. If prominent erosions, short course of PO prednisone 40 to 60 mg PO. Clobetasol suppositories for vaginal lesions. Pelvic floor physical therapy for vaginal dilator therapy.
LSC (eczema)	Appearance depends on whether patients rubs or scratches. Typically has localized thickening of the vulvar skin or erosions. Typically unilateral. Not found in the vagina. Does not scar	Chronic pruritus	Medium- to high-potency topical steroid 2–3×/d for 6 or more weeks
Vulvar psoriasis	Red moist lesions; often nonspecific with poor margins and slight scaling. May find more classic psoriasis with well-demarcated heavy scaling on the elbows, knees, or scalp	Asymptomatic or sometimes pruritus	Medium-potency topical steroids similar to LSC, UV light. May need ongoing maintenance treatment

LSC, lichen simplex chronicus.

hormonal influences. Classic changes involve white hypopigmented plaques on the vulva, perineum, and perianal areas. The vagina is not affected by LS. The resulting atrophy can cause loss of vulvar architecture including resorption of the labia minora, labial fusion, occlusion of the clitoris, and stenosis of the vaginal introitus (Fig. 13-7). LS is a chronic disorder with a waxing and waning course.

Lichen planus is an uncommon inflammatory skin condition that can affect the nails, scalp, and skin mucosa. Vulvovaginal LP is an erosive disease characterized by red shiny **pruritic papules nondescript erosive** lesions of the vulva, vagina, and/or mouth. It often has white stria or white epithelium similar to LS. Patients may also complain of pruritis, burning, irritation, and painful intercourse. LP is thought to be an **autoimmune, cell-mediated disease** of older women. This inflammatory dermatosis results in chronic eruption of shiny purple papules with white striae on the vulva. Similar lesions are often found on the flexor surfaces, and mucous membrane of the oral cavity. LP can be associated with vaginal adhesions and with erosive vaginitis. It generally occurs in women in their 50s or 60s, and it is associated with a 3% to 5% risk of vulvar skin cancer.

Vulvar psoriasis may be a feature of psoriasis—a very common skin rash that affects up to 2% of the population. There are several different types, but the usual form appears as silvery-red scaly patches over the elbows and knees. Other areas of the skin can be affected including the scalp and nails. Vulvar psoriasis can occur as part of more general disease but in some people, it affects only the vulva. It may present with nonspecific, **poorly demarcated redness** with fine scaling. It may be associated with a **secondary yeast infection**. The etiology is unknown.

FIGURE 13-7. A late case of lichen sclerosis. Note the thin, white, atrophic epithelium, and the labial fusion. (From Rubin E, Farber JL. *Pathology*, 3rd ed. Philadelphia, PA: Lippincott Williams & Wilkins; 1999.)

Lichen simplex chronicus is characterized by thickened skin with accentuated skin markings and excoriations because of **chronic itching and scratching**. This disorder may begin with something that simply rubs, irritates, or scratches the skin, such as clothing. Or, intense pruritis may develop secondary to atopic dermatitis, psoriasis, neuropathic pain, or psychologic disorders. This may cause the person to rub or scratch the affected area. The itching leads to more scratching and can trigger a **scratch–itch cycle**. The constant scratching causes an **inflammatory reaction** with subsequent **skin thicken**ing. The appearance depends on whether the patient rubs the area (lichenfication) or scratches the area (excoriations).

CLINICAL MANIFESTATIONS
History
Patients with vulvar and vaginal dermatoses present with a variety of complaints including vulvar itching, irritation, and burning. They may also report dysuria, dyspareunia, and vulvar pain, and feel that the skin of their vulva is tender, bumpy, irritated, or thickened.

Physical Examination
These disorders range in appearance from erythematous plaques to hyperkeratotic white plaques to erosions and ulcers (Table 13-1). Occasionally, petechiae and/or ecchymoses are present as a result of trauma from scratching.

DIAGNOSTIC EVALUATION
Diagnosis of these disorders may be made clinically. Histologic confirmation with **vulvar biopsy** (Fig. 13-8) is often required for identification purposes and to rule out premalignant and malignant disease. Indications for definite biopsy include ulceration, unifocal lesions, uncertain suspicion of LS, unidentifiable lesions, and lesions or symptoms that recur or persist after conventional therapy. Colpoposcopy and directed biopsy can also be used to evaluate and identify vulvar and vaginal lesions.

DIFFERENTIAL DIAGNOSIS
The differential diagnosis of vulvar and vaginal dermatoses depends on the physical findings. **Erosive disorders** may include LP, pemphigus vulgaris, blistering erythema multiforme. **Ulcerations** may be seen with aphthous ulcers, Behçet syndrome, Crohns disease, erythema multiforme, bullous pemphigoid, and plasma cell vulvitis. Vulvovaginal irritation and **pruritis** may be seen in yeast, folliculitis, trichomoniasis, contact dermatitis, and drug reactions. The differential diagnosis also includes **premalignant and malignant** disease such as vulvar and vaginal intraepithelial neoplasia, squamous cell carcinoma, and Paget disease of the vulva. Biopsies should therefore be performed, whenever there is uncertainty.

TREATMENT
For all of these lesions, healthy **vulvar and vaginal hygiene practices** are recommended. Patients should avoid tight-fitting clothes; pantyhose; panty liners; scented soaps and detergents; bubble baths;

FIGURE 13-8. Vulvar biopsy. (From Beckman CRB, Ling FW, Laube DW, et al. *Obstetrics and Gynecology*, 4th ed. Baltimore, MD: Lippincott Williams & Wilkins; 2002.)

washcloths; and feminine sprays, douches, and powders. Patients should wear loose-fitting cotton underwear and loose-fitting clothing. They should use mild, unscented detergents and soaps such as Dove or Cetaphil, and take morning and evening tub baths without additives.

High-potency topical steroids such as clobetasol can be used to treat LS or LP and severe LSC, and low- to medium-potency steroids should be used for mild cases of dermatosis (Table 13-1). The frequency of use ranges from once per week to one to two times a day. Treatment of LSC and atopic dermatitis is often limited. However, LS and LP are chronic conditions and require **long-term maintenance** with topical steroid application, one to three times per week.

In general, there is no role for topical estrogens or testosterone in the treatment of these disorders; however, low-dose vaginal estrogen is an effective treatment for concomitant **genital urinary syndrome of menopause**. Similarly, surgical management is generally not indicated in treatment of these disorders. An exception is cases of LP, where postinflammatory sequelae can include vaginal adhesions and introital stenosis. Likewise, surgical procedures to enlarge the introitus and open adhesions in LS may be necessary if attempts at intercourse have been unsuccessful following conservative measures.

BENIGN CYSTS AND TUMORS OF THE VULVA AND VAGINA

A variety of cysts and tumors can arise on the vulva and vagina. Cysts can originate from occlusion of pilosebaceous ducts, sebaceous ducts, and apocrine sweat glands. Treatment of benign cystic and solid tumors is needed only if the lesions become symptomatic or infected.

EPIDERMAL INCLUSION CYSTS

Epidermal inclusion cysts are the **most common** tumor found on the vulva. These cysts usually result from occlusion of a pilosebaceous duct or a **blocked hair follicle**. They are lined with squamous epithelium and contain tissue that would normally be exfoliated. These solitary lesions are normally small and asymptomatic; however, if these become superinfected and developed into abscesses, incision and drainage or complete excision is the treatment.

SEBACEOUS CYSTS

When the duct of a sebaceous gland becomes blocked, a sebaceous cyst forms. The normally secreted sebum accumulates in this cyst. Cysts are often multiple and asymptomatic. As with any cyst, these can become superinfected with local flora and require treatment with incision and drainage.

APOCRINE SWEAT GLAND CYSTS

Sweat glands are found throughout the mons pubis and labia majora. They can become occluded and form cysts. **Fox-Fordyce disease** is an infrequently occurring chronic pruritic papular eruption that localizes to areas, where apocrine glands are found. The etiology of Fox-Fordyce disease currently is unknown. **Hidradenitis suppurativa** is a skin disease that most commonly affects areas bearing apocrine sweat glands or sebaceous glands, such as the underarms, breasts, inner thighs, groin, and buttocks. Initial treatment for hidradenitis includes antimicrobial skin washes and antibiotic ointments. As in the axillary region, if these cysts become infected and form multiple abscesses, **excision or incision and drainage** are the treatments of choice. If an overlying cellulitis is present, antibiotics are often used as well.

SKENE'S DUCT CYSTS

Skene's glands, or paraurethral glands, are located bilaterally on either side of the urethral meatus. (Fig. 13-9). Chronic inflammation of the Skene's glands can cause obstruction of the ducts and result in cystic dilation of the glands. When conservative

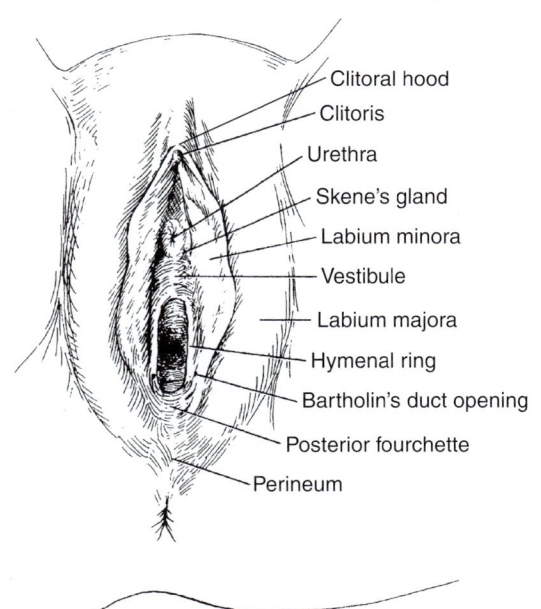

FIGURE 13-9. Vulvar and perineal anatomy. (From Beckman CRB, Ling FW, Laube DW, et al. *Obstetrics and Gynecology*, 4th ed. Baltimore, MD: Lippincott Williams & Wilkins; 2002.)

measures fail, persistent or recurrent paraurethral cysts can be treated with simple marsupialization or excision.

BATHOLIN'S DUCT CYST AND ABSCESS

The Bartholin's glands are located bilaterally at approximately **4-o'clock and 8-o'clock positions** on the posterior–lateral aspect of the vaginal orifice (Fig. 13-9). They are mucus-secreting glands with ducts that open just external to the hymenal ring. Obstruction of these ducts leads to cystic dilation of the Bartholin's duct, whereas the gland itself is unchanged (Fig. 13-10). If the cyst remains small (1 to 2 cm) and is asymptomatic, it can be left untreated and will often resolve on its own or with sitz baths. When a Bartholin's duct cyst first presents in a woman older than 40 years, a biopsy should be performed to rule out the rare possibility of Bartholin's gland carcinoma.

Although many Bartholin's cysts will resolve with minimal treatment, some cysts can become quite large and cause pressure symptoms such as local pain, dyspareunia, and difficulty walking. If these cysts do not resolve, they can become infected and lead to a **Bartholin's gland abscess**. These abscesses are the result of polymicrobial infections, but they are also occasionally associated with sexually transmitted infections. These abscesses can become quite large, causing exquisite pain and tenderness and associated cellulitis. Bartholin's abscesses or symptomatic cysts should be treated like any other abscess: by incision and drainage. However, simple incision and drainage can often lead to recurrence; therefore, one of the two methods can be used.

Word catheter placement is commonly performed in the emergent setting or in the office. This method involves making a small incision (5 mm) to drain and irrigate the cyst or abscess. Then, a Word catheter with a balloon tip is placed inside the remaining cyst and inflated to fill the space (Fig. 13-11). The balloon is left in place for 4 to 6 weeks, being serially reduced in size, while epithelialization of the cyst and tract occurs.

Marsupialization is usually done for recurrent Bartholin's duct cysts or abscesses. The entire abscess or cyst is incised, and the cyst wall is sutured to the vaginal mucosa to prevent reformation of the abscess (Fig. 13-12).

With either treatment, warm sitz baths several times per day are recommended both for pain relief and to decrease healing time. Adjunct antibiotic therapy is only recommended when the drainage is positive for *Neisseria gonorrhoeae*, which occurs approximately 10% of the time. Concomitant cellulitis or an abscess that seems refractory to simple surgical treatment should also be treated with antibiotics that cover skin flora, primarily *Staphylococcus aureus*.

GARTNER'S DUCT CYSTS

Gartner's duct cysts are remnants of the mesonephric ducts of the Wolffian system. They are found most commonly in the **anterior lateral aspects** of the **upper part of the vagina**. Most are asymptomatic. However, patients may present in adolescence with dyspareunia or difficulty inserting a tampon. These cysts are typically **treated by excision**. When the

FIGURE 13-10. Gross appearance of a Bartholin's cyst of the vulva. (From LifeART image copyright © 2006 Lippincott Williams & Wilkins. All rights reserved.)

FIGURE 13-11. Word catheter (**A**) before inflation and (**B**) after inflation. *1.* The balloon-tipped end is placed into the incision site on the Bartholin's cyst. *2.* A small-gauge needle is inserted into the opposite end and 2 to 4 mL of water is injected. *3.* The inflated balloon remains inside the cyst for 4 to 6 week until an epithelialized tract is formed to prevent blockage of the duct to recur.

FIGURE 13-12. Incision, drainage, and marsupialization of a Bartholin's abscess. (From LifeART image copyright © 2006 Lippincott Williams & Wilkins. All rights reserved.)

removal is necessary, an intravenous pyelogram and cystoscopy should be performed preoperatively to locate the position of the bladder and ureters relative to the cyst. Urethral diverticula, ectopic ureters, and vaginal and cervical cancer should be ruled out. Because of the potential for significant bleeding during excision, vasopressin may be used to maintain hemostasis during the procedure.

BENIGN SOLID TUMORS OF THE VULVA AND VAGINA

There are many benign solid tumors of the vulva and the vagina. Some of the most common include lipomas, hemangiomas, and urethral caruncles. Lipomas are soft pedunculated or sessile tumors composed of mature fat cells and fibrous strands. These tumors do not require removal unless they become large and symptomatic. Cherry hemangiomas are elevated soft red papules, also known as Campbell De Morgan spots or senile angiomas; they contain an abnormal proliferation of blood vessels.

Urethral caruncles and urethral prolapse present as small, red, fleshy tumors found at the distal urethral meatus. These occur almost exclusively in postmenopausal women as a result of **genital urinary syndrome of menopause**. This results in formation of an ectropion at the posterior urethral wall. These lesions are usually asymptomatic, and no treatment is required. When bloody spotting results, a short course of **topical estrogen** is appropriate. Rarely, surgical excision may be needed.

BENIGN CERVICAL LESIONS

CONGENITAL ANOMALIES

Isolated congenital anomalies of the cervix are rare. In case of a uterine didelphys with a double vagina, a **double cervix** (bicollis) may be found, but this does not arise in isolation. However, 25% of women who were exposed **in utero to diethylstilbestrol (DES)** have an associated abnormality of the cervix. These benign abnormalities include cervical hypoplasia, cervical collars (Fig. 13-13), cervical hoods, cock's comb cervix, and pseudopolyps. These women are also at increased risk of cervical insufficiency in pregnancy. Women who have been exposed to DES in utero are also at increased risk of a very rare **clear cell adenocarcinoma** of the cervix and vagina. This cancer is seen in young women under the age of 20 but only occurs in 0.1% of DES-exposed patients.

CERVICAL CYSTS

Most cervical cysts are mucus-filled retention cysts called **nabothian cysts** (Fig. 13-14). These are caused by intermittent blockage of an endocervical gland and usually expand to no more than 1 cm in diameter. Nabothian cysts are more commonly found in menstruating women and are usually asymptomatic. Most often, nabothian cysts are discovered on routine gynecologic examination and require no treatment.

Cervical cysts can also be mesonephric cysts. These are remnants of the mesonephric (Wolffian) ducts that can become cystic. These cysts differ from nabothian cysts in that they tend to lie deeper

FIGURE 13-13. Congenital cervical abnormalities due to in utero diethylstilbestrol (DES) exposure. Other characteristic DES-associated cervical anomalies include cervical ectropion, cervical ridges, and hypoplastic cervix. (From Bickley LS, Szilagyi P. *Bates' Guide to Physical Examination and History Taking*, 8th ed. Philadelphia, PA: Lippincott Williams & Wilkins; 2003.)

FIGURE 13-14. Nabothian cysts of the cervix. (From Bickley LS, Szilagyi P. Bates' *Guide to Physical Examination and History Taking,* 8th ed. Philadelphia, PA: Lippincott Williams & Wilkins; 2003.)

in the cervical stroma and on the external surface of the cervix.

Finally, in rare instances, **endometriosis** can implant on or near the cervix. These cysts tend to be red or purple in color, and the patient will often have associated symptoms of endometriosis such as cyclic pelvic pain and dyspareunia.

CERVICAL POLYPS

True cervical polyps are benign growths that may be pedunculated (Fig. 13-15) or sessile (broad based); these can arise anywhere on the cervix and are often asymptomatic. When symptomatic, cervical polyps usually cause **intermenstrual or postcoital spotting** rather than pain. Although cervical polyps are not usually considered a premalignant condition, they are generally removed to decrease the likelihood of masking irregular bleeding from another source such as cervical cancer, fibroids, adenomyosis, endometrial polyps, endometrial-intraepithelial neoplasia, and endometrial cancer. The **removal** of pedunculated cervical polyps is typically quick and easily performed in the office. However, sessile (broad based) polyps or larger polyps may require removal with electrocautery in the office or the operating room. Hysteroscopy may also be helpful in distinguishing cervical polyps from endometrial polyps.

CERVICAL FIBROIDS

Leiomyomas (myomas or fibroids) are common benign tumors of the uterine corpus but may also arise in the cervix or **prolapse into the cervical or vaginal canal** from the endometrial cavity. Cervical leiomyomas can cause symptoms of intermenstrual bleeding similar to both uterine fibroids and cervical polyps. Depending on their location and size, these can also cause dyspareunia and bladder or rectal pressure. Fibroids of the cervix can cause problems in pregnancy and may lead to hemorrhage, poor dilation of the cervix, malpresentation, or obstruction of the birth canal. When evaluating an asymptomatic cervical fibroid, the possibility of cervical cancer should be ruled out, and then the fibroid can be followed with routine gynecologic care. Symptomatic fibroids can be surgically removed but, depending on their location and size, hysterectomy rather than myomectomy may be required.

CERVICAL STENOSIS

Cervical stenosis can be due to congenital anomaly, infection, atrophy, or scarring (from cervical surgical manipulation or radiotherapy). Less frequently, cervical stenosis can result from obstruction with a neoplasm, polyp, or fibroid. Cervical stenosis is typically **asymptomatic** and does not affect menstruation or fertility. In these settings, no treatment is indicated. However, if egress from the uterus is completely or partially blocked, oligomenorrhea, amenorrhea, dysmenorrhea, or an enlarged uterus may result. Cervical stenosis can also impede access to the endocervical and endometrial canals for diagnostic and therapeutic procedures. And, it can result in cervical dystocia during labor. When symptoms are present or access to the endocervical or endometrial canals is needed, cervical stenosis can be treated by **gentle dilation** of the cervix or by performing a cruciate incision over the external os. Prolonged patency can be improved by leaving a catheter in the cervical canal for a few days after the stenosis is relieved. Any obstructive lesions should be removed.

FIGURE 13-15. Cervical polyp. (From Bickley LS, Szilagyi P. *Bates' Guide to Physical Examination and History Taking,* 8th ed. Philadelphia, PA: Lippincott Williams & Wilkins; 2003.)

KEY POINTS

- Labial fusion may be the result of excess androgen exposure or an enzymatic deficiency, most commonly 21-hydroxylase deficiency leading to congenital adrenal hyperplasia and ambiguous external genitalia.
- Patients with imperforate hymen and transverse vaginal septa commonly present with primary amenorrhea at puberty and cyclic abdominal pain. Both can be repaired surgically.
- Vaginal agenesis is seen in patients with MRKH who have an absent vagina and partial uterus and tubes. Patients are genetically female with normal ovarian function and normal secondary sexual characteristics.
- Vulvar itching and lesions can be secondary to a variety of atopic and atrophic skin changes, irritants, and allergens. Lesions can become hypertrophic secondary to chronic irritation and pruritus.
- Diagnosis of vulvar lesions is made by palpation, visualization, magnified vulvoscopy, and biopsy. Cancer should always be excluded by biopsy.
- Treatment involves hygiene practices, avoidance of irritants, and the use of medium- to high-potency topical steroids. There is a limited role for vaginal estrogens and surgery in the treatment of these disorders.
- A variety of cysts can arise on the vulva and vagina from occlusion of pilosebaceous ducts, sebaceous ducts, and apocrine sweat glands.
- Treatment of benign cystic and solid skin tumors is only needed if the lesions become symptomatic or infected. This can generally be achieved with incision and drainage or excision.
- Bartholin's cysts and abscesses are located at 4-o'clock and 8-o'clock positions on the labia majora. Cysts are usually asymptomatic and resolve on their own.
- When a Bartholin's cyst first appears in a woman older than 40 years, the cyst wall should be biopsied to rule out the rare possibility of Bartholin's gland carcinoma.
- Large symptomatic Bartholin's cysts and Bartholin's abscesses should be appropriately drained along with placement of a Word catheter or marsupialization. Antibiotics are generally not indicated.
- Congenital anomalies of the cervix are rare and may be associated with abnormalities of the upper genital tract and/or in utero exposure to DES.
- Cervical polyps and fibroids are typically benign and can be removed if symptomatic.
- Cervical stenosis may be congenital or idiopathic and may result from scarring from infection or surgical manipulation. When symptomatic, the stenosis can be treated with gentle dilation of the cervical canal.

CLINICAL VIGNETTES

VIGNETTE 1

A 26-year-old G0 patient comes in with a problem visit for a complaint of an intermittent painless mass on her vulva near the introitus. It seems to be aggravated by intercourse, but usually goes away on its own. She has had two lifetime sexual partners and has been with her last partner for 5 years. She has always had normal periods and Pap smears, and has never had a sexually transmitted infection. You examine her and find a 3 cm nontender mass in the area described.

1. What type of abnormality is this most likely to be?
    a. Skene's gland cyst
    b. Gartner's duct cyst
    c. Bartholin's duct cyst
    d. Cystocele
    e. Epidermal inclusion cyst

2. What treatment would you recommend for this patient?
    a. Expectant management
    b. Word catheterization
    c. I&D (incision and drainage)
    d. Marsupialization
    e. Excision

3. Two years later she comes in with a recurrent cyst. This time it is tender, red, and growing. She is having difficulty sitting at work, and has

not been able to exercise for 3 days due to pain. She denies fever or chills. What treatment do you recommend?
- a. Expectant management
- b. Word catheterization
- c. I&D
- d. Marsupialization
- e. Excision

4. If this patient had been 46 years old at the first onset of her cyst, what would be required?
- a. Biopsy of the cyst wall
- b. Word catheterization
- c. I&D
- d. Marsupialization
- e. Excision of the cyst

VIGNETTE 2

Your next patient is a 65-year-old G2P2 new patient who has been referred from her primary care provider for recurrent yeast vaginitis. Review of her outside medical records reveals five episodes of vulvar pruritus that were treated with oral and vaginal antifungal medication. The patient says these helped minimally, but her intense pruritus has been persistent for more than a year. She was married for 35 years, but is now widowed and has not been sexually active in 3 years. You examine her and find a thin white atrophic epithelium and a contracted, small introitus. There is loss of the normal architecture of the labia minora. An area of hypopigmentation surrounds the labia and the anus in a figure-of-eight pattern. Wet prep shows a pH of 5.5, rare pseudohyphae, no lactobacilli, no WBC or RBC, and rare clue cells.

1. What would you do next?
   - a. Collect fungal cultures
   - b. Screen for gonorrhea and chlamydia
   - c. Prescribe a longer course of oral fluconazole (Diflucan)
   - d. Check a fasting glucose level
   - e. Perform a vulvar biopsy

2. Most likely the diagnosis is:
   - a. atrophic change
   - b. lichen simplex
   - c. lichen sclerosus
   - d. lichen planus (LP)
   - e. vulvar psoriasis

3. How would you counsel this patient regarding her treatment options?
   - a. Expectant management
   - b. Topical estrogen
   - c. Topical high-potency steroids
   - d. Oral steroids
   - e. Surgical excision

VIGNETTE 3

Although on call you are paged to the emergency department to see a 16-year-old G0 adolescent girl with cyclic pelvic pain. She has never had a menstrual cycle. She denies any history of intercourse. She is afebrile, and her vital signs are stable. Her pregnancy test is negative. On physical examination, she has age-appropriate breast and pubic hair development and normal external genitalia. However, when attempting the pelvic examination, you are unable to locate a vaginal introitus. You obtain a transabdominal ultrasound, which reveals a hematocolpos and hematometra.

1. What is the most likely diagnosis?
   - a. Transverse vaginal septum
   - b. Vertical vaginal septum
   - c. Imperforate hymen
   - d. Vaginal agenesis (Mayer–Rokitansky–Küster–Hauser [MRKH])
   - e. Bicornuate uterus

2. You explain to the patient and her mother that further evaluation is needed. Evaluation would most likely include all except which of the following?
   - a. Intravenous pyelogram (IVP)
   - b. Ultrasound
   - c. MRI
   - d. Removal of streak ovaries
   - e. Karyotyping

3. What are the treatment options for this condition?
   - a. Patient education
   - b. Vaginal dilators
   - c. Creation of a neovagina
   - d. Psychological support
   - e. All of the above

VIGNETTE 4

Your next patient is a 13-year-old adolescent girl who presents with cyclic pelvic pain. She has never had a menstrual cycle. She denies any history of intercourse. She is afebrile, and her vital signs are stable. On physical examination, she has age-appropriate breast and pubic hair development and normal external genitalia. However, you are unable to locate a vaginal introitus. Instead, there is a tense bulge, where the introitus would be expected. You obtain a transabdominal ultrasound, which reveals a hematocolpos and hematometra.

1. What is the most likely diagnosis?
   - a. Transverse vaginal septum
   - b. Longitudinal vaginal septum
   - c. Imperforate hymen
   - d. Vaginal atresia (MRKH)
   - e. Bicornuate uterus

2. Symptoms that support this include:
   a. absent vaginal lumen
   b. tense bulging hymen
   c. cyclic pelvic pain
   d. increasing abdominal girth
   e. all of the above

3. Appropriate treatment option is:
   a. I&D
   b. high-dose steroid application
   c. topical estrogen application
   d. excision of the extra tissue and evacuation of accumulated material
   e. creation of a neovagina when ready for intercourse

ANSWERS

VIGNETTE 1 Question 1
1. Answer C:
This describes the classic location of the Bartholin's glands. These glands, located at 4-o'clock and 8-o'clock positions near the introitus, provide lubrication of the vagina. The ducts of Bartholin's glands can become blocked, resulting in a cyst formation. The Skene's glands can be identified as small openings on either side and just below the urethral meatus. Gartner's duct cysts are remnants of Wolffian system. They are found in the upper one-third of the vagina on the anterior vaginal wall. A cystocele is a prolapse of the bladder into the vagina. It typically appears as a midline protrusion of the anterior vaginal wall into the vagina and, if severe, through the introitus. Cystoceles and other pelvic organ prolapse occur most commonly in older women and in women who have had multiple vaginal deliveries. This patient has neither of those traits. The mass could represent an epidermal inclusion cyst. However, these are the most common causes of cutaneous cysts and are typically small and solitary. They can be asymptomatic or become enlarged or inflamed.

VIGNETTE 1 Question 2
2. Answer A:
In this case, where the cyst is largely asymptomatic, and there is no sign of abscess or superinfection, expectant management is appropriate.

VIGNETTE 1 Question 3
3. Answer B:
Expectant management is appropriate for an asymptomatic Bartholin's duct cysts. However, for a painful, large Bartholin's, a Word catheter is placed to relieve the obstruction. Leaving the Word catheter in place for several weeks gives the new tract time to reepithelialize hopefully resulting in a means of long-term drainage. I&D is insufficient for the management of a symptomatic Bartholin's duct cyst or of an abscess. Marsupialization is typically reserved for patients in whom the Word catheter has failed. Excision of the entire gland is rarely indicated.

VIGNETTE 1 Question 4
4. Answer A:
When a patient over 40 years of age presents with a new onset Bartholin's duct cyst, a biopsy of the cyst wall is necessary to rule out the rare possibility of Bartholin's cyst carcinoma. If benign, treatment would then depend on the status of the cyst. As above, Word catheter is most commonly used. For recurrent symptomatic cysts, marsupialization may be necessary. Excision of the Bartholin's gland is rarely indicated and often complicated by bleeding from the many venous complexes in the vulvar tissue.

VIGNETTE 2 Question 1
1. Answer E:
Although yeast infections are a common cause of vaginitis in women, this patient has been adequately treated for yeast vaginitis, but still has persistent symptoms. Her wet prep does also not support the diagnosis of yeast infection because minimal pseudohyphae are found. Therefore, it would not be reasonable to check fungal futures, prescribe a long course of antifungal, or to check a fasting glucose level to look for diabetes as a reason for recurrent yeast infections. Instead, this patient needs a vulvar biopsy to determine the source of her pruritus. This would be the best way to look for a source of the pruritus and to also rule out vulvar intraepithelial neoplasia and cancer. She has not been sexually active in 3 years, and her primary complaint is vulvar pruritus, so is unlikely to have chlamydial infection or gonorrhea.

VIGNETTE 2 Question 2
2. Answer C:
Although this patient was diagnosed with recurrent yeast infections, it is likely that she was misdiagnosed. The findings noted are consistent with lichen sclerosis. Lichen sclerosis is a chronic and progress benign condition characterized by vulvar inflammation and epithelial thinning. Symptoms include intense pruritus, pain, and anogenital hypopigmentation (whitening—often in a "keyhole" fashion around the perineum and anal

region). When left untreated, it can result in distortion of vulvar architecture (loss of labia minora, constriction of the introitus, fissures, labial fusion, and scarring). Despite its benign nature, vulvar biopsy is still required to rule out underlying atypia or malignancy.

VIGNETTE 2 Question 3
3. Answer C:
The treatment of lichen sclerosis includes patient education, vulvar hygiene, cessation of scratching, and high-potency topical corticosteroid use (e.g., clobetasol). The goal of treatment is to reduce the symptoms (itching, burning, and irritation) and to avoid progression of the disease, which could result in loss of vulvar architecture, introital constriction, labial fusion, and scarring. Of note, the classic whitening or hypopigmentation of the skin, atrophy, and scarring is often permanent and should not be used as a measurement of treatment success. Expectant management is not appropriate because treatment is needed to avoid progression of the disease even in asymptomatic patients. Surgical resection of lichen sclerosis is rarely indicated. Vaginal estrogen is used to treat atrophic vaginitis.

VIGNETTE 3 Question 1
1. Answer D:
Vaginal agenesis, also known as MRKH syndrome, is the congenital absence of the vagina along with some variable uterine development. Transverse vaginal septum is also obstructive, but a normal introitus is usually identifiable. The imperforate hymen typically presents with a tense vaginal bulge at birth or during menarche. A bicornuate uterus is nonobstructing and may be diagnosed only during pregnancy or incidental imaging.

VIGNETTE 3 Question 2
2. Answer D:
In addition to the absence of the vagina, MRKH patients can also have agenesis of the cervix, and most (95%) will have a rudimentary nonfunctioning uterus. Because most (75%) will have normal ovaries, normal female karyotype, and normal ovarian function. Patients typically have normal secondary sex characteristics. Many (25% to 50%) will have associated genitourinary anomalies such as horseshoe kidney, pelvic kidney, duplication of the collecting system, and bladder exstrophy. Evaluation most typically involves a full physical examination, pelvic/abdominal ultrasound, and MRI for better delineation of the anatomy. The genitourinary system can be evaluated with KUB, ultrasound, MRI, and IVP if needed. Streak ovaries are generally found in cases of gonadal dysgenesis (most commonly Turner syndrome) and sometimes in cases of ambiguous genitalia and premature ovarian failure. They are not typically seen in patients with MRKH.

VIGNETTE 3 Question 3
3. Answer E:
Treatment of MRKH is often multifaceted involving gynecologic, urologic, plastics surgery, and psychiatric specialists. When correction is desired, a neovagina can be created using nonsurgical (vaginal dilators) or, least commonly, surgical techniques (vaginoplasty). Psychological support and education are critical components of treatment plans for any congenital malformation.

VIGNETTE 4 Question 1
1. Answer C:
In this young patient with a tense perineum, hematocolpos, and hematometra, the most likely diagnosis is imperforate hymen. MRKH can present similarly, but these patients have a congenitally absent vagina (vaginal atresia); therefore, their clinical presentation does not include a hematocolpos or bulging perineum. A transverse vaginal septum and bicornuate uterus are typically nonobstructing malformations. The blood is able to escape so you do not see a hematocolpos or hematometra. This also explains why these diagnoses are made comparatively later—most typically at the start of pelvic examinations (vaginal septum) or when pregnancy is desired (bicornuate uterus).

VIGNETTE 4 Question 2
2. Answer E:
An imperforate hymen can be diagnosed in the newborn period if the infant is noted to have a bulging introitus. This can develop if maternal estrogen stimulates production of vaginal secretions in the infant resulting in a mucocolpos. If the imperforate hymen is not diagnosed in infancy, the mucus is reabsorbed, and the patient is asymptomatic until menarche. At this time, if the hymen is completely imperforate, blood cannot escape from the upper reproductive system. This can result in all of the signs and symptoms mentioned in the question. Other symptoms can include chronic pelvic pain and primary amenorrhea.

VIGNETTE 4 Question 3
3. Answer D:
The treatment of imperforate hymen is surgical repair under anesthesia. This involves excising the membrane, evacuating the obstructed materials, and suturing the vaginal mucosa to the hymenal ring. This can be performed at any age, but the repair is improved if done when the tissue has been estrogenized—in the newborn, postpubertal, or premenarchal periods. I&D is not an appropriate treatment for an imperforate hymen. Vaginal estrogen would be used to treat **genital urinary syndrome of menopause**. High-potency steroid trials are often given for benign epithelial disorders like lichen sclerosis or LP. Creation of a neovagina is reserved for the cases of vaginal agenesis (MRKH) or agenesis of the lower vagina.

14 | Benign Disorders of the Upper Genital Tract

CONGENITAL MÜLLERIAN ANOMALIES

PATHOGENESIS

All reproductive structures arise from the **müllerian system** except the ovaries (which arise from the genital ridge) and the lower one-third of the vagina (which arises from the urogenital diaphragm). Specifically, the superior vagina, cervix, uterus, and fallopian tubes are formed by fusion of the paramesonephric (müllerian) ducts (see Fig. 13-1). Uterine anomalies arise during embryonic development, generally as a result of incomplete fusion of the ducts, incomplete development of one or both ducts, or degeneration of the ducts (müllerian agenesis). These anomalies (Table 14-1) can vary in scope and severity from the presence of simple septums to bicornuate uterus to complete duplication of the entire female reproductive system (Fig. 14-1). Of the disorders not related to drugs, the most common condition is the septumste uterus owing to malfusion of the paramesonephric ducts. Many anatomic uterine abnormalities may also be associated with inguinal hernias and urinary tract anomalies (unilateral renal agenesis, pelvic or horseshoe kidneys, or irregularities in the collecting system) (Fig. 14-2).

EPIDEMIOLOGY

Anatomic anomalies of the uterus are extremely rare. Several years ago, the incidence was estimated to be 0.5% (1 in 201) of the female population. There is an increased incidence of müllerian anomalies in women who were exposed in utero to **diethylstilbestrol (DES)** from 1940 to 1971 (Fig. 14-3). DES was a synthetic nonsteroidal estrogen that was indicated for gonorrheal vaginitis, atrophic vaginitis, menopausal symptoms, postpartum lactation, miscarriage prevention, and for advanced prostate and breast cancer.

CLINICAL MANIFESTATIONS

History

Most congenital anomalies are discovered incidentally in the workup for common obstetric and gynecologic complaints at the onset of menarche, onset of coitus, or attempts at childbearing. Some uterine anomalies are asymptomatic and may never be discovered. Some symptoms associated with anomalies of the uterus include menstrual abnormalities, dysmenorrhea, dyspareunia, cyclic and noncyclic pelvic pain, infertility, and recurrent miscarriage.

TABLE 14-1. Classification of Müllerian Anomalies

Class I. Segmented müllerian agenesis or hypoplasia
A. Vaginal
B. Cervical
C. Fundal
D. Tubal
E. Combined

Class II. Unicornuate uterus
A. With a rudimentary horn
  1. With a communicating endometrial cavity
  2. With a noncommunicating cavity
  3. With no cavity
B. Without any rudimentary horn

Class III. Uterus didelphis

Class IV. Bicornuate uterus
A. Complete to the internal os
B. Partial
C. Arcuate

Class V. Septumste uterus
A. With a complete septum
B. With an incomplete septum

Class VI. Uterus with internal luminal changes

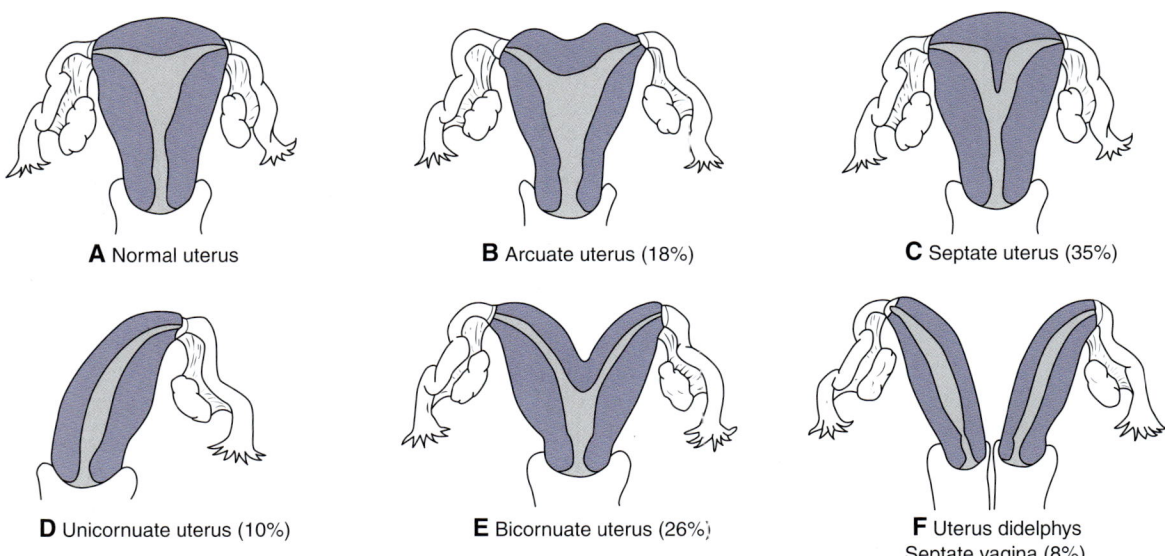

FIGURE 14-1. Examples of anatomic anomalies of the uterus. (**A**) Normal uterus. The most common uterine anomalies include (**B**) arcuate uterus, (**C**) septumste uterus (failure of dissolution of the septum), (**D**) unicornuate uterus (failure of formation of one müllerian duct), (**E**) bicornuate uterus (failure of fusion of the mid-müllerian ducts), and (**F**) uterine didelphys (complete failure of fusion).

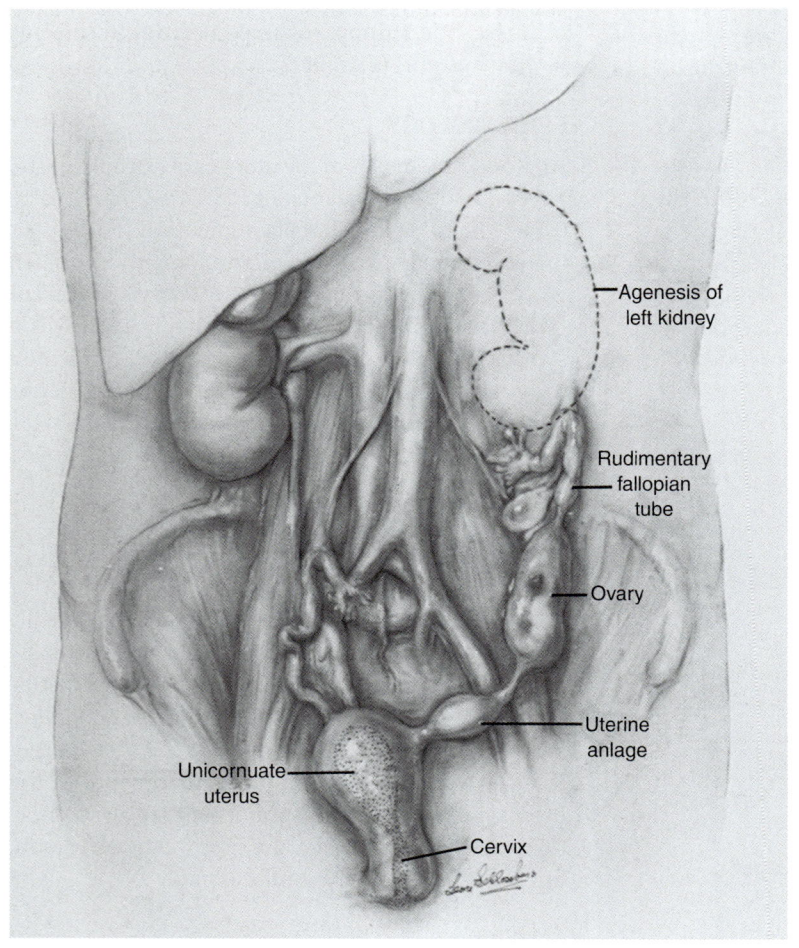

FIGURE 14-2. A congenital uterine anomaly (unicornuate uterus) and associated renal anomaly (agenesis of the kidney on the left). (Image from Rock J, Jones H. *TeLinde's Operative Gynecology*, 10th ed. Philadelphia, PA: Lippincott Williams & Wilkins; 2008.)

FIGURE 14-3. Uterine anomalies associated with in utero diethylstilbestrol (DES) exposure. Others include hypoplastic uterine cavity, shortened upper uterine segment, and transverse septums. The classic anomaly is a T-shaped uterus. (From Speroff L, Fritz M. *Clinical Gynecologic Endocrinology and Infertility,* 7th ed. Philadelphia, PA: Lippincott Williams & Wilkins; 2005.)

Uterine septums are positioned vertically and can vary in length and thickness (Fig. 14-1). They are primarily composed of collagen fibers and often lack an adequate blood supply to facilitate placentation and maintain a growing pregnancy. Thus, 25% of women with uterine septums may suffer from recurrent first-trimester **pregnancy loss**. A **bicornuate uterus** (Fig. 14-1), however, is more commonly complicated by the limited size of the uterine horn (similar to a unicornuate uterus) rather than by blood supply. As such, bicornuate and unicornuate uteri are associated with second-trimester pregnancy loss, malpresentation, intrauterine growth restriction, and **preterm labor and delivery**. Müllerian agenesis or hypoplasia (Mayer–Rokitansky–Küster–Hauser syndrome) results in absence of the vaginal with variable uterine development and presents as primary amenorrhea (Chapter 13).

Diagnostic Evaluation
The primary investigative tools for uterine abnormalities are pelvic ultrasound, computerized tomography (CT), MRI, sonohysterogram, hysterosalpingogram (HSG), hysteroscopy, and laparoscopy. Keep in mind that uterine septums and bicornuate uteri may appear identical on hysteroscopic evaluation (Fig. 14-4). The two can be better distinguished using **MRI or laparoscopy** to evaluate the uterine fundus. Because there is an increased incidence of **renal anomalies** (unilateral renal agenesis, pelvic or horseshoe kidneys, or irregularities in the collecting system), additional radiologic evaluation of the renal anatomy should be pursued when congenital mullerian anomalies are found.

Treatment
Many uterine anomalies require no treatment. However, when the defect causes significant symptoms such as pain, menstrual irregularities, or infertility, treatment options should be explored. Uterine septums can be excised with **operative hysteroscopy**, once bicornuate uterus has been ruled out. Many women with a bicornuate uterus are able to carry a pregnancy to fruition, although preterm labor and delivery is a significant risk. When a viable pregnancy cannot be achieved in a patient with a bicornuate uterus, viable pregnancies have been achieved with surgical unification procedures. These patients will require delivery via cesarean section to decrease the risk of uterine rupture.

UTERINE LEIOMYOMA

Uterine leiomyomas, also called *fibroids* or *uterine myomas*, are benign proliferations of smooth muscle cells of the myometrium. Fibroids typically occur in women of childbearing age and then regress during menopause. These benign tumors constitute the most common indication for surgery for women in the United States. Approximately one-third of all

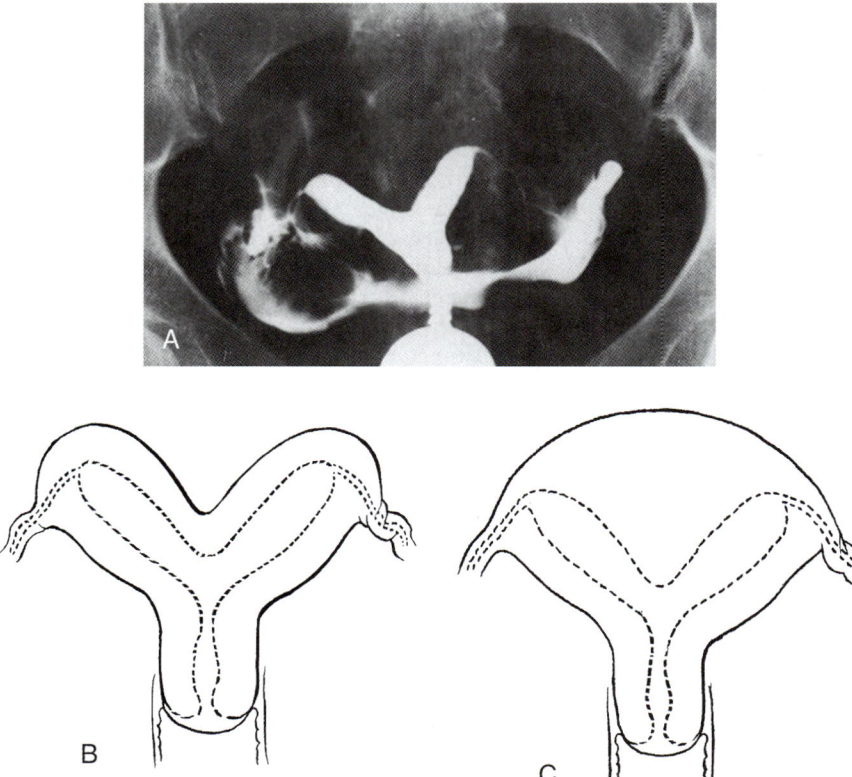

FIGURE 14-4. (**A**) A hysterosalpingogram of a double uterus. (**B**) A bicornuate uterus and (**C**) a septumste uterus are types of double uteri. Visualization of the fundus is required to determine the type of uterine anomaly. (Image from Rock J, Jones H. *TeLinde's Operative Gynecology*, 10th ed. Philadelphia, PA: Lippincott Williams & Wilkins; 2008.)

hysterectomies performed are for uterine fibroids. Most fibroids, however, cause no major symptoms and require no treatment. Generally, fibroids become problematic only when their location results in heavy or irregular bleeding or reproductive difficulties. Fibroids may also be identified, when they become large enough to cause a mass effect on other pelvic structures resulting in pelvic pain and pressure, urinary frequency, or constipation.

PATHOGENESIS

The cause of uterine leiomyomas is unclear. Fibroids are **benign monoclonal tumors**, with each tumor resulting from propagation of a single muscle cell. The normal myocytes are transformed to abnormal myocytes, which are then stimulated to grow into tumors. Genetic predisposition, steroid hormone factors, growth factors, and angiogenesis may all play a role in the formation and growth of uterine fibroids.

Fibroids can vary in size from microscopic to the size of a full-term pregnancy. Fibroids are also hormonally responsive to both estrogen and progesterone, but the relationship is complex. In reproductive-age women, individual fibroids can grow and shrink at differing rates in the same woman. During menopause, the tumors usually stop growing and may atrophy in response to naturally lower endogenous estrogen levels.

Uterine fibroids are classified by their location in the uterus (Fig. 14-5). The typical classification includes **submucosal** (beneath the endometrium), **intramural** (in the muscular wall of the uterus), and **subserosal** (beneath the uterine serosa). Intramural leiomyomas are the most common type, and submucosal fibroids are commonly associated with **heavy or prolonged bleeding**. Both submucosal and subserosal fibroids may become pedunculated. A parasitic leiomyoma is a pedunculated fibroid that becomes attached to the pelvic viscera or omentum and develops its own blood supply.

Fibroids contain a large quantity of extracellular matrix (fibronectin, collagen, and proteoglycan) and are surrounded by a **pseudocapsule** of compressed areolar tissue and smooth muscle cells. This pseudocapsule contains very few blood

FIGURE 14-5. Common locations of uterine fibroids.

vessels and lymphatic vessels. This pseudocapsule distinguishes fibroids from adenomyosis, which tends to be more diffusely organized in the myometrium (see Chapter 15). As leiomyomas enlarge, they can outgrow their blood supply, infarct, and degenerate, causing pain.

It is unclear whether fibroids have any malignant potential. From the available evidence, it is thought that benign leiomyomas and leiomyosarcomas can coexist in the same uterus but with rare exception, they are independent entities. Leiomyosarcomas are thought to represent separate new neoplasias rather than malignant transformation of an existing benign fibroid.

EPIDEMIOLOGY

The lifetime risk of fibroids is 70% in Caucasian women. Greater than 80% of African American women will develop leiomyoma by age 50. African American women are more likely to be younger at the time of diagnosis, have larger fibroids and a greater number of fibroids, heavier bleeding, and more severe anemia.

RISK FACTORS

Uterine fibroids are more commonly associated with **African American heritage**, nonsmoking, early menarche, nulliparity, perimenopause, increased alcohol use, and hypertension. Generally, low-dose oral contraceptive pills (OCPs) are protective against the development of new fibroids but may stimulate existing fibroids. The exception to this may be in women who start OCPs between the ages of 13 and 16. The use of hormone replacement in postmenopausal women with fibroids is associated with fibroid growth but typically does not result in clinical symptoms. The risk of fibroids decreases with increasing parity, with oral contraception use, and injectable depot-medroxyprogesterone acetate use.

CLINICAL MANIFESTATIONS
History

Most women with fibroids (50% to 65%) have no clinical symptoms. Of those who do (Table 14-2), **abnormal uterine bleeding** is by far the most common symptom. This is due most commonly to submucosal

TABLE 14-2.	Clinical Symptoms of Uterine Leiomyomas (Mnemonic: FIBROIDS)
F: Frequency and retention of urine, hydronephrosis	
I: Iron-deficiency anemia	
B: Bleeding abnormalities (menorrhagia, metrorrhagia, menometrorrhagia, postcoital spotting), bloating	
R: Reproductive difficulties (dysfunctional labor premature labor/delivery, fetal malpresentation, increased need for cesarean delivery)	
O: Obstipation and rectal pressure	
I: Infertility (failed implantation, spontaneous abortion)	
D: Dysmenorrhea, dyspareunia	
S: Symptomless (most common)	

fibroids impinging on the endometrial cavity (Fig. 14-5). The abnormal bleeding typically presents as increasingly heavy periods of longer duration (formerly menorrhagia). Fibroids can also cause spotting after intercourse (postcoital spotting), bleeding between periods (formerly metrorrhagia), or heavy irregular bleeding (formerly menometrorrhagia). Blood loss from fibroids can lead to **chronic iron-deficiency anemia**, dizziness, weakness, and fatigue.

In general, **pelvic pain** is not usually part of the symptom complex, unless vascular compromise is present. This is most common in subserosal pedunculated fibroids. Patients may, however, experience secondary **dysmenorrhea** with menses, particularly when heavy and/or prolonged bleeding are present. Pressure-related symptoms (pelvic pressure, constipation, hydronephrosis, and venous stasis) vary depending on the number, size, and location of leiomyomas. If a fibroid impinges on nearby structures, patients may complain of constipation, urinary frequency, or even urinary retention because the space within the pelvis becomes more crowded.

Submucosal fibroids can impact implantation, placentation, and ongoing pregnancy. Resection of submucosal fibroids in patients diagnosed with infertility does lead to increased conception rates. Intramural and subserosal fibroids are unlikely to affect conception or pregnancy loss, except when multiple fibroids are present. The vast majority of women with fibroids, however, are **able to conceive without any difficulties**. When fibroids are multiple, large (5 to 10 cm), or located behind the placenta, they may contribute to increased rates of preterm labor and delivery, fetal malpresentation, dysfunctional labor, and cesarean delivery. The antepartum and intrapartum complication rate is 10% to 40%.

Physical Examination

Depending on their location and size, uterine leiomyomas can sometimes be **palpated on bimanual pelvic examination** or on abdominal examination. Bimanual examination often reveals a nontender irregularly enlarged uterus with "lumpy-bumpy" or cobblestone protrusions that feel firm or solid on palpation.

DIAGNOSTIC EVALUATION

The differential diagnosis for uterine leiomyoma depends on the patient's symptoms (Table 14-3). Because most women with leiomyomas are asymptomatic, the diagnosis is sometimes made only as an incidental finding.

Pelvic ultrasound is the most common means of diagnosis. Fibroids can be seen as areas of hypoechogenicity among normal myometrial material. HSG, saline infusion sonogram (sonohysterogram), and hysteroscopy are additional tools for imaging the location and size of uterine fibroids. These tools can be valuable in identifying submucosal fibroids and in distinguishing fibroids from polyps within the uterine cavity. MRI is especially helpful in distinguishing fibroids from adenomyosis (Chapter 15) as well as for surgical planning.

TREATMENT

Most cases of uterine fibroids do not require treatment, and **expectant management** is appropriate. However, the diagnosis of leiomyoma must be unequivocal. Other pelvic masses should be ruled out, and the patient with actively growing fibroids should be followed every 6 months to monitor the size and growth.

When leiomyomas result in severe pain, heavy or irregular bleeding, infertility, or pressure symptoms, treatment should be considered. When fibroids show evidence of postmenopausal or extremely rapid growth, surveillance should be initiated, and treatment should be considered. The choice of treatment depends on the patient's age, pregnancy status, desire for future pregnancies, and size and location of the fibroids.

There are multiple medical therapies for the symptoms of leiomyomas (Table 14-4). **Nonhormonal options**, which include nonsteroidal anti-inflammatory drugs and antifibrinolytics (tranexamic acid), are limited at treating symptoms of dysmenorrhea, heavy or prolonged bleeding, and anemia.

TABLE 14-3. Differential Diagnosis for Uterine Fibroids

Abnormal bleeding

Structural	Adenomyosis, endometrial polyps, endometrial intraepithelial neoplasia
	Cancer: endometrial cancer, cervical cancer, vaginal cancer
Endocrinopathies	Thyroid disease, hyperprolactinemia, polycystic ovarian syndrome, Cushing disease
Anovulation or oligo-ovulation	Idiopathic, stress, exercise, obesity, rapid weight changes, polycystic ovarian syndrome, or endocrinopathy
Infections	Endometritis, cervicitis, vaginitis
Drugs	Hormonal contraception, progestins, anticoagulants, corticosteroids, psychopharmacologic agents, anticonvulsants digitalis, chemotherapy
Coagulopathies	Thrombocytopenia (due to idiopathic thrombocytopenic purpura, hypersplenism, chronic renal failure), von Willebrand disease, acute leukemia, advanced liver disease
Trauma	Sexual intercourse, sexual abuse, foreign bodies, pelvic trauma

Pelvic mass or uterine enlargement

Gynecologic	Pregnancy, adenomyosis, ovarian cyst, ovarian neoplasm, tubo-ovarian abscess, leiomyosarcoma, uterine cancer, ectopic pregnancy, hydrosalpinx
Abdominal	Peritoneal cyst, ectopic (abdominal) pregnancy, aortic aneurysm
Gastrointestinal	Phlegmon due to ruptured appendix, ruptured diverticulum, bowel malignancy, pancreatic phlegmon
Genitourinary	Urinoma, kidney tumor (including pelvic kidney)

Any of these conditions can coexist with fibroids.

TABLE 14-4. Medical Therapies for Uterine Leiomyomas (Mnemonic: GO PAN AM)

G: GnRH agonists (nafarelin acetate, leuprolide acetate depot, and goserelin acetate)

O: Oral contraceptive pills

P: Progestins (medroxyprogesterone acetate, Mirena IUD, norethindrone acetate)

A: Antifibrinolytics (tranexamic acid)

N: Nonsteroidal anti-inflammatory drugs

A: Androgenic steroids (danazol and gestrinone)

M: Mifepristone (Mifeprex, Korlyn, RU-486)

GnRH, gonadotropin-releasing hormone; IUD, intrauterine device.

Hormonal options include combined OCPs, progestins (medroxyprogesterone acetate, Mirena intrauterine device (IUD), and norethindrone acetate), mifepristone, androgenic steroids (danazol and gestrinone), and gonadotropin-releasing hormone (GnRH) agonists (nafarelin acetate, leuprolide acetate depot, and goserelin acetate). As with the nonhormonal treatment options, the hormonal options are limited to treatment of dysmenorrhea and abnormal bleeding with the exception of GnRH agonists. GnRH agonists have been found to shrink fibroids and decrease bleeding by decreasing circulating estrogen levels. Unfortunately, the tumors usually resume growth after the medications are discontinued. For women nearing menopause, these treatments may be used as a **temporizing measure** until their own endogenous estrogens decrease naturally. Likewise, GnRH agonists may be used to shrink fibroid size, stop bleeding, and increase the hematocrit prior to surgical treatment of uterine fibroids.

Uterine artery embolization (UAE) is being used with greater frequency as a less invasive surgical approach for treating symptomatic fibroids. The procedure is usually performed by an interventional radiologist who catheterizes the femoral artery under local anesthesia in order to inject an embolizing agent into each uterine artery (Fig. 14-6). The goal is to decrease the blood supply to the fibroid, thereby causing ischemic necrosis, degeneration, and reduction in fibroid size. Because the therapy is not specific to a given fibroid, the blood supply to the uterus and/or ovaries can be compromised. UAE should not be used in women who are planning to become pregnant after the procedure. This

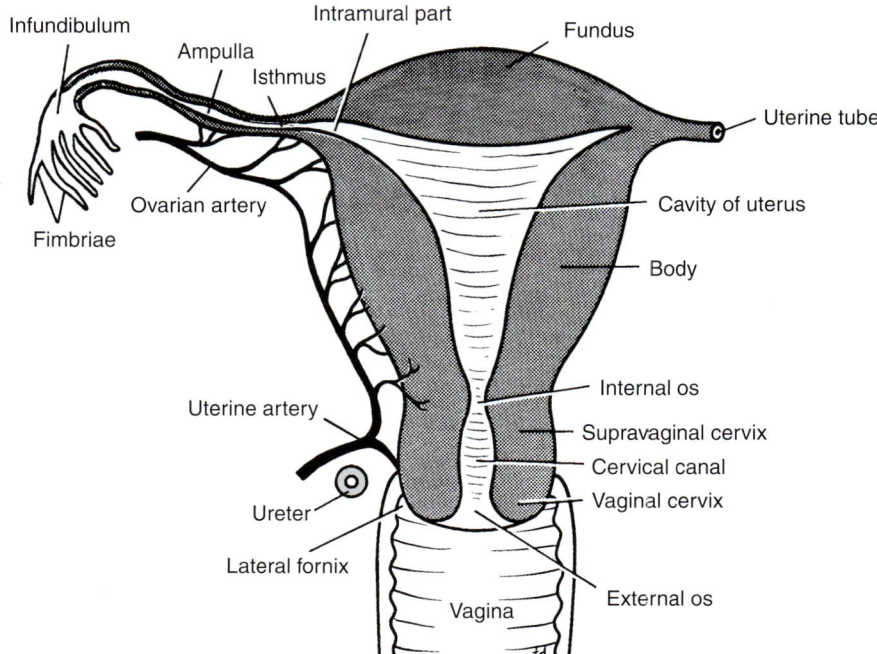

FIGURE 14-6. Uterine artery embolization (UAE) for the treatment of uterine fibroids. The uterine artery, shown here, can be catheterized through a femoral approach under fluoroscopy. The catheter is guided to the uterine artery, where polyvinyl alcohol (PVA) microspheres are injected. As a result, there is decreased blood flow to the fibroids, causing necrosis and devascularization of the fibroids.

treatment option is not recommended for large and pedunculated fibroids.

One of the newest options for uterine fibroids is the use of **Magnetic-Resonance-Guided Focused Ultrasound Surgery (MRgFUS)** (e.g., ExAblate 2100). This uses MRI to locate individual fibroids that are then thermoablated with high-intensity ultrasound waves. The technique is typically reserved for premenopausal women who have completed childbearing and wish to retain their uterus. The procedure can be performed in an outpatient setting, but is expensive and not widely available at this time.

The indications for surgical intervention for fibroids are listed in Table 14-5. A **myomectomy** is the surgical resection of one or more fibroids from the uterine wall. Myomectomy is usually reserved for patients with symptomatic fibroids who wish to preserve their fertility or who choose not to have a hysterectomy. Myomectomies can be performed hysteroscopically, laparoscopically with and without robotic assistance, or abdominally. The primary disadvantage of myomectomy is that fibroids recur in more than 60% of patients in 5 years, and adhesions frequently form that may further complicate pain and infertility.

TABLE 14-5. Indications for Surgical Intervention for Uterine Leiomyomas

Abnormal uterine bleeding, causing anemia
Severe pelvic pain or secondary amenorrhea
Uncertainty if mass is a fibroid or another type of tumor
Urinary frequency, retention, or hydronephrosis
Growth after menopause
Recurrent miscarriage or infertility
Rapid increase in size

Hysterectomy is the definitive treatment for leiomyomas. Vaginal and laparoscopic hysterectomy can be performed for small myomas, and abdominal hysterectomy is generally required for large or multiple myomas. If the ovaries are diseased or if the blood supply has been damaged, then oophorectomy should be performed as well. Otherwise, the ovaries should be preserved in women younger than 65 years with normal-appearing ovaries. Because of the potential for hemorrhage (owing to increased blood supply), surgical intervention should be avoided during pregnancy, although myomectomy or hysterectomy may be necessary at some point after delivery.

Women who undergo minimally invasive myomectomies and hysterectomies that utilize **power morcellation** to remove the specimen have a small risk of spreading an **undiagnosed uterine sarcoma**—including leiomyosarcomas. For this reason, the American College of Obstetricians and Gynecologists (ACOG) issued a special report stressing the importance of patient counseling, informed consent, and preoperative evaluation of patients prior to undergoing procedures utilizing intraperitoneal power morcellation.

FOLLOW-UP

When hysterectomy is not indicated for a patient with fibroids, careful follow-up should take place to monitor the size and location of the tumors. Rapid growth of a tumor in postmenopausal women may be a sign of leiomyosarcoma (extremely rare) or other pelvic neoplasia and should be investigated immediately. Low-dose oral contraceptives and hormone replacement therapy at low doses do not appear to pose a risk of recurrence to the patient.

ENDOMETRIAL POLYPS

PATHOGENESIS

Endometrial polyps are localized benign overgrowths of **endometrial glands and stroma** over a vascular core. These polyps vary in size from millimeters to several centimeters and may be pedunculated or sessile and single or multiple. They are generally within the endometrial cavity but can also prolapse through the endocervical canal into the vagina.

EPIDEMIOLOGY

The incidence increases with age, and they are found most commonly in women 40 to 50 years old. Women taking **tamoxifen** for breast cancer prevention are at risk of developing endometrial polyps, cysts, and cancer.

CLINICAL MANIFESTATIONS
History
Women with endometrial polyps most commonly present with abnormal vaginal bleeding. Premenopausal women can present with bleeding between periods (metrorrhagia) but may also have increasingly heavy menses (menorrhagia), heavy irregular bleeding (menometrorrhagia), or postcoital bleeding. Any bleeding in a postmenopausal woman merits investigation. Endometrial polyps account for a quarter of all causes of **postmenopausal bleeding**.

Diagnostic Evaluation
Pelvic ultrasound, sonohysterogram, and hysteroscopy are the best means of evaluation for the presence, size, and number of polyps, respectively. The added benefit of hysteroscopy is the possibility of immediate treatment. As with any other etiology for abnormal bleeding, women 45 or older with abnormal bleeding from endometrial polyps should be evaluated with **endometrial biopsy** prior to removal.

TREATMENT

Although the majority of polyps are benign, they can be malignant or premalignant in approximately 5% of postmenopausal women and 1% to 2% of premenopausal women. In addition, endometrial polyps can mask bleeding from other sources such as **endometrial intraepithelial neoplasia** (EIN) (25%) or endometrial cancer (<1%). For this reason, it is generally recommended that any polyp be removed in postmenopausal patients. Premenopausal women require the removal of symptomatic polyps and asymptomatic polyps for those at risk of infertility, EIN, and endometrial cancer.

PREMALIGNANT DISEASE OF THE ENDOMETRIUM (ENDOMETRIAL INTRAEPITHELIAL NEOPLASIA)

PATHOGENESIS

Premalignant disease of the endometrium is clinically important owing to its role in abnormal uterine bleeding and the risk for progression to endometrioid adenocarcinoma.

There are currently two systems for classifying premalignant lesions in the endometrium: the World Health Organization 1994 (WHO94) schema and the more recent and preferable International Endometrial Collaboration Group diagnostic schema.

The WHO94 histology schema classifies endometrial hyperplasia based on the **complexity of the glands** of the endometrium and on the presence or absence of **cellular atypia**. It groups endometrial hyperplasia into four groups: simple hyperplasia, complex hyperplasia, simple atypical hyperplasia, and complex atypical hyperplasia (Table 14-6). The groups have a 1%, 3%, 8%, and 29% chance, respectively, of progressing to or having a coexistent endometrial cancer. Unfortunately, this classification system has poor reproducibility and does not account for the difference in malignancy risk of clinical management among the groups.

TABLE 14-6. Classification of Endometrial Intraepithelial Neoplasia and Progression to Endometrial Cancer

Architectural Type	Cytologic Atypia	Progression to Endometrial Cancer (in %)
Simple hyperplasia	Absent	1
Complex hyperplasia	Absent	3
Simple atypical hyperplasia	Present	8
Complex atypical hyperplasia	Present	29

The EIN schema more reliably categorizes the pathologic changes into clinically meaningful and prognostic groups. This system uses three major categories for endometrial disease: **benign** (benign endometrial hyperplasia), **premalignant** (EIN), and **malignant** (endometrial adenocarcinoma carcinoma).

Endometrial proliferation is a normal part of the menstrual cycle that occurs during the follicular (proliferative) estrogen-dominant phase of the cycle. Simple proliferation is an overabundance of histologically normal endometrium. When the endometrium is exposed to **continuous endogenous or exogenous estrogen** stimulation in the absence of progesterone, simple endometrial proliferation can advance to hyperplasia and EIN. This unopposed estrogen stimulation may be from exogenous or endogenous sources. The most common exogenous source is **estrogen hormone replacement without progesterone** in women with a uterus. In obese women, excess adipose tissue results in increased **peripheral conversion** of androgens (androstenedione and testosterone) to estrogens (estrone and estradiol) by aromatase in the adipocytes.

This excess estrogen stimulation can then stimulate overgrowth of the endometrium resulting in benign hyperplasia, EIN, or cancer. The changes do not necessarily involve the entire endometrium, but rather may develop **focal patches** among normal endometrium or **coexistent endometrial carcinoma**. EIN carries a higher risk of progression to endometrial cancer and may have coexistent endometrial cancer as often as 27% to 52% of the time.

EPIDEMIOLOGY

EIN typically occurs in the menopausal or perimenopausal woman, but may also occur in premenopausal women who have chronic anovulation and/or obesity such as those with polycystic ovarian syndrome (PCOS). Most women with complex atypical hyperplasia or endometrial intraepithelial neoplasia (EIN) are either perimenopausal or postmenopausal.

RISK FACTORS

Patients at risk for EIN, like those at risk for endometrial carcinoma, typically have some form of **unopposed estrogen exposure** (Table 14-7). This includes women with obesity, nulliparity, late menopause, and exogenous estrogen use without progesterone. Chronic anovulation, PCOS, and estrogen-producing tumors such as granulosa-theca cell tumors also put women at an increased risk for EIN. Because it has weak estrogenic agonist activity, **tamoxifen** use increases the risk of EIN by stimulating the endometrial lining. Both hypertension and diabetes mellitus are independent risk factors for EIN. Women with Lynch II syndrome (hereditary nonpolyposis colorectal cancer—HNPCC) have more than a 10-fold increased lifetime risk of EIN and cancer.

CLINICAL MANIFESTATIONS
History

Patients with EIN typically present with long periods of **chronic anovulation or amenorrhea** followed by

TABLE 14-7. Risk Factors for Endometrial Intraepithelial Neoplasia (Mnemonic: ENDOMETRIUM)

E: Excess exogenous estrogen use without progesterone
N: Nulliparity
D: Diabetes mellitus
O: Obesity
M: Menstrual irregularity
E: Elevated blood pressure
T: Tamoxifen use
R: Rectal cancer (personal history of hereditary nonpolyposis colorectal cancer)
I: Infertility history
U: Unopposed estrogen
M: Menopause late (>age 55)

irregular or excessive uterine bleeding. Uterine bleeding in a postmenopausal woman should raise suspicion of EIN or carcinoma (Chapter 29) until proven otherwise.

Physical Examination

Occasionally, the uterus will be enlarged from EIN. This is attributed to both the increase in the mass of the endometrium and to the growth of the myometrium in response to continuous estrogen stimulation. More commonly, the **pelvic examination is unremarkable**. Patients may also have stigmata associated with chronic anovulation such as abdominal obesity, acanthosis nigricans, acne, and/or hirsutism.

Diagnostic Evaluation

EIN is most commonly diagnosed as part of an evaluation for abnormal uterine bleeding. After a history and physical examination, imaging with pelvic ultrasound is typically performed. The **pelvic ultrasound** may reveal a diffusely thickened endometrial stripe or focal lesion. However, **tissue diagnosis is required** for the diagnosis of EIN. This would be obtained for any women >45 years old with abnormal uterine bleeding (AUB), and for any postmenopausal woman with recurrent bleeding or with an endometrial stripe ≥4 mm. A woman with AUB who is high risk for endometrial cancer should have an endometrial sampling **regardless of age**. An endometrial biopsy is the first modality for endometrial sampling. However, if the sample is inadequate or cannot be obtained owing to patient discomfort or cervical stenosis, of if a diagnosis of EIN is made, **a hysteroscopy with dilation and curettage** should be performed given the risk for coexistent cancer.

TREATMENT

The treatment of premalignant endometrial disease depends on the histologic class. The goal of treatment is to control abnormal bleeding and to prevent progression of disease. Benign endometrial hyperplasia (simple and complex hyperplasia without atypia) can be treated medically with **progestin therapy**. Progestins reverse benign endometrial hyperplasia by counterbalancing the mitogenic effects of estrogen, activating progesterone receptors to stimulate stromal decidualization and thinning of the endometrium. Standardized schedules and dosing for progestin therapy have not been established.

Typically, **oral medroxyprogesterone acetate** (Provera) or **megestrol acetate** (Megace) is used at doses that will inhibit and eventually reverse benign endometrial hyperplasia. Side effects of progestin therapy can include irregular bleeding, bloating, headaches, irritability, and depression. Micronized vaginal progesterone (Prometrium), levonorgestrel intrauterine system (Mirena), norethindrone (Aygestin), and injectable (Depo-Provera) are alternative treatment modalities. The progestin is usually administered in cyclic or continuous fashion for 3 to 6 months, and then a repeat endometrial biopsy is performed to evaluate for regression of disease. The progestin therapy may be repeated at a higher dose or in concert with a levonorgestrel-containing IUD, if residual disease is found on repeat biopsy. Once the benign endometrial hyperplasia has been treated, preventative therapy should be initiated with regular cyclic or continuous progestin to prevent recurrence.

Hysterectomy is the treatment of choice for women with EIN (atypical endometrial hyperplasia) who are poor surgical candidates or who do not desire future fertility. Although unproven, **oral and intrauterine progestins** have been used with success in this patient population along with serial endometrial sampling. Endometrial ablation, power morcellation, and supracervical hysterectomy should not be used in patients with EIN.

OVARIAN CYSTS AND ADNEXAL MASSES

OVERVIEW

Cystic adnexal masses of the ovaries, fallopian tubes, and surrounding tissues can be gynecologic or nongynecologic in origin and benign or malignant in nature. Factors such as the location of the mass, age and reproductive status of the patient, and family history can help to determine the nature of this common OB/GYN occurrence. Although the majority of adnexal masses are benign, a chief goal is to rule out malignancy. **Postmenopausal women**, women with a **strong family history** of breast and/or ovarian cancer, and women with a **hereditary ovarian cancer syndrome** are at highest risk for an ovarian cancer.

PATHOGENESIS

In general, cystic adnexal masses can be divided into functional cysts and neoplastic growths. Benign and malignant neoplasms of the ovary are discussed in detail in Chapter 30. **Functional cysts** of the ovaries result from normal physiologic functioning of the ovaries (Chapter 20) and are divided into **follicular cysts** and **corpus luteum cysts**.

Follicular cysts are the most common functional cysts. They arise after failure of a follicle to rupture

FIGURE 14-7. Laparoscopic view of a large ovarian cyst. *C*, ovary with cyst; *U*, uterus; *O*, normal ovary. (From Emans J, Laufer M, Goldstein DP. *Pediatric and Adolescent Gynecology,* 5th ed. Philadelphia, PA: Lippincott Williams & Wilkins; 2005.)

during the follicular maturation phase of the menstrual cycle. Functional cysts may vary in size from **3 to 8 cm** and are **classically asymptomatic** and usually unilateral (Fig. 14-7). Large follicular cysts can cause a tender palpable ovarian mass and can lead to **ovarian torsion** when greater than 4 cm and less than 8 cm in size. Most follicular cysts **resolve spontaneously** in 60 to 90 days. Simple cysts smaller than 2.5 cm are typically physiologic.

Corpus luteum cysts are common functional cysts that occur during the luteal phase of the menstrual cycle. Most corpus luteum cysts are formed when the corpus luteum fails to regress after 14 days and becomes enlarged (>3 cm) or hemorrhagic (corpus hemorrhagicum). These cysts can cause a **delay in menstruation** and dull **lower quadrant pain**. Patients with a ruptured corpus luteum cyst can present with acute pain and signs of hemoperitoneum late in the luteal phase.

Theca lutein cysts are large bilateral cysts filled with clear, straw-colored fluid. These ovarian cysts result from stimulation by abnormally high β-human chorionic gonadotropin (e.g., from a molar pregnancy, choriocarcinoma, or ovulation induction therapy).

Endometriomas arise from the growth of ectopic endometrial tissue within the ovary. These cysts are also called "**chocolate cysts**," which comes from the thick brown old blood contained in them. Patients can present with the symptoms of endometriosis such as pelvic pain, dysmenorrhea, dyspareunia, and infertility.

EPIDEMIOLOGY

More than 75% of ovarian masses in women of reproductive age are **functional cysts** and less than 25% are **nonfunctional neoplasms**.

RISK FACTORS

Although functional ovarian cysts can be found in females of any age, they most commonly occur between puberty and menopause. **Women who smoke** have a twofold increase for functional cysts.

The risk of ovarian cancer in the **general population is 1.6%** or 1 in 70. The risk is higher in nulliparous women, women with primary infertility or endometriosis, and in women with early menarche or late menopause. The risk of ovarian cancer increases to 5% in a woman with a **family history of ovarian cancer** in a first degree family member (mother, sister, or daughter). Women who carry the *BRCA1* **mutation** have a 41% to 46% chance of developing ovarian, fallopian tube, or primary peritoneal cancer by age 70. The risk is 10% to 27% in women known to have the *BRCA2* **gene mutation**. Women with **Lynch syndrome** (formerly HNPCC) carry a lifetime ovarian cancer risk of 5% to 10%.

CLINICAL MANIFESTATIONS

History

Patients with functional cysts present with a variety of symptoms depending on the type of cyst. Follicular cysts tend to be **asymptomatic** and only occasionally cause menstrual disturbances such as prolonged intermenstrual intervals or short cycles. Larger follicular cysts can cause achy **pelvic pain, dyspareunia, and ovarian torsion**. Corpus luteum cysts may cause local pelvic pain and either **amenorrhea or delayed menses**. Acute abdominal pain may result from a hemorrhagic corpus luteum cyst, a torsed ovary, or a ruptured follicular cyst. Patients with an infectious etiology may report fever or chills.

A menstrual and sexual history as well of a family and personal history of breast or ovarian cancer and familial cancer syndromes should be elucidated in patients with adnexal masses.

Physical Examination

The initial examination of a patient with a cystic adnexal mass or adnexal pain should include an assessment of vital signs, general appearance, along with an **abdominal and inguinal lymph node examination**. The findings on **bimanual pelvic examination** vary with the type of cyst, but should include an evaluation of the vulva, vagina, cervix, uterus, and adenexa. Follicular cysts tend to be less than 8 cm and simple or unilocular in structure. Lutein cysts are generally larger than follicular cysts and often feel firmer or more solid on palpation. A ruptured cyst can cause pain on palpation, acute abdominal pain, and rebound tenderness. When an ovarian cyst results in a torsed adnexa, the patient may have an acute abdomen, nausea, and vomiting.

Diagnostic Evaluation

Laboratory tests should be guided by the findings on history and physical. A urine or serum **pregnancy test** can rule out normal or abnormal pregnancy, while a **complete blood count** may provide evidence of an infectious or hemorrhagic process. Screening for **gonorrhea and chlamydia and for urinary tract infection** should be obtained as indicated.

The primary imaging tool for the workup for cystic adnexal masses is the **transvaginal pelvic ultrasound**. Ultrasonography allows for better characterization of the cyst that can guide the workup and treatment. Table 14-8 and Chapter 30 review the ultrasound findings associated with benign versus malignant cystic adnexal masses. Benign cystic masses tend to be unilateral, <10 cm, and simple in appearance with thin, smooth walls. Some benign complex masses such as endometriomas and dermoid cysts have classic sonographic appearances. Malignancy is suggested by a complex mass greater than 10 cm with mural irregularities, septations, papillary or solid components, internal blood flow, and/or associated ascites.

Because most functional cysts will spontaneously resolve over 60 to 90 days, serial ultrasounds at that interval may be used to check for cyst resolution. **Computerized tomography (CT) and MRI** are typically reserved for secondary evaluation of concerning abdominal processes, complex masses, and suspected malignancy. These may provide assessment of nearby structures and look for evidence of ascites, lymph node enlargement, and metastatic disease.

A **CA-125 level** is often obtained from patients who are at high risk for ovarian cancer. However, in premenopausal women, CA-125 level can be elevated for a myriad of benign reasons (endometriosis, infection, chronic inflammation, etc.). For this reason, this serum tumor marker should be used solely as a means of evaluating the treatment response to chemotherapy and not as a diagnostic or screening test per the American College of Obstetrics and Gynecology (ACOG) guidelines (see Chapter 30).

TABLE 14-8. Management of a Cystic Adnexal Mass

Age	Type	Size of Cyst (cm)	Management
Premenarchal	Any	>2 cm	Surgical evaluation
Reproductive	Simple	≤5	No follow-up necessary
		>5 and ≤7	Repeat ultrasound in 1 y
		>7	Further imaging or surgical evaluation if change
	Hemorrhagic	≤5	No follow-up necessary
		>5	Repeat ultrasound in 6–12 wk
	Endometrioma	Any	Repeat ultrasound in 6–12 wk. Then if not surgically removed, follow yearly
	Nodule without flow or multiple thin septations	Any	MRI and/or surgical evaluation
Postmenopausal	Simple	<1	No follow-up necessary
		>1 and ≤7	Repeat ultrasound in 1 y
		>7	Further imaging or surgical evaluation
	Hemorrhagic		Early menopause: repeat ultrasound in 6–12 wk
			Late menopause: surgical evaluation
	Nodule without flow or multiple thin septations	Any	Surgical evaluation or MRI

Any cystic mass that contains thick septations, nodules/solid components with abnormal Doppler flow, and cyst wall thickening or has presence of ascites and of omental/peritoneal masses merits surgical evaluation owing to increased suspicion for malignancy. Referral to GYN oncology is appropriate.

This chapter also covers the use of other **serum tumor markers** in the setting of adnexal masses.

DIFFERENTIAL DIAGNOSIS

The differential diagnoses for cystic adnexal masses include ectopic pregnancy, hydrosalpinx, pelvic inflammatory disease, torsed adnexa, tubo-ovarian abscess, endometriomas, dermoid cysts, cystadenomas, pedunculated fibroids, and müllerian anomalies. Urologic and gastrointestinal sources such as ureteral or bladder diverticula, pelvic kidney and diverticular abscess are less common. Metastatic disease from the breast and GI system can also present as adnexal masses.

Treatment

Treatment of cystic adnexal masses depends on the age of the patient and the characteristics of the cyst. Most **follicular cysts** should resolve spontaneously within 60 to 90 days. During this observation period, patients are often started on oral contraceptives. This is not a treatment for existing cysts but rather to suppress ovulation in order to prevent the formation of future cysts.

Although there is no absolute cut off for observation based on ovarian size, nearly all **simple ovarian cysts** are benign and will resolve spontaneously, even those over 10 cm or in postmenopausal women. Given that <1% of simple cysts will be malignant, observation with **periodic ultrasound imaging** is a reasonable approach in the absence of symptoms or major risk factors. The optimal interval and duration of surveillance has not been determined.

Observation is also indicated for **complex masses** that are asymptomatic and presumed benign, such as dermoid cysts, endometriomas, and hydrosalpinx. The same is true for women who are **poor surgical candidates**. Periodic reimaging with ultrasound or MRI may be more appropriate for these patients, where surgical risk is high, and concern for malignancy is low.

Surgical intervention is indicated in patients who are acutely symptomatic with pain, infection, hemorrhage, or torsion. Surgical removal should be performed if a mass under observation becomes symptomatic or shows growth. When possible, **minimally invasive procedures** should be used in order to decrease OR time, length of stay, perioperative morbidity, and recovery time. Similarly, when possible, an attempt should be made to maximize **preservation of ovarian function**.

If malignancy is suspected in a patient with a cystic adnexal mass, referral to a gynecologic oncologist is appropriate.

KEY POINTS

- Anatomic anomalies of the uterus are extremely rare and result from problems in the fusion of the paramesonephric (müllerian) ducts. Therefore, they are often associated with urinary tract and renal anomalies.
- If present, symptoms of uterine anomalies include amenorrhea, dysmenorrhea, cyclic pelvic pain, infertility, recurrent pregnancy loss, and premature labor.
- Anomalies are diagnosed by physical examination, pelvic ultrasound, CT, MRI, HSG, hysteroscopy, and laparoscopy.
- Uterine septums can be treated with surgical excision if symptomatic.
- Fibroids are benign, estrogen-sensitive, smooth muscle tumors of unclear etiology found in >70% of reproductive-age women.
- Fibroid incidence is three to nine times higher in African American women than in Caucasian, Asian, and Hispanic women. The risk is also increased in obese, nonsmoking, and perimenopausal women.
- Fibroids may be submucosal, intramural, or subserosal and can grow to great size, especially during pregnancy. They are asymptomatic in 50% to 65% of patients; when symptomatic, they can cause heavy or prolonged bleeding (most common), pressure, pain, and infertility (rare).
- Fibroids are typically diagnosed by pelvic ultrasound. In most cases, no treatment is necessary. However, abnormal bleeding can be temporized with hormonal contraceptives, progestins, tranexamic acid or GnRH analogs. Myomectomy can be used when future fertility is desired. Endometrial ablation, UAE and MRgFUS may be used when fertility is no longer desired.
- Fibroids are treated definitively by hysterectomy in the case of severe pain, when large or

- multiple, when causing pressure symptoms, or when there is evidence of postmenopausal or rapid growth.
- Pathologic changes in the endometrium are best characterized as benign endometrial hyperplasia, premalignant endometrial intraepithelial neoplasia (EIN), or endometrial adenocarcinoma.
- EIN is caused by prolonged exposure to exogenous or endogenous estrogen in the absence of progesterone. Risk factors include chronic anovulation, obesity, nulliparity, late menopause, and unopposed estrogen use.
- The risk of coexistent malignancy or progression to malignancy in the setting of EIN is 27% to 52%.
- If EIN is diagnosed by endometrial biopsy, a hysteroscopy with endometrial sampling should be done.
- Benign endometrial hyperplasia is usually treated medically with oral or intrauterine progestin therapy for 3 to 6 months, followed by resampling of the endometrium.
- The recommended treatment for atypical complex intraepithelial neoplasia is total hysterectomy. Supracervical hysterectomy, endometrial ablation, and power morcellation should not be used in the setting of EIN or endometrial cancer.
- Follicular cysts result from unruptured follicles. These are usually asymptomatic unless torsion occurs. Management includes observation with or without oral contraceptives to suppress future cyst formation, followed by repeat pelvic ultrasound.
- Corpus luteum cysts result from an enlarged and/or hemorrhagic corpus luteum. These may cause a missed period or dull lower quadrant pain. When ruptured, these cysts can cause acute abdominal pain and intra-abdominal hemorrhage. Corpus luteum cysts should resolve spontaneously or may be suppressed with oral contraceptives if recurrent.
- The differential diagnoses for cystic adnexal masses include ectopic pregnancy, pelvic inflammatory disease, torsed adnexa, tubo-ovarian abscess, endometriosis, fibroids, and ovarian neoplasms.
- Functional ovarian cysts and presumed benign complex cysts will typically resolve in 60 to 90 days.
- Simple ovarian cysts can be observed as long as the patient is low risk, asymptomatic. The same is true for asymptomatic complex cysts, which are presumed benign such as endometriomas, dermoids, and hydrosalpinx.
- Surgical intervention with minimally invasive procedures and optimization of fertility preservation should be used for symptomatic cystic adnexal masses, and those which show active growth or are suggestive of malignancy.
- If ovarian cancer is suspected, patients should be referred to a gynecologic oncologist.

CLINICAL VIGNETTES

VIGNETTE 1

A mother brings her 13-year-old daughter in to see you because she is experiencing cyclic lower abdominal pain every month that lasts for about 4 days. She is also concerned that the patient has not started her period like most of her classmates, and wants to know if you think this is normal. Physical examination reveals Tanner stage 4 breast and pubic hair development. Vaginal examination shows a fenestrated hymen and a small, nulliparous cervix without lesions.

1. All of the following are formed by the paramesonephric ducts *except*:
   a. superior vagina
   b. cervix
   c. ovaries
   d. uterus
   e. fallopian tubes

2. In addition to a detailed evaluation of her uterus, you perform an additional workup knowing that all of the following are commonly associated with uterine anomalies *except*:
   a. Unilateral renal agenesis
   b. Pelvic or horseshoe kidney
   c. Inguinal hernia
   d. Imperforate anus
   e. Ureteral duplication

3. Which of the following is the most common müllerian anomaly?
   a. Bicornuate uterus
   b. Septate uterus
   c. Uterine didelphys
   d. Unicornuate uterus
   e. Arcuate uterus

4. You see another patient following the one previously described. She is a 22-year-old who has been diagnosed with a septate uterus. You counsel her that she is at highest risk for which of the following complications of pregnancy?
   a. Recurrent first-trimester pregnancy loss
   b. Placental abruption
   c. Fetal genitourinary anomalies
   d. Second-trimester fetal loss
   e. Premature rupture of membranes

VIGNETTE 2

A 30-year-old African American G0 woman comes to your office for her annual examination. During the history assessment, she reports increased pelvic pressure, constipation, and progressively heavy and prolonged menses. During menstrual cycles, she is using about 10 large pads per day with her heaviest flow and passing "quarter sized" blood clots.

On physical examination, you palpate a nontender, irregularly enlarged uterus with a lumpy-bumpy, firm contour. Her cervix appears normal, and she has no evidence of ascites or other abnormal physical findings. You suspect that she has uterine fibroids.

1. Which of the following tests is most commonly used for diagnosis of uterine fibroids?
   a. Computerized tomography (CT) scan
   b. Pelvic X-ray
   c. Pelvic ultrasound
   d. MRI
   e. Hysterosalpingogram (HSG)

2. All of the following medical therapies can be used to treat heavy and prolonged menses in women with uterine fibroids *except*:
   a. combined oral contraceptive pills (OCPs)
   b. antifibrinolytic agent (tranexamic acid)
   c. nonsteroidal anti-inflammatory drugs
   d. progestin only pills
   e. opioid agonists

3. Which of the following fibroid locations is most commonly associated with abnormal uterine bleeding?
   a. Submucosal
   b. Intramural
   c. Subserosal
   d. Pedunculated
   e. Parasitic

4. All of the following are risk factors for uterine fibroids *except*:
   a. African American heritage
   b. multiparity
   c. early menarche
   d. perimenopause
   e. hypertension

VIGNETTE 3

A 53-year-old G0 woman comes to your office to report that her menses have returned. She underwent menopause 4 years ago, and had not experienced any bleeding until the last 3 months. She reports several episodes of bleeding. She has a normal Pap smear history and had a normal pap and negative high-risk human papillomavirus screen performed 2 years ago. She has been taking over-the-counter medications and supplements for hot flashes, but cannot recall the names of them. She is in a monogamous relationship with her husband of 20 years. Further history reveals that she has type 2 diabetes and has a lifelong history of oligomenorrhea with heavy or prolonged bleeds, when she does have a cycle. She had a prior laparoscopic cholecystectomy 8 years ago as her only surgical history. Physical examination reveals the following: BP: 150/85 mm Hg; BMI: 48; general characteristics: obese female with moderate acanthosis over posterior neck, inner thighs and inguinal area, moderate hirsutism over chin/neck area; abdomen: well-healed laparoscopic scars; GU: uterus mobile, 9 weeks' sized (mildly enlarged), limited palpation of adnexa due to habitus, overall nontender, without discrete masses.

1. In addition to a thorough physical examination, which of the following is the next best step in evaluation of this patient?
   a. Transvaginal ultrasound
   b. CT scan of pelvis
   c. HSG
   d. Pelvic MRI
   e. Cervical bacterial culture

2. In addition to a complete examination and additional workup as chosen above, which of the following is the next best step in evaluation?
   a. Cystourethroscopy
   b. Endometrial biopsy (EMB)
   c. Colonoscopy
   d. Diagnostic laparoscopy
   e. Serum follicle-stimulating hormone (FSH)

3. You are concerned that she is at high risk for endometrial intraepithelial neoplasia (EIN) or carcinoma. You explain to her the risk factors for EIN include all of the following *except*:
   a. chronic anovulation
   b. obesity

c. multiparity
d. late menopause
e. unopposed estrogen exposure

4. Her pathology returns with evidence of EIN. When you counsel her about the different types of EIN, which histologic type do you tell her has the highest risk of progression to endometrial cancer and the highest rate of coexistent cancer?
   a. Simple endometrial hyperplasia without atypia
   b. Simple endometrial hyperplasia with atypia
   c. Complex endometrial hyperplasia without atypia
   d. Complex endometrial hyperplasia with atypia
   e. Mixed EIN

VIGNETTE 4

An 18-year-old G0 young woman presents to your office for routine gynecologic examination. She reports that her last menstrual period began about 23 days ago. It was light in flow, and lasted 4 days in length. She has minimal dysmenorrhea. She denies any history of sexually transmitted infections, and has been sexually active with two male partners in the last 2 weeks. She was given a prescription for oral contraceptives 3 months ago; however, she has not started taking these. She has no other complaints or medical/surgical history.

During her pelvic examination, you obtain a wet prep, which has normal squamous cells, rare WBCs, and no yeast. On bimanual examination, you palpate a 6 cm nontender left adnexal mass that is mobile. She has no rebound tenderness or guarding.

1. You suspect that she has an ovarian cyst. Which of the following is the most common diagnosis in a patient with this presentation?
   a. Theca lutein cyst
   b. Functional ovarian cyst
   c. Ectopic pregnancy
   d. Tubo-ovarian abscess
   e. Endometrioma

2. You determine that she does indeed have an ovarian cyst on ultrasound. She calls your office 3 days later to report acute onset of sharp left abdominal pain with waxing and waning pain, nausea, and vomiting. An ovarian cyst of which size is concerning for torsion?
   a. 2.5 cm
   b. >1 cm
   c. <4 cm
   d. >4 cm
   e. 3 cm

3. Repeat ultrasound reveals that there is excellent flow to and from the ovary. However, the ovary now has a small amount of free fluid surrounding it. Her pain subsides, and her hematocrit is stable. You diagnose a ruptured hemorrhagic cyst. She and her mother ask about options for preventing further cysts from occurring. You advise:
   a. expectant management
   b. removal of the cyst
   c. removal of the ovary
   d. progesterone-containing intrauterine device (IUD) (Mirena)
   e. combination estrogen and progesterone contraceptive

ANSWERS

VIGNETTE 1 Question 1
1. Answer C:
All reproductive structures arise from the müllerian system except the ovaries (which arise from the genital ridge) and the lower one-third of the vagina (which arises from the urogenital diaphragm). Specifically, the superior vagina, cervix, uterus, and fallopian tubes are formed by fusion of the paramesonephric (müllerian) ducts (see Fig. 13-1). Uterine anomalies are generally a result of incomplete fusion of the ducts during embryologic development, incomplete development of one or both ducts, or degeneration of the ducts (müllerian agenesis).

VIGNETTE 1 Question 2
2. Answer D:
Imperforate anus is commonly associated with other birth defects such as vertebral, cardiovascular, tracheoesophageal fistulae, esophageal atresia, and renal or limb defects (VACTERL). Müllerian anomalies are commonly associated with inguinal hernias or urinary tract anomalies (unilateral renal agenesis, pelvic or horseshoe kidney, and irregularities in the collecting system).

VIGNETTE 1 Question 3
3. Answer B:
Septumste uterus is the most common müllerian anomaly owing to malfusion of the paramesonephric

(müllerian) ducts, and is usually recognized in women presenting during routine evaluation for obstetric or gynecologic reasons. The others listed are less common than septumste uterus. Many uterine anomalies require no treatment, unless there is a concern for significant future pregnancy complication, or if the patient is symptomatic, for example, from bleeding into a noncommunicating uterine horn or nonpatent vaginal septum.

VIGNETTE 1 Question 4
4. Answer A:
Uterine septums can vary in thickness and are composed of collagen fibers and often lack an adequate blood supply to facilitate and support placental growth. For this reason, recurrent pregnancy loss is the most common complication for these patients. Once a pregnancy is successful beyond the first trimester in these women, they usually do not have further complications. Placental abruption, second-trimester fetal loss, and premature rupture of membranes occur more often in patients with bicornuate or unicornuate uteri. Fetal genitourinary anomalies are not associated with isolated maternal müllerian anomalies.

VIGNETTE 2 Question 1
1. Answer C:
Pelvic ultrasound is relatively inexpensive and delineates female pelvic anatomy as well as an MRI. It is the first-line imaging for evaluation of gynecologic conditions and does not require the use of contrast dye for enhanced imaging, such as CT scan. Pelvic X-ray is best used to differentiate calcified components and air fluid levels, but does not outline pelvic anatomy. HSG is similar to a plain film X-ray with added use of intrauterine contrast and fluoroscopy to demonstrate uterine cavity shape and tubal patency (with spill into the peritoneum). This is usually only reserved for workup of infertility or to confirm tubal occlusion following permanent sterilization.

VIGNETTE 2 Question 2
2. Answer E:
Opioid agonists are narcotic medications used to treat pain. These have no role in the treatment of heavy bleeding in women with uterine fibroids. Combined OCPs, antifibrinolytics, and progestin therapy (oral, injectable, or IUD) help to reduce the amount of menstrual bleeding, which can also aid in reduction of pain during menstruation. Nonsteroidal anti-inflammatory drugs reduce levels of prostaglandin, which are produced by the uterus during menses and cause uterine contractions that augment pain from the fibroids. These are commonly used to treat dysmenorrhea associated with menses in women with and without uterine fibroids.

VIGNETTE 2 Question 3
3. Answer A:
Several mechanisms of fibroid-induced menorrhagia have been described. It is well-known that submucosal fibroids can mechanically distort the endometrial lining, prohibiting it from building an organized endometrial layer. Other effects could be related to altered vascular growth owing to expression of angiogenic growth factors by the fibroids themselves. Intramural fibroids involve the myometrial layer of the uterus, and the most common symptom is dysmenorrhea. Subserosal fibroids are on the surface of the uterus and typically are asymptomatic. Parasitic fibroids are pedunculated off of the uterine serosa and grow within the peritoneal cavity. They recruit additional blood supply from nearby organs, but do not directly affect endometrial blood flow. All of the different types of fibroids can cause pressure and pain symptoms if their sizes are significantly increased and result in mass effect in the pelvis.

VIGNETTE 2 Question 4
4. Answer B:
Uterine fibroids are more commonly associated with nulliparity. Other known risk factors include African American heritage, nonsmoking status, early menarche, increased alcohol use, and hypertension. Generally, low-dose OCPs do not cause growth of fibroids, and depot-medroxyprogesterone acetate (Depo-Provera) is protective against fibroid formation. The use of hormone replacement in postmenopausal women with fibroids can be associated with fibroid growth, but typically does not result in clinical symptoms.

VIGNETTE 3 Question 1
1. Answer A:
A transvaginal ultrasound is the initial best imaging test for postmenopausal bleeding. This will discern if there are any uterine leiomyomas, potential masses or polyps, and evaluate the thickness of the endometrium. This has lower specificity in regard to diagnosing polyps when compared with hysteroscopy (direct visualization of the endometrial cavity), but hysteroscopy is more invasive and may need to be performed in the operating room. CT scan and MRI of the pelvis are costly and not used in the initial workup of a postmenopausal female with vaginal bleeding. HSG is used to assess the shape and contour of the endometrial cavity. Radiopaque contrast medium is injected through the cervical canal, and fluoroscopy is used to image the uterine cavity and fallopian tubes. Tubal patency is determined by spillage into the peritoneal cavity. This test will not evaluate the myometrium or endometrial thickness, and is not used for postmenopausal vaginal bleeding. Cervical culture (i.e., gonorrhea, chlamydia testing) is indicated

VIGNETTE 3 Question 2
2. Answer B:
It is prudent that you consider endometrial polyps, intraepithelial neoplasia, and endometrial carcinoma in the differential diagnosis of patients presenting with abnormal menstrual bleeding, including those older than 45 years, but especially in postmenopausal women with any bleeding. EMB is the first-line test for evaluating endometrial pathology. It is up to 95% accurate and should be performed in all postmenopausal women with a thickened endometrial stripe (>4 mm) or with persistent vaginal bleeding. It is performed in the office without the use of anesthesia. A cystourethroscopy will not aid in determination of the cause of her vaginal bleeding at this time because it evaluates the bladder and urethra. Given her age of greater than 50, she does need a colonoscopy for routine colorectal cancer screening; however, this is not used in the initial gynecologic workup for postmenopausal bleeding. Diagnostic laparoscopy is an invasive test and will not help to determine the pathologic nature of her endometrial cavity, which is causing the heavy bleeding. Serum FSH would confirm that this patient is postmenopausal, but would not give information about the endometrial lining.

VIGNETTE 3 Question 3
3. Answer C:
Nulliparity (instead of multiparity) is a known risk factor for EIN. Chronic anovulation, which can be caused by polycystic ovarian syndrome (PCOS) and obesity, allows for unopposed estrogen that causes excess stimulation of the endometrial lining without shedding in a systematic fashion. This can lead to disordered endometrial glandular growth and subsequently EIN or carcinoma. Late menopause has also the same effect as continued estrogen exposure to the endometrial lining. Unopposed estrogen exposure is the underlying cause in the majority of cases of intraepithelial neoplasia and even most endometrial carcinomas. This is seen in various clinical situations, including peripheral conversion of androgens to estrogen by adipocytes in obese women or in women who are taking exogenous estrogen without progesterone to help stabilize the endometrium and prevent overgrowth. This patient has multiple risk factors in her history including chronic anovulation, obesity, and hirsutism—likely PCOS—and is taking an unknown over-the-counter hormone replacement supplement, which could simulate unopposed estrogens in some situations.

VIGNETTE 3 Question 4
4. Answer D:
Atypical complex intraepithelial neoplasia is the most severe form of EIN. It progresses to carcinoma in approximately 30% of untreated cases. The histologic variations of EIN and their rates of progression to cancer are outlined in Table 14-6. Simple and complex refer to glandular crowding of cytologically normal cells, and atypia describes the cytologically abnormal cells in more severe EIN. These cytologic changes include large nuclei with lost polarity, increased nuclear-to-cytoplasmic ratios, prominent nuclei, and irregular clumped chromatin. Simple intraepithelial neoplasia without atypia is the simplest form of intraepithelial neoplasia, less than 1% of these lesions progress to carcinoma. Complex intraepithelial neoplasia without atypia consists of abnormal proliferation of the glandular endometrial elements without proliferation of the stromal elements. The glands are crowded in a back-to-back fashion and are of varying shapes and sizes. Approximately 3% of these lesions progress to carcinoma if left untreated. Simple intraepithelial neoplasia with atypia involves cellular atypia and mitotic figures in addition to glandular crowding and complexity and progresses to carcinoma in about 10% of cases if untreated. As many as 17% to 52% of patients with complex intraepithelial neoplasia with atypia have coexistent cancer at the time of diagnosis. Mixed EIN is not a histologic diagnosis.

VIGNETTE 4 Question 1
1. Answer B:
This patient is asymptomatic. Functional ovarian cysts are classically asymptomatic, unilateral, and arise after failure of a follicle to rupture during the follicular maturation phase of the menstrual cycle. Theca lutein cysts are large bilateral cysts with clear fluid that result from stimulation by abnormally high β-human chorionic gonadotropin. Ectopic pregnancies are often tender to palpation, and her menstrual history suggests that she may not be pregnant with the recent menstrual cycle; however, a pregnancy test is still indicated for this patient who is sexually active and not using any contraception. Implantation or first-trimester bleeding in pregnancy can sometimes be mistaken for a "light" menstrual cycle. Endometriomas are present in patients with endometriosis. Her asymptomatic menstrual history does not suggest endometriosis because she does not report dysmenorrhea. An ultrasound will aid in diagnosis of the cyst appearance and internal components. Tubo-ovarian abscess is present in patients with pelvic inflammatory disease. You would suspect this in someone with abundant WBCs on wet prep, tenderness on examination, or other systemic signs such as abdominal pain or fever.

VIGNETTE 4 Question 2

2. Answer D:
When cysts reach a size of greater than 4 cm, they are at risk for torsion. This is somewhat determined by the contents of the cyst, with mature teratomas having a slightly higher risk of torsion if solid internal components are present to act as a leading edge of the fulcrum for torsion. Acute pain in a gynecologic situation could also be caused by ruptured hemorrhagic corpus luteum cyst, a torsed ovary, or a ruptured follicular cyst. Emergent evaluation of this patient is recommended because she is at risk for ovarian necrosis if torsion is present. It is also important to counsel your patients who have a large ovarian cyst of this risk and to encourage early evaluation if pain arises.

VIGNETTE 4 Question 3

3. Answer E:
Combination estrogen and progesterone contraceptives such as OCPs, the Nuvaring, and the Ortho Evra patch work to prevent formation of future cysts by suppressing ovulation. These medications provide steady estrogen levels (as opposed to the fluctuating levels in a patient who is not on these medications). Therefore, the immature follicles never develop, there is no ovulation, and the probability of a functional cyst is decreased. Women with recurrent ovarian cysts are often placed on combination estrogen–progesterone contraceptives to prevent the formation of new cysts. Of note, these medications do not *treat* current cysts, but *prevent* future cysts by suppressing ovulation. In this clinical setting, expectant management is reasonable but will not help to prevent cyst formation. Surgical removal of the cyst and ovary is much too invasive and is not indicated for a benign functional cyst that is not torsed and is not bleeding. The progesterone-containing IUD (Mirena) has only results in a partial inhibition of follicular cyst formation and ovulation. Therefore, most women (75%) using this contraceptive method can still get functional cysts.

15 | Endometriosis and Adenomyosis

ENDOMETRIOSIS

PATHOGENESIS

Endometriosis is a chronic disease marked by the presence of endometrial tissue **(glands and stroma)** outside the endometrial cavity. Endometrial tissue is most commonly found in the pelvis (the posterior uterus, ovary, broad ligament, the uterosacral ligaments, and fallopian tubes) (Fig. 15-1) but can be found in the bowel, bladder, and diaphragm. Endometriosis in the ovary commonly appears as a cystic collection known as an **endometrioma**. Rarely, endometriosis has been identified as far away as the breast, lung, and brain.

There are several theories about the pathogenesis of endometriosis. They congregate around two main themes: endometriosis implants that arise from ectopic endometrium and implants that arise from tissues separate from the endometrium. The Halban theory proposes that endometrial tissue is transported via the **lymphatic system** to various sites in the pelvis, where it grows ectopically. Meyer proposed that multipotential cells in peritoneal tissue undergo **metaplastic transformation** into functional endometrial tissue. Finally, Sampson suggests that endometrial tissue is transported through the fallopian tubes during **retrograde menstruation**, resulting in intra-abdominal pelvic implants.

There is increasing evidence that women who develop endometriosis may have genetic and epigenetic factors that result in an **altered immune system** that is less likely to recognize and attack ectopic endometrial implants. These women often have an increased concentration of inflammatory cells in the peritoneum that contribute to the growth and stimulation of the endometrial implants (Fig. 15-2). Endometrial implants cause symptoms by disrupting normal tissue, forming adhesions and fibrosis, and causing severe inflammation. Interestingly, **the severity of symptoms does not necessarily correlate with the amount of endometriosis**. Women with widely disseminated endometriosis or a large endometrioma may experience little pain, whereas women with minimal disease in the cul-de-sac may suffer severe chronic pain.

EPIDEMIOLOGY

The estimated prevalence of endometriosis among reproductive age women is approximately 5% to 15%. Because **surgical confirmation** is necessary for the diagnosis of endometriosis, the true prevalence of the disease is unknown. It is found almost exclusively in women of reproductive age and is one of the most common reasons for hospitalization of women in this age group. Approximately 20% of women with **chronic pelvic pain** and 30% to 40% of women with **infertility** have endometriosis.

RISK FACTORS

Nulliparity, early menarche, prolonged menses, and müllerian anomalies are associated with an increased risk of diagnosis with endometriosis. Women with **first-degree relatives** (mother or sisters) with endometriosis have a 7% chance of developing the disorder compared to a 1% chance in women without an affected first-degree relative. A relationship has also been observed between endometriosis and increased rates of some **autoimmune inflammatory disorders** (including lupus and thyroiditis) and certain types of **epithelial ovarian cancers** (clear cell, endometrioid and low-grade serous). For unclear reasons, endometriosis is identified less often in Black and Hispanic women.

CLINICAL MANIFESTATIONS

History

The hallmark of endometriosis is **cyclic pelvic pain** beginning before menses, **peaking 1 to 2 days before**

FIGURE 15-1. Potential sites for endometriosis. The most common sites (indicated by *blue dots*) include the ovaries, the anterior and posterior cul-de-sacs, the uterosacral ligaments, the posterior uterus, and the posterior broad ligaments.

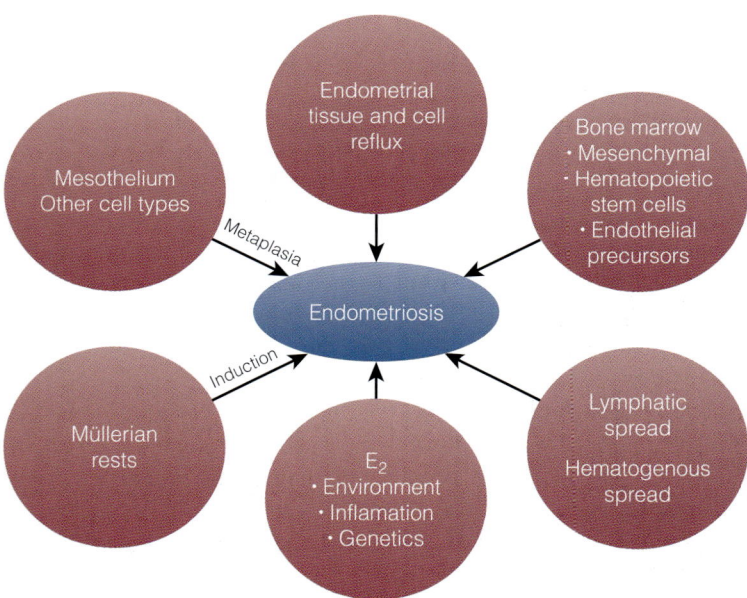

FIGURE 15-2. Theories regarding endometriosis pathogenesis. (Adapted from Burney RO, Giudice LC: Pathogenesis and pathophysiology of endometriosis. *Fertil Steril* 98[3]:511–519, 2012.)

the onset of menses, and subsiding at the onset of menses or shortly thereafter. Women with chronic endometriosis and teenagers with endometriosis may not demonstrate this classic pain pattern. Other symptoms associated with endometriosis are **dysmenorrhea, dyspareunia, abnormal bleeding, bowel and bladder symptoms**, and **subfertility**. Endometriosis is one of the most common diagnoses in the evaluation of infertile couples.

Symptoms of endometriosis vary depending on the anatomic structures involved. Over 75% of women with symptomatic endometriosis will have pelvic pain and/or dysmenorrhea. **Dysmenorrhea** often begins in the second decade, worsens with age, and can progress to chronic pelvic pain. **Dyspareunia** is usually associated with deep penetration that can aggravate endometrial lesions in the cul-de-sac or on the uterosacral ligaments.

Endometriosis is also a cause of **infertility**. Although the exact mechanism is unclear, moderate to severe endometriosis can cause dense adhesions, which can distort the pelvic architecture, interfere with tubal mobility, impair oocyte release, and cause tubal obstruction.

Physical Examination

The physical findings associated with early endometriosis may be **subtle or nonexistent**. To maximize the likelihood of physical findings, the physical examination should be performed during early menses when implants are likely to be largest and most tender. When more disseminated disease is present, the clinician may find **uterosacral nodularity** and tenderness on rectovaginal examination or a **fixed retroverted uterus**. Pain with movement of the uterus can often be seen. When the ovary is involved, a tender, **fixed adnexal mass** may be palpable on bimanual examination or viewed on pelvic ultrasound (Fig. 15-3).

Diagnostic Evaluation

When the clinical impression and initial evaluation are consistent with endometriosis, **empiric medical therapy** is often favored over surgical intervention as a safe approach to management. However, the only way to definitively diagnose endometriosis is through **direct visualization** with laparoscopy or laparotomy. When surgical intervention is used, endometrial implants vary widely in terms of size, texture, and appearance. They may appear as red vesicular lesions, dark brown to black powder-burn lesions, white fibrotic plaques, or peritoneal defects known as Allen–Masters windows. The areas may be surrounded by reactive fibrosis that can lead to dense adhesions in **deep infiltrating endometriosis**

FIGURE 15-3. Transvaginal ultrasound of an endometrioma of the ovary. Note the characteristic "ground glass" appearance of the endometrioma on ultrasound. (From Berek JS. *Berek & Novak's Gynecology*, 14th ed. Philadelphia, PA: Lippincott Williams & Wilkins; 2006.)

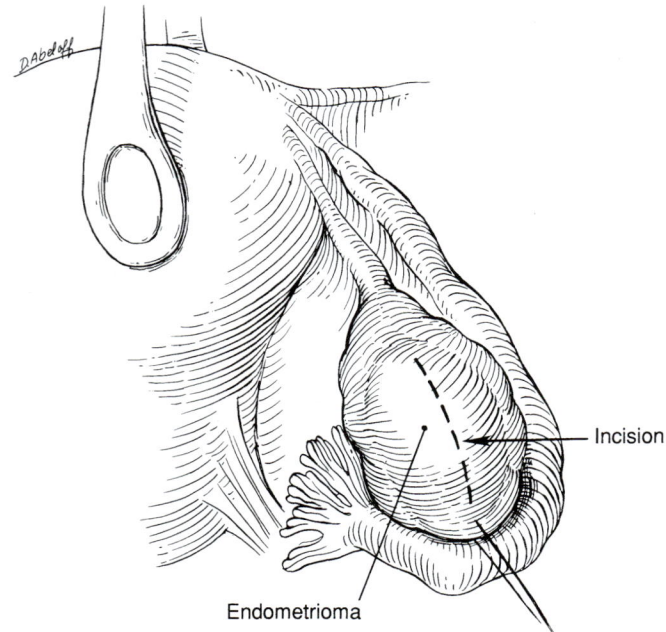

FIGURE 15-4. Endometrioma. (From LifeART image copyright © 2006 Lippincott Williams & Wilkins. All rights reserved.)

(DIE). The ovary itself can develop large cystic collections of endometriosis filled with thick, dark, old blood and debris known as **endometriomas or chocolate cysts** (Fig. 15-4). **Peritoneal biopsy** is recommended for histologic confirmation of the diagnosis of endometriosis.

Once the diagnosis of endometriosis is confirmed, the anatomic location and extent of the disease can be used to properly classify the operative findings. In general, endometriosis is categorized by how diffuse it is and whether or not it is superficial or deep. The American Fertility Society's revised classification schema is reproduced in Table 15-1. Although not commonly used, this classification method uses a point system to stage endometriosis based on the location, depth, and diameter of lesions, and density of adhesions.

DIFFERENTIAL DIAGNOSIS

The differential diagnosis for endometriosis includes other chronic processes that result in recurring pelvic pain or an ovarian mass, such as pelvic inflammatory disease, adenomyosis, irritable bowel syndrome, pelvic floor dysfunction, interstitial cystitis, pelvic adhesions, functional ovarian cysts, ectopic pregnancy, and ovarian neoplasms.

TREATMENT

The treatment of choice for patients with endometriosis depends on the extent and location of disease, the severity of symptoms, and the patient's desire for future fertility. Treatment should be embarked upon with the mindset that the endometriosis is a chronic disease that may require long-term management and multiple interventions. **Expectant management** may be used in patients with minimal or nonexistent symptoms. For other patients, both medical and surgical options are available. In the case of severe or chronic endometriosis, a multidisciplinary approach incorporating medical and surgical management as well as pain center involvement and psychiatric support may provide the most comprehensive care.

Medical treatment for endometriosis is aimed at **suppression and atrophy of the endometrial tissue**. Although medical therapies can be quite effective, these are temporizing measures rather than definitive treatments. Endometrial implants and symptoms often recur following cessation of treatment. **There is a minimal role for medical management in patients attempting to conceive**. Medical management does not improve conception rates and will delay attempts at conception. Surgical treatment has been shown to improve conception rates.

Current medical regimens for the treatment of endometriosis include **nonsteroidal anti-inflammatory drugs (NSAIDs)**, **cyclic or continuous estrogen–progestin contraceptives** (pills, patches, rings), and **menstrual suppression with progestins** (oral, injectable, or intrauterine). These treatments induce

TABLE 15-1. Classification of Endometriosis

American Society for Reproductive Medicine Revised Classification of Endometriosis

Patient's name_____ Date_____

Stage I (minimal) 1–5

Stage II (mild) 6–15   Laparoscopy_____ Laparotomy_____

Photography_____

Stage III (moderate) 16–40 Recommend treatment_____

Stage IV (severe) >40_____

Total_____ Prognosis_____

Tube	Endometriosis	<1 cm	1–3 cm	<3 cm
	Superficial	1	2	4
	Deep	2	4	6
Ovary R	Superficial	1	2	4
	Deep	4	16	20
L	Superficial	1	2	4
	Deep	4	16	20
	Posterior Cul-de-sac Obliteration	Partial 4		Complete 40
	Adhesions	<1/3 Enclosure	1/3–2/3 Enclosure	>2/3 Enclosure
Ovary R	Filmy	1	2	4
	Dense	4	8	16
L	Filmy	1	2	4
	Dense	4	8	16
R	Filmy	1	2	4
	Dense	4[a]	8[a]	16
L	Filmy	1	2	4
Peritoneum	Dense	4[a]	8[a]	16

Denote appearance of superficial implant types as red ([R], red, red-pink, flame-like, vesicular blobs, clear vesicles), white ([W], opacifications, peritoneal defects, yellow-brown), or black ([B] black, hemosiderin deposits, blue). Denote percent of total described as R__%, W__%, and B__%. Total should equal 100%.

[a] If the fimbriated end of the fallopian tube is completely enclosed, change the point assignment to 16.

---

a state of **"pseudopregnancy"** by suppressing both ovulation and menstruation and by decidualizing the endometrial implants, thereby alleviating the cyclic pelvic pain and dysmenorrhea. These options are best for patients who are not currently seeking to conceive.

Patients who have failed or cannot tolerate the treatments noted previously can also be placed in a reversible state of **pseudomenopause** with the use of danazol (Danocrine), an androgen derivative, or gonadotropin-releasing hormone (GnRH) agonists, such as leuprolide acetate (Lupron) and nafarelin (Synarel). Both classes of drugs suppress follicle-stimulating hormone and luteinizing hormone. As a result, the ovaries do not produce estrogen, resulting in decreased stimulation of endometrial implants. Subsequently, existing endometrial implants atrophy, and new implants are prevented. More recently, **aromatase inhibitors**, such as anastrozole (Arimidex) and letrozole (Femara), have been used *off-label* to treat severe endometriosis. These medications lower circulating estrogen levels by blocking conversion of androgens to estrogens in the ovary, brain, and periphery. These have not been approved for use in endometriosis; can cause bone loss, hot flashes, and nausea and vomiting; and must be used with combination oral contraceptive pills (OCPs) or GnRH agonists to prevent development of follicular cysts.

Side effects associated with OCPs and progestin agents include irritability, depression, breakthrough bleeding, and bloating. The drawback to danazol is that patients may experience some **androgen-related**, anabolic side effects, including acne, oily skin, weight gain, edema, hirsutism, and deepening of the voice. GnRH agonists, such as Lupron, result in **estrogen deficiency**. The side effects of these medications are similar to those seen during menopause, including hot flashes, decreased bone density, headaches, and vaginal atrophy and dryness. Moreover, these treatments can be costly and often have limited insurance coverage. Therefore, the use of these medications is generally limited to 6 months.

Fortunately, newer treatment regimens known as **add-back therapy** have been designed for use in conjunction with GnRH agonists. These regimens add a small amount of progestin with or without estrogen to the GnRH agonist to minimize the symptoms caused by estrogen deficiency, such as hot flashes and bone density loss. With add-back therapy, the patient receives the benefits of the GnRH agonist (endometriosis suppression and relief of pelvic pain and dysmenorrhea), while the small dose of progestin with or without estrogen minimizes the adverse effects of hypoestrogenation allowing the treatment to be continued up to 1 year.

Women with DIE, endometriomas, and infertility may be best served by surgical management. Surgical treatment for endometriosis can be classified as either conservative or definitive. **Conservative surgical therapy** typically involves laparoscopy and fulguration or excision of any visible endometrial implants. Endometriomas are best treated using laparoscopic cystectomy with removal of as much of the cyst wall as possible (Fig. 15-5). With conservative therapy, the uterus and ovaries are left in situ. For these women, the pregnancy rate after conservative surgical treatment depends on the extent of the disease at the time of surgery (Table 15-2). For patients with pain who do not desire immediate pregnancy, pain control can be optimized and recurrences delayed by starting or **restarting medical therapy** immediately after surgical treatment.

Definitive surgical therapy includes total hysterectomy and bilateral salpingo-oophorectomy

FIGURE 15-5. Resection of endometrioma. The cyst wall is removed, and the ovarian defect is closed or left to heal spontaneously. (From LifeART image copyright © 2006 Lippincott Williams & Wilkins. All rights reserved.)

TABLE 15-2. Conception Rates After Ablation of Endometrial Implants

Extent of Disease	Stage of Disease	Conception Rates (%)
Mild	1 and 2	75
Moderate	3	50–60
Severe	4	30–40

(typically by abdominal or laparoscopic approach), lysis of adhesions, and removal of any visible endometriosis lesions. This therapy is reserved for cases in which childbearing is complete and for women with severe disease or symptoms that are refractory to conservative medical or surgical treatment. Some experts have advocated for sparing the ovaries at the time of hysterectomy if they are not involved by endometriosis, and all other visible endometriosis is removed. If postsurgical **hormone replacement** therapy (HRT) is started after hysterectomy and oophorectomy, some providers will still employ combination estrogen–progestin HRT because of the theoretical possibility of stimulating transformation of residual implants into an endometrial cancer by the use of estrogen-only replacement therapy.

ADENOMYOSIS

PATHOGENESIS

Adenomyosis is the **presence of endometrial tissue (glands and stroma) within the myometrium** (Fig. 15-6). The pathogenesis is uncertain, but adenomyosis is closely associated with endometriosis and leiomyomas (Table 15-3).

The cause of adenomyosis is not known. One theory proposes that **the endometrium directly invades the myometrium.** The mechanism is unknown but may be related to weakness in the myometrium and excess estrogen. The myometrium may be weakened by placental invasion during pregnancy or secondary to uterine surgery. Reactive hyperplasia of the basalis layer occurs and penetrates into the myometrium. This mechanism has been postulated because the adenomyosis occurs more frequently in parous women and in those who have had uterine surgery. Higher expression of estradiol receptors in adenomyosis has been demonstrated, which may enhance the penetration and growth into the myometrium. Another theory is that adenomyosis develops de novo from **metaplastic transformation** of müllerian rest cells located within the myometrium.

Adenomyosis causes the uterus to become diffusely enlarged and globular owing to **hypertrophy and hyperplasia** of the myometrium *adjacent to* the ectopic endometrial tissue. The adenomyotic changes are usually most extensive in the **fundus and posterior uterine wall**. Adenomyosis may also present as a well-circumscribed, isolated region known as an **adenomyoma**. Adenomyomas contain smooth muscle cells as well as endometrial glands and stroma. These nodular growths may be located in the myometrium or extend into the endometrial cavity. Unlike uterine fibroids, which have a characteristic pseudocapsule, individual areas of adenomyosis are **not encapsulated**. Instead, adenomyosis can infiltrate throughout the myometrium giving the uterus a characteristic boggy feel on palpation.

EPIDEMIOLOGY

The incidence of adenomyosis is generally estimated to be about 20%. However, up to 65% of hysterectomy specimens contain some evidence of adenomyosis. Adenomyosis generally develops in parous women in their late 30s or early 40s. It occurs infrequently in nulliparous women. However, because the diagnosis

FIGURE 15-6. Adenomyosis. (From Rubin E, Farber JL. *Pathology,* 3rd ed. Philadelphia, PA: Lippincott Williams & Wilkins; 1999.)

TABLE 15-3.	Terminology of Aberrant Endometrial and Myometrial Tissue
Adenomyosis	The presence of endometrial tissue in the uterine myometrium leading to abnormal bleeding and pain. The uterus becomes soft and globular. Progestin-containing IUD or hysterectomy is the most effective treatment.
Adenomyoma	A well-circumscribed collection of endometrial tissue within the uterine wall. They may also contain smooth muscle cells and are not encapsulated. Adenomyomas can also prolapse into the endometrial cavity similar to a classic endometrial polyp.
Endometriosis	The presence of endometrial cells outside the uterine cavity. The hallmark of this chronic disease is cyclic pelvic pain. These estrogen-sensitive lesions can be treated with NSAIDs, OCPs, progestins, GnRH agonists, or surgery.
Endometrioma	A cystic collection of endometrial cells, old blood, and menstrual debris on the ovary; also known as "chocolate cysts."
Leiomyoma	Local proliferations of smooth muscle cells within the myometrium, often surrounded by a pseudocapsule. Also known as fibroids, these benign growths may be located on the intramural, subserosal, or submucosal portions of the uterus.

NSAIDs, nonsteroidal anti-inflammatory drugs.

is typically made at hysterectomy, there is a potential for bias in establishing the association between parity and adenomyosis. More recent reports using MRI have suggested that adenomyosis may also be present in younger women experiencing pelvic pain and dysmenorrhea.

RISK FACTORS

Adenomyosis, **endometriosis**, and **uterine fibroids** frequently coexist. About 15% to 20% of patients with adenomyosis also have endometriosis, and 50% to 60% of patients with adenomyosis also have uterine fibroids. Patients with dyspareunia, dyschezia, and menorrhagia or menometrorrhagia have an increased probability of having adenomyosis.

CLINICAL MANIFESTATIONS

History

Thirty percent of patients with adenomyosis are **asymptomatic** or have symptoms minor enough that medical attention is not sought. Symptomatic adenomyosis occurs most often in parous women between age 35 and 50 years. When symptoms do occur, the most common are **secondary dysmenorrhea** (30%), **heavy or prolonged menstrual bleeding** (50%), or both (20%). Patients typically present with increasingly heavy or prolonged menstrual bleeding (menorrhagia). They may also complain of increasingly severe dysmenorrhea that may begin up to 1 week before menses and last until cessation of bleeding. Other patients may only experience pressure on the bladder or rectum because of an enlarged uterus.

Physical Examination

The pelvic examination of a patient with adenomyosis may reveal a **diffusely enlarged globular uterus**. The uterus is usually less than 14 cm. The consistency of the uterus is typically softer and boggier than the firmer, rubbery uterus containing fibroids. The adenomyomatous uterus may be mildly tender just before or during menses but should have normal mobility and no associated adnexal pathology.

DIAGNOSTIC EVALUATION

Prior to treating adenomyosis, any patient aged 45 years or older with change in menstrual quantity or pattern should have a thyroid stimulating hormone (TSH) test, pelvic ultrasound, and an endometrial biopsy to rule out other causes of abnormal uterine bleeding. **MRI is the most accurate imaging tool** for identifying adenomyosis. However, because the cost of MRI can be prohibitive, **pelvic ultrasound** is the most common imaging modality. MRI is then used if adenomyosis is suggested by pelvic ultrasound by an indistinct endometrial–myometrial junction or glandular tissue within the myometrium. MRI is usually reserved for situations where myomectomy is being planned, and it is important to distinguish adenomyosis that is non-resectable from uterine fibroids that are typically surgically resectable. Ultimately, hysterectomy is the only definitive means of diagnosing adenomyosis.

DIFFERENTIAL DIAGNOSIS

The differential diagnosis for adenomyosis includes disease processes resulting in uterine enlargement, menorrhagia, and/or dysmenorrhea, including uterine fibroids, polyps, menstrual disorders, endometrial intraepithelial neoplasia (EIN), endometrial cancer, and pregnancy.

TREATMENT

The treatment for adenomyosis depends on the severity of the dysmenorrhea and heavy or prolonged menstrual bleeding. Women with minimal symptoms or those near menopause may be expectantly managed or managed with analgesics alone. **NSAIDs**, cyclic or **continuous estrogen–progestin contraceptives** (pills, patches, rings), and menstrual suppression with **progestins** (oral, injectable, or intrauterine) have also been found to be temporarily helpful. Short-term relief has also been achieved using endometrial ablation; however, pain and bleeding may recur more frequently when adenomyosis is present. The **levonorgestrel-containing intrauterine device (IUD)** has been found to be the most effective temporary means of managing the symptoms of adenomyosis. It has been shown to improve dysmenorrhea, heavy menstrual bleeding, and quality of life. However, there are limited long-term data suggesting worsening of symptoms after the first year of use.

Hysterectomy is the only definitive treatment for adenomyosis. Endometrial biopsy should be performed to rule out concomitant EIN and cancer in women aged >45 years before a hysterectomy is performed for adenomyosis. Prior to the surgery, it is also particularly important to distinguish adenomyosis from uterine fibroids. If adenomyosis is mistaken for uterine fibroids, a surgeon attempting a myomectomy may find only diffuse adenomyosis and be forced to perform a hysterectomy instead.

KEY POINTS

- Endometriosis is the presence of endometrial tissue outside the endometrial cavity, most often in the pelvic peritoneum. It occurs in 10% to 15% of women of reproductive age.
- The hallmark of endometriosis is cyclic pelvic pain, which is at its worst 1 to 2 days before menses and subsides at the onset of flow or shortly thereafter.
- The severity of symptoms (dysmenorrhea, dyspareunia, abnormal bleeding, and infertility) may not correlate with extent of disease.
- Complications of endometriosis include intra-abdominal inflammation and bleeding that can cause scarring, pain, and adhesion formation, which can lead to infertility and chronic pelvic pain.
- Direct visualization with diagnostic laparoscopy or laparotomy (preferably with histologic confirmation with biopsy) is the only way to definitively diagnose endometriosis.
- Endometriosis can be treated medically (NSAIDs, OCPs, progestins, danazol, GnRH agonists) to reduce pain, but these methods are used mainly as temporizing agents.
- Medical management does not improve conception rates and may delay attempts at conception.
- Endometriosis can be treated surgically with conservative therapy to ablate or excise implants and lyse adhesions while preserving the uterus and ovaries. Surgery should be followed immediately by medical therapy to delay the recurrence of endometrial implants and pain.
- Endometriosis can be treated definitively with surgery, including total hysterectomy (often with bilateral salpingo-oophorectomy), lysis of adhesions, and removal of endometriosis lesions.
- Adenomyosis is the presence of endometrial tissue in the myometrium making the uterus diffusely enlarged, boggy, and globular. It occurs in 20% of women, most of whom are parous and in their late 30s or early 40s.
- Patients typically present with increasing secondary dysmenorrhea and/or heavy or prolonged menstrual bleeding; 30% of patients are asymptomatic.
- Adenomyosis may be suggested on pelvic ultrasound. MRI can best distinguish between adenomyosis and fibroids.
- Patients aged 45 years or older who have abnormal uterine bleeding should also have an endometrial biopsy to rule out EIN and cancer prior to beginning treatment.
- Minimal symptoms may be treated with analgesics, NSAIDs, OCPs, or progestins, although adenomyosis is less responsive to hormonal management than endometriosis.
- The levonorgestrel-containing IUD is the most effective temporary means of treating the symptoms of adenomyosis.
- Hysterectomy is the only definitive means of diagnosing and treating adenomyosis.

CLINICAL VIGNETTES

VIGNETTE 1

A 25-year-old G0 woman complains of increasing pelvic pain with her menses over the last year since she stopped her OCPs. She has noticed more pain on her left side in the last couple of months and has begun to have pain with deep penetration during intercourse. She started OCPs as a teenager for painful irregular cycles but stopped them a year ago, when her insurance changed. She has had only one lifetime sexual partner and no history of sexually transmitted infections. She would like to preserve fertility. On examination, she has no abnormal discharge, but her uterus is tender as well as her left adnexa. You appreciate a fullness that you suspect may be a mass. On pelvic ultrasound, she has a 5-cm cystic ovarian mass thought to be an endometrioma. It persists in repeat ultrasound 8 weeks later, and the patient is still symptomatic.

1. What would be the most appropriate next step in her care?
   a. Refer her to a gynecologic oncologist
   b. Prescribe a GnRH agonist (i.e., Depo-Lupron)
   c. Prescribe an NSAID for her pain and repeat the ultrasound in 6 to 8 weeks
   d. Schedule diagnostic laparoscopy with left ovarian cystectomy
   e. Resume an oral contraceptive

2. You perform a laparoscopic left ovarian cystectomy and note that the cyst is a "chocolate cyst." She also has other superficial implants of endometriosis on the uterosacral ligaments. The final pathology report is consistent with an endometrioma. At your patient's postoperative visit 2 weeks after surgery, she tells you that her pain is resolved, and she is feeling well. What do you recommend for the continued postoperative management of her endometriosis?
   a. Because endometriosis cannot be cured medically, she should undergo total hysterectomy with bilateral salpingo-oophorectomy
   b. You were able to completely remove the cyst, so she does not need any further therapy at this time
   c. Initiate therapy with a combined oral contraceptive or a progestin to delay the return of her previous symptoms
   d. Wait for 9 months, and then repeat laparoscopy to make sure that there is no further endometriosis to be treated
   e. Endometrial ablation, because that will destroy her endometrium and decrease the risk of new implants developing from retrograde menstruation

3. Your patient would like to know more about the GnRH agonist, Depo-Lupron. You explain how it works and that the side effects include all of the following *except*:
   a. deepening of the voice
   b. headaches
   c. decreased bone density
   d. weight gain
   e. hot flashes

VIGNETTE 2

A couple presents because they have been trying to conceive for 2 years. During the interview, you learn that the man has fathered a child in a previous relationship and is in good health. The woman is 28 years old and reports that she has had painful menses for the past 4 or 5 years.

1. You begin to suspect that she may have endometriosis. All the information below would increase that suspicion *except*:
   a. she has experienced dyspareunia with deep penetration for several years
   b. she reports that a maternal cousin has a history of endometriosis
   c. her ethnicity is Caucasian
   d. she reports the development of abnormal bleeding in the last year
   e. her menarche began at age 9 years

2. You explain to your patient that you need to perform an examination before making any recommendations. You mention that there are certain findings that are associated with endometriosis. During your examination, which of the findings listed below would NOT increase your suspicion that she has endometriosis?
   a. A fixed deviated uterus
   b. Uterosacral nodularity on rectovaginal examination
   c. Tender adnexa
   d. A fixed adnexal mass
   e. An enlarged irregular uterus

3. On examination, you did find uterosacral nodularity, and you discuss with your patient your concern that she has endometriosis. You recommend that as part of her ongoing evaluation and treatment she undergo a diagnostic laparoscopy with ablation or excision of endometriosis if it is found. Your patient is very concerned about the diagnosis and

wonders what percent of women with infertility have endometriosis. You tell her:
a. 70%
b. 30%
c. 90%
d. 10%
e. 50%

VIGNETTE 3

A 46-year-old G2P2 obese woman is referred from her primary-care physician because of increasingly heavy and painful menses over the last 18 months. She has tried an oral contraceptive with some improvement of her bleeding but no improvement in her pain. She has never had an abnormal Pap smear and states she has never had any infections "down there." Her only medical problems are her obesity and hypertension. On examination, you note normal external genitalia, vagina, and cervix. However, her uterus is slightly enlarged, mildly tender, and softer than you expected. She has no adnexal mass or tenderness.

1. Which of these diagnoses is the least likely choice to keep in your differential?
   a. Irritable bowel syndrome
   b. Adenomyosis
   c. Leiomyoma
   d. Endometrial intraepithelial neoplasia (EIN)
   e. Endometriosis

2. You explain to your patient that you think adenomyosis is most likely causing her symptoms. However, you would like to make sure whether or not she has fibroids as well. Which imaging study listed below would best differentiate between adenomyosis and uterine fibroids?
   a. Pelvic ultrasound
   b. Pelvic CT
   c. Sonohysterogram
   d. Pelvic MRI
   e. Hysterosalpingogram

3. After further evaluation suggesting adenomyosis, your patient wants to proceed with hysterectomy because she is tired of bleeding and experiencing pain. You explain to her that she needs to undergo a test prior to scheduling her hysterectomy. What test does the patient need to undergo?
   a. Wet prep
   b. Mammogram
   c. Endometrial biopsy
   d. Colonoscopy
   e. Chest X-ray

VIGNETTE 4

A 39-year-old G2P2 woman with 12 months of heavy menses and worsening dysmenorrhea comes to you for a second opinion. She underwent a pelvic ultrasound that suggested adenomyosis, and her gynecologist recommended a hysterectomy. She states that she does not trust the ultrasound results and wants to know if there is anything else that can be done to confirm the diagnosis.

1. What would be the most appropriate next step?
   a. Review the ultrasound results and reassure her that her gynecologist is correct
   b. Repeat the pelvic ultrasound
   c. Tell her that hysterectomy is the only thing that will help to clarify her diagnosis
   d. Examine her and recommend obtaining a pelvic MRI
   e. Suggest a 3-month trial of an oral contraceptive pill

2. After you complete your evaluation, you agree that she likely has adenomyosis. She wants to avoid surgery for several months. You recommend one or a combination of the options listed *except*:
   a. levonorgestrel-containing IUD
   b. NSAID
   c. oral contraceptive pill
   d. progestin therapy
   e. doxycycline for 14 days

3. When discussing hysterectomy and the timing for surgery, she tells you that she has a younger sister who is a 29-year-old G0. She would like to know if her younger sister is likely to develop adenomyosis and menorrhagia or dysmenorrhea. You explain that all of the following may increase the risk for developing adenomyosis *except*:
   a. parous women
   b. fibroids
   c. endometriosis
   d. menopause
   e. age 30 to 50 years

ANSWERS

VIGNETTE 1 Question 1
1. Answer D:
This patient's history, examination, and ultrasound findings are consistent with endometriosis. Because of her significant symptoms and the findings of a persistent endometrioma, laparoscopy with planned cystectomy is the best option for her. Large endometriomas are not likely to resolve on their own with time in contrast to functional ovarian cysts. They are also unlikely to respond to medical management with an oral contraceptive or GnRH agonist. In this young woman with findings consistent with an endometrioma, referral to an oncologist would not be necessary because of low risk of malignancy and high sensitivity with ultrasound to correctly diagnose endometriomas.

VIGNETTE 1 Question 2
2. Answer C:
For patients with pain who do not desire pregnancy, pain control can be optimized and recurrence delayed by starting medical therapy immediately after surgical treatment. For patients who desire fertility in the future, hysterectomy is not an appropriate option. Even though removal of the cyst significantly decreases the risk of endometrioma recurrence, the patient is at increased risk of the return of her symptoms and the development of new implants with expectant management compared with medical therapy to suppress recurrent endometriosis and symptoms. Because of the risks of surgery and unlikely return of symptoms within 9 months, medical therapy would be the most appropriate initial step. Endometrial ablation is not recommended for those desiring pregnancy in the future and has not been shown to decrease the risk of recurrent symptoms from endometriosis.

VIGNETTE 1 Question 3
3. Answer A:
Deepening of the voice occurs with an androgen derivative, danazol, which initiates a pseudomenopause state. However, this symptom is not associated with the GnRH agonists. Hot flashes, headaches, decreased bone density, and weight gain can all occur secondary to GnRH agonists, such as Lupron that initiate a medical pseudomenopause and create a relatively estrogen deficient state, which helps to prevent the development of new foci of endometriosis.

VIGNETTE 2 Question 1
1. Answer B:
Genetic factors probably are associated with the risk of developing endometriosis, and an increased risk of developing endometriosis has been observed in first-degree relatives. However, this association has not been observed in third-degree relatives. Other risk factors include Caucasian ethnicity when compared with Black or Hispanic ethnicity and early menarche. The reports of deep dyspareunia, dysmenorrhea, and abnormal menstrual bleeding are all symptoms that are associated with endometriosis.

VIGNETTE 2 Question 2
2. Answer E:
An enlarged irregular uterus is typically associated with leiomyomas and not necessarily with endometriosis, although the two can be found concomitantly. Physical findings with early-stage endometriosis can be subtle or nonexistent. However, with more disseminated disease, a clinician may find uterosacral nodularity on rectovaginal examination, a fixed often retroverted uterus, tender adnexa, and/or a fixed adnexal mass when a large endometrioma is present.

VIGNETTE 2 Question 3
3. Answer B:
Approximately 30% to 40% of women who have infertility also have the diagnosis of endometriosis. The overall incidence of endometriosis in the US population is thought to be approximately 5% to 15%.

VIGNETTE 3 Question 1
1. Answer A:
Although irritable bowel syndrome is associated with pelvic pain and is likely underdiagnosed, it is not associated with heavy or prolonged menstrual bleeding or dysmenorrhea in particular. Leiomyomas are commonly associated with heavy or prolonged menstrual bleeding and sometimes dysmenorrhea. Two of the hallmarks for adenomyosis are heavy or prolonged menstrual bleeding and dysmenorrhea, especially when it develops in women who are 30 to 50 years of age. EIN must be considered in an obese woman with hypertension and abnormal bleeding, especially if she is older than 45 years. Endometriosis would be less likely due to the age of the onset of symptoms of abnormal bleeding and dysmenorrhea. Typically, these begin to present in the second and third decades. However, adenomyosis, endometriosis, and leiomyomas often coexist.

VIGNETTE 3 Question 2
2. Answer D:
Pelvic MRI is the most accurate imaging tool for identifying adenomyosis. Because the cost of MRI can be

prohibitive, ultrasound is the most common means of diagnosis. If there is difficulty in differentiating between uterine fibroids and adenomyosis, then MRI is used. CT imaging is not a helpful tool in evaluating for adenomyosis. Sonohysterography is typically used to screen for intracavitary lesions, such as endometrial polyps or submucosal fibroids. Hysterosalpingography is typically used to evaluate the uterine cavity and the patency of the fallopian tubes.

VIGNETTE 3 Question 3
3. Answer C:
Because of her abnormal bleeding, age older than 45, and obesity, endometrial biopsy should be performed prior to scheduling hysterectomy to rule out concomitant EIN or carcinoma. A screening wet prep is not necessary prior to hysterectomy and only needs to be performed if the patient is complaining of symptoms consistent with bacterial vaginosis. Mammography is suggested every 1 to 2 years for women in their 40s but is not required prior to scheduling a hysterectomy. Routine colorectal cancer screening with colonoscopy begins at age 50 in people at average risk and at age 45 in African-Americans. The patient is not having other symptoms that would require a colonoscopy. Routine chest X-rays are not necessary prior to a major gynecologic procedure and should be reserved for those where there is concern for cardiopulmonary disease.

VIGNETTE 4 Question 1
1. Answer D:
Both the examination and the pelvic MRI can increase or decrease the likelihood of adenomyosis and would be the most appropriate next step. Repeat ultrasound is unlikely to add new information to the initial ultrasound. Although hysterectomy may be eventually necessary and ultimately provides tissue to make the definitive diagnosis, MRI is a noninvasive method that is fairly sensitive in this patient who is looking for a second opinion. An oral contraceptive is used for a number of conditions, including adenomyosis. A response or lack of response to it would not necessarily help clarify the diagnosis of adenomyosis.

VIGNETTE 4 Question 2
2. Answer E:
If you suspected an underlying chronic endometritis or if endometritis was found on endometrial biopsy, then doxycycline may be appropriate. It would not typically be effective for management of her heavy or prolonged menstrual bleeding and dysmenorrhea. NSAIDs can be used alone with mild symptoms or in combination with either an oral contraceptive or a progestin. Other than hysterectomy, the levonorgestrel-containing IUD is the most effective treatment for the symptoms of adenomyosis.

VIGNETTE 4 Question 3
3. Answer D:
Menopause is not associated with the development of adenomyosis, and often, symptoms related to adenomyosis will resolve at menopause. Women in their late reproductive years who are parous have an increased risk of developing adenomyosis compared with younger nulliparous women. Endometriosis and fibroids have also been associated with adenomyosis.

16 | Infections of the Lower Female Reproductive Tract

URINARY TRACT INFECTIONS

Urinary tract infections (UTIs) are one of the most common infections of the lower genitourinary tract treated by clinicians. Approximately 50% of women will be diagnosed with a UTI during their lives. There is an incidence of approximately 1% per year in adult women, and 5% will have recurrent episodes. Women commonly present with symptoms of urethritis (discomfort or pain at the urethral meatus or a burning sensation throughout the urethra with micturition) or cystitis (pain in the midline suprapubic region and/or frequent urination). UTIs are most common in sexually active women and increased in women with obesity, increasing age, anatomic or neurologic abnormalities, diabetes mellitus, and sickle-cell disease. The rates are higher in women than men secondary to the shorter length of the urethra and its proximity to the vagina and rectum.

DIAGNOSIS

When a woman presents with dysuria, urinary urgency, and frequency, the diagnosis of UTI should lead the differential. In fact, symptoms alone have a 90% sensitivity for UTI, and some guidelines recommend treating based on symptoms alone. For additional confirmation, a clean voided midstream urine sample can be sent for urinalysis and microscopic examination. Hematuria, leukocytes, leukocyte esterase, or nitrates in the absence of a vaginal infection are indicative of a UTI. In particular, nitrates are specific and sensitive for gram-negative pathogens. To distinguish contamination from true infection, the urinalysis and microscopic examination can be repeated with urine collected via catheterization. Patients are often diagnosed and treated for UTI in the setting of a positive urinalysis with concomitant symptoms of dysuria and urinary frequency. The diagnosis of a UTI can be confirmed with a urine culture but is not required in uncomplicated cases. Each patient who presents with symptoms should also have a physical examination to rule out **pyelonephritis** with evaluation for fevers and costovertebral angle tenderness.

The role of culture in diagnosing and managing a UTI is controversial. Some recommend sending cultures with only complicated UTI or pyelonephritis, whereas others recommend sending cultures for all patients. Approximately 80% to 85% of UTIs are caused by *Escherichia coli* and other organisms that colonize the gastrointestinal (GI) tract. Other common organisms that cause UTIs are *Staphylococcus saprophyticus, Proteus mirabilis, Klebsiella pneumoniae*, and Enterococcus. If the urine culture is negative, the diagnosis should be reconsidered. In patients with symptoms consistent with urethritis, organisms such as *Chlamydia trachomatis* and *Neisseria gonorrhoeae* should be considered and screened for using a midstream collection. Another etiology of urethritis is herpes simplex virus (HSV) infection. In patients with recurrent symptoms of cystitis, but a negative culture, the diagnosis of overactive bladder or painful bladder syndrome (interstitial cystitis) should be entertained.

TREATMENT

Most uncomplicated UTIs can be treated with oral antibiotics. It is important for both begin treatment on initial diagnosis and follow-up culture sensitivities to be certain that the pathologic organisms are treated adequately. Initial treatment is often begun with trimethoprim–sulfamethoxazole, nitrofurantoin, or a fluoroquinolone for 3 to 7 days. Ampicillin or cephalexin has also been used; however, more recently, beta-lactams have become less effective in the treatment of uncomplicated UTIs. The local sensitivities of common organisms should be known. For example, the rates of ampicillin-resistant *E. coli* can range from 5% to 35% in different hospitals. Patients with symptoms consistent with pyelonephritis are usually treated as an inpatient with IV antibiotics. Outpatient management has been studied and is used increasingly in reliable patients without other medical issues. A 14-day antimicrobial therapy should be completed.

THE EXTERNAL ANOGENITAL REGION

Various infectious diseases affect the external genitalia. In the female patient, the entire perianal area and mons should be considered in addition to the vulva. The skin overlying these areas is subject to the same infections that can occur anywhere on the epidermis, but the exposure and environment differ and must be considered when discussing these infections. There are also a variety of focal and systemic processes that can cause lesions or symptoms in this region. Anogenital lesions are usually categorized as ulcerative or nonulcerative, and common symptoms include pain and itching.

VULVITIS

The most common cause of vulvitis, and usually of vulvar pruritus, is **candidiasis**. It is also a common cause of vaginitis and is discussed in greater detail later in this chapter. A candidal vulvitis usually presents with vulvar erythema, pruritus, and small satellite lesions. If the vulvitis does not respond to the usual treatment with topical or systemic antifungals, symptoms may be because of other causes, such as allergic reaction, chemical or fabric irritants, and vulvar dystrophies. Malignancy should always be ruled out in the setting of chronic vulvar irritation.

ULCERATED LESIONS

Many primary vulvar ulcers are caused by sexually transmitted infections (STIs) (Table 16-1), such as **herpes, syphilis, chancroid**, and **lymphogranuloma venereum (LGV)**. However, even with a diagnosis of an infectious process, these lesions can be associated with malignant processes as well. Up to 25% of patients with genital ulcers will not have a laboratory-confirmed diagnosis. Treatment should be based on history and clinical findings.

Of note, there are conditions other than infections that can lead to vulvar ulcerations. Crohn disease can have linear "knife-cut" vulvar ulcers as its first manifestation, preceding GI or other systemic manifestations by months to years. Behçet disease leads to tender and highly destructive vulvar lesions that often cause fenestrations in the labia and extensive scarring.

SYPHILIS

Syphilis is a chronic systemic infection caused by the spirochete *Treponema pallidum*. It is transmitted primarily through direct sexual contact; however, infections can also occur transplacentally during pregnancy. The incidence of primary and secondary syphilis in the United States increased through the 1980s until 1990, when the CDC noted a peak of 50,223 cases, a rate of 20 cases per 100,000 persons in 1990. This peak was followed by an almost 90% decrease between 1990 and 2000 to 5,979 reported cases. Unfortunately, between 2001 and 2015, there has been a steady increase in reported cases of primary and secondary syphilis with 74,702 cases reported in 2015. This was predominantly driven by increases in cases in men. However, between 2013 and 2015,

TABLE 16-1. Infectious Causes of Ulcerated Lesions

	Syphilis	Herpes	Chancroid	LGV
Incubation period (days)	7–14	2–10	4–7	3–12
Primary lesion	Papule	Vesicle	Papule/pustule	Papule/vesicle
Number of lesions	Single	Multiple	1–3, occasionally more	Single
Size (mm)	5–15	1–3	2–20	2–10
Painful	No	Yes	Yes	No
Diagnostic test	Dark-field microscopy, RPR/microhemagglutination assay for *Treponema pallidum* (MHA-TP)/FTA-ABS	Viral culture	Gram stain with "school of fish" appearance	Complement fixation
Treatment	Penicillin	Acyclovir	Ceftriaxone or azithromycin	Doxycycline

FTA-ABS, fluorescent treponemal antibody absorption; RPR, rapid plasma reagin.

the first increase in cases in women was reported, with a 27% rise in women from 2014 to 2015. Along with this, there has been an increase in congenital syphilis with 487 cases in 2015 (in comparison there were 128 vertical HIV-transmission cases).

Syphilis is divided into different stages of disease to help guide treatment and follow up. *T. pallidum* most likely enters the body through minute abrasions in the skin or mucosal surface and replicates locally. Initial lesions, therefore, commonly occur on the vulva, vagina, cervix, anus, nipples, or lips. The initial lesion that characterizes primary syphilis is a painless, red, round, firm ulcer, approximately 1 cm in size with raised edges known as a **chancre** (Fig. 16-1). It develops approximately 3 weeks after inoculation and is usually associated with concomitant regional adenopathy. Because it is painless, approximately 20% of these will be unrecognized. The lesions develop primarily from the patient's immune response and will heal without therapy. Material expressed from the chancre usually reveals motile spirochetes under dark-field microscopy.

Secondary syphilis is a systemic disease that occurs as *T. pallidum* disseminates and begins around 1 to 3 months after the primary stage resolves. Patients typically develop flu-like symptoms with fever and myalgias. Classically, a maculopapular rash may appear on the palms of the hands or soles of the feet. Moist papules and mucous patches can also occur. The dermatologic manifestations of secondary syphilis are why syphilis is known as the "great imitator." There may be other organ system involvement with meningitis, osteitis, nephritis, or hepatitis. All lesions resolve spontaneously, and this stage can be entirely asymptomatic. After resolution of this stage, the infection enters a latent phase that can last for years. Latent syphilis is further divided as early (acquired <1 year) or late (acquired >1 year) based on the time of initial symptoms.

Tertiary syphilis is quite uncommon today but is characterized by granulomas (gummas) of the skin and bones; cardiovascular syphilis with aortitis; and neurosyphilis with meningovascular disease, paresis, and tabes dorsalis.

Diagnosis

Screening for *T. pallidum* may be performed with nontreponemal anticardiolipin antibodies. Two types of nontreponemal serologic tests for syphilis are available: the Venereal Disease Research Laboratory (VDRL) test and the rapid plasma reagin (RPR) test. These tests remain positive for 6 to 12 months after treatment of primary syphilis, usually with progressively decreasing antibody titers. In primary syphilis, serologic assays may be negative during early infection, resulting in a lower sensitivity. These tests will become positive several weeks after the initial visit and should, therefore, be repeated 1 to 3 months after appearance of the ulcer in the compliant patient in whom the diagnosis cannot be made at first presentation. False-positive nontreponemal tests can occur with various autoimmune conditions, other infections, malignancy, pregnancy, and IV drug use. Therefore, a positive result must be confirmed with specific treponemal antibody studies, such as the fluorescent treponemal antibody absorption (FTA-ABS) test, *T. pallidum* particle agglutination assay (TPPA), enzyme immunoassays, or rapid treponemal assay. False-positive results in confirmatory testing occur less than 1% of the time. For this reason, some providers are performing a "reverse sequencing" algorithm and are initially screening with treponemal tests. The utility of this reverse screening is an area of active research. Primary, secondary, tertiary, and neurosyphilis can be diagnosed by the presenting signs and symptoms described earlier. However, patients who are asymptomatic with a positive titer are considered to be in early latent (acquired <1 year) or late latent (acquired >1 year) syphilis.

Treatment

Penicillin remains the drug of choice for treatment of syphilis. Primary, secondary, or early latent syphilis can be treated with benzathine penicillin G 2.4 million units IM one time. For late latent or latent of unknown duration syphilis, treatment consists of penicillin G 2.4 million units IM weekly for 3 weeks. For penicillin-allergic, nonpregnant patients with primary or secondary syphilis, several alternative regimens might be effective, including doxycycline 100 mg orally twice a day for 14 days, tetracycline 500 mg orally four times a day for 14 days, ceftriaxone 1 g IM or IV daily for 10 to 14 days, or azithromycin 2 g single oral dose. However, data to support the use of alternative regimens are still limited and close follow-up is essential. If compliance is of concern in penicillin-allergic individuals, then desensitization and treatment with penicillin are recommended. Penicillin remains the only recommended treatment in pregnancy, with sufficient evidence demonstrating efficacy for preventing maternal syphilis transmission to the fetus and for treating fetal infection.

Neurosyphilis is a more serious infection and requires aqueous crystalline penicillin G 3 to

FIGURE 16-1. (A) Slightly indurated primary chancre of 2 days duration that was neither painful nor tender. It points to the need for a high index of suspicion concerning all genital lesions. Dark-filled microscopy prevents diagnostic error and embarrassment. **(B)** Papulosquamous secondary syphilis involving the palm. **(C)** Typical coppery-red papules in secondary syphilis. **(D)** Healing gumma. Delay in diagnosis is suggested by widespread pigmentation and scarring. Response to treatment was slow, and the final scarring led to permanent edema of the foot, sometimes called paradoxical healing. (Reproduced with permission from Champion RH. *Textbook of Dermatology,* 5th ed. Oxford: Blackwell Science; 1992:2852.)

4 million units IV every 4 hours for 10 to 14 days. In individuals in whom compliance may be ensured, procaine penicillin 2.4 million units IM once daily plus probenecid 500 mg orally four times a day both for 10 to 14 days is recommended as a treatment alternative for neurosyphilis. Some authorities recommend treating neurosyphilis with an additional course of benzathine penicillin 2.4 million units IM weekly for 3 weeks after completion of either regimen. Patients with penicillin allergy in whom compliance issues are of concern will, therefore, require desensitization. Treatment success can be verified by following RPR or VDRL titers at 6, 12, and 24 months. Titers should decrease fourfold by 6 months and become nonreactive by 12 to 24 months after completion of treatment.

The Jarisch–Herxheimer reaction is an acute febrile reaction, frequently accompanied by fever, chills, headache, myalgia, malaise, pharyngitis, rash, and other symptoms that usually occur within the first 24 hours (generally within the first 8 hours) after any therapy for syphilis. This reaction was initially recognized in the treatment of neurosyphilis but can be seen with any syphilitic treatment, most commonly with early syphilis. Antipyretics may be used, but they have not been proven to prevent this reaction. The Jarisch–Herxheimer reaction might induce preterm contractions or cause changes to the fetal heart rate in pregnant women, but this should not prevent or delay therapy. This transient inflammatory reaction is not considered a drug reaction, but is related to the treatment of syphilis, and can be seen with the treatment of other spirochetes as well, such as Lyme disease, when injured or dead organisms release endotoxins into the circulation marked by systemic release of cytokines.

GENITAL HERPES

HSV infections are quite common in the perioral and genital regions. Although only about 5% of women report a history of genital herpes infection, as many as 25% to 30% have antibodies on serologic testing. Although some women have the classic severe presentation of genital herpes with painful genital ulcers, many women have a mild initial presentation or are entirely asymptomatic. Because of the asymptomatic nature of many initial presentations, it is difficult to get an estimate on the true incidence of disease; however, there has been a steady increase in patient visits to a clinician for herpes over the past two decades, with approximately 300,000 office visits in 2014. Although the majority

FIGURE 16-2. Genital herpes.

of genital herpes lesions are caused by HSV-2, up to 80% of new cases of genital HSV are attributable to HSV-1, particularly among adolescent and young adult populations. HSV is transmitted through direct contact of the virus with an incubation period of 2 to 10 days after exposure. Primary infections usually begin with flu-like symptoms, including malaise, myalgias, nausea, diarrhea, and fever. Vulvar burning and pruritus precede the multiple vesicles that appear next and usually remain intact for 24 to 36 hours before evolving into painful genital ulcers (Fig. 16-2). These ulcers can require a mean of 10 to 22 days to heal. After the primary outbreak, the herpes virus travels to the dorsal root ganglion of the nerve and can reactivate to cause recurrences, which can occur as frequently as one to six times per year. Recurrence is more frequent in HSV-2 infections. Symptoms tend to be less severe than the initial outbreak. It is important to note that subclinical or asymptomatic shedding can occur and is more frequent during the first 6 months after acquisition and immediately before or after recurrent outbreaks. Because of the possibility of frequent recurrence and the devastating consequences of neonatal herpes, pregnant women should have vaginal examinations around the time of delivery. Those with lesions should be delivered by cesarean section.

Diagnosis

Clinical diagnosis is often made with an examination of the vesicles and ulcers in conjunction with a sexual history. However, this modality has suboptimal sensitivity and specificity. Therefore, clinical diagnosis should be confirmed with laboratory testing. Viral cultures are used as the gold standard for diagnosis; however, sensitivity of culture is low, especially in recurrent or healing lesions. Nucleic Acid Amplification Testing (NAAT), including Polymerase Chain reaction (PCR) test, is the primary method of diagnosing genital HSV. Viral shedding can be intermittent, and a negative result does not always indicate absence of herpes virus. Negative results with a high index of clinical suspicion and positive results should be confirmed by serology. A PCR test cannot detect the serotype of HSV, but serology testing can subtype HSV. Type-specific antibodies for HSV-1 and HSV-2 IgG may be used to determine whether the patient has a primary infection as well as the serotype of the causative organism. Caution should be taken in patients who have had positive viral serologies without a history of genital ulcers because this can also indicate oropharyngeal colonization. Historically, a **Tzanck smear** prepared of the lesions and examined for multinucleated giant cells with a characteristic appearance may reveal typical cytologic changes, but this study is also neither sensitive nor specific and is rarely performed.

Treatment

Although many palliative treatments have evolved over the years, such as sitz baths for comfort and analgesics to reduce the pain, there is no cure for herpes. For a **primary infection**, acyclovir 200 mg five times per day, acyclovir 400 mg three times per day, famciclovir 250 mg three times per day, and valacyclovir 1 g twice a day orally for 7 to 10 days are recommended therapies in the treatment of first clinical outbreak, reducing the length of infection and the length of time a patient has viral shedding. With severe HSV infections, such as those that occur in immunocompromised patients, IV acyclovir should be used at a dose of 5 to 10 mg/kg every 8 hours. Oral acyclovir 400 mg three times daily or 800 mg twice daily for 5 days may be used for the treatment of recurrent lesions. For individuals with frequent recurrences, prophylactic or suppression therapy of 400 mg orally twice daily is recommended and can reduce recurrences by 80%. Alternatively, more costly antiviral medications may also be used, such as valacyclovir, particularly for easier dosing regimens. Additionally, daily treatment with valacyclovir 500 mg in the infected partner has been demonstrated to decrease the rate of HSV-2 transmission in discordant, heterosexual couples in whom the source partner has a history of genital HSV-2 infection.

CHANCROID

Chancroid is caused by ***Haemophilus ducreyi***. Globally, it is a common STI, although the incidence in North America has declined steadily since 1987, with just 11 reported cases in 2015. Reported cases are likely to grossly underestimate true incidence because *H. ducreyi* is difficult to culture. Males are affected more than females by ratios of 3:1 to 25:1. Chancroid is a cofactor for HIV transmission; high rates of HIV infection among patients who have chancroid occur in the United States and other countries. Additionally, approximately 10% of persons who have chancroid that was acquired in the United States are coinfected with *T. pallidum* or HSV.

Chancroid appears as a painful, demarcated, nonindurated ulcer located anywhere in the anogenital region. There is often concomitant painful suppurative inguinal lymphadenopathy. Usually, just a single ulcer is present, but multiple ulcers and occasionally extragenital infections have been known to occur.

Diagnosis

Diagnosis is a challenge because *H. ducreyi* is difficult to culture. A definitive diagnosis of chancroid requires the identification of *H. ducreyi* on special culture media that are not widely available from commercial sources; even when these media are used, sensitivity is less than 80%. Often, transporting the culture swab in Amies or Stuart transport media or chocolate agar can aid in the culture. Direct Gram stains have not been a consistent method of diagnosis, and FDA-approved PCR test for *H. ducreyi* is also not available in the United States. The diagnosis is, therefore, often made clinically by ruling out other sources of infection, such as HSV and syphilis.

Treatment

Treatment regimens include ceftriaxone 250 mg IM once, azithromycin 1 g orally once, ciprofloxacin 500 mg orally twice a day for 3 days, or erythromycin 500 mg four times a day for 7 days. As with most other STIs, sexual partners should be treated as well.

LYMPHOGRANULOMA VENEREUM

The *C. trachomatis* L-serotypes (L1, L2, or L3) cause the systemic disease **lymphogranuloma venereum** (LGV). The primary stage of this illness is often a local lesion that may be either a papule or a shallow ulcer and is often painless, transient, and can go unnoticed. The secondary stage (inguinal syndrome) occurs 2 to 6 weeks after the primary lesion and is characterized by painful inflammation and enlargement of the inguinal nodes (typically unilateral). Systemic manifestations include fever, headaches, malaise, and anorexia. Rectal exposure can result in the tertiary stage (anogenital syndrome), which is characterized by proctocolitis, rectal stricture, rectovaginal fistula, and elephantiasis (lymphatic filariasis). Initially, an anal pruritus will develop with a concomitant mucous rectal discharge. Although diagnosis is generally made per clinical suspicion, genital and lymph node specimens may be tested for *C. trachomatis* by culture, direct immunofluorescence, or nucleic acid detection.

Treatment
Treatment of LGV includes doxycycline 100 mg orally twice a day or erythromycin 500 mg orally four times a day for 21 days. With persistent illness, the antibiotic regimen can be repeated. If the external genitalia and rectum are disfigured and scarred, surgical measures may be required.

NONULCERATIVE LESIONS

One of the most common nonulcerative lesions is the condyloma (Fig. 16-3). **Condyloma acuminata** are warty lesions that occur anywhere in the anogenital region and are considered an STI. Other nonulcerative lesions include **molluscum contagiosum**, caused by a pox virus, and lesions caused by *Phthirus pubis*, the crab louse, and *Sarcoptes scabiei*, the itch mite.

Finally, when considering nonulcerative lesions, folliculitis should always be included in the differential

FIGURE 16-3. Extensive external condylomata acuminata. These fleshy, exophytic growths are covered with small, papillary surface projections. Some of the lesions are pedunculated; others are sessile. (Reproduced with permission from Blackwell RE. *Women's Medicine.* Cambridge, MA: Blackwell Science; 1996:317.)

diagnosis because the skin in the pubic region has hair follicles. In rare cases, folliculitis can lead to larger lesions, such as boils, carbuncles, and abscesses. The usual source of these infections is skin flora, primarily *Staphylococcus aureus*. Factors contributing to these lesions in the anogenital region include shaving, tight undergarments, sanitary pads, poor hygiene, diabetes, and immunosuppression.

HUMAN PAPILLOMAVIRUS

The most clinically evident results of infection with human papillomavirus (HPV) are **condyloma acuminata** or **genital warts**. Approximately 5.6% of sexually active adults aged 18 to 59 years self-reported a history of genital warts, and approximately 450,000 visits to a U.S. physician's office were for a primary diagnosis of genital warts in 2014. However, of more significance in terms of morbidity and mortality, HPV is associated with cervical cancer and other squamous cell malignancies of the female and male reproductive tracts. It is estimated that the incidence of HPV has been increasing in the United States, with an estimated prevalence between 20% and 45%. It is clearly an STI with 60% to 80% of partners being affected.

Although genital warts often occur throughout the lower reproductive tract, patients usually present with anogenital lesions that they have identified or that have become pruritic or caused bleeding. An estimated 90% of genital warts are caused by serotypes 6 and 11, whereas cervical cancer is more often associated with serotypes 16, 18, and 31. HPV testing is not indicated for patients with genital warts.

Diagnosis
Genital warts are typically asymptomatic but can be painful or pruritic. The diagnosis is usually made via clinical examination. The wart has a raised papillomatous or spiked surface. Initially, the lesions are small, 1- to 5-mm diameter lesions, but these can evolve into larger pedunculated lesions and eventually into cauliflower-like growths, particularly in immunocompromised patients. In addition to the vulva, perineal body, and anogenital region, these lesions can also arise in the anal canal, on the walls of the vagina, and on the cervix. When uncertain of diagnosis or for lesions that are unresponsive to therapy, a biopsy of the lesion can be made for definitive diagnosis.

Treatment
Treatment of the lesions includes local excision, cryotherapy, topical trichloroacetic acid, topical 25%

podophyllin, and 5-fluorouracil cream (efudex 5%). The medical treatments are usually repeated weekly by the clinician until all lesions are gone. For motivated patients with uncomplicated condyloma that can be reached, both imiquimod (Aldara) and podofilox (Condylox) can be used. Imiquimod is used three times per week and needs to be washed off after 6 to 10 hours, whereas podofilox is applied twice a day for 3 days and left in place followed by no treatment for 4 days; this therapy regimen may be repeated up to four cycles. These patients can self-treat and follow up with clinicians every 3 to 4 weeks until the lesions have resolved. For larger condylomas or those unresponsive to medical treatment, CO_2 laser may be used to vaporize the lesion or surgical excision may be required. Regardless of treatment modality, a recurrence rate of approximately 20% is seen in all patients.

For prevention of HPV, a 9-valent vaccine (Gardasil-9) protects against serotypes 6, 11, 16, 18, 31, 33, 45, 52, and 58 and is FDA approved for girls and women as well as boys and men aged 9 to 26 years. It is recommended as part of routine vaccinations for children aged 11 to 12 years.

MOLLUSCUM CONTAGIOSUM

Molluscum contagiosum is caused by a pox virus that is spread via close contact with an infected person or via autoinoculation. The lesion is a small, 1- to 5-mm, domed papule with an umbilicated center (Fig. 16-4). Also known as *water warts*, these lesions contain a waxy material that reveals intracytoplasmic molluscum bodies under microscopic examination when stained with Wright stain or Giemsa stain. Molluscum lesions can occur anywhere on the skin except on the palms of the hands and soles of the feet. These lesions are often asymptomatic and generally resolve on their own. Diagnosis is generally made clinically; however, diagnosis may be confirmed with lesion biopsy for histologic or electron microscopic examination. These can be removed via local excision and/or treatment of the nodule base with trichloroacetic acid or cryotherapy.

PHTHIRUS PUBIS AND SARCOPTES SCABIEI

The nonulcerative lesions caused by **Phthirus pubis**, the crab louse, and **Sarcoptes scabiei**, the itch mite, are similar. Signs and symptoms of these two infections include pruritus, irritated skin, vesicles, and burrows. The primary difference is that lesions from *P. pubis*, or **pediculosis**, are usually confined to the pubic hair, whereas **scabies** may spread throughout the body. Thus, treatment is site specific: pediculosis can be cured with therapy application to specific areas, whereas it is more effective to treat scabies by applying treatment over the entire body. Pediculosis is generally sexually transmitted. Treatment includes permethrin 1% cream rinse applied to affected areas and washed off after 10 minutes or pyrethrins with piperonyl butoxide applied to the affected area and washed off after 10 minutes. Scabies is commonly sexually transmitted in adults and transmitted by direct contact in children. Treatment for scabies includes permethrin cream (5%) applied to all areas of the body from the neck down and washed off after 8 to 14 hours or ivermectin 200 mcg/kg orally, repeated in 2 weeks.

VAGINAL INFECTIONS

Symptoms related to vaginal infections are the leading cause of visits to a gynecologist. The vagina provides a warm, moist environment that can be colonized by various organisms. Imbalance of microflora in the vagina caused by antibiotics, diet, systemic illness; the introduction of a pathogen; or the overgrowth of one variety of organism can lead to symptoms, including itching, pain, discharge, burning, and odor. Common organisms that cause symptoms with overgrowth include *Candida* (Fig. 16-5), and the most common pathogenic protozoan is *Trichomonas*. These can each be easily diagnosed and treated quite effectively with antimicrobials. However, any chronic vaginitis

FIGURE 16-4. Two typical molluscum lesions, one of which shows a mosaic appearance.

FIGURE 16-5. *Candida albicans*, KOH mount of skin scraping. (Reproduced with permission from Crissey JT. *Manual of Medical Mycology*. Boston, MA: Blackwell Science; 1995:90.)

with pruritus, pain, bleeding, and/or ulcerated lesions that do not respond to drug therapy should be investigated to rule out malignancy.

BACTERIAL VAGINOSIS

The vagina is commonly colonized with multiple bacteria, predominantly *Lactobacillus* sp. that generally maintains the vaginal pH below 4. **Bacterial vaginosis** (BV) can develop when there is a shift in the predominant bacterial species in the vagina (Fig. 16-6). Although BV is likely to be polymicrobial, one of the most common organisms present in culture is *Gardnerella vaginalis*. BV is quite common, with prevalence rates of 5% of college populations and as high as 60% in STI clinics. Risk factors include new or multiple sexual partners, douching, lack of vaginal lactobacilli after antibiotic use, female sexual partners, and cigarette smoking. BV is associated with acquisition of other STIs, complications after gynecologic surgery, complications of pregnancy (preterm birth), and recurrence.

Diagnosis

Symptoms of BV are required for diagnosis, and patients complain of a profuse nonirritating discharge, often with a malodorous, fishy amine odor. Diagnosis can be made using Amsel criteria, which requires that three of the four following criteria are present: presence of thin, white, homogeneous discharge coating the vaginal walls; an amine odor noted with addition of 10% KOH ("whiff" test); pH greater than 4.5; or presence of >20% of clue cells (vaginal epithelial cells that are diffusely covered with bacteria) on microscopic examination. Gram stain with examination of bacteria in the vaginal discharge is considered the gold standard diagnostic test for BV.

Vaginal culture or rapid test for *G. vaginalis*, *Bacteroides*, and other anaerobes is generally not recommended because this is not a specific diagnostic method. Therefore, the clinical diagnosis is usually made from vaginal preps.

Treatment

Treatment of BV includes either metronidazole 500 mg orally twice a day for 7 days or clindamycin 300 mg orally twice a day for 7 days. Both antibiotics are also available as gel or cream and can be used topically (metronidazole gel 0.75% one applicator intravaginally daily for 5 days or clindamycin cream 2% one applicator intravaginally daily for 7 days). A metronidazole 2 g single-dose therapy has been studied. However, it is less than 75% effective in BV when compared with 85% to 90% cure rates for the week-long treatment. Patients should be advised to avoid alcohol consumption during metronidazole treatment because of its antabuse effect. Up to 30% of women will have recurrence of BV within 3 months.

YEAST INFECTIONS

Candidiasis probably causes 30% of the vaginitis that leads women to be seen by a gynecologist. Nearly 75% of women will report having a vulvovaginal candidal infection or "yeast infection" in their life. Many of these infections are treated by women using over-the-counter (OTC) preparations. Candidiasis is caused by *Candida albicans* in 80% to 90% of all cases, with the remaining cases caused by other candidal species. Predisposing factors for candidal overgrowth include the use of broad-spectrum antibiotics, diabetes mellitus, and decreased cellular immunity as seen in AIDS patients or those on immunosuppressive therapies. Yeast infections are

FIGURE 16-6. Bacterial vaginosis.

also associated with intercourse and may increase during the late luteal phase of the menstrual cycle.

Diagnosis

Typical symptoms of genital candidiasis include vulvar and vaginal pruritus, burning, dysuria, dyspareunia, and vaginal discharge. On physical examination, there is vulvar edema and erythema with a scant vaginal discharge. Only approximately 20% of patients display the characteristic white plaques adherent to the vaginal mucosa or thick curdy vaginal discharge. Diagnosis is usually made by microscopic examination of a 10% KOH preparation of the vaginal discharge, which improves visualization of characteristic branching hyphae and spores compared with saline preparation alone. However, the KOH preparation is estimated to have a sensitivity of 25% to 80%. Other diagnostic options include Gram stain and culture. Clinically, treatment is often instituted on the basis of clinical signs and symptoms. In recurrent vaginal yeast infections (more than four symptomatic episodes in 1 year), vaginal culture should be obtained to identify non-*albicans* species, such as *Candida glabrata* that may be less responsive to azole therapy.

Treatment

Treatment includes a short course (1 to 3 days) of any of the azole agents via topical applications or vaginal suppository, including miconazole as an OTC preparation or terconazole by prescription. Nystatin suppositories are less effective. Oral therapy includes fluconazole (Diflucan) 150 mg orally once, which has been shown to be as effective as any of the local treatments. Longer duration of therapy, such as 7 to 14 days of topical regimen or two to three doses of fluconazole oral therapy every 72 hours, is recommended for the treatment of recurrent cases or complicated infections (women who are immunosuppressed, diabetic patients, pregnant women, or women with severe symptoms). First-line maintenance therapy for recurrent cases consists of oral fluconazole weekly for 6 months. In non-*albicans* candidiasis, treatment with 600 mg vaginal boric acid capsules daily for 14 days is 70% effective.

TRICHOMONAS VAGINALIS

Trichomonas vaginalis is a unicellular, anaerobic flagellated protozoan that can cause vaginitis. It inhabits the lower genitourinary tracts of women and men. It is considered the most common STI with estimated 3.7 infections annually in the United States. The disease is sexually transmitted, with 75% of sexual partners possessing positive cultures. It is often retransmitted with approximately 20% of patients diagnosed being rediagnosed within 3 months after completion of therapy.

Diagnosis

The signs and symptoms of *T. vaginalis* infection include a profuse discharge with an unpleasant odor. The discharge may be yellow, gray, or green in color and may be frothy in appearance. Vaginal pH is in the 6 to 7 range. Vulvar erythema, edema, and pruritus can also be noted. The characteristic erythematous, punctate epithelial papillae, or "strawberry" appearance of the cervix is apparent in only 10% of cases. Symptoms are usually worse immediately after menses because of the transient increase in vaginal pH at that time. Up to 70% of cases are asymptomatic.

Diagnosis of *Trichomonas* is made via wet prep microscopic examination of vaginal swabs. The protozoan is slightly larger than a WBC with three to five flagella. Often, active movement of the flagella and propulsion of the organism can be seen (Fig. 16-7). However, microscopy has only 60% to 70% sensitivity. Other more sensitive tests are available, including nucleic acid probe study and

FIGURE 16-7. Scanning electron micrograph of ***Trichomonas vaginalis***. The undulating membrane and flagella of *Trichomonas* are its characteristic features. (Reproduced with permission from Cox FEG, ed. *Modern Parasitology: A Textbook of Parasitology*, 2nd ed. Oxford: Blackwell Science; 1993:9.)

immunochromatographic capillary flow dipstick technology. The diagnosis can be confirmed when necessary with culture, which is the most sensitive and specific study.

Treatment

The mainstay of treatment for *T. vaginalis* infections is metronidazole (Flagyl) 2 g orally or tinidazole 2 g orally in a single dose. As opposed to BV management, this regimen has been found to be as effective as the more traditional 500 mg oral dose twice a day for 7 days. However, metronidazole resistance may be present in 2% to 5% of vaginal trichomoniasis cases. In cases of metronidazole single-dose treatment failure, metronidazole 500 mg orally twice a day for 7 days is prescribed. If this treatment is unsuccessful, then tinidazole or metronidazole 2 g orally daily for 5 days, consultation with specialist, and *T. vaginalis* susceptibility through the CDC should be considered. Because of the high rate of concomitant infections in sexual partners, both partners should be treated to prevent reinfection. Patients should also be told to abstain from sex for 7 days after the resolution of treatment or symptoms.

INFECTIONS OF THE CERVIX

The organisms that most commonly cause cervicitis and infections of the upper reproductive tract differ from those that most commonly cause infections of the lower reproductive tract. *N. gonorrhoeae* and *C. trachomatis* are the two most common organisms that cause cervicitis and the only organisms shown to cause mucopurulent cervicitis. Clinically, cervicitis is diagnosed as cervical motion tenderness in the absence of other signs of pelvic inflammatory disease (PID).

Other organisms can also cause infections of the cervix, including HSV, HPV, and *Mycoplasma genitalium* as well as organisms causing BV. HSV causes either herpes lesions or a white plaque that resembles cervical cancer. Infection with HPV leads to condyloma and, depending on the subtype, is also an etiology of cervical cancer. Additionally, frequent douching may also cause cervicitis.

NEISSERIA GONORRHOEAE

Gonococcal infections remain the second leading reported STIs in the United States. In 2009, a historic low of 98 per 100,000 persons was reported but has increased since then with 124 cases per 100,000 persons reported in 2015 for a total of 395,116 cases. The rising incidence of gonococcal infections is influenced by region, with a 92% increase in the West and a 9% increase in the South from 2011 to 2015. Most cases occur in the 15- to 24-year-old group with the highest rates between ages 20 and 24 years.

Multiple risk factors have been associated with gonococcal infections, including low socioeconomic status, urban residence, nonwhite and non-Asian race/ethnicity, early age of first sexual activity, illicit drug use, being unmarried, and history of STIs. Condoms, diaphragms, and spermicides decrease the risk of transmission. There are also seasonal variations in the incidence of gonorrhea in the United States with a peak observed in late summer.

Transmission between the sexes is unequal, with male-to-female transmission estimated at 80% to 90% compared with an estimated 20% to 25% female-to-male transmission rate after a single sexual encounter. This difference in transmission is most likely related to the type of epithelium exposed in the different sexes. In males, the external surface of the penis is primarily keratinized epithelium, whereas females receive primary contact with mucosa of the vagina and the nonkeratinized epithelium of the cervix. Furthermore, male ejaculation increases the amount of exposure time in women, which supports the use of condoms as an exceptional prophylactic measure against gonococcal transmission.

Gonococcus can infect the anal canal, the urethra, the oropharynx, and Bartholin glands, in addition to the more commonly reported cervicitis, PID, or tubo-ovarian abscess (TOA). Up to 50% of women with gonorrhea are asymptomatic, and screening is recommended for all women <25 years and for older women with additional risk factors. Gonococcal exposure in neonates can cause conjunctivitis. As many as 1% of recognized gonococcal infections may proceed to a disseminated infection. This infection begins with fevers and erythematous macular skin lesions and proceeds to a tenosynovitis and septic arthritis.

Diagnosis

Identification of the causative organism, *N. gonorrhoeae*, a gram-negative diplococcus resembling paired kidney beans, is necessary for definitive diagnosis. Isolation using the modified Thayer–Martin chocolate agar has a sensitivity of 96% in endocervical cultures and provides the option of antimicrobial susceptibility identification. However, specific NAAT for both gonorrhea and chlamydial infection has largely supplanted the use of culture. NAAT yields high sensitivity and specificity and provides increased female specimen testing options, including urine, endocervical swabs, and vaginal swabs.

Treatment

In 1986, the Gonococcal Isolate Surveillance Project was established to monitor trends in antimicrobial resistance of *N. gonorrhoeae* isolates. Resistance to antibiotics continues to increase nationwide and dictates changes in guidelines for antimicrobial therapy. In 2015, the CDC recommended that treatment for uncomplicated gonococcal infection is ceftriaxone 250 mg IM once or cefixime 400 mg orally once with 1g of azithromycin. The addition of azithromycin to both potentiates the treatment of the cephalosporin as well as treats any coinfection with *C. trachomatis*. It is recommended to have dual treatment at all times, including if the patient has a negative test for chlamydia.

CHLAMYDIA TRACHOMATIS

C. trachomatis is a pathogen that causes ocular, respiratory, and reproductive tract infections. In the United States, its transmission is primarily via sexual contact, although vertical transmission from a mother to a newborn is also seen. Chlamydial infection is the most prevalent bacterial STI with 1,526,658 cases reported in 2015 at a rate of 480 cases per 100,000 persons. There has been a steady increase in chlamydial infections, which is most likely secondary to the advent of NAAT for *C. trachomatis* (traditionally difficult to diagnose because they are obligate intracellular organisms and culture poorly) and aggressive screening programs of sexually active women. Prevalence is estimated at 3% to 5% in asymptomatic women, and 5% to 7% of pregnant women have had positive chlamydia tests. Epidemiologically, *C. trachomatis* infections are parallel to those of *N. gonorrhoeae*, with higher rates seen among women 15- to 24-year old, with earlier age of first coitus and greater number of sexual partners.

Another reason for the higher prevalence of chlamydial infections is that carriers of both sexes are often entirely asymptomatic. Up to 70% of women are asymptomatic. If left untreated, approximately 10% to 15% of women will develop PID that may result in infertility or increased risk of ectopic pregnancies. Because of these devastating effects, the CDC recommends annual *Chlamydia* screening for sexually active women aged 25 years or younger, older women with risk factors for chlamydial infections (those with new sexual partners or multiple sexual partners), and all pregnant women. Common sites of infection include the endocervix, urethra, and rectum. Clinical manifestations of symptomatic chlamydial infections are often quite similar to those of *N. gonorrhoeae* and include symptoms of cervicitis, urethritis, and PID. As previously discussed, the L-serotypes of *C. trachomatis* can cause the systemic disease LGV.

Treatment

Treatment of choice for chlamydial infections is azithromycin 1 g orally single dose or doxycycline 100 mg orally twice a day for 7 days. Alternative regimens include erythromycin 500 mg orally four times a day for 7 days. For LGV, the treatment regimen consists of doxycycline 100 mg orally twice a day for 3 weeks.

KEY POINTS

- Syphilis is screened for with treponemal and nontreponemal tests.
- Benzathine penicillin is the drug of choice for treating syphilis. Neurosyphilis requires IV penicillin.
- Patients being treated for syphilis may experience the Jarisch–Herxheimer reaction, seen most commonly in the treatment of secondary syphilis.
- Up to 80% of newly acquired genital herpes infections are caused by HSV-1.
- Primary herpes infection classically appears as multiple vesicles that develop into painful ulcers.
- Treatment of genital herpes is usually palliative, although acyclovir can reduce the length of primary infection and suppressive therapy may decrease the number of recurrences.
- Chancroid manifests as a painful genital ulcer and usually concomitant lymphadenopathy but can be difficult to diagnose; neither cultures nor Gram stain has been particularly consistent.
- Treatment of chancroid can include a variety of antibiotics; the simplest are single doses of PO azithromycin or IM ceftriaxone.
- HPV causes condylomata and cervical dysplasia. BV is an imbalance of bacteria and is diagnosed using Amsel criteria.

- The first-line treatment for BV is metronidazole (Flagyl) for a 7-day course.
- Seventy-five percent of sexual partners of those with *Trichomonas* will also be colonized and should be presumptively treated with first-line metronidazole 2 g oral single dose.
- *N. gonorrhoeae* is the second most common reported STD, and sequelae include cervicitis, PID, and TOA. Treatment for uncomplicated gonorrhea infections is ceftriaxone 250 mg IM or cefixime 400 mg oral single dose with azithromycin 1 g orally once.
- Up to 70% of chlamydial infections are entirely asymptomatic.
- Treatment of chlamydial infections is a one-time 1 g oral dose of azithromycin.

CLINICAL VIGNETTES

VIGNETTE 1

An 18-year-old nulligravid woman presents to the student health clinic with a 4-week history of yellow vaginal discharge. She also reports vulvar itching and irritation. She is sexually active and monogamous with her boyfriend. They use condoms inconsistently. On physical examination, she is found to be nontoxic and afebrile. On genitourinary examination, vulvar and vaginal erythema is noted along with a yellow, frothy, malodorous discharge with a pH of 6.5. The cervix appears to have erythematous punctuations. There is no cervical, uterine, or adnexal tenderness. The addition of 10% KOH to the vaginal discharge does not produce an amine odor. Wet prep microscopic examination of the vaginal swabs is performed.

1. What would you expect to see under microscopy?
   a. Branching hyphae
   b. Multinucleated giant cells
   c. Scant WBC
   d. Flagellated, motile organisms
   e. Epithelial cells covered with bacteria

2. Which of the following is the most likely causal organism?
   a. *Treponema pallidum*
   b. *Neisseria gonorrhoeae*
   c. *Trichomonas vaginalis*
   d. *Gardnerella vaginalis*
   e. *Haemophilus ducreyi*

3. What is the best initial treatment for this patient?
   a. Metronidazole 2 g orally once
   b. Doxycycline 100 mg orally twice daily for 7 days
   c. Azithromycin 1 g orally once
   d. Clindamycin 300 mg orally twice daily for 7 days
   e. Metronidazole gel 0.75% one applicator intravaginally for 5 days

4. What is another important component of the treatment plan?
   a. Performing a test of cure in 3 months
   b. *T. vaginalis* susceptibility testing
   c. Treatment of sexual partner(s)
   d. Empiric treatment for chlamydial infection
   e. No further action is needed

5. The patient returns in 3 weeks with continued symptoms. She reports compliance with her initial treatment. Infection recurrence is confirmed on microscopy. Which of the following is the most appropriate treatment option?
   a. Tinidazole 2 g orally daily for 5 days
   b. Metronidazole 500 mg orally twice daily for 7 days
   c. Consultation with infectious disease specialist
   d. *T. vaginalis* susceptibility testing
   e. Clindamycin 300 mg orally twice daily for 7 days

VIGNETTE 2

A 16-year-old girl presents to the physician for annual examination. She denies any current symptoms or concerns. She has been sexually active for 1 year and is using Depo-Provera for contraception. She does not use condoms. On urogenital examination, she has a moderate amount of yellow mucopurulent discharge from the endocervix. There is no cervical motion, adnexal, or uterine tenderness. Microscopy of the vaginal discharge was normal except greater than 10 WBCs per high-power field. Vaginal pH is normal.

1. What is the most appropriate next step in the management?
   a. Perform a Pap smear with reflex human papillomavirus testing
   b. Order a pelvic ultrasound
   c. Treat for presumptive chlamydial infection and gonorrhea
   d. Send vaginal discharge for culture and Gram stain
   e. Perform nucleic acid amplification test (NAAT) for chlamydial infection and gonorrhea

2. Test results confirm the diagnosis of gonorrhea. What is the best initial treatment for this patient?
   a. Ceftriaxone 125 mg IM once
   b. Ceftriaxone 125 mg IM once plus azithromycin 1 g orally once
   c. Doxycycline 100 mg orally twice daily for 7 days
   d. Ciprofloxacin 500 mg orally once
   e. Clindamycin 300 mg orally twice daily for 7 days

3. If left untreated, this patient would be at risk for developing:
   a. Cervicitis
   b. Pelvic inflammatory disease (PID)
   c. Tubo-ovarian abscess (TOA)
   d. Disseminated gonorrhea
   e. All of the above

VIGNETTE 3

A 21-year-old nulligravid woman presents to her gynecologist with a 3-day history of painful genital ulcer. Last week she had a low-grade fever and generalized malaise, which has since resolved. She denies any history of genital ulcers. She has had four new sexual partners in the last year and uses oral contraceptives. She reports using condoms inconsistently. On genitourinary examination, several 1- to 2-mm painful vesicles are noted on the left labia minora. There is no inguinal lymphadenopathy.

1. Which of the following is the most likely causal organism?
   a. *Treponema pallidum*
   b. Herpes simplex virus (HSV)
   c. *Trichomonas vaginalis*
   d. *Chlamydia trachomatis* L1, L2, or L3
   e. *H. ducreyi*

2. Which of the following tests should be performed to make the diagnosis?
   a. *Treponema pallidum* particle agglutination assay (TPPA)
   b. *H. ducreyi* culture
   c. HSV-1 IgG
   d. HSV-1 and HSV-2 PCR
   e. Wet mount to look for *Trichomonas vaginalis*

3. What is the best initial treatment for this patient?
   a. Ceftriaxone 250 mg IM once
   b. Imiquimod (Aldara) applied to affected area three times per week
   c. Acyclovir 200 mg orally five times daily for 7 days
   d. Benzathine penicillin G 2.4 million units IM once
   e. Doxycycline 100 mg orally twice daily for 21 days

4. The patient returns to clinic 3 months later for an annual examination. She is wondering how her diagnosis might impact her future health. You counsel her that:
   a. condom use will prevent sexual transmission
   b. there is no way to reduce recurrent outbreaks
   c. recurrence is more frequent with HSV-1
   d. asymptomatic viral shedding is an important mode of transmission
   e. she will need a cesarean section for future pregnancies

VIGNETTE 4

A 36-year-old G2P2 woman presents to her gynecologist with a 3-week history of vaginal irritation and fish-smelling vaginal discharge. She recently tried an over-the-counter antifungal treatment without any improvement in her symptoms. She is sexually active in a monogamous relationship with a male partner of 5 years, and she uses a contraceptive ring (NuvaRing). Genitourinary examination shows a thin white discharge. The remainder of her examination is normal. Microscopic evaluation of a saline "wet prep" of the vaginal secretions reveals decreased lactobacilli, a few WBCs, and 40% of the vaginal epithelial cells have a stippled appearance.

1. Which of the following additional test(s) would support the diagnosis?
   a. Branching hyphae on 10% KOH prepared microscopic examination
   b. Positive NAAT for *Chlamydia*
   c. Vaginal pH less than 4.5
   d. Amine odor noted with the addition of 10% KOH
   e. None of the above

2. What is the best initial treatment for this patient?
   a. Metronidazole 2 g orally once
   b. Doxycycline 100 mg orally twice daily for 7 days
   c. Azithromycin 1 g orally once
   d. Metronidazole 500 mg orally twice daily for 7 days
   e. Fluconazole 150 mg orally once

3. Women diagnosed with this condition should be counseled regarding which of the following?
   a. There is a 30% risk of recurrence
   b. It is a sexually transmitted infection (STI)
   c. Sexual partner(s) should be treated
   d. Treatment should include empiric treatment for chlamydial infection
   e. Treatment should be initiated for both symptomatic and asymptomatic women

4. Risk factors for developing this condition include all of the following *except*:
   a. multiple sexual partners
   b. cigarette smoking
   c. douching
   d. contraceptive ring (NuvaRing)
   e. lack of vaginal lactobacilli

ANSWERS

VIGNETTE 1 Question 1
1. Answer D:
The symptoms and findings are most consistent with *Trichomonas*. Symptomatic patients report a frothy vaginal discharge that may be yellow, gray, or green. Vaginal pH is typically 6 to 7, and vulvar or vaginal mucosa is erythematous. The classical cervical findings include erythematous, punctate epithelial papillae, or "strawberry" appearance. Motile, flagellated protozoans are visible on wet prep microscopic examination.

Branching hyphae is seen with yeast infections. Symptoms include vaginal burning; pruritus; and increased thick, white, curdy vaginal discharge. Multinucleated giant cells can be seen on Tzanck smear preparation of herpetic lesions. Genital herpes is typically described as multiple 1- to 3-mm painful vesicles. You would expect to see increased WBCs with *Trichomonas*. Epithelial cells covered with bacteria, also known as clue cells, are seen with bacterial vaginosis (BV). Typical findings of BV include pH greater than 4.5 as well as an increased thin, white, malodorous, fishy vaginal discharge coating the vaginal walls. The addition of 10% KOH to the vaginal discharge typically produces a fishy amine odor. BV does not usually cause vaginal inflammation.

VIGNETTE 1 Question 2
2. Answer C:
Trichomoniasis is caused by *Trichomonas vaginalis*. Syphilis is caused by *Treponema pallidum*. Syphilis is divided into different stages. Primary syphilis is characterized by a nontender, red, round, firm ulcer approximately 1 cm in size with raised edges, known as a chancre. None of these findings were present in this patient. *N. gonorrhoeae* causes gonorrhea. Approximately 50% of women with gonorrhea are asymptomatic. *N. gonorrhoeae* is a common cause of mucopurulent cervicitis and PID. This patient does not have clinical findings of either of these conditions. BV is typically caused by *G. vaginalis*. *H. ducreyi* causes chancroid, which is an ulcerated genital lesion. This patient did not present with an ulcerated lesion.

VIGNETTE 1 Question 3
3. Answer A:
A single-dose regimen with metronidazole or tinidazole is the mainstay treatment of trichomoniasis. An alternative multidose regimen is metronidazole 500 mg orally twice daily for 7 days. Compliance may be improved with the single-dose therapy. Doxycycline can be used to treat chlamydial infections. Azithromycin can be used to treat chlamydial infections and chancroid. Clindamycin can be used as an alternative regimen for the treatment of BV. Metronidazole gel is considerably less efficacious for the treatment of trichomoniasis. The use of topical antimicrobial preparation is unlikely to achieve therapeutic levels in the perivaginal glands and is not recommended.

VIGNETTE 1 Question 4
4. Answer C:
Because of the high rate of concomitant *Trichomonas* infections in sexual partners, all partners should be treated to prevent reinfection. No data support the rescreening for *T. vaginalis* at 3 months following initial infection. This is likely because of the high efficacy of nitroimidazole drugs, with a 90% to 95% cure rate. *T. vaginalis* susceptibility testing is available through the CDC. It is only recommended for refractory cases after multiple treatment failures. Reinfection and noncompliance should be ruled out. Empiric treatment for chlamydial infection is not recommended with the diagnosis of *Trichomonas* infections. On the other hand, empiric treatment of chlamydial infection is recommended in patients infected with *N. gonorrhoeae* because of the high frequency of coinfection (unless chlamydial coinfection has been ruled out by NAAT). Sexual partners should receive treatment.

VIGNETTE 1 Question 5
5. Answer B:
Metronidazole 500 mg orally twice a day for 7 days is recommended for cases of metronidazole single-dose treatment failure. Treatment with tinidazole 2 g orally daily for 5 days is recommended after treatment failure with both the single-dose and the multidose metronidazole regimens. Consultation with infectious disease specialist is recommended only for refractory cases after multiple treatment failures. Reinfection, abstaining from intercourse, and noncompliance should be ruled out. *T. vaginalis* susceptibility testing is available through the CDC. It is recommended only for refractory cases after multiple treatment failures. Reinfection and noncompliance should be ruled out. Clindamycin can be used as an alternative regimen for the treatment of BV. Nitroimidazoles are the only class of drugs useful for the treatment of *Trichomonas* infections.

VIGNETTE 2 Question 1
1. Answer E:
In patients with mucopurulent discharge, an NAAT for chlamydial infection and gonorrhea should be performed. In addition, the CDC recommends annual screening of all sexually active women aged 25 years and younger.

Screening for cervical cancer is not indicated in this patient. Pap smears should begin at 21 years of age regardless of age at first intercourse. A pelvic ultrasound is not indicated based on lack of current symptoms and physical examination findings. A diagnosis of chlamydial infection or gonorrhea should be made prior to treatment. Vaginal cultures are typically not a useful diagnostic tool because they are nonspecific. Vaginal cultures can be useful if yeast or trichomoniasis is suspected, and microscopy is normal. Gram stain can be useful in diagnosing BV. The sensitivity of Gram stain to the diagnosis of chlamydial infection or gonorrhea is low. In addition, the patient has no findings consistent with BV, yeast, or trichomoniasis. Performing NAAT for chlamydial infection and gonorrhea is the most appropriate next step.

VIGNETTE 2 Question 2
2. Answer B:
In patients with a confirmed diagnosis of gonorrhea without a chlamydial coinfection, the correct treatment is ceftriaxone 125 mg IM once with 1 g azithromycin orally once. Doxycycline 100 mg orally twice daily for 7 days is the correct treatment for chlamydial infection. Because of increasing resistance, fluoroquinolones are no longer recommended in the United States for the treatment of gonorrhea. Clindamycin can be used as an alternative regimen for the treatment of BV.

VIGNETTE 2 Question 3
3. Answer E:
If left untreated, this patient would be at risk for developing cervicitis, PID, TOA, or disseminated gonorrhea. Cervicitis is most commonly caused by chlamydial infection and gonorrhea. PID occurs in approximately 10% to 40% of women with cervical gonorrhea. Estimates of the progression to TOA occur in approximately 3% to 16% with PID. Disseminated gonorrhea occurs in 0.5% to 3% of *N. gonorrhoeae* infections.

VIGNETTE 3 Question 1
1. Answer B:
Genital herpes classically presents with painful clusters of small vesicles and ulcers. Moreover, primary infections usually begin with flu-like symptoms, including malaise, myalgias, nausea, diarrhea, and fever. *Treponema pallidum* causes syphilis. Syphilis is divided into different stages. Primary syphilis is characterized by a nontender, red, round, firm ulcer approximately 1 cm in size with raised edges, known as a chancre. The vesicles described in this case are different than that typically seen in primary syphilis. *Trichomonas vaginalis* typically causes vaginitis, not genital ulcers. Symptomatic patients report a frothy vaginal discharge that may be yellow, gray, or green. Vaginal pH is typically elevated, and vulvar or vaginal mucosa is erythematous. The classic cervical findings include erythematous, punctate epithelial papillae, or "strawberry" appearance. Motile, flagellated protozoans are visible on wet prep microscopic examination. *C. trachomatis* L-serotypes (L1, L2, or L3) cause lymphogranuloma venereum (LGV). The primary stage of LGV is characterized by nontender papules or shallow ulcers, which heal quickly and often go unnoticed. Painful inguinal lymphadenopathy typically occurs 2 to 6 weeks after the primary lesion. The vesicles described in this case are different than that typically seen in primary LGV. *H. ducreyi* causes chancroid. The lesion presents initially as an erythematous papule, which evolves to a pustule and ulcer. The ulcer is painful with an erythematous base and irregular, well-demarcated borders.

VIGNETTE 3 Question 2
2. Answer D:
A definitive diagnosis of genital herpes should be made through viral culture or PCR testing. This is most reliable at the time of primary outbreak, with new lesions that have not crusted. An HSV viral culture is used to diagnose genital herpes in this case but cannot be used to diagnose latent herpes. A positive *Treponema pallidum* particle agglutination assay (TPPA) would be diagnostic for syphilis. A positive *H. ducreyi* culture would be diagnostic for chancroid. This patient has a primary genital herpes infection. The majority of these infections are attributed to HSV-1, not HSV-2. HSV-1 serology would also have a risk of being false positive for oral herpes. The patient does not have characteristic signs of *Trichomonas vaginalis*, and a wet mount is not indicated.

VIGNETTE 3 Question 3
3. Answer C:
For primary genital herpes infections, acyclovir 200 mg orally five times daily for 7 to 10 days is recommended to reduce the length of infection and the length of time a patient has viral shedding. Other options include a 7- to 10-day oral treatment with acyclovir 400 mg three times per day, famciclovir 250 mg three times per day, or valacyclovir 1 g twice per day. Ceftriaxone is used to treat chancroid and gonorrhea. Imiquimod (Aldara) is used to treat genital warts. Benzathine penicillin G is used to treat primary, secondary, or early latent syphilis. Extended regimens of doxycycline can be used to treat LGV caused by *C. trachomatis* L-serotypes (L1, L2, or L3).

VIGNETTE 3 Question 4
4. Answer D:
Viral shedding can occur both with and without genital herpes symptoms. It is important to counsel patients that they can transmit the virus even if they

are asymptomatic. Subclinical viral shedding appears to be highest in the first 6 months following acquisition and is more common immediately before and after a clinical outbreak. Condom use can reduce the risk of transmission of genital herpes but will not prevent the transmission. Both symptomatic and asymptomatic viral shedding can occur in genital areas not covered or protected by a condom. Recurrent outbreaks can be reduced through the use of daily suppressive antiviral drugs. Suppressive therapy prevents approximately 80% of recurrences. Recurrence is more frequent with HSV-2. Cesarean delivery is recommended only for those pregnant patients with active genital lesions or prodromal symptoms.

VIGNETTE 4 Question 1

1. Answer D:

This patient most likely has BV. BV is caused by an overgrowth of anaerobic bacteria *Prevotella* sp., *Mobiluncus* sp., *G. vaginalis, Ureaplasma, Mycoplasma*, and numerous fastidious or uncultivated anaerobes. With this shift in vaginal flora, there is an accompanied decrease in lactobacilli. Patients usually complain of an increased vaginal discharge that often has a malodorous, fishy amine odor. Diagnosis of BV can be made with three of the following findings: presence of thin, white, homogeneous discharge coating the vaginal walls; an amine odor noted with addition of 10% KOH ("whiff" test); pH of greater than 4.5; or presence of clue cells (vaginal epithelial cells that are diffusely covered with bacteria) on microscopic examination.

Branching hyphae on 10% KOH prepared microscopic examination would support the diagnosis of candidiasis. This patient does not have any major risk factor for chlamydial infection. Her examination findings do not reveal a mucopurulent discharge or any signs of cervicitis or PID. A vaginal pH greater than 4.5 would support the diagnosis of BV.

VIGNETTE 4 Question 2

2. Answer D:

Metronidazole 500 mg orally twice daily for 7 days is the correct treatment for BV. Alternatives include clindamycin 300 mg twice daily for 7 days or topical formulations of these antibiotics. Metronidazole 2 g orally once is only 75% effective in treating BV. However, it is the correct treatment for *T. vaginalis*. Doxycycline 100 mg orally twice daily for 7 days is the correct treatment for chlamydial infection. Azithromycin 1 g orally once is also the correct treatment option for chlamydial infection. Fluconazole 150 mg orally once is the treatment for candidiasis.

VIGNETTE 4 Question 3

3. Answer A:

There is a high risk of BV recurrence after treatment, reported up to 30%. Women should be advised to return for evaluation if symptoms recur. BV is not an STI. It is associated with the acquisition of other STIs as well as multiple sexual partners. However, women who have never been sexually active can also be affected. Treatment of sexual partners is not recommended with BV. Clinical trials indicate that treatment of sexual partners has not been beneficial in preventing BV recurrence. Although BV is associated with acquisition of some STIs, empiric treatment for chlamydial infection is not recommended. On the other hand, empiric treatment of chlamydial infection is recommended in patients infected with *N. gonorrhoeae* owing to the high frequency of coinfection (unless chlamydial coinfection has been ruled out by NAAT). Treatment for BV is recommended only for symptomatic women.

VIGNETTE 4 Question 4

4. Answer D:

Risk factors for BV include new or multiple sexual partners, douching, lack of vaginal lactobacilli, female sexual partners, and cigarette smoking. The use of the contraceptive ring (NuvaRing) has not been associated with an increased risk of BV.

17 | Infections of the Upper Female Reproductive Tract and Systemic Infections

THE UPPER FEMALE REPRODUCTIVE TRACT

Women experience more upper reproductive tract, pelvic, and abdominal infections compared to men because of the absence of a mucosal lining or epithelium between these spaces and the external body in the female patient. Although defenses such as ciliary movement creating flow and cervical mucus exist, there is essentially an open tract between the vagina, the pelvis, and abdomen. This can lead to ascending infections of the uterus, fallopian tubes, adnexa, pelvis, and abdomen. This open ascending tract may also lead to the acquisition of toxic shock syndrome (TSS). Further, because the vaginal epithelium is easily abraded during intercourse, transmission of systemic infections such as HIV and hepatitis B and C is more common from men to women than the converse.

ENDOMETRITIS

Pathogenesis

Endometritis is an infection of the uterine endometrium; if the infection invades into the myometrium, it is known as **endomyometritis**. Endometritis and endomyometritis are included in a spectrum of inflammatory disorders of the upper female genital tract that comprise pelvic inflammatory disease (PID). The risk factors include retained products of conception, sexually transmitted infections (STIs), intrauterine foreign bodies or growths, and instrumentation of the intrauterine cavity. It is seen most commonly after cesarean delivery, but also after vaginal deliveries and surgical pregnancy terminations. Endometritis is an uncommon complication of minimally invasive transcervical gynecologic procedures such as hysteroscopy, endometrial ablation, endometrial biopsy, and intrauterine device (IUD) placement. In such cases, routine use of antibiotic prophylaxis is not recommended. However, antibiotic prophylaxis is recommended for cesarean sections, surgical terminations of pregnancy, and hysterosalpingography or sonohysterography in women with a history of pelvic infection, or if dilated tubes are demonstrated. Nonpuerperal endometritis is not commonly recognized but is probably coexistent with 70% to 80% of PID. Its etiology is related to ascent of infection from the cervix, which then proceeds to the fallopian tubes to cause acute salpingitis and, eventually, widespread PID. Diagnosis of endomyometritis is made in the clinical settings described earlier with a bimanual examination revealing uterine tenderness, as well as fever and elevated white blood cell (WBC) count.

Chronic endometritis is often asymptomatic but is clinically significant because it leads to other pelvic infections and, uncommonly, endomyometritis. It is often a polymicrobial infection with a variety of pathogens, including skin and gastrointestinal flora in addition to the usual flora colonizing the lower reproductive tract. Mycobacterium tuberculosis is a rare cause of chronic endometritis in the developed countries but is a leading cause of infertility in endemic countries. Chronic endometritis can be suspected in patients with chronic irregular bleeding, discharge, and pelvic pain. The diagnosis can be made in a nonpuerperal patient with endometrial biopsy showing plasma cells.

Treatment

Treatment of severe endomyometritis unrelated to pregnancy is the same as treatment for PID. For postpartum endomyometritis, treatment consists of clindamycin 900 mg IV every 8 hours and gentamicin loaded with 2 mg/kg IV and then maintained with 1.5 mg/kg IV every 8 hours. Single daily IV dosing of gentamicin (5 mg/kg every 24 hours) may be substituted for 8-hour dosing. Single antibiotic agent treatment of endometritis may also be considered, including cephalosporins such as cefoxitin 2 g IV every 6 hours. Treatment course continues until clinical improvement and afebrile status for 24 to 48 hours. Oral antibiotic therapy is not required following successful parenteral treatment. In nonpuerperal infections where chlamydial infection may be the suspected cause, doxycycline should be added to the regimen for a total of 14 days. Chronic endometritis, on the other hand, is treated with a 10- to 14-day course of doxycycline 100 mg PO BID.

PELVIC INFLAMMATORY DISEASE

Pelvic inflammatory disease (PID) is an infection of the upper female genital tract including any combination of endometritis, salpingitis, tubo-ovarian abscess (TOA), and pelvic peritonitis. It is the most common serious complication of STIs. An estimated 750,000 to 1 million cases occur annually in the United States. The annual expense of initial treatment is estimated at $3.5 to $5 billion, which does not account for possible future treatment for the principal sequelae, including infertility and increased ectopic pregnancies. PID is strongly associated with infertility. Specifically, infertility risk increases with the number of PID episodes: 12% with one episode, approximately 20% with two episodes, and 40% with three or more episodes. Additionally, the risk of ectopic pregnancy is increased as much as 7- to 10-fold, and approximately 20% of women develop chronic pelvic pain during their lifetime. Sequelae, including chronic pelvic pain, dyspareunia, and pelvic adhesions, may also require surgical therapy, contributing to the economic costs and morbidity of this disease.

Among sexually active women, the incidence of this disease is highest in the 15- to 25-year-old age group (at least three times greater than in the 25- to 29-year-old age group). This may be attributed to higher risk behavior of this age group. It may also be related to decreased immunity to STI agents in younger women, although the pathophysiology is unclear. Finally, the younger age group is less likely to have regular gynecological care or to seek medical attention until bacterial vaginosis or cervicitis has progressed to the more symptomatic PID (Fig. 17-1).

Other risk factors for PID include nonwhite and non-Asian ethnicity, multiple partners, recent history of douching, prior history of PID, and cigarette smoking. IUDs are considered a risk factor for PID, when insertion occurs in the setting of concurrent chlamydial infection or gonorrhea, where the prevalence of STIs is high, and when aseptic conditions cannot be assured. In contrast, barrier contraceptives have been shown to decrease the incidence of PID, and the use of oral contraceptives appears to diminish the severity of PID.

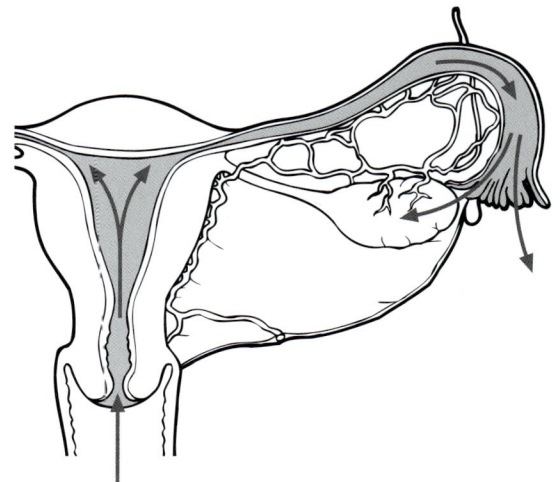

FIGURE 17-1. Route of intra-abdominal spread of gonorrhea and other pathogenic bacteria.

Clinical Manifestations

The principal symptom of acute salpingitis is abdominal or pelvic/adnexal pain. The character of the pain can range from burning, cramping, and stabbing and can be unilateral or bilateral. Pain may also be absent in what has been deemed "silent" PID. Other associated symptoms include increased vaginal discharge, abnormal odor, abnormal bleeding, gastrointestinal disturbances, and urinary tract symptoms. Fever is a less common symptom, seen in only 20% of women with PID.

Diagnosis

Because untreated PID can lead to serious sequelae (e.g., infertility), a low threshold for diagnosis and treatment should be maintained. Minimum criteria for empiric treatment include pelvic or lower abdominal pain in sexually active young women or women at risk for STIs, and one or more of the following: cervical motion tenderness, uterine tenderness, or adnexal tenderness. Additional diagnostic criteria that support the diagnosis of PID include fever (>38.3°C), abnormal cervical or vaginal mucopurulent discharge, abundant WBC on saline microscopy of vaginal secretions, elevated erythrocyte sedimentation rate (ESR), elevated C-reactive protein, and cervical *Neisseria gonorrhoeae* or *Chlamydia trachomatis* infections. Cervical cultures are performed to find a causative organism but, because of the disease's polymicrobial nature, should not dictate the treatment regimen. The definitive diagnosis is made via laparoscopy, endometrial biopsy, or pelvic imaging with PID findings. In practice, a more invasive diagnostic laparoscopic surgical procedure is usually performed only when appendicitis cannot be ruled out by clinical examination or when there is a poor response to treatment with antibiotics. Occasionally, PID is complicated by **Fitz-Hugh-Curtis syndrome** (Fig. 17-2). This is a perihepatitis from the ascending infection resulting in right upper quadrant pain and tenderness and liver function test elevations.

PID has been traditionally associated with *N. gonorrhoeae* and *C. trachomatis* infections, and it is thought that these infections lead to local inflammation and allow for polymicrobial passage to the upper genital tract. Yet, likely due to early detection, these two organisms are associated with PID <50% of the time. Cultures from women with PID are likely to be polymicrobial, including anaerobic organisms such as *Bacteroides* species and facultative bacteria such as *Gardnerella*, *Escherichia coli*, *Haemophilus influenzae*, and streptococci.

Treatment

Because of the high rate of ambulatory treatment failures and the seriousness of sequelae, patients are often hospitalized for treatment of PID. In particular, hospitalization is recommended for teenagers, nausea and vomiting, pregnant women, follow-up or ability to take medications as an outpatient, those with a high fever, or who have been refractory to outpatient therapy. PID is usually treated with a broad-spectrum cephalosporin, such as cefoxitin 2 g IV every 6 hours or cefotetan 2 g IV every 12 hours plus doxycycline 100 mg IV or orally every 12 hours because of its polymicrobial nature. The IV antibiotic regimen is continued until the patient demonstrates clinical improvement for 24 hours, and doxycycline 100 mg orally twice a day is continued for a total 14-day course. In patients allergic to cephalosporins, IV clindamycin and gentamicin can be used. On an outpatient basis, a single dose of ceftriaxone 250 mg IM or cefoxitin 2 g IM plus 1 g of probenecid orally along with oral doxycycline 100 mg orally twice a day for 14 days is used with close follow-up for resolution of symptoms. If patients have Bacterial Vaginosis (BV) or *Trichomonas*, then metronidazole 500 mg orally twice a day for 14 days must be added. PID is rare in pregnant patients; because tetracyclines and fluoroquinolones are avoided in pregnancy, clindamycin and gentamicin are the treatment of choice during pregnancy. Additionally, because of the emergence of fluoroquinolone-resistant *N. gonorrhoeae* in the United States, fluoroquinolones are no longer recommended by the CDC for treatment of gonorrhea or of PID cases in which *N. gonorrhoeae* may be a causative agent.

TUBO-OVARIAN ABSCESS

Persistent PID can lead to the development of TOA (Fig. 17-3). Most so-called TOAs are actually tubo-ovarian complexes (TOCs), the difference being

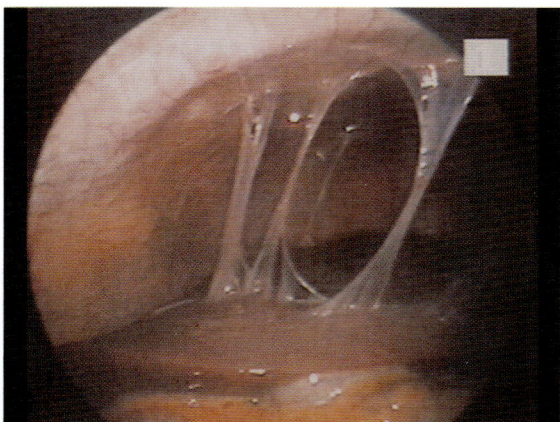

FIGURE 17-2. Fitz-Hugh-Curtis syndrome. (From Sweet R, Gibbs R. *Atlas of Infectious Diseases of the Female Genital Tract*, Philadelphia, PA: Lippincott Williams & Wilkins; 2005.)

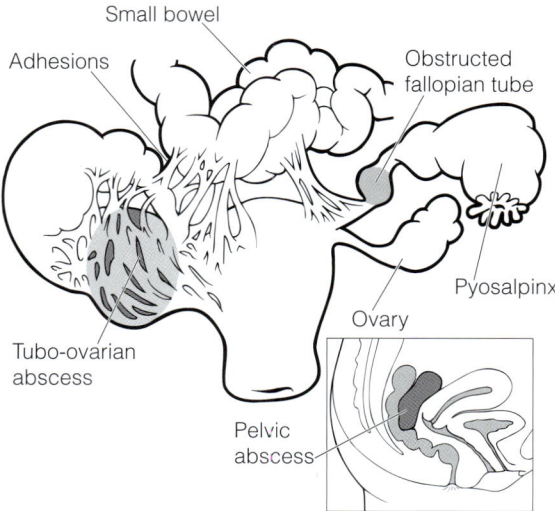

FIGURE 17-3. Findings associated with chronic pelvic inflammatory disease, including tubo-ovarian abscess, adhesions, pyosalpinx, and an abscess located in the posterior cul-de-sac.

that complexes are not walled off like the true abscess and are thus more responsive to antimicrobial therapy. Estimates of the progression from PID to TOA range from 3% to 16%; thus, any PID not responsive to therapy should be investigated further to rule out TOA. Furthermore, HIV-infected women with PID are at increased risk of development of TOA.

Diagnosis
The diagnosis of TOA can be made clinically in the setting of PID and the appreciation of an adnexal or posterior cul-de-sac mass or fullness. Most patients will endorse abdominal and/or pelvic pain (90%) and demonstrate fever and leukocytosis (60% to 80%). WBC count is usually elevated with a left shift, and the ESR is often elevated as well. Cultures should include endocervical swabs and blood cultures to rule out sepsis. Culdocentesis that reveals gross pus is diagnostic but has been used less because advances in imaging studies have been made. Although most TOAs are appreciated by clinical examination, a negative examination does not rule out a TOA. Ultrasound is the imaging study of choice to diagnose TOAs and is able to distinguish between TOAs and TOCs. However, pelvic CT may be required, particularly in obese patients for whom ultrasound use is limited. Finally, laparoscopy can lead to a definitive diagnosis but is usually used only when the clinical picture is unclear.

Treatment
Although treatment of TOAs can be medical or surgical, a trial of medical management with broad-spectrum antibiotics in an inpatient setting is frequently the first step. Unless the abscess is ruptured and causing peritoneal signs or is impenetrable by antibiotics, surgical treatment can often be avoided. Treatment is the same as that for the parenteral treatment for PID and includes broad-spectrum cephalosporin (cefotetan 2 g IV every 12 hours or cefoxitin 2 g IV every 6 hours) plus doxycycline (100 mg PO or IV every 12 hours). Clindamycin (900 mg every 8 hours) plus gentamicin (loading dose of 2 mg/kg, followed by 1.5 mg/kg IV every 8 hours or 5 mg/kg IV every 24 hours) with or without ampicillin (3 g IV every 6 hours) is another recommended regimen. The course of this disease can be monitored by symptoms, clinical examination, temperature, WBC count, and, if these are equivocal, imaging studies. Typically, a repeat pelvic examination is performed after the patient has been afebrile for 24 to 48 hours to monitor for improvement and eventual resolution of tenderness. If responsive to medical management, the patient can be converted to oral antibiotics to complete a 10- to 14-day course with doxycycline plus clindamycin or metronidazole.

For more serious TOAs, either unresponsive to antibiotic therapy or with gross rupture, surgical intervention is necessary. Drainage of TOA using ultrasound guidance or laparoscopy may be considered in patients who do not respond to 48 hours of medical therapy. Unilateral salpingo-oophorectomy is considered as a curative therapy for the unilateral TOA by some authorities. For bilateral TOAs, often a total abdominal hysterectomy and bilateral salpingo-oophorectomy may be necessary.

TOXIC SHOCK SYNDROME

Toxic shock syndrome (TSS) reached its peak in the United States in 1980, when the rate was 6 to 12 per 100,000 menstruating women. Since 1984, the incidence has decreased dramatically with only 59 cases reported in 2014. Initially, TSS was correlated with high-absorbency tampons and menstruation in approximately 50% to 70% of cases over the last two decades. Of note, the proportion of menstrual-related TSS has been decreasing over time. Nonmenstrual-related TSS has been associated with vaginal infections, vaginal delivery, cesarean section, postpartum endometritis, miscarriage, and laser treatment of condylomata.

Diagnosis
TSS is caused by colonization or infection with specific strains of *Staphylococcus aureus* that produce an epidermal toxin—toxic shock syndrome toxin-1 (TSST-1). This toxin and other staphylococcal toxins are likely to cause most of the symptoms of TSS. Symptoms include high fever (>38.9°C or 102°F), hypotension, diffuse erythematous macular rash, desquamation of the palms and soles 1 to 2 weeks after the acute illness, and multisystem involvement of three or more organ systems. Gastrointestinal disturbances (abdominal pain, vomiting, and diarrhea), myalgias, mucous membrane hyperemia, increased blood urea nitrogen and creatinine, platelet count less than 100,000, and alteration in consciousness can also be seen. Blood cultures are often negative, possibly because the exotoxin is absorbed through the vaginal mucosa.

Treatment
Because of the seriousness of the disease (2% to 8% mortality rate), hospitalization is always indicated. For more severe cases in which patients are hemodynamically unstable, admission to an intensive

care unit may be necessary. Of highest priority is supportive treatment of hypotension with IV fluids and pressors if needed. Because this disease is caused by the exotoxin, treatment with IV antibiotics does not often shorten the length of the acute illness. Antibiotic therapy consists of clindamycin plus vancomycin for empiric treatment, when specific *S. aureus* isolate sensitivity is unknown, clindamycin plus vancomycin or linezolid in MRSA TSS cases, and clindamycin plus nafcillin or oxacillin in MSSA TSS cases. Treatment duration is generally 10 to 14 days. Currently, there is a lack of controlled studies to support the use of IV immune globulin or corticosteroid therapy.

HUMAN IMMUNODEFICIENCY VIRUS

HIV is the causative agent of AIDS. HIV is transmitted via sexual contact, via parenteral inoculation, and vertically from mothers to infants via a transplacental route, during birth from direct exposure, and via breast milk. There were an estimated 8,300 women newly diagnosed with HIV infection in 2014. Women account for 19% of all new cases, and 85% of this is through heterosexual sexual transmission. Women of color are disproportionally affected at all stages of HIV infection. In 2014, African American women were diagnosed with HIV with a rate 17× higher than Caucasian or Asian women. Similarly, Latina women had a rate 3.5 times that of Caucasian or Asian women. From 2010 to 2014, the proportion of infections defined as AIDS had continued to decrease. Women account for approximately 25% of all patients with AIDS diagnoses in the United States. Yet, worldwide, women represent a far more substantial proportion of those affected with HIV. According to UN AIDS, women account for 47% of new diagnoses and 50% of HIV infections globally. Worldwide, the number of new HIV infections, mother-to-child transmission of HIV, and AIDS-related deaths is decreasing. The effects of antiretrovirals are especially evident in sub-Saharan Africa since 2004 with the expansion of antiretroviral therapy (ART).

Infection with HIV—a retrovirus—leads to decreased cellular immunity because various cells carrying the CD4 antigen become infected, including helper T cells, B cells, monocytes, and macrophages. Initially, the infection is entirely asymptomatic, although the individual is a carrier of the disease; this stage can last from 5 to 7 years. This disease may appear initially with the AIDS-related complex, which includes lymphadenopathy, night sweats, malaise, diarrhea, weight loss, and unusual recurrent infections such as oral candidiasis, varicella zoster, or herpes simplex. Because the infection further decreases cellular immunity, full-blown AIDS develops when opportunistic infections such as *Pneumocystis carinii* pneumonia, toxoplasmosis, *Mycobacterium avium-intracellulare*, cytomegalovirus, and various malignancies such as Kaposi sarcoma and non-Hodgkin lymphoma are identified.

Diagnosis

The diagnosis of HIV infection is made initially via a screening test. Most commonly, the test is an enzyme-linked immunosorbent assay (ELISA), using HIV antigens, to which patient serum is added. A positive test results when antigen–antibody complexes form. This test does have false-positive results, which, in low-risk populations, may occur more often than true-positive results. Positive tests are therefore confirmed by a Western blot. Another level of confirmation may be obtained, if a viral load is sent and is positive. Viral loads and CD4 cell counts are used to follow the progression of disease. The CDC currently recommends routine HIV screening as a normal part of medical practice for nonpregnant patients and as a normal part of prenatal screening for pregnant women. Of note, as HIV frequently coexists with other STIs, annual screening of HIV-positive patients is recommended for syphilis, gonorrhea, chlamydia, and trichomonas. Initial testing for hepatitis C is also now recommended.

Treatment

There is no known cure for HIV or AIDS. The approach to this disease is prevention of transmission, prophylaxis of opportunistic infections, and prolonging the lives of infected patients by slowing progression of disease with antiretroviral agents. All patients with the diagnosis of HIV are recommended to be started on combination antiretroviral therapy (cART). Great efforts are being directed toward prevention of HIV transmission by encouraging modification of risky behavior and with pre-exposure prophylaxis. In 2012, the Food and Drug Administration approved of the combination medication, tenofovir disoproxil fumarate plus emtricitabine, for use as "pre-exposure prophylaxis" among adults at risk for HIV transmission (HIV-infected partner, IV drug users, etc.) to reduce their risk of becoming infected. Condoms are recommended for sexually active patients. IV drug users should avoid sharing needles and use clean needles. With improved screening methods, the risk of HIV infection from blood transfusion is currently estimated at less than 1:1,000,000.

Prophylaxis and treatment of the opportunistic infections in HIV-positive patients are discussed in *Blueprints Medicine*. Delaying the progression of the disease is accomplished primarily with nucleoside analogs and protease inhibitors. The nucleoside analogs—zidovudine (AZT), lamivudine (3TC), abacavir, didanosine, and stavudine—act to inhibit reverse transcriptase and interfere with viral replication. Protease inhibitors (lopinavir, atazanavir, indinavir, saquinavir, ritonavir) interfere with the synthesis of viral particles and have been effective in increasing CD4 counts and decreasing viral load. Because the mechanisms of action of these two groups differ, a synergistic effect is seen with combination therapy known as highly active antiretroviral therapy. Multi-agent therapy also decreases drug resistance. Other antiretroviral drug classes include nonnucleoside reverse transcriptase inhibitors, and newer drug classes including entry inhibitors, CCR5 receptor antagonists, and integrase inhibitors.

Beyond this simple review of HIV management, there are issues regarding HIV infection in women that deserve special emphasis. First, obstetric care of the HIV patient demands attention to both the ongoing care of the patient and the prevention of vertical transmission to the fetus. Second, the high incidence of invasive cervical cancer in this population requires more aggressive screening than in the general population. Third, there are specific considerations in cART in women that deserve attention in this population.

In the United States, approximately 7,000 infants are born annually to mothers who are infected with HIV. With no treatment, approximately 25% of infants born to HIV-infected mothers will become infected with HIV. Increased transmission can be seen with higher viral burden or advanced disease in the mother, rupture of the membranes, and invasive procedures during labor and delivery that increase neonatal exposure to maternal blood. Vertical transmission can occur intrauterine (20% to 50%), intrapartum (50% to 80%), or postpartum (15%). In 1994, Pediatric AIDS Clinical Trials Group (PACTG) protocol 076 demonstrated that a three-part regimen of **zidovudine** (ZDV) administered during pregnancy and labor and to the newborn could reduce the risk of perinatal transmission by two thirds in women. Additionally, with the use of cART to further decrease viral load with potent regimens, the rate of transmission can be further decreased to less than 1% to 2% with an undetectable viral load. Currently, cART in pregnancy is any regimen that reduces viral load effectively, Zidovudine/Lamivudine/Ritonavir/Lopinavir is a recommended regimen. A cART regimen is continued throughout all of pregnancy and through the intrapartum course. Cesarean delivery has been shown to lower transmission rates by roughly two thirds compared to vaginal delivery in women on no therapy and particularly without onset of labor or rupture of membranes or in the setting of high viral load. However, in women with viral loads less than 1,000 copies/mL, there is no additional benefit of cesarean delivery versus vaginal delivery in HIV perinatal transmission. Therefore, cesarean delivery should be considered in HIV-infected pregnant women with viral loads greater than 1,000 copies/mL and without longstanding onset of labor or rupture of membranes. Because of the effective interventions in HIV-positive women to decrease vertical transmission, it is recommended that HIV screening be offered to all pregnant women at their first prenatal visit and again in the third trimester, if the woman has specified risk factors for HIV infection. Furthermore, in resource-rich nations, where safe bottle feeding alternatives are available, breastfeeding is contraindicated in HIV-infected women as the virus is found in breast milk and is responsible for HIV transmission to the infant. Postnatal HIV transmission from breast milk at 2 years may be as high as 15%. Furthermore, studies are lacking regarding the efficacy of maternal ART for prevention of transmission of HIV through breast milk and the toxicity of antiretroviral exposure of the infant via breast milk.

Of note, there are several considerations for cART regimens to women. In particular, Efavirenz (category D) has been associated with increase in neural tube defects, and women who are interested in becoming pregnant should be on an alternate regimen. Moreover, in women who are using oral contraceptives, the metabolism can be increased by several protease inhibitors and NNRRTIs leading to decreased efficacy of the OCPs. All LARC methods are safe and recommended for HIV-positive patients. In patients who want to use OCPs, the specific drug interaction and metabolic pathways should be checked.

The high incidence of invasive cervical cancer in HIV-infected women is an important issue in gynecologic outpatient management. Studies confirm the synergistic association of HIV and human papillomavirus (HPV), the causative agent in squamous cell carcinoma of the cervix. There are both increased frequency of abnormal Pap smears and increased progression to carcinoma in HIV-positive women. The American College of Obstetricians and Gynecologists currently recommends routine Pap smear within 1 year of initial diagnosis or with first sexual encounter. Thereafter, yearly Pap smears are recommended without HPV testing for women under the age of 30 with history of negative results. Women over the age of 30 who are HIV positive should have a Pap smear and HPV cotest. In any patient with an abnormal Pap smear (including atypical squamous cells of undetermined significance), colposcopy and biopsy are recommended.

KEY POINTS

- Endomyometritis occurs most commonly after a delivery or instrumentation of the endometrial cavity.
- Diagnosis of endomyometritis is made clinically with findings of uterine tenderness, fever, and elevated WBC count.
- Endomyometritis unrelated to pregnancy is treated the same as PID. Endomyometritis related to pregnancy is treated with broad-spectrum antibiotics such as IV clindamycin and gentamicin or IV cephalosporins.
- There may be as many as 1 million cases of PID reported annually.
- Twelve percent of patients with one episode of PID will become infertile.
- Minimal diagnosis criteria for PID consist of pelvic or lower abdominal pain, plus uterine, adnexal, or cervical motion tenderness.
- Because of the seriousness of this disease and its sequelae, patients are often hospitalized and treated with IV antibiotics.
- Chronic or acute PID can lead to TOAs.
- Diagnosis of TOA is most likely, when there is an adnexal mass in the setting of PID symptoms. Confirmation is usually achieved with an imaging study such as pelvic ultrasound or CT.
- TOA treatment includes hospitalization and broad-spectrum IV antibiotics. For TOAs not responsive to antibiotics, surgical drainage of TOA is recommended.
- TSS peaked in 1984; since then the incidence has decreased dramatically.
- TSS symptoms, which include fever, rash, and desquamation of palms and soles, are most likely caused by an *S. aureus* toxin, TSST-1.
- Because of the seriousness of TSS, patients are hospitalized and treated with IV antibiotics and, if necessary, hemodynamic support.
- HIV is transmitted via sexual contact, shared IV needles, and any activity, where infected blood is introduced to a noninfected host.
- HIV infection is screened for with the ELISA test and confirmed with a Western blot.
- There is currently no cure for HIV infection, so treatment focuses on antiretroviral agents such as nucleoside analogs and protease inhibitors and treatment of the multiple opportunistic infections.
- Vertical transmission rates during pregnancy have been shown to decrease with antiretroviral treatment and are positively associated with viral load.
- HPV and HIV are synergistic in causing cervical dysplasia, and Pap smears occur at a different frequency and interval in HIV-positive patients.

CLINICAL VIGNETTES

VIGNETTE 1

A 28-year-old G1P1 presents to the emergency department 4 days after primary cesarean section with complaints of fever, malaise, and increased lower abdominal pain for the last 6 hours. Her labor course was complicated by prolonged rupture of membranes and stage 2 arrest because of cephalopelvic disproportion resulting in a cesarean delivery. Her postoperative course was uncomplicated, and she had been discharged home stable the day prior to presentation. Her temperature is 38.1°C (100.6°F), pulse rate is 102/min, respirations are 20/min, and BP is 110/70 mm Hg. Abdominal examination shows fundal tenderness. The incision is intact without erythema, warmth, or discharge. On pelvic examination, there is foul-smelling lochia. Her WBC count is elevated, and there is moderate blood on urine analysis.

1. Which of the following is the leading differential diagnosis?
   a. Pyelonephritis
   b. Endomyometritis
   c. Chorioamnionitis
   d. Septic pelvic thrombophlebitis
   e. Cellulitis

2. Which of the following is the most appropriate next step in management?
   a. Dilation and curettage
   b. Discharge home with oral doxycycline
   c. Exploratory laparotomy
   d. CT scan of abdomen and pelvis
   e. Administer IV clindamycin and gentamicin

3. What is the most important risk factor for developing postpartum endomyometritis?
   a. Route of delivery
   b. Multiple vaginal examinations
   c. Prolonged rupture of membranes
   d. Internal fetal monitoring
   e. Low socioeconomic status

VIGNETTE 2

A 20-year-old nulligravid young woman presents to the emergency department 4 hours after the onset of nausea, vomiting, and moderate lower abdominal pain. Her last menstrual period was 2 weeks ago. She reports three new sexual partners in the last 6 months and uses condoms intermittently. She denies any history of sexually transmitted infections (STIs). Her temperature is 38.0°C (100.4°F), pulse rate is 96/min, respirations are 20/min, and BP is 110/60 mm Hg. Examination shows a soft abdomen and lower quadrant tenderness without guarding or rebound. On pelvic examination, there is a mucopurulent cervical discharge, moderate cervical motion tenderness, and uterine tenderness. Bilateral adnexa are nontender and without enlargement.

1. What is the most likely diagnosis?
   a. Ectopic pregnancy
   b. Pelvic inflammatory disease (PID)
   c. Ovarian torsion
   d. Pyelonephritis
   e. Cervicitis

2. All of the following support the patient's diagnosis except:
   a. cervical motion tenderness and uterine tenderness
   b. mucopurulent cervical discharge
   c. abundant lactobacilli on saline prepared microscopy
   d. elevated C-reactive protein
   e. elevated erythrocyte sedimentation rate (ESR)

3. What is the best initial treatment for this patient?
   a. Ceftriaxone 250 mg IM once plus doxycycline 100 mg orally twice daily for 14 days
   b. Ceftriaxone 250 mg IM once plus doxycycline 100 mg orally twice daily for 14 days plus metronidazole 500 mg orally twice daily for 14 days
   c. Doxycycline 100 mg orally twice daily for 14 days
   d. Cefoxitin 2 g IV every 6 hours plus doxycycline 100 mg IV every 12 hours
   e. Clindamycin 900 mg IV every 8 hours

4. What is this patient's future risk of infertility?
   a. 1%
   b. 12%
   c. 20%
   d. 40%
   e. 60%

5. Which of the following has been demonstrated to be protective against PID?
   a. Condoms
   b. Diaphragm with spermicide
   c. Oral contraceptive pill
   d. All of the above
   e. None of the above

VIGNETTE 3

A 32-year-old primigravid woman at 8 weeks' gestation presents to establish prenatal care. She was diagnosed with HIV 6 years ago and is currently on combination antiretroviral therapy (cART). Four months ago, her HIV viral load was 7,000 copies/mL, and her CD4 count was 850 cells/mm^3. This is a planned and desired pregnancy.

1. What is the best initial treatment for this patient?
   a. Continue cART and repeat viral load and CD4 count
   b. Add Efavirenz to the current regimen
   c. Stop cART and follow CD4 count and start cART only if viral load is less than 500 cells/mm^3
   d. Start AZT at 36 weeks regardless of viral load and medication regimen
   e. None of the above

2. During what time period is vertical transmission of HIV most likely to occur?
   a. Early antepartum
   b. Late antepartum
   c. Intrapartum/labor and delivery
   d. Postpartum
   e. All of the above confer equal risk of vertical transmission

3. The patient presents to triage with painful contractions. On vaginal examination, her cervix is dilated to 6 cm with a bulging bag of water. She is admitted to labor and delivery triage. Last week, her viral load was found to be 450 copies/mL. Which of the following is the most appropriate next step?
   a. Start zidovudine IV and expectantly manage labor
   b. Perform an urgent cesarean section
   c. Continue her antenatal antiretroviral therapy and expectantly manage labor
   d. Check CD4 count
   e. Start zidovudine IV and then artificially rupture membranes to expedite labor

4. The patient is wondering if it is safe for her to breastfeed. Which of the following is the most appropriate recommendation?
   a. Breast and bottle feed
   b. Breastfeed as long as she remains on cART
   c. Bottle feed only
   d. Breastfeed as long as her viral load is low
   e. None of the above

VIGNETTE 4

A 34-year-old G2P2 woman comes to the emergency department with 8 hours of increasing right lower quadrant pain, inability to tolerate orals, and nausea. She is sexually active and uses Depo-Provera for contraception. She was treated for gonorrhea and reports compliance with treatment. Her temperature is 38.5°C (101.3°F), pulse rate is 114/min, respirations are 22/min, and BP is 110/70 mm Hg. On examination, her abdomen is soft with right lower quadrant tenderness. Voluntary guarding is present without rebound. Pelvic examination shows no cervical motion tenderness or uterine tenderness. The right adnexa are exquisitely tender, and fullness is appreciated. Her WBC count is 17,000 cells/μL, and there are 15% bands. Urine human chorionic gonadotropin (hCG) is negative.

1. What is the most likely diagnosis?
   a. Ovarian torsion
   b. Appendicitis
   c. Tubo-ovarian abscess (TOA)
   d. Cervicitis
   e. Ectopic pregnancy

2. Which of the following is the most appropriate next step in management?
   a. Pelvic ultrasound
   b. Abdominal X-ray
   c. Measurement of serum β-hCG concentration
   d. Dilation and curettage
   e. Discharge home on oral antibiotics

3. What is the best initial treatment for this patient?
   a. Ceftriaxone 250 mg IM once plus doxycycline 100 mg orally twice daily for 14 days
   b. Gentamicin 5 mg/kg IV every 24 hours
   c. Doxycycline 100 mg orally twice daily for 14 days
   d. Cefoxitin 2 g IV every 6 hours plus doxycycline 100 mg IV every 12 hours
   e. Clindamycin 900 mg IV every 8 hours

4. After 48 hours, the patient is found to be in moderate distress. Her temperature is 39.1°C (102.4°F), pulse rate is 130/min, respirations are 26/min, and BP is 105/55 mm Hg. On examination, her abdomen is diffusely tender with guarding and rebound present. Which of the following is the most appropriate next step in management?
   a. Exploratory laparotomy
   b. Repeat pelvic ultrasound
   c. Add metronidazole 500 mg IV twice daily
   d. Consult infectious disease specialist
   e. Perform a CT scan of abdomen and pelvis

ANSWERS

VIGNETTE 1 Question 1

1. Answer B:
One of the most common causes of postpartum fever is endomyometritis. The diagnosis is largely made clinically with findings of fever and uterine tenderness in a postpartum woman. Other findings that support the diagnosis are foul-smelling lochia, lower abdominal pain, and elevated WBC count.

Pyelonephritis should be suspected in a patient with fever, flank pain, and costovertebral angle tenderness. Urinalysis should reveal pyuria and bacteriuria. The hematuria in this patient is likely due to contamination from the lochia postpartum. Chorioamnionitis or intra-amniotic infection is a maternal febrile morbidity exclusive to the intrapartum period. Septic pelvic thrombophlebitis is often a diagnosis of exclusion and should be considered in the setting of persistent unexplained fever in the postpartum period. This patient has a normal appearing incision making wound cellulitis very unlikely.

VIGNETTE 1 Question 2

2. Answer E:
Postpartum endomyometritis is typically a polymicrobial infection involving both aerobes and anaerobes from the genital tract. After diagnosing endomyometritis,

treatment should be initiated with broad-spectrum parenteral antibiotics such as IV clindamycin plus gentamicin or cephalosporins. Treatment course continues until clinical improvement and afebrile status for 24 to 48 hours. Oral antibiotic therapy is not required following successful parenteral treatment.

Although retained products of conception can cause endomyometritis, performing a dilation and curettage is not the most appropriate next step. In patients refractory to broad-spectrum parenteral antibiotics, additional imaging should be performed to look for other causes of fever. If retained tissue is found, a dilation and curettage may be necessary to remove the necrotic material. Patients with postpartum endomyometritis should be treated with broad-spectrum parenteral antibiotics. Oral doxycycline is typically used to treat chronic endometritis and chlamydial infections. Exploratory laparotomy is not indicated in a patient with postpartum endomyometritis. The diagnosis of postpartum endomyometritis is largely based on clinical findings. Imaging studies can be helpful in patient refractory to broad-spectrum parenteral antibiotics to look for an abscess, retained products, or septic pelvic thrombophlebitis.

VIGNETTE 1 Question 3
3. Answer A:
Cesarean delivery is the most important risk factor for developing postpartum endomyometritis. In the absence of prophylactic antibiotics, there is a 30% rate of developing postpartum endomyometritis after a nonelective cesarean delivery versus 3% for a vaginal delivery. Additional risk factors may include multiple vaginal examinations, prolonged rupture of membranes, internal fetal monitoring, low socioeconomic status, manual removal of the placenta, and prolonged labor.

VIGNETTE 2 Question 1
1. Answer B:
PID should be suspected in sexually active young women or women at risk for STIs who have pelvic or lower abdominal pain and one or more of the following: cervical motion tenderness, uterine tenderness, or adnexal tenderness. By using condoms intermittently, this patient is at risk for pregnancy. However, clinical manifestations of ectopic pregnancies typically appear 6 to 7 weeks after the last normal menstrual period. Women also typically have vaginal bleeding, pain, and symptoms of early pregnancy. Women with ovarian torsion typically complain of a sudden onset of sharp lower abdominal pain. Intermittent nausea and vomiting are often present. Fever and mucopurulent discharge are unlikely findings. Pyelonephritis should be suspected in a patient with fever, flank pain, and costovertebral angle tenderness. Cervicitis should be suspected in women with mucopurulent discharge and cervical motion tenderness in the absence of other signs of PID. In this case, the patient is febrile and with concurrent uterine tenderness.

VIGNETTE 2 Question 2
2. Answer C:
Lactobacilli are part of the normal flora of the female genital tract and are not indicative of an infection. Minimal criteria are used to diagnose PID. The CDC recommends that empiric treatment for PID be initiated in sexually active young women or women at risk for STIs who have pelvic or lower abdominal pain and one or more of the following: cervical motion tenderness, uterine tenderness, or adnexal tenderness. Additional diagnostic criteria that support the diagnosis of PID include fever (>38.3°C), abnormal cervical or vaginal mucopurulent discharge, abundant WBC on saline microscopy of vaginal secretions, elevated ESR, elevated C-reactive protein, and cervical *Neisseria gonorrhoeae* or *Chlamydia trachomatis* infection.

VIGNETTE 2 Question 3
3. Answer D:
This patient should be admitted for treatment of PID with parenteral antibiotics owing to her inability to tolerate PO. PID is usually treated with a broad-spectrum cephalosporin, such as cefoxitin 2 g IV every 6 hours or cefotetan 2 g IV every 12 hours plus doxycycline 100 mg IV or orally every 12 hours because of its polymicrobial nature. For those patients who are candidates for outpatient treatment of PID, the recommended treatment is ceftriaxone 250 mg IM once plus doxycycline 100 mg orally twice daily for 14 days. For those patients who are candidates for outpatient treatment of PID and who have been diagnosed with BV or *trichomonas*, the recommended treatment is ceftriaxone 250 mg IM once plus doxycycline 100 mg orally twice daily for 14 days plus metronidazole 500 mg orally twice daily for 14 days. Doxycycline 100 mg orally twice daily for 14 days is the treatment regimen for chronic endometritis. For those patients with a cephalosporin allergy, clindamycin can be used with gentamicin. Using clindamycin as a single agent to treat PID is not recommended.

VIGNETTE 2 Question 4
4. Answer B:
PID is strongly associated with infertility. Specifically, infertility risk increases with the number of PID episodes: 12% with one episode, approximately 20% with two episodes, and 40% with three or more episodes.

VIGNETTE 2 Question 5
5. Answer D:
Barrier contraceptives, such as the condom or diaphragm, have been shown to reduce the risk of STIs

and PID. The use of oral contraceptives appears to diminish the severity of PID.

VIGNETTE 3 Question 1
1. Answer A:
cART in pregnancy is generally continued through pregnancy. In the United States, all patients are recommended to be on cART regardless of viral load. This is no different for pregnant patients. Efavirenz is category D and should be avoided. AZT should be given intrapartum not at 36 weeks.

VIGNETTE 3 Question 2
2. Answer C:
Approximately 50% to 80% of vertical transmission of HIV occurs intrapartum. Twenty percent to 50% of transmissions occur during the antepartum period, as early as 8 to 15 weeks' gestation. Fifteen percent of transmissions occur postpartum through breastfeeding.

VIGNETTE 3 Question 3
3. Answer A:
In women with viral loads less than 1,000 copies/mL, there is no additional benefit of cesarean delivery versus vaginal delivery in HIV perinatal transmission. This patient is a candidate for a trial of labor. The use of zidovudine IV during labor and delivery has been proven to reduce the risk of perinatal transmission. Invasive procedures including artificial rupture of membranes and use of fetal scalp electrodes should be avoided.

Women with a viral load greater than 1,000 copies/mL should be offered and recommended a cesarean section. These women are at increased risk of vertical transmission of HIV. Women should continue on their antepartum cART during labor. However, intrapartum zidovudine IV should also be added because it has been proven to reduce the risk of perinatal transmission. The CD4 count was recently checked, and repeating this test is not needed in managing this patient.

VIGNETTE 3 Question 4
4. Answer C:
In resource-rich nations, breastfeeding is contraindicated in HIV-infected women, regardless of viral load or use of cART. Postnatal HIV transmission from breast milk at 2 years may be as high as 15%. The use of concurrent breast and bottle feeding is not recommended because it has been shown to have higher rates of postnatal HIV transmission from breast milk.

VIGNETTE 4 Question 1
1. Answer C:
This patient most likely has a TOA. The diagnosis of TOA can be made clinically in the setting of PID and the appreciation of an adnexal or posterior cul-de-sac mass or fullness. The diagnosis is further supported by a fever, leukocytosis, and bandemia.

Women with ovarian torsion typically complain of a sudden onset of sharp lower abdominal pain. Intermittent nausea and vomiting are often present. Fever, adnexal tenderness, and fullness are unlikely findings. Appendicitis should be suspected in any patient with right lower quadrant pain. However, this patient has a recent gonorrhea infection and has adnexal tenderness and fullness on examination that supports the diagnosis of TOA. Cervicitis should be suspected in women with mucopurulent discharge and cervical motion tenderness in the absence of other signs of PID. In this case, the patient is febrile with adnexal tenderness and fullness. An ectopic pregnancy is essentially ruled out with a negative urine hCG.

VIGNETTE 4 Question 2
2. Answer A:
Pelvic ultrasound is the imaging study of choice to diagnose TOAs. In addition, it is able to distinguish between TOAs and tubo-ovarian complexes (TOCs). TOCs are not walled off like the true abscess and are thus more responsive to antimicrobial therapy. An abdominal X-ray is a poor imaging technique for female reproductive organs. A negative urine hCG is very accurate and sufficient to rule out pregnancy. Performing a dilation and curettage will provide no therapeutic or diagnostic utility for TOAs. This patient needs to be treated with broad-spectrum parenteral antibiotics owing to her inability to tolerate PO.

VIGNETTE 4 Question 3
3. Answer D:
A trial of medical management with broad-spectrum antibiotics in an inpatient setting is frequently the first step in the treatment of TOAs. Treatment options include a broad-spectrum cephalosporin like cefoxitin 2 g IV every 6 hours plus doxycycline 100 mg IV every 12 hours. Other options include clindamycin plus gentamicin with or without ampicillin. The patient should be monitored with a repeat pelvic examination after the patient has been afebrile for 24 to 48 hours. If the patient is responsive to medical management, the patient can be converted to oral antibiotics with doxycycline plus clindamycin or metronidazole for 10 to 14 days.

Ceftriaxone 250 mg IM once plus doxycycline 100 mg orally twice daily for 14 days is the outpatient treatment for PID. Gentamicin can be used for the treatment of TOAs but only in conjunction with clindamycin to provide coverage for anaerobic bacteria. Ampicillin can also be added to this regimen to increase coverage for gram-positive bacteria. Doxycycline 100 mg orally twice daily for 14 days is the treatment regimen for chronic endometritis. Clindamycin can be used for the treatment of TOAs but only in conjunction with gentamicin to provide coverage for gram-negative bacteria. Ampicillin can also be added to this regimen to increase coverage for gram-positive bacteria.

VIGNETTE 4 Question 4
4. Answer A:
This patient has a clinical picture concerning for a ruptured TOA. Surgical management is necessary at this time. A delaying surgery will lead to further deterioration and septic shock. Repeat imaging would delay surgical management. Change in antibiotic regimen is not indicated. Consulting infectious disease specialist is not appropriate in a potentially unstable patient. Repeat imaging would delay surgical management.

18 | Pelvic Organ Prolapse

PATHOGENESIS

As shown in Figure 18-1, normal structural support of the pelvic organs is provided by a complex interaction between the muscles of the pelvic floor and connective tissue attachments to the bony pelvis. This network of **muscles** (e.g., levator ani muscles), **fascia** (e.g., urogenital diaphragm, endopelvic fascia including the pubocervical and rectovaginal), **nerves**, and **ligaments** (e.g., uterosacral and cardinal ligaments) provides support on which the pelvic organs rest. This is most often described using the DeLancey levels of vaginal support (Table 18-1). Damage to any one of these structures can potentially result in a weakening or loss of support to the pelvic organs (Fig. 18-2). It is helpful to think of pelvic organ prolapse in the same way one views abdominal hernias; a break in the structural fascia leads to the bulging of structures normally held in by that fascia. These vaginal defects are named by what structures presumably lie beneath them. Damage to the anterior vaginal wall pubocervical fascia can result in herniation of the bladder (**cystocele**) and/or urethra (**urethrocele**) into the vaginal lumen. Injuries to the endopelvic fascia of the rectovaginal septum in the posterior vaginal wall can result in herniation of the rectum (**rectocele**) into the vaginal lumen. Injury or stretching of the uterosacral and cardinal ligaments can result in descensus, or prolapse, of the uterus (**uterine prolapse**). After hysterectomy, some women may experience prolapse of the small intestine (**enterocele**) or the apex of the vagina (**vaginal vault prolapse**) secondary to loss of the support structures after removal of the uterus and cervix.

Pelvic organ prolapse presents with a variety of symptoms including **pelvic pressure** and discomfort, **dyspareunia**, difficulty evacuating the

FIGURE 18-1. Normal structural support of the pelvic floor as seen from above.

TABLE 18-1. DeLancey Levels of Vaginal Support

	Components	Function	Result if Damaged
Level I	Cardinal and uterosacral ligaments	Suspends the vaginal apex	Apical prolapse
Level II	Endopelvic fascia, arcus tendineus fasciae pelvis, levator ani muscle fascia	Lateral attachments of the midvagina	Cystocele, rectocele
Level III	Perineal body (connection between the bulbospongiosus, transverse perinei, and external anal sphincter muscles)	Distal support	Perineocele, urethrocele

bowels and bladder, and low back discomfort. These clinical symptoms are often associated with a visible or **palpable bulge in the vagina**. It is not typical for patients to report pain. Pelvic support is most commonly compromised by pregnancy and subsequent delivery (especially operative vaginal delivery); chronic increases in intra-abdominal pressure from obesity, chronic cough (COPD and emphysema), or chronic heavy lifting; connective tissue disorders; and atrophic changes owing to aging or estrogen deficiency.

EPIDEMIOLOGY

Pelvic relaxation is especially apparent in the **postmenopausal** population. This increase is attributed to **decreased endogenous estrogen**, the effects of gravity over time, and normal aging in the setting of previous pregnancy and vaginal delivery. **Atrophy** is associated with compromised elasticity, diminished vascular support, and laxity in anatomical structures. Tissues become less resilient to forces of gravity and increased intra-abdominal pressure, and accumulative stresses on the pelvic support system take effect. The Women's Health Initiative showed that approximately 40% of women will develop some degree of pelvic organ prolapse during their lifetime. Population-based surgical intervention studies report an 11% to 19% lifetime risk for undergoing surgery for symptomatic prolapse. Previous studies have asserted that lower rates of prolapse are seen in African American women compared to Caucasian women, but this has not been consistently demonstrated in the literature. Because pelvic organ prolapse is, for the most part, a quality of life issue for patients, it is likely that its prevalence is underreported and, therefore, undertreated.

RISK FACTORS

Risk factors for pelvic organ prolapse include **advancing age**, **menopause**, and **parity**. The incidence of pelvic relaxation increases four- and eightfold with the first two **vaginal deliveries**, respectively. Obstructed labor and **traumatic delivery** are also risk factors for pelvic organ prolapse as are conditions that result in chronically **elevated intra-abdominal pressure**. This pressure differential can be seen in the setting of obesity, chronic cough, chronic obstructive pulmonary disease (COPD), chronic constipation, repeat heavy lifting, and large pelvic tumors. Additionally, a surgical history of **hysterectomy** is associated with an increase in apical prolapse because part of the normal anatomic scaffolding has been removed.

Cystocele   Rectocele   Enterocele

FIGURE 18-2. Anatomic defects in pelvic relaxation.

CLINICAL MANIFESTATIONS

History

The symptoms reported with pelvic relaxation vary depending on the structures involved and the degree of prolapse (Table 18-2). With small degrees of pelvic relaxation, patients are often asymptomatic; however, prolapse severity and symptoms are not always well correlated. When symptomatic, patients often complain of **pelvic pressure**, heaviness in the lower abdomen, or a **vaginal bulge** that may worsen at night or become aggravated by prolonged standing, vigorous activity, or lifting heavy objects.

Women with prolapse often experience concurrent **urinary dysfunction** with complaints ranging from incomplete bladder emptying and obstructed voiding to overactive bladder. Paradoxically, stress incontinence can appear to "improve" as the prolapse worsens. As the support for the anterior vaginal wall weakens and the bladder descends, a kink is introduced into the urethra. It is a mechanical obstruction that masquerades as "improvement." For these women, it is important that any occult stress urinary incontinence is diagnosed prior to surgery so that one problem (prolapse) is not replaced with another (incontinence).

Defecatory issues can be associated with prolapse of the apical and posterior aspects of the vaginal wall and include incomplete emptying, fecal urgency, or constipation. Some patients perform a maneuver known as "**splinting**" to aid in evacuation of stool. This refers to the application of manual pressure (usually by a finger) to the perineum or posterior vaginal wall.

Although dyspareunia and pelvic pain are usually not attributable to prolapse per se, **sexual dysfunction** can occur as a consequence of embarrassment or fear of discomfort. These symptoms can impact daily activities, and can have a detrimental impact on body image, sexuality, and relationships.

Physical Examination

Pelvic relaxation is best observed by separating the labia and viewing the vagina while the patient coughs or strains, performing a Valsalva maneuver. A **split-speculum examination** should be performed by using a Sims speculum or the lower half of a Graves speculum to provide better visualization of the anterior vaginal wall, posterior vaginal wall, and apex individually. Using this method, the speculum is used to retract the posterior vaginal wall, and a **cystocele** may cause a downward movement of the anterior vaginal wall, when the patient strains (Fig. 18-3). Similarly, **rectoceles** and **enteroceles** result in an upward bulging of the posterior vaginal wall, when the patient strains with the split speculum placed upside down retracting the anterior vaginal wall (Fig. 18-4). This laxity in the rectovaginal wall can also be demonstrated on **rectal examination**. A

TABLE 18-2. Symptoms That May Be Manifested in Pelvic Organ Prolapse
Vaginal/sexual symptoms
Pelvic pressure and/or heaviness and/or discomfort
Palpable or visible vaginal bulging
Backache
Urinary symptoms
Urinary frequency
Urinary urgency
Incomplete, interrupted, or double voiding
Difficulty starting urinary stream
Urinary incontinence
Bowel symptoms
Obstructed defecation
Constipation
Painful defecation
Incomplete defecation
Splinting[a]

[a]Placing fingers in or around the vagina/perineum to aid in defecation.

FIGURE 18-3. A cystocele (*seen here via split-speculum examination*) is the bulging of the bladder into the anterior vaginal wall. It is usually caused by an acquired defect in the anterior endopelvic fascial anatomy. It can be repaired with an anterior colporrhaphy.

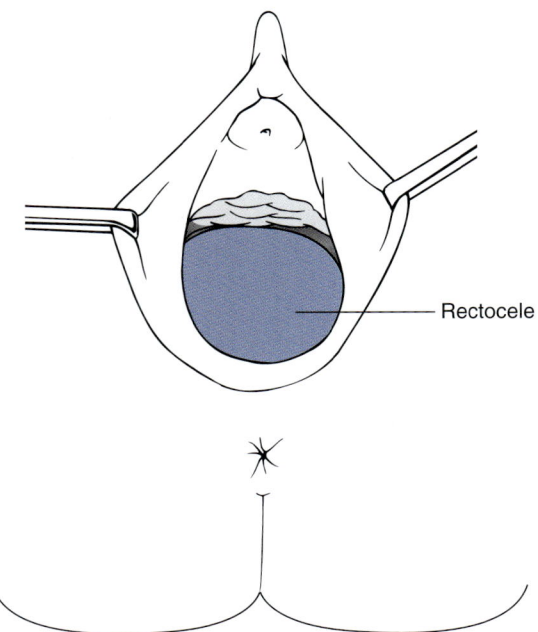

FIGURE 18-4. A rectocele is the bulging of the rectum into the posterior vaginal wall. It is usually caused by an acquired defect in the posterior endopelvic fascial anatomy. It can be repaired with a posterior colporrhaphy.

prolapsed uterus can also be viewed on split-speculum examination or by bimanual pelvic examination. **Procidentia** refers to complete eversion of the vagina with the entire uterus prolapsing outside the vagina (Fig. 18-5). In the absence of a uterus, this is called complete vaginal vault prolapse.

Many clinicians formerly used the **Baden-Walker Half-way Scoring System** for quantifying pelvic organ prolapse. It records the amount of descent of the structure (bladder, rectum, etc.) using a four-point system with the hymen as a fixed point of reference (Fig. 18-6).

More commonly, however, the **Pelvic Organ Prolapse Quantitative scale** (POP-Q) is used as an objective, site-specific system for describing, quantifying, and staging pelvic support in women (Fig. 18-7). There are six points measured in centimeters along the vagina with respect to a fixed point: the hymen. Points above the hymen are negative numbers and points below the hymen are positive numbers (Table 18-3). POP-Q is particularly helpful in both the clinical and research settings for comparing patients' examinations over time and among different examiners.

DIAGNOSTIC EVALUATION

The diagnosis of pelvic organ prolapse depends primarily on an accurate history and thorough physical examination. Other tools that may be useful in the diagnosis and preoperative evaluation of cystoceles and urethroceles include urine cultures, cystoscopy, urethroscopy, and urodynamic studies, if indicated.

FIGURE 18-5. Complete procidentia (prolapse) of the uterus and vagina. (From Sweet R, Gibbs R. *Atlas of Infectious Diseases of the Female Genital Tract*, Philadelphia, PA: Lippincott Williams & Wilkins; 2005.)

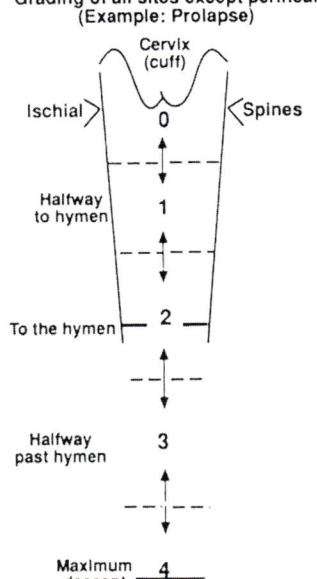

FIGURE 18-6. Baden-Walker halfway system for grading pelvic organ prolapse. In general, Grade 1 is given to a defect that descends at least half-way to the hymenal ring. Grade 2 is given to a defect extending to the hymenal ring. Grade 3 is given to a defect extending half-way beyond the hymenal ring. Grade 4 is given if the uterus is completely outside of the vagina. (Image from Rock J, Jones H. *TeLinde's Operative Gynecology*, 10th ed. Philadelphia, PA: Lippincott Williams & Wilkins; 2008.)

When a rectocele is suspected from a history of chronic constipation and difficulty passing stool, obstructive lesions should be ruled out using anoscopy or sigmoidoscopy. A defecography study (similar to a barium enema) may also help to show a rectocele or enterocele but is not essential to diagnosis.

TABLE 18-3.	POP-Q Staging
Stage 0	No prolapse
Stage I	Most distal portion >1 cm above the level of the hymen
Stage II	Most distal portion <1 cm above or below the level of the hymen
Stage III	Most distal portion >1 cm below the level of the hymen
Stage IV	Complete eversion

FIGURE 18-7. Schematic of the quantified pelvic organ prolapse (POP-Q) system. Six sites (points Aa, Ba, C, D, Bp, and Ap), genital hiatus (gh), perineal body (pb), and total vaginal length (tvl) are used to quantify the degree of pelvic organ prolapse. The vagina and hymenal ring are shown in *blue*.

DIFFERENTIAL DIAGNOSIS

Although rare in comparison, the differential diagnosis for cystocele and urethrocele includes urethral diverticula, Gartner cysts, Skene's duct cysts, and tumors of the urethra and bladder. When a rectocele is suspected, obstructive lesions of the colon and rectum (lipomas, fibromas, sarcomas, and adenocarcinomas) should be investigated. Cervical elongation, prolapsed cervical polyp, prolapsed uterine fibroid, and prolapsed cervical and endometrial tumors may be mistaken for uterine prolapse as can lower uterine segment fibroids.

TREATMENT

Prolapse is generally a benign condition, therefore evaluation and treatment are guided by the patient's goals for improvement in her quality of life. Thus, asymptomatic prolapse (typically POP-Q Stage I or II) can be monitored but does not require any further treatment, and **expectant management** is acceptable. For those patients who have significant bother from their prolapse symptoms, intervention is appropriate. Regardless of the etiology, symptomatic pelvic organ prolapse is essentially a **structural problem** and therefore requires therapies that reinforce the lost support to the pelvis.

Conservative modalities begin with exercises to strengthen the pelvic floor musculature (**Kegel exercises**). Mechanical support devices (**pessaries**) may be used to manage prolapse and the associated symptoms, or the defect may be **repaired surgically**. In postmenopausal women, **low-dose vaginal estrogen cream** can be an important supplemental treatment, improving tissue tone and facilitating reversal of atrophic changes in the vaginal mucosa.

In motivated patients with mild symptoms, a first-line therapy involves the use of Kegel exercises to strengthen the pelvic musculature. These exercises involve the tightening and releasing of the levator ani muscles repeatedly to strengthen the muscles and improve pelvic support. **Pelvic floor physical therapy with biofeedback** is often used in conjunction to ensure that the patient is performing these exercises appropriately. Although these may play a protective role in the prevention of prolapse, the available literature does not support the notion that these measures reverse or treat existing symptomatic prolapse.

The mainstay of conservative management is the use of **vaginal pessaries**. Pessaries act as mechanical support devices to replace the lost structural integrity of the pelvis and to diffuse the forces of descent over a wider area. Pessaries are indicated for any patient that desires nonsurgical management, and those in whom surgery is contraindicated. Pessaries are often used in pregnant and postpartum women as well. These devices are fitted in the vagina, positioned like a diaphragm, and serve to hold the pelvic organs in their normal position (Fig. 18-8). Pessaries come in a variety of shapes and sizes depending on the anatomy of a particular patient, so it is not uncommon for patients to try several pessaries before finding one that

FIGURE 18-8. Placement of a vaginal pessary to treat pelvic organ prolapse.

corrects their problem and is comfortable to wear. Studies suggest that certain physical characteristics such as longer vagina, smaller introitus, and lower weight are associated with more successful pessary placement. The use of vaginal pessaries requires a highly motivated patient who is willing to accept an intravaginal device and the small risks of pain, ulcerations, bleeding, leukorrhea, and infection. Pessaries may be used intermittently (interval removal and self-replacement) or may remain inside the vagina for up to 3 to 6 months at a time. Close follow-up with removal, vaginal examination, cleaning, and replacement ensures proper placement and hygiene, and minimizes the small associated risks.

Symptomatic patients who are not happy with nonoperative approaches may require **surgical correction**. In general, surgical repair for pelvic relaxation produces good results, although the recurrence rate over time may be as high as 30%. As outlined in Table 18-4, correction of cystoceles and rectoceles can be accomplished by **anterior and posterior colporrhaphy**, respectively. These procedures repair the **fascial defect** through which the herniation occurred (see Figs. 18-9 to 18-11). **Enteroceles**, which represent the herniation of small bowel into the vaginal canal, can be repaired along with the reinforcement of the rectovaginal fascia and the posterior vaginal wall. The key to the repair of any and all compartments is the re-establishment of the normal connection of the respective fascial layers to each other and the support ligaments. With significant uterine prolapse, **hysterectomy** may be indicated, although the removal of the uterus in and of itself is not curative for descent. In addition to

TABLE 18-4. Surgical Treatment of Pelvic Organ Prolapse

Anatomical Defect	Repair Procedure	Details of Repair
Cystocele	Anterior colporrhaphy	Plication (reinforcement) of the endopelvic fascia and reattachment to the apex or uterine cervix (if present) to resuspend the anterior vaginal wall and bladder
Rectocele	Posterior colporrhaphy	Similar to anterior colporrhaphy, except the posterior endopelvic fascia is identified and reattached to the apical support or uterine cervix (if present) and distally to the perineal body
Enterocele	Vaginal enterocele repair	The enterocele is repaired along with the reattachment of the rectovaginal fascia to the apex or uterine cervix (if present)
Uterine prolapse	Hysterectomy (abdominal or vaginal) and McCall culdoplasty	Hysterectomy followed by attachment of the resulting vaginal cuff to the uterosacral ligaments to decrease the risk of future vault prolapse
Vaginal vault prolapse (after hysterectomy)	Sacrospinous/uterosacral ligament fixation or Abdominal sacral colpopexy	The vaginal apex is suspended to the named ligaments via a vaginal approach Uses mesh to attach the vaginal apex to the sacrum via an abdominal, laparoscopic, or robotic approach

the hysterectomy, an **apical suspension procedure** is often performed to prevent later prolapse of the vaginal vault.

In women who have prolapse of the vaginal vault after hysterectomy, the **vaginal vault prolapse** is corrected by suspension of the vaginal apex to fixed points within the pelvis such as the sacrum (abdominal sacral colpopexy), the uterosacral ligaments (high uterosacral ligament suspension), or sacrospinous ligaments (sacrospinous ligament fixation). The degree of success depends on the skill of the surgeon, the degree of pelvic relaxation, and the age, weight, and lifestyle of the patient.

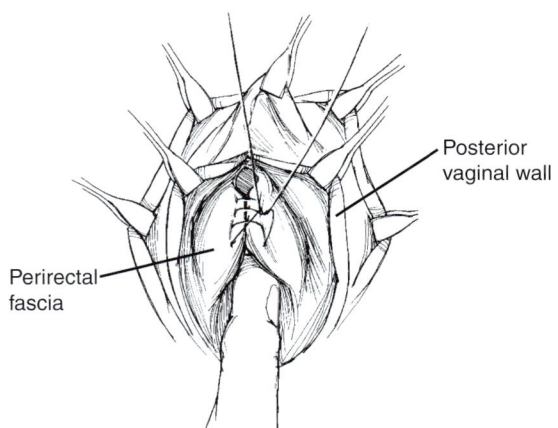

FIGURE 18-10. The rectocele is reduced by plicating (reinforcing) the perirectal fascia to the midline. (From Bourgeois FJ. *Obstetrics & Gynecology Recall*, 3rd ed. Philadelphia, PA: Lippincott Williams & Wilkins; 2008.)

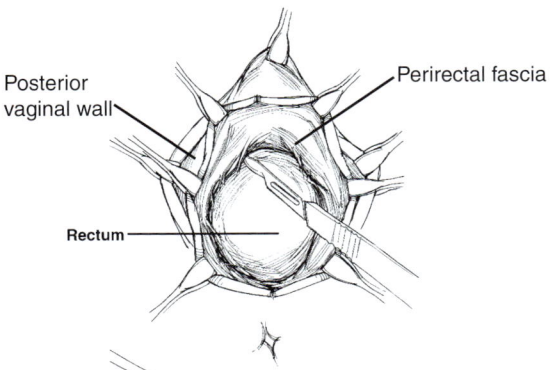

FIGURE 18-9. The posterior vaginal wall and rectovaginal fascia are incised and reflected. (From Bourgeois FJ. *Obstetrics & Gynecology Recall*, 3rd ed. Philadelphia, PA: Lippincott Williams & Wilkins; 2008.)

Similar to general surgeons repairing abdominal hernias with mesh, transvaginal mesh came to be used frequently in the repair of vaginal fascial defects in the 1990s and early 2000s. This synthetic, nonabsorbable material made sense as a replacement for the lost integrity and strength of the native vaginal tissues. Initial reports examining the efficacy of transvaginal mesh were promising, and it came to be widely used for this purpose, but not always by subspecialty-trained pelvic surgeons. Although the recurrence of vaginal prolapse was low in patients treated with mesh, other

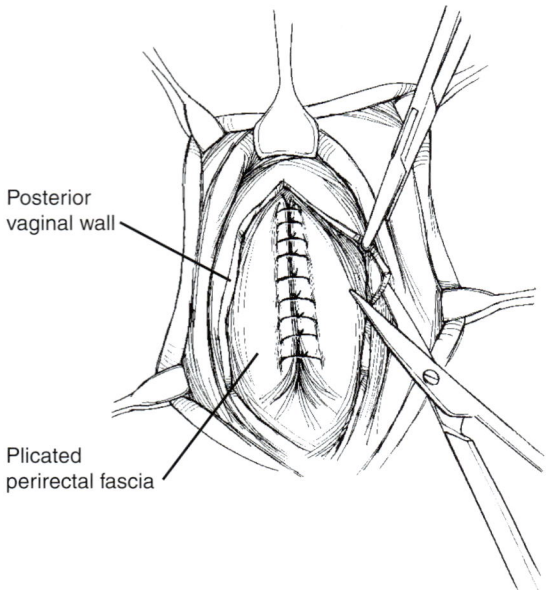

FIGURE 18-11. The excess vaginal mucosa is trimmed from the posterior vaginal wall, and the vaginal incision is closed in the midline. (From Bourgeois FJ. *Obstetrics & Gynecology Recall,* 3rd ed. Philadelphia, PA: Lippincott Williams & Wilkins; 2008.)

complications including pain, mesh exposure, vaginal discharge and bleeding, dyspareunia, and the need for reoperation were more common. The Food and Drug Administration (FDA) issued a **Public Health Notice** on the use of transvaginal mesh in 2008. After further investigation, the FDA confirmed their recommendations in 2012 that transvaginal mesh should be used only by providers with specialized training and in specific patients deemed to be appropriate candidates. However, the legal outcry over these complications created a stigma around mesh, and its use has largely fallen out of favor. Of note, although initially lumped together with transvaginal mesh used in **pelvic organ prolapse**, midurethral slings for **stress urinary incontinence** are exempt from the FDA's recommendation.

Women who are poor surgical candidates and who no longer plan vaginal intercourse may be offered a colpocleisis. This is a vaginal obliterative procedure that closes off the vaginal canal as a means of treating symptomatic pelvic organ prolapse. These procedures are less invasive with a shorter operative time, fewer complications and recurrences, and a high patient satisfaction rate.

KEY POINTS

- Pelvic organ prolapse is a general term used to denote a herniation of the anterior, apical, or posterior vaginal walls into the vaginal lumen.
- Traditionally, these were named by the organ presumed to be behind the prolapse including bladder (cystocele), urethra (urethrocele), rectum (rectocele), small bowel (enterocele), and/or uterus (uterine prolapse).
- Vaginal vault prolapse occurs most commonly in patients who have undergone hysterectomy. The vagina can then invert into the vaginal canal and potentially prolapse outside the body in its most severe form.
- Debate exists as to the exact contribution of individual risk factors for prolapse but risk factors include obstetric trauma, chronic elevations in intra-abdominal pressure, hypoestrogenic state, and inherent poor tissue quality, such as associated with musculoskeletal syndromes.
- Pelvic organ prolapse primarily manifests as pelvic pressure and vaginal bulging, although urinary, defecatory, and sexual dysfunction can be present.
- Pelvic organ prolapse is diagnosed primarily by history and physical examination, but may also require urine cultures, cystoscopy, urethroscopy, urinary dynamic studies, anoscopy, sigmoidoscopy, and defecography as indicated.
- Both the POP-Q and the Baden-Walker systems are used for the quantification of pelvic organ prolapse. POP-Q is used more commonly now, especially in areas of research.
- Treatment of pelvic organ prolapse is guided by the severity of symptoms. Pelvic organ prolapse can be treated nonsurgically with Kegel exercises, pelvic floor physical therapy, and biofeedback. Vaginal pessary use is the mainstay of nonsurgical management of pelvic organ prolapse.
- Surgical treatment options for pelvic organ prolapse include anterior and posterior colporrhaphy for cystoceles and rectoceles, respectively. These procedures repair the fascial defect and strengthen the existing vaginal wall support.
- Uterine prolapse is most commonly treated with abdominal or vaginal hysterectomy with apical suspension of the vault. Vaginal vault prolapse is repaired by resuspending the vaginal vault to a fixed structure in the pelvis.

CLINICAL VIGNETTES

VIGNETTE 1
A 69-year-old woman with pelvic pressure and palpable bulge presents for evaluation. She recalls some mention of a cystocele diagnosis, given by her primary care provider. Today, she requests formal evaluation by a gynecologist.

1. When performing the physical examination, what is one type of staging system to describe prolapse?
    a. Pelvic Organ Prolapse Quantification Scale (POP-Q)
    b. Gray scale
    c. Visual analog scale
    d. Breslow scale
    e. Clark scale

2. In discussing her symptoms, the patient points out that her voiding function has changed because the prolapse has grown in severity. Initially, the patient reported stress urinary incontinence, but as the prolapse worsened, the incontinence improved. Although she is happy with the resolution of her incontinence, she currently experiences incomplete bladder emptying, which is improved upon manual reduction of the prolapse. How do you counsel her about her risk of incontinence after an isolated anterior wall repair (with no other concomitant surgery)?
    a. High likelihood of de novo urgency and urge urinary incontinence
    b. High likelihood of urinary frequency
    c. High likelihood that her stress incontinence will be cured by anterior repair
    d. High likelihood that an anterior repair will unmask and potentially "worsen" her stress urinary incontinence symptoms
    e. High likelihood of de novo fecal incontinence

3. In assessing the above patient, you also find a posterior vaginal wall defect. What is a common symptom that is associated with rectoceles?
    a. Urinary urgency
    b. Hematuria
    c. Incomplete evacuation of stool that may require splinting
    d. Vaginal bleeding
    e. Vaginal wall erosion

VIGNETTE 2
A 53-year-old woman presents for counseling and management of her Stage II anterior wall prolapse. She is only symptomatic on days, when she has engaged in heavy lifting or particularly strenuous activity. She is morbidly obese and would like to begin a formal weight loss program. She is curious about management options.

1. Of the following, which do you recommend?
    a. Conservative management (may include pelvic floor exercises, weight loss, or pessary)
    b. Colpocleisis obliterative procedure
    c. Gellhorn space occupying pessary
    d. Round ligament suspension
    e. Hysterectomy

2. She agrees to a trial with a pessary. You choose a supportive pessary and counsel her regarding pessary insertion, removal, cleaning, etc. Which of the following are factors associated with a successful pessary fitting?
    a. Wide introitus
    b. Long vaginal length
    c. Obesity
    d. History of traumatic vaginal deliveries
    e. Menopausal state

VIGNETTE 3
An 89-year-old female patient with multiple, serious medical comorbidities presents to discuss options for treatment of her Stage III prolapse. The prolapse is externalized and becoming ulcerated from friction against her undergarments. She cannot tolerate a pessary. Her main priority is to "fix or get rid of this thing," but her primary care provider has cautioned against a lengthy or open abdominal procedure. She is not interested in future intercourse.

1. What can you offer this patient?
    a. Nothing can be done
    b. Open abdominal sacral colpopexy
    c. Robot-assisted laparoscopic sacral colpopexy
    d. Hysterectomy with anterior and posterior colporrhaphy, vault suspension
    e. Colpocleisis

2. After counseling the patient about her options, she expresses concern about losing her potential for future intercourse. She is not ready to proceed with any surgical repairs. She asks about the use of topical estrogen cream. Which of the following is NOT a contraindication to estrogen administration?
    a. Endometrial cancer
    b. Stroke
    c. Active arterial thromboembolic disease (i.e., myocardial infarction)
    d. Concomitant progestin use
    e. Hormone receptor positive breast cancer

VIGNETTE 4

A 29-year-old G2P1 woman is 22 weeks' pregnant with reports of pelvic bulge and bothersome pressure. Physical examination reveals cervical prolapse, approaching the opening of the vaginal introitus. She is worried that the prolapse will worsen as the pregnancy progresses.

1. What can you offer this patient for her symptomatic prolapse?
    a. Pessary trial
    b. Reassessment after delivery but no treatment during the pregnancy
    c. Cervical cerclage
    d. Hysteropexy (resuspension of the prolapsed uterus)
    e. Uterosacral ligament fixation

2. The patient also complains of occasional small volume stress incontinence with coughing or sneezing, only during her pregnancy. How would you counsel this patient on incontinence treatment during pregnancy?
    a. Offer trial of anti-cholinergic medication
    b. Offer a sling procedure
    c. Offer periurethral bulking injections
    d. Offer reassurance, encourage expectant management
    e. Offer the Burch procedure (retropubic bladder suspension)

ANSWERS

VIGNETTE 1 Question 1
1. Answer A:
Both the Baden-Walker system and the POP-Q are used to describe prolapse and quantify the degree of descent. In the past, the Baden-Walker Halfway Scoring System was in wide use among gynecologic providers. Conversely, initially the POP-Q system was regarded as being useful for research purposes, but with the documentation of nine separate points, it has become one of the most clinically used systems for grading POP. The gray scale simply refers to non–color-Doppler sonographic images. The Breslow and Clark classifications refer to staging for melanoma.

VIGNETTE 1 Question 2
2. Answer D:
Typically, symptoms of urgency and frequency are related to urge urinary incontinence and not to pelvic organ prolapse. However, with the spectrum of pelvic floor relaxation and its associated disease processes, it is not uncommon to diagnose patients with both prolapse and stress urinary incontinence. With advanced anterior wall prolapse, the urethra may be kinked upon itself, thus introducing a dynamic barrier to the frank leakage of urine. This is sometimes referred to as "occult" stress urinary incontinence. These patients may relay a history of stress incontinence that improved as the prolapse worsened. With reconstruction of the anterior vaginal wall and restoration of normal anatomy, this mechanical obstruction is removed, and the outflow tract is restored. In other words, once the kink is removed—it may be easier for the urine to pass freely, thus exacerbating the symptoms of stress urinary incontinence.

VIGNETTE 1 Question 3
3. Answer C:
Prolapse can be a dynamic entity with symptoms waxing and waning with level of activity, time of day, etc. Also, severity of symptoms may not necessarily correlate with the extent of prolapse. Further, compounding the issue of obtaining an accurate patient history is the sensitive nature of the involved anatomy; therefore, patients may not always readily offer a full account of symptoms. In consideration of the above, the provider should make specific inquiries about voiding, defecatory, and sexual function. With a posterior vaginal defect, incomplete or difficulty with evacuation of the bowels is a common finding, and some patients manually apply pressure (i.e., "splint") to aid in defecation. Rectoceles are not routinely associated with any of the other answer choices.

VIGNETTE 2 Question 1
1. Answer A:
Treatment for pelvic organ prolapse is guided by the patient's request and desire for symptom control. As with many other areas of medicine, the least invasive modality is recommended with escalation to more invasive methods if resultant improvement is not achieved. Although there are no strong data to support the role of pelvic floor muscle exercises in preventing progression of prolapse, there is evidence that it may improve concurrent issues such as stress urinary incontinence. Additionally, weight loss has been shown to improve pelvic floor pathology. Colpocleisis is generally not considered a first-line option, because this obliterative procedure closes off the vaginal introitus

and permanently removes the potential for vaginal intercourse. Round ligament suspensions are not effective. A Gellhorn pessary is a space-occupying device and is usually used in high-grade prolapse. With low-grade prolapse, a smaller, supportive pessary might be a better option. A hysterectomy, in and of itself without an apical suspension procedure, will not correct the prolapse.

VIGNETTE 2 Question 2
2. Answer B:
There are some data to suggest that a longer vaginal length (>7 cm), and a narrower introitus (<4 finger breadths) may influence the success of pessary fitting. None of the other answer choices routinely benefit pessary fitting or positively impact continuation rates in the short term. Pessaries are offered as first-line therapy for all types of prolapse and can be fitted regardless of stage or dominant compartment (cystocele vs. rectocele). Pessaries are available in many shapes and sizes, and many patients will maintain use after a successful fitting (41% to 67%).

VIGNETTE 3 Question 1
1. Answer E:
Because reconstructive surgery for pelvic organ prolapse is considered an elective procedure (as opposed to surgeries that are vital to survival), the severity of a patient's medical comorbidities may preclude a surgical approach, especially one that requires an open abdominal incision, insufflation of the abdomen, or steep Trendelenburg positioning. In poor surgical candidates, first-line therapy will entail noninvasive modalities such as pessaries or expectant management. However, if conservative management has been exhausted and the patient desires to proceed with surgery, a colpocleisis is one procedure that may be offered. Appropriate candidates are those who no longer desire the potential for vaginal intercourse and understand the anatomical consequences of an obliterative procedure. This procedure essentially closes off the vaginal opening by approximating the anterior and posterior walls, thereby reducing the prolapse in the process. The peritoneal cavity is never entered, operative time is short, and recovery is rapid. Generally, satisfaction rates are very high, and recurrence rates are exceedingly low.

VIGNETTE 3 Question 2
2. Answer D:
A strict contraindication or "warning" has been issued against all of the above answer options except for D (i.e., progestin use). In fact, unopposed estrogen can be dangerous in women who have not undergone hysterectomy; progesterone is *recommended* to offset the hyperplastic potential of unopposed systemic estrogen. However, very low systemic levels of estrogen can be detected in women using low-dose vaginal estrogen cream for treatment of atrophy; therefore, its use does not require similar concomitant use of a progestin.

VIGNETTE 4 Question 1
1. Answer A:
If the patient is asymptomatic, evaluation and management can be deferred until after the delivery, but this patient reports discomfort. A pessary can be used during pregnancy for symptomatic prolapse. Similar to nongravid patients, women should be counseled regarding removal, cleaning, and maintenance. This patient should be followed to monitor for vaginal erosions, lesions, or ulcerations. A cerclage is indicated for cervical insufficiency and will not address pelvic floor relaxation or descent. A hysteropexy is not an effective procedure for prolapse; furthermore, operative manipulation of the uterus during the pregnant state is not recommended, especially for an elective procedure. An uterosacral ligament fixation during pregnancy is not recommended for several reasons, including laxity of these ligaments during pregnancy, and because the enlarged uterus will interfere with access to these structures. Lastly, elective procedures should be deferred until completion of the pregnancy and postpartum recovery for both maternal and fetal safety.

VIGNETTE 4 Question 2
2. Answer D:
Secondary to the anatomic changes of an expanding uterus in pregnancy, the incidence of stress incontinence can be quite high. In many cases, incontinence resolves after recovery from the peripartum period. If the patient has incontinence that is both persistent and bothersome after delivery, formal evaluation can be undertaken after healing is complete. No elective invasive procedures are recommended during the pregnancy itself, especially with the risk of blood loss associated with the engorged pelvic vasculature. Anticholinergic medication is indicated for urge incontinence.

19 Urinary Incontinence

URINARY INCONTINENCE OVERVIEW

EPIDEMIOLOGY

The involuntary loss of urine is common, affecting an estimated 18.3 million American women in 2010, with an expected 55% increase to 28.4 million in 2050. Nearly 50% of all women experience occasional urinary incontinence, and 44% of women older than 65 years are affected daily. Urinary incontinence is often a major reason for placing individuals in nursing homes, with some 70% of nursing home residents suffering from urinary incontinence. In a large survey study of noninstitutionalized US women, 49.6% reported incontinence symptoms, of which 49.8% reported stress incontinence, 34.3% reported mixed incontinence, and 15.9% reported pure urgency incontinence. It is estimated that more than $17 billion are spent on the treatment of stress incontinence and $76 billion on the treatment for urgency incontinence and overactive bladder annually.

Urinary incontinence is failure of the bladder to store and empty urine appropriately (Table 19-1). There are three main types of urinary incontinence: stress, urgency, and mixed. The most common type is **stress (urinary) incontinence**, which is characterized by involuntary urine loss on effort or physical exertion (e.g., sporting activities), or on sneezing or coughing. The annual incidence of stress incontinence is estimated to be approximately 10%; however, studies involving postmenopausal patients show this to be up to 20%. **Urgency (urinary) incontinence**, the complaint of involuntary loss of urine associated with unpredictable urge or "gotta go" sensation, may be associated with detrusor overactivity and occurs in 5% to 10% of women at least monthly. Many women will suffer from a combination of urgency and stress incontinence; this is known as **mixed (urinary) incontinence**.

TABLE 19-1. Types of Urinary Incontinence

Stress (urinary) incontinence	
Involuntary loss of urine on effort or physical exertion, or on sneezing or coughing	
Urgency (urinary) incontinence	
Involuntary loss of urine associated with urgency	
Mixed (urinary) incontinence	
Involuntary loss of urine associated with urgency and also with effort or physical exertion or on sneezing or coughing	
Overflow (urinary) incontinence	
The loss of urine due to poor or absent bladder contractions or bladder outlet obstruction that leads to urinary retention with overdistension of the bladder and overflow incontinence	
Continuous (urinary) incontinence	
The loss of urine at all times, possibly due to a urinary fistula secondary to surgery, radiation, or obstructed labor	
Functional (urinary) incontinence	
The loss of urine due to a physical or psychological (e.g., dementia) inability to respond to voiding cues. Often seen in nursing home patients and geriatric patients	

There are several other less common conditions that lead to involuntary loss of urine (Table 19-1). **Urinary retention** secondary to detrusor underactivity, an acontractile detrusor, or bladder outlet obstruction can result in urinary incontinence; this is often referred to as **overflow (urinary) incontinence** and is much more common in men. Conditions that may be associated with this type of incontinence include diabetes, neurologic diseases, severe genital prolapse, and postsurgical obstruction from urinary continence procedures. Bypass (urinary) incontinence or **continuous (urinary) incontinence** is typically the result of a **urinary fistula** formed between the urinary tract and the vagina, but can also be the result of a urethral diverticulum or ectopic ureter. In the United States, almost all cases of urinary fistula result from pelvic surgery or pelvic radiation; whereas in developing countries, the etiology is usually obstetric birth trauma and obstructed labor. **Functional (urinary) incontinence** can result when a woman has any condition that interferes with her ability to reach a toilet in a timely fashion or attend to her toileting needs; this includes cognitive, psychological, or physical impairments. This type of incontinence is often seen in the elderly with limited mobility and those with dementia.

RISK FACTORS

Age is an important risk factor for all types of urinary incontinence. The prevalence of urinary incontinence increases as women age. Stress incontinence is more predominant in younger and middle-aged women, whereas urgency incontinence and mixed incontinence are more predominant in older women. The effect of **menopause and hormonal status** on urinary incontinence has been investigated in several studies with conflicting results. In postmenopausal women, low estrogen levels may contribute to urinary incontinence. Treatment with local (vaginal) estrogen was shown to improve symptoms, whereas oral hormone replacement therapy worsened symptoms. **Obesity** has been shown to be a significant risk factor for urinary incontinence in multiple large-scale studies, with a greater impact on stress incontinence compared with urgency and mixed incontinence. **Type 2 diabetes mellitus** is a strong independent risk factor for urinary incontinence, particularly urgency incontinence. Pregnancy, vaginal delivery, pelvic surgery, medication (e.g., α-blockers), smoking, and genetic factors have also all been implicated as risk factors for urinary incontinence. Table 19-2 delineates the risk factors specific to stress urinary incontinence.

PATHOPHYSIOLOGY

Understanding the anatomy and physiology of the lower urinary tract and pelvic floor is crucial to understanding the mechanism behind each type of urinary incontinence. The bladder, or **detrusor muscle**, is a meshwork of smooth muscle layers ending in the trigone area at its base (Fig. 19-1). The **internal sphincter** is at the junction of the bladder and the urethra. This is also known as the **urethrovesical junction**. The urethra is also made of smooth muscle. It is suspended by the pubourethral ligaments that originate at the lower pubic bone and extend to the middle third of the urethra to form the **external sphincter**.

Urinary continence at rest is possible because the **intraurethral pressure** exceeds the **intravesical pressure**. Continuous contraction of the internal sphincter is one of the primary mechanisms for maintaining continence at rest. The external sphincter provides about 50% of urethral resistance and is the second line of defense against incontinence. When the urethrovesical junction is in its proper position, any sudden increase in intra-abdominal pressure is transmitted equally to the bladder and proximal third of the urethra. Therefore, as long as the intraurethral pressure exceeds the intravesical pressure, continence is preserved.

TABLE 19-2. Risk Factors for Urinary Stress Incontinence

Age
Obesity
Diabetes mellitus
Pregnancy and vaginal delivery
Genetics
Hormonal status
Pelvic surgery
Smoking
Chronic cough
Medications

FIGURE 19-1. Location of various structures along the urethra. (From Kursh ED, McGuire EJ. *Female Urology*, Philadelphia, PA: J. B. Lippincott Company; 1994.)

In addition to the internal and external sphincters, continence is also maintained via the action of the muscles of the pelvic floor and the **submucosal vasculature** of the urethra. When this vasculature complex fills with blood, the intraurethral pressure is increased, thus preventing involuntary loss of urine.

Neurologic control of the bladder and urethra is provided by both the **autonomic system** (sympathetic and parasympathetic) and the **somatic nervous system** (Fig. 19-2). The sympathetic nervous system provides continence and prevents micturition by contracting the bladder neck and internal sphincter via α-1 adrenoreceptors. Sympathetic control of the bladder is achieved via the **hypogastric nerve** originating from T10 to L2 of the spinal cord. The parasympathetic nervous system allows micturition to occur by contraction of the detrusor muscle via β-2 adrenoreceptors and muscarinic acetylcholine M_3 receptors. Parasympathetic control of the bladder is supplied by the **pelvic nerve** derived from S2, S3, and S4 of the spinal cord. Finally, the somatic nervous system aids in voluntary prevention of micturition by innervating the striated muscle of the external sphincter and pelvic floor through the **pudendal nerve**.

During micturition, the bladder releases its contents under voluntary control through a series of coordinated activities, resulting in urethral relaxation and bladder contraction. Stretch receptors in the bladder wall send a signal to the central nervous system to begin voluntary voiding. This triggers inhibition of the sympathetic sacral and pudendal nerves, thereby causing relaxation of the urethra, external sphincter, and levator ani muscles. This is closely followed by the activation of the parasympathetic pelvic nerve, resulting in contraction of the detrusor muscle, and micturition begins.

HISTORY

Care of all patients with urinary incontinence should begin with obtaining a thorough medical and surgical history. Terminology developed by the International Continence Society (ICS) and International Urogynecological Association (IUGA) can be helpful in

FIGURE 19-2. Innervation of the lower urinary tract.

TABLE 19-3. IUGA/ICS Terminology for Symptoms of Pelvic Floor Dysfunction

Urinary incontinence symptoms		
Incontinence	Positional	Insensible (unaware)
Stress incontinence	Nocturnal	Coital incontinence
Urge incontinence	Continuous	Mixed symptomatology
Bladder storage symptoms		
Daytime frequency	Urgency	Nocturia
Sensory symptoms		
Increased bladder sensation	Reduced bladder sensation	Absent bladder sensation
Voiding symptoms		
Hesitancy	Straining	Immediate revoiding
Slow stream	Spraying	Postvoid leakage
Intermittency	Incomplete emptying	Position-dependent voiding
Dysuria	Retention	
Prolapse symptoms		
Vaginal bulging	Bleeding, discharge, infection	Low back pain
Pelvic pressure	Splinting/digitation	
Sexual dysfunction		
Dyspareunia	Deep dyspareunia	Vaginal laxity
Introital dyspareunia	Obstructed intercourse	Other symptoms
Anorectal dysfunction		
Anal incontinence	Straining	Rectal prolapse
Fecal incontinence	Incomplete evacuation	Rectal bleeding/mucus
Fecal urgency	Diminished rectal sensation	Coital fecal incontinence
Fecal urgency	Constipation	Passive fecal incontinence
Lower urinary tract pain/pelvic pain		
Bladder pain	Vulvar pain	Perineal pain
Urethral pain	Vaginal pain	Pelvic pain
Lower UTI		
UTI	Recurrent UTI	Hematuria

UTI, urinary tract infection.
From Haylen BT, de Ridder D, Freeman RM, et al. An International Urogynecological Association (IUGA)/International Continence Society (ICS) joint report on the terminology for female pelvic floor dysfunction. *Int Urogynecol J.* 21:5–26, 2010.

obtaining and documenting the patients symptoms. These include symptoms discreetly categorized into a comprehensive, user-friendly, female-specific, clinically based system (Table 19-3).

PHYSICAL EXAMINATION

The physical examination should include both internal and external pelvic examinations. Pelvic organ prolapse is often found in patients with urinary incontinence and should be evaluated and documented. Because the innervation of the lower urinary tract is closely associated with the innervation of the lower extremities and rectum, patients should receive a thorough **neurologic examination**. In particular, deep tendon reflexes, anal reflex, pelvic floor contractions, and the bulbocavernosus reflex should be elicited.

DIAGNOSTIC EVALUATION

Fortunately, a variety of diagnostic tests are available for the evaluation of urinary incontinence. The scope of this text precludes an exhaustive compilation of every diagnostic modality. In general, the goal of

Number of pads changed today: 1
Type of pad used: Maxi pad

	Urinate in toilet (time and amount)		Accident (time)	Activity during accident	Fluid intake (time, type, amount)
To Bed →	2200	240 cc			1 glass water
	0300	660 cc	0300	Leak on way to bathroom	
	0500	540 cc	0500	Preparing to urinate	
Up For Day →	0700	150 cc			16 oz coffee 1 cup water
	0845	35 cc			
	1145	160 cc			
	1200				16 oz lemonade
	1540	60 cc			
	1800	100 cc			2 glasses wine 2 cups water
	1940	60 cc			16 oz diet coke 1 glass water

FIGURE 19-3. Voiding diary (also called bladder chart). This patient's diary demonstrates urinary frequency, nocturia, urge incontinence, and greater consumption of fluid, caffeine, and alcohol in the evening. (From Berek JS. *Berek & Novak's Gynecology*, 14th ed. Philadelphia, PA: Lippincott Williams & Wilkins; 2006.)

diagnostic testing is to distinguish between stress incontinence and urgency incontinence because the treatments for these two conditions are very different. Initial tests typically include the stress test, the cotton-swab test, cystometrogram, and uroflowmetry. More complex urodynamic studies can be obtained when indicated (considering surgery, patient 65 years or older, complicated history, prior urogynecologic surgery, underlying neurologic disease, etc.).

A voiding diary or bladder chart (Fig. 19-3) can be used to document the specific circumstances of the patient's voiding habits (e.g., intake, amount voided, leak volume, associated activity, and urgency presence). A **urinalysis** with microscopy and **urine culture** should be obtained to rule-out infection as a cause of incontinence.

A **stress test** is performed by filling the bladder with up to 300 mL of normal saline or sterile water through a catheter. The patient is asked to cough, and the clinician observes to verify the loss of urine. This can be done standing or in the lithotomy position. If urine leakage is witnessed by the clinician, the patient is then said to have **genuine stress incontinence**. A **postvoid residual** (PVR) is obtained by catheterization of the bladder after voiding. This specimen can then be used to rule-out urinary retention and infection. An alternative is to measure the PVR with an ultrasound bladder scanner. The upper limits of a normal PVR have been reported as 50 to 100 mL.

The purpose of the **cotton-swab test** is to diagnose a hypermobile urethra associated with stress incontinence. The clinician inserts a lubricated cotton swab into the urethra to the angle of the urethrovesical junction (Fig. 19-4). When the patient strains as if urinating, the urethrovesical junction descends, and the cotton swab moves upward. The change in cotton-swab angle is normally less than 30° (Fig. 19-4A), and a value of greater than 30° is consistent with a hypermobile urethra (Fig. 19-4B). This factor becomes important when considering different treatment modalities later on.

Urodynamics, the functional study of the lower urinary tract, is usually reserved for patients contemplating surgery and for those in whom a clear diagnosis cannot be made on preliminary tests. This test is performed in the clinic, while the patient is positioned in a special uroflow or "birthing" chair and takes approximately one hour to complete. Small pressure catheters are placed in the bladder, the urethra, and the rectum or vagina (Fig. 19-5). The rectal or vaginal pressure catheter acts as an approximation of the intra-abdominal pressure. Detrusor

A: During the cotton swab test, a swab is placed in the urethra to the bladder neck. Normal movement of the UVJ with Valsalva (straining) should be less than 30°.

B: When pelvic relaxation results in hypermobility of the bladder neck, there is a large change (30° to 60°) of the UVJ with Valsalva (straining).

FIGURE 19-4. (**A, B**) Cotton-swab test. UVJ, urethrovesical junction.

FIGURE 19-5. Complex cystometry. (From Wall LL, Norton PA, DeLancy JOL. *Practical Urogynecology*, Baltimore, MD: Williams & Wilkins; 2003.)

pressure is calculated by subtracting the abdominal pressure from the intravesical pressure. The three major components of urodynamic studies include evaluation of **urethral function** (urethrocystometry and urethral pressure profilometry), **bladder filling** (cystometry), and **bladder emptying** (uroflowmetry and voiding cystometry or pressure flow studies).

As part of urodynamic testing, **cystometry** measures the pressure and volume relationship of the bladder during filling and/or pressure flow study during voiding. It also assesses bladder sensation, bladder capacity, detrusor activity, and bladder compliance. The sensation to void typically occurs after the bladder is instilled with 150 mL of fluid. Normal bladder capacity is 400 to 600 mL.

Urodynamic measurements may also include **uroflowmetry**, which measures the rate of urine flow and flow time through the urethra, when a patient is asked to spontaneously void while sitting on an uroflow chair. Uroflowmetry is useful in diagnosing outflow obstruction and abnormal bladder reflexes, especially in patients complaining of hesitancy, incomplete bladder emptying, poor stream, and urinary retention.

STRESS INCONTINENCE

PATHOGENESIS

Stress incontinence is the involuntary loss of urine through the intact urethra in response to an increase in **intra-abdominal pressure** such as coughing, sneezing, or exercise. In many cases, patients with stress incontinence will have a **hypermobile urethra**. As a result, increases in intra-abdominal pressure are no longer transmitted equally to the bladder and urethra. Instead, increases in intra-abdominal pressure are transmitted primarily to the bladder. Therefore, because intravesical pressures exceed intraurethral pressure, urinary stress incontinence occurs (Fig. 19-6). In 1990, the **integral theory** was introduced by

FIGURE 19-6. Patient with urinary stress incontinence.

Petros and Umsten. This landmark theory proposes that the control of urethral closure is mainly the interplay of the pubourethral ligaments, suburethral vaginal hammock, and pubococcygeus muscles. This theory led to the development of midurethral slings. DeLancey introduced the hammock theory in 1994, which states that the urethra lies on the supportive layer of the endopelvic fascia and anterior vaginal wall. This supportive layer gains structural support through its lateral attachments to the arcus tendineus fascia and levator ani muscles. During a cough, the urethra is compressed against this hammock-like supportive layer with a resultant increase in urethral closure pressure. Therefore, women in whom this structure has been compromised will report symptoms of stress urinary incontinence. In a smaller percentage of women, stress urinary incontinence may be due to weakness in the internal urethral sphincter known as **intrinsic sphincter deficiency** (ISD).

HISTORY

Patients with stress incontinence may present with a complaint of involuntary loss of urine with coughing, laughing, sneezing, exercise, or straining. With more severe stress incontinence, urine leakage may occur with activities that cause even small increases in intra-abdominal pressure, such as walking, standing, or changing positions.

DIAGNOSTIC EVALUATION

Leakage of urine with an increase in intra-abdominal pressure (coughing, jumping, and Valsalva effort) during either a simple stress test or more complex urodynamics can be used to make the diagnosis of stress incontinence. Urodynamics are not necessarily indicated, when genuine stress urinary incontinence is demonstrated on examination and should be reserved for elucidating more complex presentations of incontinence.

TREATMENT

Treatment of stress incontinence includes a multi-faceted approach, including lifestyle and behavioral modifications, and medical and surgical managements.

Lifestyle and behavioral modifications include weight loss, caffeine restriction, fluid management, bladder training, pelvic floor muscle exercises (**Kegel exercises**), and physical therapy (biofeedback, magnetic therapy, and electrical stimulation). Pelvic floor muscle exercises result in an increase in resting and active muscle tone and thereby increase urethral closing pressure.

Medical therapy for the treatment of stress incontinence is limited, and no mediations are Food and Drug Administration (FDA) approved for this purpose. The use of **systemic estrogen** to treat stress incontinence has been studied, but has not been shown to improve the symptoms and may worsen or lead to the development of stress incontinence in some women. Low-dose **vaginal estrogen** does appear to be helpful in management of stress urinary incontinence in peri- and postmenopausal women.

Incontinence pessaries and other intravaginal devices are used to physically elevate and support the urethra, which restores normal anatomic relationships. As a result, increases in intra-abdominal pressures are transmitted equally to the bladder and urethra, and continence is maintained. Incontinence pessaries differ from pessaries for pelvic organ prolapse in that incontinence pessaries have added features to specifically support the urethra (Fig. 19-7). Because pessaries are noninvasive, they are useful in patients for whom surgery is contraindicated (elderly, ill, or pregnant women). These devices require close medical supervision to avoid infection of the vaginal epithelium or damage to the vaginal tissues. Patients are often given vaginal estrogen cream to decrease the risk of vaginal trauma and ulceration.

Surgery is frequently the treatment of choice for stress incontinence. Several approaches have been employed with roughly equal success. These include the abdominal retropubic urethropexies (Burch procedures), bladder neck slings, and **tension-free midurethral slings** (tension-free vaginal tape and transobturator tape). Most of the abdominal procedures and bladder neck slings aim to resuspend the hypermobile urethra to its normal anatomic position (Fig. 19-8), whereas the aim of the **tension-free midurethral sling** is to provide reinforcement at the midurethra to the pubic bone, suburethral vaginal hammock, and pubococcygeus muscles. Disadvantages of surgery include the risks of an invasive procedure and the risk of failure with resumption of symptoms over time.

The most widely performed surgery for stress urinary incontinence is the tension-free midurethral sling because of its ease of placement, short operative time, small incisions, and quick patient recovery time. It is important to note that although this procedure does include the implantation of a permanent mesh in the vagina, this is different than the transvaginal mesh used in the treatment of pelvic organ prolapse. The mesh for midurethral slings is exempt from the FDA's **Public Health Notice** on transvaginal

FIGURE 19-7. Vaginal incontinence pessaries for treating stress urinary incontinence. Incontinence pessaries differ from more common prolapse pessaries in that most incontinence pessaries have a portion of the device specifically designed to support the bladder neck. (From Berek JS. *Berek & Novak's Gynecology,* 14th ed. Philadelphia, PA: Lippincott Williams & Wilkins; 2006.)

FIGURE 19-8. Suburethral sling. The sling is supporting the urethra and bladder neck, and the ends are anchored within the patient's own tissue. (From Berek JS. *Berek & Novak's Gynecology,* 14th ed. Philadelphia, PA: Lippincott Williams & Wilkins; 2006.)

FIGURE 19-9. Periurethral injection of collagen or other material around the urethra just distal to the bladder neck. (Image from Rock J, Jones H. *TeLinde's Operative Gynecology*, 10th ed. Philadelphia, PA: Lippincott Williams & Wilkins; 2008.)

mesh because it has not shown the same worrisome complication rate and is still considered the gold standard treatment of stress urinary incontinence. To clarify this point to both providers and patients, the American Urogynecologic Society (AUGS) and the Society of Urodynamics, Female Pelvic Medicine, and Urogenital Reconstruction (SUFU) released a Position Statement on this topic in 2014, which has recently been endorsed by several other major medical and patient advocacy groups.

Patients with stress urinary incontinence as a result of **ISD** may benefit from periurethral or transurethral placement of bulking agents to improve sphincter tone (Fig. 19-9). Of course, a risk with all of these procedures is overcorrection of the problem, which leads to urinary retention and the need for Foley catheter placement or clean intermittent self-catheterization. Generally, this retention is temporary and will resolve within a few weeks of the procedure.

URGENCY INCONTINENCE

PATHOGENESIS

Urgency incontinence is the involuntary loss of urine associated with a sudden, strong need to urinate and has traditionally been associated with detrusor overactivity; however, a patient may have urgency incontinence without discernible detrusor overactivity. Most detrusor overactivity is **idiopathic**, but it is important to rule-out other causes first. Some conditions known to cause involuntary bladder contractions include urinary tract infections (UTIs), bladder stones, bladder cancer, urethral diverticula, and foreign bodies (Fig. 19-10). Neurologic disorders such as stroke, spinal cord injury, Parkinson's disease, multiple sclerosis, and diabetes mellitus can also cause detrusor overactivity (Table 19-4).

CLINICAL MANIFESTATIONS

Patients with urgency incontinence usually present with a history of involuntary urine loss and urgency, whether or not the bladder is full. Many women complain of not being able to reach the bathroom in time or of dribbling or leaking triggered by just seeing a bathroom, hearing car keys jingle, or being near running water. Detrusor overactivity presents with symptoms including urinary urgency, frequency, and nocturia. Given the wide differential for detrusor overactivity, patients should also be asked about neurologic symptoms, history of previous anti-incontinence surgery, and hematuria (suggestive of cancer, stones, or infection).

DIAGNOSTIC EVALUATION

The diagnosis of urgency incontinence is clinical and does not require specialized testing. Urodynamic studies should be reserved for cases resistant to initial treatment, complex cases, or if surgery is planned.

TREATMENT

The treatment of urge incontinence will depend on the etiology of disease. In cases, where an underlying etiology like those listed in Table 19-4 is identified, it should be treated appropriately. **Idiopathic urgency incontinence**, the most common type, is managed with a combination of lifestyle and behavior modifications, medication, and sometimes surgery. Lifestyle and behavioral modifications include weight loss, caffeine restriction, smoking cessation, fluid management, bladder training, pelvic floor muscle exercises (Kegel exercises), and physical therapy (biofeedback, magnetic therapy, and electrical stimulation).

There are several different medications indicated for the treatment of urgency incontinence (Table 19-5). The most commonly used medications are **anticholinergic drugs** with antimuscarinic effects. Anticholinergic drugs act by increasing bladder capacity and decreasing urgency resulting in decreased incidences of incontinence and decreased voids overall. The effect may take up to four weeks, and therefore, premature

FIGURE 19-10. Causes of detrusor overactivity.

TABLE 19-4. Common Causes of Detrusor Overactivity
Non-neurologic causes
UTIs
Urethral obstruction
Urethral obstruction (previous surgery)
Bladder stones
Bladder cancer
Suburethral diverticula
Foreign bodies
Neurologic causes
Cerebrovascular accident
Alzheimer disease
Parkinsonism
Multiple sclerosis
Diabetes
Peripheral neuropathies
Autonomic neuropathies
Cauda equina lesions
UTI, urinary tract infection.

TABLE 19-5. Medications Indicated for Urgency Incontinence
Antimuscarinic
Oxybutynin (Ditropan) 5 mg PO BID to QID
Oxybutynin extended release (Ditropan XL) 5, 10, 15, 20, 25, and 30 mg PO QD
Oxybutynin transdermal patch (Oxytrol) one 3.9 mg/day patch twice weekly
Oxybutynin gel 10% (Gelnique) one 100 mg/g sachet QD
Tolterodine (Detrol) 2 mg PO BID
Tolterodine extended release (Detrol LA) 4 mg PO QD
Fesoterodine (Toviaz) 4 and 8 mg PO QD
Solifenacin (Vesicare) 5 and 10 mg PO QD
Trospium (Sanctura) 20 mg PO BID
Trospium extended release (Sanctura XR) 60 mg PO QD
Darifenacin (Enablex) 7.5 and 15 mg PO QD
β-3 Agonist
Mirabegron (Myrbetriq) 25 and 50 mg PO QD

discontinuation and dose changes should be avoided before this time. Side effects of anticholinergic drugs include dry mouth, blurred near vision, tachycardia, drowsiness, decreased cognitive function, and constipation. They are contraindicated in patients with gastric retention and angle-closure glaucoma. Anticholinergic drugs should be avoided or used with caution in patients with dementia, because they may worsen this condition. A newer medication called mirabegron (Myrbetriq) is a **β-3 agonist drug** and is a good option for patients who cannot tolerate anticholinergics. Studies have shown that mirabegron has a similar efficacy to anticholinergics and a more tolerable side effect profile. It should not be used in patients with poorly controlled hypertension or a history of cardiac arrhythmia.

Surgical treatments for urgency incontinence include sacral and peripheral neuromodulation, bladder injections, and augmentation cystoplasty. The FDA has approved **sacral neuromodulation** for the treatment of urinary retention and the symptoms of overactive bladder, including urinary urge incontinence and significant symptoms of urgency frequency alone or in combination, in patients who have failed or could not tolerate more conservative treatments. **Percutaneous tibial nerve stimulation** has been approved for urinary frequency, urinary urgency, and urgency incontinence. **Botulinum toxin**, which is now FDA approved for this purpose, is injected into the detrusor muscle for the treatment of urgency incontinence. Rarely, **augmentation cystoplasty** is required in patients with severe refractory urgency incontinence.

OVERFLOW INCONTINENCE

PATHOGENESIS

Overflow incontinence in women is usually due to an **underactive** or **acontractile detrusor muscle**. As a result, bladder contractions are weak or nonexistent, causing incomplete voiding, urinary retention, and overdistension of the bladder (Fig. 19-11). The causes of overflow incontinence owing to detrusor underactivity vary widely from fecal compaction, to use of certain medications, to neurologic diseases such as spinal cord injuries and multiple sclerosis (Table 19-6).

Bladder outlet obstruction, typically due to surgical procedures that result in urethral kinking, stenosis, or obstruction, can also cause bladder overdistension and overflow incontinence, but it is rarely seen in women. **Postoperative overdistension** of the bladder owing to unrecognized urinary retention and the use of epidural anesthesia are common causes of overflow incontinence.

FIGURE 19-11. Overdistended bladder with overflow incontinence.

Neurogenic loss of detrusor function causes emptying phase abnormality, resulting in overflow incontinence. Bladder empties when capacity is exceeded.

CLINICAL MANIFESTATIONS

Patients with overflow incontinence may present with a wide variety of symptoms including frequent or **constant urinary dribbling**, along with the symptoms of stress incontinence and urge incontinence. Outflow obstruction (rare) involves a history of urinary retention, straining to void, poor stream, and incomplete emptying. Bladder outlet obstruction may occur following continence procedures, such as bladder neck and midurethral slings.

TREATMENT

Medications to treat overflow incontinence are rarely used in women because the target for most of these medications, the prostate, is obviously absent. Cholinergic agents (bethanechol) can be used to increase bladder contractility. Intermittent self-catheterization is usually indicated in overflow incontinence to avoid chronic urinary retention and infection.

TABLE 19-6. Causes of Overflow Incontinence

Neurogenic causes
Lower motor neuron disease
Spinal cord injuries
Diabetes mellitus (autonomic neuropathy)
Multiple sclerosis

Obstructive causes
Postsurgical urethral obstruction
Postoperative overdistension
Pelvic masses
Fecal impaction

Pharmacologic causes
Anticholinergic drugs
α-Adrenergic agonists
Epidural and spinal anesthesia

Other causes
Cystitis and urethritis
Psychogenic (psychosis or severe depression)
Idiopathic

Abnormal communication between bladder and vagina results in urine loss (vesicovaginal fistula).

FIGURE 19-12. Vesicovaginal fistula.

Patients with overflow incontinence owing to bladder outlet obstruction caused by a continence procedure such as a sling benefit from surgical correction of the obstruction. Postoperative overdistension of the bladder is typically temporary and may be managed by continuous bladder drainage for 24 to 48 hours.

CONTINUOUS URINARY INCONTINENCE (URINARY FISTULAS)

PATHOGENESIS

Urinary fistulas can be a cause of urinary incontinence. **Continuous urinary incontinence** is typically the result of a **urinary fistula** formed between the bladder and the vagina (vesicovaginal fistula), as shown in Figure 19-12, or between the urethra and the vagina (urethrovaginal fistula), or between the ureter and the vagina (ureterovaginal fistula).

A urinary fistula will result in extra urethral leakage of urine, which is usually reported by the patient as continuous incontinence. Pelvic radiation and pelvic surgery account for more than 95% of urinary fistula incontinence cases in the United States. In particular, simple abdominal hysterectomy and vaginal hysterectomy alone account for more than 50% of **vesicovaginal fistulas**. **Urethrovaginal fistulas** may also occur as complications of surgery for urethral diverticula, anterior vaginal wall prolapse, or stress urinary incontinence. **Ureterovaginal fistulas**, as seen after 1% to 2% of radical hysterectomies, are usually due to devascularization rather than direct injury. Obstetric injuries associated with operative vaginal deliveries (forceps and vacuum) were once the leading cause of urinary fistulas but are now rare causes of urinary fistula in the United States, Canada, and western Europe. In many developing nations, a urinary fistula often results from **birth trauma** and **obstructed labor**. Ectopic ureters and urethral diverticula may also produce total incontinence.

RISK FACTORS

The incidence of fistula formation after surgery is higher if the patient has a history of preoperative radiation, endometriosis, pelvic inflammatory disease, or previous pelvic surgery. In developing countries, risks for urinary fistula are linked to obstructed labor and may include absent or untrained birth attendants, inadequate pelvic dimensions (secondary to early childbearing, chronic disease, and malnutrition), inadequate labor, malpresentation, hydrocephalus, and introital stenosis secondary to female genital cutting and circumcision.

HISTORY

Patients with a urinary fistula usually present with a history of painless and continuous loss of urine, usually after pelvic surgery, pelvic radiation, or obstetric trauma. Fistulas due to surgery usually become clinically apparent within 14 postoperative days.

DIAGNOSTIC EVALUATION

Medications can be used to change the color of urine to be more obvious when attempting to localize the fistula. **Oral phenazopyridine** or **IV indigo carmine** is most frequently used for this purpose. If the fistula is very small and difficult to visualize, a tampon can be placed in the vagina following the administration of the medication; the dye will stain the tampon if a fistula is present. **Cystourethroscopy** and the **voiding cystourethrogram** can be used to identify the number and location of the fistulas. Intravenous pyelogram and retrograde pyelogram may also be used to localize urinary fistulas as well.

TREATMENT

Surgery is the primary treatment for urinary fistulas. It is typical to wait 3 to 6 months before attempting to repair **postsurgical fistulas**. This waiting period allows inflammation to decrease and vascularity and pliability of the area to increase. **Antibiotics** for urinary infection and **estrogen** for postmenopausal women are also used during this period.

KEY POINTS

- Under normal circumstances, urinary incontinence is maintained due to the complex system of muscles, ligaments, sphincters, and nerves that keep the intraurethral pressure greater than the intravesical pressure.
- Diagnostic evaluation includes a thorough history and physical examination, urine analysis with microscopy and culture, stress test, cotton-swab test, and use of a voiding diary. Urodynamics (cystometrogram and uroflowmetry) can be used as indicated (e.g., prior to surgery, mixed incontinence).
- Risk factors for urinary incontinence include age, hormonal status, obesity, diabetes, impaired functional status, and some neurologic disorders.
- Stress incontinence is characterized by leaking with physical activity such as coughing, sneezing, lifting, or exercising.
- Stress incontinence can be treated with lifestyle and behavioral modifications, incontinence pessaries, and surgical management. Common surgical treatments include supportive slings for the urethra and bladder neck.
- Urgency incontinence is characterized by leaking associated with urgency and may exhibit detrusor overactivity. Most cases of detrusor overactivity are idiopathic. Other cases are caused by UTI, bladder stones, cancer, diverticula, and neurologic disorders (stroke, multiple sclerosis, and Alzheimer disease).
- The goal of treatment for urgency incontinence is to relax the bladder, suppress involuntary bladder contractions, and enhance urine storage. This can be achieved with lifestyle and behavioral modifications as well as anticholinergic or β-3 agonist medication. Surgical procedures include sacral and peripheral nerve stimulation, bladder injections, and augmentation cystoplasty.
- Overflow incontinence is most commonly due to decreased detrusor contractions caused by medications or neurologic disease; obstruction and postoperative overdistension occur less frequently in women.
- The primary symptom of overflow incontinence is urinary retention with continuous dribbling. It is usually treated with self-catheterization or surgery.
- The most common causes of urinary fistulas in the United States are pelvic radiation and pelvic surgery. In developing countries, total incontinence is attributable to obstetric trauma, often leading to urinary fistula.

CLINICAL VIGNETTES

VIGNETTE 1

A 56-year-old G3P3 woman is referred to the urogynecology clinic for urinary leakage by her primary care provider (PCP). She has leaked urine when coughing, sneezing, and jogging for the last 3 years. She denies leakage of urine with urgency. Her BMI is 33. She uses three pads per day for urinary leakage. Urinalysis and urine cultures done in her PCP's office 1 week ago were negative.

1. Which of the following is NOT a first-line treatment for this patient?
   a. Pelvic floor muscle exercises (Kegel exercises)
   b. Caffeine restriction
   c. Oxybutynin (anticholinergic medication)
   d. Bladder training
   e. Weight loss

2. After trying behavioral and lifestyle modifications, the patient continues to be symptomatic. Urodynamic studies are done to further evaluate the incontinence. Cystometry reveals leakage of urine with increases in intra-abdominal pressure during Valsalva effort and coughing. No involuntary detrusor contractions are seen. Bladder compliance is normal. The pressure flow pattern is continuous and normal with a void initiated by urethral relaxation and a normal detrusor contraction. What type of urinary incontinence does this patient most likely have?
   a. Stress incontinence
   b. Urgency incontinence
   c. Overflow incontinence
   d. Mixed incontinence
   e. Functional incontinence

3. After trying conservative management with behavioral and lifestyle modifications, the patient has not had complete resolution of her symptoms and is still bothered by the loss of urine with coughing, sneezing, and exercise. After appropriate counseling, she opts to proceed with surgery. Which of the following is an appropriate surgical choice for her?
   a. Vaginal hysterectomy
   b. Midurethral sling
   c. Cystourethroscopy
   d. Sacral neuromodulation (InterStim)
   e. Colpocleisis

4. Following surgery for urinary incontinence, the patient complains of difficulty starting a stream of urine, a weak and interrupted stream, and feeling because if she is not completely empty. She is also experiencing urinary leakage. A postvoid residual (PVR) measured with a catheter is 250 mL. What is the most likely diagnosis?
   a. Urgency incontinence
   b. Continuous incontinence
   c. Stress incontinence
   d. Bladder outlet obstruction with overflow urinary incontinence
   e. Functional incontinence

VIGNETTE 2

A 45-year-old G5P5 woman who had three vaginal deliveries and two caesarian sections underwent an abdominal hysterectomy for large symptomatic fibroids 3 months ago. On postoperative day 10, she began leaking urine continuously, even at night. She is wearing adult diapers (Depends) and protective pads all of the time and sleeps with an additional pad under her at night. Urinalysis and urine cultures are negative.

1. From this history, you are suspicious that this patient may have:
   a. Overflow incontinence
   b. Stress incontinence
   c. Continuous incontinence secondary to a urinary fistula
   d. Urgency incontinence
   e. Functional incontinence

2. On pelvic examination, the vagina is well-healed, and you do not see any lesions or active leaking of urine into the vagina. Further testing at this time may include:
   a. Cystourethroscopy
   b. Dye testing with PO phenazopyridine (Pyridium)
   c. IV dye testing with indigo carmine
   d. All of the above
   e. None of the above

VIGNETTE 3

An 82-year-old G3P2 woman is brought to your office by her caregiver from a local retirement home. She has a diagnosis of dementia that has been worsening over the last year. She is followed closely by her PCP and saw him recently for her general conditions. She is communicative but has a poor memory. Her history is obtained from her caregiver. She is ambulatory with minimal assistance and is able to follow commands. Her BMI is 23.5. Her caregiver tells you that over the last year she has had an increase in the number of urinary leakage episodes. She wears adult diapers (Depends), which have to be changed at least two times per day due to leakage. In the morning, she wakes up with a wet pad. Her pelvic examination is normal except for atrophic vaginitis (consistent with menopause).

1. Which of the following laboratory tests would you order on this patient?
   a. Urinalysis with culture and sensitivity
   b. Urine eosinophils
   c. Urine cytology
   d. Serum creatinine
   e. All of the above

2. Your test results are negative. What is the most likely diagnosis for this patient?
   a. Stress incontinence
   b. Urgency incontinence
   c. Functional incontinence
   d. Overflow incontinence
   e. Continuous incontinence secondary to fistula

3. What is the initial management of this patient?
   a. Pelvic floor muscle exercises, 3 sets of 10 per day
   b. Bladder training, she should be instructed to empty her bladder every 2 to 3 hours
   c. Weight loss
   d. Incontinence pessary
   e. Expectant management

VIGNETTE 4

A 63-year-old G3P2 woman is referred to the urogynecology clinic for evaluation of urinary incontinence. Urinalysis and urine culture done by her PCP 1 week earlier were negative. Her medical history is positive for hypertension and osteoarthritis. She is complaining of leakage of urine following an overwhelming need to void. She runs to the bathroom, but leaks a large amount before she makes it to the toilet. She also has urinary frequency and empties her bladder every 1 to 1.5 hours during the day and gets up four times at night to void. She denies loss of urine with cough, sneeze, and exercise.

1. From this patient's history, what is your initial diagnosis?
   a. Urgency incontinence
   b. Overflow incontinence
   c. Stress incontinence
   d. Mixed incontinence
   e. Continuous incontinence secondary to a urinary fistula

2. What is the most likely cause of this patient's urinary incontinence?
   a. Neurogenic bladder
   b. Bladder outlet obstruction
   c. Idiopathic urgency incontinence
   d. Urinary fistula
   e. Pelvic mass

3. On physical examination, she has mild pelvic organ prolapse that is not bothersome, vaginal atrophy, and her BMI is 32. Which of the following would you recommend for this patient as initial management for her condition?
   a. Midurethral sling
   b. Sacral neuromodulation
   c. Lifestyle and behavioral modifications including, weight loss, caffeine restriction, smoking cessation, fluid management, bladder training, pelvic floor muscle exercises, and physical therapy
   d. Botulinum toxin A
   e. Vaginal hysterectomy

4. The patient returns for a follow-up appointment, she has implemented your suggestions and has noticed a moderate improvement in her urinary incontinence, urgency, and frequency. You suggest that she begin which treatment?
   a. Sacral neuromodulation
   b. Botulinum toxin A injections
   c. Detrol LA (anticholinergic medication)
   d. Percutaneous tibial nerve stimulation
   e. Midurethral sling

ANSWERS

VIGNETTE 1 Question 1
1. Answer C:
This patient has a history consistent with stress incontinence. Her initial treatment should include behavioral and lifestyle modifications such as weight loss, caffeine restriction, fluid management, bladder training, and pelvic floor muscle exercises (Kegel exercises). Oxybutynin is an anticholinergic medication used to treat urgency incontinence.

VIGNETTE 1 Question 2
2. Answer A:
Urodynamic studies support the history of stress incontinence given by this patient. The loss of urine with increases in abdominal pressure and no increase in detrusor pressure during cystometry is consistent with the diagnosis of stress incontinence. Urgency incontinence is usually a clinical diagnosis, but can be associated with detrusor overactivity on urodynamics;

this patient does not give a history of or demonstrate urgency incontinence. Overflow incontinence is associated with either an underactive/acontractile detrusor or outlet obstruction; this patient has a normal detrusor contraction when voiding and a normal urine flow pattern. Mixed incontinence is a combination of urgency and stress incontinence. Functional incontinence is attributed to factors outside the lower urinary tract including physical or mental impairments that prevent the patient from being able to response normally to cues to void.

VIGNETTE 1 Question 3
3. Answer B:
A midurethral sling, such as tension-free transvaginal sling or transobturator approach midurethral sling, would be the treatment of choice for stress incontinence in this patient. Vaginal hysterectomy is not a procedure for stress incontinence. Cystourethroscopy is an endoscopic procedure used to evaluate the interior of the bladder and urethra and is not a procedure for the treatment of urinary incontinence. Sacral neuromodulation (InterStim) is used for the treatment of urgency incontinence, not stress incontinence. Colpocleisis is a vaginal obliteration procedure used to treat pelvic organ prolapse in patients who are poor surgical candidates and no longer plan on vaginal intercourse.

VIGNETTE 1 Question 4
4. Answer D:
Bladder outlet obstruction with overflow urinary incontinence is the most likely diagnosis given the patient's incomplete emptying and large PVR. Urodynamics with pressure flow studies can help to better evaluate her problem. The treatment for bladder outlet obstruction from a midurethral sling would be surgical release/revision of the sling.

VIGNETTE 2 Question 1
1. Answer C:
This patient's history of continuous urinary incontinence following an abdominal hysterectomy is consistent with a urinary fistula. She has risk factors for fistula, including prior pelvic surgery and large uterine fibroids. She has no history of surgery for urinary stress incontinence or of an underactive bladder, making overflow incontinence unlikely. Stress incontinence is characterized as involuntary urine loss on effort or physical exertion (e.g., sporting activities) or on sneezing or coughing. She also does not have the complaint of involuntary loss of urine associated with urgency. Functional incontinence is due to physical or mental impairments that prevent the patient from being able to response normally to cues to void.

VIGNETTE 2 Question 2
2. Answer D:
Oral phenazopyridine and IV indigo carmine can be given to help visualize leaking through the fistula into the vagina. If the fistula is very small and difficult to see, a tampon can be placed in the vagina; the dye will stain the tampon if a fistula is present. Cystourethroscopy and further imaging such as a voiding cystourethrogram, intravenous pyelogram, and retrograde pyelogram can then be used to identify the number and location of the fistulas.

VIGNETTE 3 Question 1
1. Answer A:
Urinary tract infection is a reversible cause of urinary incontinence and should always be ruled out in a patient with urinary incontinence. Urine eosinophils are typically seen in acute interstitial nephritis. Urine cytology looks at cells is the urine to rule-out evidence of malignancy. Serum creatinine is a blood test used to assess kidney function.

VIGNETTE 3 Question 2
2. Answer C:
Functional incontinence is attributed to factors outside the lower urinary tract including physical or mental impairments that prevent the patient from being able to respond normally to cues to void. These are particularly common in nursing home residents and in geriatric patients in general. Factors such as physical immobility, dementia, delirium, medications, and systemic illness can all contribute to functional incontinence. To make the diagnosis of functional incontinence, a history of the other types of urinary incontinence such as stress or urgency incontinence should be ruled out. It is possible that this patient is also experiencing other types of incontinence; however, with the information given, functional incontinence is the most likely diagnosis at this time.

VIGNETTE 3 Question 3
3. Answer B:
Instructing the patient to void on a schedule every 2 to 3 hours is one of the first interventions to recommend in this patient. Management of her fluid and caffeine intake should also be encouraged. This patient is probably not capable of performing pelvic floor muscle exercises. She does not need to lose weight; her BMI is in the normal range. A pessary is used to treat stress incontinence and will not benefit a patient with functional incontinence. Expectant management is insufficient because she is symptomatic and capable of following instructions.

VIGNETTE 4 Question 1
1. Answer A:
This patient meets the definition of urgency incontinence—involuntary urine loss and urgency whether or not the bladder is full. Many women complain of not being able to reach the bathroom in time or of dribbling or leaking triggered by just seeing a bathroom.

VIGNETTE 4 Question 2

2. Answer C:
Idiopathic urgency incontinence is the most common cause of urgency incontinence. There is no reason to believe that this patient is experiencing neurogenic bladder, bladder outlet obstruction, urinary fistula, or a pelvic mass.

VIGNETTE 4 Question 3

3. Answer C:
The initial first-line therapy in a patient with urgency incontinence should include lifestyle and behavioral modifications. Midurethral sling is a surgical treatment for stress incontinence. Sacral neuromodulation and botulinum toxin A are treatments for medication refractory urgency incontinence. There are no indications for hysterectomy described here.

VIGNETTE 4 Question 4

4. Answer C:
An anticholinergic medication such as Detrol LA would be the next most logical treatment to try in this patient for the treatment of urgency incontinence, frequency, and nocturia. Sacral neuromodulation, botulinum toxin A injections, and percutaneous tibial nerve stimulation are reserved for patients refractory to medications. A midurethral sling is one treatment for stress incontinence.

20 | Puberty, the Menstrual Cycle, and Menopause

PUBERTY

Puberty describes the series of events in which a child matures into a young adult. It encompasses a series of neuroendocrine and physiologic changes, which result in the ability to ovulate and menstruate. These changes include the development of secondary sex characteristics, the growth spurt, and achievement of fertility. Before any perceived phenotypic change, **adrenarche** occurs with regeneration of the zona reticularis in the adrenal cortex and production of androgens and ultimately stimulates the appearance of pubic hair. **Gonadarche** describes the activation of the hypothalamic–pituitary–gonadal axis, which involves pulsatile gonadotropin-releasing hormone (GnRH) secretion stimulating the anterior pituitary to produce luteinizing hormone (LH) and follicle-stimulating hormone (FSH). These, in turn, trigger the ovary to produce estrogens (Fig. 20-1).

The **pubertal sequence** includes accelerated growth, breast development (thelarche), development of pubic and axillary hair (pubarche), and onset of menstruation (menarche). These stages usually occur in that order (Fig. 20-2). Concerned parents can be reassured by knowing that, on average, the length of time from breast bud development to menstruation is typically 2.5 years.

ADRENARCHE AND GONADARCHE

Adrenarche occurs between ages 6 and 8 years when the adrenal gland begins regeneration of the zona reticularis. This inner layer of the adrenal cortex is responsible for the secretion of sex steroid hormones. As a result of the regeneration, the adrenal gland produces increased quantities of the androgens dehydroepiandrosterone sulfate (DHEAS), DHEA, and androstenedione. Production of these **androgenic steroid hormones** increases from age 6 to 8 years

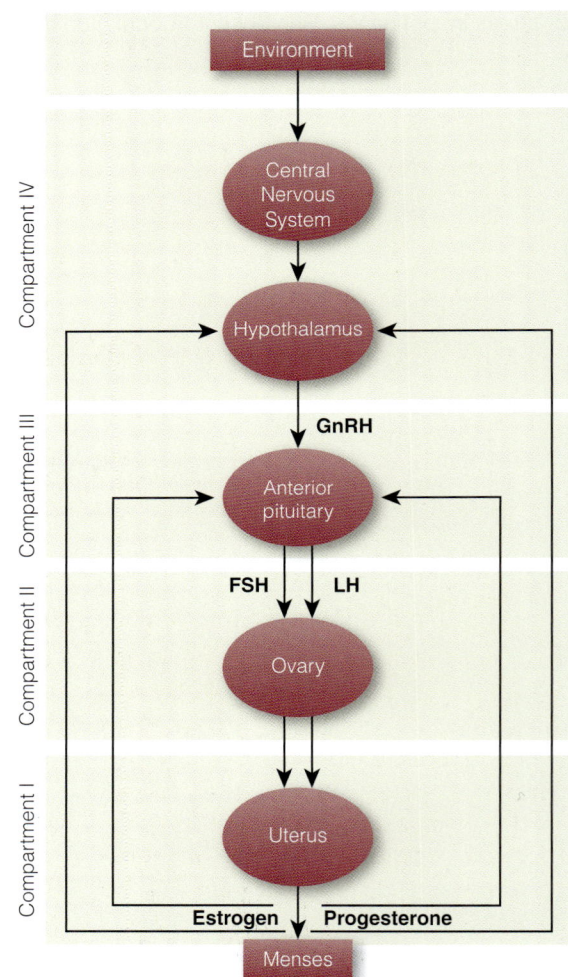

FIGURE 20-1. Basic principles of menstrual function. The hypothalamic–pituitary–ovarian axis can be segmented into distinct compartments; each is necessary for normal menstrual function. (From Bourgeois FJ. *Obstetrics & Gynecology Recall,* 3rd ed. Philadelphia, PA: Lippincott Williams & Wilkins; 2008.). FSH, follicle-stimulating hormone; GnRH, gonadotropin-releasing hormone; LH, luteinizing hormone.

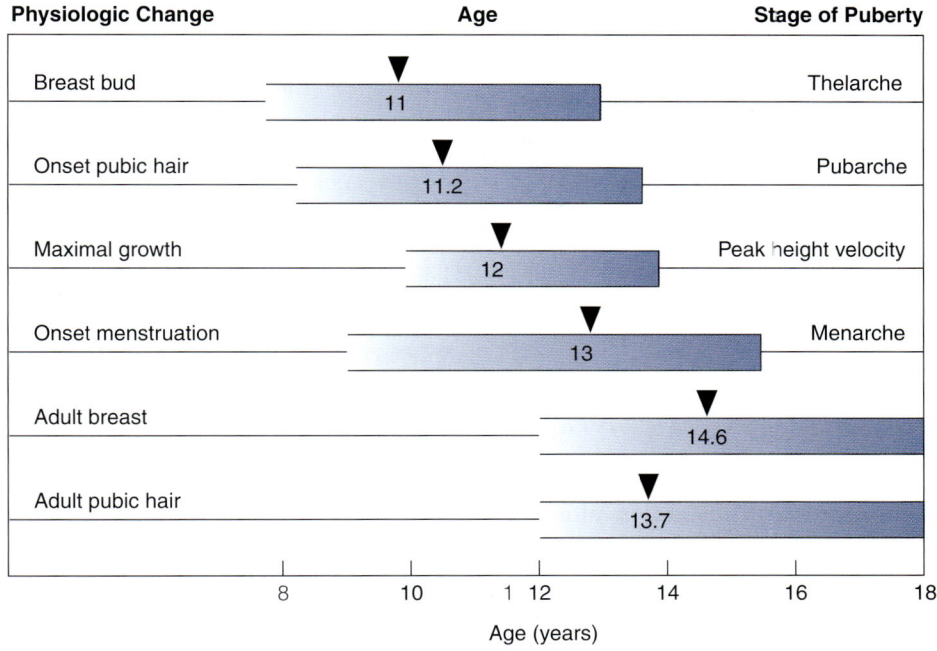

FIGURE 20-2. Average age and age range for the onset of the major physical changes associated with puberty.

up until age 13 to 15 years. The primary stimulus of adrenarche is unknown.

Gonadarche is independent of adrenarche and begins around age 8 years, when **pulsatile GnRH** secretion from the hypothalamus is increased. There is also a changing sensitivity of the neuroendocrine system to negative feedback by gonadal hormones. This leads to subsequent pulsatile **secretion of LH and FSH** from the anterior pituitary. Initially, these increases occur mostly during sleep and fail to lead to any phenotypic changes. As a girl enters early puberty, the LH and FSH pulsatility lasts throughout the day, eventually leading to stimulation of the ovary and subsequent estrogen release. This, in turn, triggers the characteristic **breast bud development** associated with puberty. The positive feedback of estradiol also results in the initiation of the LH surge and the ability to ovulate.

ACCELERATED GROWTH

The growth spurt is characterized by an **acceleration in the growth rate** around age 9 to 10 years, leading to a mean peak growth velocity of about 9 cm/year around age 12 years. The increased rate of growth is because of the direct effect of sex steroids on epiphyseal growth and because of the increased pituitary **growth hormone secretion** in response to sex steroids (Fig. 20-2).

THELARCHE

The first stage of thelarche, the development of breast buds, usually occurs around age 10 years. Thelarche is usually the first phenotypic sign of puberty and occurs in response to the increase in levels of circulating estrogen. Concomitantly, there is estrogenation of the vaginal mucosa and **growth of the vagina and uterus**. Further **development of the breast** will continue throughout puberty and adolescence, as described by Marshall and Tanner (Table 20-1 and Fig. 20-3).

PUBARCHE

The onset of **growth of pubic hair** (Fig. 20-3) usually occurs around age 11 years and is often accompanied by **growth of axillary hair**. Pubarche usually follows thelarche, but a normal variant may occur with pubarche preceding thelarche, particularly in African American girls. The growth of pubic and axillary hair is likely secondary to the increase in circulating androgens.

MENARCHE

The average age at onset of menstruation is between 12 and 13 years or 2.5 years after the development of breast buds. As **gonadal estrogen production** increases during puberty, it increases sufficiently

TABLE 20-1.	The Tanner Stages of Breast Development
Stage 1	Preadolescent: elevation of papilla only
Stage 2	Breast bud stage: elevation of breast and papilla, areolar enlargement
Stage 3	Further enlargement of breast and areola without separation of contours
Stage 4	Projection of areola and papilla to form a secondary mound
Stage 5	Mature stage: projection of papilla only as areola recesses to breast contour

Adapted from Speroff L, Glass RH, Kase NG. *Clinical Gynecologic Endocrinology and Infertility*, 5th ed. Baltimore, MD: Williams & Wilkins; 1994:377.

to stimulate **endometrial proliferation**, ultimately resulting in the start of menses. The adolescent menstrual cycle is usually **irregular for the first 1 to 2 years after menarche**, reflecting anovulatory cycles. On average, it takes about 2 years after menarche before **regular ovulatory cycles** are achieved. Failure to achieve a regular menstrual cycle after this point may represent a reproductive disorder. Menarche is often delayed in gymnasts, distance runners, and ballet dancers. Some theories propose that this is because of an insufficient percentage of body fat that may result in hypothalamic anovulation and amenorrhea. Others postulate that the exercise and stress on the body may inhibit ovulation through positive effects on norepinephrine and GnRH, thus interfering with menarche.

ABNORMAL PUBERTY

Precocious puberty is defined as pubarche or thelarche before 7 years of age in Caucasian girls and before 6 years of age in African American girls. Absent or incomplete breast development by the age of 12 years is defined as **delayed puberty** and also needs further workup. The initial workup for both includes a careful history, physical examination, hormone assessment, and bone age determination.

THE MENSTRUAL CYCLE

The hypothalamus, pituitary, ovaries, and uterus are all involved in maintaining the menstrual cycle (Fig. 20-1). The menstrual cycle is divided into two 14-day phases: the **follicular and luteal phases**, which describe changes in the ovary over the length of the cycle, and the **proliferative and secretory phases**, which describe concurrent changes in the endometrium over the same period of time (Fig. 20-4).

During the follicular phase, the release of FSH from the pituitary gland results in development of a **primary ovarian follicle**. The ovarian follicle produces estrogen, which causes the uterine lining to proliferate. At mid cycle—approximately day 14—there is an LH spike in response to a preceding estrogen surge, which stimulates ovulation, the release of the ovum from the follicle (Fig. 20-4). After ovulation, the luteal phase begins. The remnants of the follicle left behind in the ovary develop into the corpus luteum. This **corpus luteum** is responsible for the **secretion**

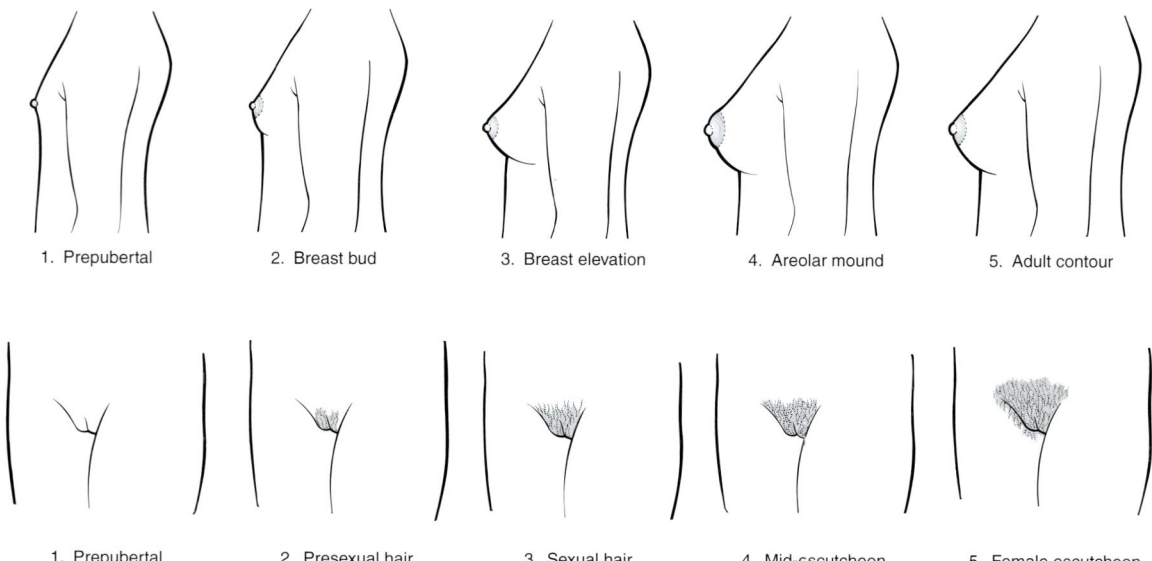

FIGURE 20-3. Tanner stages of thelarche (breast development) and of pubarche (onset of pubic hair growth).

FIGURE 20-4. Normal menstrual cycle, day 1 to day 28. The cyclic changes of FSH and LH and the resultant changes in the ovarian histology (follicular and luteal phases) in estrogen and progesterone levels, in basal body temperature, and the endometrial histology (proliferative and secretory phases) are shown. Note how the LH surge near day 14 of a 28-day cycle triggers ovulation and a rise in basal body temperature, signifying the time of maximum fertility during the cycle. FSH, follicle-stimulating hormone; LH, luteinizing hormone.

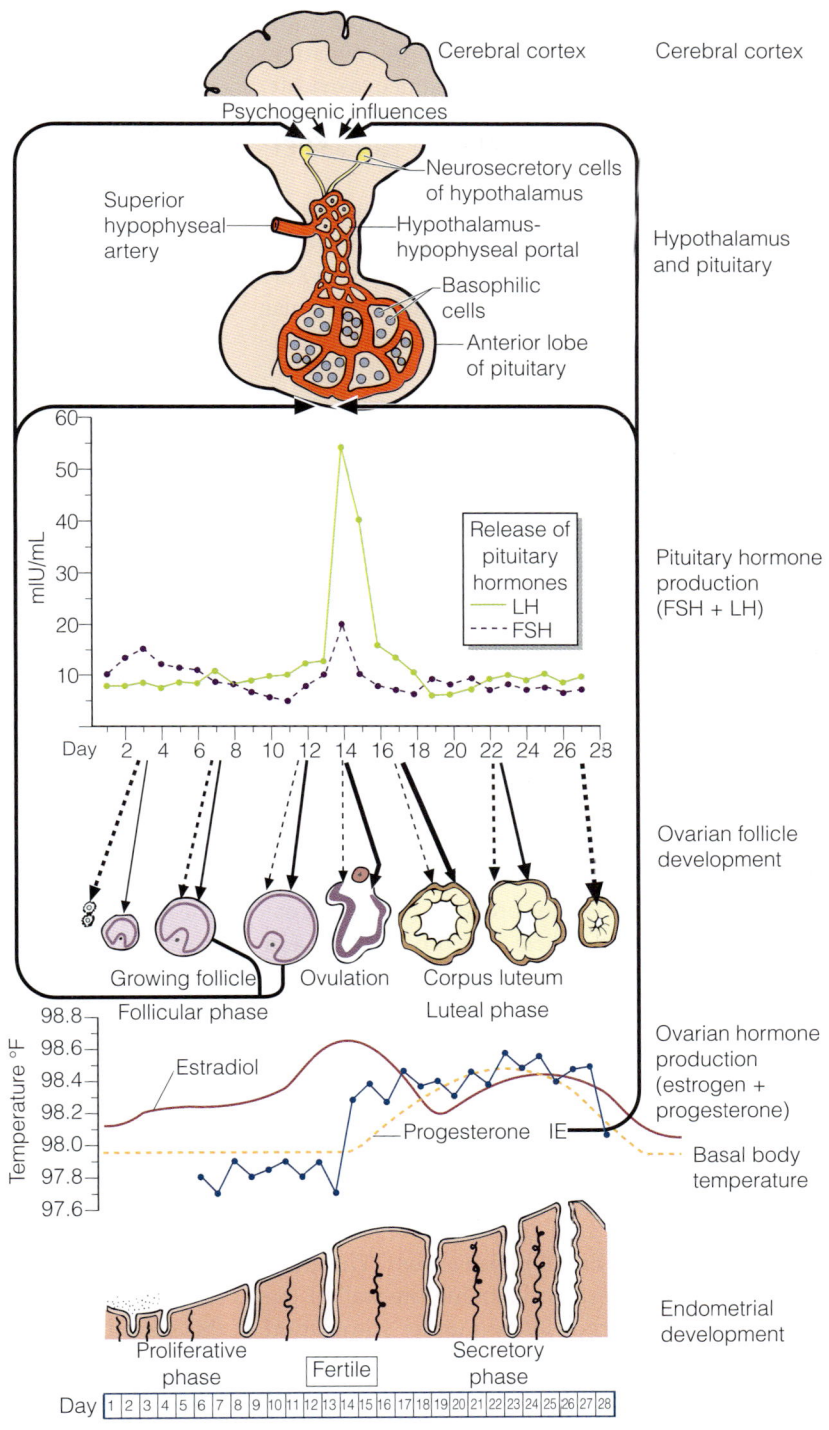

of **progesterone**, which maintains the endometrial lining in preparation to receive a fertilized ovum. If fertilization does not occur, the corpus luteum degenerates, and progesterone levels fall. Without progesterone, the endometrial lining is sloughed off, which is known as **menstruation** (Fig. 20-4).

FOLLICULAR PHASE

The withdrawal of estrogen and progesterone during the luteal phase of the prior cycle causes a gradual **increase in FSH**. In turn, FSH stimulates the growth of approximately 5 to 15 **primordial ovarian follicles**, initiating the follicular phase again. Of these primordial follicles, one becomes the **dominant follicle** and develops and matures until ovulation. The developing dominant follicle, destined to ovulate, produces estrogen that enhances follicular maturation and increases the production of FSH and LH receptors in an autocrine fashion.

Estrogen synthesis is based on a theory known as the **two-cell theory** or **the two-cell, two-gonadotropin theory**. This theory postulates the role of both FSH and LH (two gonadotropins) on ovarian follicular maturation and the production of estrogens involving both theca and granulosa cells (two cells). In the two-cell theory, **LH stimulates production of androgens** (androstenedione) from cholesterol and pregnenolone in the theca cells. The androgens are then transported into the granulosa cells where **FSH stimulates the conversion of androgens to estrogens** (estrone). As rising estrogen levels have negative feedback on pituitary FSH secretion, the dominant follicle is protected from the decrease in FSH by its increased number of FSH receptors (Fig. 20-5).

OVULATION

Toward the end of the follicular phase, estrogen levels eventually surge to reach a critical level that triggers the anterior pituitary to release an LH spike. The **LH surge** triggers the resumption of meiosis in the oocyte and induces production of progesterone and prostaglandins within the follicle. The progesterone and prostaglandins, in turn, are responsible for the rupture of the follicular wall with **release of the mature ovum or ovulation** (Fig. 20-5). The ovum usually passes into the adjoining fallopian tube and is swept down to the uterus by the cilia lining the tube. This process takes 3 to 4 days. **Fertilization** of the ovum must occur within 24 hours of ovulation or it degenerates.

LUTEAL PHASE

After ovulation, the **luteal phase** ensues. The granulosa and theca interna cells lining the wall of the follicle form the corpus luteum under stimulation by LH. The corpus luteum synthesizes **estrogen and significant quantities of progesterone**, which cause the endometrium to become more glandular and secretory in preparation for implantation of a fertilized ovum (Fig. 20-5). If fertilization occurs, the developing trophoblast synthesizes **human chorionic gonadotropin** (hCG)—a glycoprotein very similar to LH—which maintains the corpus luteum, so that it can continue production of estrogen and progesterone to support the endometrium.

This continues until the placenta develops its own synthetic function at 8 to 10 weeks of gestation. If fertilization, with its concomitant rise in hCG, does not occur, the corpus luteum degenerates, progesterone levels fall, the endometrium is not maintained, and menstruation occurs.

MENSTRUATION

The endometrium of the uterus undergoes cyclical changes during the menstrual cycle (Fig. 20-4). During the follicular phase, the endometrium is in the **proliferative phase**, growing in response to estrogen. During the luteal phase, the endometrium enters the **secretory phase,** as it matures and is prepared to support implantation. If the ovum is not fertilized, the corpus luteum degenerates after approximately 14 days, leading to a fall in estrogen and progesterone levels. The **withdrawal of progesterone** causes the endometrium to slough, initiating the menstrual phase. At the same time, FSH levels begin to slowly rise in the absence of negative feedback, and the follicular phase starts again. A menstrual cycle less than 24 days or longer than 35 days or a menses that lasts more than 7 days merits further evaluation.

PERIMENOPAUSE

The menopausal transition or perimenopause is the transition from normal ovulatory cycles to menopause because of **progressive ovarian failure**. Symptoms can begin from 2 to 8 years prior to the final menstrual period (FMP). The time from the FMP and beyond is considered postmenopausal. The menopausal transition and early postmenopausal years are when women have their most **significant symptoms**. Vasomotor symptoms (VMS), including night sweats and daytime hot flashes, mood swings, including irritability and depression, insomnia, and sleep disturbances, are reported by up to 80% of women at some point during this transition. Physiologically, in this period, inhibin B secretion from granulosa cells falls because of the diminished follicular numbers, and as a result, FSH rises, and progesterone levels are low. Estradiol levels fluctuate greatly but, in general, are preserved until late perimenopause when both estradiol and FSH can fluctuate. Perimenopausal women may ovulate and are considered fertile until a full 12 months of amenorrhea has been attained. **Contraceptive services** and counseling should be provided to perimenopausal women who do not wish to become pregnant.

FIGURE 20-5. Cyclic changes in ovarian follicle development over the menstrual cycle. Under the influence of FSH, the primordial follicle matures into the preantral follicle and then into the graafian follicle. During the last few days of the growing period, the estrogen produced by the follicular and theca cells stimulates the formation of LH in the pituitary. The LH surge triggers ovulation, and the oocyte is discharged from the ovary together. During the luteal phase of the cycle, the follicular cells remaining inside the collapsed follicle differentiate into luteal cells. The corpus luteum is formed by hypertrophy and accumulation of lipid in the granulose and theca interna cells. The remaining cavity of the follicle is filled with fibrin. If pregnancy does not occur, the corpus luteum then degenerates into the corpus albicans and menstruation begins. (From Eroschenko VP. *Di Fiore's Atlas of Histology, with Functional Correlations,* 9th ed. Baltimore, MD: Lippincott Williams & Wilkins; 2000.). FSHRF, follicle stimulating hormone releasing factor; LHRF, luteinizing hormone releasing factor; FSH, follicle-stimulating hormone; LH, luteinizing hormone.

MENOPAUSE AND POSTMENOPAUSE

Menopause is defined by **12 months of amenorrhea after the FMP** in the absence of any other pathologic or physiologic causes. At this point, nearly all the oocytes have undergone atresia, although a few remain and can be found on histologic examination. Menopause is characterized by complete, or near complete, **ovarian follicular depletion** and **absence of ovarian estrogen** secretion. The estrogen and FSH levels stabilize 2 years after the FMP. Symptoms generally begin to dissipate at this time.

The average age at menopause in the United States is 51 years (range 45 to 55 years). Five percent of women will have **late menopause** (occurring after age 55 years) and another 5% of women have **early menopause** (occurring between ages 40 and 45 years). Early age at menopause is more common in women with a history of cigarette smoking, short menstrual cycles, nulliparity, type 1 diabetes, and family history of early menopause. Women with a history of hysterectomy or tubal ligation are at increased risk of early menopause. This is thought to be because of decreased vascular supply to the ovaries after these procedures. **Primary ovarian insufficiency (POI)**, formerly premature ovarian failure, is the onset of spontaneous menopause before the age of 40 years and requires further testing. POI is usually **idiopathic or autoimmune**. If it occurs before age 30 years, chromosomal studies can be ordered to rule out a genetic basis (e.g., mosaicism). Approximately 6% of women with POI are found to have premutations of the *FMR1* gene, and another 3% will have autoimmune or adrenal abnormalities.

Various physiologic changes also occur during this period, resulting from the decrease in estrogen. Table 20-2 covers **classic symptoms** of menopause, including VMS; emotional changes, including anxiety and depression; and sleep disturbances. Forty to eighty percent of women will begin having mild symptoms during perimenopause, and 50% will experience an increase in frequency and intensity of symptoms during menopause transition. Often, the symptoms are the most intense during the late perimenopause phase. Gradually, most women will see a reduction in severity of these symptoms over time. Average medial duration of reported VMS symptoms from the Study of Women's Health Across the Nation (SWAN) clinical trials is 7.5 years, increased from the previously estimated 5 years. Up to 25% of women will have **persistent VMS**, however, and other physiologic etiologies need to be ruled out.

TABLE 20-2. Menopausal Symptoms and Long-Term Effects (Mnemonic: FSH > 40 IU/L)

F	Flushes, forgetful (Alzheimer disease)
S	Sweats at night, sad (depression) stroke, skeletal changes (accelerated bone loss leading to osteoporosis), skin changes, sexual dysfunction
H	Headaches, heart disease
I	Insomnia
U	Urinary symptoms (stress and urge incontinence), urogenital atrophy (loss of pelvic floor muscles)
L	Libido decreases

Remember that an FSH level >40 IU/L is the blood test to confirm menopause.
FSH, follicle-stimulating hormone.

SWAN data show a highest reported incidence of Vasomotor symptoms (VMS) in African American, followed by Caucasian and then Asian populations.

The term **genital urinary syndrome of menopause (GSM)** was adopted by North American Menopause Society (NAMS) and International society for the Study of Women's Sexual Health in 2014 and includes symptoms of **vulvovaginal atrophy** (VVA), such as dryness with itching, discharge, dyspareunia, and urinary system changes, such as **incontinence and dysuria**. GSM is seen in late peri- and postmenopausal women. GSM results from low-estrogen levels. Unlike VMS symptoms, the changes seen with GSM will, if untreated, become **more severe over time**. It is known that over half of the women do not report symptoms of GSM to their health-care provider despite the negative impact it has on their sexual health and quality of life overall. Menopause represents the end of a woman's reproductive viability. Beliefs regarding menstruation, childbearing, sexual activity after menopause, and demographic variation, such as religion and ethnicity, all are key components to how women perceive the menopause transition.

ETIOLOGY

Menopause is generally heralded by menstrual irregularity because the number of oocytes decreases, resulting in increasingly sporadic ovulation. It is commonly believed that, as part of the natural aging process, the onset of menopause is caused by a disruption in the function of the hypothalamic–pituitary–ovarian axis and **gradual oocyte depletion (follicular atresia)**. This causes a decrease in estrogen production and an increase in FSH and LH.

DIAGNOSIS

The diagnosis of menopause can usually be made by history and physical examination. Patients classically present between **ages 48 and 52 years (average age is 51 years)** complaining of irregular menses or amenorrhea and Vasomotor symptoms, mood changes, depression or anxiety, insomnia, and vaginal dryness or dyspareunia, which may be associated with a loss of desire for sexual intimacy or activity.

On **physical examination**, there may be a decrease in breast size and change in texture. Increases in abdominal circumference and upper **abdominal weight gain** are common findings. Findings consistent with VVA may be present because the lower estrogen levels result in a thinning of the superficial vaginal epithelium. The vagina will be pale and smooth and shows a loss of rugation. Vaginal pH levels are elevated (>5 to 6), and there is a decrease in lactobacillus.

Other exam findings include **increase in the BMI** (weight gain of approximately 5 lbs), which is common. **Skin changes** including rapid onset of a loss of elasticity of the skin and loss of thickness and collagen in the skin are common. **Hair changes** that may include loss of pubic hair, female pattern baldness, androgenic alopecia, and excessive growth of terminal facial hair are frequent findings. Complaints of dry eyes and increase in periodontal disease are common findings as well.

During perimenopause, **FSH levels** may vary greatly and are not required to diagnose menopause. The absence of menses for 1 year with consistently elevated FSH levels > 40 IU/L is considered diagnostic of menopause. FSH levels above 40 IU/L do not, however, correlate with when a woman will have the FMP. Laboratory analysis looking for a reliable and predictive marker for the FMP is ongoing. **Estradiol levels** fluctuate greatly during late perimenopause and early postmenopause and are not helpful in diagnosis or clinical management.

PATHOGENESIS

Although menopause is a naturally occurring event, there are two important **long-term consequences** of the estrogen-deficient state of menopause (Fig. 20-6). First, from a cardiovascular standpoint, the protective benefits of estrogen on the lipid profile (increased HDL, decreased LDL and triglycerides) and on the vascular epithelium (decreased atherogenesis, increased vasodilation, decreased platelet adherence) are lost. As a result, menopausal women are at **increased risk for coronary artery disease**. Second, with menopause, bone resorption increases, which can lead to **low bone density** (formally known as osteopenia) and potentially osteoporosis.

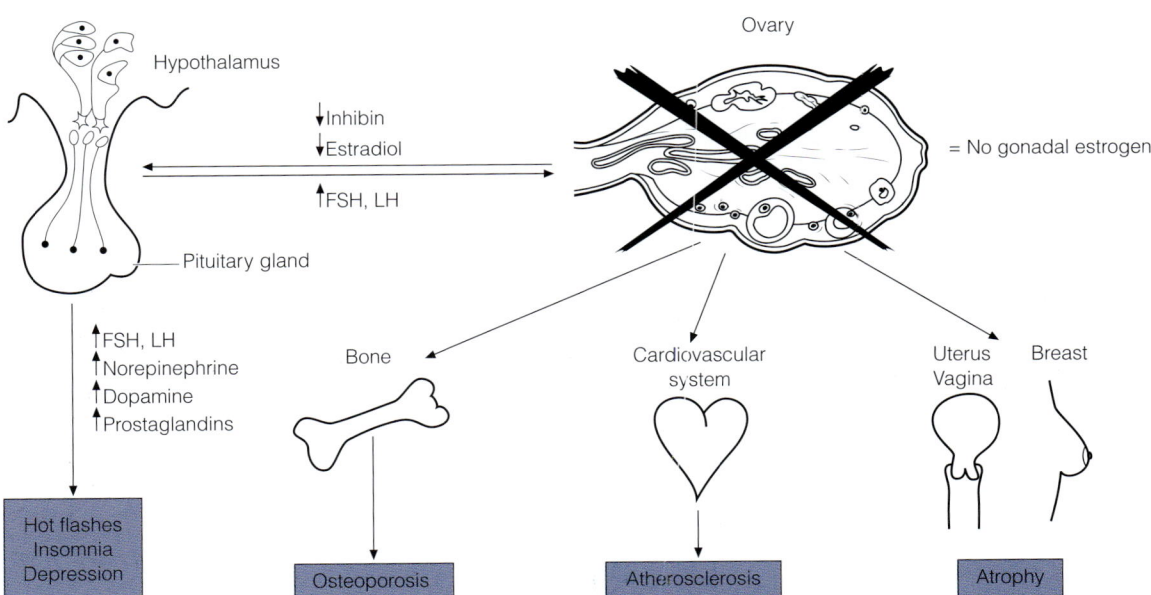

FIGURE 20-6. Changes in both the ovary and the hypothalamus contribute to the physiologic changes of menopause. FSH, follicle-stimulating hormone; LH, luteinizing hormone.

MENOPAUSAL HORMONE THERAPY

The term menopausal hormone therapy (MHT) includes both estrogen therapy (ET) and estrogen + progesterone therapy (EPT). Both ET and EPT successfully treat the bothersome symptoms of menopause. Efficacy rates are commonly seen in the 90% range. ET is reserved for women without an intact uterus. The use of **unopposed estrogen is contraindicated in women with a uterus** and requires the addition of a suitable progestin to prevent increased incidence of endometrial intraepithelial neoplasia (EIN), endometrial hyperplasia, and endometrial cancer. Almost all versions of ET and EPT available are approved by the FDA for treatment of VMS. Treatment options include oral medications and topical medications, including gels, patches, and sprays. Vaginal rings and injections are available and FDA approved. In women with an intact uterus who desire contraception, the **levonorgestrel-releasing intrauterine system** may be an appropriate option.

New treatments available include **selective estrogen receptor modulators** (SERMs) and **tissue-specific estrogen complex** (TSEC). Duavee (combination conjugated equine estrogen (CEE) 0.45 mg and bazedoxifene (BZE) 20 mg) is the first TSEC, FDA approved to treat VMS and prevent osteoporosis in women with a uterus. This medication does not require the addition of a progesterone. SERMs each have a unique pattern of both agonistic and antagonistic effects on other tissues, including heart, bone, uterus, and breast. Only bazedoxifene (BZE) has been shown to have an adequate antagonistic effect on the uterus; therefore, it does not require additional progesterone therapy when paired with an estrogen.

The risks and benefits of MHT have been the subject of numerous studies over the past 30 years. These trials have been designed to evaluate the most common causes of death, disability, and poor quality of life in postmenopausal women, including cardiovascular disease, venous thromboembolism, cancer, osteoporosis, and loss of cognitive function. Among the studies contributing to our knowledge of the safety and efficacy of hormone replacement therapy (HRT) and estrogen replacement therapy (ERT) were the Heart and Estrogen/Progestin Replacement Studies (**HERS I and II**), Postmenopausal Estrogen/Progestin Interventions (**PEPI**) Trial, the WHI Memory Study (**WHIMS**), and the Women's Health Initiative (**WHI**). Although initially some epidemiologic studies suggested a cardioprotective effect or HRT with preservation of cognitive function and prevention of dementia, later data from WHI, HERS I and II, and others did not support these conclusions. The collective findings from the major studies are summarized in Table 20-3.

TABLE 20-3. Summary of the Major Studies on the Benefits and Risk of Estrogen and Progesterone Therapy (EPT) and Estrogen Therapy (ET)

Outcome	Estrogen and Progesterone	Estrogen Only
Heart attack	↑	↔
Stroke (ischemic)	↑	↑
Deep vein thrombosis (DVT)	↑	↑
Pulmonary embolus (PE)	↑	↔
Invasive breast cancer	↑	↔
Colorectal cancer	↓	↑
Osteoporotic hip fracture	↓	↓
Osteoporotic vertebral fracture	↓	↓
Cognitive functioning	↔	↔
Dementia	↑	↑
Hot flashes, night sweats	↓	↓

↑, increased risk with hormone therapy use.
↓, decreased risk with hormone therapy use.
↔, no change in risk with hormone therapy use.

Benefits of MHT

In general, MHT use results in excellent control of menopausal symptoms, including reduction of VMS, improvement in mood and sleep dysfunction, prevention and treatment of GSM, and improvement in skin and muscle tone. Women who begin MHT before age 60 years or within 10 years of the FMP obtain the largest benefit in **control of vasomotor symptoms** and **prevention of bone loss**. The more remote a woman is from menopause (over 10 years from FMP and over 60 years of age), the less favorable the outcomes become. Increased rates of stroke, deep vein thrombosis (DVT), CVD, and dementia are seen in this population.

Risks of MHT

Conversely, both ET and EPT use **increased DVTs, pulmonary emboli (PE), and ischemic strokes**. This risk appears by 1 to 2 years of use and decreases over time. This risk is rare in women ages 50 to 59 years. Large studies show that this risk is lower when a transdermal delivery method is used. Head-to-head clinical trials are needed to confirm. An **increased risk of invasive breast cancer** in women who used conjugated equine estrogen + medroxyprogesterone acetate (0.625 mg CEE + 2.5 mg MPA) was seen in WHI after 3 to 5 years. The risk decreases after hormone therapy is stopped. ET use was associated with fewer invasive breast cancers after 7 years. Observational data suggest a trend toward increased risk at 10 to 15 years. EPT use but not ET was associated with higher rates of death from non–small-cell lung cancer, neither was associated with an incidence of lung cancer. Increased cases of dementia were diagnosed in women ages 65 to 79 years in the WHIMS data.

The major limitation of the WHI trials is that the participants were much older (average age of 63 years) and had higher BMIs (average BMI of 34), and the sample had a higher percentage of smokers than subjects in most epidemiologic studies. This makes it more difficult to generalize the findings to healthy, younger, newly menopausal women with symptoms for whom the benefits of short-term use often far outweigh the risks.

Recommendations and Contraindications

NAMS recommendations for MHT use:

- For women with **moderate to severe VMS or GSM** and no contraindication to estrogen, MHT is the recommended treatment.
- MHT is recommended for the **prevention of osteoporosis** but not for the treatment of osteoporosis.
- For women whose only symptoms relate to GSM, local, **low-dose vaginal estrogens** should be recommended.
- Doses used should be **lowest effective dose** in keeping with the goals of treatment. Individualization is crucial for management of menopause symptoms. The route of administration, the type of estrogen and progesterone used, or use of a TSEC or SERM should all be considered when individualizing therapy.
- **Extended therapy** (longer than 3 to 5 years for EPT and 7 years for ET) may be appropriate for women with persistent symptoms who understand the risks and benefits and desire treatment continuation. Longer therapy may be used in women at risk for osteoporosis and osteoporotic fractures who cannot tolerate treatment with other medications.

As a result of cumulative studies, the current national recommendation is that MHT is a suitable option for women with bothersome symptoms of menopause, including vasomotor and genital urinary symptoms (in the absence of any contraindication). **Contraindications to MHT** include chronic liver impairment, known estrogen-dependent neoplasm (breast, ovary, and endometrium), active thromboembolic disease, and undiagnosed uterine bleeding. The results are most favorable for women who begin MHT before age 60 years and within 10 years of menopause. Treatment must be considered carefully, however, particularly in older women. MHT should not be used for the prevention of other chronic diseases such as cardiovascuar disease, coronary heart disease, or dementia. Treatment options should be individualized and carefully considered. Patient education and informed consent are crucial components of MHT use.

NONHORMONAL TREATMENT OF MENOPAUSAL SYMPTOMS

Alternative regimens for postmenopausal women who are unable or unwilling to take MHT or who have completed short-term ET or EPT should be targeted toward the individual's symptoms and treatment goals (Table 20-4).

TABLE 20-4. Treatment Options to Address the Various Symptoms/Conditions of Menopause

Menopausal Symptom	Treatment Option
Cardiovascular changes	BP and lipid control medications, smoking cessation, weight loss, exercise
Osteoporosis prevention	MHT, calcium, Vitamin D, bisphosphonates, calcitonin, SERMs, weight-bearing exercise, and decrease smoking and caffeine and alcohol intake
VMS (hot flashes, night sweats)	MHT, SSRIs, SNRIs, gabapentin, clonidine, behavioral changes (cooling pillow, sweat-wicking pajamas, fan)
Genital menopausal symptoms (vaginal dryness, dyspareunia, incontinence, dysuria)	Low-dose vaginal estrogen, water-based lubricant, vaginal moisturizers
Mood disturbances	MHT, SSRIs, SNRIs, counseling

MHT, menopausal hormone therapy; SERMs, selective estrogen receptor modulators; SSRIs, selective serotonin reuptake inhibitors; SNRIs, serotonin–norepinephrine reuptake inhibitors; VMS, vasomotor symptoms.

Hot flashes and night sweats may be managed in women who either choose not to or cannot take ET. The only FDA approved nonhormonal medication to treat VMS in menopausal women is **paroxetine sulfate** (Brisdelle 7.5 mg). Other selective serotonin reuptake inhibitors (**SSRIs**) **and** serotonin–norepinephrine reuptake inhibitors (**SNRIs**), including citalopram and venlafaxine, have shown efficacy. Low doses of gabapentin or clonidine have also been shown to have beneficial effects in clinical trials. **Cognitive behavior therapy** has also been shown to be an effective tool to manage hot flashes. Behavioral changes including avoidance of triggers, use of fans, use of cooling sleep pillow, or sweat-wicking sleepwear also offer symptomatic relief. Risks, benefits, onset of action, and side effects vary with each of these medications and may include sexual side effects, drowsiness, or nausea making patient education a critical component to success.

Where indicated, **other causes for hot flashes,** such as thyroid disease, autoimmune disorders, carcinoid, and pheochromocytoma tumors, SERMs (tamoxifen/raloxifene, ospemifene) use should be ruled out. **Complementary and alternative therapies** (soy, black cohosh, phytoestrogens, dong quai, evening primrose oil) have not been found to be more effective than placebos in the treatment of VMS. Each of these over-the-counter therapies may have side effects as well and is not recommended.

Vaginal and urogenital atrophy can be treated using vulvovaginal lubricants and moisturizers. Low-dose vaginal estrogen can have excellent local effects on vaginal and urethral atrophy with only minimal systemic absorption. When used at low vaginal dosing, these estrogen sources **do not require opposing progestin** use in women with an intact uterus. Emerging treatment options in the field of vaginal rejuvenation are becoming more available, including the use of thermal and CO_2 lasers. These may be excellent choices for women who have contraindications to ET; however, more research is needed on these products.

With respect to **cardiovascular health**, improvement in lifestyle and diet are key factors, as well as optimal blood pressure and weight control to decrease morbidity and mortality.

OSTEOPOROSIS

EPIDEMIOLOGY

Osteoporosis is one of the major long-term complications of menopause. It occurs five times more among women than men and carries significant implications for morbidity, mortality, and quality of life for women. Women have twice the fracture rate of men, with 80% of hip fractures occurring among elderly women. Fifteen percent of women older than 50 years will be diagnosed with osteoporosis and 50% with low bone density (formerly osteopenia). In fact, a woman can lose 20% of her original bone density in the first 5 to 7 years after menopause. Subsequently, menopausal patients are at risk of **hip and vertebral fractures**, chronic pain, loss of height, immobility, and loss of function.

RISK FACTORS

Family history and **age** are major determinants of lifelong bone density. Risk also varies by **race and ethnicity**, with Caucasian and Asian women being at higher risk than Mexican American woman and African American women being at lowest risk. Table 20-5 identifies other **major risk factors** for osteoporosis. An additional risk factor is **prolonged use of medications,** such as depot medroxyprogesterone acetate, GnRH agonists, glucocorticoids ($\geq$5 mg/day prednisone for >3 months), and aromatase inhibitors.

PATHOGENESIS

The pathophysiology of osteoporosis is a combination of a **decline in estrogen levels** and an increase in reactive oxygen species with aging, which results in the **increased rate of resorption** and the **decreased rate of osteoblastogenesis**.

Women achieve the **maximum bone density** between age 20 and 25 years. Therefore, achieving

TABLE 20-5.	Risk Factors Mnemonic for Osteoporosis SHATTERED Family
S	Steroid use (>5 mg/d of prednisone)
H	Hyperthyroidism/hyperparathyroidism/hypercalciuria
A	Alcohol (>3/d) and tobacco (active or passive) use
T	Thin (BMI < 22; weight < 127 lbs)
T	Testosterone low, hypogonadism
E	Early menopause
R	Renal or liver failure
E	Erosive/inflammatory bone disease (e.g., rheumatoid arthritis and myeloma)
D	Dietary Ca low/malabsorption or diabetes mellitus type I
Family	Family history/genetics

TABLE 20-6.	The Institutes of Medicine (IOM) Recommended Dietary Allowance for Calcium and Vitamin D
Age	**Dosage**
Calcium	
9–18 y old	1,300 IU
19–50 y old	1,000 IU
Over 50 y old	1,200 IU
Vitamin D	
Almost everyone	600 IU
Over 70 y old	800 IU

TABLE 20-7.	World Health Organization Criteria for Diagnosing Osteoporosis by DXA Bone Densitometry
Diagnostic Interpretation	**T-score**[a]
Normal	≥ -1.0
Low bone mass (osteopenia)	< -1.0 to > -2.5
Osteoporosis	≤ -2.5

DXA, dual-energy X-ray absorptiometry.
[a]T-score is the number of standard deviations above or below the mean average bone density result for young adult women.

maximum bone density is critical to the care for female patients at all ages. Low vitamin D can result in osteomalacia in adults and rickets in children, and diets low in calcium are associated with low bone mineralization. In 2011, the Institutes of Medicine (IOM) changed its recommended dietary allowance for **calcium intake** to a range of 1,000 to 1,300 mg/day depending on age (Table 20-6). There has been controversy over high intake of supplemental calcium and its potential risk of coronary artery calcification. For this reason, the use of dietary calcium is preferred over the use of supplementation by some providers. In 2011, the IOM also decreased recommended dietary allowance for **vitamin D intake**, lowered to 600 IU/day for most women and 800 IU/day for women over age 70 years. Routine screening for vitamin D deficiency should be limited to patients with medical conditions or medication use placing them at high risk of vitamin D deficiency. **Vitamin D levels of >30 ng/dL** were associated with a decreased risk of bone fracture.

DIAGNOSIS

Bone mineral density (BMD) screening should begin at age 65 years for all women. Postmenopausal women under the age of 65 years should be screened if they have significant risk factors including history of fragility fracture, weight <127 lbs, parent with a history of hip fracture, current smoking, alcoholism, or rheumatoid arthritis (Table 20-5).

The gold standard for diagnosing osteoporosis is a **dual-energy X-ray absorptiometry (DXA)** of the lumbar spine and hip. Table 20-7 shows the World Health Organization's criteria for diagnosis of osteoporosis using the T-Score. Osteoporosis is defined as a T-Score ≤ 2.5. The Z-score is reserved for use in children, teens, premenopausal women, and younger men in the rare instances when bone density testing is indicated in these groups. Repeat BMD screenings are performed no more frequently than every 2 years unless a patient's response to medication is being evaluated. **FRAX, a fracture risk assessment tool**, can help to further predict a person's risk of hip fracture or major osteoporotic fracture in the next 10 years. FRAX is based on risk factors, such as age, BMI, history of fracture, daily alcohol intake, and whether or not a patient smokes, has rheumatoid arthritis, or has any other secondary causes of osteoporosis. In the United States, the FRAX tool is used most often in postmenopausal women with low bone density (osteopenia) than DXA to decide on treatment initiation. A **clinical diagnosis** of osteoporosis can be made when a patient suffers a low-trauma (fragility) fracture as a result of normal activities like falling from a standing height or less.

TREATMENT

Once the diagnosis of osteoporosis is made, **consider secondary causes** and work up prior to initiating treatment. Likewise, women with osteoporosis and those at risk for osteoporosis should be encouraged to make **lifestyle changes** to decrease their risk. **Weight-bearing exercise** (such as walking, hiking, and stair climbing) and muscle-strengthening exercise have been found to decrease the risk of falls and fractures. These groups should also be counseled regarding adequate calcium and vitamin D intake. Reduction in active and passive smoking and alcohol intake (<3/day) has also been shown to lower the rate of bone loss. Women should also be encouraged to use fall prevention strategies to limit the risk of falls and fractures.

Medications approved for the prevention of osteoporosis include bisphosphonates (Fosamax, Actonel, Boniva), zoledronic acid (Reclast), raloxifene (Evista), and MHT.

There are many medications for treatment of osteoporosis, including bisphosphonates, partial estrogen agonists and antagonists, denosumab (Prolia), teriparatide (Forteo), calcitonin, parathyroid hormone, and MHT. **Bisphosphonates** are the leading treatment, and the mechanism of action is **inhibition of osteoclast resorption of bone**. Partial estrogen agonists and antagonists, also known as SERMs, inhibit bone resorption. **Denosumab is** a human monoclonal antibody to the receptor activator of nuclear factor-κB ligand, which blocks proliferation and differentiation of osteoclasts, resulting in decreased bone resorption and increased BMD. **Calcitonin** is an antiresorptive treatment. **Parathyroid hormone** stimulates osteoblastic activity.

KEY POINTS

- The typical order of the events in puberty is accelerated growth, thelarche (breast development), pubarche (pubic hair development), and menarche (onset of menstruation).
- During the normal menstrual cycle, the ovary goes through follicular and luteal phases, and at the same time, the endometrium goes through the proliferative and secretory phases.
- Ovulation occurs in response to the LH surge signaling the cascade for the mature follicle to break open and release the mature oocyte. Fertilization of the ovum must occur within 24 hours of ovulation.
- Menstruation occurs as the result of decreasing progestin levels, resulting in the sloughing of the endometrium.
- Perimenopause can begin 2 to 8 years prior to menopause. It is characterized by irregular menstrual cycles and milder, less frequent symptoms that are associated with menopause, such as hot flashes, night sweats, and mood swings.
- Menopause marks the termination of the reproductive phase of a woman's life. It is characterized by the cessation of menses and the onset of an estrogen-deficient state.
- The average age of menopause is 51 years. Menopausal patients present with amenorrhea, hot flashes, vaginal atrophy, and mood and sleep changes; all consistent with decreased levels of estrogen.
- Menopause can be diagnosed after 12 months of amenorrhea and consistently elevated FSH level levels > 40 IU/L. Menopausal symptoms may also be present. It can be confirmed by elevated levels of FSH.
- Women who wish to use MHT for menopausal symptoms and who still have a uterus in place should use EPT. This decreases the risk of endometrial hyperplasia, EIN and endometrial cancer from unopposed estrogen exposure.

- Major benefits of ET and EPT are the prevention of bone loss and osteoporosis and the relief of symptoms associated with menopause.
- Combination EPT has been associated with an increased risk of heart attacks, strokes, DVTs, PE, and invasive breast cancer.
- When used alone, ERT has been associated with an increased risk of strokes and DVTs.
- When used, MHT should be reserved for the treatment of moderate to severe VPS and GSM. Its benefit is greatest in women who are <60 years old and are within 10 years of FMP. In general, MHT at the lowest effective dose is used to treat symptoms.
- Contraindications to MHT include chronic liver disease, undiagnosed abnormal uterine bleeding (AUB), active thromboembolic disorder, pregnancy, and known estrogen-dependent neoplasm.
- If MHT is completed, not tolerated, or not desired, alternative therapies are available to address each of the symptoms and side effects of menopause.
- Osteoporosis is one of the major long-term complications of menopause. It can be diagnosed with a DXA T-Score ≤ −2.5 or clinically in the setting of a low-trauma (fragility) fracture.
- Screening should include the use of DXA beginning at age 65 years or earlier in postmenopausal women with significant risk factors. The FRAX tool is used most often in postmenopausal women with low bone density (osteopenia) in determining whether to start therapy.
- Major risk factors for osteoporosis include increasing age, female gender, family history, low-estrogen status, weight < 127 lbs. and certain medications among others.
- Prevention and treatment options include calcium, vitamin D, weight-bearing exercise, MHT, bisphosphonates, SERMs, Prolia, Forteo, Reclast and calcitonin.

CLINICAL VIGNETTES

VIGNETTE 1
An 8-year-old African American girl is brought to your office by her parents concerned that she has started developing breasts too soon. Physical examination reveals a Tanner stage II breast and pubic hair growth.

1. Breast bud development is the beginning of what stage of puberty?
   a. Thelarche
   b. Adrenarche
   c. Pubarche
   d. Menarche
   e. Accelerated growth

2. You reassure the parents that this is normal. What is typical pubertal sequence?
   a. Menarche, pubarche, thelarche, accelerated growth
   b. Pubarche, thelarche, accelerated growth, menarche
   c. Thelarche, pubarche, accelerated growth, menarche
   d. Accelerated growth, thelarche, pubarche, menarche
   e. Pubarche, accelerated growth, thelarche, menarche

3. When can the patient expect her first menses?
   a. At 14 years of age
   b. At 12 years of age
   c. At 11 years of age
   d. At 13 years of age
   e. It is impossible to tell from the data provided

VIGNETTE 2
A 28-year-old patient is in your office to discuss the possibility of getting pregnant. As part of her history, you take thorough menstrual history. She states that she had menarche at age 12 years. Initially, her menses was irregular, but since she was 14 years, her menses has been every 30 days and last for 5 days. She uses four to five tampons a day and denies dysmenorrhea.

1. The menstrual cycle is divided into which two phases when describing the endometrium?
   a. Follicular and secretory phases
   b. Follicular and luteal phases
   c. Proliferative and luteal phases
   d. Proliferative and secretory phases
   e. Atrophic and menstrual

2. Which of these structures does NOT produce progesterone?
   a. Placenta
   b. Endometrium
   c. Corpus luteum
   d. Follicle
   e. Adrenal cortex

3. The patient comes back to your office, and she is pregnant. What hormone does the developing trophoblast produce?
   a. Human chorionic gonadotropin (hCG)
   b. Progesterone
   c. Androstenedione
   d. Luteinizing hormone (LH)
   e. Estrogen

VIGNETTE 3
A 51-year-old woman presents to your office with amenorrhea for the past year. Since she has not had any hot flashes, she is wondering if she is menopausal.

1. What blood test would confirm the diagnosis of menopause?
   a. Follicle-stimulating hormone (FSH)
   b. Estrogen
   c. Testosterone
   d. hCG
   e. Prolactin

2. Early menopause is more common in all of the following except:
   a. in nulliparous women
   b. women with hypertension
   c. women who smoke
   d. women with type 1 diabetes
   e. women with family history of early menopause

3. Which of the following is NOT a classic symptom of menopause?
   a. Hot flashes
   b. Insomnia
   c. Visual changes
   d. Vaginal atrophy
   e. Night sweats

VIGNETTE 4
A 51-year-old woman presents to your office to discuss menopausal hormone therapy (MHT). She has been amenorrheic for more than a year. She reports hot flashes multiple times a day and daily night sweats. These symptoms are interfering with her concentration and sleep.

1. Which of the following is NOT a contraindication to MHT?
   a. History of a deep vein thrombosis (DVT)
   b. History of breast cancer
   c. Cirrhosis
   d. Current smoking history
   e. History of pulmonary emboli (PE)

2. What is an acceptable indication for MHT use?
   a. Osteoporosis treatment
   b. Isolated vaginal dryness treatment
   c. Hot flashes and night sweats interfering with quality of life
   d. Cardiovascular disease prevention
   e. Dementia prevention

3. The patient still has her uterus. If the patient is started on estrogen therapy (ET), what other hormone also needs to be prescribed?
   a. A progestin
   b. FSH
   c. hCG
   d. Testosterone
   e. Vaginal estrogen cream

ANSWERS

VIGNETTE 1 Question 1
1. Answer A:
The first stage of thelarche is breast bud development and is the first phenotypic sign of puberty. Adrenarche is when the adrenal gland begins regeneration of the zona reticularis, which is responsible for the secretion of sex steroid hormones. Pubarche is the onset of pubic hair growth. Menarche is the first menses.

VIGNETTE 1 Question 2
2. Answer D:
The normal pubertal sequence is initiated with accelerated growth. Breast development (thelarche) is next, followed by appearance of pubic hair (pubarche). Onset of menstruation (menarche) is at the end. A normal variant seen most commonly with African American girls is that pubarche precedes thelarche.

VIGNETTE 1 Question 3
3. Answer C:
Average length of time from breast bud development to menstruation in typically 2.5 years, and so you would expect her to have her menses between 10 and 11 years of age. The other ages are all later than you would expect.

VIGNETTE 2 Question 1
1. Answer D:
The menstrual cycle is divided into the follicular and luteal phases in respect to changes in the ovary over the length of the cycle. The proliferative and secretory phases describe the concurrent changes in the endometrium. Options A and C are both wrong because these describe a phase in respect to both the ovary and endometrium. Atrophic and menstrual are terms used to describe the status of the endometrium, but this terminology is not used for phases of the menstrual cycle.

VIGNETTE 2 Question 2
2. Answer B:
The endometrium does not produce progesterone. The corpus luteum produces progesterone to maintain the endometrium until the placenta takes over at 8 to 10 weeks of gestation. In the absence of fertilization, the corpus luteum degenerates, and the progesterone levels fall, so the endometrium is unable to be maintained, resulting in a menstruation. The follicle produces progesterone in response to the LH surge and results in ovulation. This follicle then becomes the corpus luteum after ovulation.

VIGNETTE 2 Question 3
3. Answer A:
The trophoblast produces hCG to maintain the corpus luteum. Without this rise in hCG, it signals to the corpus luteum that fertilization has not occurred and triggers the cascade that results in menstruation. The follicle produces progesterone in response to the LH surge and results in ovulation. This follicle then becomes the corpus luteum after ovulation. The corpus luteum produces progesterone to maintain the endometrium until the placenta takes over at 8 to 10 weeks of gestation. Androstenedione is produced by the theca interna cells. LH is produced by the anterior pituitary gland.

VIGNETTE 3 Question 1
1. Answer A:
An FSH level greater than 40 IU/L is diagnostic of menopause. Estrogen levels do not consistently predict menopause, especially if there is peripheral conversion of estrogen in the morbidly obese patient. Testosterone has no role in predicting menopause. If there is a presence of hCG at this age, pregnancy (though unlikely) and gestational trophoblastic disease must be ruled out. Prolactin is produced in the anterior pituitary and causes milk secretion from the breast and preventing ovulation in lactating women. High prolactin levels (hyperprolactinemia) may result in galactorrhea and/or amenorrhea. It is not diagnostic of menopause.

VIGNETTE 3 Question 2
2. Answer B:
The average age of menopause is 51 years, with 90% of women experiencing this change between ages 45

and 55 years. Hysterectomy and tubal ligation are associated with a slightly earlier menopause (1 to 2 years). Early menopause is defined as occurring between ages 40 and 45 years. Early menopause is more common in women with a history of cigarette smoking, short cycles, nulliparity, type 1 diabetes, in utero exposure to diethylstilbestrol, and family history of early menopause. Hypertension has not been shown to increase the risk of early menopause. Menopause occurring before age 40 years is considered premature ovarian insufficiency (previously termed premature ovarian failure).

VIGNETTE 3 Question 3
3. Answer C:
Hot flashes, insomnia, and vaginal atrophy are all common symptoms of menopause and are a result of the diminished estrogen production. Visual changes are age related and not a direct effect of menopause.

VIGNETTE 4 Question 1
1. Answer D:
Contraindications to MHT include chronic liver impairment, pregnancy, known estrogen-dependent neoplasm (breast, ovary, uterus), history of thromboembolic disease (DVT, PE, CVA), and unevaluated vaginal bleeding. Oral contraceptives, but not hormone replacement therapy (HRT), are contraindicated in female smokers >35 years of age. However, the principal conclusion of the Women's Health Initiative (WHI) study was that the lowest dose possible should be chosen, especially in patients with an increased cardiovascular risk, as is the case in smokers.

VIGNETTE 4 Question 2
2. Answer C:
Currently, the only clinical indication for MHT is moderate to severe vasomotor symptoms (VMS), including hot flashes and night sweats. An added benefit of MHT is the prevention of osteoporosis; however, HRT should not be a first-line therapy for the treatment of osteoporosis. HRT use should be limited to the lowest dose necessary to control VMS and for the shortest period of time needed. If isolated vaginal dryness is the primary symptom, this patient would best be treated with vaginal lubricants and moisturizers first, followed by low-dose vaginal estrogen, so that there is a minimal systemic absorption. MHT should not be used to treat or prevent cardiovascular disease or dementia.

VIGNETTE 4 Question 3
3. Answer A:
When estrogens are being used to treat menopausal symptoms in women who still have uterus in situ, progestins must be used to decrease the risk of benign endometrial hyperplasia, endometrial intraepithelial neoplasia, and endometrial cancer. None of the other options would be protective of the endometrium.

21 | Amenorrhea

Amenorrhea—the absence of menses—is classified as either primary or secondary. **Primary** amenorrhea is the absence of menarche (first menses) by age 15 in the presence of normal growth and secondary sexual characteristics. **Secondary** amenorrhea is the absence of menses for 3 months in women with previously regular cycles or 6 months in women with a history of irregular cycles. The pathophysiology underlying these two processes differs greatly, as do the differential diagnoses.

PRIMARY AMENORRHEA

The diagnosis of primary amenorrhea is the absence of menses by age 15 in the presence of normal growth and secondary sexual characteristics. If, however, at age 13, there is complete absence of secondary sexual characteristics and no menarche, an evaluation for primary amenorrhea should be initiated. In the United States, the prevalence of primary amenorrhea is 1% to 2%. The causes of primary amenorrhea include congenital and chromosomal abnormalities, hormonal aberrations, hypothalamic–pituitary disorders, and the variety of causes of secondary amenorrhea that may present before menarche. Primary amenorrhea can be divided into three categories: outflow tract obstruction, end-organ disorders, and central regulatory disorders (Table 21-1).

OUTFLOW TRACT ANOMALIES
Imperforate Hymen
During fetal development, the hymen may fail to canalize, remaining a solid membrane across the vaginal introitus. If the hymen is imperforate, it will not allow egress of menstrual blood or menses. Thus, despite having begun to menstruate, patients appear to have primary amenorrhea. After a time, patients present with pelvic or abdominal pain from the accumulation and subsequent dilation of the vaginal vault and uterus by menses. On physical examination, these patients have a bulging membrane just inside the introitus, often with purple-red discoloration behind it consistent with hematocolpos. The treatment of imperforate hymen is surgical; usually a cruciate incision is made, and the hymen is sewn open to allow the passage of menstrual flow.

Transverse Vaginal Septum
A transverse vaginal septum may result from failure of the Müllerian-derived upper vagina to fuse with the urogenital sinus-derived lower vagina. The result of this failed fusion, an imperforate transverse vaginal septum, is commonly found at the level of the midvagina, and its persistence may lead to primary amenorrhea by obstruction. The clinical history may include a young woman who presents with primary amenorrhea with cyclic pelvic pain. Diagnosis is made on careful examination of the female genital tract, examining for a bulging septum consistent with hematocolpos. The diagnosis is commonly mistaken as imperforate hymen, and can be differentiated by the presence of a hymeneal ring below the septum. Surgical correction involves resection of the septum.

Vaginal Agenesis
Patients with **Mayer–Rokitansky–Kuster–Hauser** syndrome have Müllerian agenesis or dysgenesis. They may have complete vaginal agenesis and the absence of a uterus or partial vaginal agenesis with a rudimentary uterus and distal vagina. This differs from **vaginal atresia**, where the Müllerian system is developed, but the distal vagina is composed of fibrosed tissue. Diagnosis is made with physical examination that reveals no patent vagina, chromosomes that are 46,XX, and ovaries visualized on ultrasound. With partial vaginal agenesis or vaginal atresia, a rectal examination may reveal a pelvic mass consistent with a

TABLE 21-1. Etiologies of Primary Amenorrhea

Outflow tract abnormalities
Imperforate hymen
Transverse vaginal septum
Vaginal agenesis
Vaginal atresia
Testicular feminization
Uterine agenesis with vaginal dysgenesis
MRKH syndrome

End-organ disorders
Ovarian agenesis
Gonadal agenesis 46,XX
Swyer syndrome/gonadal agenesis 46,XY
Ovarian insufficiency
Enzymatic defects leading to decreased steroid biosynthesis
Savage syndrome—ovary fails to respond to FSH and LH
Turner syndrome

Central disorders
Hypothalamic
Local tumor compression
Trauma
Tuberculosis
Sarcoidosis
Irradiation
Kallmann syndrome—congenital absence of GnRH
Pituitary
Damage from surgery or radiation therapy
Hemosiderosis deposition of iron in pituitary

MRKH, Mayer–Rokitansky–Kuster–Hauser; FSH, follicle-stimulating hormone; LH, luteinizing hormone; GnRH, gonadotropin-releasing hormone.

uterus. The uterus can be visualized with ultrasound, CT, or MRI. A neovagina can be created either by serial dilation of the perineal body by the patient over an extended period of time or by reconstructive surgery. In true vaginal atresia, the neovagina created may be connected with the upper genital tract.

Testicular Feminization

Testicular feminization, also known as androgen insensitivity syndrome, results from a dysfunction or the absence of the testosterone receptor that leads to a phenotypical female with 46,XY chromosomes. This syndrome occurs in 1 in 50,000 women. Because these patients have testes, **Müllerian inhibiting factor** (MIF) is secreted early in the development, and these patients therefore have an absence of all Müllerian-derived structures. Of note, the testes may be undescended or may have migrated down to the labia majora. The diminished testosterone sensitivity commonly leads to an absence of pubic and axillary hair. Usually estrogen is produced, and these patients develop breasts but present with primary amenorrhea because they have no uterus. Patients commonly have a vagina that ends as a blind pouch. For those patients with the absence of or a foreshortened vagina, therapy involves creating a neovagina for sexual function; however, these patients are unable to reproduce. Additional health consequences may include testicular cancer and complex psychosocial issues.

END-ORGAN DISORDERS

Ovarian Insufficiency

Primary ovarian insufficiency (POI) results in low levels of estradiol but elevated levels of gonadotropins termed **hypergonadotropic hypogonadism**. There are a variety of causes of POI (Table 21-2). **Savage syndrome** is characterized by failure of the ovaries to respond to follicle-stimulating hormone (FSH) and luteinizing hormone (LH) secondary to a receptor defect. In **Turner syndrome** (45,XO), the ovaries undergo such rapid atresia that by puberty, there are usually no primordial oocytes. Defects in the enzymes involved in steroid biosynthesis, particularly 17-hydroxylase, can result in amenorrhea and the absence of breast development given the lack of estradiol.

Gonadal Agenesis with 46,XY Chromosomes

If there is a defect in the enzymes that are involved in testicular steroid production—**17-α-hydroxylase** or **17,20 desmolase**—testosterone production will be absent. However, MIF will still be produced; hence, there will be no female internal reproductive organs. These patients will otherwise be phenotypically female, usually without breast development. Patients with an absence of or defect in the testosterone receptor develop testicular feminization syndrome.

Although testicular feminization results from peripheral effects of diminished or absent sensitivity of testosterone receptors, another situation in which the patient is genetically male, but phenotypically female is gonadal agenesis. The congenital absence of the testes in a genotypical male, **Swyer syndrome**, results in a phenotypical picture similar to that of ovarian agenesis. Because the testes never develop, MIF is not released, and these patients have both internal and external female genitalia. However, without estrogen, they will not develop breasts.

CENTRAL DISORDERS

Hypothalamic Disorders

The pituitary will not release FSH and LH if the hypothalamus is unable to produce gonadotropin-releasing

TABLE 21-2.	Causes of Primary Gonadal Failure (Hypergonadotropic Hypogonadism)

Idiopathic premature ovarian failure
Steroidogenic enzyme defects (primary amenorrhea)
Cholesterol side-chain cleavage
3β-ol-Dehydrogenase
17-Hydroxylase
17-Desmolase
17-Ketoreductase
Testicular regression syndrome
True hermaphroditism
Gonadal dysgenesis
Pure gonadal dysgenesis (Swyer syndrome) (46,XX and 46,XY)
Turner syndrome (45,XO)
Turner variants
Ovarian resistance syndrome (Savage syndrome)
Autoimmune oophoritis
Postinfection (e.g., mumps)
Postoophorectomy (also wedge resections)
Postirradiation
Postchemotherapy

Adapted from DeCherney A, Pernoll M. *Current Obstetric and Gynecologic Diagnosis and Treatment*. Norwalk, CT: Appleton & Lange; 1994:1009.

hormone (GnRH), transport it to the pituitary, or release it in a pulsatile fashion. Anovulation and amenorrhea result from this hypogonadotropic hypogonadism. **Kallmann syndrome** is one form of hypogonadotropic hypogonadism, which involves the congenital absence of GnRH and is commonly associated with anosmia. In Kallmann syndrome, the normal migration of the GnRH neurons is disrupted in their travel from the olfactory placode to the hypothalamus, and the olfactory bulbs also do not form, leading to the combination of hypogonadotropic hypogonadism and anosmia. Other ways that GnRH transport may be disrupted include compression or destruction of the pituitary stalk or arcuate nucleus. This can result from tumor mass effect, trauma, sarcoidosis, tuberculosis, irradiation, or Hand–Schuller–Christian disease. Finally, there may be defects in GnRH pulsatility in cases of anorexia nervosa, extreme stress, athletes, hyperprolactinemia, hypothyroidism, rapid or severe weight loss, and constitutionally delayed puberty.

Pituitary Disorders

Primary defects of the pituitary are a rare cause of primary amenorrhea. Pituitary dysfunction is usually secondary to hypothalamic dysfunction. It may be caused by tumors, infiltration of the pituitary gland, or infarcts of the pituitary. Surgery or irradiation of pituitary tumors may lead to decreases in or absence of LH and FSH. Hemosiderosis can result in iron deposition in the pituitary, leading to destruction of the gonadotrophs that produce FSH and LH.

DIAGNOSIS

A patient who presents with primary amenorrhea can be worked up based on the phenotypic picture (Table 21-3 and Fig. 21-1). Lack of a uterus is seen in males because of the release of MIF by the testes and in females with Müllerian agenesis. Breast development is dependent on estradiol secretion by the ovaries. Patients who have neither a uterus nor breasts are generally 46,XY males with steroid synthesis defects or varying degrees of gonadal dysgenesis, in which adequate MIF is produced by gonadal tissue, but androgen synthesis is insufficient.

If breasts are present but no uterus, the etiologies can include congenital absence of the uterus (Müllerian agenesis) in the female or testicular feminization in the male. In the latter case, estradiol from direct testicular secretion as well as peripheral conversion of testosterone and androstenedione leads to breast development. The presence of a normal amount and distribution of pubic hair supports Müllerian agenesis, whereas absent or scant pubic hair indicates androgen insensitivity.

TABLE 21-3. Diagnosis of Etiology of Primary Amenorrhea		
	Uterus Absent	**Uterus Present**
Breasts absent	Gonadal agenesis in 46,XY	Gonadal failure/agenesis in 46,XX
Breasts present	Enzyme deficiencies in testosterone synthesis	Disruption of hypothalamic–pituitary axis
	Testicular feminization	Hypothalamic, pituitary, or ovarian pathogenesis similar to that of secondary amenorrhea
	Müllerian agenesis or MRKH	Congenital abnormalities of the genital tract

MRKH, Mayer–Rokitansky–Kuster–Hauser.

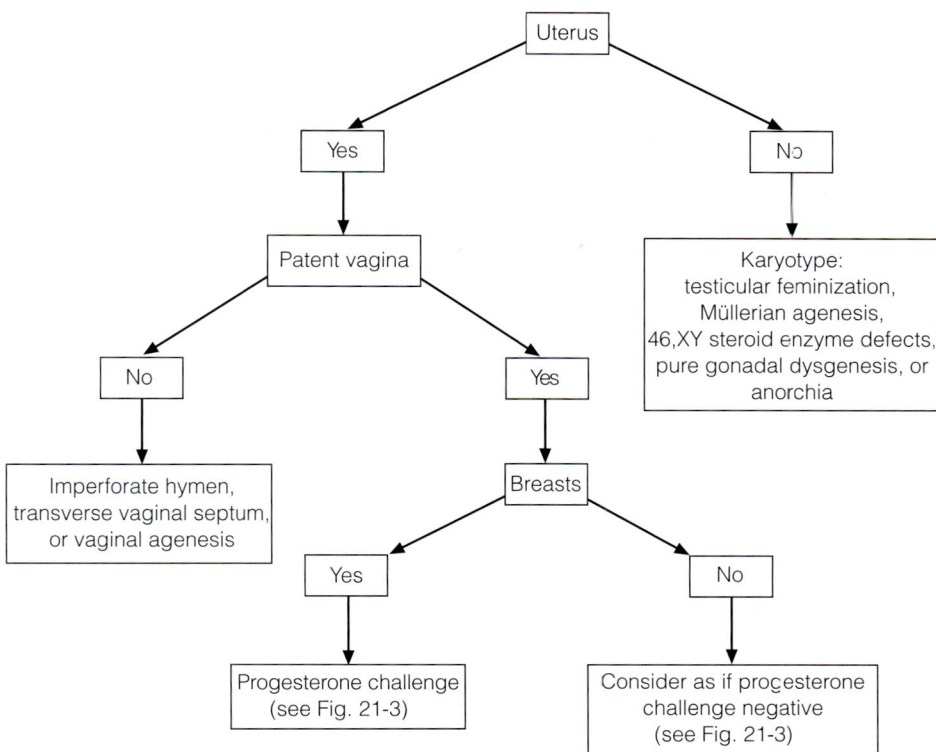

FIGURE 21-1. Diagnostic flowchart for patients with primary amenorrhea.

For patients who have a uterus but breast development is absent, the differential includes hypergonadotropic hypogonadism, as seen in gonadal dysgenesis in both sexes, and with defects in steroid pathways in 46,XX patients and hypogonadotropic hypogonadism, which is seen in central nervous system (CNS), hypothalamic, and pituitary dysfunction. A serum FSH level differentiates between these two, with elevation seen in hypergonadotropic hypogonadism.

The workup for amenorrhea in phenotypic females with the absence of either a uterus or breasts should include a karyotype analysis, followed by testosterone and FSH assays. Further biochemical and hormonal assays may be performed to elucidate specific enzyme defects. Patients with both a uterus and the breast development should be evaluated to determine whether there is a patent outflow tract from the uterus. If the vagina, cervix, and uterus are continuous, these can be evaluated as if the patient was presenting with secondary amenorrhea.

TREATMENT

Patients with congenital abnormalities may be treated surgically with reconstructive procedures to allow egress of menses in those with a functional uterus or to create a functional vagina. Patients with an absent uterus and breasts can be treated with estrogen replacement to effect breast development and prevent osteoporosis. Patients who have breast development, but an absent uterus may not require medical intervention.

Patients with a uterus but without breast development and with hypergonadotropic hypogonadism often have irreversible ovarian insufficiency and will require estrogen replacement therapy. Patients with hypogonadotropic hypogonadism require further workup as patients with secondary amenorrhea.

SECONDARY AMENORRHEA

Secondary amenorrhea is the absence of menses for three months in women with previously regular cycles or six months in women with a history of irregular cycles. **The most common cause of secondary amenorrhea is pregnancy.** Other causes can be categorized as anatomic abnormalities, ovarian dysfunction, prolactinoma and hyperprolactinemia, and CNS or hypothalamic disorders.

ANATOMIC ABNORMALITIES

The common anatomic causes of secondary amenorrhea are Asherman syndrome and cervical stenosis. **Asherman syndrome** is the presence of intrauterine synechiae or adhesions, usually secondary to intrauterine surgery or infection. The potential etiologies of Asherman syndrome include dilation and curettage, myomectomy, cesarean delivery, or endometritis. **Cervical stenosis** can manifest as secondary amenorrhea and dysmenorrhea. It is usually caused by scarring of the cervical os secondary to surgical or obstetric trauma.

OVARIAN FAILURE

Ovarian failure may result from ovarian torsion, surgery, infection, radiation, or chemotherapy. **Primary ovarian insufficiency** (POI), previously called premature ovarian failure, is often idiopathic. It is defined as the development of hypergonadotropic hypogonadism before the age of 40 and occurs in 1 in 250 women by age 35 and 1 in 100 by age 40. Menopause occurring before age 35 should prompt a chromosomal analysis to evaluate for a genetic basis of POI. Patients with either idiopathic POI or a known cause of early ovarian failure are generally treated with supplemental estrogen to decrease the risk of cardiovascular disease and osteoporosis.

POLYCYSTIC OVARY SYNDROME

Polycystic ovary syndrome (PCOS) was first described in 1935 and is now known as one of the most common hormonal disorders in women, with a prevalence of 5% to 10% in the United States and developed world. Diagnosis is made when women meet two of the following: oligo or anovulation, clinical or laboratory evidence of hyperandrogenism, and polycystic ovaries on ultrasound. Clinical evidence of hyperandrogenism may include excessive hair growth (hirsutism) and male pattern hair loss as well as acne. It is not entirely clear what precipitates the disease, but once it begins, a self-perpetuating cycle occurs.

In the case of PCOS, chronic anovulation leads to elevated levels of estrogen and androgen. The increased androgen released from the ovaries and the adrenal cortex is converted peripherally in the adipose tissue into estrone. Further, the elevated androgens lead to a decrease in the production of sex hormone–binding globulin, resulting in even higher levels of free estrogens and androgens. This hyperestrogenic state leads to an increased LH:FSH ratio, atypical follicular development, anovulation, and increased androgen production. Once again, the androgens are peripherally converted to estrogens, leading to a cyclical propagation of the disease. Many patients with PCOS who are hyperandrogenic and obese also develop insulin resistance and hyperinsulinemia. Not surprisingly, the incidence of Type 2 diabetes mellitus is increased in these patients.

Treatment of these patients depends on the particular symptoms and the desires of the patient. For patients desiring pregnancy, ovulation induction may be performed using clomiphene citrate (Clomid) or Letrozole. Patients with PCOS may be particularly resistant to ovulation induction, even with medication. Further, there is evidence that the probability of ovulation can be significantly increased by weight loss; therefore, patients are strongly encouraged to take an active role in maintaining or losing weight prior to pregnancy. In patients with hyperinsulinemia and insulin resistance, metformin may increase spontaneous ovulation, and in the least will improve insulin resistance and may help with weight loss. For patients who are not currently interested in fertility, the goal of therapy is menstrual cycle control. Oral contraceptive pills (OCPs) not only will assist in cycle regulation and reduce risk of endometrial hyperplasia or carcinoma, but also may improve symptoms of acne and arrest further development of hirsutism by decreasing circulating levels of androgens. If estrogen is contraindicated, or patient preference indicates, progestin therapy alone in the form of a levonorgestrel intrauterine device, oral pills (Provera), or injectable medications (Depo-Provera) will similarly decrease their risk of endometrial disease. Again, obese patients should be strongly urged to lose weight. Similar to the metabolic syndrome, patients with PCOS have increased risk of hypertension, obstructive sleep apnea, coronary artery disease, insulin resistance, and Type 2 diabetes. Weight loss can decrease these risks as well as break the cycle of anovulation. Most clinicians would recommend that patients undergo a screen for Type 2 diabetes mellitus and ensure that they are connected with a primary care physician for monitoring other health disorders associated with PCOS as listed earlier.

HYPERPROLACTINEMIA-ASSOCIATED AMENORRHEA

Excess prolactin leads to amenorrhea and galactorrhea. Menstrual irregularities often result from abnormal gonadotropin (FSH and LH) secretion owing to alterations in dopamine levels typically seen in hyperprolactinemia. The etiologies and consequences of excess prolactin are numerous. Prolactin release is inhibited by dopamine and stimulated by serotonin and thyrotropin-releasing hormone (TRH). Because of the constant suppression of prolactin release by hypothalamic release of dopamine, any disturbance in this process by a hypothalamic or pituitary lesion can lead to disinhibition of prolactin secretion.

Hyperprolactinemia has several possible etiologies (Table 21-4). Primary hypothyroidism that leads to elevated thyroid-stimulating hormone (TSH) and TRH can cause hyperprolactinemia. Medications that increase prolactin levels (by a hypothalamic–pituitary effect) include dopamine antagonists (Haldol, Reglan, and phenothiazine), tricyclic antidepressants, estrogen, monoamine oxidase inhibitors, and opiates. A prolactin-secreting pituitary adenoma leads to elevated prolactin levels. The empty sella syndrome, in which the subarachnoid membrane herniates into the sella turcica, causing it to enlarge and flatten, is another cause of hyperprolactinemia. Other conditions associated with high prolactin include pregnancy and breastfeeding. Any patient with an elevated prolactin level should have an imaging study to rule out prolactinoma.

DISRUPTION OF THE HYPOTHALAMIC–PITUITARY AXIS

As in the hypothalamic and pituitary causes of primary amenorrhea, disruption in the secretion and transport of GnRH, the absence of pulsatility of GnRH, or acquired pituitary lesions will all cause hypogonadotropic hypogonadism (Table 21-5). Common causes of hypothalamic dysfunction include stress, exercise, anorexia nervosa, and weight loss.

Diagnosis

The approach to secondary amenorrhea always begins with a beta human chorionic gonadotropin (β-hCG) assay to **rule out pregnancy** often before a formal history is taken. If this is negative, the standard

TABLE 21-4. Differential Diagnosis of Galactorrhea–Hyperprolactinemia

Pituitary tumors secreting prolactin
Macroadenomas (>10 mm)
Microadenomas (<10 mm)

Hypothyroidism

Idiopathic hyperprolactinemia

Drug-induced hyperprolactinemia
Dopamine antagonists
    Phenothiazines
    Thioxanthenes
    Butyrophenone
    Diphenylbutylpiperidine
    Dibenzoxazepine
    Dihydroindolone
    Procainamide derivatives
Catecholamine-depleting agents
False transmitters (α-methyldopa)

Interruption of normal hypothalamic–pituitary relationship
Pituitary stalk section

Peripheral neural stimulation
Chest wall stimulation
    Surgery (e.g., mastectomy)
    Burns
    Herpes zoster
    Bronchogenic tumors
    Bronchiectasis/chronic bronchitis

Nipple stimulation
Stimulation of nipples
Chronic nipple irritation

Spinal cord lesion
Tabes dorsalis
Syringomyelia

CNS disease
Encephalitis
Craniopharyngioma
Pineal and hypothalamic tumors
Hypothalamic tumors
Pseudotumor cerebri

CNS, central nervous system.

TABLE 21-5. Differential Diagnosis of Hypoestrogenic Amenorrhea (Hypogonadotropic Hypogonadism)

Hypothalamic dysfunction
Kallmann syndrome
Tumors of hypothalamus (craniopharyngioma)
Constitutional delay of puberty
Severe hypothalamic dysfunction
Anorexia nervosa
Severe weight loss
Severe stress
Exercise

Pituitary disorder
Sheehan syndrome
Panhypopituitarism
Isolated gonadotropin deficiency
Hemosiderosis (primarily from thalassemia major)

Adapted from DeCherney A, Pernoll M. *Current Obstetric and Gynecologic Diagnosis and Treatment.* Norwalk, CT: Appleton & Lange; 1994:1013.

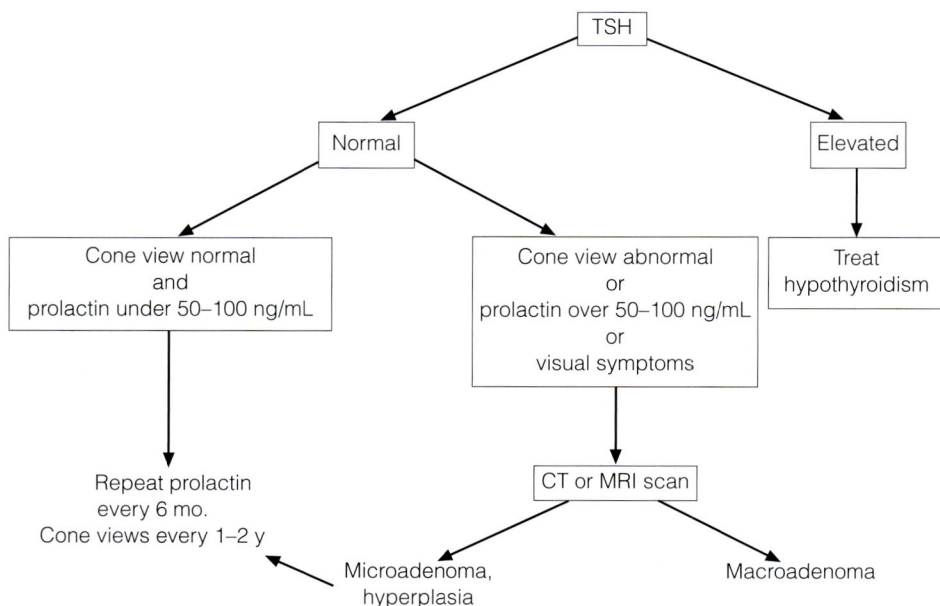

FIGURE 21-2. Diagnostic flowchart for patients with amenorrhea–galactorrhea–hyperprolactinemia. TSH, thyroid-stimulating hormone.

history should include focused questions toward hypothyroidism (e.g., lethargy, weight gain, and cold intolerance), hyperprolactinemia (e.g., nipple discharge and usually bilateral), and hyperandrogenism (e.g., recent changes in hirsutism, acne, or virilism; see Chapter 23). **TSH** and **prolactin** levels should then be checked to rule out hypothyroidism and hyperprolactinemia, both of which can cause amenorrhea. If both are elevated, the hypothyroidism should be treated, and the prolactin level can be checked after thyroid studies have normalized to verify resolution.

If the prolactin level is elevated and TSH is normal, a workup for the other causes of prolactinemia should ensue (Fig. 21-2). In the diagnostic evaluation of the patient, a careful history should be taken, including a complete list of medications and clear documentation of the onset of symptoms. A thorough physical examination should include visual fields, cranial nerves, breast examination, and an attempt to express milk from the nipple. An MRI can rule out a hypothalamic or pituitary lesion.

If the prolactin level is normal, a **progesterone challenge test** (10 mg orally for 7 to 10 days to mimic progesterone withdrawal) can be performed to assess the adequacy of endogenous estrogen production and the outflow tract. Withdrawal bleeding occurring after the progesterone challenge indicates the presence of estrogen and an adequate outflow tract. In this case, amenorrhea is usually secondary to anovulation, which can be caused by a variety of endocrine disorders that alter pituitary/gonadal feedback such as polycystic ovaries, tumors of the ovary and adrenals, Cushing syndrome, thyroid disorders, and adult-onset adrenal hyperplasia (Table 21-6).

TABLE 21-6. Differential Diagnosis of Eugonadotropic Eugonadism (Progesterone Challenge Positive)

Mild hypothalamic dysfunction
Emotional stress
Psychologic disorder
Weight loss
Obesity
Exercise induced
Idiopathic
Hirsutism-virilism
Polycystic ovary syndrome
Ovarian tumor
Adrenal tumor
Cushing syndrome
Congenital and adult-onset adrenal hyperplasia
Systemic disease
Hypothyroidism
Hyperthyroidism
Addison disease
Chronic renal failure
Many others seen in other chronic diseases

Adapted from DeCherney A, Pernoll M. *Current Obstetric and Gynecologic Diagnosis and Treatment*. Norwalk, CT: Appleton & Lange; 1994:1013.

The absence of withdrawal bleeding in response to progesterone alone must then be evaluated with estrogen and progesterone administration. If there is still no menstrual bleeding, an outflow tract disorder such as Asherman syndrome or cervical stenosis is suspected. If menstrual bleeding does occur in response to estrogen and progesterone administration, this suggests an intact and functional uterus without adequate endogenous estrogen stimulation. Measurement of FSH and LH will help differentiate between a hypothalamic–pituitary disorder (low/normal FSH and LH levels) and ovarian failure (high FSH and LH levels) (Fig. 21-3).

Treatment

Patients with hypothyroidism are treated with thyroid hormone replacement. Those with pituitary macroadenomas are treated with surgical resection. Some patients with macroadenomas and most with microadenomas are treated with bromocriptine, a dopamine agonist that often causes tumor regression and the resumption of ovulation. Other hyperprolactinemic patients can also be treated with bromocriptine in order to resume ovulation. Further, this treatment should be followed with serial prolactin levels and cone view radiographs to diagnose development of a macroadenoma.

Patients who respond to a progesterone challenge should be withdrawn with progesterone on a regular basis to prevent endometrial hyperplasia. OCPs are useful in this case and may be beneficial in the management of hirsutism. However, if the patient is a smoker and older than 35 years, progesterone alone is indicated because of the increased risk of cerebrovascular accidents and venous thromboembolism with estrogen usage in these patients.

For patients who are hypoestrogenic, consideration should be given to estrogen and progesterone replacement for the effects these have on bone density and genital atrophy. OCPs are often used for women younger than 35 years or nonsmokers older than 35 years. For other patients, a regimen of 0.625 mg of conjugated estrogen cycled with 5 to 10 mg of medroxyprogesterone acetate is suitable. These patients should also receive 1.2 g of elemental calcium supplementation per day.

Ovulation Induction

Ovulation induction with bromocriptine can be used in patients with hyperprolactinemia. If the cause of hyperprolactinemia is medication related, discontinue or decrease the medication if possible. Patients who respond to the progesterone challenge have evidence of estrogenation. Any specific cause of this amenorrheic state should be corrected. If menses do not resume, ovulation induction may be performed with clomiphene citrate (Clomid), which acts as an antiestrogen to stimulate gonadotropin

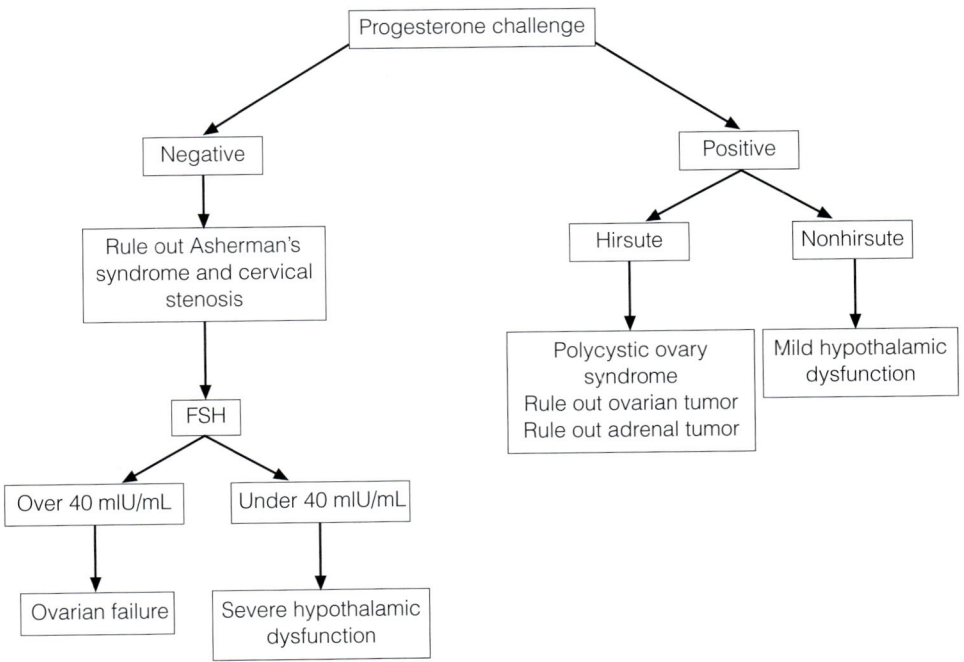

FIGURE 21-3. Diagnostic flowchart for patients with secondary amenorrhea. FSH, follicle-stimulating hormone.

release. Patients with elevated androgens may need therapy with Clomid.

Patients who do not respond to progesterone alone are presumed to have low estrogen levels; however, these patients will occasionally respond to Clomid as well. For patients who do not respond to Clomid, human menopausal gonadotropin or recombinant GnRH can be used to stimulate ovulation. Careful monitoring with ultrasound and estradiol levels should be done in the case of gonadotropin ovulation induction because of the risk of ovarian hyperstimulation.

KEY POINTS

- Primary amenorrhea is the absence of menarche by age 15.
- Primary amenorrhea can be caused by congenital abnormalities of the genital tract, chromosomal abnormalities, enzyme or hormonal deficiencies, gonadal agenesis, ovarian insufficiency, or disruption of the hypothalamic–pituitary axis.
- The workup of primary amenorrhea is usually organized into four categories based on the presence or absence of a uterus and the presence or absence of breast development.
- In the absence of both uterus and breasts, karyotype usually reveals 46,XY.
- In the absence of a uterus and presence of breasts, karyotype will differentiate between Müllerian agenesis and testicular feminization.
- In the absence of breasts and presence of a uterus, FSH will differentiate between hypergonadotropic and hypogonadotropic hypogonadism. Karyotype may be necessary to rule out gonadal agenesis in a 46,XY.
- Patients with both a uterus and breasts should be evaluated as if presenting with secondary amenorrhea.
- Anatomic abnormalities including Asherman syndrome and cervical stenosis may lead to secondary amenorrhea. These patients fail to respond to estrogen and progesterone withdrawal.
- Hyperprolactinemia is a common cause of secondary amenorrhea.
- Patients with normal prolactin levels may be given a progesterone challenge to investigate whether or not the endometrium is estrogenized.
- With progesterone challenge failure, the differential diagnosis becomes hypergonadotropic or hypogonadotropic hypogonadism that can be differentiated by an FSH measurement.
- For patients not seeking current fertility, it is important to treat the specific cause of amenorrhea and to consider hormone replacement in the hypoestrogenic patient.
- For patients who desire fertility, ovulation induction can usually be achieved. Patients with hyperprolactinemia require bromocriptine, whereas patients with other forms of hypogonadism may respond to clomiphene and gonadotropins.

CLINICAL VIGNETTES

VIGNETTE 1

An 18-year-old young woman presents to your office with a complaint of amenorrhea. She notes that she has never had a menstrual period, but that she has mild cyclic abdominal bloating. She reports normal breast development starting at age 12. She reports that she has become sexually active, but she finds intercourse painful. Her past medical and surgical history is unremarkable. On physical examination, you note normal appearing axillary and pubic hair. Her breast development is normal. Pelvic examination reveals normal appearing external genitalia, and a shortened vagina ending in a blind pouch.

1. Which of the following tests would be your first step in determining the diagnosis?
   a. Karyotype
   b. Pelvic ultrasound
   c. Serum follicle-stimulating hormone (FSH)
   d. Diagnostic laparoscopy

2. You perform a bedside ultrasound and find normal appearing bilateral ovaries as well as an absent uterus and fallopian tubes. What is your most likely diagnosis?
   a. Imperforate hymen
   b. Transverse vaginal septum
   c. Müllerian agenesis
   d. Androgen insensitivity syndrome (AIS)

3. Which additional organ system should you be evaluating in a patient with this disorder?
   a. Pancreas and duodenum
   b. Cerebral circulation
   c. Olfactory system
   d. Renal and urinary collecting system

4. Your patient's concerned mother calls you later that afternoon. "How will my daughter be able to start a family?" You wisely counsel her about her options, which include:
   a. intrauterine insemination
   b. uterine transplant
   c. in vitro fertilization (IVF) with gestational carrier
   d. the patient will not be able to reproduce using her genetic material

VIGNETTE 2

A 32-year-old G1P1001 woman presents to your office with the chief complaint of amenorrhea since her most recent vaginal delivery 1 year ago. She notes that she had an uncomplicated pregnancy, followed by the delivery of a healthy baby boy. Her delivery was complicated by an intra-amniotic infection as well as a postpartum hemorrhage requiring a postpartum dilation and curettage (D&C). After her delivery, she breastfed for 6 months, and during this time, she had scant and irregular vaginal bleeding. After stopping breastfeeding 6 months ago, she notes the absence of menses, but instead has monthly painful cramping, which seems to be getting worse. She remarks that prior to her pregnancy, she had normal, regular menses, which were not too heavy or painful. She and her husband would like to have another child, and have been having unprotected intercourse for the last 6 months without achieving a pregnancy. Your review of systems is otherwise negative. You perform a physical examination, which is normal other than a slightly enlarged, tender uterus. A urine pregnancy test in the office is negative.

1. What is the most likely diagnosis?
   a. Sheehan syndrome
   b. Lactational amenorrhea
   c. Asherman syndrome
   d. Primary ovarian insufficiency (POI)

2. You suspect Asherman syndrome, and perform a hysterosalpingogram, which reveals multiple synechiae within the uterus, confirming your suspicions. Your next step in therapy is which of the following?
   a. Diagnostic and operative hysteroscopy
   b. Provera 10 mg daily for 5 days in an attempt to achieve a withdrawal bleed
   c. IVF
   d. Place an intrauterine device (IUD)
   e. Inform your patient that unfortunately, she is "barren" and will not be able to carry a pregnancy again

3. What obstetrical complication might you be concerned about for your patient in her next pregnancy?
   a. Preterm labor
   b. Cervical insufficiency
   c. Preeclampsia
   d. Placenta accreta

VIGNETTE 3

A 15-year-old female adolescent presents to your office with primary amenorrhea. She notably has short stature, a webbed neck, and widely spaced nipples. She has noticed that she has not developed breasts or pubic hair like her friends at school have, and this is frustrating to her. She is not sexually active. Physical examination confirms the absence of secondary sex characteristics, and auscultation of the chest reveals a harsh systolic murmur. Pelvic examination reveals normal appearing female external genitalia and a normal vagina, with a palpable uterus on bimanual examination.

1. To confirm your suspected diagnosis, which test would you first order?
   a. Pelvic ultrasound
   b. Serum FSH and luteinizing hormone (LH)
   c. Karyotype
   d. Serum estradiol

2. Suddenly you remember from medical school that there are other medical predispositions that Turner patients have, and you order all of the following tests except:
   a. thyroid function testing
   b. echocardiogram
   c. basic metabolic panel
   d. antiendomysial antibody test
   e. DEXA scan

3. The patient and her family are surprised about her diagnosis, but glad to have an explanation for her symptoms. The patient notes that what bothers her most is her lack of breasts and absent pubic hair. What therapy can you offer for her delayed puberty?
   a. Growth hormone therapy
   b. Gonadotropin therapy (FSH and LH)
   c. Estrogen plus progesterone
   d. Estrogen alone

4. Five years later, at age 20, your patient returns to your clinic for an infertility consultation. She has had surgical repair of her aortic coarctation, and has been on oral contraceptive pills for the last 2 years for hormone replacement. She is followed by an internist who reports that all other systems (hepatic, renal, etc.) have been stable. What advice might you give your patient about attempting pregnancy?
   a. None, she is not a good candidate for pregnancy
   b. Stop the birth control pills because they are preventing spontaneous conception
   c. Clomid ovulation induction
   d. IVF

VIGNETTE 4

A 19-year-old female college freshman presents with amenorrhea for the last 8 months. She states that she had normal menarche at age 12, and initially had irregular menses for the first few cycles, but they became regular quickly, and had been normal until 8 months ago. She denies sexual activity, has had no sexually transmitted infections, and is otherwise healthy with no past medical problems or surgeries. She reports that she eats a healthful diet and has been running approximately 15 miles/week with her cross-country team for the past year. She states that running is her "passion" and sometimes she puts in a few extra miles to blow off stress from her classes. Physical examination reveals a thin, athletic female with normal breast development and normal secondary sex characteristics. Pelvic examination reveals normal external genitalia and on bimanual examination, you palpate a small, anteverted uterus with no adnexal masses.

1. Which test would you first perform?
   a. Pelvic ultrasound
   b. Urinary LH test strips
   c. Serum FSH
   d. Serum beta human chorionic gonadotropin (β-hCG)
   e. Prolactin
   f. Thyroid-stimulating hormone (TSH)

2. You perform a serum β-hCG that is negative, and subsequently test FSH, prolactin, and TSH. Prolactin and TSH are within normal limits. FSH is low. What is your suspected diagnosis?
   a. POI
   b. Exercise-induced amenorrhea
   c. Lactational amenorrhea
   d. Anorexia nervosa
   e. Bulimia nervosa
   f. Iatrogenic amenorrhea

3. What findings would you expect to see on laboratory testing in a patient with POI?
   a. Elevated TSH, normal FSH, low estradiol
   b. Normal TSH, elevated FSH, normal estradiol
   c. Normal TSH, elevated FSH, low estradiol
   d. Elevated TSH, elevated FSH, elevated estradiol

4. Another similar patient presents to your office with secondary amenorrhea, but she also reports galactorrhea and headache. Your laboratory findings include an elevated prolactin of 120 ng/mL, normal FSH, and normal TSH. What is your next step in diagnosis?
   a. MRI of the head
   b. Pelvic ultrasound
   c. Serum estradiol
   d. Serum testosterone
   e. No further testing is necessary

5. What therapy would you first initiate with this patient?
   a. Transsphenoidal resection
   b. Dopamine agonist
   c. Radiation
   d. Chemotherapy

ANSWERS

VIGNETTE 1 Question 1

1. Answer B:
A pelvic ultrasound should be the first step, aimed to determine the presence or absence of the uterus, tubes, and ovaries. Given the presence of normal thelarche (breast development appears normal) and adrenarche (pubic hair is present), a random FSH would not be helpful. A karyotype and diagnostic laparoscopy may also be helpful in determining a final diagnosis, but an ultrasound should be the next step.

VIGNETTE 1 Question 2
2. Answer C:
Müllerian agenesis (also known as Mayer–Rokitansky–Kuster–Hauser syndrome) refers to the congenital absence of the uterus, tubes, and upper vagina. Variants of Müllerian agenesis may include rudimentary uterine horns with or without a functional endometrium, and may lead to cyclic abdominal pain.

Imperforate hymen and transverse vaginal septum typically would present with cyclic abdominal pain and evidence on examination of hematocolpos. AIS patients would have scant or absent pubic hair, but otherwise may present in a similar fashion—primary amenorrhea with normal appearing breast tissue in a young phenotypical female adult.

VIGNETTE 1 Question 3
3. Answer D:
Embryologically speaking, development of the uterus, cervix, and vagina is closely tied with the development of the urinary system. The Müllerian ducts (also known as the paramesonephric ducts) form bilaterally and fuse to form the uterus, tubes, cervix, and upper vagina in the female. Abnormalities in Müllerian duct fusion have been associated with renal agenesis or hypoplasia, ectopic kidney, and horseshoe kidney.

Other systems that may be involved include skeletal, auditory, and cardiac systems. The gastrointestinal tract, cerebral circulation, and olfactory system have not been associated.

VIGNETTE 1 Question 4
4. Answer C:
Although this patient will not be able to reproduce spontaneously because of her absent uterus, tubes, and cervix, she does have normal ovaries. With the addition of assisted reproductive technologies, she will be able to entertain the possibility of biological children. When she is interested in childbearing, she may opt to undergo stimulation of her ovaries with injectable gonadotropins followed by retrieval of her oocytes, fertilization with her partner's sperm, and embryo transfer to a gestational carrier.

Intrauterine insemination is not an option for her, given her absent uterus. Uterine transplant has occurred only in rare circumstances, and subsequent pregnancy would be high risk (and likely contraindicated) given immunosuppressive medications needed for the success of the transplant; this is not currently an available therapy for women with Müllerian agenesis.

VIGNETTE 2 Question 1
1. Answer C:
This patient has secondary amenorrhea and the most likely cause given her clinical presentation is Asherman syndrome. Intrauterine adhesions caused by prior obstetric procedures (typically D&C) obstruct the uterine cavity and cause cyclic pain and (in some cases) secondary amenorrhea. More commonly it presents as dysmenorrhea.

Lactational amenorrhea is unlikely given that she is no longer breastfeeding. Sheehan syndrome is panhypopituitarism secondary to infarction of the pituitary gland caused by postpartum hemorrhage and relative hypotension: this is less likely given her ability to breastfeed without difficulty for 6 months after delivery. The patient's symptoms of cyclic pain make premature ovarian failure less likely given your suspicion that she is ovulatory (cyclic pain), although it is additionally a possibility.

VIGNETTE 2 Question 2
2. Answer A:
The correct answer is to offer surgical management with hysteroscopy to resect the scar tissue within her uterine cavity, which would allow the patient relief from her cyclic pain (by releasing the obstructed menstruation), and additionally would assist her in attaining a more hospitable uterine cavity for future pregnancy.

Inducing a withdrawal bleed with Provera would not improve her obstructed flow or increase her fertility. Although IVF may be an option in future should operative intervention fail, it is not the first step in management. Placement of an IUD may prove challenging given her intrauterine scar tissue, and furthermore may cause increased pain and most importantly will not reduce her scar tissue. An intrauterine Foley catheter or IUD is frequently placed at the end of a hysteroscopic resection of scar to reduce reformation of scar tissue, but the IUD should not be used as first line therapy.

VIGNETTE 2 Question 3
3. Answer D:
Because the endometrial surface is thought to be denuded in the setting of Asherman syndrome, leading to the formation of scar tissue, patients are at risk for placenta accreta in a subsequent pregnancy. Placenta accreta is the abnormal implantation of the placenta past the decidual layer of the endometrium and into the myometrium. It leads to abnormal adherence of the placenta to the uterus, which in some cases can lead to placenta increta (deep invasion into the myometrium) and placenta percreta (invasion through the uterine serosa and into other pelvic organs such as the bladder or rectum).

Preterm labor is unlikely to be increased in a subsequent pregnancy if the scar tissue is adequately resected, and the uterine cavity is normal prior to pregnancy. Cervical insufficiency is the premature shortening and sometimes dilation of the cervix. A patient may be at risk for this secondary to prior cervical procedures (loop electrocautery excisional procedures and cold knife cones) as well as D&C, but in this setting of Asherman the most correct answer is placenta accreta. There is no known association between Asherman syndrome and preeclampsia.

VIGNETTE 3 Question 1
1. Answer C:
A karyotype in this case would confirm your suspected diagnosis of Turner syndrome, with a result of 45,X. Clues that led to this diagnosis include primary amenorrhea in the setting of absent secondary sex characteristics, physical examination findings of short stature, webbed neck, and widely spaced nipples (also known as "shield chest"). Additionally, her murmur is likely secondary to coarctation of the aorta, one of the more common cardiac anomalies patients with Turner syndrome may have. Other characteristic findings include "streak gonads," which are often nonfunctional, and subsequent pregnancy is rare.

Pelvic ultrasound would likely reveal a normal appearing uterus, and may or may not identify streak gonads; it is less helpful in definitive diagnosis. Serum FSH and LH would likely be elevated and estradiol low for a patient with Turner syndrome, but this would be less helpful in confirming her diagnosis.

VIGNETTE 3 Question 2
2. Answer E:
Although patients with Turner syndrome commonly develop osteoporosis secondary to POI, at age 15, this is less likely, therefore you would not order a DEXA scan at this age.

It is reasonable to check a thyroid function panel, because patients are at increased risk of Hashimoto thyroiditis. You heard a murmur on your physical examination, which prompts you to order an echocardiogram, especially in light of your knowledge that Turner syndrome carries an increased risk for aortic coarctation, bicuspid aortic valve, and aortic dissection. You look for hyperglycemia and abnormal renal function on your basic metabolic panel, given known increased risk of diabetes and renal disease in Turner syndrome. You ordered antiendomysial antibodies to check for Celiac disease, which is also associated with this syndrome, although less commonly than the above disorders.

VIGNETTE 3 Question 3
3. Answer C:
The patient, now at age 15, is likely to have reached her full growth potential; therefore, initiation of estrogen therapy is indicated. Given the presence of a uterus (and risk for endometrial hyperplasia or carcinoma with unopposed estrogen), you would also administer a cyclic or daily progestin to protect her endometrium. Initially, estrogen is started at a low (prepubertal) dose and increased gradually over 3 to 4 years to physiologic adult levels. Estrogen and progesterone therapy should continue until she reaches the age of menopause.

Growth hormone therapy would be indicated if she had presented at an age prior to the fusion of her distal epiphyses, in order to maximize her height. In this setting, however, it would not be of assistance. Gonadotropin therapy would likely affect puberty as would estrogen and progesterone, but it should be given in a subcutaneous manner. The ease of oral estrogen and progestin with good effects makes use of gonadotropins in this setting cumbersome and contraindicated.

VIGNETTE 3 Question 4
4. Answer D:
IVF using donor eggs and most likely a gestational carrier are her options for conceiving a pregnancy. Given that most likely her gonads do not have functional tissue (from her presentation with absent breast development at age 15), most likely they also do not have functional follicles. Ovulation induction for IVF therefore would likely fail and may put her health at risk. The patient's most safe route for pregnancy would be the use of donor eggs (with her partner's sperm) and a gestational carrier. The option for her to carry the pregnancy in her own uterus may be possible, but only after careful collaboration with a perinatologist and an infertility specialist.

In this case, birth control pills are functioning for hormone replacement rather than contraception. Clomid ovulation induction would also be contraindicated given her likely lack of functional ovarian follicles in her streak gonads.

VIGNETTE 4 Question 1
1. Answer D:
Although this patient reports no sexual activity, it is of utmost importance to rule out pregnancy in any case of secondary amenorrhea (and most cases of primary amenorrhea). A negative β-hCG test rules out the most common cause of secondary amenorrhea: pregnancy.

A pelvic ultrasound would not be useful in this setting, because the patient is without symptoms of pain (no concern for obstructive cause of amenorrhea). Urinary LH test strips are used for patients attempting to test for evidence of ovulation. Given that this patient is not menstruating, it follows that she is likely not ovulating, therefore urinary LH testing would not be helpful. Serum FSH, prolactin, and TSH would be helpful in your workup, but only after pregnancy has been ruled out.

VIGNETTE 4 Question 2
2. Answer B:
The most likely diagnosis is exercise-induced amenorrhea (hypogonadotropic hypogonadism), which

would carry a normal prolactin and TSH, with a low FSH. Women who are involved in strenuous exercise commonly have menstrual irregularity, and this may progress to amenorrhea as the intensity and/or duration of the exercise increases. Exercise-induced amenorrhea occurs, when the reduction of weight below a threshold is achieved. It is hypothesized that when the body weight is low, and physical exertion is high for these extended periods, the pulsatile nature of GnRH is disturbed such that normal stimulation of the ovaries by FSH and LH is absent, and therefore, anovulation and amenorrhea ensue. This process is reversible by decreasing exercise or increasing caloric intake.

The laboratory findings are not consistent with POI. The patient is not currently lactating; therefore, she does not have lactational amenorrhea. Anorexia and bulimia nervosa may result in similar laboratory findings, but this patient gives no history of eating disorder. It is important, however, that during your evaluation you screen her for evidence of abnormal eating patterns and unusual weight control habits. Iatrogenic amenorrhea refers to medication-induced amenorrhea, as with Depo-Lupron or oral contraceptives. The patient gives no history of use of these medications.

VIGNETTE 4 Question 3
3. Answer C:
POI, previously known as premature ovarian failure, is one type of hypergonadotropic hypogonadism, which presents as secondary amenorrhea at an age less than 40. Laboratory studies would show a markedly elevated FSH with low estradiol. TSH is not affected in this setting. Causes of POI may include chromosomal abnormalities and genetic disorders (Fragile X), although in most cases, a definitive cause is not found. Young women with this diagnosis understandably may be devastated by these findings, particularly if they had planned childbearing. Fertility options include in vitro fertilization with their own eggs, but most likely they will require egg donation, depending on the level of depletion of their own follicles. They will benefit from estrogen and progesterone replacement to reduce their risk of osteoporosis and improve their long-term cardiovascular health—this should be strongly recommended to them in your counseling. The three other combinations of laboratory tests earlier are not consistent with POI.

VIGNETTE 4 Question 4
4. Answer A:
Because of this patient's elevated prolactin, headache, and galactorrhea, you are most suspicious of a prolactinoma, therefore you order an MRI. Prolactinomas are the most common type of pituitary adenoma. Amenorrhea occurs secondary to inhibition of GnRH secretion, which causes decreased FSH and LH secretion leading to anovulation and another form of "hypogonadotropic hypogonadism."

A pelvic ultrasound would not be helpful in this case because it would likely be normal, with normal appearing ovaries and a thin endometrial stripe (secondary to lack of stimulation by ovulating ovaries). You more highly suspect a prolactinoma because of the serum prolactin. Estradiol and testosterone testing also would not be diagnostic in this case.

VIGNETTE 4 Question 5
5. Answer B:
You suspect that this is a microadenoma given the PRL level is less than 200, so you opt to initiate therapy with a dopamine agonist. The two medications in use today include bromocriptine and cabergoline, both of which are highly effective in reducing the size of the adenoma. Many providers try bromocriptine before cabergoline because of the increased risk for valvular heart disease with cabergoline. Initiation of treatment with either drug should start at a low level, and slowly titrate up. You would follow serum prolactin levels to determine the final effective dose, and would additionally repeat the MRI in 3 to 6 months to evaluate for treatment effect.

Transsphenoidal resection is a treatment option for patients who do not respond to dopamine agonists or who cannot tolerate the treatment; however, this would not be your first line therapy given increased risk of surgery as well as risk of treatment failure (and persistently present prolactinoma cells). Radiation therapy is primarily used for women who fail resection or who have large adenomas refractory to other treatment. There is no role for chemotherapy in treating a prolactinoma.

22 | Abnormalities of the Menstrual Cycle

Characteristics of the menstrual cycle vary from woman to woman. Normal variances include a cycle length between 21 and 35 days, bleeding for up to 7 days, as well as mild to moderate cramping, often relieved with over-the-counter (OTC) medications. Additionally, rare women also may have spotting to light bleeding at mid cycle as a result of a slight decline in estrogen levels that precede ovulation. Bleeding that occurs outside of these parameters is defined as abnormal uterine bleeding (AUB) and is a common reason to consult a gynecologist. This chapter will describe common abnormalities of the menstrual cycle, including appropriate diagnostic evaluation and treatment options.

DYSMENORRHEA

Dysmenorrhea is defined as pain and cramping during menstruation that **interferes with normal activities** and requires OTC or prescription medication. Mild pain during menses is normal. Fifty percent of menstruating women suffer from dysmenorrhea, and 10% of these are incapacitated for 1 to 3 days each month.

Dysmenorrhea is classified as primary or secondary. Primary dysmenorrhea is idiopathic menstrual pain without identifiable pathology, often occurring with the initiation of ovulatory menstrual cycles; secondary dysmenorrhea is painful menses due to underlying pathology (endometriosis, fibroids, adenomyosis, pelvic inflammatory disease (PID), cervical stenosis).

PRIMARY DYSMENORRHEA

Primary dysmenorrhea usually occurs before age 20 years. Because primary dysmenorrhea is almost always associated with **ovulatory cycles**, it is usually diagnosed in late teens rather than at menarche when cycles are often anovulatory. Although there is no obvious organic cause, primary dysmenorrhea is thought to result from **increased levels of endometrial prostaglandin production** derived from the arachidonic acid pathway. Additionally, there may be a psychological component involved for some patients that depends on attitudes toward menstruation learned from mothers, sisters, and friends.

Diagnosis

The diagnosis of primary dysmenorrhea is made on the basis of history and the **absence of organic causes**. The most common misdiagnosis of primary dysmenorrhea is endometriosis. Often, the pain of dysmenorrhea occurs with ovulatory cycles on the first or second day of menstruation, whereas pain from endometriosis may begin 1 to 2 days to weeks before menstruation, worsens 1 to 2 days before menstruation, and is relieved at or right after the onset of menstrual flow (Chapter 15). Associated symptoms of primary dysmenorrhea include nausea, vomiting, and headache. On physical examination, there are no obvious abnormalities except a generalized tenderness throughout the pelvis.

Treatment

The first-line medical treatment for primary dysmenorrhea is **nonsteroidal anti-inflammatory** drugs (NSAIDs). The most commonly used agents include aspirin, ibuprofen, ketoprofen, and naproxen. These drugs are all available without prescription; however, to best control symptoms, education around initiation, duration, and dosing of medications is critical to success. Patients may need **prescription-strength dosages** to obtain adequate symptom relief. Because antiprostaglandins work by blocking prostaglandin synthesis and metabolism, these medications should be taken with the onset of menses, continued for 1 to 3 days, and then taken as needed. COX-2 inhibitors, such as Celebrex (celecoxib), are another class of NSAIDs that have been shown to be effective in the treatment of primary dysmenorrhea. However, potential side effects have limited their use in the United States.

Oral contraceptive pills (OCPs) are the second line of treatment for women who do not get adequate pain relief from antiprostaglandin agents and NSAIDs alone or who cannot tolerate these drugs. More than 90% of women with primary dysmenorrhea find adequate pain relief with the use of oral contraceptives given in a continuous (preferred) or cyclic fashion. The same is true for other estrogen/progestin combination contraceptives, such as the Ortho Evra patch and NuvaRing. The mechanism of relief is either secondary to the cessation of ovulation or because of the **decrease in endometrial proliferation** leading to **decreased prostaglandin production**. Most patients who have been cycled for 1 year on OCPs experience a reduction in symptoms even if the OCPs are discontinued. For women who cannot tolerate estrogens, several **progestin-only contraceptives** also provide excellent relief, including Depo-Provera, Nexplanon, and levonorgestrel-containing intrauterine devices (IUDs).

Nonmedical options for the treatment of primary dysmenorrhea include the use of heating pads and patches to the lower abdomen, exercise, massage, acupuncture, and hypnosis. The use of transcutaneous electrical nerve stimulation (TENS) has also been shown to relieve or decrease pain in women suffering from primary dysmenorrhea.

Surgical therapies, including cervical dilation, uterosacral ligament ligation, and presacral neurectomy, have been used in the past but **have little use in current management** of true primary dysmenorrhea. Often, primary dysmenorrhea will decrease throughout a patient's 20s and early 30s. In addition, a pregnancy carried to viability will usually decrease the symptoms of primary dysmenorrhea. Very rarely, a patient with true primary dysmenorrhea may require hysterectomy to relieve her pain. Prior to this, a **thorough evaluation**, possibly including questioning about childhood molestation or sexual assault, pelvic ultrasound, MRI, and laparoscopy, should be performed to look for secondary causes of dysmenorrhea.

SECONDARY DYSMENORRHEA

Secondary dysmenorrhea is menstrual pain with an identifiable etiology. It can be attributed to a number of causes (Fig. 22-1). Structural causes include müllerian anomalies, cervical stenosis, fibroids, adenomyosis, endometrial polyps, ovarian or fallopian

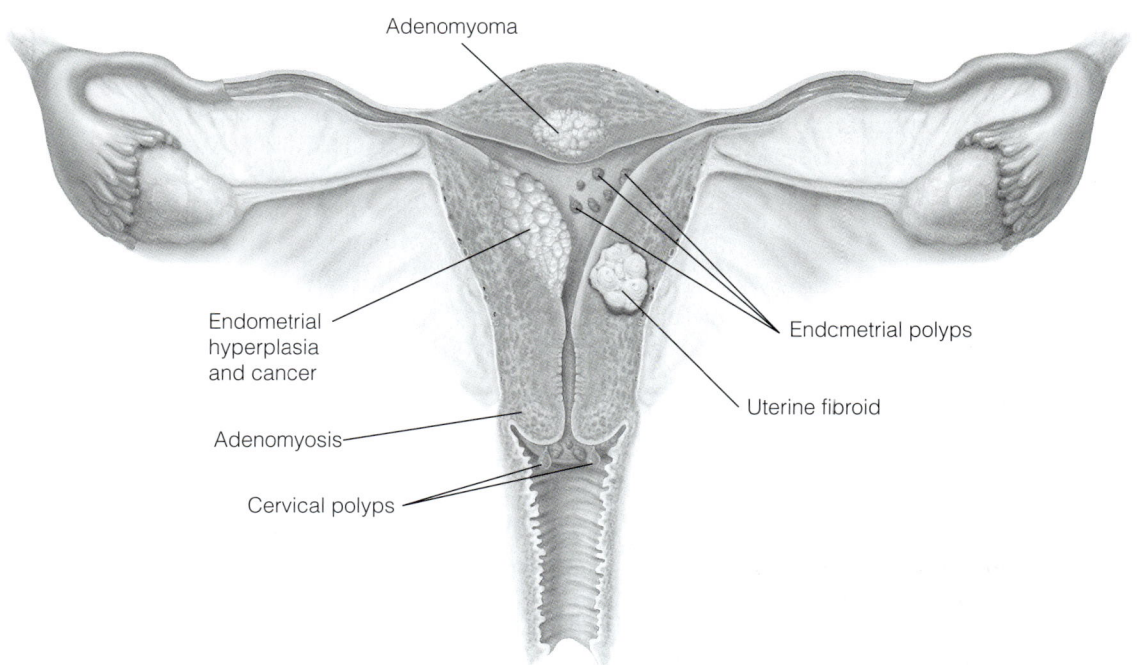

FIGURE 22-1. Common causes of abnormal vaginal bleeding. (From Anatomical Chart Co.)

tube neoplasms, as well as inflammatory changes and adhesions related to pelvic infections, prior surgical procedures, and endometriosis. Endometriosis and adenomyosis (Chapter 15) and uterine fibroids (Chapter 14) are discussed in other chapters, refer to those particular chapters for detailed management.

Pelvic ultrasound, and the more recently available 3D pelvic ultrasound, is a common initial diagnostic tool, able to diagnose most structural abnormalities and neoplasms of the upper genital tract. Adhesions, pelvic infection, and endometriosis are most commonly diagnosed with direct visualization at laparoscopy or laparotomy. Cervical cultures can be used to rule out sexually transmitted infections (STIs).

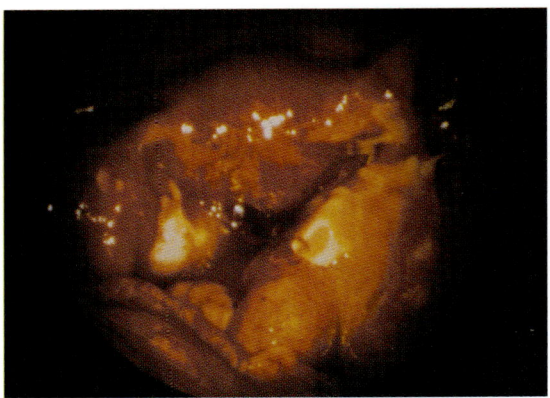

FIGURE 22-2. Laparoscopic view of adult pelvic inflammatory disease. (From Sweet R, Gibbs R. *Atlas of Infectious Diseases of the Female Genital Tract*. Philadelphia, PA. Lippincott Williams & Wilkins; 2005.)

Cervical Stenosis

Cervical stenosis causes dysmenorrhea by obstructing blood flow during menstruation. The stenosis can be **congenital** or secondary to **scarring from infection, trauma, or surgery**. Patients often complain of scant or prolonged light menses associated with severe cramping pain that is relieved with increased menstrual flow. On physical examination, there may be an obvious scarring of the external os; often, the clinician is unable to pass a uterine sound through the cervical canal.

Treatment

Cervical stenosis is treated by dilation of the cervix. Either a **mechanical dilation** can be performed or laminaria tents can be used. Surgical dilation is usually performed in the operating room but can be attempted in the office with a paracervical block and misoprostol prophylaxis to soften the cervix. Progressively, larger dilators are placed through the cervical canal until it becomes patent. Ultrasound guidance can be helpful in avoiding creation of a false passage or uterine perforation.

Laminaria osmotic dilators may be placed in the cervix in the office setting. Made from seaweed, these dilate over a 24-hour period by absorbing water from the surrounding tissue. Slow dilation of the cervix results from expansion of the laminaria. Dilation will provide relief; however, symptoms often recur, requiring multiple dilations. Pregnancy with vaginal delivery often leads to a permanent cure.

Pelvic Adhesions

Patients with a history of pelvic infections, including cervicitis, PID (Fig. 22-2), or tubo-ovarian abscess, may have symptoms of dysmenorrhea secondary to adhesion formation. Patients with other local inflammatory diseases (appendicitis, endometriosis, or Crohn disease) or prior pelvic surgery (especially myomectomy) may also have adhesions leading to dysmenorrhea. If a patient has a history of any of these problems and reports pain associated with movement or activity, pelvic adhesions should be suspected. In some patients, pelvic adhesions can be so extensive as to "cement" the uterus into a fixed position, which may be noted on pelvic examination. Adhesions are **not visible on traditional imaging modalities**, such as pelvic ultrasound, MRI, or CT.

Treatment

Patients with pelvic adhesions will occasionally respond to the antiprostaglandins prescribed for primary dysmenorrhea. When suspicions are high and the pain necessitates treatment, pelvic adhesions can be both **diagnosed and treated via laparoscopy**. Occasionally, the adhesions may be so dense as to necessitate laparotomy for safe lysis. However, the patient should be aware that surgery can lead to further adhesions and further problems with dysmenorrhea, infertility, and/or chronic pelvic pain.

PREMENSTRUAL SYNDROME AND PREMENSTRUAL DYSPHORIC DISORDER

Premenstrual syndrome (PMS) and its more severe variant, premenstrual dysphoric disorder (PMDD), are characterized by a constellation of physical and/or behavioral changes that occur in the second half of the menstrual cycle. These changes might include headache, weight gain, bloating, breast tenderness, mood fluctuation, restlessness, irritability, anxiety, depression, fatigue, and a feeling of being out of control. To meet criteria for diagnosis, these symptoms must occur in the **2 weeks prior to menstruation** and **resolve following onset of menses**. Likewise, there must be at least a **7-day symptom-free interval** in the first half of the menstrual cycle. Symptoms must occur in at least two consecutive cycles for the diagnosis to be made.

About 75% of women suffer from some recurrent PMS symptoms; of these, 30% report significant problems, and 5% of women are incapacitated or severely distressed by PMDD at some point during their cycle. The highest incidence occurs among women in their late 20s to early 30s.

PATHOGENESIS

The exact etiology of PMS and PMDD is unknown but is likely multifactorial and includes both physiologic and psychological causes. Past hypotheses have included abnormalities in estrogen–progesterone balance, disturbances in the renin–angiotensin–aldosterone pathway, excesses in prostaglandin and prolactin production, and psychogenic factors. Recent studies also suggest that PMS and PMDD may be caused by the interaction between the neurotransmitter serotonin and cyclic changes in the ovarian steroids. The serum concentrations of estrogen and progesterone are no different in patients with PMS/PMDD and those without. However, studies have suggested that although women with PMS and PMDD have normal levels of estrogen and progesterone, they may have **an abnormal response to normal hormonal changes**.

TREATMENT

Effective treatments for PMS and PMDD have been identified after systematic reviews. The **selective serotonin reuptake inhibitors** (SSRIs) have demonstrated clear efficacy in treating both the physical and mood symptoms of these disorders. Prozac (fluoxetine) has been approved by the U.S. FDA for the treatment of PMDD. Other drugs in this category, including Celexa (citalopram), Paxil (paroxetine), and Zoloft (sertraline), have also been shown to be effective. SSRIs are the **first line of treatment for PMDD**. These medications may be given every day or limited to use during the first 2 weeks of the cycle.

The **serotonin and norepinephrine reuptake inhibitors**, Effexor (venlafaxine) and the benzodiazepine Xanax (alprazolam), have also shown efficacy in treating these disorders. However, care should be used with alprazolam given its potential for addiction. In small trials, both Lupron (leuprolide acetate) and Danocrine (danazol) have shown efficacy in treating PMS and PMDD. Side effects of these medications, however, prevent widespread use of these options.

A number of additional medications may have possible efficacy in the treatment of PMS and PMDD. Several older studies showed **oral contraceptives** to have **no greater efficacy** than placebo in managing PMS and PMDD. Yaz, which is formulated with low-dose estrogen and uses **drospirenone** (a spironolactone with antimineralocorticoid and antiandrogenic activity) as its progestin, has been FDA-approved for the treatment of PMDD but is not indicated for the treatment of PMS. Spironolactone itself has not consistently shown to be effective. There is some suggestion that **exercise and relaxation techniques** may improve the symptoms of PMS and PMDD.

Several studies have looked at **vitamin supplementation** as a treatment for PMS and PMDD. There appears to be some role for the use of calcium (600 mg BID), vitamin D (800 IU/day), vitamin B_6 ($\leq$100 mg/day), magnesium (200 to 360 mg/day), and chasteberry extract (one tablet per day) in the treatment of these disorders. Several studies have also showed that complex carbohydrate-rich beverage consumption improved both the psychological symptoms and appetite cravings. This is thought to work by modulating tryptophan and serotonin synthesis.

Other supplements, such as evening primrose oil, essential fatty acids, and ginkgo biloba extract, have not been found to be effective nor has the use of progesterone and progestins.

ABNORMAL UTERINE BLEEDING

The normal menstrual cycle consists of cyclic bleeding approximately **every 28 days** (normal range, 21 to 35 days), lasting **3 to 5 days** with about **30 to 50 mL** of blood loss per cycle. AUB refers to any departure from the norm in the menstrual cycle or bleeding perceived by the patient to be abnormal. AUB may also refer to inappropriate unscheduled bleeding (bleeding between periods, postcoital spotting, and postmenopausal bleeding). The most common causes of AUB are covered briefly in this chapter and in more detail in other chapters of this book (Fig. 22-1).

The term **dysfunctional uterine bleeding (DUB)** was used in the past to describe idiopathic heavy and/or irregular bleeding that **could not be attributed to another cause** following a complete evaluation. Use of this terminology is no longer recommended.

Amenorrhea—complete absence of periods for at least 6 consecutive months—is discussed in Chapter 21.

PALM-COEIN SYSTEM OF ABNORMAL UTERINE BLEEDING

The typical patterns of AUB are summarized in Table 22-1. It is generally agreed that these definitions to describe different types of AUB in nonpregnant reproductive-aged women have been inconsistent and confusing. Efforts have been ongoing to simplify the terminology. This new classification system known by the acronym **PALM-COEIN** (pronounced "palm coin") was introduced in 2011 by the International Federation of Gynecology and Obstetrics (FIGO) and is supported by the American College of OB/GYN (ACOG). This new nomenclature system (Fig. 22-2) classifies AUB in nonpregnant reproductive-aged women by both the **pattern of bleeding** and the **etiology of the bleeding**. The PALM-COEIN system divides AUB into patterns of bleeding, including heavy menstrual bleeding (HMB) and intermenstrual bleeding (IMB). In terms of etiologies of AUB, the system uses **PALM** to represent the structural causes of AUB, including **P**olyps, **A**denomyosis, **L**eiomyomas, and **M**alignancy and hyperplasia. **COEIN** delineates the nonstructural causes of AUB, including **C**oagulopathy, **O**vulatory dysfunction, **E**ndometrial and **I**atrogenic causes, and those etiologies that are **N**ot yet classified.

PATTERNS OF ABNORMAL UTERINE BLEEDING

Heavy Menstrual Bleeding

Patients with HMB (formerly menorrhagia) have regularly timed menstrual cycles, but the flow is either excessive in its duration (>7 days) or in its volume (>80 mL/cycle). Most gynecologists define HMB as soaking through a pad every 1 to 2 hours, interfering with work or activities, awakening a patient from sleep, or staining clothing or sheets. However, it is now generally accepted that if a patient perceives her bleeding to be heavy, her symptoms should be evaluated, and treatment should be offered as indicated. Patients with HMB occasionally describe the

TABLE 22-1. Patterns of Uterine Bleeding

Bleeding Pattern	Description	Timing of Cycle	Flow Amount
Normal menstrual cycle	Regular bleeding, average Q 28 d (range, 21–35), lasting 3–5 d, bleeding on average 30–50 mL/cycle	Regular	Normal
Heavy menstrual bleeding (formerly menorrhagia)	Heavy (>80 mL/cycle) or prolonged (>7 d) menstrual flow occurring at regular intervals	Regular	Heavy
Light menstrual bleeding (formerly hypomenorrhea)	Regularly timed menses but light flow	Regular	Light
Intermenstrual bleeding (formerly metrorrhagia)	Any bleeding between normal menses, usually lighter than normal menstrual bleeding	Irregular	Normal–light
Heavy irregular bleeding (formerly menometrorrhagia)	Excessive or prolonged bleeding at irregular intervals	Irregular	Heavy
Infrequent menstrual cycles (oligomenorrhea)	Irregular cycles >35 d apart	Irregular	Varies
Polymenorrhea	Frequent regular cycles but <21 d apart	Regular	Normal
Amenorrhea, secondary	No menses for 6 or more consecutive months	N/A	N/A
Amenorrhea, primary	No menses by age 14 y in the absence of secondary sexual characteristics *or* No menses by age 16 y in the presence of secondary sexual characteristics	N/A	N/A

blood as flooding or gushing and may have blood clots along with their excessive flow. HMB is most commonly caused by uterine fibroids, adenomyosis, endometrial polyps, and less commonly by endometrial intraepithelial neoplasia (EIN) or cancer or cervical polyps or cancer (Fig. 22-1). Teenagers with HMB should be evaluated for primary bleeding disorders, such as von Willebrand disease, idiopathic thrombocytopenic purpura, platelet dysfunction, and thrombocytopenia from malignancy. Nearly 20% of adolescents hospitalized for AUB will have an underlying coagulopathy.

Intermenstrual Bleeding

IMB is characterized by bleeding that occurs between regular menstrual periods (formerly metrorrhagia). This bleeding is usually less than or equal to normal menstrual volume. Primary causes include cervical lesions (polyps, ectropions, and carcinoma) and endometrial polyps and carcinoma. Heavy irregular bleeding (formerly menometrorrhagia) is excessive (>80 mL) or prolonged bleeding at irregular intervals. The usual causes include uterine fibroids, adenomyosis, endometrial polyps, EIN, and cancer (Fig. 22-1). Thyroid disorders can result in increased or decreased flow or no change in menstrual flow.

OTHER PATTERNS OF ABNORMAL UTERINE BLEEDING

Infrequent Menstrual Cycles

Patients with periods **greater than 35 days apart** are described as having infrequent menses (oligomenorrhea). Those with no period in 3 to 6 months are said to have amenorrhea. The causes include disruption of the hypothalamic–pituitary–gonadal axis or systemic diseases, such as hyperprolactinemia and thyroid disorders (Chapter 21). The most common causes of oligomenorrhea are **polycystic ovarian syndrome (PCOS), chronic anovulation, and pregnancy.** When a patient has no period for 6 consecutive months, secondary amenorrhea is diagnosed.

Light Menstrual Cycles

Patients with decreased menstrual volume (formerly hypomenorrhea) have regularly timed menses but an unusually light amount of flow. This is commonly caused by hypogonadotropic hypogonadism, which is seen most commonly in anorexic patients and athletes. Atrophic endometrium can also occur in the case of Asherman syndrome (intrauterine adhesions or synechiae), congenital malformations, infection, and intrauterine trauma. Patients on **OCPs, Depo-Provera, and the progestin-containing IUDs** can have endometrial atrophy resulting in light menses as can women who have undergone endometrial ablation. Outlet obstruction secondary to cervical stenosis or congenital abnormalities can also result in decreased menstrual volume.

Regular Menstrual Cycles with Increased Frequency

Frequent regular periods (formerly polymenorrhea) describe regular periods that occur less than 21 days apart. Frequent menstrual cycles can be confused with IMB. However, if all of the bleeding episodes are similar in amount and fewer than 21 days apart, frequent menstrual cycles should be considered. This is usually caused by **anovulation**.

EVALUATION OF ABNORMAL UTERINE BLEEDING

The workup for AUB includes a careful history and physical examination followed by diagnostic tests to determine the underlying etiology. The **history** should include questions about the timing, quantity, and amount of bleeding, and any associated symptoms. A GYN, OB, menstrual, sexual, surgical, and contraceptive history should be obtained. It should also include risk factors for endometrial cancer as well as a family history of bleeding disorders, particularly, if HMB occurs at menarche.

On **physical examination**, care should be taken to look for sequelae of PCOS (hirsutism, acne, truncal obesity, acanthosis nigricans), thyroid disease (thyromegaly, thyroid nodule, skin changes, diaphoresis, increased pulse), bleeding disorders (bruising, petechiae, skin pallor, swollen joints), hirsutism (excessive male-pattern facial and body hair), and less commonly, virilization (deepening of the voice, temporal balding, breast atrophy, changes toward a male body habitus, and/or clitoromegaly). On **pelvic examination**, rectal, urethral, vaginal, and cervical causes of bleeding should be ruled out. The **bimanual examination** may reveal uterine or adnexal masses consistent with fibroids, adenomyosis, pregnancy, or cancer. A **Pap test**, with or without high-risk human papillomavirus (HPV) screening as indicated, is used to screen for cervical neoplasia and cancer, and cervical cultures should be taken to rule out infection. Testing for **chlamydia trachomatis** is indicated for those at high risk of infection.

Initial **laboratory evaluation** should be tailored to the type of menstrual irregularity. For light or skipped cycles, evaluation would include a **pregnancy test, thyroid stimulating hormone (TSH), prolactin**

(PRL) and follicle stimulating hormone (FSH) levels if menopause or primary ovarian insufficiency (POI, formerly premature ovarian failure–PMOF) is suspected. **Ovulatory status** is most commonly evaluated using a mid-luteal, days 21 to 23 serum progesterone level. This can also be accomplished with ovulation prediction kits, which are at-home tests for detecting the luteinizing hormone (LH) surge from urine samples. The spectra of hormonal tests that can be performed are included in the discussions of the evaluations of amenorrhea, PCOS, and PMOF elsewhere in the text.

For heavy, frequent, or prolonged cycles, appropriate initial laboratory tests would include a **pregnancy test, TSH,** and complete blood count **(CBC)**. A primary bleeding disorder evaluation should be done when HMB presents at menarche, in teenagers or in women with symptoms suggestive of a systemic or hematologic etiology, such as easy bruising (>5 cm), frequent nosebleeds, bleeding gums, and excessive bleeding after surgery, dental extraction, or childbirth. Evaluation for these women might include a **CBC, including platelet count** and differential **prothrombin time (PT)/partial thromboplastin time (PTT), factor VIII, and von Willebrand factor antigen and activity**.

Importantly, any woman older than 45 years with AUB (excessive or insufficient) should undergo an office **endometrial biopsy (EMB)** as a first-line test to rule out benign endometrial hyperplasia, EIN, and endometrial cancer even if other testing reveals a potential explanation for the AUB. Patients with a history of **unopposed estrogen exposure** (e.g., obese patients with prolonged oligomenorrhea) should also undergo EMB even if they are younger than 45 years. These women are at increased risk of EIN and endometrial cancer because of the peripheral conversion of androgens into estrogens in their adipose cells. Similarly, women younger than 45 years of age with **persistent AUB** and those who have **failed medical management** should also undergo EMB.

A **pelvic ultrasound** can be used to identify endometrial polyps, fibroids, EIN, cancers, and adnexal masses. If intrauterine pathology is suspected on pelvic ultrasound, a 3D ultrasound, saline-infused sonohysterogram (SIS), or hysterosalpingogram can be performed to show intrauterine defects. **MRI** is expensive but useful in distinguishing adenomyosis from uterine fibroids. **Hysteroscopy** in the office or operating room allows for direct visualization of the intrauterine cavity. A dilation and curettage **(D&C)** provides tissue for diagnosis and sometimes treatment of AUB.

TREATMENT
Treatment of Structural Causes of AUB

The treatment of AUB depends on the specific underlying etiology. The most common causes and treatments are detailed in Table 22-2. In general, **structural etiologies for AUB** (PALM from the PALM-COEIN system) generally require surgical correction. However, for ovulatory AUB with heavy regular menstrual bleeding, it is reasonable to attempt a trial of medical management. Nonhormonal therapy with NSAIDs (e.g., 800 mg ibuprofen TID for 5 days) has been shown to decrease menstrual blood loss by 20% to 50%. This therapy may be used alone or in conjunction with hormonal contraception therapy, including the use of **combination estrogen and progesterone** in the form of OCPs, Ortho Evra patch, or NuvaRing. These may be dosed in a continuous (preferred) or cyclic fashion depending on the patient's desire. Numerous extended cycle formulations are also available that reduce menstrual cycles to every 3 months in most cases. In patients in whom the use of estrogen is contraindicated (women with hypertension, thrombophilias, and history of deep vein thrombosis (DVT) or pulmonary embolus (PE) and those 35 years and older who smoke), or those who prefer an alternative to estrogen/progestin combination, similar cycle control can be achieved using **progestin-only options**. These include cyclic progestin administration (10 mg medroxyprogesterone acetate per day for 10 consecutive days each month) or progesterone in the form of Depo-Provera, levonorgestrel-releasing intrauterine device (Mirena), or Nexplanon. The latter three are likely to result in light menses or amenorrhea over time. **Tranexamic acid (Lysteda)**, an antifibrinolytic agent, has been shown to decrease menstrual blood loss and is FDA approved for the treatment of HMB. Because it promotes clotting, it is contraindicated in women using combination hormonal contraception and in those with active thromboembolic disease (DVT, PE) or a history of thromboembolism.

Although some women will respond to medical management of AUB due to structural causes, many will eventually require surgical management. **Polyps (AUB-P)** can typically be removed via hysteroscopic resection. Women with multiple or recurrent polyps may opt for definitive management with hysterectomy (Chapter 14).

Adenomyosis (AUB-A) is occasionally responsive to hormonal contraceptives. However, the levonorgestrel-containing IUD (Mirena) has been found to substantially decrease the bleeding and pain associated with adenomyosis. Endometrial

TABLE 22-2. Common Causes and Treatments for Abnormal Uterine Bleeding

Bleeding Disorder	Bleeding Amount	Typical Treatment
Neoplasms		
Uterine fibroids	Heavy	Hormonal management, tranexamic acid, uterine artery embolization, myomectomy, endometrial ablation, hysterectomy
Adenomyosis	Heavy	Hormonal management, Mirena IUD, endometrial ablation hysterectomy
Cervical polyps	Light	Polypectomy
Endometrial polyps	Heavy	Hysteroscopy, polypectomy ± D&C, endometrial ablation, hysterectomy
Benign endometrial hyperplasia and endometrial intraepithelial neoplasia (EIN)	Varies	Progestin therapy (if no atypia or desires fertility), hysteroscopy with D&C followed by hysterectomy if EIN is present
Endometrial cancer	Heavy	Hysterectomy, bilateral salpingo-oophorectomy (BSO), ±radiation
Pregnancy problems		
Pregnancy	Varies	Expectant management vs. delivery
Miscarriage	Heavy	Expectant management, medical induction, manual vacuum evacuation, D&C
Ectopic pregnancy	Varies	Methotrexate vs. surgical management (usually salpingotomy vs. salpingectomy)
Hormonal problems		
Hypothyroidism	Varies	Thyroid hormone replacement
Hyperprolactinemia	None	Dopamine agonists
Anovulation	Varies	Combined estrogen/progestin pills, patch, or ring; or cyclic progestin; levonorgestrel IUD

D&C, dilation and curettage.

ablation can be used in patients with symptomatic adenomyosis, although there may be an increased incidence of post-ablation pain and recurrent abnormal bleeding in women with adenomyosis who undergo ablation. In patients with refractory pain and/or bleeding, hysterectomy may be required for the treatment of adenomyosis after ruling out EIN and endometrial cancer (Chapter 15).

Leiomyomata (AUB-L) can be managed medically with hormonal contraceptives or levonorgestrel-containing IUD or surgically with hysteroscopic resection for submucosal fibroids (AUB-L$_{SM}$), or with endometrial ablation, uterine artery embolization, and uterine myomectomy or hysterectomy (Chapter 14).

Benign endometrial hyperplasia (AUB-M) is most commonly managed with progestin therapy if no cytologic atypia is present (i.e., no EIN). The treatment of choice for EIN is total hysterectomy (Chapter 14). Endometrial ablation and supracervical hysterectomy are not acceptable for patients with EIN or endometrial cancer.

Treatment of Nonstructural Causes of AUB

Therapy for **nonstructural causes of AUB** (COEIN from the PALM-COEIN System) should be directed at treatment of the underlying cause when a cause is identifiable (Table 22-2). Patients with inherited and acquired **coagulopathies (AUB-C)** are typically evaluated and managed by a hematologist. These patients most often have a pattern of heavy regular cycles. They can generally be managed with hormonal contraception, levonorgestrel-containing IUD, or global endometrial ablation. Rarely, hysterectomy may be indicated.

Patients with AUB due to **ovulatory disorders (AUB-O)** most commonly have irregular bleeding patterns marked by weeks to months of no bleeding followed by weeks to months of heavy and/or prolonged bleeding. This most common cause of AUB-O is anovulation due to PCOS, extremes in reproductive age (adolescence, perimenopause), and endocrine disorders (thyroid disease, hyperprolactinemia, hyperandrogenism, hypothalamic hypogonadism, or POI). Once identified, the primary cause should be addressed when possible. After this, menstrual regulation can often be achieved with the use of hormonal contraceptives or cyclic progestins. The levonorgestrel-containing IUD can provide bleeding control while also protecting the endometrium from premalignant and malignant disease. Treatment for symptoms of POI and perimenopause is directed toward relief of specific symptoms and long-term sequelae of low estrogen levels (Chapter 20).

AUB, especially IMB, may be because of nonstructural **endometrial sources (AUB-E)**. These include infection and inflammation due to STI, chronic PID, and endometritis as well as alterations in prostaglandins, resulting in disorders impacting local endometrial hemostasis. Again, treatment should be aimed at addressing the underlying source. When the source is not clearly definable and infection has been ruled out, hormonal contraceptives, levonorgestrel-containing IUD, and endometrial ablation offer symptom management. Rarely, hysterectomy is indicated.

AUB due to **iatrogenic etiologies (AUB-I)** includes medications that impact coagulation, ovulation, the endometrium, and the hypothalamic–pituitary–ovarian axis. Examples include anticoagulants, hormonal contraceptives, estrogens, progestins, and androgens, as well as both medicated and inert IUDs. The most common cause of AUB-I is unscheduled bleeding, or so called "break-through-bleeding," due to the use of contraceptives. In most cases, medication adjustments will resolve the symptoms. This should include education on avoiding skipped, delayed, or erratic administration of contraceptive agents. When endometrial atrophy is suspected, high-dose NSAIDs (ibuprofen 800 mg TID for 5 days), combination hormonal contraception, or an estradiol patch (0.1 mcg for 1 month) may be used to stabilize the endometrium.

Other rare or ill-defined entities can result in AUB but have **not yet been classified (AUB-N)**. Examples include chronic endometritis, arteriovenous malformations, Cesarean scar defect, and myometrial hypertrophy. In these cases, treatment should be geared toward the specific etiology.

Treatment of Acute Hemorrhage

In the case of acute hemorrhage, therapy to stop the bleeding should be initiated immediately. Intravenous estrogen (25 mg conjugated estrogen every 4 hours up to 24 hours) not only provides a quick response but also carries an increased risk of venous thromboembolic events (DVT, PE). For patients with excessive blood loss who are hemodynamically stable, high-dose oral estrogens can control the bleeding within 24 to 48 hours. A typical dose of estradiol might be 2.5 mg every 4 hours for 14 to 21 days, followed by medroxyprogesterone acetate 10 mg/day for 7 to 10 days. Instead of this sequential hormone therapy, an OCP taper can be used for endometrial stabilization. A typical taper would use a monophasic pill containing 35 mcg ethinylestradiol given three times a day for 3 days, then two times a day for 2 days, and then daily for the remainder of the pack.

Surgical intervention may be required for patients with AUB who do not respond to medical therapy. Hysteroscopy with **D&C** may be both diagnostic and therapeutic, but the result is typically temporary.

Hysterectomy is the definitive surgery for acute hemorrhage but should be reserved for those cases refractory to all other treatments or for women for whom childbearing is complete. Hysterectomy may be performed laparoscopically, vaginally, or abdominally. The patient's personal risk factors and age may be used to determine if the ovaries and/or cervix is left in situ or removed.

POSTMENOPAUSAL BLEEDING

Menopause is marked by 12 months of amenorrhea after the final menstrual period (Chapter 20). Postmenopausal bleeding, then, is any vaginal bleeding that occurs more than 12 months after the last menstrual period. **Any postmenopausal bleeding is abnormal** and should be investigated given the increased risk of reproductive cancers in women in this age group. The most common cause of postmenopausal bleeding, however, is **endometrial and/or vaginal atrophy**, not cancer (Table 22-3). Premalignant and malignant endometrial disease is responsible for only 10% to 15% of all postmenopausal vaginal bleeding (PMVB).

TABLE 22-3. Causes of Postmenopausal Bleeding

Etiology	Percentage
Vaginal/endometrial atrophy	30
Exogenous estrogens	30
Endometrial cancer	10
Endometrial polyps	10
Benign endometrial hyperplasia or endometrial intraepithelial neoplasia (EIN)	10
Other	10

ETIOLOGIES

Bleeding in postmenopausal women can be because of nongynecologic etiologies, lower and upper genital tract sources, reproductive tumors, or exogenous hormonal stimulation. **Nongynecologic causes** include rectal bleeding from hemorrhoids, anal fissures, rectal prolapse, and lower gastrointestinal tumors. Urethral caruncles are another source of bleeding in the postmenopausal woman. These disorders can be identified by history and physical examination, anoscopy, fecal immunoassay test, barium enema, or colonoscopy.

The most common cause of postmenopausal bleeding from the lower genital tract is **genitourinary atrophy** caused by low estrogen levels. The thin vaginal mucosa is easily traumatized and, therefore, likely to bleed. Other causes of **lower genital tract** bleeding are benign and malignant lesions of the vulva, vagina, or cervix.

Other causes of postmenopausal bleeding from the **upper genital tract** include endometrial polyps, EIN, and endometrial cancer. Fibroids themselves do not directly cause PMVB, but rather, bleeding is caused by atrophic endometrium that overly the fibroids. Estrogen-secreting tumors of the ovary can cause stimulation of the endometrium that presents as postmenopausal bleeding. Each of these disorders can be identified with a combination of Pap screen and high-risk HPV, EMB, and pelvic ultrasound.

The use of **exogenous hormones** is another common cause of postmenopausal uterine bleeding. Despite the occurrence of bleeding with the use of menopausal hormone therapy (50% in the first year of use), thorough evaluation of the postmenopausal patient with PMVB is still required to rule out benign endometrial hyperplasia, EIN, and cancer.

DIAGNOSIS

A careful history is important. Physical examination should include a careful inspection of the external anus, urethra, vulva, vagina, and cervix. A **Pap test** and **high-risk HPV screen** should be performed if indicated as well as a digital rectal examination and fecal immunoassay test. Laboratory tests might include a **CBC, TSH, prolactin, and FSH levels**. If an ovarian mass is identified, tumor markers (Ca-125, LDH, hCG, AFP, CEA, inhibin, and estradiol) should also be considered.

A **pelvic ultrasound, SIS, and MRI** can be useful in the evaluation of the endometrial stripe and uterine cavity. In the postmenopausal woman, the endometrial stripe should be thin and less than or equal to 4 mm. **Office EMB** should be performed in a postmenopausal patient with an endometrial stripe greater than 4 mm or if the bleeding is recurrent or persistent. This is done to rule out EIN and cancer even if there is another identifiable source of postmenopausal bleeding. Hysteroscopy—either in the office or operating room—can further elucidate intrauterine abnormalities, such as endometrial polyps and fibroids. **D&C** can be both diagnostic and therapeutic for some lesions of the uterus and cervix. If the office EMB cannot be obtained, **hysteroscopy with D&C** should be performed.

TREATMENT

Treatment of postmenopausal bleeding should be directed at **treating the causal agent**. Lesions of the vulva and vagina should be biopsied and treated accordingly. Lacerations of the vaginal mucosa should be repaired. **Genital urinary syndrome of menopause** can be treated with low-dose topical or vaginal estrogen preparations (cream, pill, ring).

Endometrial polyps may be removed by hysteroscopic resection or D&C (Chapter 14). Benign endometrial hyperplasia can be treated with progestin therapy if no atypia is present. However, hysterectomy is the treatment of choice for EIN. Endometrial cancer is usually treated by total hysterectomy and bilateral salpingo-oophorectomy (TAHBSO) performed in conjunction with radiation if indicated.

KEY POINTS

- Primary dysmenorrhea is severe pain with menses that cannot be attributed to any identifiable cause. It is thought to be because of increased levels of prostaglandins.
- Most primary dysmenorrhea is managed with NSAIDs and/or contraceptive steroids in pill, patch, or ring form. TENS units, heating pads, exercise, massage, acupuncture, and hypnosis may also help. There is a little role for surgery in the management of primary dysmenorrhea.
- Secondary dysmenorrhea is painful menses owing to an identifiable cause, such as adenomyosis, endometriosis, fibroids, cervical stenosis, or pelvic adhesions. The treatment should be tailored to the cause.
- PMS and PMDD represent a multifactorial disease spectrum with physiologic and psychological components, including headache, weight gain, bloating, breast fluctuation, irritability, fatigue, and a feeling of being out of control.
- In order to make the diagnosis of PMS/PMDD, symptoms must be in the second half of the menstrual cycle with at least a 7-day symptom-free interval during the first half of the menstrual cycle. Symptoms must occur in at least two consecutive cycles.
- Although the cause of PMS/PMDD is unknown, a variety of treatments offer relief, including SSRIs (Prozac, Zoloft) and OCPs, as do diet modification, exercise, and vitamin supplementation (calcium, vitamin D, vitamin B_6, and magnesium).
- The normal menstrual cycle occurs, on average, every 28 days (range, 21 to 35 days) and lasts 3 to 5 days with 30 to 50 mL of blood loss per cycle.
- HMB (formerly menorrhagia) is regular bleeding that is heavy or prolonged as perceived by the patient. IMB (formerly metrorrhagia) is bleeding between periods. The most common causes of heavy or prolonged bleeding include polyps, fibroids, infection, cancer, and pregnancy complications.
- The most common causes of oligomenorrhea (periods >35 days apart) include chronic ovulation, PCOS, and pregnancy.
- PALM-COEIN is the new classifications denoting structural (polyps, adenomyosis, leiomyomas, malignancy, and premalignancy) and nonstructural (coagulopathy, ovulatory dysfunction, endometrial, iatrogenic, not yet classified) causes of AUB in non-gravid reproductive-aged women.
- The initial evaluation of AUB should include a history and physical examination, laboratory tests (pregnancy test, TSH, prolactin, ±FSH), EMB (for women >45 and those at high risk of EIN and endometrial (EM) cancer), and pelvic ultrasound. Treatment should be directed at the cause of the abnormal bleeding.
- Most women with HMB can achieve menstrual regularity using a daily monophasic birth control pill, patch, ring, or by use of cyclic progestins when estrogens are contraindicated. Lysteda is another option in patients with no history of venous thromboembolism (VTE).
- IV estrogens and high-dose oral estrogens can be used to stop acute bleeding. Acute hemorrhage that is not responsive to medical therapy may require surgical treatment with D&C, Mirena IUD, endometrial ablation, or, rarely, hysterectomy.
- The most common cause of postmenopausal bleeding is genital urinary syndrome of menopause. Other causes include cancer of the upper and lower genital tract, endometrial polyps, exogenous hormonal stimulation, and bleeding from nongynecologic sources.
- Postmenopausal bleeding should always be investigated to rule out premalignant and malignant endometrial disease. The evaluation of postmenopausal bleeding should include a thorough history and physical examination, TSH, and other laboratory tests as indicated. A pelvic ultrasound should be performed to look for structural abnormalities.
- All postmenopausal women with an endometrial stripe >4 mm or persistent or recurrent bleeding should have an EMB to rule out premalignant and malignant endometrial disease.

CLINICAL VIGNETTES

VIGNETTE 1

A 58-year-old G3P3003 Caucasian, postmenopausal woman comes to your office. She has been menopausal since age 50 years. She has a negative past medical and surgical history. She took hormone replacement for about 2 years but stopped due to concerns of an increased risk of cancer that she heard about from friends. Prior to the onset of menopause, she had a history of normal and regular menses. She has had annual GYN care with you and has never been diagnosed with cervical dysplasia. Her last Pap smear with HPV was obtained last year, and both were negative. She has recently become sexually active with a new partner and has noted some spotting with intercourse. She also reports some intermittent spotting when she wipes and occasional mild low abdominal cramping over the past 2 to 3 months. She complains of a general feeling of vaginal dryness and does have pain and dryness with intercourse. She has no other complains whatsoever.

1. Her most likely diagnosis is:
   a. endometrial cancer
   b. cervical cancer
   c. genitourinary syndrome of menopause
   d. bleeding disorder
   e. uterine fibroids

2. On examination, she has normal appearing external female genitalia. She has a normal appearing rectum, and a fecal immunoassay test is negative for blood. On speculum examination, she has pale, thin vaginal epithelium without lesions, blood, or discharge. Her cervix is pale and stenotic but without lesions. A bimanual examination reveals a small, nontender mid-position uterus, with no adnexal masses. The most appropriate testing includes:
   a. endometrial biopsy (EMB)
   b. transvaginal ultrasound
   c. sexually transmitted infection (STI) testing (gonorrhea and chlamydia)
   d. all of the above
   e. none of the above

3. You perform an examination testing for gonorrhea and chlamydial infection as well as perform an EMB. In addition, you order a pelvic ultrasound. Sexually transmitted disease (STD) testing is negative. Her EMB returns with inactive, atrophic endometrium, negative for hyperplasia, endometrial intraepithelial neoplasia (EIN), or malignancy. Her transvaginal ultrasound reveals a normal appearing uterus with evidence of a 2-cm intracavitary lesion, consistent with an endometrial polyp. Ovaries are normal; there is no free fluid present in the peritoneal cavity. The next most appropriate step in the management of this patient is:
   a. reassurance and follow up in 1 year
   b. reassurance and follow up ultrasound in 1 year
   c. outpatient hysteroscopy D&C with polypectomy
   d. treat the urogenital atrophy with systemic or vaginal estrogens and follow up in 3 months
   e. no additional follow up is indicated

VIGNETTE 2

An 18-year-old college student is referred to you for worsening pain with her menses. She had onset of menses at age 14. She describes irregular periods until age 16 when her periods became more regular but also more painful. At this time, she is missing classes 1 or 2 days each month because of symptoms. She has tried over-the-counter Midol and Tylenol without significant relief of her pain. She has a negative past medical and surgical history. She denies sexual activity, is on no medications, and has no allergies. Although she does not seem very clear about her family history, she is unaware of any significant medical conditions, heritable cancers, or other conditions. She has never been pregnant and has never seen a gynecologist. She does not smoke, drink, or use alcohol or illicit drugs.

1. What is the best initial treatment for this patient?
   a. Trial of scheduled nonsteroidal anti-inflammatory drugs (NSAIDs)
   b. Trial of oral contraceptive
   c. Diagnostic laparoscopy
   d. Transvaginal ultrasound
   e. Endometrial ablation

2. You prescribe naproxen sodium 500 mg PO every 12 hours at onset of menses taken as a scheduled medication for the first 3 days of her period followed by PRN administration. On follow up, she endorses partial relief of her symptoms. Although she is able to attend class, she continues to have significant pain for 3 to 4 days during her cycle. She also admits to being sexually active (she was afraid to discuss this at her first visit) and to using condoms infrequently. Her first sexual encounter occurred 2 months ago. At this point, what additional evaluation would you perform?
   a. Pap smear and HPV testing
   b. STI screening
   c. Transvaginal ultrasound
   d. Both options a and b
   e. EMB

3. The patient's screening returns as negative. An in-office pregnancy test is also negative. At this point, what would you offer to your patient for treatment of her dysmenorrhea?
   a. Continued use of NSAIDs
   b. Combination oral contraceptive pills (OCPs)
   c. Tranexamic acid
   d. Hydrocodone and acetaminophen
   e. Both options a and b

VIGNETTE 3

A 26-year-old G1P1001 woman presents to your office with a concern that she has premenstrual syndrome (PMS). She states that she feels very "hormonal" most months in the week or so before her menses. She has been told that she is on edge and loses her temper easily with coworkers and at home with her family during these times. She does not feel like leaving the house or even getting dressed some days, has not been sleeping well, and is gaining weight due to overeating. Her menstrual cycles are regular; she is single and not sexually active. She has one child, born by SVD at term without complications. She recalls some depression following the delivery but was never treated and her symptoms resolved. Her past medical and surgical histories are negative. She wants to know what you can do to help her.

1. What diagnostic evaluation would you offer this patient at this visit?
   a. Reassurance and general stress reduction/healthy lifestyle tips
   b. Send her to see her primary care provider (PCP)
   c. Ask her to fill out a symptom calendar for 2 months and return
   d. Send a complete blood count (CBC), TSH, and prolactin
   e. Start her on a daily selective serotonin reuptake inhibitor (SSRI)

2. The patient returns to your office in 2 months with a symptom calendar. Her calendar does show that her menstrual cycles are regular and occur every 30 days. She documented that her symptoms of emotional lability, sleep disturbances, "emotional eating," and decreased interest in activities are most prominent for about 10 days prior to the onset of a period. Her symptoms dissipate 2 to 3 days after the start of her menstrual cycle. She feels well in general for about 2 weeks, although not completely symptom free on all days. Her severe symptoms begin to return 10 days prior to the next cycle. You diagnose PMS and outline her treatment options. These include:
   a. vitamin supplementation with calcium, vitamin E, vitamin B_6, and magnesium
   b. fluoxetine (Prozac)
   c. oral contraceptive Yaz
   d. exercise and relaxation techniques
   e. any of the above

3. The patient chooses to start vitamin supplements, and has taken calcium, vitamin E, vitamin B_6, and magnesium for the past 2 months, while continuing to keep a symptom calendar. You see her in follow up. She states that her symptoms prior to the onset of menses are somewhat improved but not sufficiently to allow her to feel like "herself" and to perform as she would like at work and in her home. You examine her calendar and note that she continues to have symptoms throughout the month, with rare isolated symptom-free days. At this point, what do you recommend?
   a. Stop the vitamin supplements and continue to keep a symptom calendar
   b. Continue the vitamin supplements and continue to keep a symptom calendar for two more months
   c. Start progestin therapy
   d. Add an SSRI, such as Prozac (dosed for PMS during the luteal phase only)
   e. Consider treatment for underlying depression

VIGNETTE 4

A 27-year-old G0P0 woman presents to your office with a history of amenorrhea. She has a history of infrequent menstrual cycles in high school but she had regular withdrawal bleeds in college and medical school while on oral contraceptive pills. She stopped her birth control pills about 7 months ago and her period never resumed and she developed mild hirsutism along with a 10 lbs weight gain. She is sexually active with a male partner and uses condoms for contraception. She has a history of seasonal allergies, no prior surgeries, and no prior pregnancies.

1. Additional significant history that you might want to ask about includes:
   a. the type/brand of oral contraception she was taking
   b. her typical diet and exercise pattern
   c. family history of amenorrhea
   d. age at first coitus
   e. does she desire future fertility

2. When you question her about her general diet and activity, she states that she is a vegetarian. She is a resident, so often eats on the run or skips meals but does eat one to two meals per day and has no prior history of an eating disorder. She exercises when she can, about one to two times per week. She typically jogs or goes for a walk with her dog. Her BMI is elevated at 30. Which of the following tests are most appropriate to order at this visit?
   a. TSH, prolactin, and β-hCG
   b. 17-OH progesterone, dehydroepiandrosterone sulfate (DHEAS), and testosterone
   c. Transvaginal ultrasound
   d. Hysterosalpingogram to look for intrauterine adhesions
   e. All of the above

3. Her pregnancy tests as well as tests for thyroid and prolactin disorders are all negative. She has an elevated fasting insulin as well as a high normal fasting glucose. Her androgens (testosterone and DHEAS) are elevated but not in the range that you would be concerned for an androgen-producing tumor. You make a diagnosis of polycystic ovarian syndrome (PCOS). You discuss the importance of a continued healthy balanced diet (and watching that she limits simple carbohydrate intake) as well as continued regular exercise. Additional appropriate treatment includes adding the following:
   a. Oral contraceptives
   b. Spironolactone
   c. Mirena IUD
   d. Weight reduction
   e. Any of the above

ANSWERS

VIGNETTE 1 Question 1
1. Answer C:
Genitourinary syndrome of menopause (GSM) refers to changes in the epithelium of the lower urinary and genital tract because systemic levels of estrogen decline, as is seen in menopause. There is a thinning of the epithelium that can cause fragility, decreased compliance, and abrasions or tearing sufficient to cause clinically evident bleeding.

Endometrial cancer is the most common gynecological cancer in the United States. Although there are well-known associations and risk factors, including anovulation, obesity, nulliparity, hypertension, and diabetes, a second subset of women with endometrial cancer lack these associated risks. This patient has no historical risks that place her at increased risk of endometrial cancer. Additionally, she does give symptoms that correlate with GSM, including general dryness and pain with intercourse.

Cervical cancer is similarly unlikely in a woman with a normal findings on life-long history of Pap smear (cervical cytology) and, more recently, HPV testing. With a negative Pap smear and HPV test in the prior 12 months, the chance of a clinically relevant cervical lesion is so low that our current screening guidelines do not recommend repeat testing for 5 years from the last screening.

Although it is possible for uterine fibroids to cause such symptoms, she has no history of fibroids, and fibroids often shrink in response to decreased estrogen levels during menopause. Although hormonal replacement therapy can cause fibroids to grow, they typically do not cause clinical symptoms in menopause.

This patient has no prior past medical history of a bleeding disorder, and no additional history suggesting this diagnosis currently (frequent nose bleeds, bleeding gums, easy bruising). Although it is appropriate to consider in the differential diagnosis, it would be less likely than urogenital atrophy.

VIGNETTE 1 Question 2
2. Answer D:
In this case scenario, it is appropriate to consider all of the diagnostic tests listed. Although not always neoplastic or cancerous, all occurrences of postmenopausal bleeding do need to be thoroughly evaluated.

Transvaginal ultrasound is appropriate to evaluate for structural lesions of the cervix, uterus, or adnexa, including endometrial polyps, fibroids, and ovarian cysts or tumors. The endometrial thickness (EMS) can also be measured and reported. An EMS of less than or equal to 4 mm in a woman not taking hormone replacement is less likely to be associated with EIN or malignancy, whereas an EMS of greater than 4 mm is associated with an increased risk of endometrial abnormalities. In women with an EMS greater than 4 mm and those with persistent postmenopausal bleeding, endometrial sampling with office-based EMB or dilation and curettage is needed to rule out endometrial hyperplasia, EIN, and cancer.

Any woman who is sexually active should undergo basic screening that includes a risk assessment for the acquisition of STIs including HIV on an annual basis. In this patient with a new sexual partner, STI testing is appropriate. Cervicitis from chlamydial infection or gonorrhea can cause irregular vaginal bleeding.

VIGNETTE 1 Question 3
3. Answer C:
Endometrial polyps are common; often, benign neoplasms arising from the endometrial cavity. Although they are most commonly identified in women of reproductive age, they can present well into the menopausal years. Although the clinical course of smaller polyps may include spontaneous regression in younger women, the finding of endometrial polyps in postmenopausal women is of sufficient concern and risk to recommend removal for patients who are candidates for an outpatient surgical procedure. It is possible to find benign endometrial hyperplasia, EIN, and/or endometrial cancer in the base of an otherwise benign-appearing endometrial polyp.

Although this patient clearly has symptoms and physical findings associated with GSM, the addition of exogenous estrogens is contraindicated in any woman with unexplained vaginal bleeding. Moreover, genitourinary syndrome of menopause (GSM) is not an indication for systemic menopausal hormone therapy (MHT). Following polypectomy, she would likely benefit from low-dose vaginal estrogen to treat her atrophy.

VIGNETTE 2 Question 1
1. Answer A:
This patient's clinical presentation is classic for primary dysmenorrhea. Often, women begin to experience pain with menses in the late teens and early twenties because cycles become ovulatory. NSAIDs are considered first-line treatment for primary dysmenorrhea, particularly in women who do not otherwise need contraception.

If the patient was at risk for pregnancy, or one whose pain is not controlled with NSAIDs, contraceptive steroids (pills, patch, or ring) would also be a good choice. In addition to inhibiting ovulation, OCPs limit the growth of endometrial tissue and, secondarily, limit the production of prostaglandin in endometrial tissue. With such a straightforward history, neither pelvic ultrasound nor laparoscopy is warranted at this time. Endometrial ablation is used to treat heavy menstrual bleeding (HMB) in patients who have completed childbearing. It would be contraindicated in this case.

VIGNETTE 2 Question 2
2. Answer B:
Annual STI screening in indicated in all sexually active women ≤24 years of age. Current recommendations for cervical screening with cytology include first Pap smear at age 21 years regardless of the age of first intercourse. Previous recommendations to start at age 21 years or 3 years from the first sexual intercourse have now been dropped. In this patient who is 18 years old, a Pap smear is not indicated. Although she has only had a partial response to the trial of NSAIDs, as long as there are no obvious abnormalities on physical examination, it is not yet necessary to consider imaging. EMB is generally reserved for ruling out benign endometrial hyperplasia, EIN, and cancer in women 45 years or older and who have abnormal uterine bleeding. There is no indication for EMB in this patient. Most providers would consider an alternate first-line medication prior to conducting a more in-depth evaluation.

VIGNETTE 2 Question 3
3. Answer E:
Given that the patient is in need of contraception and needs additional management of her dysmenorrhea, a trial of oral contraceptives is an ideal option. This can be used alone or in combination with NSAIDs. Given that she has had only partial relief of her symptoms with a trial of NSAIDs, using both might provide her with greater relief. Hydrocodone (Lortab, Vicodin, Norco) is a potentially addictive opioid analgesic and is not indicated for the routine treatment of dysmenorrhea. These medications should be reserved for the short-term treatment of severe pain. Tranexamic acid is an antifibrinolytic agent used to treat HMB. It is not indicated in the treatment of dysmenorrhea.

VIGNETTE 3 Question 1
1. Answer C:
This patient is presenting with symptoms that are interfering with her activities of daily living and appear to be affecting her overall quality of life, so evaluation and considering treatment options is appropriate for her. Although general counseling regarding healthy lifestyle is important and may be helpful to women with a diagnosis of PMS, the severity of symptoms in this patient's presentation warrants a more assertive approach. This initial evaluation is within the scope of an OB/GYN provider.

Given the timing of symptoms relative to her menses, PMS is high on the differential. Diagnosis relies upon demonstrating that symptoms worsen in the luteal phase (1 to 2 weeks prior to the onset of menses) and resolve completely with the start or shortly following the onset of menses. This is the most common way that a provider can differentiate between PMS and an underlying mood disorder, such as anxiety or depression.

PMS is a clinical diagnosis based upon analysis of a patient's symptoms and signs. There are no laboratory tests that support the diagnosis. Although SSRIs have been very effective in the treatment of PMS and other conditions, further evaluation of this patient is needed before starting medications.

VIGNETTE 3 Question 2
2. Answer E:
The etiology of PMS is largely unknown and is likely because of a combination of physiological, psychological, and other causes. No single treatment is known, and dozens have been suggested, some of which work for some women but not in all. Reviews of PMS treatment studies have identified a few agents that appear to significantly decrease symptoms associated with PMS. Studies have shown that the use of SSRIs, such as Prozac, Paxil, Celexa, and Zoloft, is effective for treating both the physical and mood symptoms associated with PMS. Prozac is FDA approved for this use.

Older studies do not show OCPs to be effective in treating PMS symptoms. However, newer formulations using the progestin drospirenone (a spironolactone with antimineralocorticoid and antiandrogenic activity) and a 4-day rather than 7-day pill-free interval have been shown to be effective in the treatment of PMDD.

Several studies have shown that the use of vitamin supplements, including high-dose calcium, vitamin D, vitamin E, vitamin B$_6$, and magnesium, is effective in the treatment of PMS. In small studies, exercise and relaxation techniques have been shown to decrease PMS symptoms.

VIGNETTE 3 Question 3
3. Answer E:
If following 2 months of treatment with vitamin supplementation the patient does not see improvement of symptoms, additional time with this treatment plan is unlikely to work. Similarly, abandoning treatment would not help when the patient continues to complain of significant symptoms. In the past, progesterone was commonly used for the treatment of PMS. However, studies show that they are no more effective than placebo. They are no longer used in the management of PMS. Considering another therapeutic approach with a SSRI is an option; however, there is an additional clue in the patient's presentation at this visit. Review of the symptom calendar reveals that she is having symptoms throughout the cycle, and no longer appears to have complete resolution of symptoms following onset of a period. In light of this new information, it is appropriate to revisit the initial diagnosis and consider an underlying mood disorder, such as depression. Although medications in the SSRI category are very effective in the treatment of mood disorders, to treat mood disorders, they must be given on a daily basis and not limited to the luteal phase as is often done in the treatment of PMS.

VIGNETTE 4 Question 1
1. Answer B:
A common cause of amenorrhea in young women is hypothalamic hypogonadism, which is seen most frequently in athletes who engage in vigorous daily exercise as well as in women with eating disorders, including anorexia and bulimia. Inquiring about her daily exercise and diet is the most correct answer in this situation.

Although it is important to obtain a thorough history of all medications, including type and dose of oral contraceptives in this patient, any of the OCPs can induce "post-pill amenorrhea," which can last for up to 6 months following discontinuation.

Family history, as well, is an important part of any new-patient evaluation. Amenorrhea is not strictly known to be a heritable condition. Some causes of amenorrhea, such as PCOS, can be seen to run in families. Knowing that there are other women in this patient's family who are affected by amenorrhea would not alter the course of this patient's evaluation.

Obtaining a detailed sexual history, including use of hormonal and barrier contraceptives, the frequency of intercourse, number or partners, their gender, as well as the timing of most recent exposure, is an important part of all gynecologic evaluations. In a woman with oligo/amenorrhea and who is sexually active, a pregnancy test is always indicated regardless of the timing of her most recent intercourse because bleeding patterns can be unreliable in determining if a given woman is pregnant.

VIGNETTE 4 Question 2
2. Answer A:
In this patient, you are suspicious for anovulation because of her history of amenorrhea following discontinuation of her oral contraceptives. The most common etiologies for anovulation include PCOS, pregnancy, hypo- or hyperthyroidism, and hyperprolactinemia. 17-OH progesterone, DHEAS, and testosterone are typically used to look for causes of hirsutism. In this case, she is not hirsute, and these tests would not be indicated at this point.

Because she has a history of withdrawal bleeds on oral contraceptives, she is unlikely to have a structural or congenital defect (absence of a uterus or ovaries, imperforate hymen, or vaginal septum). An ultrasound can be used in supporting a diagnosis of PCOS by identifying multiple immature ovarian follicles ("string of pearls"); however, it is not sufficient nor is it required to diagnose the condition. An ultrasound might be used later in the evaluation of this patient but is not an appropriate initial test. Similarly, with a history of normal withdrawal bleeds on OCPs, and no intervening pregnancy, trauma, surgery or infection, it would be unusual to have a diagnosis of intrauterine adhesions.

VIGNETTE 4 Question 3
3. Answer E:
In women with PCOS, chronic anovulation often results in oligomenorrhea or amenorrhea, with occasional, irregular episodes of bleeding that can be heavy and prolonged. Prolonged stimulation of the endometrium by estrogen without regular exposure to progesterone (at ovulation) can lead to EIN as well as endometrial cancer. The choice of a treatment modality depends on a woman's current desire for contraception. If hoping to become pregnant, we prescribe medication to induce ovulation, such as clomiphene citrate or Glucophage. In addition to these medications, general counseling about weight loss is important, because a reduction in BMI alone can lead to a resumption of normal ovulation and regular menses. Weight loss has also been shown to improve insulin resistance, hirsutism, and hyperlipidemia.

In women who desire contraception, options include combination OCPs, as well as progestin-only methods, such as the Mirena IUD, progestin-only pills, Nexplanon, or Depo-Provera. Exposure to progesterone in a cyclic or continuous fashion will protect the endometrium from developing benign endometrial hyperplasia, EIN, and cancer. Caution should be taken with the use of Depo-Provera and possibly Nexplanon, because these agents have been associated with weight gain (in women with a predisposition to gain weight) and may not be the best choice in the overall treatment of obese women with PCOS. Another option in women who do not need contraception but are not trying to become pregnant is the use of intermittent progestins administered for 12 to 14 days per month to induce regular bleeding and protect the endometrium from hyperplasia and cancer.

23 | Hirsutism and Virilism

Adults have two types of hair: vellus and terminal. Vellus hair is nonpigmented and soft, and covers the entire body. Terminal hair is, on the other hand, pigmented and thick, and covers the scalp, axilla, and pubic area. During puberty, androgens are responsible for the conversion of vellus to terminal hair resulting in the development of pubic and axillary hair. An abnormal increase in terminal hair is due to androgen excess or increased 5α-reductase activity; this enzyme converts testosterone to the more potent dihydrotestosterone (DHT). DHT is believed to be the main stimulant of terminal hair development.

Hirsutism refers to the increase in terminal hair on the face, chest, back, lower abdomen, and inner thighs in a woman. It can also be characterized by the development of pubic hair as a male escutcheon, which is diamond shaped, as opposed to the triangular female escutcheon. Whereas hirsutism describes a pattern of masculine hair growth, **virilization** refers to the development of male features, such as deepening of the voice, frontal balding, increased muscle mass, clitoromegaly, breast atrophy, and male body habitus.

The evaluation of hirsutism and virilism in the female patient is complex and requires the understanding of pituitary, adrenal, and ovarian function, with detailed attention to the pathways of glucocorticoid, mineralocorticoid, androgen, and estrogen synthesis.

NORMAL ANDROGEN SYNTHESIS

The adrenal gland is divided into two components: the adrenal cortex, which is responsible for glucocorticoid, mineralocorticoid, and androgen synthesis, and the adrenal medulla, which is involved in catecholamine synthesis. The adrenal cortex is composed of three layers: the zona glomerulosa, the zona fasciculata, and the zona reticularis. The outermost **zona glomerulosa** layer produces aldosterone via the enzyme **aldosterone synthase** and is regulated primarily by the renin–angiotensin system. In contrast, the inner layers of the adrenal cortex, the **zona fasciculata** and the **zona reticularis**, produce both cortisol and androgens because of the presence of the 17α-hydroxylase enzyme. These two inner zones are highly regulated by adrenocorticotropic hormone (ACTH).

ACTH regulates the conversion of cholesterol to pregnenolone by hydroxylation and side-chain cleavage. Pregnenolone is then converted to progesterone and eventually to aldosterone or cortisol or shunted over to the production of sex steroids (Fig. 23-1).

In the adrenal glands, androgens are synthesized from the precursor 17α-hydroxypregnenolone, which is converted to **dehydroepiandrosterone** (DHEA) and its sulfate (DHEA-S), androstenedione, and finally to testosterone. DHEA and DHEA-S are the most common adrenal androgens, whereas only others are secreted only in small amounts.

In the ovaries, the theca cells are stimulated by luteinizing hormone (LH) to produce androstenedione and testosterone. Both androstenedione and testosterone are then aromatized to estrone and estradiol, respectively, by the granulosa cells in response to follicle-stimulating hormone (FSH). Elevations in the ratio of LH to FSH may therefore lead to elevated levels of androgens.

PATHOLOGIC PRODUCTION OF ANDROGENS

Elevation of androgens can be due primarily to adrenal or ovarian disorders. Because synthesis of steroid hormones in the adrenal cortex is stimulated by ACTH at a nondifferentiated step, elevated ACTH levels increase all the steroid hormones, including the androgens. If enzymatic defects are present, the precursor proximal to the defect accumulates and

FIGURE 23-1. Biosynthesis of androgens, estrogens, and corticosteroids. (Reproduced with permission from Mishell DR, Davajan V, Lobo RA. *Infertility, Contraception, and Reproductive Endocrinology,* 3rd ed. Cambridge, MA: Blackwell Science; 1991.)

is shunted to another pathway. Thus, enzymatic blockade of either cortisol or aldosterone synthesis can lead to increased androgen production. Because DHEA-S is derived almost entirely from the adrenal glands, its elevation is used as a marker for adrenal androgen production.

In the ovary, any increase in LH or in the LH:FSH ratio appears to lead to excess androgen production. Further, tumors of both the adrenal gland and the ovary can lead to excess androgens. Regardless of the source, elevated androgens lead to hirsutism and possibly virilism.

ADRENAL DISORDERS

The adrenal disorders leading to virilization in a woman are divided into two categories: nonneoplastic and neoplastic etiologies. Androgen-producing adrenal tumors may be either adenomas or carcinomas. Adrenal adenomas typically cause glucocorticoid excess and virilizing symptoms are rare. Carcinomas, on the other hand, can be more rapidly progressive and lead to marked elevations in glucocorticoid, mineralocorticoid, and androgen steroids.

CUSHING SYNDROME

Cushing syndrome is characterized by excess production of cortisol. Because the intermediates in production are androgens, there will be a concomitant hyperandrogenic state. Cushing syndrome may be caused by pituitary adenoma, ectopic sources of ACTH, and tumors of the adrenal gland. The most common cause of Cushing syndrome (other than exogenous glucocorticoid intake) is **Cushing disease**, which refers to a pituitary adenoma that hypersecretes ACTH. Paraneoplastic syndromes, such as nonpituitary ACTH-secreting tumors, may also lead to increased ACTH levels. Adrenal gland tumors usually result in decreased levels of ACTH secondary to the negative feedback from the increased levels of adrenal steroid hormones. All three of these situations lead to the glucocorticoid excess characteristic of Cushing syndrome, as well as hirsutism, acne, and menstrual irregularities related to adrenal androgen production.

When Cushing syndrome is suspected, it can be diagnosed with one of the following first-line tests: late-night salivary cortisol (two measurements), 24-hour urinary free cortisol (two measurements), or the overnight dexamethasone suppression test (DST). In patients with a high index of suspicion, it is recommended to do two of the above first-line tests. If using the 24-hour urinary free cortisol, a result of three times the upper limit of normal indicates hypercortisolism. The low-dose DST is performed by administering 1 mg of dexamethasone at 11 p.m. to 12 a.m. and then measuring a serum cortisol level at 8 a.m. the next morning. Essentially, if there is normal negative feedback from exogenous steroid hormone, then the adrenal gland should decrease production in response to the dexamethasone. A plasma cortisol level of <1.8 mcg/dL (50 nmol/L) would indicate that the patient does not have Cushing syndrome. It is important to recognize that using a stringent cut off of 1.8 mcg/mL optimizes the sensitivity of diagnosing Cushing syndrome but decreases the specificity of the test, and this test should be used in conjunction with the other tests discussed earlier in confirming the diagnosis.

CONGENITAL ADRENAL HYPERPLASIA

Congenital adrenal hyperplasia (CAH) refers to a constellation of enzyme deficiencies involved in steroidogenesis. The most common disorder is 21α-hydroxylase deficiency. As seen in Figure 23-1, an enzymatic block at this step will lead to the accumulation of 17α-hydroxyprogesterone (17-OHP), which is then shunted to the androgen pathway. Patients with CAH do not synthesize cortisol or mineralocorticoids and thus present with salt wasting and adrenal insufficiency at birth. Female infants will have ambiguous genitalia because of androgen excess. In milder or adult-onset forms, the degree of deficiency can vary, and often the only presenting sign is mild virilization and menstrual irregularities.

The other types of CAH that can be associated with virilization include 11β-hydroxylase and 3β-hydroxysteroid dehydrogenase (3β-HSD) deficiencies. Patients with 11β-hydroxylase deficiency present with similar symptoms of androgen excess because accumulated precursors are shunted to androstenedione and testosterone production pathways. Patients with 3β-HSD deficiency actually accumulate DHEA because they are unable to convert pregnenolone to progesterone or DHEA down the androgen synthesis pathway. DHEA and its sulfate, DHEA-S, both have mild androgenic effects. Importantly, because this defect is also present in gonadal steroidogenesis, males have feminization, and females have hirsutism and virilization. All patients have impaired cortisol synthesis and varying degrees of either mineralocorticoid excess or deficiency, depending on the location of the enzymatic block.

When CAH is suspected, a 17-OHP level should be checked because 21α-hydroxylase deficiency is the most common etiology. If 17-OHP is elevated (>200 ng/dL), the diagnosis can be confirmed with an ACTH stimulation test in which Cortrosyn (ACTH) is given IV, and a 17-OHP level is checked after 1 hour. A marked increase in 17-OHP is consistent with CAH, with lower elevated values being seen in late-onset CAH and heterozygote carriers for the 21α-hydroxylase deficiency.

FUNCTIONAL OVARIAN DISORDERS

The ovarian disorders leading to virilization are divided into nonneoplastic and neoplastic etiologies. Polycystic ovaries, theca lutein cysts, stromal hyperplasia, and stromal hyperthecosis all involve nonneoplastic lesions. Neoplastic lesions vary and often cause rapid onset of virilization.

NONNEOPLASTIC OVARIAN DISORDERS
Polycystic Ovarian Syndrome
Polycystic ovarian syndrome (PCOS), previously known as the Stein-Leventhal syndrome, is one of the most common endocrine/metabolic disorders affecting reproductive age women with a prevalence of up to 10%. PCOS is characterized by androgen excess, ovulatory dysfunction, and/or polycystic ovaries. Patients present with a constellation of symptoms, including hirsutism, virilization, anovulation, amenorrhea, and obesity. There is also an increased incidence of hyperinsulinemia, diminished insulin sensitivity, and Type 2 diabetes mellitus in this population. PCOS is now thought to be a complex genetic trait similar to Type 2 diabetes or cardiovascular disease. The cause of androgen excess appears to be related to altered and excess LH stimulation leading to cystic changes in the ovaries and increased ovarian androgen secretion. PCOS patients have higher serum LH concentrations when compared to matched controls and exhibit overexpression of LH receptors in theca and granulosa cells. Genetic variations in the LH β subunit of PCOS patients have also been reported. It appears that any number of factors may be involved in this cycle, including obesity, insulin resistance, and excessive adrenal androgen production. PCOS is diagnosed using the Rotterdam criteria and requires the presence of two out of three of the following: olio- and/or anovulation, clinical and/or biochemical signs of hyperandrogenism, and polycystic ovaries (seen on ultrasound). In addition, other conditions that mimic PCOS such as thyroid disease, conclastic CAH, hyperprolactinemia, and androgen secreting tumors must be ruled out.

Theca Lutein Cysts
The **theca cells** of the ovary are stimulated by LH to produce androstenedione and testosterone. These androgens are normally shunted to the **granulosa cells** for aromatization to estrone and estradiol. Theca lutein cysts produce an excess amount of androgens that are secreted into the circulation. These cysts may be present in either normal or molar pregnancy. The ovaries are enlarged, and patients present with hirsutism and, occasionally, virilization. Diagnosis is made by ovarian biopsy. These cysts are more common with elevated levels of β-hCG during molar pregnancy, multiple pregnancies, and during gonadotropin stimulation with infertility treatment.

Stromal Hyperplasia and Hyperthecosis
Stromal hyperplasia is common between ages 50 and 70 and can cause hirsutism. The ovaries are uniformly enlarged. **Stromal hyperthecosis** is characterized by foci of utilization within the hyperplastic stroma. It is more likely than simple hyperplasia to result in virilization because the utilized cells continue to produce ovarian androgens. The ovaries typically appear enlarged and fleshy, with the more florid cases seen in younger patients.

NEOPLASTIC OVARIAN DISORDERS
Functional Ovarian Tumors
Sex cord-stromal tumors and Germ cell tumors are types of functional ovarian tumors that can produce varying amounts of androgens. Sex cord-stromal tumors include granulosa cell tumors (which can differentiate toward female characteristics), fibrothecomas, and Sertoli-Leydig cell tumors (which can differentiate toward male characteristics). Granulosa-stromal cell tumors include granulosa cell tumors, thecomas, and fibromas. Granulosa cell and theca cell tumors are hormonally active, fibromas are not. Sertoli-Leydig cell tumors usually occur in young women and account for less than 1% of all ovarian neoplasms. Hilar cell tumors are even rarer than Sertoli-Leydig cell tumors and are usually seen in postmenopausal women. These tumors may secrete androgens, leading to hirsutism and virilism.

Pregnant women may develop a luteoma—a benign tumor that grows in response to human chorionic gonadotropin. This tumor can result in high levels of testosterone and androstenedione and virilization in 25% of patients. There will also be virilization of 65% of female fetuses. These findings should resolve in the postpartum period.

Nonfunctional Ovarian Tumors

Androgen excess can also occur in the case of nonfunctional ovarian tumors (e.g., a cystadenoma or Krukenberg tumor). Although these tumors do not secrete androgens themselves, they do stimulate proliferation in the adjacent ovarian stroma, which in turn may lead to increased androgen production.

DRUGS AND EXOGENOUS HORMONES

A variety of drugs can affect the circulating levels of sex hormone-binding globulin (SHBG). SHBG is one of the major proteins that binds circulating testosterone, leaving a small proportion of free testosterone to interact at the cellular level. Androgens and corticosteroids decrease SHBG, leaving a greater percentage of free testosterone circulating. Patients who use anabolic steroids often present with hirsutism and virilization. In addition, drugs such as minoxidil, phenytoin, diazoxide, cyclosporin, and valproate will cause hirsutism without using androgenic pathways.

IDIOPATHIC HIRSUTISM

Hirsutism is considered idiopathic in the absence of adrenal or ovarian pathology, an exogenous source of androgens, or use of the above-listed drugs. Patients may actually have occult androgen production, but many will have normal circulating androgen levels. There may be an increase in peripheral androgen production owing to elevated 5α-reductase activity at the level of the skin and hair follicles.

Clinical Manifestations

A detailed history including time of onset, progression, and symptoms of virilization/hirsutism should be obtained, as well as a pubertal, menstrual, and reproductive history. Because various medications can affect androgen levels by affecting SHBG or intrinsic androgenic activity, a detailed drug history should be obtained. A family history is also important in order to look for genetic disorders such as CAH.

Physical Examination

On physical examination, the hair pattern should be noted, with attention to facial, chest, back, abdominal, and inner thigh hair, as well as the presence of frontal balding. The body habitus and the presence or absence of female contours should be described. Breast examination may reveal atrophic changes, and a careful pelvic examination should include inspection of the escutcheon (pattern of pubic hair), clitoris (for clitoromegaly), and palpation for ovarian masses. Cushingoid features should be ruled out and inspection for acanthosis nigricans (velvety, thickened hyperpigmentation) in the axilla and nape of the neck should be performed because this dermatologic finding is often associated with insulin resistance, which can be seen in polycystic ovary syndrome.

Diagnostic Evaluation

Laboratory evaluation should include free testosterone, 17-OHP, and DHEA-S, the latter of which is normally exclusive to the adrenal gland. An elevation in free testosterone confirms androgen excess, and a concomitant elevation in DHEA-S suggests an adrenal source. An elevated 17-OHP is suggestive of CAH. If an adrenal source is suspected, an abdominal CT should be performed to rule out an adrenal tumor, as well as further tests to diagnose Cushing syndrome or CAH.

If the DHEA-S is normal or minimally elevated, an ovarian source should be considered, and a pelvic ultrasound or CT should be performed to rule out an ovarian neoplasm. An elevation in the LH:FSH ratio greater than 3 is suggestive of PCOS. However, most obstetrician–gynecologists do not diagnose PCOS with the LH:FSH ratio any longer. Rather, polycystic ovary syndrome is a diagnosis of exclusion—when two out of the three Rotterdam criteria are met: secondary amenorrhea/oligomenorrhea, evidence of hyperandrogenism, or evidence of polycystic ovaries as assessed by ultrasound.

Rapid onset of virilization and testosterone levels >200 ng/dL may indicate an ovarian neoplasm. At times, the source of androgen excess is not readily evident, and further diagnostic tests such as abdominal MRI and selective venous sampling need to be done for localization. In the hirsute woman with normal free testosterone, an assay for 5α-reductase activity is performed to determine whether increased peripheral enzymatic activity is responsible for the development of hirsutism.

Treatment

Adrenal nonneoplastic androgen suppression can be achieved with glucocorticoid administration, such as prednisone 5 mg nightly. Finasteride inhibits the 5α-reductase enzyme, and thus diminishing peripheral conversion of testosterone to DHT. Antiandrogens such as spironolactone have been helpful as well, but are temporizing at best. In the case of ovarian or adrenal tumors, the underlying disorder should be treated. Often surgical intervention is required.

In general, ovarian nonneoplastic androgen production can be suppressed with oral contraceptives that will suppress LH and FSH as well as increase SHBG. Progesterone therapy alone may help patients with contraindications to estrogen use. Progesterone decreases levels of LH and thus androgen production; further, the catabolism of testosterone is increased, resulting in decreased levels. Gonadotropin-releasing hormone (GnRH) agonists can also be used to suppress LH and FSH. However, this leads to a hypoestrogenic state and requires concomitant estrogen replacement.

Patients using exogenous androgens or other drugs leading to increased androgens or hair growth should be advised to discontinue use. For patients with idiopathic hirsutism or contraindications to hormonal use, waxing, depilatories, and electrolysis will often provide cosmetic improvement.

KEY POINTS

- Hirsutism is excess hair growth with a male pattern on the face, back, chest, abdomen, and inner thighs, usually in response to excess androgens.
- Virilism is a constellation of symptoms including hirsutism, deepening of the voice, frontal balding, clitoromegaly, and increased musculature.
- Primary causes of hirsutism and virilization include PCOS, ovarian tumors, adrenal tumors, CAH, and Cushing syndrome.
- Diagnosis is made by history and physical, serum assays for testosterone, DHEA-S, and 17-OHP, and imaging studies.
- Management involves primary treatment for the underlying cause; hormonal therapy with oral contraceptive pills, GnRH, or progestins; and cosmetic treatment of hirsutism.

CLINICAL VIGNETTES

VIGNETTE 1

A 16-year-old female presents to your office with her mother, who is concerned that she is pregnant. Over the last 3 months, the patient and her mother have noticed a swelling in her lower abdomen. The patient notes a sensation of fullness, and occasional left lower pelvic pain. The patient reports that she does have a male partner, but they have not yet been sexually intimate. She reports irregular menses over the last 6 months, but thought it was secondary to stress. She has noted increased hair over her chin and breasts, and her acne seems to have worsened and spread onto her chest and back, whereas it used to be only on her face. Her mother attributes this to "normal puberty stuff." She is otherwise healthy, with no other known medical problems or prior surgeries. She is normotensive, and vital signs are normal. On physical examination, you notice a few dark colored hairs over her upper lip, and several beneath her chin. Her breast development is normal. Pelvic examination reveals a prominent, enlarged clitoris, and bimanual examination reveals a 17-cm, mobile, smooth left adnexal mass. An in-office urine pregnancy test is negative.

1. What set of laboratory tests would you first perform to aid in your diagnosis?
   a. Serum testosterone and DHEA-S
   b. TSH, free T4
   c. 24-hour urine collection for metanephrines
   d. Plasma aldosterone and renin

2. Your laboratory tests confirm your suspicions, and you perform a pelvic ultrasound, which reveals a 15 × 16 × 17 cm^3 solid left ovarian mass. Which of the following is the most likely diagnosis?
   a. Polycystic ovary syndrome
   b. Sertoli-Leydig cell tumor
   c. Luteoma of pregnancy
   d. Cushing syndrome

3. You opt to proceed with excision of her left adnexal mass. What procedure do you recommend?
   a. Total abdominal hysterectomy, bilateral salpingo-oophorectomy and staging procedure
   b. Total abdominal hysterectomy, bilateral salpingo-oophorectomy with intraoperative frozen section followed by staging
   c. Laparotomy, left ovarian cystectomy and possible oophorectomy with intraoperative frozen section
   d. Neoadjuvant chemotherapy

4. Another patient presents for her 18-week anatomy ultrasound. She is a 19-year-old African American G1P0 who has had an uncomplicated pregnancy. On your ultrasound, you find normal fetal anatomy in a female appearing fetus. However, you do note bilateral 6 cm masses that appear homogenous. You suspect bilateral ovarian luteomas and perform serum testing of the mother, which reveals elevated testosterone and androstenedione. A subsequent examination of the patient reveals evidence of hirsutism. The patient shrugs and states, "I thought that was normal in pregnancy." What obstetric and perinatal complication is her fetus at risk for?
   a. Preeclampsia
   b. Abruption
   c. Virilization of the fetus
   d. Preterm premature rupture of membranes (PPROM)

VIGNETTE 2

A 31-year-old obese woman presents to your office for an infertility consultation. She and her husband have been attempting pregnancy for the preceding 18 months. She states that her menses are irregular, occurring every 25 to 47 days, and sometimes she skips menses altogether. They are sometimes heavy, other times light with just brown spotting. She notes that her menses have always been this way, ever since menarche at age 12. She denies any history of sexually transmitted infections, and her husband has proven paternity with a previous wife. She notes that she has never been pregnant. On further questioning, she admits to plucking and shaving excessive hair from her chin, around her navel, and on her lateral thigh. She also admits to bothersome acne and extreme difficulty with weight loss. Physical examination reveals obesity with BMI 31, normal breast development, and the presence of excessive hair as described by the patient. Pelvic examination reveals normal external genitalia and unremarkable bimanual examination.

1. What additional information do you need to make your diagnosis?
   a. Day 3 serum follicle-stimulating hormone (FSH) and estradiol
   b. Pelvic ultrasound
   c. Serum testosterone, DHEA-S, and prolactin
   d. None of the above

2. What test might you perform to determine whether this patient is ovulatory in any given month?
   a. Urinary ovulation predictor kits
   b. Day 3 progesterone
   c. Day 28 progesterone
   d. Luteal phase endometrial biopsy

3. The patient is grateful to have a syndrome to explain her symptoms; however, she is anxious to hear what you may offer to her in terms of fertility treatment—getting pregnant is all she can really think about now. In addition to starting a prenatal vitamin with folic acid, you recommend:
   a. Attempted weight loss with a sensible diet and regular vigorous exercise
   b. Insulin therapy
   c. Clomiphene citrate ovulation induction
   d. In vitro fertilization
   e. a and c
   f. a, b, and c
   g. a, b, and d

4. Your patient goes on to successfully conceive a pregnancy and delivers a healthy baby boy. During her 6-week postpartum visit, you discuss birth control options. Which of the following contraceptive choices will improve her symptoms of hirsutism and acne?
   a. Condoms
   b. Depo-Provera
   c. Levonorgestrel intrauterine device (IUD)
   d. Combined estrogen and progestin contraceptive pill

5. Two years later, your patient returns to your clinic for her annual examination. She is now 35 years old and mentions to you that she decided to use condoms for the past few years because she did not like the oral birth control pills you suggested. She admits to very heavy menstrual flow over the past year (lasting 8 days and filling 10 pads on 5 of the 8 days), and her menses continue to be irregular. She has not lost much of her "baby weight" after her delivery and currently has a BMI of 36. She is unsure if she desires more children in the future. You again discuss birth control and suggest the placement of a levonorgestrel IUD, which the patient accepts. What further testing or evaluation would you recommend for her at this time?
   a. Glucose tolerance test and fasting lipid screening test
   b. Thyroid function testing and complete blood count
   c. Endometrial biopsy and pelvic ultrasound
   d. a and b
   e. a, b, and c

VIGNETTE 3

A patient presents to your office for a return OB visit. She is a 25-year-old G5P2204 at 20 weeks 5 days by first trimester ultrasound. She presented with symptoms of excessive weight gain, acne, abdominal and upper extremity striae, migraine headache, fatigue, and muscle weakness. So far she has gained 60 lb this pregnancy without significant dietary changes. She complains of facial swelling, bruising, and "stretch marks." She reports excessive hair growth since the onset of this pregnancy and states that she has "furry cheeks, breasts, and arms." The hair is notably darker and of greater quantity than normal for her. This hair growth is also associated with significant worsening of her acne. Regarding her stretch marks—she states that in prior pregnancies, they were a whitish color, while these are purple and extremely pruritic. Migraine headaches are not new for her but worsened during this pregnancy to nearly daily episodes, whereas prior to pregnancy she had a migraine one to two times weekly. She is otherwise a healthy female with no prior history of medical illness (including history of hypertension or diabetes). Regarding her gynecologic history, she reports normal, monthly menses since menarche at age 13. On physical examination, she was noted to have an elevated systolic blood pressure of 140/90, and is tachycardic in the 110 to 120s. Fetal heart tones are 144 beats/minute. Physical examination confirms the above reported hirsutism, acne, bruising, and abdominal striae. Additionally, she has increased fat deposition on her posterior neck. She has a fundal height of 19 cm, and there are no pelvic masses on sterile vaginal examination.

1. You suspect Cushing syndrome. What is the first step in your workup?
   a. 24-hour urinary free cortisol excretion
   b. Late-night salivary cortisol level
   c. Dexamethasone suppression test (DST)
   d. a, b, and c
   e. Plasma adrenocorticotropic hormone (ACTH) concentration
   f. Abdominal ultrasound

2. An ultrasound is performed and reveals an enlarged right adrenal mass, measuring 5.7 × 5.6 × 4.4 cm with well-defined margins. The radiologist tells you that the characteristics of the mass do not appear consistent with a pheochromocytoma; however, because of your patient's additional complaints of worsening headaches, and additionally her hypertension and tachycardia, you are concerned about this rare possibility. To rule out pheochromocytoma, you order the following tests:
   a. 24-hour urine protein collection
   b. Plasma metanephrines
   c. 24-hour urine metanephrines and catecholamines
   d. Complete metabolic panel

3. Another patient with a known diagnosis of Cushing syndrome secondary to chronic glucocorticoid treatment to prevent flares of her rheumatoid arthritis presents to your clinic requesting treatment for her hirsutism. She is a 32-year-old G1P1001 and had a healthy term pregnancy 3 years ago. She has already tried depilatory lotions and plucking with only mild improvement. Which therapeutic option might you offer her initially?
   a. Shaving, plucking, waxing
   b. Oral contraceptive pills
   c. Spironolactone
   d. Gonadotropin-releasing hormone (GnRH) agonists

VIGNETTE 4

A 19-year-old female presents to your clinic with her mother for evaluation regarding possible vaginoplasty. She has classic "salt wasting" CAH and has been moderately controlled with her pediatric endocrinologist. She is controlled on fludrocortisone and prednisone daily. When she was 18 months old, she underwent a U-flap vaginoplasty and clitoroplasty for ambiguous genitalia, which is now stenotic because of lack of use. She reports oligomenorrhea with menses approximately every 4 months. She does have some anxiety, for which she has seen a counselor every 2 weeks regarding anxiety as well as her sexuality. She reports that at this point in her life, she has had relationships with both men and women, and is equally attracted to both. However, she and her mother feel that her lack of a normal vagina inhibits her ability to be fully intimate with a male, therefore inhibiting her from fully exploring her sexuality. On physical examination, the patient is well appearing, with normal breast development. She has a muscular build and is noted to have multiple bruises on her body. Pelvic examination is notable for a prominent clitoris. A normal appearing anus is noted. Between the clitoris and rectum, there is a single small opening that is a urogenital sinus, allowing efflux of both menstrual flow and urine. No additional vaginal opening is present. Rectal examination confirms the presence of a uterus.

1. Which protein is deficient in a patient with classic "salt wasting" congenital adrenal hyperplasia (CAH)?
   a. 21-Hydroxylase
   b. 11β-Hydroxylase
   c. 3β-Hydroxysteroid dehydrogenase (3β-HSD)
   d. Aromatase
   e. None of the above

2. Your physical examination and a bedside ultrasound confirm the presence of a uterus and ovaries. The presence of a normal appearing uterus and tubes is surprising, given this patient's clitoromegaly and absent lower vagina. However, this is embryologically explained by the fact that females with CAH have:
   a. Testicles and concomitant development of the uterus and tubes
   b. Ovaries and the lack of testicular derived Müllerian-inhibiting substance (MIS)
   c. Absent Sertoli cells
   d. Absent 5α-reductase enzyme, which prevents synthesis of DHT

3. What is the most likely reason this patient is having oligomenorrhea?
    a. Oligo-ovulation secondary to polycystic ovary syndrome
    b. Premature ovarian failure
    c. Exercise-induced hypothalamic hypogonadotropic hypogonadism
    d. Inadequate glucocorticoid therapy, leading to relative hyperandrogenemia

4. You decide to proceed with surgical intervention and trial of vaginoplasty. What serious complication is she at risk for during the procedure?
    a. Intractable hemorrhage
    b. Sudden cardiac death
    c. Adrenal crisis
    d. Cerebrovascular accident
    e. Disseminated intravascular coagulopathy (DIC)

ANSWERS

VIGNETTE 1 Question 1
1. Answer A:
Although each of these tests may be helpful, the first set of testing you should consider is a serum testosterone and DHEA-S, both of which are measurements of serum androgen. If testosterone is elevated, this confirms androgen excess. A DHEA-S level assists with determining if the source of the androgens is adrenal in origin.

Thyroid testing is not helpful in this setting given that the patient has signs and symptoms of virilization rather than hypothyroidism or hyperthyroidism. Because the patient does not display evidence of hypercortisolism, the 24-hour urine collection and plasma aldosterone and renin are not likely to be helpful.

VIGNETTE 1 Question 2
2. Answer B:
The presence of an adnexal mass on examination and the absence of pregnancy make a Sertoli-Leydig cell tumor, although rare, the most likely diagnosis. These are sex cord-stromal tumors of the ovary, which may be benign or malignant. These tumors commonly secrete androgens and building blocks of androgens (testosterone, androstenedione, and 17-OHP), which lead to the virilizing features seen clinically (in this case, hirsutism, acne, and clitoromegaly). Definitive diagnosis is made histologically after surgical excision of the mass.

Polycystic ovary syndrome does not typically present with an abdominal mass; the polycystic ovaries are typically multiple, small peripheral cysts instead. Luteoma may cause similar symptoms, but this would be the case in a patient with a current or recent pregnancy, neither of which fits this clinical scenario. Cushing syndrome would cause hirsutism and virilization, but typically also presents with evidence of hypercortisolism.

VIGNETTE 1 Question 3
3. Answer C:
Given this patient's young age, a fertility sparing procedure is ideal if possible. Knowing that Sertoli-Leydig cell tumors can be benign or malignant, you correctly elect to have a frozen section performed at the time of your procedure. Because the mass approaches 17 cm, laparoscopic removal is not possible in this case, and she needs an open procedure. You counsel your patient that the best procedure for her would be a laparotomy with left ovarian cystectomy and possible oophorectomy.

Although you should discuss with your patient before going to the operating room the possibility of finding a malignancy, in which case proceeding with hysterectomy and full staging is necessary, your goal will be to preserve her fertility. The most likely scenario is that she will have a benign neoplasm, and oophorectomy alone will be required. There is no role for neoadjuvant chemotherapy in this case.

VIGNETTE 1 Question 4
4. Answer C:
This patient has bilateral luteomas of pregnancy that are ovarian masses and are thought to be caused by elevated circulating levels of β-hCG. They are typically asymptomatic other than mild symptoms of maternal virilism in some but not all cases. Serum studies typically show elevated levels of circulating androgens. This fetus is at risk of virilization in utero. Typically, the masses regress postpartum without need for intervention.

Preeclampsia, abruption, and PPROM are not known to be associated with ovarian luteomas of pregnancy.

VIGNETTE 2 Question 1
1. Answer D:
The diagnostic criteria for polycystic ovary syndrome (PCOS) are the Rotterdam criteria, which were established in 2003. These maintain that the diagnosis of PCOS is made on the basis of meeting two out of the following three criteria: oligo/anovulation, clinical or laboratory evidence of hyperandrogenism, and polycystic ovaries on ultrasound. For the patient in this scenario,

she already meets the criteria for oligo-ovulation (irregular and skipped menses) and clinical evidence of hyperandrogenism (acne and hirsutism).

Thus, the addition of a pelvic ultrasound, testosterone, DHEA-S, and prolactin is unnecessary to make the diagnosis. However, the knowledge of the values from these tests may rule out additional disorders and are often checked as well. Day 3 FSH and estradiol may be helpful in determining the underlying quality of her remaining oocytes in terms of her fertility, but are not necessary in making the diagnosis of PCOS.

VIGNETTE 2 Question 2
2. Answer A:
Because this patient's menstrual cycles have been irregular, predicting ovulatory cycles is more difficult than a patient with regular cycles. The use of daily urinary ovulation predictor kits starting at cycle day 11 or 12 can aid in predicting ovulation and timing intercourse for conception. Ovulation predictor kits detect the luteinizing hormone (LH) surge, which occurs approximately 24 to 36 hours prior to ovulation. They can unfortunately be falsely positive in patients with PCOS, however, because of elevated baseline circulating levels of LH.

Measurement of progesterone in the luteal phase may indicate that ovulation has occurred (although it will not help with predicting ovulation in order to time intercourse). In a woman with normal 28-day cycles, it is typically measured on cycle day 21, when you would expect elevated levels secondary to progesterone production by the corpus luteum after ovulation. Neither a Day 3 nor a Day 28 progesterone would be helpful. In the case of a woman with irregular menses, it is also difficult to determine the accuracy of a progesterone level, and therefore, this test may be less useful in this particular case. In years past, an endometrial biopsy used to be performed to evaluate for evidence of decidualization of the endometrium as evidence of progesterone effect. This is no longer a standard procedure in the workup of anovulation because there are other, less painful, methods to determine ovulation.

VIGNETTE 2 Question 3
3. Answer E:
The first step in attempting to achieve pregnancy is to attempt weight loss through diet and exercise, and consider the addition of ovulation induction with clomiphene citrate (Clomid). Many women will start to ovulate spontaneously with as little as 10% weight reduction. Clomid is an antiestrogen that increases the probability that ovulation occurs by removing the negative feedback of circulating estrogen to the brain, thereby increasing circulating levels of FSH seen by the ovary. Administration usually starts with the lowest dose, 50 mg daily starting on cycle day 3 or 5, continuing for 5 days of therapy. Patients should be counseled regarding increased risk of multiple pregnancy (secondary to multiple oocytes released in one cycle) as well as risk of ovarian hyperstimulation. An effective alternative to Clomid is letrozole, an aromatase inhibitor, also used for ovulation induction in women with PCOS. In obese women (BMI $\geq$ 30), letrozole results in higher cumulative live birth rates when compared to Clomid, and it is becoming the preferred drug of choice for ovulation induction in obese PCOS patients.

Although patients with PCOS have increased risk of diabetes, initiating insulin therapy without a diagnosis of diabetes is contraindicated. Although this patient may eventually require ovulation induction with other medications or injectable gonadotropins, in vitro fertilization is not yet indicated.

VIGNETTE 2 Question 4
4. Answer D:
Combined oral contraceptive pills (OCPs) are the first-line therapy for helping to decrease circulating androgens, and may prevent progressive hirsutism and acne. This is achieved by increasing the levels of sex hormone-binding globulin (SHBG) concentrations, in turn decreasing circulating free androgen levels and their stimulatory effect on hair follicles.

Condoms have no effect on SHBG and therefore would not prevent worsening or reduce current levels of circulating androgens. Depo-Provera and the levonorgestrel IUD work well to decrease heavy bleeding and for contraception, but will not be of help in reducing symptoms of hyperandrogenism.

VIGNETTE 2 Question 5
5. Answer E:
Provided that this patient presented today for her annual examination, and your knowledge that she meets the criteria for polycystic ovary syndrome, you astutely test her for diabetes and hyperlipidemia because you know that she is at increased risk for both of these diseases as well as cardiovascular disease. Because of her heavy menstrual flow, you opt to screen her for hypothyroidism and evaluate for the possibility of anemia. Finally, because you know that she is at increased risk for endometrial hyperplasia and carcinoma from chronic anovulation and elevated levels of circulating estrogens, you recommend a pelvic ultrasound and an endometrial biopsy.

VIGNETTE 3 Question 1
1. Answer D:
The first step in the evaluation of this patient is to determine whether she truly meets the criteria for Cushing syndrome, and the next is to determine the

etiology. Current recommendations are to start with at least two of the three "first-line" tests, which include a 24-hour urinary free cortisol test, late-night salivary cortisol measurement, and a DST. The urinary and salivary cortisol measurements should be obtained at least twice, and the diagnosis of Cushing syndrome is confirmed, when there are two abnormal tests. Because of the low specificity for these tests, if any of them come back equivocal, additional testing should be performed prior to confirming the diagnosis.

Plasma ACTH testing is used to determine the cause of Cushing syndrome after the diagnosis is made. A low ACTH indicates that the syndrome is caused by ACTH independent disease (for example, an adrenal adenoma), whereas an elevated value is indicative of pituitary or ectopic secretion of ACTH. An abdominal ultrasound may be useful in evaluating for the presence of an adrenal adenoma, but a CT scan is more sensitive and more commonly used. In this particular case, an ultrasound may be used first given increased risks of radiation to the fetus with a CT scan compared with an abdominal ultrasound.

VIGNETTE 3 Question 2
2. Answer C:
The collection of a 24-hour urine sample and testing for metanephrines and catecholamines is felt to be the first-line test for evaluating for pheochromocytoma, followed closely by plasma metanephrines. Plasma metanephrines have high sensitivity for pheochromocytoma, but poor specificity.

A 24-hour urine protein collection and complete metabolic panel may enlighten you to other metabolic or renal derangements, but will not aid in diagnosis of a pheochromocytoma.

Your patient undergoes a CT scan, which is concerning for an adrenal adenoma and given that she is at 20 weeks of gestation, she is taken to the operating room for a unilateral adrenalectomy that is uncomplicated. She goes on to have an uncomplicated pregnancy and delivers her infant at term.

VIGNETTE 3 Question 3
3. Answer B:
The patient is presenting to your office already having tried some depilatory strategies, so your first option for treatment would be an OCP. The OCP will reduce circulating levels of androgens by stimulating production of SHBG and in turn decreasing circulating levels of androgens. This method should be tried for at least 6 months before trying another method. Your patient should be counseled that while the pill should improve symptoms of acne and prevent additional hair growth, it will not reduce the already present hirsutism. Waxing, plucking, and shaving may decrease her current unwanted hair, and the pill may reduce new hair growth.

Spironolactone (as well as other antiandrogen medications) acts as an androgen receptor antagonist. It is best used in conjunction with combined oral contraceptives after a trial of oral contraceptives alone has failed. GnRH agonists (such as leuprolide) essentially cause a state of menopause, effectively decreasing serum androgen levels as well as serum estrogens. They are very effective in treating hirsutism, but should not be used as a first-line agent given their side-effect profile.

VIGNETTE 4 Question 1
1. Answer A:
Classic "salt wasting" CAH is caused by a deficiency in 21-hydroxylase, leading to elevated levels of 17-OHP. Female infants present with ambiguous genitalia, as in the above patient, as well as adrenal insufficiency. All infants in the United States are screened at birth by measuring levels of 17-OHP in the blood. The absence of 21-hydroxylase causes decreased cortisol synthesis and therefore increased stimulation of the adrenals by ACTH. This in turn leads to increased androgen production, leading to virilization of females.

There are other, more mild forms of CAH, in which the enzymes 11β-hydroxylase and 3β-HSD are absent. Aromatase deficiency can lead to virilization of a female fetus, but is not related to the CAH spectrum.

VIGNETTE 4 Question 2
2. Answer B:
Female patients with CAH are chromosomally 46,XX, and develop ovaries. The internal genitalia in both males and females initially develop by means of wolffian and müllerian ducts in both sexes. In males, the presence of testicles and Sertoli cells within them initiates secretion of MIS, which causes regression of the müllerian ducts (which would have otherwise fused to form the uterus, tubes, and upper vagina). Because this patient is genetically 46,XX, she will by default (and by the absence of MIS) develop a uterus.

The case in which a patient appears to have testicular tissue with a present uterus and tubes may be gonadal dysgenesis or testicular regression (in which testicular function is inadequate or absent). Absent Sertoli cells would lead to absent MIS as well, causing a persistent müllerian system. Additionally, mutations in the gene for MIS may lead to persistence of the müllerian ducts with externally appearing male genitalia. The lack of DHT would lead to abnormal development of external genitalia in a male.

VIGNETTE 4 Question 3
3. Answer D:
The most likely cause of her oligomenorrhea is inadequate control of her CAH, leading to elevated levels of circulating androgens, leading to anovulation.

Premature ovarian failure is unlikely in this setting, because the more likely explanation is her CAH. Although exercise-induced amenorrhea is possible, she does not give a history of excessive vigorous exercise, and again, the more likely explanation is her CAH. PCOS is a diagnosis of exclusion; therefore it is not the correct answer, given that the patient already carries a diagnosis of CAH.

VIGNETTE 4 Question 4
4. Answer C:
This patient is at risk for adrenal crisis. Because of her underlying adrenal insufficiency, she is unable to mount a response to the stress of surgery. Signs and symptoms of adrenal crisis include hypotension, hyponatremia, hypoglycemia, and shock. She will need "stress dose steroids," which for her age would require 100 mg hydrocortisone IV once prior to induction followed by 50 mg every 8 hours for 24 hours and then a taper over the following several days, in addition to her regular doses of fludrocortisone and prednisone.

Hemorrhage and DIC are unlikely if preoperative coagulation studies are normal and she has been well controlled in terms of her medications, as long as no additional surgical complications present. Surgical risk for sudden cardiac death and cerebrovascular accidents is not increased above her baseline risk with CAH.

24 | Contraception and Sterilization

Approximately 90% of women of childbearing age use some form of contraception. Despite this, in the United States, **nearly 50% of pregnancies are unintentional**. Of these, 43% result in live births, 13% in miscarriages, and 44% end in elective abortion. In weighing the risks and benefits of contraceptive methods, couples must keep in mind that no contraceptive or sterilization method is 100% effective. Table 24-1 outlines relative failure rates or the number of women likely to become pregnant within the first year of using a particular method. Theoretical efficacy rate refers to the efficacy of contraception when used exactly as instructed. Actual efficacy rate refers to efficacy when used in real life, assuming variations in the consistency of usage.

NATURAL METHODS

The methods of contraception described in this section—periodic abstinence, coitus interruptus, and lactational amenorrhea—are physiology-based methods that use neither chemical nor mechanical barriers to contraception. Many couples, for religious, philosophical, or medical reasons, prefer these methods to other forms of contraception. However, these are the least effective methods of contraception and should not be used if pregnancy prevention is a high priority.

PERIODIC ABSTINENCE
Method of Action
Periodic abstinence (the rhythm or calendar method) is a physiologic form of contraception that emphasizes **fertility awareness and abstinence** shortly before and after the estimated ovulation period. This method requires instruction on the physiology of menstruation and conception and on methods of determining ovulation. It also requires the woman to have **regular, predictable menstrual cycles**. Ovulation assessment methods may include the use of ovulation prediction kits, basal body temperature measurements (Fig. 24-1), menstrual cycle tracking, cervical mucus evaluation, and/or documentation of any premenstrual or ovulatory symptoms.

Effectiveness
The average effectiveness of periodic abstinence is relatively low (55% to 80%) compared with other forms of pregnancy prevention.

Advantages and Disadvantages
Periodic abstinence uses neither chemical nor mechanical barriers to conception and is, therefore, the method of choice for many couples for various reasons. However, this method requires a highly motivated couple willing to learn reproductive physiology, predict ovulation, and abstain from intercourse. Periodic abstinence is **relatively unreliable** compared with the more traditional methods of contraception. This low reliability may require prolonged periods of abstinence and regular menstrual cycles, making it less desirable for some couples.

COITUS INTERRUPTUS
Method of Action
Coitus interruptus, or withdrawal of the penis from the vagina before ejaculation, is one of the oldest methods of contraception. With this method, the majority of semen is deposited outside of the female reproductive tract with the intent of preventing fertilization.

Effectiveness
The failure rate for coitus interruptus is quite high (27%) compared with other forms of contraception. Failure can be attributed to the deposition of semen

TABLE 24-1. Failure Rates for Various Contraceptive Methods During the First Year of Use in the United States

Method	Percentage of Women Who Become Pregnant	
	Theoretical Failure Rate (%)	Actual Failure Rate (%)
No method	85.0	85.0
Periodic abstinence		
Calendar	9.0	25.0
Ovulation method	3.0	25.0
Symptothermal	2.0	25.0
Post ovulation	1.0	25.0
Withdrawal	4.0	27.0
Lactational amenorrhea	2.0	15.0–55.0
Condom		
Male condom	2.0	15.0
Female condom	5.0	21.0
Diaphragm with spermicide	6.0	16.0
Cervical cap with spermicide		
Parous women	26.0	32.0
Nulliparous women	9.0	16.0
Spermicide alone	18.0	29.0
Intrauterine devices		
Copper T IUD (ParaGard)	0.6	0.8
Levonorgestrel IUS (Mirena)	0.1	0.1
Combination estrogen and progesterone		
Combination pill	0.1	3.0
Transdermal patch (Ortho Evra)	0.3	0.8
Vaginal ring (NuvaRing)	0.3	0.8
Progesterone-only methods		
Progestin-only pill (POPs)	0.5	8.0
Depo-Provera	0.3	0.3
Subdermal implant (Implanon/Nexplanon)	0.4	0.4
Surgical sterilization		
Female sterilization	0.5	0.5
Male sterilization	0.1	0.15

IUD, intrauterine device.

(pre-ejaculate) into the vagina before orgasm or the deposition of semen near the introitus after intracrural intercourse.

Advantages and Disadvantages

The primary disadvantage of coitus interruptus is its high failure rate. Other disadvantages include the need for sufficient self-control to withdraw the penis before ejaculation.

LACTATIONAL AMENORRHEA

Method of Action

Continuation of breastfeeding has long been a widespread method of contraception for many couples. After delivery, the restoration of ovulation is delayed because of a breastfeeding-induced hypothalamic suppression of ovulation. Specifically, there is a **prolactin-induced inhibition of pulsatile**

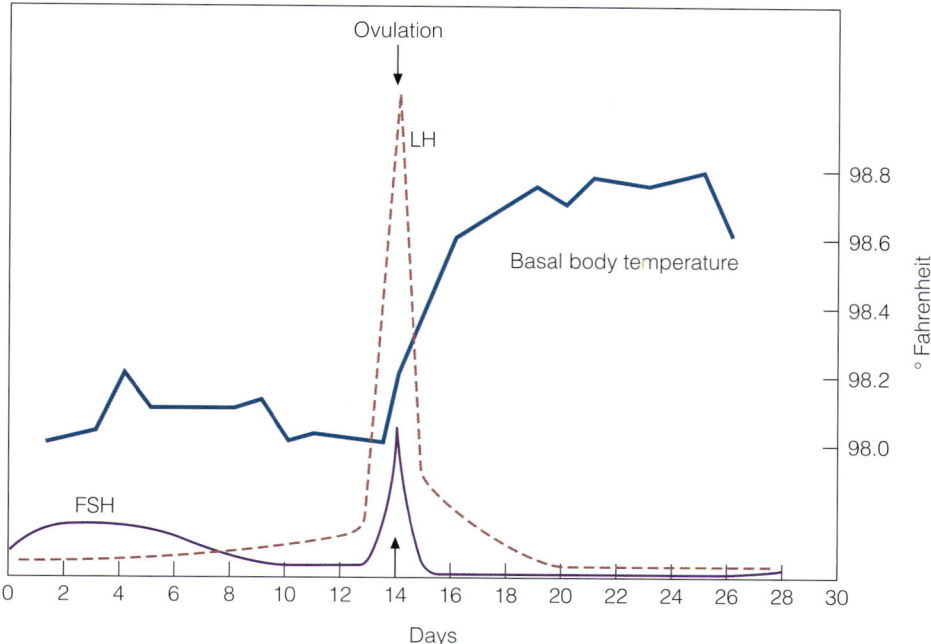

FIGURE 24-1. The relationship between ovulation and basal body temperature. FSH, follicle-stimulating hormone; LH, luteinizing hormone.

gonadotropin-releasing hormone (GnRH) from the hypothalamus resulting in suppression of ovulation.

Effectiveness

The duration of ovulatory suppression during breastfeeding is highly variable. In fact, 50% of lactating mothers will begin to ovulate between 6 and 12 months after delivery, even while breastfeeding. Importantly, **return of ovulation occurs before the return of menstruation**. As a result, 15% to 55% of mothers using lactation for contraception subsequently become pregnant.

The effectiveness of lactational amenorrhea as a short-term method of contraception can be enhanced by following certain principles. First, breastfeeding should be the only form of nutrition for the infant. Second, this method of contraception should be used only as long as the woman is experiencing amenorrhea and, even then, it should only be used for a maximum of 6 months after delivery. Following these guidelines, lactational amenorrhea as a method of contraception can have a much lower failure rate. In practice, however, most mothers are not able to meet these stringent requirements.

Advantages and Disadvantages

Lactational amenorrhea has no effect on breastfeeding and is safe, simple, convenient, and free. Studies show that babies who receive breast milk have increased body contact and bonding, have a lower risk of infections, and benefit from exposure to maternal antibodies. The use of lactational amenorrhea is limited to the immediate 6 months after delivery and can result in vaginal dryness for some women. Also, while the theoretical failure rates are reasonable, the failure rates for actual practice are so high as to make this an unacceptable and unreliable sole means of contraception.

BARRIER METHODS AND SPERMICIDES

These contraceptive methods work by preventing sperm from entering the endometrial cavity, fallopian tubes, and peritoneal cavity. Figure 24-2 shows the various barrier method contraceptives and spermicides.

MALE CONDOMS

Method of Action

Condoms are latex sheaths placed over the erect penis before ejaculation. They prevent the ejaculate from being released into the reproductive tract of the woman.

Effectiveness

When properly used, the condom can be 98% effective in preventing conception. The **actual efficacy rate in the population is 85% to 90%**. To maximize

FIGURE 24-2. Barrier methods and spermicides.

effectiveness and decrease the risk of condom breakage, it is important to leave a well at the tip of the condom to collect the ejaculate and to avoid leakage of semen as the penis is withdrawn. Efficacy is also increased by use of spermicide-containing condoms or by using a spermicide along with condoms.

Side Effects
Some individuals may experience a hypersensitivity to the latex, lubricant, or spermicide in condoms.

Advantages and Disadvantages
Condoms are widely available for a moderate cost and carry the added benefit of preventing the transmission of many sexually transmitted infections (STIs). Condoms are the only method of contraception that offers protection against human immunodeficiency virus (HIV). Drawbacks of the male condom include coital interruption and possible decreased sensation or hypersensitivity.

FEMALE CONDOMS
Method of Action
The female condom (FC2 Female Condom), also known as an internal condom, is a pouch made of synthetic nitrile (previously polyurethane) that has a flexible ring at each end. One ring is silicon based and lubricated. It is inserted into the depth of the vagina, and the other ring stays outside the vagina near the introitus (Fig. 24-3). The female condom may also be inserted into the anus.

Effectiveness
The theoretical failure rate of the female condom is 5%. However, studies show that the actual failure rate of the female condom is 20% to 25%, somewhat higher than that of the male condom. However, these were short-term studies and may not reflect the failure rate with long-term usage.

Advantages and Disadvantages
By covering the vagina or anus, female condoms **protect against STIs**, while also placing the control of contraception with the female partner. Efforts are underway to develop a latex female condom and to make the female condom more accessible in developing countries. The female condom is also hormone free and relatively easy to obtain without a prescription. Because of its design, it will stay in place even if the male erection is lost. Major drawbacks include **cost and overall bulkiness**. Some users report decreased sensation during intercourse. The nitrile and lubricant may also cause irritation of the penis, vagina, anus, or vulva. The acceptability rating is somewhat higher for the male partner (75% to 80%) than for the female partner (65% to 70%).

DIAPHRAGM
Method of Action
The vaginal diaphragm is a dome-shaped shallow cup made of a soft silicone or latex (rubber) sheet which is stretched over a thin coiled rim. Spermicidal gel, foam

FIGURE 24-3. Placement of the female condom.

FIGURE 24-4. **(A)** Insertion of the vaginal diaphragm. **(B)** Checking to ensure the diaphragm covers the cervix. (From Beckmann C, Ling F. *Obstetrics & Gynecology*, 5th ed. Philadelphia, PA: Lippincott Williams & Wilkins; 2006.)

or cream is placed on the rim and on either side of the diaphragm, and it is placed into the vagina, so that it covers the cervix (Fig. 24-4). The diaphragm and spermicide should be placed in the vagina before intercourse and left in place for a minimum of 6 hours (maximum of 30 hours) after intercourse. If further intercourse is to take place within 6 to 8 hours after the first episode of intercourse, additional spermicide should be placed in the vagina without removing the diaphragm.

Effectiveness
The theoretical effectiveness of the diaphragm approaches 94%. The actual effectiveness rate of the diaphragm with spermicide is 80% to 85%.

Side Effects
Possible side effects include bladder irritation, which can lead to urinary tract infections. If the diaphragm is left in place too long, colonization by *Staphylococcus aureus* may lead to the development of **toxic shock syndrome**. Some women also experience a hypersensitivity to the rubber, latex, or spermicide.

Advantages and Disadvantages
The diaphragm is a safe, effective, and convenient method of contraception. It must be fitted and prescribed by a clinician, making its initial cost significantly higher than over-the-counter methods of contraception. The diaphragm should be replaced every 2 years or when the patient gains or loses more than 20% of her body weight. Fit should also be checked after each pregnancy. Women who are not comfortable with inserting and removing the diaphragm, or who cannot be properly fitted because of pelvic relaxation defects are poor candidates for the diaphragm, as are women who are at high risk of HIV. Because <1% of women in the United States rely on a diaphragm for birth control, there are fewer options on the market and fewer gynecologists have experience with fitting diaphragms.

CERVICAL CAP
Method of Action
The cervical cap (FemCap, Lea Shield) is a small, soft, silicone cap that fits directly over the cervix (Fig. 24-5). It is held in place by suction and acts as a barrier to sperm. The cap must be **fitted by a clinician** and must be used with a spermicidal gel, foam or cream. Because of the variability in cervix size, proper fit and usage of the cap are essential to its effectiveness. Although it is widely used in Britain and Europe, the cervical cap is **not widely available in the United States**.

Effectiveness
The actual efficacy rate of the cervical cap is 68% to 84% (16% to 32% failure rate), depending on the woman's parity. There is an increased risk of failure in parous women. Dislodgment is the most common cause of failure.

Advantages and Disadvantages
The cervical cap is small and immediately effective. It does not interfere with endogenous hormones and

FIGURE 24-5. Insertion of the cervical cap.

can be used while breastfeeding. Another advantage of the cervical cap is that it can be inserted up to 6 hours prior to intercourse, so it does not interrupt the sex act. The cap **can be left in place for 1 to 2 days**. However, a foul discharge often develops after the first day. The cap must be refitted after a pregnancy or in the event of large weight change. Also, many women have a difficult time mastering the placement and removal techniques for the cervical cap; as a result, the **continuation rate is low** (30% to 50%).

SPERMICIDES
Method of Action
Spermicidal agents come in varying forms, including vaginal creams, gels, films, suppositories, and foams (Fig. 24-2). The most widely used spermicides are nonoxynol-9 and octoxynol-9. Other agents, such as menfegol and benzalkonium chloride, are used around the world but are not available in the United States. Nonoxynol-9 and octoxynol-9 both **disrupt the cell membranes** of the spermatozoa and also act as a mechanical barrier to the cervical canal. In general, spermicides should be placed in the vagina at least 30 minutes before intercourse to allow for dispersion throughout the vagina. Spermicides may be used alone but are far more effective when used in conjunction with condoms, cervical caps, diaphragms, or other contraceptive methods.

Effectiveness
When properly and consistently used with condoms, spermicides can have an effectiveness rate as high as 95%. However, in actual usage, the efficacy of spermicides when used alone is only 70% to 75%. This effectiveness is further reduced by failure to wait long enough for the spermicide to disperse in the vagina prior to intercourse.

Side Effects
Spermicides can irritate the vaginal mucosa and external male and female genitalia.

Advantages and Disadvantages
Spermicidal agents are widely available in a variety of forms and are relatively inexpensive. Some formulations can also be messy to use.

In addition to providing contraception, it was initially thought that spermicides might provide some protection against STIs. However, it now appears that these agents **do not** confer any protection against STIs. They may, in fact, make the user **more susceptible to STIs**, including HIV by causing vaginal irritation. For this reason, **spermicides should not be used by women with HIV** or at high risk of contracting HIV. This is of special significance in developing nations where contraception and STI prevention are paramount. For the general public, it is strongly recommended that **consistent condom use** be employed whenever protection against STIs is desired.

INTRAUTERINE DEVICES

Intrauterine devices (IUDs) have been used to prevent pregnancy since the 1800s. In the 1960s and 1970s, IUDs became extremely popular in the United States. However, legal ramifications stemming from pelvic infections associated with one particular IUD—the Dalkon shield—resulted in consumer fear and limited availability of all IUDs. Currently, five IUDs are available in the United States: four of which are **levonorgestrel (LNG) intrauterine systems** (Mirena, Skyla, Liletta, and Kyleena) and one that is **hormone free and contains copper** (TCu389A or ParaGard) (Fig. 24-6). Despite previous fears, there are nearly 100 million IUD users globally, making the IUD **the most widely used method of reversible**

FIGURE 24-6. Intrauterine devices (IUD). (**A**) ParaGard Copper T (TCu-380A). (**B**) Mirena (Levonorgestrel IUD). (**C**) Lippes loop (used throughout the world but not available in the United States). (From Speroff L, Fritz M. *Clinical Gynecologic Endocrinology and Infertility*, 7th ed. Philadelphia, PA: Lippincott Williams & Wilkins; 2005.)

and also used in postmenopausal women receiving estrogen therapy. The three newer forms of LNG IUDs (Skyla, Liletta, and Kyleena) do not have specific indications for use other than contraception at this time. Absolute and relative contraindications for IUD use are outlined in Table 24-2.

METHOD OF ACTION

IUDs are introduced into the endometrial cavity by the clinician using a cervical cannula (Fig. 24-8). IUDs have two monofilament strings that extend through the cervix where they can be checked to detect expulsion or migration (Fig. 24-8). The strings also facilitate removal of the device by the clinician.

The mechanism of action for IUDs is not completely understood, but they are known to act mainly by **killing sperm** (spermicidal) and **preventing fertilization**. Specifically, the primary method of action is to elicit a **sterile inflammatory response**, resulting in sperm being engulfed, immobilized, and destroyed by inflammatory cells. The IUD is also thought to **reduce tubal motility** that in turn inhibits sperm and blastocyst transport. IUDs do not affect ovulation, nor do they act as abortifacients. Their

contraception in the world (Fig. 24-7). IUD use in the United States has grown from <2% to just over 10% in the past decade.

The IUD is especially indicated for women in whom oral contraceptives are contraindicated, those who are at low risk for STIs, and in **monogamous women of any age**. The LNG-containing IUD (Mirena) can also be used to treat menorrhagia, dysmenorrhea,

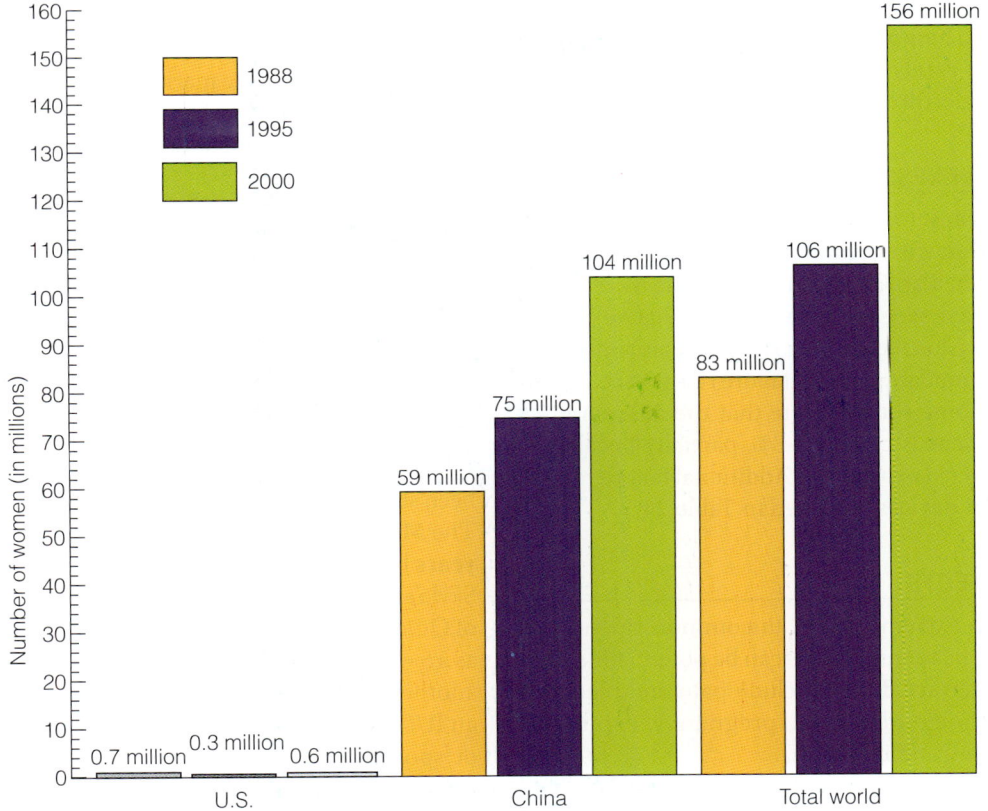

FIGURE 24-7. Use of the intrauterine devices (IUDs) in the United States, China, and the rest of the world.

TABLE 24-2. Contraindications for Intrauterine Device (IUD) Use
Absolute contraindications
Known or suspected pregnancy
Undiagnosed abnormal vaginal bleeding
Acute cervical, uterine, or salpingeal infection
Copper allergy or Wilson disease (for ParaGard only)
Current breast cancer (for Mirena only)
Relative contraindications
Prior ectopic pregnancy
History of STIs in past 3 mo
Uterine anomaly or fibroid distorting the cavity
Current menorrhagia or dysmenorrhea (for ParaGard only)
STI, sexually transmitted infection.

presumed mechanisms of action are augmented by the addition of LNG in the Mirena, Skyla, Liletta, and Kyleena IUDs and copper in the ParaGard IUD. Progesterone in the LNG devices **thickens the cervical mucus** and **atrophies the endometrium** to prevent implantation. Copper in the ParaGard is thought to **hamper sperm motility and capitation**, so sperm rarely reach the fallopian tube and are unable to fertilize the ovum.

EFFECTIVENESS

The efficacy for IUDs rivals that of permanent sterilization with prolonged use. The failure rate is 0.8% for the ParaGard and 0.2% for the Mirena IUD within the first year of use. The cumulative 10-year failure rate for the ParaGard is approximately 1.9%, and the cumulative 5-year failure rate for the Mirena is 0.7%. Some sources state that the failure rate in the first year is closer to 3%, partially because of unrecognized expulsions. Additional failure rates of the newer devices are listed in Table 24-3.

SIDE EFFECTS

Although extremely safe, uncommon side effects and complications of IUDs can be potentially severe and dangerous. These include pain and bleeding, intrauterine and ectopic pregnancy, expulsion, perforation, and infection.

Placement of IUDs in women with cervical infections can lead to **insertion-related pelvic inflammatory disease** (PID). This increased risk is now believed to be due to contamination of the endometrial cavity at the time of insertion. Otherwise, pelvic infection is rarely seen beyond the first 20 days after insertion. **Antibiotic prophylaxis is not needed** for IUD insertion, nor is it indicated for bacterial endocarditis prophylaxis. Instead, emphasis should be placed on appropriate patient selection and screening women for gonorrhea and *Chlamydia* prior to insertion of the IUD. Moreover, studies show that women using LNG IUDs have a **decreased risk of PID** owing to the protection of progesterone-induced cervical mucus thickening. Given these findings, IUDs are being used more liberally in younger women, women who have not completed childbearing, and nulliparous women.

The pregnancy rate with IUD use is very low; however, when pregnancy does occur, the spontaneous abortion rate is increased to 40% to 50% for women who become pregnant with an IUD in place. Given this, if intrauterine pregnancy occurs while an IUD is in place, the device **should be removed by gentle traction on the string**. If the device cannot be removed with gentle traction, it should be left in situ during the pregnancy. The risk of life-threatening spontaneous septic abortion has only been seen with the Dalkon shield, which had a braided polyfilament tail that wicked bacteria into the uterus placing the user at risk for PID, sepsis, and infertility. The Dalkon shield was taken off the market in 1975, 4 years after its introduction. IUDs are not associated with any increased risk of congenital abnormalities.

ADVANTAGES AND DISADVANTAGES

The IUD must be prescribed, inserted, and removed by a clinician. However, once in place, it is highly effective, cost-effective, long-lasting, and rapidly reversible. The user is encouraged to do a monthly string check to ensure the device has not been expelled. This improves coital spontaneity and decreases fear of pregnancy. In the United States, the **ParaGard IUD has been approved for use for 10 years** but has been shown to maintain its effectiveness for 12 years. The **Mirena IUD has been approved for use for 5 years** but is effective for at least 7 years. Liletta and Skyla are currently approved for use up to 3 years. As of October 2016, a new device, *Kyleena*, is approved as a 5-year LNG IUD. One IUD can be removed and another one can be inserted on the same visit. Also, an IUD may be inserted immediately after induced or spontaneous first trimester abortions without increased risk of infection or perforation. **ParaGard is also approved for emergency contraception (EC)** when placed within 72 hours of unprotected

FIGURE 24-8. (**A**) Placement of a ParaGard intrauterine device (IUD). (**B**), Insertion device for a levonorgestrel IUD.

intercourse or contraceptive failure. The ParaGard IUD can be inserted immediately postpartum (within 10 minutes of placental delivery) with an increased risk of expulsion but no increased risk of infection or perforation. All of the current IUDs can be used safely at **6 weeks postpartum** and are safe in breastfeeding women.

In general, because IUDs are so effective at preventing pregnancy, **the risk of ectopic pregnancy is reduced** in IUD users compared with that of noncontraceptive users. In the rare event that a woman does become pregnant with an IUD in place, however, **the risk of ectopic pregnancy may be as high as 30% to 50%** of those patients. Although controversial, the IUD is an acceptable form of contraception for women with a **prior history of ectopic pregnancy**, remote PID (none in past >3 months), history of cervicitis, and HIV.

The Mirena IUD has been found to decrease menorrhagia (90% less blood loss) and dysmenorrhea. It is also as equally or more effective than oral progestins in treating endometriosis, benign

TABLE 24-3. Intrauterine Device Comparisons

Device Name	Size (Width × Length)	Years of Use	Failure Rate (Cumulative)	Indication	Amenorrhea
Copper device					
ParaGard (T 380A Copper)	32 × 36 mm	10 y	1.9% (10 y)	Pregnancy prevention; Emergency contraception	N/A
Levonorgestrel devices					
Mirena (52 mg LNG)	32 × 32 mm	5 y	0.7% (5 y)	Pregnancy prevention; Treatment of heavy bleeding[b]	(~60% at 5 y[a])
Skyla (13.5 mg LNG)	28 × 30 mm	3 y	0.9% (3 y)	Pregnancy prevention	12% at 3 y
Liletta (52 mg LNG)	32 × 32 mm	3 y	0.55% (3 y[c])	Pregnancy prevention	38% at 3 y
Kyleena (19.5 mg LNG)	28 × 30 mm	5 y	0.37% (5 y)	Pregnancy prevention	23% at 5 y

Table information based on product labeling/prescribing information specific to each product.
[a]Five-year rates available for Mirena device in post market studies.
[b]In women who choose to use intrauterine contraception as their method of contraception.
[c]Calculated cumulative pregnancy rate (3-year life table), 1 year rate 0.15%.
LNG, Levonorgestrel.

endometrial hyperplasia, and endometrial cancer. It also protects the user from PID with a lower rate of PID than found in women who use no contraception. As a result, this decreases the number of surgeries (D&Cs, endometrial ablations, hysterectomies) needed for pelvic pain and bleeding. About 60% of women will experience amenorrhea while using the Mirena IUD at 5 years. The other LNG IUDs also reduce bleeding and dysmenorrhea in some capacity.

Most of the IUDs are MRI compatible, but certain circumstances exist. It is recommended that the product labeling be referenced for MRI specific settings.

HORMONAL CONTRACEPTIVE METHODS

Hormonal contraceptives are **the most commonly used reversible means of preventing pregnancy** in the United States and consist of combined (estrogen and progesterone) and progesterone-only methods. Currently, combined hormonal methods are available in oral, transdermal, and vaginal forms, whereas progesterone-only methods are available in oral, injectable, implantable, and intrauterine forms. At this time, there are several hormonal contraceptives in various stages of the FDA approval process in the United States, including new formulations for oral use, new subdermal implants, vaginal delivery systems, self-injectables, and male hormonal methods.

COMBINED ESTROGEN AND PROGESTIN METHODS

Oral Contraceptive Pills

Method of Action

Oral contraceptive pills (OCPs) are composed of **progesterone alone** or a **combination of progesterone and estrogen**. (The progesterone-alone pill is described later in the section Progesterone-Only Contraception.) Over 150 million women worldwide—including one-third of sexually active women in the United States—use oral contraceptives.

Oral contraceptives place the body in a pseudopregnancy state by interfering with the pulsatile release of follicle-stimulating hormone (FSH) and luteinizing hormone (LH) from the anterior pituitary. This pseudopregnancy state **suppresses ovulation** and prevents pregnancy from occurring. Figure 24-9 illustrates the serum levels of FSH and LH during the normal menstrual cycle, and Figure 24-10 shows FSH and LH levels during a cycle on the combination pill. The estrogen component of OCPs inhibits FSH secretion thereby suppressing formation of the dominant follicle. The progestin component of OCPs suppresses LH secretion, thus preventing the LH surge and ovulation. The progestin also induces a **thin decidualized endometrium** that is not receptive to implantation, while also **thickening the cervical mucus** making it less permeable to sperm. The bleeding that takes place during the hormone-free interval is actually

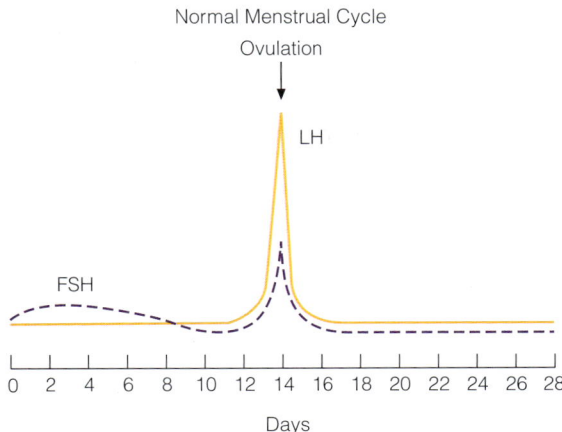

FIGURE 24-9. Serum levels of FSH and LH during a normal menstrual cycle. FSH, follicle-stimulating hormone; LH, luteinizing hormone.

a bleed due to the **withdrawal of hormone** rather than a menstrual period induced by endogenous hormone fluctuation.

Monophasic (Fixed Dose) Combination Pills

Monophasic combination pills contain a fixed dose of estrogen and a fixed dose of progestin in each tablet. In most cases, contemporary pills contain between 20 and 35 mcg of ethinyl estradiol (EE). **"Low dose"** OCPs are those which contain 10 or 20 mcg of EE rather than 30 or 35 mcg. **"High dose"** OCPs generally refer to formulations containing 50 mcg of EE. **Multiphasic pills** provide a varying amount of estrogen and/or progestin over the course of the cycle.

There are over 35 different branded and generic OCP formulations available in the United States. Newer formulations provide for shortened placebo length, extended cycles and continuous cycles. In general, the selection of a particular pill depends on the individual side effects, risk factors and goals for each patient.

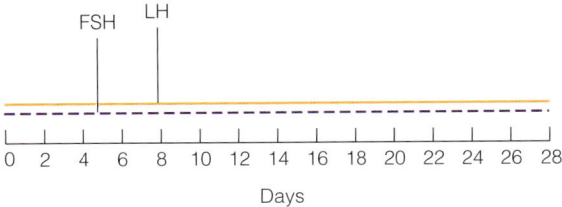

FIGURE 24-10. Serum levels of FSH and LH during the intake of monophasic oral contraceptive pills. FSH, follicle-stimulating hormone; LH, luteinizing hormone.

The traditional combination pill containing both estrogen and progestin is taken for the first 21 days out of a 28-day monthly cycle. During the last 7 days of the cycle, a placebo pill or no pill is taken. Bleeding should begin within 3 to 5 days of completion of the 21 days of hormones. Newer formulations are now available that **shorten the placebo time and cycle length** by giving 24 days of hormone (rather than the traditional 21 days) followed by a 4-day hormone-free interval. The so-called "24/4 regimens" result in a shorter 3- to 4-day menstrual cycle for most users. **Continuous regimens** (such as Lybrel) with a daily hormone pill and no hormone free interval have been found to be safe and effective. Pills that contain **iron and folic acid supplementation** are also available, as well as **chewable tablets**.

Women with **menstrual-related disorders** (such as endometriosis, heavy menstrual periods, anemia, dysmenorrhea, menstrual irregularity, menstrual migraines, premenstrual syndrome [PMS], polycystic ovary syndrome [PCOS], or ovarian cysts) may benefit from extending the number of consecutive days of hormonal pills taken from 21 days to 1, 2, or 3 months, thus increasing the length of continuous hormonal suppression and decreasing the number of withdrawal bleeds. These **extended or long-cycle regimens** (such as Seasonale and Seasonique) provide continued suppression of ovulation and decreased menstrual-related symptoms (such as pain, heavy bleeding, cysts, anemia, and headaches) for their users. These are also options for women who prefer to have fewer withdrawal bleeds while taking OCPs.

Multiphasic (Dose Varying) Combination Pills

Multiphasic oral contraceptives differ from monophasic pills only in that they **vary the dosage of estrogen and/or progestin** in the active hormone pills in an effort to mimic the menstrual cycle. The advantage of the multiphasic dosing is that it may provide a lower level of estrogen and progestin overall, but is still highly effective at preventing pregnancy. **Triphasic** (e.g., Trivora-28) and even **quadriphasic** (e.g., Natazia) formulations are available. These formulations contain three or four different levels, respectively of estrogen and/or progestin within the pack.

Effectiveness

OCPs are remarkably effective in preventing pregnancy. In fact, the theoretical failure rate for the first year of use is less than 1%. However, the failure rate with **actual real-life usage is closer to 8%**. Nausea, breakthrough bleeding, and the necessity of taking the pill every day are often cited as reasons for discontinuing the pill.

TABLE 24-4. Interactions of Oral Contraceptives with Other Medications

Medications That Reduce the Efficacy of Oral Contraceptives	Medications Whose Efficacies Are Changed by Oral Contraceptives
Barbiturates	Chlordiazepoxide (Librium)
Carbamazepine (Tegretol)	Diazepam (Valium)
Griseofulvin	Hypoglycemics
Phenytoin (Dilantin)	Methyldopa
Rifampin	Phenothiazines
St. John wort	Theophylline
Topiramate (Topamax)	Tricyclic antidepressants

Several medications are thought to interact with oral contraceptives, resulting in reduced effectiveness of the pill. Despite common belief, the only antibiotic that lowers the effectiveness of OCPs is Rifampin. Conversely, oral contraceptives can also reduce the efficacy of many medications (Table 24-4).

Side Effects

Table 24-5 lists some of the cardiovascular, neoplastic, and biliary complications associated with oral contraceptive use.

Oral contraceptives with estrogen doses greater than 50 mcg can increase coagulability, leading to higher rates of myocardial infarction (MI), stroke, deep vein thrombosis (DVT), and pulmonary embolism (PE), particularly in women who smoke. Even at lower doses of estrogen (35 mcg or less), women older than 35 years who smoke more than 15 cigarettes a day are still at increased risk of heart attack, stroke, DVT, and PE if they use OCPs. The progestins in oral contraceptives have been found to raise low-density lipoproteins, while lowering high-density lipoproteins in pill users smoking more than one pack per day. For these reasons, oral contraceptives are **contraindicated in women older than 35 years who smoke 15 or more cigarettes a day**. The advent of new progestins and lower estrogen doses has led to pill formulations that are essentially neutral in terms of cardiovascular effect. However, combination oral contraceptive use is still contraindicated in women older than 35 years who smoke. These women often benefit from progesterone-only contraception (depo-provera, Nexplanon), hormonal and inert IUDs or permanent female or male sterilization.

Neoplastic complications of oral contraceptive use are rare. The effect of long-term oral contraceptive use on breast cancer has been studied extensively with no conclusive findings. There is, however, an **increased incidence of gall bladder disease** and **benign hepatic tumors** associated with oral contraceptive use.

Table 24-6 outlines both the absolute and relative contraindications to oral contraceptive use.

TABLE 24-5. Complications Associated with Oral Contraceptives

Cardiovascular[a]

Deep vein thrombosis (DVT)
Pulmonary embolism (PE)
Stroke (CVA)[b]
Myocardial infarction (MI)[b]
Hypertension

Other

Cholelithiasis
Cholecystitis
Benign liver adenomas (rare)
Cervical adenocarcinoma (rare)
Retinal thrombosis (rare)

[a]These complications occur mainly in smokers.
[b]Most MIs and CVAs occur in users of high-dose estrogen products.

TABLE 24-6. Contraindications to Combination Estrogen–Progesterone Contraceptives

Absolute Contraindications	Relative Contraindications
Thromboembolism	Uterine fibroids
Pulmonary embolism	Lactation
Coronary artery disease	Diabetes mellitus
Cerebrovascular accident	Sickle-cell disease or sickle C disease
Smokers older than 35 y	Hepatic disease
Breast/endometrial cancer	Hypertension
Unexplained vaginal bleeding	Lupus (SLE)
Abnormal liver function	Age 40 years and older and high risk for vascular disease
Known or suspected pregnancy	Migraine headaches
Severe hypercholesterolemia	Seizure disorders
Severe hypertriglyceridemia	Elective surgery

SLE, systemic lupus erythematosus.

The Centers for Disease Control and Prevention (CDC) has developed a comprehensive list of recommendations on contraceptive use for men and women with various medical conditions (Table 24-7). These guidelines also include use of contraceptives with various medications, such as anticonvulsants and antiretrovirals within this resource. This is a very helpful reference and can be accessed through the CDC website in table and written format. (This information is also available for download as a cellular phone app http://www.cdc.gov/reproductivehealth/contraception/usmec.htm.)

A sample of medical conditions is listed in an abbreviated format in Table 24-7. The number categories correspond to the proposed risk of using that particular contraceptive mechanism for the specified condition. The chart goes further into detail with guidance on the risk/benefit ratio of initiating versus continuing a particular method.

Advantages and Disadvantages

The major advantages of OCPs include their extremely high efficacy rates and the noncontraceptive health benefits including decreased menstrual flow, anemia, dysmenorrhea, and ovarian cysts. These benefits also include a reduced incidence of ovarian cancer, endometrial cancer, ectopic pregnancy, PID, and benign breast disease (Table 24-8). By taking OCPs, nearly 50,000 women avoid hospitalizations; of these, 10,000 avoid hospitalization for life-threatening illnesses.

Disadvantages to OCP use include cardiovascular complications, increased gallbladder disease, increased incidence of benign hepatic tumors, and the need to take a medication every day. Because they contain estrogen, combination OCPs are not suitable for many women. Many women also complain of nausea, headaches, breakthrough bleeding, and weight gain associated with OCP use. Most of these symptoms are generally mild and transient.

Transdermal Hormonal Contraception—Ortho Evra patch

Mechanism of Action

The transdermal contraceptive patch (Ortho Evra, Xulane) contains both progesterone and estrogen.

TABLE 24-7. Sample from Summary Chart of US Medical Eligibility Criteria for Contraceptive Use (CDC 2016)

Condition	Sub-Condition	CHC I/C	POP I/C	DMPA I/C	Implant (progestin) I/C	LNG-IUD I/C	Cu-IUD I/C
Headaches	a. Nonmigraine (mild or severe)	1	1	1	1	1	1
	b. Migraine						
	i. Without aura (including menstrual migraine)	2	1	1	1	1	1
	ii. With aura	4	1	1	1	1	1
Hypertension	a. Adequately controlled	3	1	2	1	1	1
	b. Elevated Blood Pressure						
	i. Systolic 140–159 or diastolic 90–99	3	1	2	1	1	1
	ii. Systolic ≥160 or diastolic ≥ 100	4	2	3	2	2	1
	c. Vascular disease	4	2	3	2	2	1
Liver tumors	a. Benign						
	i. Focal nodular hyperplasia	2	2	2	2	2	1
	ii. Hepatocellular adenoma	4	3	3	3	3	1
	b. Malignant (hepatoma)	4	3	3	3	3	1

CHC, combined hormonal contraceptives (including pills, patch, and vaginal ring); POP, progestin-only pill; DMPA, depot medroxyprogesterone acetate; I, initiation of contraceptive method; C, continuation of method.
Risk stratification: *1*, no restriction (method can be used); *2*, advantages generally outweigh theoretical or proven risks; *3*, theoretical or proven risks usually outweigh the advantages; *4*, unacceptable health risk (method not to be used).
See complete guidelines for clarification of each classification. Adapted from table: http://www.cdc.gov/reproductivehealth/contraception/pdf/summary-chart-us-medical-eligibility-criteria_508tagged.pdf.

TABLE 24-8. Noncontraceptive Health Benefits of Oral Contraceptives

Decrease risk of serious diseases
- Ovarian cancer
- Endometrial cancer
- Ectopic pregnancy (combination pills only)
- Severe anemia
- Pelvic inflammatory disease
- Salpingitis

Improve quality-of-life problems
- Iron deficiency anemia
- Dysmenorrhea
- Functional ovarian cysts
- Benign breast disease
- Osteoporosis (increased bone density)
- Rheumatoid arthritis

Treat/manage many disorders
- Dysfunctional uterine bleeding
- Control of bleeding in bleeding disorders and anovulation
- Dysmenorrhea
- Endometriosis
- Acne/hirsutism
- Premenstrual syndrome

FIGURE 24-11. Vaginal contraceptive ring (NuvaRing) and transdermal contraceptive patch (Ortho Evra). Both contain a combination of estrogen and progesterone, which are released over a period of 1 week and 3 weeks, respectively. (From Speroff L, Fritz M. *Clinical Gynecologic Endocrinology and Infertility,* 7th ed. Philadelphia, PA: Lippincott Williams & Wilkins; 2005.)

(Fig. 24-11). The patch releases 150 mg/day of the progestin, norelgestromin, and 35 mg/day of EE. The overall average **estrogen exposure is 60% higher** in patch users compared with women taking a standard 35 mcg OCP. Therefore, these patients should be made aware of the **increased risk of thromboembolism**, specifically DVT and PE in Ortho Evra users compared with women taking standard OCPs. There does not appear to be an increased risk of heart attack and stroke in these patients.

Women apply one patch on the same day each week (patch change day) for three consecutive weeks followed by a 1-week patch-free period where they will have a withdrawal bleed. It can be worn on the upper outer arm, abdomen, buttock, or back in a location that would not be disturbed by clothing. The patch should not be placed on the breasts. Extended dosing regimens have been studied. Again, just like combined OCPs, the primary mechanism of action is suppression of ovulation by decreasing endogenous FSH and LH levels, thickening cervical mucus, and thinning the endometrium (Figs. 24-9 and 24-10).

Effectiveness

The patch has been shown to have a 1% pregnancy rate in actual use—similar to other combination hormonal methods. The transdermal patch has been found to have a **decreased effectiveness in women weighing more than 198 lbs (90 kg)**.

Advantages and Disadvantages

The transdermal patch is safe, effective, and convenient. Bleeding is generally lighter and shorter on hormonal contraceptives. The same primary side effects and noncontraceptive health benefits of OCPs apply to the patch as well. The patch can cause skin irritation in some users. The patch has the added benefit of being **self-administered only once a week**.

Vaginal Hormonal Contraception—NuvaRing

Method of Action

The hormone-releasing vaginal ring (Fig. 24-11) with the brand name of NuvaRing releases a daily dose of 15 mcg of EE and 120 mcg of etonogestrel (the active form of desogestrel). The ring is **placed in the vagina for 3 weeks** (it is likely effective for 4 weeks), and is removed for 1 week to allow for a withdrawal bleed. This hormone-free period can be skipped to allow for continuous dosing, typically for 3 months.

Effectiveness

The vaginal ring is highly effective (1% to 2% failure rate in actual use), similar to other forms of combined hormonal contraception.

Advantages and Disadvantages

Because one size of vaginal ring fits all women, the vaginal ring does not need to be fitted by a clinician. Women place the ring in the vagina themselves for three continuous weeks and then remove it for 1 week. Because the ring is left in place continuously, it provides a low, steady release of hormone with **lower total hormone exposure** compared with other combination hormone methods. Although douching with the NuvaRing in place is discouraged, the use of antifungal agents and spermicides is permitted.

The disadvantages of the vaginal ring include a woman's (or partner's) concern with having a foreign body in the vagina and the potential for expulsion. Studies have shown that women do not feel the ring inside once placed in the vagina, and **the ring does not need to be removed for intercourse**. If it is removed for intercourse, it should be rinsed in cool to lukewarm water and replaced within 3 hours. Reasons for discontinuation include discomfort, headache, vaginal discharge, and recurrent vaginitis.

PROGESTERONE-ONLY CONTRACEPTION

Progesterone-only contraception consists of oral, injectable, implantable, and intrauterine options (the LNG IUDs are discussed in the section Intrauterine Devices). All these function primarily using the same mechanisms: **thickening the cervical mucus, inhibiting sperm motility,** and **thinning the endometrial lining**, so that it is not suitable for implantation.

Progestin-Only Oral Contraception Pills

Method of Action

Progestin-only pills (POPs, Micronor, Nor-QD) deliver a small daily dose of progestin (0.35 mg norethindrone) without any estrogen. POPs have lower progestin doses than combination pills, thus the nickname *minipills*. POPs also differ from traditional pills in that **they are taken every day of the cycle** with no hormone-free days. POPs are believed to thicken the cervical mucus making it less permeable to sperm. This effect, however, decreases after 22 hours, so the minipill must be taken at the **same time each day**. Other mechanisms of action include endometrial atrophy and ovulation suppression (50% of cycles).

Effectiveness

POPs are generally not as effective as combination hormone regimens, with **failure rates estimated at greater than 8%**. This failure rate increases if punctual dosing is not achieved.

Side Effects

Side effects of the progesterone-only OCP include irregular ovulatory cycles, breakthrough bleeding, increased formation of follicular cysts, and acne. POPs can also cause breast tenderness and irritability.

Advantages and Disadvantages

Because they contain no estrogen, POPs are ideal for **breastfeeding mothers** and **women for whom estrogens are contraindicated,** including women older than 35 years who smoke and women with hypertension, coronary artery disease, collagen vascular disorder, lupus, migraines with aura, and those with a personal history of thromboembolism. In addition to their contraceptive benefits, **POPs can be used to treat abnormal uterine bleeding in high-risk medical populations whose bleeding has been adequately evaluated** (i.e., anovulatory bleeding and benign endometrial hyperplasia in poor surgical candidates).

The disadvantages include irregular menses ranging from amenorrhea to irregular spotting. Also, POPs must be taken at the same time each day. A delay of more than 3 hours is akin to a missed pill.

Injectable Progesterone-Only Contraception—Depo-Provera

Method of Action

Although it was only approved for contraceptive use in the United States in 1992, Depo-Provera (depot medroxyprogesterone acetate, DMPA) has been used in other countries since the mid-1960s. Depo-Provera (150 mg/1 mL, intramuscular "IM") is injected IM every 3 months in a vehicle that allows the slow release of progestin over a 3-month period. A low-dose DMPA (104 mg/0.65 mL, subcutaneous "SC") is also available, although not widely used yet. This formulation carries the benefit of lower progestin levels but the same efficacy rates. Depo-Provera acts by **suppressing ovulation, thickening the cervical mucus, making the endometrium unsuitable for implantation, and reducing tubal motility**. After an injection, ovulation does not occur for 14 weeks; therefore, patients have a 2-week grace period in their every 12-week dosing.

Effectiveness

With a first-year theoretical failure rate of only 0.3%, Depo-Provera is one of the most effective contraceptive methods available. Typical use failure rates are estimated at 3%, mostly attributed to patients failing to return at scheduled times for follow-up injections.

Side Effects

The primary side effects experienced by Depo-Provera users include irregular menstrual bleeding, depression, weight gain, hair loss, and headache. Over 70% of patients experience spotting and irregular menses during the first year of use. Irregular bleeding is the primary reason for discontinuing Depo-Provera. It is anticipated that **50% of DMPA users will have amenorrhea after 1 year** of use and 80% after 5 years of DMPA use. However, the possibility of amenorrhea makes Depo-Provera a good option for women with bleeding disorders and heavy menstrual bleeding, women on anticoagulation, women in the military, and women who are mentally or physically disabled.

Women using DMPA for more than 2 years may experience a **reversible decrease in bone mineralization** similar to that seen in lactating women, due to the decrease in ovarian estradiol production. The effect of Depo-Provera use on bone mineralization is summarized in Table 24-9. Thus, calcium, vitamin D, weight-bearing and strengthening exercises, and smoking cessation should be encouraged in all women using Depo-Provera. A recent randomized controlled trial demonstrated the SC and IM forms to be similar in their effects on bone mineral density. There is no role for bone density measurement while on Depo-Provera.

TABLE 24-9. The Effects of Depo-Provera Use on Bone Mineralization

Bone density is decreased in women using Depo-Provera, because of the decrease in ovarian estradiol production
The decrease in bone density is most rapid in the first year of use
The decrease in bone density increases with length of use
The decrease in bone density is reversible and occurs over 6 mo–2 y
There is no role for the use of bone density screening in DMPA users
There is no role for the use of bisphosphonates, estrogens, and SERMs in DMPA users
Women on Depo-Provera should be encouraged to take calcium and vitamin D, stop smoking, and do regular weight-bearing exercises.

DMPA, depot medroxyprogesterone acetate; SERM, selective estrogen receptor modulator.

Advantages and Disadvantages

The primary advantages of Depo-Provera are that it is **highly effective**, acts independent of intercourse, and requires infrequent injections (**every 3 months**). Like other progestins, Depo-Provera **reduces the risk of endometrial cancer and PID** and also the amount of **menstrual bleeding**. It is also useful in the treatment of menorrhagia, dysmenorrhea, endometriosis, menstrual-related anemia, and endometrial hyperplasia. DMPA is especially useful in women who desire effective contraception, but may have concomitant medical conditions that prevent the use of estrogen-containing contraceptives, such as women with migraines with auras, seizure disorders, lupus, sickle-cell disease, hypertension, coronary artery disease, and smokers.

Irregular bleeding to DMPA use, weight gain, and mood changes are the major disadvantages. Although not contraindicated, Depo-Provera should be used with caution in patients with a history of depression, mood disorders, PMS, and premenstrual dysphoric disorder. Depo-Provera is not contraindicated in obese women, but **weight monitoring** should be used in women taking DMPA who have an increased risk for weight gain. Women who gain >10 lbs after 6 months of use should consider another contraceptive.

After discontinuation of Depo-Provera injections, some women may experience a significant delay in the return of regular ovulation (range of 6 to 18 months; average of 10 months). This is independent of the number of injections but may be directly related to the weight of the patient. Within 18 months, however, fertility rates return to normal levels.

Implantable Progesterone-Only Contraception—Nexplanon

Method of Action

Nexplanon (the newest generation of the Implanon device) is a single-rod, **subdermal progestin implant** that provides **3 years** of uninterrupted contraceptive coverage. The progestin used in Nexplanon is etonogestrel, the same progestin as used in the NuvaRing. The device is 4 cm × 2 mm, contains 68 mg of etonogestrel, and provides a slow release of hormone over 3 years. It is radiopaque and the size of a matchstick. Its applicator facilitates placement in the subdermal skin of the inner side of a woman's upper arm. When appropriate timing of placement is utilized, Nexplanon is effective 24 hours after placement and has quick return to fertility once the device is removed by a clinician. Similar to other progesterone-only contraceptives, it acts by suppressing ovulation, altering the endometrium, and thickening cervical mucus.

Effectiveness
Nexplanon is one of the **most highly effective reversible** contraceptive methods, with only a 0.5% failure rate.

Side Effects
Irregular and unpredictable light bleeding is the major side effect of Nexplanon. In the majority of cases (75%), the bleeding is lighter than a normal menstrual bleeding and requires only a panty liner or less for protection. However, irregular bleeding was the reason for approximately 15% of discontinuations, followed by headaches (approximately 12%).

Advantages and Disadvantages
The major advantage of Nexplanon is that it is implantable and provides **three uninterrupted years of contraceptive coverage**. There is no maintenance associated with the device, and thus, no interruption of sexual spontaneity.

The disadvantages include the need for a provider to insert and remove the device and the unpredictable bleeding profile. Rarely, device migration from original placement site into deeper tissue layers has been reported. If this occurs, it requires additional imaging to identify the exact location of the device followed by surgical removal.

EMERGENCY CONTRACEPTION (EC)

EC is a safe and effective means of preventing pregnancy after unprotected intercourse or in the case of contraceptive failure (condom break, patch/ring/diaphragm dislodgment, IUD expulsion, missed pill, and late Depo-Provera injection). It is used only if a woman is not already pregnant from a previous act of intercourse. The use of emergency contraceptive pills (ECPs) is not indicated in women with a known or suspected pregnancy. However, there is **no known evidence of harm** to the patient, her pregnancy, or to the fetus if ECPs are unintentionally taken during pregnancy. EC **can also be used safely** in women in whom continual estrogen might otherwise be contraindicated, such as women with a history of DVT, PE, MI, stroke, or migraines with auras.

EC works by preventing pregnancy, not by disrupting an implanted pregnancy. In fact, EC is thought to account for a 40% **decline in therapeutic abortions** in the past 10 years, while also **decreasing the number of teen pregnancies**. It is available in three forms: ECPs (also called the *post-coital* or the *morning-after pill*), an emergently inserted Copper T IUD (ParaGard), or a selective progesterone receptor modulator (SPRM, ulipristal acetate or Ella). Although mifepristone (RU 486) has been approved in the United States for the termination of pregnancy up to 49 days of gestation, its use has not been approved for EC. In the United States, EC does not require an examination by a provider, although a pregnancy test should be performed before placing a Copper IUD or giving ulipristal (Ella). The ECPs may be obtained over-the-counter **without a prescription** by men and women 17 years or older.

EMERGENCY CONTRACEPTIVE PILLS
Methods of Action
ECPs use high doses of both estrogen and progestins or progesterone alone (Plan B One Step, Next Choice) to prevent pregnancy after unprotected intercourse has taken place. Several differing regimens exist, including those using high doses of regularly prescribed OCPs and some using prepackaged brand name and generic regimens. For those using ECPs, **LNG methods are preferred over estrogen–progesterone regimens**, because LNG is more effective and has fewer side effects (decreased nausea, vomiting). Many formulations are available over-the-counter, with no age restriction and in generic form.

The most common prepackaged formulation is Plan B (progestin only). This regimen can be taken as a single 1.5 mg of LNG (Plan B One Step) or as two 0.75 mg doses taken 12 hours apart (Next Choice). Studies show that Plan B is equally effective if taken in a single dose with minimal increased side effects. Regardless of the regimen, **the first dose must be taken within 72 hours of unprotected vaginal intercourse.** There is some additional efficacy if initiated within 120 hours, although not as high as within the first 72 hours. An antiemetic is often prescribed at the same time to prevent nausea (more common in estrogen-containing regimens).

The mechanism of action for ECPs depends on the point during the cycle when the pills are taken. EC is used to prevent pregnancy by inhibiting ovulation, interfering with fertilization and tubal transport, preventing implantation, or causing regression of the corpus luteum.

Effectiveness
When taken within 72 hours of intercourse, ECPs have a failure rate of 0.2% to 3%. The sooner an ECP is taken after unprotected intercourse, the

more effective it is. The **risk of pregnancy is reduced by 75% to 90%** in women who have had unprotected intercourse during the second or third week of their menstrual cycles, when they are most likely ovulating. Of all the oral EC regimens, the progesterone-only formulations (Plan B) are the most effective and have fewer side effects. Thus, the **single dose of LNG 1.5 mg** (Plan B One Step, My Way, Next Choice One Dose) **should be used as a first choice** when it is available, rather than using a combination method.

Side Effects
The primary side effects of EC include **nausea (50%), vomiting (20%)**, headaches, dizziness, and breast tenderness. Most of these symptoms are thought to be secondary to the high doses of estrogen in the combined regimens. The side effects of the progesterone-only formulations are less severe than symptoms experienced with estrogen and progesterone-containing methods.

Although there are relative and absolute contraindications for use of oral contraceptives in women with certain medical conditions (history of stroke, heart attack, DVT, and PE), these **contraindications do not apply to women using emergency contraceptives**. However, repeated use of ECP is not recommended in this high-risk group.

Advantages and Disadvantages
ECPs are extremely effective in preventing pregnancy and are safe for the user. In 2013, the FDA approved over-the-counter dispensing of Plan B EC without a prescription for patients of any age.

The major disadvantages include the short window of time when they can be used (within 72 to 120 hours of intercourse). Additionally, these cannot be used as long-term contraception.

EMERGENCY IUD INSERTION
Method of Action
The **Copper T IUD** (ParaGard) can be inserted (Fig. 24-6A) in the uterine cavity **within 120 hours (or 5 days)** of unprotected intercourse as a form of EC. The IUD functions primarily by eliciting a **sterile inflammatory response** within the uterus, making the environment unsuitable for fertilization.

Effectiveness
Emergency Copper T IUD insertion reduces the risk of pregnancy by 99.8%; therefore, only 1 in 1,000 become pregnant after emergency IUD insertion, making it the **most effective form of EC**.

Side Effects
The side effects are the same as those discussed in the section Intrauterine Devices. Copper T is not an acceptable form of EC in women who are not candidates for IUDs, including those with active PID or STI cervicitis or a history of PID or STI cervicitis in the past 3 months, cervical or endometrial cancer, or women who have a confirmed pregnancy.

Advantages and Disadvantages
Emergency Copper T IUD insertion is extremely effective, even more effective than the oral regimens. It differs from ECPs in that it **can be continued for long-term contraception (10 years)**, whereas the ECPs have a one-time-only use. Disadvantages of the ParaGard IUD for EC are that it must be placed by a provider, it has a higher one-time cost than oral regimens, and it can potentially result in rare complications, such as infection and perforation (described in the section Intrauterine Devices). The ParaGard IUD is also associated with heavier menses and dysmenorrhea.

EMERGENCY PROGESTERONE RECEPTOR MODULATORS
Method of Action
The newest form of ECP received FDA approval in August 2010. **Ulipristal (*Ella, EllaOne*)** is a derivative of 19-norprogesterone and acts as an SPRM with agonist/antagonist effects at progesterone receptor sites. Its primary mechanism of action is to **delay ovulation (follicular rupture)** and **inhibit implantation** into the endometrial lining. It is available worldwide and is administered in a **single dose of 30 mg** within 120 hours (5 days) after unprotected intercourse. Small trials suggest that ulipristal is more effective than progestin-only regimens in preventing pregnancy when used between the 72- and 120-hour postcoital time period.

A closely related drug to ulipristal is **mifepristone (RU 486)**. Its mechanism of action is similar to ulipristal. Currently, mifepristone is not available in the United States for prevention of pregnancy, although trials have shown 99% to 100% efficacy (similar to or better than that of current ECPs). The actual dosing has not yet been determined for this indication, and its current use in the United States is limited to medical termination of pregnancy.

Effectiveness
The pregnancy rate when prescribed within the 120-hour window is about 2%.

Side Effects
The most common side effects are similar to ECPs and include self-limited headache, bleeding, nausea, and abdominal pain.

Advantages and Disadvantages
Ulipristal is **contraindicated in women who are breastfeeding** or currently pregnant, given its antiprogestin effects and potential to terminate an existing pregnancy. **A pregnancy test is required before the administration of ulipristal.** Advantages of its use include one-time dosing and relatively mild side effects.

One disadvantage is that it is available by **prescription only**. Ulipristal's use is also controversial given its potential use as an abortifacient (although not approved for this indication). This is, in contrast to progestin-only or combined estrogen/progestin ECPs, because they do not terminate an existing pregnancy nor cause teratogenic effects. For these reasons, ulipristal is not as widely prescribed when compared with other ECPs.

SURGICAL STERILIZATION

The rate of surgical sterilization as a method of contraception has increased dramatically over the past three decades. Approximately 30% of reproductive-age couples in the United States and Great Britain choose female sterilization for contraceptive purposes. The rate of sterilization is higher in women who are **married, divorced, over age 30, or African American.**

Before performing any sterilization procedure, careful counseling should be provided and informed consent obtained. The patient should understand the **permanent and largely irreversible nature** of the procedure, operative risks, chance of failure, and possible side effects. Sterilization is ideal in stable monogamous relationships where no (additional) children are desired. It is also indicated in women for whom pregnancy would be life-threatening, such as those with major cardiac issues.

TUBAL STERILIZATION
Method of Action
Tubal sterilization prevents pregnancy by surgically occluding both fallopian tubes to prevent the ovum and sperm from uniting. Tubal ligation can be performed in the immediate postpartum period (postpartum sterilization [PPS]) or outside the postpartum period via a laparoscopic approach (laparoscopic tubal ligation [LTL]) or via hysteroscopic tubal occlusion (*Essure*).

Prior to performance of permanent sterilization, women should be thoroughly counseled on the **risk of regret**, as well as alternatives such as vasectomy and long-acting reversible contraceptives (LARCs).

Tubal ligation can be performed immediately postpartum (PPS) through a small subumbilical incision using epidural or spinal anesthesia. The most commonly used method, the *modified* Pomeroy tubal ligation (aka Parkland), is illustrated in Figure 24-12. Laparoscopically, there are a number of methods by which tubal occlusion can be accomplished, including bipolar fulguration (Fig. 24-13), Silastic banding with Falope rings (Fig. 24-14), or clipping with Hulka clips or Filshie clips (Fig. 24-15).

Modern techniques have evolved to incorporate sterilization procedures in both operating room and outpatient (in office) practices that involve **non-incisional hysteroscopic approaches**. Essure was introduced in the United States in 2002. In this method, soft, flexible, 4 cm radiopaque microinserts are introduced into the proximal (uterine) portions of the fallopian tubes. An outer spring coil made of a nickel–titanium alloy and molds to the shape of the fallopian tube to anchor the microinsert across the utero-tubal junction. The inner coil contains polyethylene terephthalate (PET) fibers that incite a natural in-growth of tissue. **Over about 12 weeks, sterilization is accomplished** as in-growth of tissue around the coils results in occlusion of

FIGURE 24-12. The Parkland (modified Pomeroy) method of postpartum tubal ligation. A 2- to 3-cm segment of the tube is doubly ligated, and the intervening segment is removed. This technique is typically performed during the immediate postpartum period through a small subumbilical incision. (From Rock J, Jones H. *TeLinde's Operative Gynecology*, 10th ed. Philadelphia, PA: Lippincott Williams & Wilkins; 2008.)

FIGURE 24-13. Tubal occlusion with the bipolar electrocoagulation. A 3-cm portion of the isthmic tube is desiccated with bipolar forceps. (From Rock J, Jones H. *TeLinde's Operative Gynecology*, 10th ed. Philadelphia, PA: Lippincott Williams & Wilkins; 2008.)

FIGURE 24-15. Tubal occlusion with the Filshie clip. The clip is applied to the mid-isthmic portion of the tube about 2 cm from the cornua. The lower jaw of the clip should be visible through the mesosalpinx to ensure inclusion of the entire circumference of the tube. (From Rock J, Jones H. *TeLinde's Operative Gynecology*, 10th ed. Philadelphia, PA: Lippincott Williams & Wilkins; 2008.)

the fallopian tubes. Tubal occlusion is achieved by both the space-filling outer coil and tissue in-growth elicited by the PET fibers of the inner coil.

The advantage of the Essure procedure is that it requires **no general anesthesia or surgical incisions**. As a result, when hysteroscopic tubal sterilization/occlusion is performed, very little recuperative time is needed, and it provides a **safer, more effective,**

FIGURE 24-14. Tubal occlusion with the silicone band (Falope ring). The isthmic portion of the tube is retracted into the applicator barrel using grasping tongs. During this retraction process, the ring is rolled forward to occlude the portion of tube. The intervening "knuckle" of the tube becomes ischemic and necroses. (From Rock J, Jones H. *TeLinde's Operative Gynecology*, 10th ed. Philadelphia, PA: Lippincott Williams & Wilkins; 2008.)

hormone-free method of permanent birth control. The Essure procedure is most commonly performed in the **office setting**, making it a preferable option to surgical sterilization for all women, including obese women, women with prior abdominal surgeries, or those at risk from anesthesia use.

Because the tubal blockage is accomplished over time, the patient's current method of birth control should be continued until an Essure Confirmation Test is performed 3 months after the procedure. A modified **hysterosalpingogram** (HSG) can confirm coil location and complete tubal occlusion, whereas a **specialized transvaginal ultrasound** can verify correct micro-insert location without confirming occlusion. Most patients are reassured by this confirmatory test, whereas others are burdened by the additional step to achieving permanent sterilization. Prior to the procedure, patients should understand that tubal occlusion by this method is essentially **irreversible**.

Effectiveness

Tubal ligation has a failure rate of 0.3% but varies by method, patient age, and surgeon's experience. The highest success rates are achieved with **PPS** and **Essure tubal occlusion**. When the laparoscopic approach is undertaken, the Falope ring has been found to be most effective in women younger than 28 years. Electrocoagulation and Falope rings are equally effective in women older than 28. More recently, titanium Filshie clips have been used for tubal ligation, but long-term efficacy rates are not yet available. Essure offers the lowest rates of all of these methods when tubal occlusion is achieved (2.6/1,000 pregnancy rate over 5 years), aside from unipolar sterilization, which is no longer used due to safety concerns.

Side Effects
There are no side effects associated with tubal sterilization. Some women report pain and menstrual disturbances. This phenomenon was once described as **post-tubal ligation syndrome** but has largely been discounted by the literature. In most of these women, symptoms are due to **discontinuation of hormone-containing contraceptives**. As a result, patients may experience heavier baseline menses and dysmenorrhea. In rare circumstances, malplacement of *Essure* coils has contributed to significant pain requiring subsequent surgical coil removal, salpingectomy or, rarely, hysterectomy.

Advantage/Disadvantages
Tubal ligation/occlusion offers the advantage of permanent effective contraception without continual expense, effort, or motivation. The mortality rate of bilateral tubal ligation is 4 in 100,000 women. The major risks are those associated with surgery including the risk of infection, hemorrhage, conversion to laparotomy, viscus injury, vascular damage, and anesthesia complications.

Tubal ligation results in a very low risk of pregnancy. However, when pregnancy does occur, there is an **increased risk of ectopic pregnancy** (1 in 15,000). However, nearly 1,000 maternal lives are saved because of sterilization during the period from the time of sterilization to the end of the woman's reproductive life. The rate of ectopic pregnancy after Essure is significantly decreased compared with that of LTL. Patients may also benefit from a reduction in the risk of ovarian cancer. The reason for this is unclear, but it is speculated that tubal ligation may limit the migration of carcinogens from the lower genital tract into the peritoneal cavity.

Of women who undergo permanent sterilization, **regret is highest in women who were younger than 30 years** when the procedure was performed. However, it is estimated that less than 2% of women seek reversal of tubal sterilization. The success of reversal varies from 41% to 84% depending on the method used. The success rate of reanastomosis is highest when clips are used because they destroy a much smaller segment of the tube. When pregnancy is desired after tubal ligation, in vitro fertilization (IVF) offers a greater likelihood of pregnancy than tubal microplasty. However, when multiple future pregnancies are desired, tuboplasty may be a more economical alternative than multiple IVF cycles.

VASECTOMY
Method of Action
Vasectomy is a simple and safe option for permanent sterilization involving **ligation of the vas deferens**. This procedure may be performed in a provider's office under local anesthesia through a small incision in the upper outer aspect of each scrotum (Fig. 24-16). In 1985, the no-scalpel vasectomy technique was introduced. With this procedure, both vasa are ligated through a single small midline incision that reduces the already low rate of complications associated with vasectomy. Unlike female tubal ligations, **vasectomy is not immediately effective**. Because sperm can remain viable in the proximal collecting system after vasectomy, patients should use **another form of contraception** until azoospermia is confirmed by semen analysis, usually in 6 to 8 weeks.

Effectiveness
The failure rate for vasectomy in actual practice is 0.15%. In fact, with the exception of Essure, vasectomy is **safer, simpler, and more effective than female sterilization**. When pregnancies occur after vasectomy, many are due to having intercourse too soon after vasectomy rather than from recanalization of the vas deferens.

Side Effects
Complications after vasectomy are rare and usually involve slight bleeding, skin infection, and reactions to the sutures or local anesthesia. Fifty percent of patients form antisperm antibodies after the procedure. However, there are no long-term side effects of vasectomy.

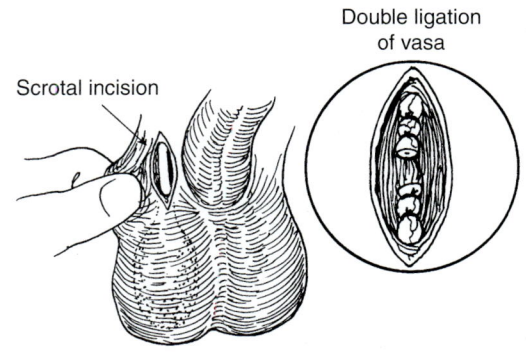

FIGURE 24-16. Sterilization by vasectomy. Typically performed in an office setting under local anesthesia. (From Beckmann C, Ling F. *Obstetrics & Gynecology,* 5th ed. Philadelphia, PA: Lippincott Williams & Wilkins; 2006.)

Advantages/Disadvantages

Vasectomy is a permanent, highly effective form of contraception with few, if any, side effects. Vasectomy is generally safer and less expensive than tubal ligation and can be performed in an outpatient under local anesthesia. Vasectomy offers male sterilization leaving the woman without contraception if she leaves the relationship. The success rate of vasal reanastomosis is 60% to 70%. Pregnancy rates after vasectomy reversal range from 18% to 60%.

KEY POINTS

- Natural family planning methods and coitus interruptus are the least effective methods of contraception and should not be used if pregnancy prevention is a high priority.
- Lactational amenorrhea provides a prolactin-induced suppression of GnRH and subsequent suppression of ovulation. It should only be used for a maximum of 6 months after delivery in an amenorrheic woman, and breastfeeding should be the only source of nutrition for the infant.
- Condoms, diaphragms, and cervical caps act as mechanical barriers between sperm and egg. Their efficacy rate is 75% to 85% with actual use.
- Male and female condoms carry the added benefit of prophylaxis against STIs.
- Efficacy of spermicides is 70% to 80%, but variability in user technique can significantly lower efficacy. Spermicides DO NOT protect against STIs and may, in fact, make the vaginal mucosa more susceptible to infections, such as HIV.
- IUDs provide long-term, highly effective, and cost-effective contraception. There are currently five IUDs in the U.S. market: ParaGard (copper-containing, 10 years of use) and four LNG (progestin)-containing devices (Mirena and Kyleena, 5 years of use; Liletta and Skyla, approved for 3 years of use).
- The primary mechanism of action for IUDs is a sterile spermicidal inflammatory response. Other mechanisms include inhibition of implantation, thickening of cervical mucus, and alteration in tubal motility. Potentially serious side effects include insertion-related PID, uterine perforation, and spontaneous abortion.
- Hormonal contraceptives have extremely low failure rates when used appropriately and are available in oral, injectable, transdermal, implantable, vaginal, and intrauterine forms.
- Combined hormonal contraception methods (OCPs, Ortho Evra patch, and NuvaRing) prevent pregnancy by suppressing ovulation, altering cervical mucus, and causing atrophic changes in the endometrium.
- Serious complications from combined hormonal contraception use occur mainly in smokers older than 35 years, including PE, stroke, DVT, and heart attack.
- An excellent reference for suitability of specific medical conditions with various contraceptive methods can be found within the 2016 CDC Medical Eligibility Criteria table.
- Benefits of combined hormonal contraception include protection from ovarian and endometrial cancer, anemia, PID, osteoporosis, dysmenorrhea, acne, hirsutism, and benign breast disease.
- Progesterone-only contraception (progestin-only OCPs, Depo-Provera, Nexplanon, and the LNG IUDs) uses progestins to suppress ovulation, thicken the cervical mucus, and make the endometrium unsuitable for implantation.
- Primary side effects of Depo-Provera include irregular bleeding, reversible bone demineralization, and a potentially significant delay in return of fertility after discontinuation. It should be used with *caution* in women with depression and obesity.
- Nexplanon is a radiopaque, single-rod, subdermal implant of etonogestrel that is placed in the upper arm of the patient. It provides 3 years of contraception without impacting the patient's bone density, weight, or mood.
- ECPs contain high doses of estrogen and progestin or progesterone alone and must be taken within 72 hours of unprotected intercourse to prevent pregnancy. These pills act to suppress ovulation and to prevent fertilization and implantation. They do not cause abortions.
- When available, a single dose of progesterone-only ECP (Plan B) should be used preferentially, given its increased effectiveness and lower rate of side effects.
- Emergency IUD insertion (Copper T only) must be performed within 120 hours of unprotected intercourse; it can then be used as long-term contraception.

- Both vasectomy and tubal occlusion are highly effective forms of permanent sterilization. Vasectomies are safer, simpler, and more easily reversed than female sterilization.
- Patients requesting sterilization should be counseled of the permanent and largely irreversible nature of the procedures. The risk of regret is highest among women younger than 30 regardless of their parity.
- The most effective tubal ligations are those done immediately postpartum or those utilizing the Essure tubal occlusion system.
- When interval laparoscopic approach is undertaken, Falope rings have the highest efficacy in women younger than 28 years. Electrocoagulation and Falope rings have equal efficacy in women 28 years and older.
- Essure offers a hysteroscopic approach to tubal ligation and the safest and most effective means of permanent birth control. It does not require a surgical incision or general anesthesia, but it does require use of a backup method for 3 months and an HSG or specialized transvaginal ultrasound to confirm complete tubal occlusion.
- Reversal rates for tubal ligation vary from 41% to 84% depending on the method used for sterilization. These procedures are costly and are associated with a higher rate of ectopic pregnancy.

CLINICAL VIGNETTES

VIGNETTE 1

A 17-year-old G0 F presents to your office for contraceptive counseling. She has never used any method of contraception before and is engaged in a monogamous sexual relationship. Gynecologic history is significant for regular, heavy menstrual cycles using up to eight pads per day, lasting up to 7 days at a time, with severe pain (dysmenorrhea). She smokes one-half pack of cigarettes per day and tells you that her mother and aunt both have Factor V Leiden disease, but that she has never been tested herself nor had a thromboembolic event. She will attend college soon and has no plans for a pregnancy in the near future. She indicates her desire for the "most reliable" method of contraception that you can offer.

1. Which of the following methods of contraception has the least efficacy?
   a. Ortho Evra patch
   b. COC pills
   c. Coitus interruptus
   d. Condoms with spermicide
   e. Levonorgestrel (LNG) IUD

2. Physical examination in the office reveals a blood pressure of 145/90 mm Hg, pulse of 80, and BMI of 40. Abdomen is soft and nontender, and genitourinary examination is unremarkable with no cervical inflammation. Which of the following would be the best choice of contraception for this patient?
   a. LNG IUD
   b. COC pills
   c. Ortho Evra patch
   d. Condoms with spermicide
   e. Coitus interruptus

3. Of course, during your discussion at this visit, you could encourage smoking cessation and recommend weight loss to help improve her overall health. You and the patient have decided to proceed with IUD placement. Prior to placement, it is important to perform which of the following tests?
   a. Follicle-stimulating hormone (FSH) level
   b. Prolactin level
   c. Urine pregnancy test
   d. Gonorrhea/Chlamydia testing
   e. Both c and d

VIGNETTE 2

A 35-year-old F G5P5 has come to your office to discuss long-term contraception. A thorough history and office examination reveal a healthy, thin female, in no acute distress. She reports seasonal allergies and has undergone one cesarean section in the past as well as four spontaneous vaginal deliveries, and no additional surgeries. She has never had an STI and is a nonsmoker. Her Pap smears and human papillomavirus (HPV) screens have all been normal and are up to date. She asks you to explain which methods will be effective for a long period of time, because she has trouble remembering to take a pill daily with five small children at home.

1. You inform her that many methods can be considered "long term," except which of the following?
   a. Tubal Ligation/Occlusion
   b. Etonogestrel rod (Nexplanon)
   c. Copper IUD (ParaGard)
   d. LNG IUD (Mirena, Skyla, Lyletta, and Kyleena)
   e. 1.5 mg LNG pill

2. She chooses to consider the options presented above, and returns 3 weeks later after discussing the methods with her husband. They have decided to undergo permanent sterilization. She is nervous about "going to sleep" under anesthesia as she's had severe nausea from this in the past, and does not want any additional abdominal scars. Which one of the following methods can be performed in the office with local anesthesia and oral pain medication, avoiding the need for general anesthesia?
   a. Falope rings
   b. Filshie clips
   c. Pomeroy method (postpartum tubal)
   d. Essure (microinsert coils)
   e. Bipolar fulguration

3. Once you have performed the chosen procedure (above) in the office, you instruct her that she will need a follow-up test in 3 months to confirm that the coils are in the correct location and that tubal occlusion has been achieved. Which of the following tests is used to confirm complete tubal occlusion?
   a. Transvaginal ultrasound
   b. Flat/upright abdominal X-ray
   c. MRI of pelvis with contrast
   d. CT scan of Pelvis without contrast
   e. Low-pressure modified hysterosalpingogram (HSG)

VIGNETTE 3

A 40-year-old F G3P3 comes to your office to discuss contraception. She has been married for 15 years and smokes one pack of cigarettes per day. She was diagnosed with systemic lupus erythematosus (SLE) at the age of 20 years and has only been hospitalized once for an acute exacerbation of joint swelling and fatigue. Her BMI is 24, and she has light to normal menstrual flow. She has no plans for a future pregnancy, but is not ready to commit to permanent sterilization.

1. You inform her that all of the following are absolute contraindications to COC pill use, except:
   a. History of or current thromboembolism
   b. Coronary artery disease
   c. Tobacco use of greater than or equal to 15 cigarettes/day over the age of 35 years
   d. Abnormal liver function
   e. Diabetes Mellitus

2. Which of the following would *not* be a reasonable method of contraception for this patient?
   a. Ortho Evra patch
   b. Depo-Provera
   c. ParaGard IUD
   d. LNG IUD
   e. Progestin-only oral pill

3. The patient decides to continue using condoms and spermicide. She is aware of the 95% effectiveness when spermicide is used. Several months later, she calls your office 36 hours after having unprotected intercourse and is very concerned about becoming pregnant. You prescribe her Plan B and tell her that it is most effective if taken within 72 hours of the event. What is the most common side effect of Plan B?
   a. Heavy vaginal bleeding
   b. Nausea/vomiting
   c. Fever
   d. Diarrhea
   e. Dizziness

VIGNETTE 4

A 23-year-old F G0 comes to your office to discuss an effective method of contraception. Her only medical condition is endometriosis—diagnosed by laparoscopy 3 years ago. She was placed on oral contraceptives shortly after her laparoscopy and fulguration of endometriosis. Unfortunately, she lost her health insurance after the surgery and was not able to refill the medication. She has not resumed care until now. She has been sexually active with the same partner for 3 years and has monthly menses with moderate flow. She has never had an STI and is not planning to become pregnant in the near future.

1. You tell her that the mechanism of action of oral contraceptives includes:
   a. Thickening of cervical mucous
   b. Making the endometrial environment unsuitable for implantation
   c. Interfering with pulsatile FSH/luteinizing hormone (LH) surges
   d. Suppressing ovulation and follicular recruitment
   e. All of the above

2. She reports severe dysmenorrhea that begins 1 week prior to each menstrual cycle, and is resolved 1 to 2 days after bleeding begins. This pain is only partially relieved with nonsteroidal anti-inflammatory drugs, and she would like to know what can be done to help with this. To reduce dysmenorrhea caused by endometriosis, you instruct her to take COC pills in the following manner:
   a. Continuous dosing—take active pills only for 3 months, then take 1 week of placebo to have withdrawal bleed
   b. Take two active pills each day, can take up to three pills per day if pain becomes severe
   c. Tapered dosing—take four pills for 4 days, then three pills for 3 days, and so on until the pack is complete, then resume from the beginning
   d. Take one pill every other day
   e. Change to a progesterone-only "mini pill" and take one each day

3. You have prescribed the appropriate COC pill regimen to the patient described in the prior question. You now see a 30-year-old F G1P0010 who presents to your office with the diagnosis of menstrual migraines without aura, and otherwise negative workup and medical history. She desires COC pills, and you prescribe the same method of use as you did to the previous patient. Taking COC pills in this manner can be used as treatment for patients with all of these conditions, except which of the following?
   a. Premenstrual syndrome (PMS)
   b. Polycystic ovary syndrome (PCOS)
   c. Ovarian cysts
   d. Endometrial hyperplasia
   e. Menstrual migraines without aura

ANSWERS

VIGNETTE 1 Question 1
1. Answer C:
Coitus interruptus has a significantly high failure rate—up to 27%. Ortho Evra patch has a 1% pregnancy rate with recommended use, which is comparable with that of COC pills. However, actual use of oral contraceptive pills has a failure rate of 8%. Condoms are 85% to 90% efficacious and up to 95% effective with addition of spermicide.

VIGNETTE 1 Question 2
2. Answer A:
The progesterone-only LNG IUDs provide a low maintenance delivery of contraception that can also be useful for the treatment of heavy menstrual bleeding. We have established the patient's family history of thromboembolic disorder, as well as obesity (BMI: 40), hypertensive, and a smoker; therefore, it is prudent to avoid an estrogen-containing method in this patient because of the increased risk of cardiovascular disease, specifically thromboembolic event. Ortho Evra patch and COC pills both contain estrogen. Condoms with spermicide would be a good alternative; however, the patient has requested the "most reliable method." LNG IUDs have a failure rate of less than 0.9%, whereas condoms with spermicide have approximately 5% failure rate. LNG IUDs also confer the added benefit of reduced menstrual flow and treatment of dysmenorrhea. Skyla and Kyleena were specifically developed and targeted to include the nulliparous population. Coitus interruptus is not a reliable method of contraception given its high rate of failure.

VIGNETTE 1 Question 3
3. Answer E:
Urine pregnancy and Gonorrhea/Chlamydia testing should be performed prior to IUD insertion in this patient. Absolute contraindications to IUD insertion include known or suspected pregnancy, undiagnosed abnormal vaginal bleeding, acute cervical/uterine/or salpingeal infection, Copper allergy or Wilson disease (for ParaGard only), or *current* breast cancer (for LNG IUD only). STI testing is indicated in any "high-risk" population (defined as age <25 years or multiple sexual partners). FSH and prolactin level tests are not necessary for this patient, because these are traditionally used in workup of abnormal bleeding and have no bearing on this patient's situation. One additional test that we would recommend to her is Factor V Leiden genetic testing, given her family history.

VIGNETTE 2 Question 1
1. Answer E:
LNG pill (Plan B) is a progestin-only method used for emergency contraception. It is available over-the-counter to those aged 17 years and older and is very effective (up to 97% success rate) when taken within 72 hours of unprotected intercourse. This method is not intended for repeated or long-term use. The Etonogestrel rod (Nexplanon), Copper IUD (ParaGard), and LNG IUD (Mirena/Skyla/Liletta/Kyleena) are all considered "Long-Acting Reversible Contraception" methods (LARCs). Nexplanon, Skyla, and Liletta can be used up to 3 years; Mirena and Kyleena up to 5 years; and ParaGard up to 10 years. Tubal ligation and tubal occlusion are permanent forms of birth control, and patients are counseled that this method is not intended to be reversed.

VIGNETTE 2 Question 2
2. Answer D:
The Essure method was approved by the FDA in 2002 and is widely available in the United States today. It consists of microinsert coils containing flexible metal alloy and induces a mild fibrotic reaction in the tubal lumen, resulting in occlusion. Advantages of this method include the ability to perform the procedure in office, thus avoiding the need for general anesthesia. It is performed transcervically, which confers less risk to adjacent organs, therefore, avoiding the need for abdominal entry (laparoscopy). Falope rings, Filshie clips, and bipolar fulguration are also commonly used methods; however, they require laparoscopic entry into the abdominal peritoneum. The Pomeroy method is

commonly performed at the time of cesarean section or through a small subumbilical incision when immediately following a vaginal delivery. During the immediate postpartum period, the uterus remains enlarged and sits just beneath the umbilicus, making the fallopian tubes accessible through this small incision.

VIGNETTE 2 Question 3
3. Answer E:
HSG is an X-ray (fluoroscopy) of the pelvis during which radiopaque contrast medium is placed via a catheter through the cervix and injected into the endometrial cavity. The course of the contrast is observed, and the tubes are confirmed to be completely occluded if there is no dye spill through the tubes into the peritoneal cavity. This test is also used during an infertility workup to evaluate tubal patency or uterine cavity shape.

Current studies are assessing the ability of ultrasonography to evaluate tubal occlusion following the Essure procedure; however, this method can only demonstrate coil placement, not tubal patency and is not recommended for confirmation of tubal closure at this time in the United States. The microcoils are radiopaque and can be seen on a flat/upright X-ray film; however, this does not tell us about their effectiveness but only location. A CT scan and MRI are not recommended to evaluate success of tubal occlusion. MRI for other diagnostic purposes is safe with Essure coils in place.

It is important that the patients have a reliable method of contraception during the 3 months after placement of the microinserts until a confirmatory test has been performed to verify correct coil location and demonstrate bilateral tubal occlusion.

VIGNETTE 3 Question 1
1. Answer E:
Diabetes mellitus is a relative contraindication to administering COC pills. It is not recommended for use in patients with long-standing or uncontrolled diabetes, especially those with vascular complications (renal and ophthalmologic involvement). A history of venous thromboembolic event is an absolute contraindication, as well as any coronary artery disease, or tobacco use (>15 cigarettes/day) over the age of 35 years. Other absolute contraindications include history of cerebrovascular accident, breast or endometrial cancer, suspected or current pregnancy, and severe hypercholesterolemia or hypertriglyceridemia. SLE is a relative contraindication; COC pills should be used cautiously in this population and avoided when possible. All of these specific conditions and contraceptive recommendations can be referenced in the United States Medical Eligibility Criteria (US MEC) available through the CDC website and an interactive app is available for download.

VIGNETTE 3 Question 2
2. Answer A:
The Ortho Evra patch is a combination contraception patch, and contains both estrogen and progesterone (EE and norelgestromin). A patch is placed on the skin weekly for 3 weeks, then removed for the fourth week at which time a withdrawal bleed should occur. It carries the same risks as oral contraceptives and should not be given to women who are smokers over the age of 35 years, as well as the other absolute contraindications listed in Vignette 3, Question 1. Its primary action is suppression of ovulation by decreasing endogenous FSH and LH levels. It should also not be given in women over 198 lb (or 90 kg). Depo-Provera, LNG IUD, and Progestin-only pills are all non-estrogen–containing methods of contraception. There is a negligible risk of thromboembolism with these methods, and they are often used for those patients who are not candidates for estrogen use. The ParaGard IUD is a Copper T device and is effective in limiting sperm and tubal motility and also creates a "sterile inflammatory environment" within the uterus. It should not be used in women with a history of menorrhagia or unexplained abnormal bleeding. Given her low BMI and no history of depression, Depo-Provera use would also be reasonable.

VIGNETTE 3 Question 3
3. Answer B:
Nausea is present in approximately 50% and vomiting in 20% of patients who take Plan B. These are slightly less severe in those taking Plan B (progestin-only, single dose) versus prior combination methods (Yuzpe method) containing estrogen. Often providers prescribe antiemetics at the same time as EC. Headaches, dizziness, and breast tenderness are also side effects, however, not the most common. There are no significant reports of fever or diarrhea when using EC. The patient should expect her menses to come a couple of days earlier than expected after using ECPs. The Copper IUD is also a method of EC when used up to 5 days after unprotected intercourse.

VIGNETTE 4 Question 1
1. Answer E:
Oral contraceptives have multiple mechanisms of action. Their primary effect is to suppress the mid-cycle surge by interfering with the pulsatile release of FSH and LH from the anterior pituitary, thus preventing follicular maturation and ovulation. The progesterone component works by thickening the cervical mucus, impairing tubal motility, and making the endometrium less suitable for implantation.

VIGNETTE 4 Question 2
2. Answer A:
Of the dosing regimens shown, the most effective would be the continuous method. Women with endometriosis,

PMS, PCOS, ovarian cysts, or menstrual migraines may benefit from extending the number of consecutive days of hormonal pills (up to 1, 2, or 3 months) and decreasing the number of withdrawal bleeds. These extended or long-cycle regimens provide continued suppression of ovulation—reducing the circulating estrogen levels and decreasing the menstrual-related symptoms (i.e., pain, heavy bleeding, anemia, cysts, and/or headaches).

Taking more than one active pill per day for extended periods of time is contraindicated and can lead to thromboembolic events, such as DVT and PEs. This method of dosing is used for very short periods of time in selected circumstances, such as for EC and abnormal uterine bleeding. The tapering method is generally reserved for management of extremely heavy and prolonged bleeding. Again, it is used for a short period of time and only in specific circumstances, not as a routine dosing method. Taking one pill every other day increases the risk of both an endometriosis flare and pregnancy.

Progestins may be effectively used in the treatment of endometriosis. The low dose (0.35 mg) of the progesterone-only contraceptive pills is less effective at suppressing ovulation and maintaining low levels of estrogen compared with COC pills. However, other progesterone-only methods are effective at treating endometriosis, including oral medroxyprogesterone acetate (Provera), depot medroxyprogesterone acetate (Depo-Provera), norethindrone acetate (2.5 to 10 mg), and the LNG IUD (Mirena Skyla, Liletta, Kyleena).

VIGNETTE 4 Question 3
3. Answer D:
Endometrial hyperplasia is an abnormal overgrowth of the endometrial cells, which can ultimately develop into endometrial cancer if left untreated. Most commonly, this is a result of excess estrogen effect with inadequate progesterone balance and is often seen in women with obesity and oligomenorrhea—such as those with PCOS or anovulatory cycles. The treatment for this would be progesterone or surgical treatment but not COCs, because these contain estrogen. Women with PMS, PCOS, ovarian cysts, or menstrual migraines without auras may benefit from extending the number of consecutive days of hormonal pills (up to 1, 2, or 3 months) and decreasing the number of withdrawal bleeds. These extended or long-cycle regimens provide continued suppression of ovulation—reducing the number of new cysts formed and decreasing menstrual-related symptoms (i.e., pain, heavy bleeding, anemia, and headaches).

25 | Termination of Pregnancy

Abortion is a **common procedure** in the United States, with 3 in 10 women having the procedure by the age of 45 years. In the United States, nearly 50% of all pregnancies are unintended and 40% of these **unintended pregnancies** end in abortion. Excluding miscarriages, 22% of all pregnancies are terminated. As such, the availability of safe and effective means of pregnancy termination is an important component of family planning and an integral part of obstetrics and gynecologic care. Of the over 1.2 million abortions performed annually in the United States, approximately 60% are performed on women in their 20s and 35% are obtained by women in their 30s. Those younger than 20 made up 12% of abortion patients representing a 32% decline between 2008 and 2014. About 60% of women undergoing abortions have one or more children and 14% are married. Caucasian women account for 39% of procedures; Black women for 28%; and Hispanic women for 25%; Asian or Pacific islander for 6%. The most common reasons women give for choosing to have an abortion include financial burden, familial obligations, interference with work or school, and desire to avoid single parenting.

The abortion procedures used in the United States are both **safe and effective**. Since the legalization of abortion in 1973, the risk of death from abortion has declined by 85%. The most recent maternal mortality rate for induced abortion in the United States ranges from 0.3 per 100,000 abortions at or <8 weeks of pregnancy to 6 per 100,000 abortions >18 weeks of gestation. This is in comparison to a maternal mortality of 18.5 per 100,000 for completed pregnancy and delivery. The major causes of abortion mortality are complications of **hemorrhage and infection**, followed by thromboembolism and anesthetic complications. In general, maternal morbidity is lowest if abortion is performed before 8 weeks of gestation (Fig. 25-1). Less than 0.05% of abortions performed in the first-trimester result in complications that require hospitalization.

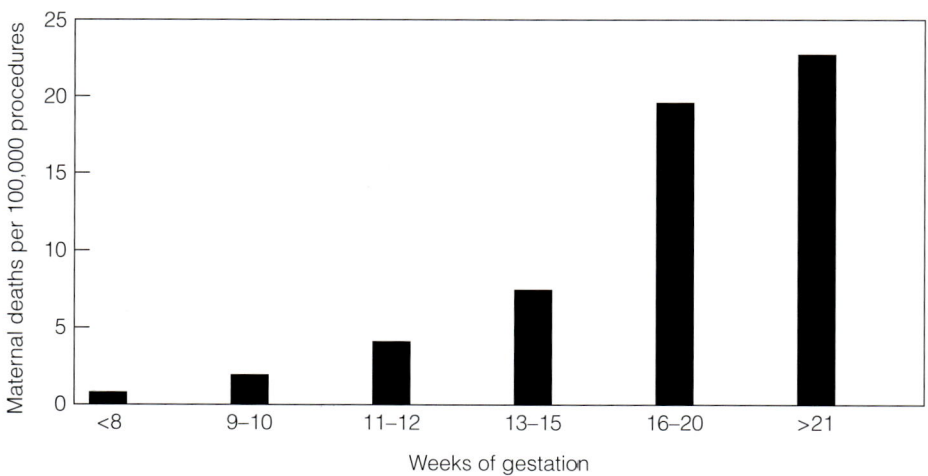

FIGURE 25-1. The effect of gestational age on maternal mortality for legal abortions.

Chapter 25 / Termination of Pregnancy • 407

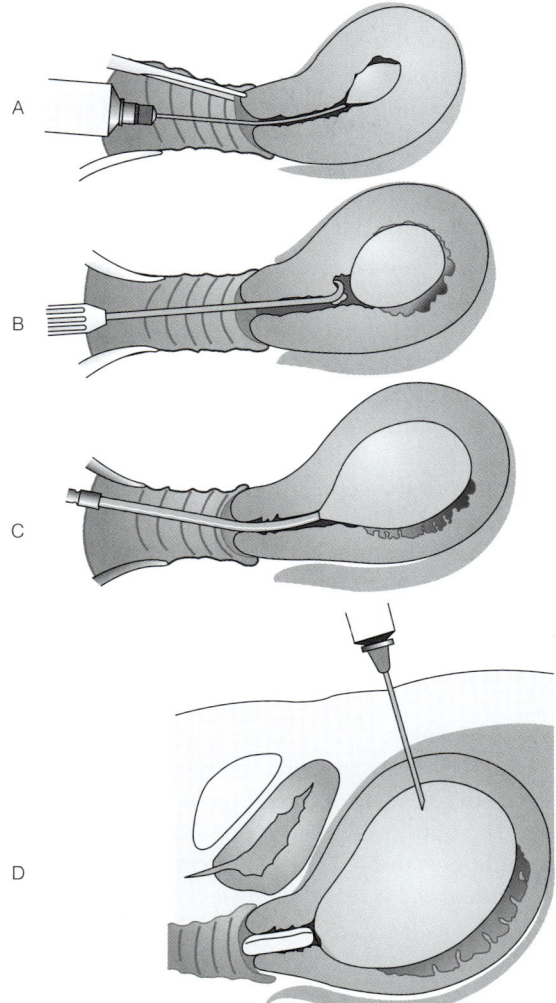

FIGURE 25-2. Various techniques used for termination of pregnancy. (**A**) Manual extraction. (**B**) Sharp curettage. (**C**) Suction dilation and curettage or evacuation. (**D**) Induction of labor by intra-amniotic instillation. (From Pillitteri A. *Maternal and Child Nursing*, 4th ed. Philadelphia, PA: Lippincott Williams & Wilkins; 2003.)

TABLE 25-1. Termination of Pregnancy Options, by Gestational Age
First-trimester terminations
Suction curettage (D&C)
Manual vacuum aspiration
Nonsurgical medication abortion[a]
Misoprostol
Mifepristone plus misoprostol
Methotrexate plus misoprostol
Second-trimester terminations
Surgical evacuation of the uterus (D&E)
Medical induction of labor
Mifepristone followed by misoprostol
Misoprostol
Pitocin
[a]Only used up to 70 days from the last menstrual period.

There are several surgical and medical procedures by which pregnancy termination can be achieved (Fig. 25-2). Evacuation of the uterus is an important technique in the field of obstetrics and gynecology. Not only is it used for elective termination of pregnancy, but it is also an integral part of managing spontaneous abortion, missed abortion, intrauterine fetal demise, retained products of conception (POCs), and gestational trophoblastic neoplasia. Approximately 92% of induced abortions are performed in the first trimester of pregnancy (66% prior to 9 weeks). Approximately, 1% of abortions occur after 21 weeks of gestation.

The options for **first-trimester abortion** include suction dilation and curettage (D&C), manual vacuum aspiration, and nonsurgical medication abortion. **Second-trimester options** include surgical evacuation of the uterus (D&E) and medical induction of labor. In general, the technique used for termination is determined by the duration of the pregnancy, provider experience, and patient preference. Table 25-1 outlines the various options available during the first and second trimesters. Laws vary from state to state, but generally, terminations are legal until viability at about 24 weeks of gestation. After this, abortions are rare owing to lethal fetal or maternal indications. Although second trimester abortions are rare, access to providers is often reported as a barrier that pushes women into having procedures beyond the first trimester. In 2000, 87% of counties in the United States had no access to an abortion provider.

Prior to termination, gestational age should be confirmed by last menstrual period (LMP), bimanual examination, and pelvic ultrasound. All Rh-negative women should receive **RhoGAM** at the time of procedure to prevent isoimmunization. Women should be counseled on reliable forms of contraception with initiation of chosen method, if appropriate. Patients may be offered **sexually transmitted infection (STI) screening** for infections such as gonorrhea and chlamydia at this time as well. Two to four weeks after completion of termination of pregnancy, the routine follow-up includes an assessment of the physical and emotional status of the patient. Clinical, laboratory, or imaging studies can be used as needed to confirm completion of the abortion and address any potential complications. This may also be an opportune time to obtain cervical cytology if the **Pap test** is not up-to-date and to provide indicated immunizations such as the human papillomavirus (HPV), rubella, or influenza vaccines.

FIRST-TRIMESTER OPTIONS

The majority of all abortions are performed before 12 weeks of gestation. Suction curettage either with **electric or manual vacuum aspiration**, and **nonsurgical medication abortions** are all methods of inducing abortion in the first trimester. Most first-trimester terminations in the United States are achieved using the suction curettage (D&C) procedure. However, an increasing number of terminations (23%) are being accomplished by nonsurgical abortions since Food and Drug Administration (FDA) approval (September 2000) of mifepristone (RU 486) for pregnancy termination in the United States. In general, the risk of complications from either surgical or medication management is small and directly proportional to the gestational age.

SUCTION CURETTAGE/MANUAL VACUUM ASPIRATION
Method
Suction curettage is both a safe and effective means of terminating a pregnancy between 6 and 14 weeks of gestation. According to Centers for Disease Control and Prevention (CDC) surveillance data, **D&C is used for 69% of all induced abortions**. D&C typically involves mechanical dilation of the cervix and removal of the POCs using a **suction cannula** (Fig. 25-3). A **sharp curettage** may then be performed if necessary. A D&C is generally performed using a **paracervical block** with a local anesthetic often in conjunction with oral or IV sedation. Less commonly, general or regional anesthesia is used. **Antibiotic prophylaxis** (doxycycline, ofloxacin, ceftriaxone, or metronidazole) is recommended to avoid the risk of postabortal upper genital tract infection.

For early pregnancies up to 12 weeks of gestation, **manual vacuum aspiration** can be performed. This technique involves insertion of a 4- to 12-mm cannula into the cervical os. The uterine contents are then manually extracted using a 50- or 60-mL self-locking vacuum syringe instead of a suction machine. Evacuation is achieved by a gentle in and out motion, while also rotating the unit to ensure clearance of all POCs. Sharp curettage is not performed in this procedure.

Effectiveness
When performed by a trained physician, the **success rate for suction curettage is 99%**. After any type of suction curettage procedure, the POCs should be examined to ensure completion. If the gestational age is less than 6 weeks, verification of

FIGURE 25-3. Suction curettage of uterine cavity for termination of pregnancy.

POCs on pathology report may be helpful. In these early pregnancies, an effort should also be made to identify gestational sac and villi after the procedure by floating the evacuated tissue in saline. If no tissue is identified, or the patient has persistent symptoms, then serial β-hCG levels can be measured to rule out ectopic pregnancy, gestational trophoblastic disease, or an ongoing pregnancy.

Complications

First-trimester termination using suction curettage (D&C) is the **safest of all surgical termination methods**. Complications of suction curettage are rare and include infection (1% to 5%), excessive bleeding (2%), uterine perforation (1%), and incomplete abortion (1%). There is virtually **no risk of long-term complications** from first-trimester induced abortion such as preterm labor, infertility, ectopic pregnancy, or low birth weight. The maternal mortality rate for D&C is 0.3 per 100,000 procedures at 8 weeks of gestation or less.

NONSURGICAL ABORTION

Mifepristone (RU 486)

The FDA approved mifepristone for use in termination of pregnancies in the United States in September 2000. Since that time, medication abortion has become increasingly utilized and now accounts for 23% of terminations prior to 10 weeks of gestation. **Mifepristone (RU 486)** is a synthetic **progesterone receptor antagonist** that binds to progesterone receptors in the uterus, thus blocking the stimulatory effects of progesterone on endometrial growth. Mifepristone thereby disrupts the pregnancy by making the endometrial lining unsuitable to sustain the pregnancy. This leads to detachment of the embryo. Mifepristone can be used up to **70 days from the last menstrual period** (LMP). The success rate of completed pregnancy is greatly improved when used in combination with a **prostaglandin analog** such as misoprostol. This is considered the gold standard for medication termination of pregnancy. The typical protocol used for termination involves a single oral dose (200 mg) of RU 486 followed by a buccal (800 mcg) or vaginal (800 mcg) dose of **misoprostol (Cytotec)** 24 to 72 hours later. Approximately 2 weeks after the procedure, the success of completion is typically confirmed with ultrasound or a serum β-hCG level.

Methotrexate

Methotrexate is a chemotherapeutic agent and **dihydrofolate reductase inhibitor** that works by interfering with DNA synthesis, thereby **preventing placental villi proliferation**. Because methotrexate has been approved for use for a variety of medical conditions including ectopic pregnancy, it has been used by clinicians on an off-label basis as an abortifacient. Like mifepristone, methotrexate is also used with a prostaglandin analog. Methotrexate is contraindicated for patients with immunodeficiency and those with hepatic or renal disease. Methotrexate is administered intramuscularly or orally **within 49 days of the LMP, followed by misoprostol (Cytotec)** 3 to 6 days later. Two weeks after the procedure, the success of completion should be confirmed with ultrasound or a serum β-hCG level.

Misopristol alone can be used to induce medical termination of pregnancy. However, alone it is much less effective (80% to 85%) than in combination with mifepristone or methotrexate.

Effectiveness

When used alone, the efficacy rate of mifepristone is approximately 65% to 85%. However, when given with misoprostol, the **success rate is 92% to 98%**. The efficacy rate of methotrexate with misoprostol for induced abortion is 94% to 96%. Methotrexate is also therapeutic for ectopic pregnancy in 90% to 95% of the cases. The efficacy rates of both mifepristone and methotrexate decline for pregnancies greater than 7 weeks of gestation. Failed medical abortions require suction D&C.

Side Effects

The most common side effects of medication abortion are **abdominal pain** and **vaginal bleeding**. Other side effects include nausea, vomiting, diarrhea, and excessive or prolonged uterine bleeding. The majority of women using misoprostol as a component of medication termination will start bleeding 4 hours after taking the prostaglandin analog. Time required for completion is typically 24 hours. Vaginal bleeding averages 10 to 17 days. The rate of endometritis for medical abortion is lower than that after surgical abortion.

Advantages/Disadvantages

Nonsurgical abortion offers the advantages of being a **highly effective noninvasive** means of termination. Also, it can be achieved on an outpatient basis in the privacy of a home setting. However, in a nonsurgical abortion, the woman must go through the experience of miscarriage, which involves uterine cramping and bleeding. Medication abortion typically requires two visits to a health provider: one to

TABLE 25-2. Contraindications of Medication Abortion

- Pregnancy >70 days from LMP
- Pregnancy with an intrauterine device in place
- Obstruction of the cervical canal
- Ectopic pregnancy
- Gestational trophoblastic disease
- Chronic systemic steroid use, chronic adrenal failure
- Bleeding disorder
- Allergy to mifepristone or misoprostol
- Inability to participate in the procedure

LMP, last menstrual period.

obtain the medication, and then a 2-week follow-up visit. The contraindications of nonsurgical abortion are presented in Table 25-2.

SECOND-TRIMESTER OPTIONS

Second-trimester terminations are performed between **14 and 24 weeks of gestation**. Options for second-trimester termination of pregnancy include **dilation and evacuation (D&E)** and **induction of labor** using systemic or intrauterine installation agents (Table 25-1). When a second-trimester termination is necessary, **D&E is the safest method** of termination of pregnancy. D&E has a lower maternal mortality and morbidity compared with second-trimester induction of labor.

DILATION AND EVACUATION
Method of Action
D&E is the general term used to describe **cervical dilation** and **evacuation of uterine** contents after 14 weeks of gestation. This method of termination is very similar to first-trimester D&C except that wider cervical dilation is required. A combination of forceps, suction, and sharp curettage may be needed to assist in complete evacuation of the uterus, especially after 16 weeks of gestation. This is generally performed using **IV conscious sedation** in combination with a paracervical block. Spinal, epidural, and general anesthesias can also be used.

Typically, D&E involves the **gradual dilation of the cervix** to accommodate the larger volume of uterine contents. Cervical preparation can be achieved with careful manual dilation, osmotic dilators, mifepristone, and/or prostaglandin agents.

Osmotic dilators can be synthetic (Lamicel, Dilapan) or natural (seaweed-based laminaria). These dilators are placed into the cervix 1 to 2 days before the procedure, and gradually dilate and soften the

FIGURE 25-4. Osmotic dilation of the cervix. Multiple laminaria are placed inside the cervix through both the internal and external os. They slowly expand by absorbing moisture from the vagina, thereby dilating the cervix.

cervix as they absorb cervical moisture (Fig. 25-4). Once dilated, a large suction cannula (14 to 16 mm) can be introduced into the uterus to extract the amniotic fluid, fetal tissue, and placenta. At more advanced gestational ages greater than 15 weeks, forceps designed to extract uterine contents are often needed in addition to suction curettage. Upon completion of the procedure, the clinician should verify completion of the procedure by **examining the POCs**. Ultrasound can be used to guide the extraction and to rule out retained POCs.

Effectiveness
When performed by a **highly experienced clinician**, the success rate for second-trimester extraction procedures is 98% to 99%.

Side Effects
Complications from D&E are uncommon but may include cervical laceration, hemorrhage, uterine perforation, infection, and retained tissues. These can be lessened by visual inspection of the fetal parts to ensure complete evacuation of the POCs. For pregnancies at 20 weeks' gestational age and less, D&E has been found to be **safer than induction of labor**.

Advantages/Disadvantages
As a method of second-trimester abortion, D&E offers the advantage of being performed on an outpatient basis, without the need to undergo induction of labor and delivery. Complications from D&E occur

at lower rates than those for induction of labor with intra-amniotic instillation or intravaginal prostaglandin. Some patients may feel that the decreased amount of time for this procedure is advantageous over an induction of labor; however, other patients may feel that the delivery of a nonintact fetus is unacceptable. Perceptions of advantages and disadvantages of these procedures depend greatly on patient preference.

INDUCTION OF LABOR
Method of Action
Termination of a second-trimester pregnancy between 13 and 24 weeks of gestation can also be achieved with **induction of labor**. In the past, installation of intrauterine abortifacient agents, such as hypertonic saline, prostaglandin F2α, or hyperosmolar urea, was a common method of inducing labor for second-trimester terminations. These methods have largely been abandoned for safer methods including D&E or induction of labor. Recommended regimens for termination through induction of labor are 200 mg **mifepristone followed by prostaglandin analogs** such as misoprostol 24 to 48 hours later or by misoprostol alone. Third line for second-trimester induction of labor is **IV Pitocin**. Feticidal agents (intra-amniotic saline or digoxin and intracardiac potassium chloride) can be used in conjunction with prostaglandins to circumvent the possibility of live birth.

Effectiveness
Depending on the regimen used, the success rate for second-trimester abortions using induction of labor is **80% to 85% at 24 hours**.

TABLE 25-3. Complications Associated with Second-Trimester Abortion by Induction of Labor

Complications	Side Effects
Retained placenta	Nausea
Incomplete abortion	Vomiting
Hemorrhage	Diarrhea
Infection	Fever
Cervical laceration	Chills

Side Effects
General complications of induction of labor for termination of pregnancy include retained placenta, uterine rupture, hemorrhage, and infection (Table 25-3). Oral and vaginal prostaglandins alone have a higher incidence of live births and significant gastrointestinal side effects (nausea, vomiting, and diarrhea), whereas instillation agents have a higher rate of retained placenta (13% to 46%). The maternal mortality rate for second-trimester induction of labor is 8 in 100,000 abortions.

Advantages/Disadvantages
Induction of labor is a longer process than D&E. It requires an inpatient admission and can be a multiday process. However, induction of labor allows for the potential delivery of an **intact fetus**. This may be emotionally important for some patients and also facilitates a more comprehensive **postmortem evaluation** of the fetus, particularly when fetal anomalies are involved, and fetopsy is requested.

KEY POINTS

- First-trimester abortion options include suction curettage, manual vacuum aspiration, and medication abortion.
- Suction curettage can be performed anytime during the first trimester but is most effective between 6 and 13 weeks of gestation.
- Complications are rare but can include infection, bleeding, and perforation of the uterus.
- Mifepristone (RU 486) is an abortifacient that blocks progesterone stimulation of the endometrial lining, thus causing detachment of the embryo.
- Methotrexate is a chemotherapeutic agent that blocks dihydrofolate inhibitor that interrupts placental proliferation.
- Both mifepristone and methotrexate are used in combination with a prostaglandin (often misoprostal) and have high efficacy rates (92% to 98%) for medical termination when used within 63 days of the LMP.
- During the second trimester, abortion may be achieved via D&E or induction of labor. D&E has lower maternal mortality and morbidity compared with induction of labor for second-trimester abortions.

- D&E is similar to suction curettage (D&C) but requires wider cervical dilation and special forceps and curettes to assist with the extraction of the larger volume of fetal parts.
- Complications of D&E include cervical laceration, hemorrhage, infection, uterine perforation, and retained tissue.
- Induction of labor techniques most commonly includes cervical ripening with a prostaglandin, and amniotomy along with induction of labor with high-dose oxytocin.
- Complications from induction of labor include retained placenta, hemorrhage, infection, and cervical laceration.
- Maternal morbidity is 4 in 100,000 abortions for D&E and 8 in 100,000 for induction of labor compared with 18.5 in 100,000 for term pregnancy and delivery.

CLINICAL VIGNETTES

VIGNETTE 1

A 36-year-old G3P2002 female presents to a family planning clinic for termination of pregnancy. She states that her last menstrual period (LMP) was 7 weeks ago. She has no significant past medical history and has had two previous full-term vaginal deliveries. She currently smokes over half a pack of cigarettes a day and has mild hypertension that is well controlled. Ultrasound confirms a single intrauterine pregnancy of 7 weeks' gestation. She reports that she is recently divorced and has a new sexual partner. She is not using any kind of contraception.

1. What is the MOST important test for this patient to have prior to her procedure?
   a. Basic metabolic panel
   b. Pulmonary function testing
   c. Rh status
   d. Hematocrit
   e. Gonorrhea and chlamydia screening

2. At 7 weeks gestational age, what methods of termination can be offered to this patient?
   a. Medication abortion
   b. D&C with suction curettage
   c. Manual vacuum aspiration
   d. D&E
   e. a, b, c

3. The patient chooses a medication abortion. She is given mifepristone (RU-486) in the office and counseled to self-administer buccal misoprostol (Cytotec) 24 to 48 hours later. What follow-up is most appropriate for this patient?
   a. No follow-up is needed
   b. She is counseled on signs of complications and instructed to call for an appointment if needed
   c. She is scheduled for 2 weeks to confirm completion of termination via ultrasound or β-hCG
   d. She is scheduled to return weekly for serum β-hCG monitoring until the levels turn negative
   e. She is counseled to return to clinic after her next period

4. The patient is interested in contraception three months later. Which type of contraception would NOT be recommended for her?
   a. Intramuscular medroxyprogesterone
   b. Levonorgestrel intrauterine device (IUD)
   c. Copper-T IUD
   d. Combined oral contraceptive pills
   e. Condoms

VIGNETTE 2

A 19-year-old woman presents to your general practice gynecology office with complaints of irregular menses. She states that she has not had a period for 2 months. Prior to this, her menses have been regular. She complains of nausea and vomiting as well as breast tenderness. She has no significant past medical history. On physical examination, she seems well-appearing, and bimanual examination revealed a slightly enlarged uterus.

1. What is the most helpful test to obtain at this point?
   a. Complete blood count (CBC)
   b. Urine pregnancy test
   c. Serum β-hCG level
   d. Basic metabolic panel
   e. Rapid plasma reagin

2. The patient's pregnancy test is positive. What is the most appropriate way to convey these results?
   a. Congratulate her on becoming a new mother
   b. Have your medical technician inform her the results, so you can continue to see other patients
   c. Tell her that her pregnancy test is positive and ask her how she feels about that

d. Hand her brochures on pregnancy and tell her you are available to answer any questions
e. Leave a message on her voice mail

3. You sit down across from the patient and tell her that her pregnancy test is positive. She is visibly upset. You ask her what her thoughts are regarding this pregnancy, and she states that she is not ready to become a parent. What is the most appropriate next step?
   a. Tell her you do not believe in abortion and that she would be making a mistake to terminate the pregnancy
   b. Present her with her options, which include carrying the pregnancy to term with parenting, adoption, and induced abortion
   c. Give her the number to a local family planning clinic
   d. Tell her you have a nurse who is interested in adoption
   e. Relate a story about your cousin who went through a similar experience

4. After considering all of her options, she chooses to terminate the pregnancy. You refer her to a local family planning clinic. What additional tests could you offer her at this time?
   a. HIV testing
   b. Human Papillomavirus vaccination
   c. Gonorrhea and chlamydia
   d. Rh status
   e. All of the above

VIGNETTE 3

A 24-year-old G2P1001 female is diagnosed with fetal anencephaly, a lethal anomaly, at her first prenatal visit at 16 weeks. She is otherwise healthy. She had a previous term vaginal delivery without complications. She wishes to terminate this pregnancy.

1. Which termination method has the lowest maternal mortality rate at this gestational age?
   a. D&E
   b. Labor induction
   c. Medication abortion
   d. Manual vacuum aspiration
   e. D&C

2. The patient is counseled on the risks and benefits of both D&E and labor induction. She opts for D&E. Which is NOT used for cervical dilation prior to the procedure?
   a. Osmotic dilators
   b. Laminaria
   c. Misoprostol
   d. High-dose IV oxytocin
   e. Foley balloon catheter

3. On the day of the procedure, she would like to talk to you about pain management. What method of pain control do you recommend?
   a. General anesthesia
   b. Spinal anesthesia
   c. IV conscious sedation combined with paracervical block
   d. Paracervical block alone
   e. Oral nonsteroidal anti-inflammatory drugs (NSAIDs) only

4. Postoperatively she does well, and there are no intraoperative complications. Two weeks later, she calls your nurse and says that she is passing large clots and having increased abdominal cramping. What is in your differential diagnosis?
   a. Uterine perforation
   b. Retained products of conception (POCs)
   c. Continuing pregnancy
   d. Postabortal endometritis
   e. b and d

VIGNETTE 4

A 30-year-old G2 P0010 female presents to a family planning clinic for termination of her current pregnancy. She has a remote history of pelvic inflammatory disease. She has had one previous spontaneous miscarriage and no other pregnancies. She states that her LMP was 4 1/2 weeks ago. She complains of left lower quadrant pain, and she has had vaginal spotting over the past few days.

1. What next steps would be appropriate in her evaluation?
   a. Physical examination
   b. Urine pregnancy test
   c. Rh status
   d. Transvaginal ultrasound
   e. All of the above

2. On physical examination, she has mild left lower quadrant tenderness, and her uterus is approximately 5 to 6 weeks in size. She has no rebound, rigidity, or guarding. Urine pregnancy test is positive. She is Rh-positive. Transvaginal ultrasound shows no gestational sac in the uterus and no adnexal masses. What do you recommend next?
   a. You counsel her that she probably has an early intrauterine pregnancy that is too small to be detected on ultrasound and that she should have a medication abortion if she desires
   b. You recommend that she have a suction D&C the same day
   c. You recommend that she have serial serum β-hCG levels starting the same day
   d. You tell her that she has an ectopic pregnancy and needs emergency surgery
   e. You schedule her to come back the next day for repeat ultrasound

3. The patient's serum β-hCG level is 600 mIU/mL. You counsel her on warning signs such as severe abdominal pain and heavy vaginal bleeding for which she should call or go to the emergency room. She returns to the clinic in 72 hours for repeat serum testing, and the level is 1,000. You schedule her to come back to the clinic in 72 hours for repeat serum testing and transvaginal ultrasound. She has an appropriate rise in her pregnancy hormone levels, and transvaginal ultrasound now detects an intrauterine pregnancy at approximately 5 1/2 weeks of gestation. She still desires pregnancy termination. What are her options?
   a. D&C with suction
   b. Manual vacuum aspiration
   c. Medication abortion
   d. D&E
   e. a, b, and c

ANSWERS

VIGNETTE 1 Question 1

1. Answer C:
It is important to determine Rh status prior to an induced abortion. Regardless of the method of termination that is chosen, all Rh-negative women should be given RhoGAM to prevent isoimmunization, which could occur if an Rh-negative woman is exposed to Rh-positive fetal blood cells. Without RhoGAM, this exposure would cause an Rh-negative woman to form antibodies to the Rh factor. Any future pregnancies with a fetus with Rh factor would be at risk for attack by those maternal antibodies. By giving RhoGAM, future pregnancies are protected from the complications of isoimmunization. There is no need to perform a basic metabolic panel or pulmonary function testing. Hematocrit and STI screening are often obtained prior to an induced abortion, but these are not mandated.

VIGNETTE 1 Question 2

2. Answer E:
At this gestational age, the patient is eligible for medication abortion, D&C, or manual vacuum aspiration. D&C with suction curettage is the most common procedure at this gestational age. Medication abortion can be administered up to 63 days of gestation. At clinics that offer options of surgical and medication abortion, she would be counseled on risks and benefits of both options to enable her to make the decision that is the best for her. Manual vacuum aspiration is a type of suction curettage that may be performed up to 10 weeks of gestation. D&E is a procedure that is used for second-trimester procedures greater than 14 weeks of gestation.

VIGNETTE 1 Question 3

3. Answer C:
Most providers prefer to have the patient return in 2 weeks to ensure completion of the abortion. Since 92% to 98% of medication abortions are successful, there will be a small percentage of women who need additional intervention to complete the procedure. It is important to identify those women in a timely fashion, so the answers A and E would not be the best choice. Although it is important to counsel a woman on the signs of complications, a 2-week follow-up appointment would be more appropriate. The correct answer would be D in the absence of an intrauterine pregnancy, when ectopic pregnancy is suspected.

VIGNETTE 1 Question 4

4. Answer D:
Estrogen-containing contraceptives are contraindicated in this patient because she has HTN, is over 35, and smokes >15 cigarettes/day. Any of the other options would be reasonable, but either the Levonorgestrel or Copper IUD would provide the most effective contraception.

VIGNETTE 2 Question 1

1. Answer B:
This patient presents with symptoms of early pregnancy. The most helpful test at this point would be to get a urine pregnancy test, because this would facilitate the most rapid diagnosis; hence, the answer is B. Answer C, serum pregnancy test would also help establish the diagnosis, but it is more expensive and would take more time to get the results. Answers A and E are included in standard prenatal laboratories, but these would not be the most helpful tests at this time prior to the establishment of the diagnosis. Unless her nausea and vomiting is severe, a basic metabolic panel (D) is not warranted.

VIGNETTE 2 Question 2

2. Answer C:
C is the correct answer because the most appropriate and patient-centered way to deliver these results is directly by the clinician and in a nonjudgmental fashion.

Answer A is incorrect because it assumes that the pregnancy is desired. Answer B is incorrect because it has another staff member tell her the results. Answer D is incorrect because the results are not given in a straightforward or sensitive manner. Answer E is incorrect because there is an appropriate way to give patient sensitive results.

VIGNETTE 2 Question 3
3. Answer B:
The correct answer is B. Providing options counseling is important because it presents the patient with all of her options without making assumptions on which decision is the best for her. Answer A imposes personal beliefs on to the patient and is judgmental. Answer C assumes that she has already made a decision. Answer D is inappropriate and unethical because it potentially takes advantage of the patient who is in a vulnerable position. Answer E is incorrect because it does not focus on the patient and her needs, but instead makes the situation about someone else.

VIGNETTE 2 Question 4
4. Answer E:
Although several of these tests would be offered to her prior to her procedure, you could order them prior to her visit and send the results. Offering STI screening, such as HIV and gonorrhea/chlamydia testing, is appropriate because she has had unprotected intercourse and is at risk. CBC would be appropriate because it would be helpful to know if she was anemic prior to any procedure that will induce bleeding. Rh status is important to protect future pregnancies from isoimmunization if she is Rh-negative.

VIGNETTE 3 Question 1
1. Answer A:
The maternal mortality rate for D&E at this gestational age is approximately 4 per 100,000 when compared with 8 per 100,000 for labor induction. Therefore, A is the correct answer. Answer C is incorrect because medication abortions cannot be offered past 63 days of gestation. Manual vacuum aspiration, answer D, is offered up to 10 weeks of gestation. D&C is generally done up to 14 weeks of gestation.

VIGNETTE 3 Question 2
2. Answer D:
D is the correct answer. IV oxytocin is used for labor induction because it stimulates uterine contractions. It is not an agent for cervical ripening. Osmotic dilators, laminaria, misoprostol, and Foley balloon catheters have all been used for cervical ripening to assist with dilation prior to second-trimester D&E. Osmotic dilators and prostaglandins, such as misoprostol (Cytotec), are most typically used.

VIGNETTE 3 Question 3
3. Answer C:
For most women having second-trimester procedures at 16 weeks of gestation, IV conscious sedation combined with a paracervical block would be the most acceptable option. General anesthesia is typically not required in this setting and introduces more risk for the patient. Spinal anesthesia could be offered in the right setting, but most women do not require such an intervention. Paracervical block alone may not be adequate. NSAIDs, although an appropriate component of postoperative pain control, would not be adequate in isolation.

VIGNETTE 3 Question 4
4. Answer E:
Uterine perforation would most likely be diagnosed at the time of the procedure and would be unlikely to cause delayed symptoms 2 weeks out from the procedure. Continuing pregnancy is unlikely, because the tissue should have been examined during the procedure. Retained POCs are a possibility because a small piece of placental tissue can cause delayed bleeding such as this. Intraoperative use of ultrasound assists in decreasing the risk of retained POCs. Postabortal endometritis can cause uterine bleeding and cramping and should be in the differential diagnosis.

VIGNETTE 4 Question 1
1. Answer E:
All of the listed answers would add useful clinical information. A physical examination would give the clinician an indication of the nature of the left lower quadrant pain as well as an estimate of uterine size. A urine pregnancy test could confirm pregnancy. Rh status is not only important because she is seeking termination, but would be important to know because she is having vaginal bleeding in the context of pregnancy. Women who are having threatened miscarriages are given RhoGAM if they are Rh-negative. Transvaginal ultrasound is important to determine location and estimated gestational age of the pregnancy.

VIGNETTE 4 Question 2
2. Answer C:
At this point, this patient has a pregnancy of unknown location. The differential diagnosis includes early intrauterine pregnancy, nonviable intrauterine pregnancy, or ectopic pregnancy. Answer C is correct because serial measurement of the pregnancy hormone level can assist in determining the location of the pregnancy. Early intrauterine pregnancies will cause at least a rise of 50% over 48 to 72 hours in serum β-hCG. Hormone levels that decline or plateau are a concern for nonviable pregnancy or ectopic pregnancy. Medication abortion is not appropriate if there is no

evidence of an intrauterine pregnancy; so A would be incorrect. Answer B would also not be correct for the same reason. Although it is possible that she has an ectopic pregnancy (D), it is not possible to diagnose this from the available data. It would be appropriate to counsel her on warning signs for ectopic pregnancy and miscarriage. Answer E is not correct because a day is not an appropriate interval to detect changes on an ultrasound. The earliest duration for repeating the ultrasound would be in 1 week.

VIGNETTE 4 Question 3

3. Answer E:

At 5 1/2 weeks gestational age, either medication abortion or manual vacuum aspiration is appropriate. Suction D&C is also an option but is more likely to miss the pregnancy at gestations of less than 7 weeks. D&E procedures are not necessary on early first trimester pregnancies.

26 | Infertility and Assisted Reproductive Technologies

Infertility is a complex medical disorder that requires the evaluation and treatment of a couple rather than an individual. **Infertility** is defined as the failure of a couple to conceive after 12 months of unprotected sexual intercourse. If the female partner is 35 years of age or older, evaluation should be initiated after 6 months of unprotected intercourse. In their National Survey of Family Growth, the Centers for Disease Control and Prevention (CDC) found that 7.4 million women in the United States (12% of women) have received infertility services during their lifetime.

Fecundability, or the ability to achieve pregnancy in one menstrual cycle, is a more accurate measurement to evaluate fertility potential. The fecundability of a typical couple who has had unprotected intercourse is approximately 20% to 25% for the first 3 months, followed by 15% during the next 9 months. This means that 60% of couples conceive within 6 months of unprotected intercourse, and 80% to 90% of couples are able to spontaneously conceive within 12 months (Table 26-1). The fecundability of the cohort decreases over time and with increasing maternal age. Distinct from fecundability, fecundity is the probability of achieving a live birth in single cycle. Fecundity will always be lower than fecundability because it factors in miscarriage. For the remaining 10% to 20% of couples who are incapable of conceiving on their own within that time frame, the factors contributing to infertility vary widely.

In couples who underwent evaluation for infertility in 2014, approximately one-third of cases are attributed to female factors, one-third to male factors, and one-third either to a combination of male and female factors or to unexplained causes (Fig. 26-1). After evaluation, 13% of couples will have no identifiable cause for their infertility (Table 26-2). Once the cause of infertility is identified, therapy is aimed at correcting reversible conditions or overcoming irreversible conditions. The overview of infertility evaluation is shown in Figure 26-2.

Since its inception in 1981 in the United States, assisted reproductive technology (ART) has become

TABLE 26-1.	Average Conception Rates for All Couples
Percentage of Couples	**Length of Time Before Conception**
20	Conceive within 1 mo
60	Conceive within 6 mo
75	Conceive within 9 mo
80	Conceive within 12 mo
90	Conceive within 18 mo

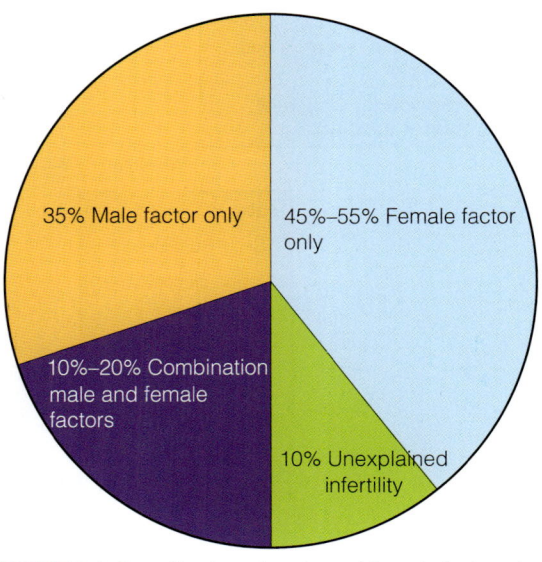

FIGURE 26-1. Contribution of male and female factors to infertility.

TABLE 26-2. Contribution of Various Male and Female Factors to the Incidence of Infertility in 2014

Etiology	Incidence (%)
Male factor	33
Hypothalamic–pituitary disease	2
Testicular disease	35
Post-testicular defects in sperm transport	15
Idiopathic	45
Female factor	45–55
Ovulatory and ovarian factors	47
Peritoneal/tubal factors	13
Endometriosis	9
Uterine and cervical factors	6
Multiple female factors	12
Combined male and female factors	17
Unexplained infertility	13

the most technical and expensive therapeutic intervention to help infertile couples. ARTs involve all therapies in which both sperm and oocytes are handled in vitro for the purpose of increasing the rate of conception. In 2014, 208,604 ART cycles were conducted in the United States, resulting in 57,323 live births (deliveries of one or more living infants) and 70,354 infants. Currently, more than 1% of all births in the United States result from ART procedures (largely in vitro fertilization [IVF]) with an average success rate of 40% depending on the age of the patient, diagnosis, and treatment.

FEMALE FACTOR INFERTILITY

The World Health Organization (WHO) task force on Diagnosis and Treatment of Infertility performed a study of 8,500 infertile couples and found that the most common identifiable female factors were ovulatory/ovarian disorders (32%); fallopian tube

FIGURE 26-2. Algorithm for evaluation and treatment of the infertile couple. 17OHP, 17α-hydroxyprogesterone; LH, luteinizing hormone; TSH, thyroid stimulating hormone; PRL, prolactin; FSH, follicle-stimulating hormone; CCCT, clomiphene citrate challenge test; DHEA-S, dehydroepiandrosterone sulfate; PID, pelvic inflammatory disease. (From Curtis M. *Glass' Office Gynecology*, 6th ed. Philadelphia, PA: Lippincott Williams & Wilkins; 2005.)

TABLE 26-3. Causes of Female Factor Infertility

Ovulatory/Ovarian
Polycystic ovarian syndrome (PCOS)
Advanced maternal age
Primary ovarian insufficiency (POI)
Hypothalamic amenorrhea
Hyperprolactinemia

Tubal factors
Pelvic inflammatory disease/salpingitis
Tubal ligation
Endometriosis
Pelvic adhesions

Uterine factors
Congenital malformations
Fibroids
Uterine polyps
Intrauterine synechiae (Asherman syndrome)

Cervical factors
Müllerian duct abnormalities
Cervical stenosis

OVULATORY/OVARIAN DISORDERS

Disruption in the hypothalamic–pituitary–gonadal axis (HPGA) (Fig. 20-1) at any level can result in menstrual disorders and infertility through impairment of folliculogenesis, ovulation, and endometrial maturation (Table 26-4). The WHO has classified ovulatory disorders into four groups: WHO group 1, hypogonadotropic hypogonadal anovulation (e.g., hypothalamic amenorrhea); WHO group 2, normogonadotropic normoestrogenic anovulation (e.g., polycystic ovarian syndrome [PCOS]); WHO group 3, hypergonadotropic hypoestrogenic anovulation (e.g., primary ovarian insufficiency [POI] and decreased ovarian reserve—the oocyte-related decline in fertility); and WHO group 4, hyperprolactinemic anovulation. The most common ovulatory disorders that lead to infertility are PCOS and decreased ovarian reserve.

Oocyte aging is an important factor affecting female fertility. During fetal life, the ovary contains the greatest number of germ cells, approximately 6 to 7 million in mid gestation. The germ cell population then begins an exponential decline through gene-mediated apoptosis, numbering 1 to 2 million at birth and 300,000 at the onset of puberty (Fig. 26-4). The number of viable follicles continues to decline throughout the reproductive years, and the rate of loss accelerates after the mid-30s. At the time of

abnormalities, including pelvic adhesions (34%); and endometriosis (15%). Other factors that cause infertility include uterine factors and genetic disorders (Table 26-3 and Fig. 26-3).

FIGURE 26-3. Causes of female factor infertility.

TABLE 26-4. Causes of Anovulatory Infertility
Central
Pituitary insufficiency (trauma, tumor, congenital)
Hypothalamic insufficiency
Hyperprolactinemia (drug, tumor, empty sella)
Peripheral defects
Gonadal dysgenesis
Primary ovarian insufficiency (POI)
Ovarian tumor
Insulin resistance
Metabolic disease
Polycystic ovarian syndrome (chronic hyperandrogenemic anovulation)
Thyroid disease
Liver disease
Obesity
Androgen excess (adrenal, neoplastic)

menopause, the ovary contains fewer than 1,000 follicles. Factors that can lead to **decreased ovarian reserve** include tobacco smoking, viruses, radiation and chemotherapy, and autoimmune and genetic disorders. When the store of oocytes decreases to the point where a woman undergoes menopause before the age of 40 years, the diagnosis is POI, formerly known as premature ovarian failure (POF).

The **age-related decrease in fecundability** is due to both the decline of quantity and quality of the oocytes. It is generally accepted that oocyte age is the single most important factor affecting the probability of success with ART. The live birth rates for nulliparous women undergoing ART using fresh non-donor eggs exponentially decline after 35 years of age. However, if donor eggs are utilized, the live birth rate is determined by the age of the donor (Fig. 26-5). The age-related decrease in fertility is mostly due to the corresponding increase in the rate of aneuploidy.

FIGURE 26-4. The number of oocytes in the ovary before and after birth and through menopause. (From Berek JS. *Berek & Novak's Gynecology*, 14th ed. Philadelphia, PA: Lippincott Williams & Wilkins; 2006.)

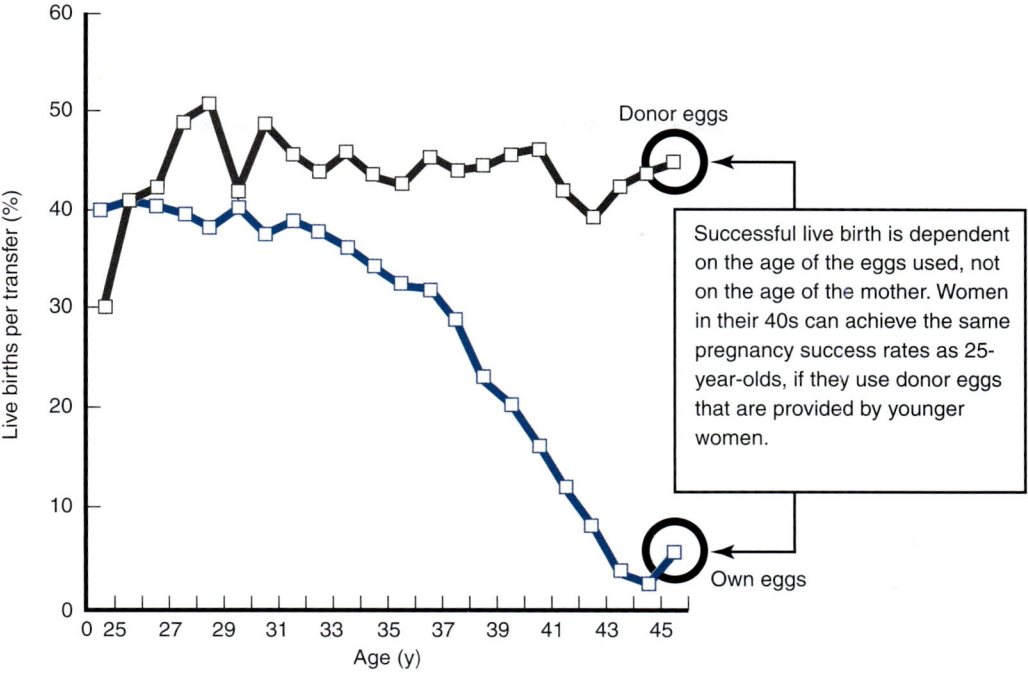

FIGURE 26-5. Live births per embryo transfer comparing use of a patient's own versus donor oocytes. (From Berek JS. *Berek & Novak's Gynecology*, 14th ed. Philadelphia, PA: Lippincott Williams & Wilkins; 2006.)

PCOS is the most common cause of oligo-ovulation and anovulation among all women and those presenting with infertility (Chapters 21 and 23). The diagnostic criteria of this syndrome have been avidly debated ever since it was first described by Stein and Leventhal in 1935. In general, most clinicians use the **Rotterdam Criteria to diagnose PCOS**. The criteria require a patient to have two of the following three findings once other causes of anovulation are ruled out: (1) menstrual irregularity caused by oligo-ovulation or anovulation, (2) clinical or biochemical evidence of hyperandrogenism (hirsutism, acne, male pattern balding, or elevated serum androgen concentrations), and/or (3) the presence of polycystic appearing ovaries.

The prevalence of PCOS in reproductive-age women in the United States is 6.5% to 8%. Risk factors include obesity, insulin resistance, diabetes, premature adrenarche, and a positive family history of PCOS among first-degree relatives.

PCOS is a complex disorder with a multifactorial etiology where multiple genetic variants and environmental factors interact, resulting in several related phenotypes. Suspected genetic variants include genes that are responsible for the regulation of gonadotropin, androgen, or insulin secretion and action (Fig. 26-6). These genetic polymorphisms interplay with diet and obesity. The end result is **hyperinsulinemia**, which contributes to hyperandrogenism by stimulating androgen biosynthesis in the ovary and decreasing the circulating level of sex hormone–binding globulin. **Hyperandrogenism** then leads to disruption of the HPGA manifest by infrequent or absent menses due to chronic anovulation.

TUBAL FACTORS

Tubal disease and pelvic adhesions (Fig. 22-2) result in infertility by preventing the transport of the oocyte and sperm through the fallopian tube (Fig. 26-7). The primary cause of tubal factor infertility is **pelvic inflammatory disease** (PID; Chapter 17). In countries where infection by gonorrhea and *Chlamydia* is increasing and treatment is limited, tubal factor infertility is on the rise. Other conditions that can interfere with normal tubal transport include severe endometriosis, history of ectopic pregnancy, and pelvic adhesions from previous surgery or nongynecologic infection, such as appendicitis or diverticulitis.

ENDOMETRIOSIS

Although the true prevalence of endometriosis is unknown, it is believed that approximately 10-15% of infertile women have endometriosis. Endometriosis is the presence of endometrial cells outside

FIGURE 26-6. A proposed mechanism for polycystic ovarian syndrome. LH, luteinizing hormone; LRH, luteinizing releasing hormone. (From Beckmann C, Ling F. *Obstetrics & Gynecology*, 5th ed. Philadelphia, PA: Lippincott Williams & Wilkins; 2006.)

the uterine cavity (Chapter 15). It can invade local tissues and cause severe inflammation and adhesions (Fig. 22-2 and Fig. 26-3).

Although the presence of endometriosis has been associated with an increased risk of infertility, the exact mechanism is not understood. Endometriosis can interfere with tubal mobility, cause tubal obstruction, or result in tubal or ovarian adhesions that contribute to infertility by holding the fallopian tube away from the ovary, obstructing the tube, or by trapping the released oocyte. However, infertility has also been diagnosed in women with minimal endometriosis and minimal to no adhesive disease. It is thought that endometriosis may stimulate the production of inflammatory mediators, which impair ovulation, fertilization, and/or implantation.

UTERINE AND CERVICAL FACTORS

Uterine and cervical factors account for less than 10% of female factor infertility cases (Table 26-2). Varying **uterine conditions** can contribute to infertility, such as submucosal fibroids, polyps, intrauterine synechiae, and congenital malformations (especially uterine septums) (Table 26-3). Similarly, endometrial abnormalities, such as hyperplasia, out-of-phase endometrium, and carcinoma, can cause infertility. These factors may distort the uterine cavity, prevent implantation, or affect endometrial development.

Risk factors for uterine factor infertility include conditions that predispose to intrauterine adhesions, such as history of PID, infection after pregnancy loss, and multiple curettages of the uterus. **Diethylstilbestrol (DES) exposure in utero** also increases uterine factor infertility (Table 26-3 and Fig. 14-3). DES was banned by the FDA in the United States in 1971. Although there was some minimal use after that date, the majority of women who had the potential for in utero exposure to DES have largely moved beyond the age of childbearing.

Cervical problems can contribute to infertility in the form of structural abnormalities of the cervix, cervicitis, and abnormal cervical mucus production. Cervical stenosis may be iatrogenic and may result from cervical scarring after loop electrocautery excision procedure (LEEP) conization, mechanical dilations (e.g., cervical dilation for miscarriage, termination of pregnancy, or hysteroscopy), and from extensive laser or cauterization of the cervix. These procedures may result in stenosis as well as destruction of the endocervical epithelium, leading to inadequate mucus production. Normal mid-cycle cervical mucus facilitates the transport of sperm into the endometrial cavity. Disruptions in normal mucus production can thereby lead to difficulty in conceiving.

OTHER FACTORS

Luteal phase defect is a controversial and poorly understood disorder. The defect may possibly begin with disruption of the HPGA (Fig. 20-1), resulting in inadequate production of progesterone by the

FIGURE 26-7. Hysterosalpingograms showing (**A**) normal uterine cavity and patent tubes, (**B**) bilateral hydrosalpinx, and (**C**) bilateral tubal occlusion. (From Beckmann C, Ling F. *Obstetrics & Gynecology*, 5th ed. Philadelphia, PA: Lippincott Williams & Wilkins; 2006.)

corpus luteum and subsequent delay in endometrial maturation. This results in impaired implantation following fertilization.

For couples in whom no other cause of infertility can be determined, infertility may be due to genetic abnormalities (trisomies, mosaics, translocations, etc.). **The most common aneuploidy associated with female infertility is 45X (Turner syndrome).**

Clinical Manifestations

History
The evaluation should begin with a thorough medical history, including a menstrual history (Fig. 26-2).

The physician should guide the interview systematically while looking for symptoms related to ovulatory/ovarian, tubal, uterine, and cervical factors, which can lead to infertility.

Patients with ovulatory dysfunction may report amenorrhea, oligomenorrhea, or menorrhagia. Additional questioning should elicit symptoms related to PCOS, thyroid dysfunction, hyperprolactinemia, and primary ovarian insufficiency. Patients with PCOS may report hirsutism, irregular menses, and/or weight changes. A detailed social history might reveal reasons for centrally mediated ovulatory dysfunction, including eating disorders, extreme exercise, or unusual stress.

Women with endometriosis often give a history of cyclic pelvic pain, dysmenorrhea, and/or dyspareunia. Pelvic adhesions may be asymptomatic or may be associated with varying degrees of pelvic pain, especially with movement or lifting.

The clinical presentation of uterine factor infertility varies with the etiology. For many of these factors, infertility may be the only symptom. Among the most common causes, endometritis may present with pelvic pain and fever, and submucosal fibroids and polyps may present with abnormal uterine bleeding. Uterine anomalies, such as uterine septum, may present with a history of recurrent pregnancy loss, cyclic pelvic pain, and/or abnormal uterine bleeding. Cervical factor infertility may present with a history of prior cryotherapy, conization, and/or cervical dilations.

Physical Examination
A physical examination should be performed to look for signs that may point toward a disorder associated with infertility. Careful evaluation may uncover signs of PCOS, such as acne, hirsutism, acanthosis nigricans (Fig. 26-8), skin tags, and central obesity (BMI > 27). Similar care should be taken while evaluating for thyroid dysfunction (goiter, changes in hair/nails, body habitus, and tachycardia). The examination should also look for breast development as a sign of past estrogen exposure.

When performing a pelvic examination, POI might present with signs of estrogen deficiency, such as vaginal atrophy. Visualization of the cervix may demonstrate cervical stenosis, signs of infection, or malformations. The findings associated with endometriosis or pelvic adhesions include a fixed or retroverted uterus, uterosacral nodularity, or tender fixed adnexa. With pelvic adhesions, the pain can sometimes be reproduced on abdominal or pelvic exam. Uterine size should be evaluated, and the physician should look for fibroids and any signs

FIGURE 26-8. Acanthosis nigricans associated with insulin resistance. (From Berek JS. *Berek and Novak's Gynecology*, 14th ed. Philadelphia, PA: Lippincott, Williams & Wilkins; 2006.)

of current or prior pelvic infection. Endometriomas and other ovarian pathology may be palpated during the pelvic examination.

Diagnostic Evaluation

The primary tests for the evaluation of ovulatory factor infertility (Fig. 26-2) involve looking for evidence of ovulation by tracking the menstrual cycle, measuring the basal body temperature (Fig. 24-1), monitoring the cervical mucus, and measuring the mid-luteal **progesterone (days 21 to 23)**. Over-the-counter **ovulation prediction kits** have made predicting the presence and timing of ovulation much easier and have largely replaced daily basal body temperature monitoring.

As it is common for women to delay childbearing, an **assessment of ovarian reserve** has become an important topic in fertility. This can also be especially useful in women over 30 years of age, and those with a history of prior ovarian surgery, one ovary, prior chemotherapy or radiation exposure and women who have had a poor response to ovulation induction (OI).

Traditionally, a **clomiphene citrate challenge test (CCCT)** can be used to assess for decreased ovarian reserve—the oocyte-related decline in fertility. The test involves administration of 100 mg of clomiphene citrate (Clomid) on days 5 through 9 of the menstrual cycle. The follicle-stimulating hormone (FSH) level is measured on days 3 and 10. Even small elevations in FSH levels correlate with decreased fecundity. However, the CCCT has largely been replaced by the use of basal FSH/estradiol testing, the antral follicle count (AFC), and the anti-mullërian hormone (AMH) assay.

Measurement of a **day 3 FSH level** is based on the notion that women with good ovarian reserve will make enough ovarian hormone early in the menstrual cycle to provide inhibition of FSH, thus keeping it at a low level. Comparatively, women with poor ovarian reserve will have insufficient ovarian hormone production early in the cycle. This insufficiency results in a reflexive increase in FSH level. In general, a day 3 FSH value less than 10 mIU/mL is indicative of adequate ovarian reserve; 10 to 15 mIU/mL is borderline ovarian reserve, and greater than 20 mIU/mL is indicative of poor ovarian reserve. The greatest value is the correlation between abnormally high levels (>20 mIU/mL) and an inability to conceive using the patient's own eggs. In these cases, the use of donor oocytes will likely be needed.

Measurement of the **day 3 estradiol level** may also be used to assess ovarian reserve by looking for elevated basal rates of estradiol. This may be indicative of premature follicle recruitment that can occur in women with poor ovarian reserve. Thus, a higher day 3 estradiol level (>80 pg/mL) is suggestive of diminished reserve, whereas a lower level (<80 pg/mL) is suggestive of adequate ovarian capacity.

Measurement of the **antral follicle count (AFC)** can also be used to assess ovarian reserve. This ultrasound test measures the number of antral follicles (2 to 10 mm in diameter) present between days 2 and 4 of the menstrual cycle. In general, the presence of 4 to 10 antral follicles is a sign of good ovarian reserve, whereas lower follicle numbers suggest poor reserve. Most recently, measurement of **anti-mullërian hormone (AMH)** has been used in predicting ovarian reserve. It is based on measurement of AMH from the primordial follicle pool. When the pool is robust, a high level of AMH is detected. As women age and the pool declines, a lower amount is found. An AMH level of greater than 0.5 ng/mL is considered adequate ovarian reserve, whereas levels less than 0.15 ng/mL are suggestive of a reduced follicle pool and decreased pregnancy rates.

Endocrine evaluation may include measurements of FSH, luteinizing hormone (LH), prolactin, thyroid function tests (TFTs), and thyroid antibodies. If Cushing syndrome is suspected, serum testosterone, dehydroepiandrosterone sulfate (DHEA-S), 17-hydroxyprogesterone, 24-hour urine cortisol levels, and an overnight dexamethasone suppression test are helpful. When intracranial lesions are suspected, MRI or CT imaging of the head should be done.

Endometriosis or pelvic adhesions may be strongly suspected based on the patient's history, but direct visualization with laparoscopy or laparotomy is necessary to confirm the diagnosis. Ovarian endometriomas (cystic collections of endometrial cells on the ovaries) can be diagnosed on pelvic ultrasound (Fig. 15-3).

Tubal patency can be demonstrated with a **hysterosalpingogram (HSG)** performed during the follicular phase (Fig. 26-7) or tubal lavage (chromopertubation) performed during laparoscopy. An HSG can also aid in the search for structural abnormalities in the endometrial cavity. This involves installation of a contrast dye transcervically to evaluate for filling defects in the cavity and to test for tubal patency.

Pelvic ultrasound is one of the primary investigative tools for evaluating the female reproductive tract for structural defects, such as fibroids, polyps, adenomyosis, ovarian cysts, and congenital anomalies. A saline sonohysterogram can complement the pelvic ultrasound by allowing better visualization of the intrauterine cavity. This is accomplished by transcervical infusion of saline into the cavity to separate the uterine walls while ultrasound examination of the uterus is being performed.

Hysteroscopy in the office or in the operating room may be used to directly visualize the endocervical canal and endometrial cavity. MRI can also be useful in better delineation of adenomyosis, leiomyomas, and uterine anomalies.

A Pap test and cervical cultures for gonorrhea and *Chlamydia* should be performed in all women undergoing an infertility evaluation because cervicitis and cervical dysplasia are often asymptomatic. Other evaluative tests, including the postcoital test, endometrial biopsy, basal body temperature measurements, karyotyping, and mycoplasma cultures, have not been found to have any value in the evaluation of infertility and are no longer routinely used.

Treatment

The underlying etiology of infertility should be identified and corrected when possible. For uncorrectable cases, OI with fertility drugs, intrauterine insemination (IUI) with sperm, or IVF can be used.

Regular ovulation can be restored in 90% of infertility cases that are due to endocrine factors by treating the underlying disorder. The most common etiology of ovulatory infertility is PCOS. For these patients, weight loss, metformin, and OI with clomiphene citrate (Clomid) or letrozole (Femara) have been effective in establishing ovulation and producing viable pregnancies. In PCOS patients, even small amounts of weight loss (5% of initial weight) can result in lowered fasting insulin, testosterone, and androstenedione levels and in restoration of spontaneous ovulation.

Metformin (Glucophage) is an oral biguanide typically used for the treatment of non–insulin-dependent diabetes mellitus. This insulin sensitizer results in inhibition of gluconeogenesis and increased peripheral glucose uptake. PCOS patients using metformin experience a decrease in fasting insulin levels and testosterone levels. These improvements can help promote the reestablishment of spontaneous ovulation in PCOS patients.

If spontaneous ovulation cannot be established, **ovulation induction** can be utilized to stimulate ovulation (Table 26-5). Of these medications, the most frequently used are Clomid and letrozole (Femara). If these treatments are unsuccessful, OI and pregnancy can be attempted with a combination of Clomid, letrozole, or human gonadotropins with IUI or IVF.

For patients with hypothalamic–pituitary failure (WHO group 1), ovulation can usually be achieved with pulsatile gonadotropin-releasing hormone (GnRH) therapy or human gonadotropins (Table 26-5). Of note, there is no treatment for WHO group 3 patients with POI because these patients lack viable oocytes. Patients with this diagnosis should be offered the options of egg donation, gestational surrogacy, or adoption.

Symptomatic relief of endometriosis can be achieved medically or surgically. However, **there is no role for medical management in the treatment of infertility caused by endometriosis**. Medical treatments, such as Danazol, Lupron, oral medroxyprogesterone (Provera), or continuous oral contraceptives, can temporarily relieve symptoms but do not increase fertility rates.

For patients with endometriosis, fertility rates can be improved by surgical ligation of periadnexal adhesions and excision, coagulation, vaporization,

TABLE 26-5. Medications Used in the Treatment of Infertility and in Assisted Reproductive Technologies

Commercial Name	Generic Name	Mechanism
Clomid Serophene	Clomiphene citrate	Antiestrogen, stimulates follicular development for ovulation induction
Glucophage	Metformin	Inhibits gluconeogenesis; insulin sensitizer; decreases glucose levels and insulin levels to a lesser extent; decreases body weight; promotes ovulation
Novarel Pregnyl Ovidrel	Human chorionic gonadotropin	Similar structure to LH, triggers ovulation after gonadotropin follicle stimulation
Lutrepulse Factrel	Pulsatile GnRH/ gonadorelin	GnRH agonist, stimulates release of FSH/LH from pituitary
Femara	Letrozole	Aromatase inhibitor, blocks androgen conversion to estrogen, stimulates follicular development for ovulatory induction

BMI, body mass index; GnRH, gonadotropin-releasing hormone; FSH, follicle-stimulating hormone; LH, luteinizing hormone.

or fulguration of endometrial implants typically via laparoscopy. Pregnancy rates after surgical treatment depend on the extent of the disease, but increased fertility through spontaneous conception and IVF has been demonstrated after surgical treatment of mild, moderate, and severe endometriosis.

Microsurgical tuboplasty with tubal reanastomosis or neosalpingostomy has proven to be effective for treating tubal occlusion caused by prior infection or from prior tubal ligation. However, because it is more effective, most couples undergo IVF rather than tuboplasty. The advantage of tuboplasty is that it allows for more than one future pregnancy without the cost and need for additional IVF cycles. When hydrosalpinges (fallopian tubes filled with fluid) result from infection or injury, reproductive endocrinologists will often remove the damaged tube(s) and use IVF to treat the patient. Removing the damaged tubes increases the likelihood of both successful IVF and a healthy pregnancy.

Operative hysteroscopy is used to treat uterine factors, such as uterine synechiae, septae, polyps, or submucosal fibroids. Following surgical ligation of synechiae or septae, estrogen therapy or intrauterine devices are often used to prevent recurrence of adhesions. Fertility is restored in 50% of these cases. Most surgeons reserve myomectomy for treatment after recurrent pregnancy loss or when symptomatic fibroids have been identified.

Treatment of cervical factor infertility varies with the cause. Cervical stenosis can often be treated with surgical or mechanical dilation of the endocervical canal. Both cervical stenosis and abnormal cervical mucus can be treated by bypassing the cervix with intrauterine insemination (IUI) (Fig. 26-9).

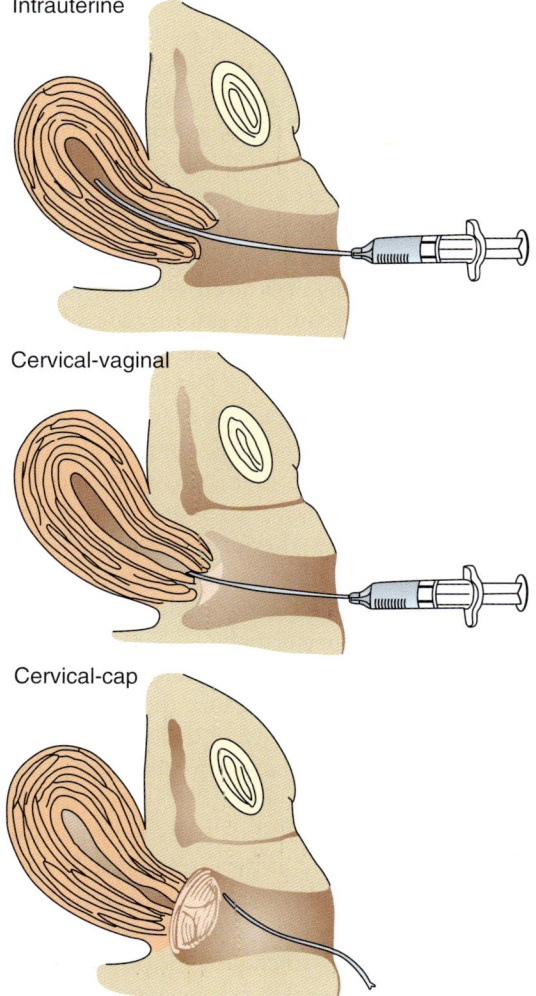

FIGURE 26-9. Techniques of artificial insemination. (From Beckmann C, Ling F. *Obstetrics & Gynecology*, 5th ed. Philadelphia, PA: Lippincott Williams & Wilkins; 2006.)

IUI appears to be the most effective treatment for cervical factor infertility. In cases that are refractory to other treatments, patients should be offered IVF.

MALE FACTOR INFERTILITY

PATHOGENESIS

There are multiple causes of male factor infertility (Table 26-6), including endocrine disorders, anatomic defects, problems with abnormal sperm production and motility, as well as sexual dysfunction. **Varicocele is the most common reversible cause of male factor infertility;** comprising 30% to 40% of infertility in men.

EPIDEMIOLOGY

Thirty-three percent of infertility in 2014 was contributed to male factors (Fig. 26-1). Of couples undergoing infertility evaluation in 2014, 17% were affected by a combination of male and female factors. It is imperative, therefore, that evaluation of the male be done concurrently with evaluation of the female.

TABLE 26-6. Common Etiologies of Male Factor Infertility

Abnormal semen
Cryptorchidism (congenital)
Mumps orchitis
Antisperm antibodies
Endocrine disorders
Hypogonadotropic hypogonadism
Thyroid disease
Environmental exposures
Radiation
Heat
Chemicals
Genetic
Klinefelter syndrome
Immobile cilia syndrome
Cystic fibrosis
Sexual dysfunction
Erectile dysfunction
Ejaculation failure
Retrograde ejaculation
Structural factors
Varicocele
Testicular torsion
Vasectomy
Unexplained
No identifiable cause
Idiopathic abnormal semen

TABLE 26-7. Drugs that Decrease Semen Quality and Quantity

Medications		Exogenous Exposures
Cimetidine	Metoclopramide	Anabolic steroids
Sulfasalazine	Chemotherapeutic agents	Marijuana
Spironolactone	β Blockers	Alcohol abuse
Antidepressants	Nitrofurans	Heroin/cocaine abuse

RISK FACTORS

Men with occupational or environmental exposure to chemicals, radiation, or excessive heat are at increased risk for infertility, as are those with a history of varicocele, mumps, hernia repair, pituitary tumor, marijuana use, anabolic steroid use, testicular injury, and impotence. Certain medications have also been found to depress semen quantity and quality, cause erectile dysfunction, or result in ejaculation failure (Table 26-7).

CLINICAL MANIFESTATIONS

History

The physician should ask about previous pregnancies fathered by the patient; sexual functioning; environmental exposures; medications; recreational drugs; and any history of sexually transmitted infections (STIs), mumps orchitis, hernia repair, and surgery or trauma to the genitals.

Physical Examination

The physical examination for suspected or confirmed male infertility is typically performed by a urologist and includes identification of the urethral meatus; measurement of testicular size; and a search for signs of varicocele, hernias, and congenital absence of a testicle or the vas deferens. Testosterone deficiency may be evidenced by increased body fat; decreased muscle mass; loss of pubic, axillary, and facial hair; decreased skin oil and fine facial wrinkles.

DIAGNOSTIC EVALUATION

A **semen analysis** is the primary investigative tool for male factor infertility. The semen sample is analyzed for sperm count, volume, motility, morphology, pH, and white blood cell count (Table 26-8). In the

TABLE 26-8.	Semen Analysis Normal Parameters
Volume	>2.0 mL
pH	7.2–7.8
Concentration	>20 million/mL
Morphology	>30% normal forms
Motility	>50% with forward progression
WBC	<1 million/mL

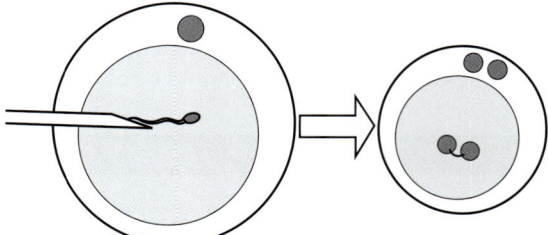

FIGURE 26-10. Intracytoplasmic sperm injection (ICSI). A spermatid or spermatozoon is collected by ejaculation or aspiration from the epididymus or testis. One sperm is injected directly into each harvested egg. The embryos are then transferred back into the uterine cavity via in vitro fertilization.

case of an abnormal semen analysis, an **endocrine evaluation** should include testosterone, prolactin, LH, and FSH (to assess for parenchymal damage to testes and hypogonadism). In cases of azoospermia (absence of sperm in the semen), a karyotype and a Y-chromosome microdeletion genetic testing should be ordered.

The postcoital test is *rarely performed* but can be used to examine the interaction between the sperm and the cervical mucus. An abnormal postcoital test, sperm agglutination, and reduced sperm motility may be suggestive of the presence of antisperm antibodies. Several tests are presently available to detect such antibodies.

TREATMENT

In general, the probability of conception can be enhanced by improvements in coital practice. This includes having intercourse every other day near ovulation. Men should avoid the use of tight underwear; saunas and hot tubs; and unnecessary environmental exposures, such as radiation, excess heat, and medications that decrease semen quality or quantity (Table 26-7).

Treatment of male factor infertility depends on the etiology. Hypothalamic–pituitary failure can be treated with injections of human menopausal gonadotropins (hMGs), and varicoceles can be repaired by ligation.

ARTs can be used to overcome an abnormal semen analysis, when treating the underlying disorder is not effective. Low semen volume, low sperm density, and low sperm motility are most often treated by washed sperm for IUI (Fig. 26-9).

In cases with severe male factor, intracytoplasmic sperm injection (ICSI) can be used. ICSI is another option for patients with low sperm density or impaired motility and has revolutionized the treatment of male factor infertility (Fig. 26-10). This method involves individually injecting a single sperm directly into an egg, to help achieve fertilization. The sperm can be retrieved from the male by ejaculation, or by direct aspiration from the testis (testicular sperm extraction [TSE]) or epididymis either microscopically (microsurgical epididymal sperm aspiration [MESA]) or percutaneously (PESA).

In cases of absolute male factor infertility, that is, when no sperm is available, artificial insemination with donor sperm is highly effective.

UNEXPLAINED INFERTILITY

Among those couples who complete an initial assessment, as many as 25% find no cause for their infertility and are diagnosed with unexplained infertility (Fig. 26-1). When the initial infertility evaluation reveals no cause, the problem often involves abnormalities in sperm transport, the presence of antisperm antibodies, or problems with penetration and fertilization of the egg. When problems in sperm transport, motility, or functional capacity are identified, IVF and ICSI may be used for treatment. If this fails, the use of donor sperm may result in pregnancy.

When no cause for infertility is identified after in-depth testing, studies show that **most therapies for unexplained infertility have no higher success rates than no treatment at all**. Although some patients with unexplained infertility may undergo three to six cycles of gonadotropin stimulation with IUI followed by IVF cycles, many opt for no treatment. The eventual pregnancy rate for couples with unexplained infertility who receive no treatment approaches 60% over 3 to 5 years. Other options include use of donor sperm, gestational surrogacy, adoption, or acceptance of childlessness.

ASSISTED REPRODUCTIVE TECHNOLOGIES

Since their inception, the treatment of infertility with ARTs has progressed rapidly and now includes not only fertility drugs that stimulate multiple follicular development but also technologies that combine OI agents with IUI, IVF, or ICSI. Oocytes may also be obtained via natural, nonstimulated cycles, but the number of eggs per cycle is increased by OI. About 85% to 90% of infertility cases can be treated with drug therapy or surgery. Less than 3% require advanced reproductive technologies like IVF.

OVULATION INDUCTION

Clomiphene citrate (Clomid) is a selective estrogen receptor modulator (SERM) that competitively binds to estrogen receptors in the hypothalamus. In doing so, it blocks the negative feedback effect of endogenous estrogen. This results in increased pulsatile GnRH frequency. Subsequently, FSH and LH production is increased, leading to follicular growth and ovulation (Table 26-5). Clomid is generally administered orally to women with absent or infrequent ovulation, starting on day 3 or 5 of the follicular phase of the menstrual cycle for approximately 5 days. Ovulation generally occurs 5 to 12 days after the last day of Clomid.

Letrozole (Femara) is an aromatase inhibitor that decreases the conversion of androgens (testosterone and androstenedione) to estrogens (estradiol and estrone) (Table 26-5). Lower estrogen levels reduce the negative feedback effect on the hypothalamus and pituitary, which leads to an increase of FSH and follicular development. Its use for OI is off-label in the United States.

Absent or infrequent ovulation in women with PCOS or mild hypothalamic amenorrhea is the major indication for Clomid and Femara. Specific causes of anovulation should be ruled out first, and patients should have normal thyroid stimulating hormone (TSH), FSH, and prolactin levels. Although Clomid is used as a first-line therapy in couples with unexplained infertility, it has no use in patients with POI. These women typically require donor oocytes in order to conceive.

The other major category of OI agents is hMGs. These are best used when the pituitary gland fails to secrete sufficient FSH and LH to stimulate follicular maturation and ovulation and when Clomid is also incapable of stimulating ovulation. Patients with mild to severe hypothalamic dysfunction fall into this category and often require hMGs for OI.

The hMGs (Table 26-5) often come in combined preparations of FSH and LH or of FSH alone. They are administered via intramuscular injection during the follicular phase of the menstrual cycle. The patient's response to OI should be monitored closely through serial estrogen levels and pelvic ultrasounds to measure the number of follicles, size of follicles, and the total estrogen production level. Monitoring decreases the risk of both multiple gestations and ovarian hyperstimulation.

Each means of OI can potentially produce multiple follicles. Once ovulation occurs, fertilization may be attempted by intercourse or IUI. Conversely, after OI, oocyte retrieval may be accomplished with transvaginal aspiration (Fig. 26-11). The oocytes are then fertilized via IVF (Fig. 26-12) or ICSI (Fig. 26-10). Selected embryos are then transferred into the uterus under ultrasound guidance. Progesterone is often used to promote endometrial receptivity beginning after embryo transfer and lasting through the first trimester. Any remaining embryos are saved using cryopreservation techniques for future cycles, embryo donation, or research.

Effectiveness

Clomiphene citrate is successful in inducing ovulation in 80% of correctly selected patients, but <50% will become pregnant. If pregnancy does not occur after three to six cycles of Clomid where ovulation is

FIGURE 26-11. Transvaginal ultrasound-guided needle aspiration of oocytes. Following ovulation induction, multiple eggs are removed from the ovaries by placing a vaginal probe into the vagina. A fine needle is guided toward the ovary while the physician visualizes the follicles on ultrasound. Fluid around the follicles is then collected through a needle connected to a test tube.

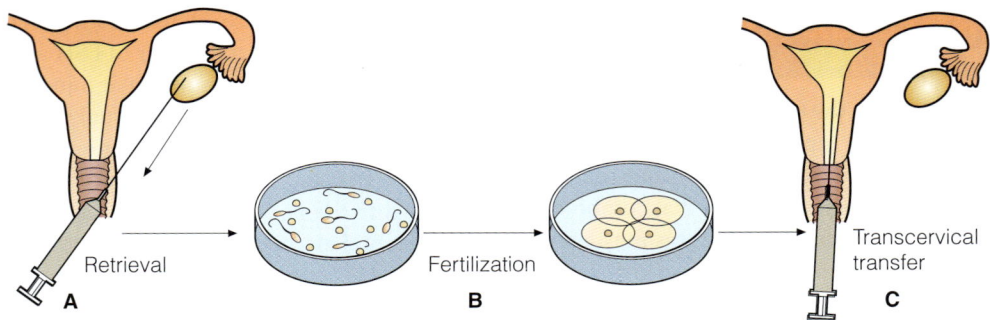

FIGURE 26-12. In vitro fertilization (IVF). (**A**) After ovulation induction, oocytes are harvested transvaginally. (**B**) The egg and sperm are placed together in the laboratory and fertilization takes place. (**C**) The fertilized embryos are transferred into the uterine cavity through the cervix.

achieved, then more aggressive therapies are needed. Gonadotropins have an 80% to 90% ovulation success rate and a 10% to 40% pregnancy success rate per cycle depending on the diagnosis (recall fecundity is only 20% to 25% in the general population). Gonadotropins carry a much higher risk of ovarian hyperstimulation (1% to 3%) and multiple gestation pregnancy (20%) than do Clomid and Femara.

Side Effects and Complications
The potential side effects of Clomid are related to its antiestrogen effects: hot flashes, abdominal distension and bloating, and emotional lability. These side effects are mostly mild and disappear after discontinuation of the medication. Although there is some controversy about the risk of teratogenesis with aromatase inhibitors, care should be taken to rule out pregnancy prior to induction of ovulation for this off-label indication.

Multiple gestation pregnancy is a major side effect of OI and ARTs. Multiple gestation pregnancies occur in 8% of Clomid-induced pregnancies and in 20% of pregnancies from gonadotropins.

The other major complication of OI with gonadotropins is **ovarian hyperstimulation syndrome** (OHSS). This is a potentially life-threatening condition caused by overstimulation of the ovaries occurring in 1% to 3% of patients undergoing OI. This completely iatrogenic disorder can range from ovarian enlargement and minimal symptoms to significant ovarian enlargement, torsion, or rupture. This may be complicated by ascites, pleural effusions, hemoconcentration, hypercoagulability, electrolyte disturbances, renal failure, and even death.

The risk of both multiple gestations and OHSS can be mediated by careful monitoring of estradiol production and follicle growth during OI and by limiting the number of embryos placed during IVF.

ADVANCED REPRODUCTIVE TECHNOLOGIES (IVF, ICSI, PGD)

Method of Action
ARTs have advanced the treatment of infertility by allowing physicians to successfully bypass the normal mechanisms of gamete transportation and fertilization. In conjunction with OI, multiple oocytes may be harvested from the ovary using ultrasound (Fig. 26-11).

During **IVF**, the oocytes are allowed to mature briefly in vitro before washed sperm are added. Fertilization is verified 14 to 18 hours later by the presence of two pronuclei. In the case of IVF, the conceptuses (day 3 embryos or day 5 blastocysts) are then placed into the uterus through the cervix using a catheter (Fig. 26-12), making IVF a relatively noninvasive procedure.

ICSI has revolutionized the treatment of male factor infertility by allowing a single spermatid or sperm to be directly injected into the cytoplasm of a harvested oocyte (Fig. 26-10). The resulting embryos can then be placed back into the uterus for implantation.

Preimplantation genetic diagnosis (PGD) refers to the evaluation of the embryo for genetic abnormalities prior to transfer during an IVF cycle. PGD involves removing one or two cells from a six- to eight-cell embryo, and then screening the cells for common chromosomal abnormalities or genetic mutations, such as sickle-cell anemia, Tay–Sachs disease, cystic fibrosis, Down syndrome, hemophilia A, and fragile X syndrome. This technique is usually performed when a patient has a known inherited genetic disease, is a carrier of a chromosomal translocation that has resulted in recurrent miscarriages, has an affected child, or is of advanced maternal age with increased risk of aneuploidy. PGD is used in approximately 5% of ART cycles nationwide.

Effectiveness

The success rate of these advanced reproductive technologies varies from center to center. On average, with IVF, delivery is achieved in 34% of oocyte retrievals using fresh non-donor embryos and 55% of transfers using fresh donor embryos. Success rates depend on maternal age, diagnosis, the number and quality of oocytes, sperm, and embryos. The most favorable rates are seen among women younger than 35 years, those without hydrosalpinges, and women with adequate ovarian reserve. The most recent published statistics show a live birth rate of 48% in women younger than 35 years and 39% in women aged 35 to 37 years when fresh non-donor embryos are transferred. Again, keep in mind that the normal fecundity rate in a couple without infertility is approximately 20% to 25% per month.

Multiple gestation pregnancies are a major complication of ART. The Society for Assisted Reproductive Technologies reports that, in 2009, the rate of multiple gestations at delivery was 31% for IVF (29% twins, 3% triplets and higher-order multiples). This compares with a multiple-infant birth rate of slightly more than 3% in the general U.S. population. The rate of multiple gestations is important because these pregnancies are at greater risk for maternal complications (preeclampsia, gestational diabetes, placenta previa, premature delivery, and postpartum hemorrhage) and fetal and neonatal complications (intrauterine growth restriction [IUGR], respiratory distress syndrome, intraventricular hemorrhage, neonatal sepsis, low birth weight, and death). Guidelines have been established regarding the number of embryos to transfer in various clinical scenarios with the intent of minimizing the risk for multiple gestations.

KEY POINTS

- Female factor infertility is purely responsible for 45% to 55% of all infertility cases. These can be divided into ovulatory, tubal, uterine, and cervical factors.
- Female factor infertility may be due to ovulatory factors that interrupt the hypothalamic–pituitary–ovarian axis as seen in PCOS, POI, hyperprolactinemia, and thyroid diseases. The most common causes of ovulatory factor infertility are PCOS and advanced maternal age.
- Ovulatory factors are diagnosed by confirming ovulation through menstrual history, ovulation detection kits, midluteal progesterone level, along with endocrine evaluation (TSH, prolactin, FSH, and LH) and assessment of ovarian reserve (day 3 FSH and estradiol levels, AMH levels, and AFC).
- Ovulatory factors are best addressed by treating the cause of the ovulatory dysfunction. PCOS-related infertility can be treated with weight loss, metformin, and OI with Clomid or letrozole. When refractory to treatment, OI with human gonadotropins can be used along with IUI or IVF.
- The most common causes of tubal factor infertility are endometriosis and pelvic adhesions. These factors are diagnosed by history and laparoscopy and treated surgically to improve fertility rates. Tubal occlusion may be repaired with microsurgical tuboplasty, but most couples opt for IVF to bypass the fallopian tubes.
- Female infertility may be due to uterine factors, such as uterine synechiae, polyps, submucosal fibroids, congenital malformations, or endometritis. Uterine factors are diagnosed by pelvic ultrasound, HSG, saline sonohysterogram, hysteroscopy, and laparoscopy.
- Uterine factors are treated according to the cause of the infertility. Synechiae, submucosal fibroids, and polyps can be resected; endometritis is treated with antibiotics.
- Female infertility may also be due to cervical factors, such as cervical stenosis from surgical or mechanical dilation. These factors are diagnosed on physical examination and treated with surgical or mechanical dilation of the endocervical canal or IUI to bypass the cervix.
- Male factor infertility is the cause of one third of all infertility cases.
- Male factor infertility may be idiopathic or due to improper coital practices; sexual dysfunction; endocrine disorders; or abnormalities in spermatogenesis, sperm volume, density, or

mobility. The most common cause is varicocele, comprising 30% to 40% of infertility in men.
- Male factor infertility is diagnosed by semen analysis and endocrine evaluation if indicated. The treatment of male factor infertility depends on the causal agent and includes improved coital practices, repair of anatomic defects, ICSI, and the use of donor sperm.
- Over 25% of couples find no explanation for infertility after their initial assessment. When this occurs, further assessment may be done to search for problems with sperm transport, ability to penetrate and fertilize the egg, and antisperm antibodies. IVF/ICSI can be used to treat these patients with unexplained infertility.
- Most therapies for unexplained infertility have not been shown to have higher success rates than no treatment. Couples with unexplained infertility who choose no treatment will conceive up to 60% of the time over 3 to 5 years.
- Clomiphene citrate is an antiestrogen that binds to estrogen receptors in the hypothalamus to cause increased FSH and LH production, thereby promoting follicular maturation and ovulation. Letrozole is an aromatase inhibitor that decreases the conversion of androgens into estrogens, thereby lowering estrogen levels and increasing FSH and follicular development. Its use for OI is off-label in the United States.
- Clomiphene citrate is best used for OI in women with chronic anovulation or mild hypothalamic insufficiency after specific causes of hypothalamic dysfunction have been ruled out.
- hMGs are forms of FSH or combinations of FSH and LH that directly stimulate follicular maturation in patients for whom Clomid has failed or those with hypothalamic or pituitary failure or unexplained infertility.
- The primary complications of fertility drugs include ovarian hyperstimulation and multiple gestation pregnancy. These risks can be lowered with careful ultrasound and hormonal monitoring of follicular development and limiting the number of embryos or blastocysts placed in the uterus during IVF.
- IVF and ICSI may be used to bypass the normal mechanisms of gamete transport and fertilization with deliveries in about 30% of cases.
- The live birth rate of fresh non-donor embryo transfer is 48% for women younger than 35 years and 39% for women aged 35 to 37 years in the most recently available statistics.

CLINICAL VIGNETTES

VIGNETTE 1

A young couple comes in with a chief complaint of infertility. The patient is a 30-year-old G0 who has not undergone any evaluation. Her husband is 33 years old, has had a semen analysis, which was reported as normal. He has never fathered a child. The couple reports having unprotected intercourse for the past 14 months. On further history, the patient reports that her periods have been quiet irregular over the last year and that she has not had period in the last 3 months. She also reports hot flashes, vaginal dryness, and decreased libido.

1. The most likely diagnosis for this patient based on her history is
   a. Polycystic ovarian syndrome (PCOS)
   b. Primary ovarian insufficiency (POI)
   c. Endometriosis
   d. Kallmann syndrome
   e. Spontaneous pregnancy

2. To confirm your suspicion, you decide to do some lab tests. All of the following would be appropriate test of ovarian reserve, except:
   a. Anti-müllërian hormone (AMH)
   b. Day 3 follicle-stimulating hormone (FSH) level
   c. Day 3 estradiol level
   d. Day 3 progesterone level
   e. Clomiphene citrate challenge test (CCCT)

3. The patient's FSH level is 40 mIU/mL, and the estrogen level is less than 20 pg/mL. You repeat the lab tests in 4 weeks, and the findings are similar. You have the patient and her husband come back to clinic and gently give them the diagnosis. They have many questions of what this means in terms of their ability to achieve a pregnancy. You let them know that their best chances of achieving a pregnancy are with
   a. Gonadotropins/intrauterine insemination (IUI) therapy

b. In vitro fertilization (IVF) with the patient's own eggs
c. IVF with donor eggs
d. There is no way for this patient to carry a pregnancy given the diagnosis
e. Ovulation induction (OI) with aromatase inhibitors

VIGNETTE 2

A 27-year-old patient and her husband present to you with primary infertility. The patient reports regular periods every 28 to 30 days. The patient has no significant medical history and does not take any medications other than prenatal vitamins. Her husband is also in good health, is 30 years of age, and has two children from a previous marriage. When you asked the patient how long they have been trying to achieve a pregnancy, they tell you 6 months.

1. Your instructions to the couple are the following:
   a. They will likely need IVF to achieve a pregnancy
   b. They will likely need Clomid/IUI cycles
   c. Continue trying appropriately timed intercourse for 6 more months, and if no pregnancy is achieved, come back to see you
   d. Consider donor egg
   e. Consider adoption

2. The couple comes back to you after appropriately timed intercourse, not having achieved a pregnancy. At this time, you embark on a workup that includes a semen analysis, an hysterosalpingogram (HSG), and an endocrine evaluation, including FSH, E2, TSH, prolactin levels, and ovarian reserve testing. All of the tests come back normal. What will be your next recommendation?
   a. Have 6 more months of timed intercourse, and if no pregnancy is achieved, come back to see you
   b. Clomiphene citrate with IUI
   c. IVF
   d. IVF with donor egg
   e. Human gonadotropin (hMG)

3. Ovulation was induced successfully in this patient with six cycles of Clomid, three of which included IUI. However, after six cycles with ovulation while on Clomid, a pregnancy had not been achieved. How would you proceed?
   a. Have six more cycles of Clomid
   b. Aromatase inhibitors
   c. Donor egg
   d. Intracytoplasmic sperm injection (ICSI)
   e. OI with human gonadotropins (hMG) followed by IVF

ANSWERS

VIGNETTE 1 Question 1
1. Answer B:
Although the patient's irregular periods and oligomenorrhea are consistent with PCOS, her symptoms of hot flashes, vaginal dryness, and decreased libido are not. The finding of endometriosis is not typically associated with any type of amenorrhea or oligomenorrhea or any of the other symptoms described. Although Kallmann syndrome is associated with amenorrhea, it is primary amenorrhea rather than secondary amenorrhea. This patient reports a lifelong history of regular menses except for the past year. Similarly, although pregnancy could explain the lack of menses for the past 3 months, pregnancy is not associated with hot flashes, vaginal dryness, or decreased libido. The most likely diagnosis for this is patient is answer B—primary ovarian insufficiency (POI). POI, formerly called premature ovarian failure (POF), is associated with the premature marked decrease in the oocyte pool prior to the age of 40 years. This woman, although young, presents with classic menopausal symptoms associated with low estrogen levels, including hot flashes, night sweats, decreased libido, and vaginal dryness.

VIGNETTE 1 Question 2
2. Answer D:
There are several available tests for the assessment of ovarian reserve. Traditionally, the CCCT was used to assess ovarian reserve. This involves administration of 100 mg of Clomid on days 5 to 9 of the cycle. The FSH level is then measured at days 3 and 10. The CCCT is still a valid test but has largely been replaced by direct measurement of AMH, day 3 FSH, and day 3 estradiol. Measurement of a day 3 FSH level is based on the notion that women with good ovarian reserve will make enough ovarian hormones early in the menstrual cycle to provide inhibition of FSH, thus keeping it at a low level. In general, a day 3 FSH value greater than 20 mIU/mL is indicative of poor ovarian reserve. Measurement of the day 3 estradiol level assesses ovarian reserve by looking for elevated basal rates of

estradiol caused by premature follicle recruitment in women with poor ovarian reserve. Thus, a higher day 3 estradiol level measurement of AMH reflects the size of primordial follicle pool, and >80 pg/mL is suggestive of diminished reserve. As women age and the pool declines, a lower amount of AMH is found. A level of less than 0.15 ng/mL is suggestive of a reduced follicle pool and is associated with decreased pregnancy rates. Days 21 to 23 progesterone levels are used to assess ovulation for a given cycle, not ovarian reserve.

VIGNETTE 1 Question 3
3. Answer C:
The diagnosis of POI is associated with elevated FSH levels due to a markedly decreased ovarian reserve. Giving exogenous gonadotropins or aromatase inhibitors in this case would be of no benefit to this patient because they would not result in maturation of oocytes, given the patient's depleted store. Similarly, having the patient undergo IVF with her own eggs would be of no benefit because the patient's store of eggs has been mostly exhausted; although the new term primary ovarian insufficiency reflects the small, although unlikely, chance that spontaneous pregnancy can take place. Having the patient undergo IVF using an egg donor is plausible and gives her the most likely chance of a successful pregnancy. In this situation, an egg donor would undergo ovarian stimulation and egg retrieval, and the donated eggs would be combined with the patient's husband's sperm, and the resulting embryos would be transferred into the patient. D is not the correct answer because while the patient's store of eggs is depleted, POI is not typically associated with any uterine malformation, and thus these patients are typically able to carry a pregnancy to term without complications.

VIGNETTE 2 Question 1
1. Answer C:
The definition of infertility is the inability to conceive after 12 months of unprotected intercourse. Eighty percent to 90% of couples will conceive spontaneously within 12 months of unprotected intercourse. Couples in whom the woman is younger than 35 years, infertility evaluation should begin only after the couple has tried on their own for at least 12 months. If the woman is older than 35 years, or if there is a history of irregular menses, risk factors for infertility, such as endometriosis, or history of PID or uterine anomalies, evaluation might begin after 6 months of unprotected intercourse.

VIGNETTE 2 Question 2
2. Answer B:
At this point, the couple has had 12 months of unprotected appropriately timed intercourse, and hence, testing and intervention would be the next course of action; so another 6 months of timed intercourse would not be recommended. First-line treatment for infertility of unknown cause is clomiphene citrate (Clomid) with or without IUI. Clomid is one of the oldest and safest infertility drugs that is used. It is associated with a low (4% to 8%) risk of twins and very low risk of triplets or higher-order multiples (<1%). Eighty percent of appropriately selected patients will ovulate using Clomid, and 40% will become pregnant. Higher pregnancy rates are seen when Clomid is combined with IUI.

VIGNETTE 2 Question 3
3. Answer E:
As the patient successfully ovulated on Clomid and completed six cycles of Clomid, additional cycles are not indicated. Patients who ultimately conceive on Clomid usually do so in the first 3-6 ovulatory cycles. Moreover, the association between OI and ovarian cancer was primarily seen among women who completed high numbers of Clomid cycles. Donor egg would not be indicated at this time given that the patient is younger than 35 years and has adequate ovarian reserve. Similarly, with a normal semen analysis, ISCI would not be indicated. The next step for this couple would be OI with gonadotropins followed by IVF.

27 | Vulvar and Vaginal Neoplasia

Benign lesions of the vulva and vagina are discussed in Chapter 13. This chapter discusses preinvasive neoplasia and invasive cancers of the vulva and vagina, respectively (Table 27-1). It is important to distinguish between benign disease and neoplastic disease so that appropriate treatment and follow-up can be offered to patients.

PREINVASIVE NEOPLASTIC DISEASE OF THE VULVA

Preinvasive neoplastic disease of the vulva is divided into two categories: squamous (**vulvar intraepithelial neoplasia**; VIN) and nonsquamous intraepithelial neoplasias (**Paget disease, melanoma in situ**). Histologically, VIN, Paget disease, and melanoma of the vulva can all be quite similar. Therefore, immunohistochemical staining is often used to assist in the diagnosis of vulvar lesions.

VULVAR INTRAEPITHELIAL NEOPLASIA
Pathogenesis

Just as the incidence of cervical dysplasia has been rising in younger women, so has the incidence of VIN. VIN is defined as **cellular atypia** contained **within the epithelium**. It is characterized by a loss of epithelial cell maturation, cellular crowding, nuclear hyperchromatosis, and abnormal mitosis. The lesions were previously designated as VIN I (mild dysplasia), VIN II (moderate dysplasia), or VIN III (severe dysplasia), based on the depth of epithelial involvement. In 2004, the classification for VIN was revised. What was formerly VIN I became classified as **koilocytic atypia**, and VIN II and III were categorized as VIN and subdivided into two distinct clinicopathologic subtypes: **Usual VIN** and **Differentiated VIN** (Table 27-2). The 2004 classification was not widely implemented. In 2015, the classification for VIN was updated to include all types of squamous intraepithelial lesions (SILs) and to create consistency among multiple professional organizations.

The concomitant rise in VIN and cervical intraepithelial neoplasia (CIN) is not surprising because both cervical and vulvar neoplastic diseases are correlated with **human papillomavirus** (HPV) infection; 80% to 90% of VIN lesions will have DNA

TABLE 27-1. Classification of Neoplastic Diseases of the Vulva and Vagina

	Vulvar Disease	Vaginal Disease
Premalignant	VIN	VAIN
Malignant	Squamous cell (85%)	Squamous cell (90%)
		Adenocarcinomas (6%)

VIN, vulvar intraepithelial neoplasia; VAIN, vaginal intraepithelial neoplasia.

TABLE 27-2. Historic Classification of Vulvar Squamous Intraepithelial Lesions -International Society for the Study of Vulvovaginal Disease (ISSVD), 2015

Older Terminology	2004 Terminology	2015 Terminology
VIN 1	Reactive changes/HPV effect/Condyloma	LSIL
VIN 2	VIN, usual type[a]	HSIL
VIN 3	VIN, usual type[a]	HSIL
Differentiated VIN	VIN, differentiated type	Differentiated type VIN

[a]Encompasses VIN, warty type; VIN, basaloid type; and VIN, mixed (warty or basaloid) type.
VIN, vulvar intraepithelial neoplasia; HPV, human papillomavirus; LSIL, low-grade squamous intraepithelial lesion; HSIL, high-grade squamous intraepithelial lesion.

FIGURE 27-1. Severe vulvar intraepithelial neoplasia (VIN III). (From Rock J, Jones H. *TeLinde's Operative Gynecology,* 10th ed. Philadelphia, PA: Lippincott Williams & Wilkins; 2008.)

fragments from HPV, and 60% of women with VIN have cervical neoplasia as well. Additional risk factors for VIN include **cigarette smoking** and an **immunocompromised state**.

This disease has two distinct forms, which differ by the age of the patient. Younger premenopausal women are more likely to have more aggressive multifocal lesions (Fig. 27-1) that rapidly become invasive and are associated with HPV 75% to 100% of the time. Older postmenopausal women have another form that is more likely to involve focal lesions that are slow to become invasive and are not typically associated with HPV.

Epidemiology

In the past, VIN was thought of as a disorder primarily affecting postmenopausal women. However, in the last few decades, the incidence of VIN has nearly doubled. Today, the majority of cases occur in **premenopausal women (75%)**, and the median age is 40 years. Interestingly, despite the increased incidence in VIN, the incidence of vulvar cancer has stayed relatively stable over the same period of time. Risk factors for VIN include infection with **HPV types 16 and 18**, **cigarette smoking**, **immunodeficiency**, and immunosuppression. The incidence of HPV-associated VIN decreases as age increases. There is no racial predisposition to VIN.

Diagnosis

As many as 50% of patients with VIN are **asymptomatic**. This highlights the need for a thorough inspection of the vulva for masses, ulcerations, and color changes at the annual examination. When symptoms are present, the most common are vulvar pruritus or vulvar irritation. Patients may also experience a palpable abnormality, **perineal or perianal burning**, and dysuria. Often, these women would have been examined several times and diagnosed with candidiasis, but experience no relief of symptoms with antifungal treatments or topical steroids. Any time a pruritic area of the vulva does not respond to topical antifungal creams—particularly in the postmenopausal woman—further evaluation with **vulvar biopsy** should be undertaken (Fig. 13-6).

On physical examination, there may be a variety of lesions that are **discrete** and often **multifocal**. Lesions may appear white, red, or pigmented and may be raised or flat. When the patient is symptomatic and there are no obvious lesions, colposcopic-directed vulvar biopsy may be performed. Extensive colposcopy of the entire vulvar region often reveals multiple suspicious lesions that can be biopsied to make a pathologic diagnosis (Fig. 27-1). VIN appears as distinct acetowhite lesions with or without punctations. Associated vascular abnormalities are more commonly associated with invasive disease.

Treatment

Treatment depends on the degree of the disease. Unlike CIN, VIN encompasses a mixed group of lesions with **varying potential for progression** to invasive vulvar cancer. Although spontaneous regression of VIN can occur, it should be considered a premalignant condition. The options for treatment include **wide local excision**, laser ablation, or topical imiquimod (off label). Superficial skinning vulvectomy may be considered for confluent multifocal lesions. When there is no concern for invasive disease, **laser vaporization** or **imiquimod** (off label) has been used to eradicate multifocal lesions; this results in less scar tissue and decreased healing time, but it provides no pathologic specimen and should therefore only be used when previous biopsies show no invasive disease.

Follow-Up

These therapies can be curative for VIN; however, studies have reported **recurrence rates from 18% to 55%**. Recurrence is more common with multifocal lesions, high-grade squamous intraepithelial lesion (HSIL), and in patients with positive margins. Patients should undergo a thorough visual examination of the vulva 6 and 12 months after treatment and then annually.

PAGET DISEASE OF THE VULVA

Extramammary Paget disease (EMPD) is an uncommon apocrine gland neoplasia most often affecting the anogenital areas of both women and men. It typically presents between the ages of 50 and 80 years in Caucasian women. EMPD is commonly an intraepithelial disease that tends to recur locally with minimal propensity to invade. Only about 20% of patients with Paget disease will have **coexistent adenocarcinoma** underlying the outward changes. When this occurs, metastasis is common. When adenocarcinoma is not present, Paget disease can be treated locally without concern for metastases.

Diagnosis

The lesions of Paget disease are consistent with **chronic inflammatory changes**—hyperemic, sharply demarcated, and thickened with areas of excoriation and induration. Commonly, there is a long-standing pruritus that accompanies **velvety red lesions** of the skin that eventually become eczematous and scar into **white plaques**. These lesions may be focal on the labia, perineum, or perianal region or may encompass the entire region. The disease is most common in patients over age 60 years, but the symptoms of vulvar pruritus and vulvodynia can precede the diagnosis by years. Absolute diagnosis is made only with vulvar biopsy (Fig. 13-6).

Treatment

In the absence of invasion, EMPD is generally treated with **wide local excision** of the circumscribed lesion. Because microscopic Paget disease often extends beyond the obvious gross lesions, wide margins should be taken, and excised segments checked in pathology for clean margins. It is also important to rule out underlying adenocarcinoma during pathologic evaluation. Finally, even with clean margins, Paget disease has a **high recurrence rate** and may require multiple local excisions. Without nodal metastases, the disease is commonly cured with local excision; however, the disease is almost invariably fatal if it spreads to lymph nodes.

CANCER OF THE VULVA

Pathogenesis

Cancers of the vulva may arise from the skin, glandular tissue, subcutaneous tissue, or the mucosa of the lower vagina. The most common type of vulvar cancer is **squamous cell carcinoma** (SCC) which makes up 90% of the cases. The other types of vulvar cancers include malignant melanoma, Bartholin adenocarcinoma, basal cell carcinoma, soft tissue sarcomas, and verrucous carcinoma. Although lesions can appear anywhere on the vulva, most are on the labia majora. These lesions range in appearance from cauliflower-like masses to hard indurated ulcers (Fig. 27-2). The spread of disease is primarily via the lymphatics to the superficial inguinal lymph nodes, with a smaller degree of spread via direct extension to vagina, urethra, and anus. In patients without metastases to the inguinal nodes, it is rare for the disease to spread to the intra-abdominal pelvic nodes.

Epidemiology

Vulvar cancer accounts for **only 4% of gynecologic malignancies**, with over 5,000 new cases diagnosed and 1,000 deaths reported in the United States each year. Although the rate of noninvasive neoplasia of the vulva has increased dramatically over time, the rate of vulvar carcinoma has remained relatively stable. **Risk factors** for vulvar cancer include menopausal status, cigarette smoking, VIN, CIN,

FIGURE 27-2. Multifocal carcinoma of the vulva. (From Rock J, Jones H. *TeLinde's Operative Gynecology*, 10th ed. Philadelphia, PA: Lippincott Williams & Wilkins; 2008.)

HPV, immunosuppression, and history of cervical cancer. The average age of diagnosis is 65 years. Young women are more likely to have associated HPV infections and VIN. It is possible that the rate of HPV-related vulvar cancer will decrease due to currently available HPV vaccines.

Diagnosis

Annual examination of the vulva by a healthcare provider is an important component in the diagnosis of vulvar cancer. Patients with vulvar cancer often present with long histories of **vulvar pruritus**, pain, and bleeding. Focal lesions tend to be merely inflamed and erythematous in early cancers and heaped up or ulcerated in later stages. They may also present with a **vulvar mass** that may be fleshy, nodular, or warty (Fig. 27-2).

The most common location is the **labia majora**. Ninety percent of lesions are **unifocal**. Final diagnosis is made by pathologic examination of a biopsy specimen, which should be taken even if the patient is asymptomatic. Twenty percent of patients will have a secondary neoplasia (usually cervical). The presence of bleeding, discharge, or a visible mass is strongly suggestive of invasive carcinoma.

Staging

Vulvar carcinoma is **surgically staged** using the International Federation of Gynecology and Obstetrics (FIGO) staging criteria based on tumor size, level of invasion, nodal involvement, and distant metastases (Table 27-3). Staging is the most important prognostic factor for vulvar cancer. The most common surgical approach is **radical local excision** with inguino-femoral **lymph node dissection**. Patients with superficial (<1 mm invasion) and unilateral disease can forego unilateral lymph node dissection. Patients with deeper disease (>1 mm invasion), bilateral disease, or disease that crosses the midline may require ipsilateral bilateral lymph node dissection depending on the location of the lesion.

Given its method of spread, **inguinal lymph node dissection** is required to definitively stage vulvar cancer. Staging may be approximated by a thorough examination for palpable lymph nodes, although 25% of those with positive nodes will have no palpable nodes on physical examination. The use of **sentinel node biopsy**, as a means of preventing some of the complications associated with complete inguinal node dissection, is under investigation. Metastasis to the intra-abdominal pelvic lymph nodes is very unlikely if the inguinal nodes are disease-free.

TABLE 27-3. FIGO Staging of Vulvar Cancer

Carcinoma of the Vulva

Ia	Tumor confined to the vulva or perineum, ≥2 cm in size with stromal invasion ≥1 mm, negative nodes
Ib	Tumor confined to the vulva or perineum, >2 cm in size or with stromal invasion <1 mm, negative nodes
II	Tumor of any size with adjacent spread (one-third lower urethra, one-third lower vagina, and anus), negative nodes
IIIa	Tumor of any size with positive inguino-femoral lymph nodes (i) One lymph node metastasis ≥5 mm (ii) One to two lymph node metastasis(es) of <5 mm
IIIb	(i) Two or more lymph nodes metastases ≥5 mm (ii) Three or more lymph nodes metastases <5 mm
IIIc	Positive node(s) with extracapsular spread
IVa	(i) Tumor invades other regional structures (two-third upper urethra, two-third upper vagina), bladder mucosa, rectal mucosa, or fixed to pelvic bone (ii) Fixed or ulcerated inguino-femoral lymph nodes
IVb	Any distant metastasis including pelvic lymph nodes

FIGO, International Federation of Gynecology and Obstetrics.

Treatment

Prior to definitive treatment, women with vulvar cancer should undergo a complete pelvic examination including palpation of the inguinal nodes, collection of cervical cytology, and colposcopy of the cervical vagina, vulva, and perianal areas.

For a primary occurrence of invasive SCC of the vulva, **wide radical local excision** with **inguinal lymph node dissection** is the treatment of choice. Stage I disease rarely has positive contralateral lymph nodes, and thus **ipsilateral lymphadenectomy** is sufficient. Most stage II diseases can be treated with **modified radical vulvectomy** and separate inguinal incisions for resection of lymph nodes. Stage III and stage IV diseases may require radical vulvectomy, bilateral inguino-femoral lymph node dissection (Fig. 27-3), and **pelvic exenteration**. Preoperative radiation therapy and chemoradiation have been

FIGURE 27-3. Incision for radical vulvectomy with separate incisions for bilateral inguino-femoral lymph node dissection. (From Rock J, Jones H. *TeLinde's Operative Gynecology*, 10th ed. Philadelphia, PA: Lippincott Williams & Wilkins; 2008.)

used to avoid the morbidity and mortality associated with pelvic exenteration.

If lymphadenectomy reveals metastatic disease, **pelvic radiation** is used as adjuvant therapy. In patients for whom extensive surgery is contraindicated, the procedure may be confined to vulvectomy. In these patients, preoperative radiation therapy with or without radiosensitizing chemotherapy has been used to reduce tumor burden. For recurrence, secondary excision or chemoradiation therapy can be used. Recurrences are usually near the primary site.

Melanoma of the vulva occurs predominantly in postmenopausal Caucasians. It can be treated similarly to SCC, except that lymphadenectomy is rarely performed. **Depth of invasion** is the key prognostic factor. **Once the melanoma has metastasized, the mortality rate is nearly 100%**. Basal cell carcinoma can be treated with wide local excision. These lesions rarely metastasize to the lymph nodes; thus, lymphadenectomy is not required.

Prognosis
Five-year survival rates are as follows: 86% for stages I/II, 54% for stages III/IVA, and 16% for stage IVB. The most important prognostic factor is the number of positive inguinal lymph nodes.

Follow-Up
The risk of recurrence is greatest in the first year; however, long-term follow-up is required with visual inspection of the vulva and palpation of inguinal lymph nodes.

PREINVASIVE DISEASE OF THE VAGINA
Pathogenesis
Vaginal intraepithelial neoplasia (VAIN) is a **premalignant lesion** similar to that of the vulva and cervix. However, VAIN is much less common than either VIN or CIN. By definition, the squamous cell atypia seen in VAIN is limited to the epithelium. Lesions are designated as VAIN I, II, or III based on the depth of epithelium with cellular changes. VAIN I and II encompass the lower one-third and two-thirds of the epithelium, respectively. **VAIN III** involves greater than two-thirds of the epithelium as well as full thickness abnormalities (**carcinoma in situ**). VAIN occurs most commonly as **multifocal lesions** in the **vaginal apex**. VAIN is associated with CIN, cervical cancer, condyloma, and history of **infection with HPV**.

Epidemiology
The peak incidence occurs in patients in their mid- to late 40s. At least 50% to 90% of patients with VAIN will have **coexistent or prior neoplasia**, or cancer of the vulva or cervix.

Diagnosis
Patients with VAIN are **almost always asymptomatic**; however, some patients can present with vaginal discharge or postcoital spotting. Many patients are diagnosed due to an abnormality on Pap test. In particular, suspicion of vaginal neoplasia should be raised in patients with **persistently abnormal Pap tests but no cervical neoplasia** detected on colposcopy or cervical biopsy. Patients who have undergone hysterectomy for a history of high-grade CIN should continue to have routine Pap tests to screen for VAIN for 20 years.

VAIN can be diagnosed with a thorough colposcopy of the cervix (if present) and vagina using both acetic acid and Lugol solution. The identified lesions should then be biopsied to give a final pathologic diagnosis and rule out invasive disease.

Treatment
The primary treatments for VAIN are **local excision** or **laser ablation**. For focal lesions, local resection is both the curative and the only way to rule out invasive disease. If invasive disease has been ruled out with extensive biopsies, the lesions can be treated with laser ablation, which heals well and has few side effects. **Intravaginal 5-fluorouracil** (5-FU) is especially helpful in treating patients with multifocal lesions and immunosuppression. Follow-up may include **visual examination** and **Pap testing** as indicated.

CANCER OF THE VAGINA

Pathogenesis
Vaginal cancer is extremely rare and comprises only 1% to 2% of malignant neoplasms of the female genital tract. The most common histologic type of vaginal cancer is **SCC** (85%); adenocarcinoma (6%), sarcomas, and melanomas are found in a much smaller percentage of patients. In the 1970s, **clear cell adenocarcinoma** was found to be associated with **in utero exposure to diethylstilbestrol (DES)**.

SCC may appear ulcerated, nodular, or exophytic and usually involves the posterior wall and **upper one-third of the vagina**. Spread may occur via lymphatic drainage to the inguinal nodes and deep pelvic nodes or via direct extension to the bladder or rectum. Late in the disease process, hematogenous spread to liver, lungs, and bone is possible.

Epidemiology
Primary vaginal cancers make up **only 1% to 4% of all gynecologic cancers**. In fact, secondary carcinoma of the vagina is more common than primary disease. The mean age for diagnoses of squamous cell cancer of the vagina is 60 years. The cause of SCC of the vagina is unknown. Similar to vulvar and cervical cancers, vaginal cancers can be associated with **HPV infection**. However, because the vaginal mucosa is not undergoing constant metaplasia like cervical epithelium, the vagina is much less susceptible to the oncogenic effects of the virus.

Women who were exposed in utero to DES have a propensity to develop clear cell adenocarcinoma of the vagina. Even then, the incidence in DES-exposed women is only 0.1%. They can present as polypoid masses palpated on the anterior aspect of the vagina.

Diagnosis
Many patients (20%) with vaginal cancer are asymptomatic. The most common presenting symptoms are **pruritus**, **postmenopausal vaginal bleeding**, postcoital spotting, and/or watery, **blood-tinged discharge**. With more advanced disease, urinary (dysuria, hematuria, and frequency) and gastrointestinal (constipation and melena) symptoms may also be reported. As in VAIN, vaginal cancer may be diagnosed during Pap test screening and follow-up colposcopy and biopsy. The differential diagnosis for vaginal cancer includes Gartner duct cysts, endometrial implants, and cancer of the urethra, bladder, or rectum.

Staging and Treatment
Invasive SCC of the vagina is often complicated by **involvement with local structures** such as the rectum or bladder (Table 27-4). Given this, patients diagnosed with vaginal cancer should undergo preoperative chest imaging, cystoscopy, proctosigmoidoscopy, and intravenous pyelogram (IVP) to assess for disease spread. At the time of presentation, 26% of vaginal cancer patients have stage I disease, 37% have stage II, 24% have stage III, and 13% have stage IV disease.

Small stage I lesions (<2 cm) in the upper third of the vagina are amenable to **surgical resection** (radical hysterectomy, upper vaginectomy, and bilateral pelvic lymph node dissection). Lesions >2 cm, those in the lower two-thirds of the vagina, and stage III and IV lesions are treated with **external and internal radiation therapy alone** (see Table 27-4). Comprehensive treatment should also include addressing the psychosexual ramifications of treatment.

Adenocarcinoma of the vagina is **treated similarly to SCC**. However, a clear-cut therapy for clear cell carcinoma has not been established. These lesions are often treated similarly with resection of earlier staged lesions, and radiation for stage III and IV lesions and those involving the lower vagina.

Prognosis
The 5-year survival rate for SCC of the vagina is highly dependent on the clinical stage and tumor size at the time of diagnosis. Five-year survival rates by stage are: 84% for stage I, 75% for stage II, and 57% for stages III & IV. The overall survival rate for primary vaginal cancer is 45% to 55%.

TABLE 27-4. FIGO Staging for Carcinoma of the Vagina

Stage	Clinical/Pathologic Findings
Stage I	The carcinoma is limited to the vaginal wall
Stage II	The carcinoma has involved the subvaginal tissue, but has not extended to the pelvic wall
Stage III	The carcinoma has extended to the pelvic wall
Stage IV	The carcinoma has extended beyond the true pelvis or has clinically involved the mucosa of the bladder or rectum; bullous edema as such does not permit a case to be allotted to stage IV
Stage IVa	Spread of the growth to adjacent organs and/or direct extension beyond the true pelvis
Stage IVb	Spread to distant organs

KEY POINTS

- VIN is a premalignant disease confined to the vulvar epithelium.
- VIN is often asymptomatic but can present with vulvar pruritus and vulvar irritation that are unresponsive to treatment with antifungals or steroids.
- Risk factors for VIN include HPV 16 and 18, cigarette smoking, immunodeficiency, and immunosuppression.
- VIN lesions are quite varied, and vulvar biopsy is required for diagnosis and to rule out invasive disease.
- Treatments of VIN include wide local excision, simple or skinning vulvectomy, laser ablation or imiquimod (off label) with close follow-up.
- Extramammary Paget's disease (EMPD) is another preinvasive intraepithelial neoplasia of the vulva; it is rare but is associated with adenocarcinoma 20% of the time.
- EMPD lesions are often velvety red in appearance and can eventually scar into white plaques. Diagnosis is made only by biopsy.
- Treatment for EMPD is with wide local excision; there is a high recurrence rate, and close follow-up is important.
- Vulvar carcinoma is surgically staged; it makes up <4% of all gynecologic cancers. Risk factors include menopausal status, VIN, immunosuppression, smoking, HPV, HIV, and history of cervical cancer.
- Patients with vulvar cancer often present with vulvar itching, pain, and bleeding, and the diagnosis is made by vulvar biopsy.
- The most common histologic type of vulvar cancer is SCC (90%).
- Most treatments include radical local excision (stage I) or radical vulvectomy (stages II, III, and IV) and regional lymphadenectomy; pelvic exenteration or preoperative chemoradiation may also be used for advanced disease.
- Five-year survival rates for vulvar cancer range from 86% to 16% based on staging. The most important prognostic factor is the number of positive inguinal lymph nodes.
- VAIN lesions are often asymptomatic, but may present with vaginal discharge or postcoital spotting. They can also be picked up on cervical cytology.
- VAIN is much less common than CIN or VIN. Most lesions are multifocal and located in the vaginal apex. Diagnosis is made by colposcopically directed biopsy.
- At least 50% to 90% of patients with VAIN have a coexistent intraepithelial lesion or invasive lesion of the cervix or vulva.
- Local excision, laser vaporization, and topical 5-FU are common therapies for VAIN.
- Vaginal cancer is often asymptomatic, but can present with vaginal pruritus, discharge, or bleeding.
- Diagnosis is made by colposcopic-assisted vaginal biopsy. Prior to treatment, patients should undergo chest imaging, cystoscopy, proctosigmoidoscopy, and IVP to assess for the extent disease.
- Small stage I malignancies of the upper vagina can be treated with surgical excision; all other lesions are treated with internal and external radiation therapy for an overall 5-year survival rate between 45% and 55%.

CLINICAL VIGNETTES

VIGNETTE 1

A 38-year-old obese white female presents to your office with complaints of "something is not right down there. It feels like worms crawling all over." While obtaining her health history, you learn that she underwent a total vaginal hysterectomy 5 years ago for a history of high-grade cervical dysplasia and heavy menses. She says she was told that she no longer needed gynecologic care. She denies any abnormal vaginal bleeding but complains of vulvar itching and discomfort. She has smoked one pack of cigarettes per day for the past 15 years. On pelvic examination, you note a rash under her pannus and bilaterally in her groin folds, consistent with Candida. Her vulva is notable for erythema, hyperpigmentation of the labia, and small fissures. The patient declines speculum examination stating that it would be too uncomfortable.

1. What test(s) are you likely to perform at this visit?
   a. KOH wet prep of the vulva
   b. Colposcopy of the vulva with acetic acid
   c. Biopsy of the hyperpigmented lesion
   d. Referral to gynecologic oncologist
   e. Both a and c

2. A microscopic evaluation reveals yeast buds and hyphae. It is negative for WBCs. You discuss with the patient that you would like to treat her Candida and would like her to return to see you in 1 week to discuss the biopsy result. Biopsy of the vulva returns as high-grade squamous intraepithelial lesion (HSIL). Your recommendation for treatment includes:
   a. Radical vulvectomy
   b. High-dose steroid ointment
   c. Observation
   d. Wide local excision
   e. Chemoradiation

3. The patient questions how she got this because she has not been sexually active in more than 7 years. You explain that she has many risk factors for the development and persistence of VIN. Which of the following is not a risk factor?
   a. Smoking
   b. History of CIN
   c. Obesity
   d. Human papillomavirus (HPV) infection
   e. Immunosuppression

VIGNETTE 2

Your next patient is a 28-year-old African-American female with a history significant for a renal transplant 3 years ago. She presents to the clinic for a colposcopy for further evaluation of a high-grade squamous intraepithelial lesion (HSIL) Pap test. On colposcopic examination, there were no lesions seen or identified on her cervix. She returns 6 months later for another repeat Pap test, which remains HGSIL. On colposcopic examination, her results are satisfactory, and she continues to have no colposcopic changes on her cervix.

1. There are no cervical lesions to biopsy. Your next recommendation is:
   a. Perform endocervical curettage (ECC)
   b. Colposcopic examination of the entire vagina
   c. Molecular testing for HPV types
   d. All of the above
   e. Both a and b

2. You have performed an ECC and examination of the vagina. In the posterior vaginal fornix, you note a single acetowhite lesion with punctation. Your next recommendation is to:
   a. Biopsy
   b. 5-FU
   c. Loop electrosurgical excision procedure conization of the cervix
   d. Wide local excision
   e. Laser vaporization

3. The pathology report returns as VAIN III, now what is your recommendation?
   a. Imiquimod
   b. 5-FU
   c. Local excision
   d. Intravaginal clindamycin
   e. Intralesional steroid injection

VIGNETTE 3

A 75-year-old female living in a nursing home is referred to you for a velvety red vulvar lesion with associated white plaques. The lesion has been slowly expanding in size and causing burning and itching over the last 5 years. She has been treated with various topical agents without relief, although she does get some relief from the itching and pain from the use of a steroid cream.

1. Which conditions are in your differential diagnosis?
   a. Contact dermatitis
   b. Eczema
   c. Invasive vulvar cancer
   d. Paget disease
   e. All of the above

2. Her biopsy returns and shows Paget's disease of the vulva. You recommend further evaluation because she is at increased risk for:
   a. Melanoma
   b. SCC of the vulva
   c. Crohn disease
   d. Adenocarcinoma
   e. Ulcerative colitis

3. Treatment recommendations would include:
   a. Laser vaporization
   b. Wide local excision
   c. Radical vulvectomy
   d. Pelvic exenteration
   e. Chemoradiation

VIGNETTE 4

A 54-year-old female presents to the clinic with a complaint of vulvar pain for 2 years. On examination, you note a 1.5-cm lesion on her left labia majora. She does not have palpable inguinal adenopathy, and the remainder of her examination is unremarkable.

1. What is her stage?
   a. Stage I
   b. Stage II
   c. Inadequate information for staging
   d. Stage III
   e. Stage IV

2. Patient goes to the OR for a wide radical local excision with lymph node dissection, with final pathology showing a 1.5-cm lesion with depth of invasion of 1.2 mm. There are no nodal metastases. She is staged as
   a. Stage Ia
   b. Stage Ib
   c. Stage IIIc
   d. Stage 0
   e. Stage IV

3. What is the most important prognostic factor?
   a. Size of lesion
   b. Depth of invasion
   c. Number of positive lymph nodes
   d. High-risk HPV status
   e. Smoking history

ANSWERS

VIGNETTE 1 Question 1
1. Answer E:
A wet prep obtained from the vulva and groin will confirm the diagnosis of cutaneous Candida. It is also important to inspect the vulva and to biopsy the lesions for definitive diagnosis.

Colposcopy of the vulva would not be inappropriate; however, she has already commented to her provider that she has significant discomfort, and application of acetic acid would likely cause significant burning and pain. If indicated, the colposcopy may be better done at a follow-up visit once the biopsy results are available.

A referral to a gynecologic oncologist at this time would be inappropriate unless you are suspecting a cancer or have a biopsy-proven diagnosis.

VIGNETTE 1 Question 2
2. Answer D:
A radical vulvectomy is not an appropriate treatment for preinvasive disease of the vulva. A high-dose steroid ointment would not treat the vulvar HSIL or yeast. Observation of vulvar HSIL is not recommended. Although spontaneous regression of VIN can be seen in women under 40 years, the risk of progression of untreated disease may be as high as 100% in women over 40 years. Surgical therapy with wide local incision is the recommended treatment for vulvar HSIL.

VIGNETTE 1 Question 3
3. Answer C:
Although obesity has multiple comorbidities associated with it, it is not in itself considered to be a risk factor for VIN.

The patient has been a heavy smoker for many years. Smoking is a known risk factor for the development and persistence of VIN. She has a documented history of CIN. Both cervical and vulvar neoplastic diseases are correlated with HPV infection. Nearly 90% of all VIN lesions are HPV positive. Immunosuppression is also a major risk factor for VIN.

VIGNETTE 2 Question 1
1. Answer E:
Her Pap test continues to remain with a high-grade abnormality, and there are no abnormalities on her cervix. An ECC would be a helpful diagnostic tool to ensure that there are no abnormalities in the canal that you are unable to visualize. A Pap test does often pick up abnormalities in the vagina as well as cervix. Molecular testing for HPV would not be beneficial or cost effective because the result would not change our management of the current results.

VIGNETTE 2 Question 2
2. Answer A:
Biopsy is the appropriate choice at this time to obtain a histologic diagnosis. 5-FU is not a good choice because we do not have a diagnosis yet. Wide local excision would give a histologic diagnosis; however, there is more morbidity associated with it, and the finding may not require such an extensive surgery. Laser vaporization would not be a good choice again because there is no diagnosis. Moreover, based on laser criteria, there needs to be reasonable certainty that there is no microinvasive or invasive cancer.

VIGNETTE 2 Question 3
3. Answer C:
The primary treatment for VAIN is local excision or laser ablation. For focal lesions, local excision can be both curative and the only way to rule out invasive disease. Imiquimod and intravaginal clindamycin treatments are currently not approved for VAIN III. 5-FU is helpful in treating patients who have multifocal disease or are immunosuppressed.

VIGNETTE 3 Question 1
1. Answer E:
Because of its eczematoid appearance, it is not unusual for Paget disease to be misdiagnosed as eczema or contact dermatitis.

VIGNETTE 3 Question 2
2. Answer D:
Studies have shown that around 20% of patients with Paget disease have a coexistent adenocarcinoma underlying the outward changes.

VIGNETTE 3 Question 3
3. Answer B:
Current recommended first-line therapy is a wide local excision. Laser vaporization will not provide a tissue sample to rule out other pathologies. A radical vulvectomy and pelvic exenteration are not indicated for the treatment of preinvasive disease.

VIGNETTE 4 Question 1
1. Answer C:
Vulvar cancer is surgically staged, and the information provided is inadequate to properly stage her cancer.

VIGNETTE 4 Question 2
2. Answer B:
Tumor confined to the vulva or perineum, >2 cm in size or with stromal invasion >1 mm, negative nodes. Stage Ia = Tumor confined to the vulva or perineum, ≤2 cm in size with stromal invasion ≤1 mm, negative nodes. There is stage IIIc = Positive node(s) with extracapsular spread. With the International Federation of Gynecology and Obstetrics (FIGO) staging guidelines from 2009, there is no longer a stage 0, which was previously carcinoma in situ.

VIGNETTE 4 Question 3
3. Answer C:
Vulvar carcinoma is surgically staged using the FIGO staging criteria based on tumor size, depth of invasion, nodal involvement, and distant metastases (Table 27-2). The stage of the disease is the most important prognostic factor for vulvar cancer.

28 | Cervical Neoplasia and Cervical Cancer

Prior to the 20th century, cervical cancer was the most common cancer in women and the most common cause of cancer death in women in the United States. Since the advent of the Papanicolaou (Pap) smear, which gained widespread acceptance in the 1950s and 1960s, it has been easier to detect and treat premalignant changes before they develop into cancer. As a result of public health initiatives involving population-based screening, detection, and treatment, cervical cancer has dropped to the 11th leading cause of death from cancer in women in the United States, accounting for about 4,100 deaths per year (Fig. 28-1).

Further advances in detection and screening have resulted from identification of the **human papillomavirus (HPV)** as the causal agent in the vast majority of cervical intraepithelial neoplasia (CIN) lesions and cervical cancers. By allowing us to pick up premalignant changes in the cervix, the combination of Pap test screening and HPV testing reduces a woman's risk of dying of cervical cancer by 90%. Current vaccinations are up to 97% effective in reducing the risk of cervical, vaginal, and vulvar neoplasias and cancers. Cervical cancer is one of the most preventable types of cancer in women. However, because many countries lack available screening, vaccination, and treatment modalities, cervical cancer continues to be the fourth most common cancer in women worldwide and is the **number one cancer killer of women in the developing world**.

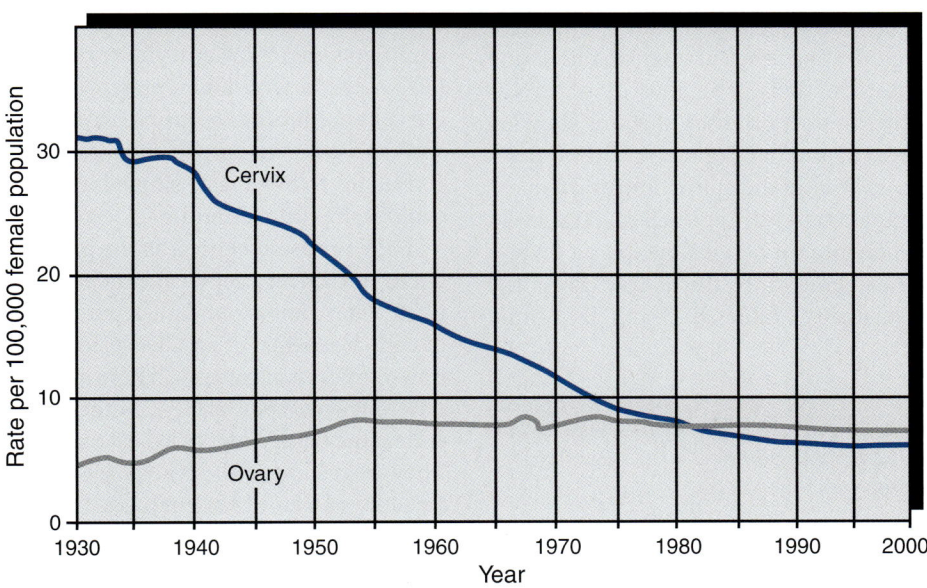

FIGURE 28-1. Declining rates of cervical cancer in the United States since the introduction of the Pap test. The Pap test was first used in the early 1930s and 1940s and became more commonly used in the 1950s. (From Beckmann CRB, Ling FW, Laube DW, et al. *Obstetrics and Gynecology,* 4th ed. Baltimore, MD: Lippincott Williams & Wilkins; 2002.)

FIGURE 28-2. Histologic classification of cervical intraepithelial neoplasia (CIN). The degree of CIN is determined by the portion of epithelium showing disordered growth and development. Changes are restricted to the lower one-third of the epithelium in CIN I. The lower two-thirds of the epithelium is involved in CIN II, and more than two-thirds of the epithelium shows abnormal changes in CIN III. If the entire epithelium is abnormal, this represents CIS, but is still within the CIN III category. In invasive cervical cancer, the abnormalities invade through the basement membrane into the cervical stroma. CIN, cervical intraepithelial neoplasia; CIS carcinoma in situ. (From Beckmann CRB, Ling FW, Laube DW, et al. *Obstetrics and Gynecology,* 4th ed. Baltimore, MD: Lippincott Williams & Wilkins; 2002.)

CERVICAL INTRAEPITHELIAL NEOPLASIA

PATHOGENESIS

Cervical intraepithelial neoplasia (CIN) refers to premalignant changes in the cervical epithelium that has the potential to progress to cervical cancer. The **histologic features** most commonly associated with cervical neoplasia include cellular immaturity, cellular disorganization, nuclear abnormalities, and increased mitotic activity. The severity of CIN is determined by the portion of epithelium showing disordered growth and development. The changes start at the basal layer of the epithelium and can expand to encompass the entire epithelium (Fig. 28-2).

The nomenclature for cervical neoplasia divides the epithelial thickness into thirds to express the degree of abnormality (Table 28-1). In CIN I (mild dysplasia), the changes are restricted to the lower one-third of the epithelium. In CIN II (moderate dysplasia), two-thirds of the epithelium is involved. In CIN III (severe dysplasia), more than two-thirds of the epithelium shows abnormal changes. The atypical cells in CIN III can expand the full thickness of the epithelium (formerly CIS or carcinoma in situ). Despite the nomenclature, CIS is still a *pre*malignant disease.

During menarche, the production of estrogen stimulates metaplasia in the transformation zone (TZ) of the cervix. When metaplasia is most active, the cells are more susceptible to oncogenic factors, such as during menarche and after pregnancy. CIN is thought to begin as a single focus in the TZ, but can develop into a multifocal lesion.

HPV is now accepted as the primary causative agent in CIN and cervical cancer. DNA fragments of HPV have been found incorporated into the DNA of cells from 80% of all CIN lesions and 99% of all invasive cervical cancers. There are more than 100 different serotypes of HPV. Serotypes 6 and 11 are among the types with the lowest oncogenic potential. They are responsible for causing 90% of condylomas. Serotypes 16 and 18 are of higher oncogenic potential and are responsible for 70% of cervical cancers.

High-risk HPV testing allows providers to more accurately predict which precancerous lesions have the potential to progress to cancer if left untreated and which will most likely spontaneously regress. Cervarix (bivalent), Gardasil (quadrivalent), and Gardasil 9 (nonavalent) are vaccines available to

TABLE 28-1. Classification of CIN
CIN I: Cellular dysplasia confined to the basal third of the epithelium (mild dysplasia)
CIN II: Cellular dysplasia encompassing the lower two-thirds of the epithelium (moderate dysplasia)
CIN III: Cellular dysplasia encompassing more than two-thirds of the epithelial thickness (severe dysplasia), including full-thickness lesions (formerly carcinoma in situ or CIS)
CIN, cervical intraepithelial neoplasiat; CIS, carcinoma in situ.

prevent certain HPV infections and reduce the risk of cervical cancer by 70% to 97%. **HPV vaccination** is recommended for males and females age 9 to 26. Cervarix immunizes against high-risk HPV types 16 and 18. Gardasil immunizes against low-risk HPV types 6 and 11 and high-risk HPV types 16 and 18. Gardasil 9 is indicated for the prevention of cervical, vulvar, vaginal, and anal cancers, and precancers caused by HPV types 16, 18, 31, 33, 45, 52, and 58; and genital warts caused by HPV types 6 and 11.

EPIDEMIOLOGY

CIN is most commonly diagnosed in women in their 20s, CIN III is diagnosed most commonly in women of age 25 to 35 years, and invasive cancer is typically diagnosed after the age of 40.

RISK FACTORS

Risk factors for cervical dysplasia include characteristics that predispose to early and multiple exposures to HPV (early intercourse, multiple sexual partners, early childbearing) and decreased access to screening and treatment (low socioeconomic status, Hispanic ethnicity). Most of these behavioral and sexual risk factors are proxies for HPV infection rather than independent risk factors in and of themselves. **High-risk HPV infection** is the most important risk factor for CIN. At least 80% of sexually active individuals will have acquired a genital HPV infection by age 50. Most will be able to clear the virus or get it down to an undetectable viral load over 6 to 24 months.

Other factors that influence CIN are cigarette smoking, immunodeficiency (**HIV infection**), and **immunosuppression** (autoimmune disorders, solid organ transplant recipients, chemotherapy administration, and chronic high-dose steroid use). **Cigarette smoking** appears to have a synergistic effect when combined with HPV infection. Approximately 10% of women with CIN have concomitant vulvar (VIN), vaginal (VAIN), or perianal (PAIN) intraepithelial lesions.

DIAGNOSIS

Pap Test Screening

Because CIN is otherwise asymptomatic, the Pap test has revolutionized our ability to identify, monitor, and treat premalignant cervical changes before cancer arises. The goal of cytologic screening is to sample the TZ, the area where transformation from squamous epithelium to columnar endocervical epithelium takes place and where dysplasia and cervical cancer arise.

FIGURE 28-3. Performing a Pap test. (**A**) Spatula. (**B**) Endocervical brush. (From Bickley LS, Szilagyi P. *Bates' Guide to Physical Examination and History Taking*, 8th ed. Philadelphia, PA: Lippincott Williams & Wilkins; 2003.)

The Pap test involves scraping endocervical and ectocervical cells from the external os of the cervix, with a spatula to sample cells from the TZ (Fig. 28-3). Because the squamocolumnar junction (SCJ) may be in the endocervical canal, it is also important to sample the endocervical canal with a cytobrush. The sample is then placed directly on a glass slide (conventional Pap smear) or into a liquid-based medium that is then used to make a slide. The prepared slides are then examined by a cytopathologist with or without aid of an automated cytology. **Liquid-based Pap tests** are most commonly used today, because they have a higher rate of CIN detection and they have the advantage of adding HPV testing. When the two tests (Pap and HPV) are combined, the testing is termed "cotesting."

Cervical Cancer Screening Guidelines

In 2012, cervical cancer screening guidelines were updated. An interim update was issued in October 2016.

Initiation of Screening: The new guidelines recommend initiation of cervical cancer screening at **age 21** (Table 28-2). With the exception of women who are infected with HIV or who are otherwise immunocompromised, women under the age of

TABLE 28-2. Cervical Cancer Screening Recommendations for Women in Typical Screening Groups and Women in Special Populations

Average-Risk Women	Screening Recommendations[a]
<21 y	No screening recommended EXCEPT if HIV positive[a] (see below)
21–29 y	Cytology alone every 3 y
30–65 y	Cotesting every 5 y with cytology and HR HPV testing is preferred; cytology alone every 3 y is acceptable
>65 y	No further screening needed if: • adequate prior screening (two consecutive negative cotest results or three consecutive negative cytology results within the previous 10 y, with the most recent within the past 5 y) AND • no history of CIN II and CIN III, no AIS in last 20 y, and no cervical cancer at any time
Women in Special Screening Groups	**Screening Recommendations**
Total Hysterectomy	No further screening needed after hysterectomy if: • uterus AND cervix are removed AND • no history of CIN II and CIN III, no AIS in last 20 y, and no cervical cancer at any point
History of CIN II/III or higher or history of AIS	Continue age appropriate screening as noted above for at least 20 y after spontaneous regression or appropriate management of abnormality
High-risk HPV vaccinated	HPV vaccination does not change screening recommendations. Follow the same age-specific guidelines as recommended for women who have not been vaccinated
History of in utero DES exposure	General consensus supports annual lifetime screening with cytology only
HIV positive or otherwise immunocompromised[a]	Initiation of screening with cytology alone • within 1 y of onset of sexual activity or, if already sexually active, within first year after HIV diagnosis but by age 21 • continue annually until three negative cytology screens then Q 3 y screening with cytology alone until age 30 Screening after age 30 • after three negative annual screens with cytology alone or one negative cotest, women may be screened over their lifetime with cytology alone every 3 y or cotesting every 3 y (do not stop screening at age 65)

[a]Refer to the ACOG Practice Bulletin #168, Cervical Cancer Screening and Prevention, for detailed screening and management recommendations for screening women who are HIV positive, women in other special populations and for screening women over age 25 using primary HPV testing alone.

CIN, cervical intraepithelial neoplasia; AIS, adenocarcinoma in situ; HR HPV, high-risk human papilloma virus; DES, diethylstilbestrol.

21 should not be screened regardless of the age of onset of sexual intercourse or the presence of high-risk behaviors. This recommendation is predicated on the fact that most HPV infection in this age group is transient and will clear its own. Subsequently, the rate of cervical cancer in this group is <1 to 2 cases per year per 1,000,000 females aged 15 to 19.

Screening Frequency and Modalities: Women aged 21 to 29 should be screened with cytology (Pap testing) every 3 years (Table 28-2). The preferred option for women aged 30 to 65 is to screen with both Pap and HPV tests (cotesting), and if both are negative, rescreening no sooner than every 5 years. Cotesting with Pap and HPV tests is 95% to 100% sensitive for CIN III. If HPV testing is unavailable, screening with Pap test done alone every 3 years is acceptable for women 30 and over.

Cessation of Screening: For women with no history of CIN II/III or higher in the last 20 years, it is recommended that cervical cancer screening be its own provided adequate prior negative screening results are evident (Table 28-2). Adequate screening is defined as three consecutive negative Pap test results or two negative cotest results in the previous 10 years provided that the most recent test is within 5 years.

- **Screening After Total Hysterectomy:** If a woman has had a total hysterectomy (removal of both the uterine corpus and the cervix) for benign indications (such as bleeding or fibroids) and she does not have a history of CIN II, CIN III, or higher, she may stop Pap screening at the time of her total hysterectomy. Importantly, women who have undergone a supracervical hysterectomy and have an intact cervix still need to continue routine Pap test screening appropriate for their age.
- **Screening After a History of CIN II/III:** Women with a history of CIN II and CIN III have a 2.8-fold increased risk of invasive cervical cancer for up to 20 years posttreatment. For this reason, women with a history of CIN II/III should continue screening for a total of 20 years after spontaneous regression or treatment even if screening extends beyond age 65 or if the patient obtains a total hysterectomy (Table 28-2). Screening should be done with cytology (Pap test) alone every 3 years for a total of 20 years.
- **Screening in Specific Populations:** Women who are infected with HIV should be screened with cytology only within 1 year of onset of sexual activity or, if already sexually active, within the first year of HIV diagnosis but no later than age 21 (Table 28-2). These women should continue to be screened throughout their entire lifetime (i.e., do not stop screening at age 65). Women with HIV infection who are <30 years of age should be **screened annually with Pap test only** (no cotesting). If these results are all negative, these women can be **screened every 3 years with Pap test only**. Women infected with HIV who are ≥30 years of age can be screened with cytology alone or with cotesting. Screening can be done every three years after initial normal annual screening (refer to ASCCP guidelines for details).

There are no major studies to guide us on screening of women who are immunocompromised because of non-HIV causes (e.g., women with solid organ transplant). However, it is reasonable to follow the same recommendations as those proposed for women with HIV infection. Women with a history of **in utero diethylstilbestrol (DES) exposure** should receive annual cervical cancer screening with cytology only (Table 28-2).

Abnormal Pap Test Management

Pap test reports may show findings consistent with normal cellular material, inflammatory changes, infection, dysplasia, or cancer. Nearly 3.5 million American women have abnormal Pap test findings each year; this represents approximately 5% to 7% of Pap tests performed. Table 28-3 presents the major classes of epithelial abnormalities as they are reported using the 2001 Bethesda classification system. The American Society for Colposcopy and Cervical Pathology (ASCCP) provides extensive written and electronic algorithms for cervical cancer screening and the **management of abnormal Pap tests (www.ASCCP.org)**. Please refer to those for more detailed management guidelines.

Cytological abnormalities occur because actively replicating HPV produces **characteristic cellular changes**, such as nuclear enlargement, multinucleation, hyperchromasia, and perinuclear cytoplasmic clearing (halos), which are detected on Pap test during cytopathologic evaluation. These cytological features are used to categorize the abnormal Pap test. Resolution of active HPV infection is associated with regression of these abnormalities.

The cellular changes ascribed to the **atypical squamous cells (ASC)** category may represent benign inflammatory response to infection or trauma, but may also herald a preinvasive neoplastic lesion. In fact, it is estimated that **10% to 15% of ASC Pap tests harbor severe dysplasia** histology that should be treated. To better differentiate Pap tests with more benign appearing features from those that are more concerning for dysplasia, the ASC category has been divided into two groups: **ASC-US** (atypical

TABLE 28-3. Major Classes of Epithelial Cell Abnormalities Found on Pap Tests

ASC-US: Atypical squamous cells of undetermined significance
ASC-H: Atypical squamous cells cannot rule out high-grade squamous intraepithelial lesion
LSIL: Low-grade squamous intraepithelial lesion
HSIL: High-grade squamous intraepithelial lesion (carcinoma in situ)
SCC: Squamous cell carcinoma
AGC: Atypical glandular cells

squamous cells of undetermined significance) and **ASC-H** (atypical squamous cells—cannot rule out high-grade intraepithelial lesion). Management of patients with ASC-US Pap results is detailed in Table 28-4.

Patients who receive an **ASC-H** or **high-grade squamous intraepithelial lesion (HSIL)** Pap test result should proceed directly to colposcopy (Table 28-4). Because of the potential for both cervical and endometrial adenocarcinoma, patients with a Pap test reading of **atypical glandular cells (AGC)** should undergo colposcopy with **endocervical sampling**. When AGCs are identified in patients aged 35 and older and those younger than 35 with risk factors for endometrial intraepithelial neoplasia (EIN) or endometrial cancer, they should also have an **endometrial biopsy** (Table 28-4).

HPV Testing

It is recommended that women aged 25 and over with an ASC-US result be tested immediately for the presence of high-risk HPV subtypes. This process is known as **reflex HPV testing**. The HPV results are added to the initial Pap test interpretation. This eliminates the need for the patient to return for repeat testing, and it allows the clinician to predict a patient's risk for a high-grade lesion with more accuracy and to better direct the plan of care. HPV

TABLE 28-4. Management of Abnormal Pap Test Results

Women aged 21–24 y	
ASC-US, LGSIL	Repeat Pap test in 12 mo (preferred), Reflex HPV testing acceptable for ASC-US only → If negative, return to routine screening; if positive, repeat cytology in 12 mo
ASC-H, HGSIL, AGC	Colposcopy with cervical biopsies if indicated; Immediate LOOP electrical excision is NOT acceptable
Women aged ≥ 25 y	
NILM pap, high-risk HPV positive (ages 30+)	Repeat cotesting in 1 y (acceptable) or obtain HPV DNA typing (preferable)
	If HPV 16 and 18 negative, repeat contesting in 1 y.
	If HPV 16 or 18 positive, then colposcopy with cervical biopsies if indicated
ASC-US, high-risk HPV not done	Repeat cytology in 1 y (acceptable) OR HPV testing (preferred) then proceed as indicated below
ASC-US, high-risk HPV negative	Repeat cotesting in 3 y
ASC-US, high-risk HPV positive	Colposcopy and cervical biopsies if indicated
LSIL, HR HPV unknown	Colposcopy and cervical biopsies if indicated
LSIL, HR HPV negative (ages 30+)	Repeat cotesting in 1 y (preferred) OR colposcopy with cervical biopsies if indicated (acceptable)
LSIL, HR HPV positive	Colposcopy and cervical biopsies if indicated
ASC-H	Colposcopy and cervical biopsies if indicated
HSIL	Colposcopy with endocervical assessment, and cervical biopsies if indicated; Immediate LOOP also acceptable
SCC	Colposcopy, HPV screen, and cervical biopsies, and potential CKC to rule out microinvasion
AGC	Colposcopy, HPV screen, cervical biopsies, endocervical sampling AND endometrial biopsy in women aged 35 or older and in women with risk factors for endometrial hyperplasia, EIN, and endometrial cancer

ECC, endocervical curettage; CKC, cold-knife conization; EIN, endometrial intraepithelial neoplasia.

testing should not be performed for women aged 21 to 24.

If a woman with an **ASC-US Pap test is positive for a high-risk HPV type**, she should be evaluated with colposcopy (Table 28-4), where directed biopsies can be performed if indicated. However, if the patient with an **ASC-US Pap test is negative for a high-risk HPV** type, she should have cotesting repeated in 3 years.

For women aged 30 or older who are screened with a pap and a high-risk HPV, a **normal pap and positive high-risk HPV screen** should be followed by repeating both the Pap and HPV screens in 12 months. If either result is subsequently abnormal, colposcopy should be performed. Conversely, in facilities where specific HPV typing is available, a patient ≥30 with **a normal pap and positive screen for high-risk HPV can be subtyped for HPV 16 and 18**. If positive for either, colposcopy should be performed. If negative for both, the Pap and HPV screens should be repeated in 1 year and managed with colposcopy if either is abnormal. High-risk HPV testing is not recommended for ASC-H, low-grade squamous intraepithelial lesion (LSIL), and HSIL, because nearly all of these lesions will be positive for high-risk HPV types.

Fortunately, many epithelial abnormalities found on Pap tests will **regress to normal** over 6 months to 2 years. Some of the abnormalities will persist at their current level, and the remainder will progress to more serious lesions or cervical cancer (Table 28-5). ASC and LSIL lesions usually represent a transient infection with HPV, so the majority will regress spontaneously over time. However, HSIL lesions are more likely to be associated with persistent infection and progression to cancer. Therefore, patients who receive an **ASC-H or HSIL Pap test result should proceed directly to colposcopy** (Table 28-4).

COLPOSCOPY AND CERVICAL BIOPSY

Once a *cytologic* diagnosis of epithelial abnormalities has been made on Pap test, a *histologic* examination is needed to make the diagnosis of cervical dysplasia or cancer. This histologic evaluation can be achieved during **colposcopy with directed biopsies** to determine the severity of dysplasia and to identify any invasive carcinoma. The colposcope gives a magnified view of the cervix, and when stained with acetic acid, cervical lesions can be better identified. Changes may include **acetowhite epithelium, mosaicism, punctations, and atypical vessels** (Fig. 28-4 and Color Plate 14). These lesions should be biopsied, and the specimens should be sent to pathology, where more definitive histologic diagnoses can be made.

Cervical dysplasia is classified as CIN I (mild), CIN II (moderate), or CIN III (severe), depending on the depth of involvement of the epithelium on cervical biopsy (Fig. 28-2). The treatment plan is then determined by the level of cervical dysplasia. In general, CIN I lesions can be followed without treatment. If biopsy-proven CIN I persists beyond 2 years, surgical excision can be considered. Because of their potential to progress to cervical cancer, CIN II and CIN III are typically treated with surgical excision.

Treatment of Cervical Dysplasia

CIN I is commonly followed with repeat Pap test or cotesting in 1 year depending on age. If any of the testing is abnormal, the patient should have a repeat colposcopy with biopsy if indicated. If the repeat Pap test or cotesting is negative, age appropriate screening is repeated in 3 years.

Women with CIN I that persists for more than 2 years, or those with CIN II are recommended to have **ablation of the TZ** with cryotherapy or laser, or may have surgical excision with loop electrosurgical excision procedure (LEEP)/ large-loop excision of the transformation zone (LLETZ). An alternative to treatment in young women (age 21 to 24) with CIN II is observation with colposcopy and Pap testing every 6 months for 24 months.

Women with CIN III are treated with surgical excision. Historically, a cold-knife conization (CKC) was performed, which removes a wedge-shaped portion of the cervical stroma and endocervical canal with a scalpel (Fig. 28-5). CKC is no longer

TABLE 28-5.	Natural History of Cervical Intraepithelial Lesions			
CIN Level	Regress Spontaneously (%)	Persist at Same Level	Progression to CIN III	Progress to Invasive Cancer
CIN I	60	30	10	<1
CIN II	40	35	20	5
CIN III	30	50	N/A	12–22

FIGURE 28-4. Colposcopic view of the cervix. Abnormalities shown include acetowhite epithelium, punctations, and mosaic patterns. (From Rubin E, Farber JL. *Pathology,* 3rd ed. Philadelphia, PA: Lippincott Williams & Wilkins; 1999.)

the standard of care for CIN; rather, it is reserved for when there is concern for cancer. The LEEP or LLETZ is now more commonly performed to treat CIN II and CIN III (Fig. 28-6A).

LEEP, loop, and LLETZ all refer to the same procedure that involves removing a cone-shaped piece of cervical portio (conization) with a cauterized fine-wire loop or with a laser (Fig. 28-6A). The LEEP can be performed as an office procedure under local anesthesia or in the operating room.

Table 28-6 describes the suggested means of surgical excision of CIN based on characteristics of the lesion or patient. For small lesions confined to the ectocervix, an **in-office LEEP** is the most common means of excision, although cryotherapy or laser therapy may be used. Lesions involving the endocervix are usually treated with **CKC or a two-stage LEEP** to allow more of the endocervix to be removed. In the two-stage LEEP procedure, the first LEEP is performed to remove the ectocervix, and a second smaller, deeper LEEP is then done to remove a portion of the endocervical canal. This is also known as a "top hat," because the resulting defect in the cervix resembles the shape of a top hat. Lesions that are large, multifocal, or those involving the vagina are often treated in combination with **laser ablation**. This allows for more precise removal of only abnormal tissue and removal of less normal cervix.

In general, cervical excisional procedures remove cervical tissue without causing extensive damage to the stroma of the cervix, although scarring of the endocervical canal may still ensue. Infrequent complications include cervical stenosis, cervical insufficiency, infection, or bleeding. The persistence rate is about 4% for CIN II and CIN III, and the recurrence rate is 10% and 15%, respectively. After cervical excision, patients with negative surgical margins should be followed with cotesting in 12 and 24 months following treatment. If CIN II or III is identified at the surgical margin, cytology and endocervical sampling are performed at 4 to 6 months posttreatment. If the results all remain normal, the

FIGURE 28-5. Cold-knife cone of the cervix.

FIGURE 28-6. Methods of cervical conization. (**A**) Cold-knife conization. (**B**) Loop electrosurgical excision procedure (LEEP)/large-loop excision of the transformation zone (LLETZ) conization procedure. (From Beckmann CRB, Ling FW, Laube DW, et al. *Obstetrics and Gynecology,* 4th ed. Baltimore, MD: Lippincott Williams & Wilkins; 2002.)

TABLE 28-6. Various Surgical Excision Options Based on Characteristics of the Lesion or Patient

Characteristics	Suggested Procedure
Confined to ectocervix	LEEP[a]
Endocervix involved	Two-stage LEEP or CKC
Large lesion	Laser conization
Upper vagina involved	Laser conization

[a]Cryotherapy is acceptable if lesion is small, limited to CIN I or CIN II, and there is no endocervical involvement.
CKC, cold-knife conization.

patient can return to routine screening for at least 20 years (Table 28-2).

CERVICAL CANCER

PATHOGENESIS

Oncogenic (high-risk) HPV is the causative agent for cervical neoplasia and cervical cancer. High-risk HPV types are also strongly linked to cancer of the vulva, and vagina in women, penile cancer in men, and cancers of the anus, mouth, and throat in both men and women. HPV is spread via skin-to-skin contact including vaginal, anal, and oral sex.

Two-thirds of all cervical cancers are caused by **HPV types 16 and 18**, although there are more than 15 serotypes that can cause cervical cancer. Although HPV is found in 99% of cervical cancers, the majority of women with HPV infection will *not* develop cervical cancer. This is because 90% of HPV infections resolve on their own in women with intact immune systems. In the small number of cases of persistent infection, the transformation from cervical dysplasia to cervical cancer typically occurs over years to decades making detection and treatment likely in women receiving routine care.

Squamous cell carcinoma (SCC) accounts for 80% to 90% of all cervical cancers. Most SCCs occur in the **transformation zone**, where the exocervix meets the endocervix. The route of metastasis is most often by direct extension (Fig. 28-7). **Adenocarcinoma** accounts for most of the remaining 10% to 20% cervical cancers. Adenocarcinomas develop from the mucus-producing glandular cells of the endocervix. One type of adenocarcinoma is clear cell carcinoma, which is correlated with **in utero**

FIGURE 28-7. Spread patterns of cervical carcinoma.

DES exposure. Almost all cervical cancers are SCCs or adenocarcinomas. Very rarely cervical sarcomas, melanomas, or lymphomas can be found.

EPIDEMIOLOGY

According to the American Cancer Society, there are approximately **13,000 new cases** of invasive cervical cancer diagnosed annually in the United States, leading to an estimated **4,100 deaths**. The majority of these women have either never been screened for cervical cancer or they have received inadequate screening for in the 5 years prior to their diagnosis. Routine Pap test screening combined with HPV typing decreases a woman's risk of cervical cancer by 90%. Over the last 30 years, cervical cancer deaths in American women have decreased by over 50%.

Fifty percent of women with cervical cancer are **diagnosed between ages 35 and 55**. The median age of diagnosis is 52, and the average is 45. Only **0.1% of cervical cancers occur before the age of 20**. This represents fewer than 1 to 2 cases per year per 1,000,000 females aged 15 to 19. Although 15% of cervical cancers occur in women over the age of 65, it rarely occurs in those women who have had routine Pap testing prior to age 65.

In the United States, the CDC reported that Hispanic women are at highest risk for cervical cancer followed by African-American and Caucasian women and Asian/Pacific Islander women. Native-American women and Alaskan natives are at lowest risk of cervical cancer in the United States.

RISK FACTORS

As noted, **high-risk HPV infection**, especially serotypes 16, 18, 31, and 45, is the most important risk factor for cervical cancer and cervical dysplasia. **Cigarette smoking** is also a risk factor for cervical cancer. **Women who smoke** are twice as likely to develop cervical cancer as women who do not smoke. The postulated mechanisms of action include the epigenetic impact of tobacco by-products from the mucus-producing cells of the endocervix and smoke-related immunosuppression.

Additionally, patients with **immunosuppression**, such as those with solid organ transplants and those being treated with corticosteroids are at increased risk of cervical cancer. Women with an intact immune system will generally clear the HPV virus in 12 to 18 months. This ability to clear an HPV infection is decreased for women who are immunocompromised. Similarly, women with poorly controlled **HIV infection** (high viral loads and low CD4 counts) have an increased persistence, progression, and recurrence of disease. In fact, cervical cancer is considered an AIDS-defining illness.

Other potential risk factors for cervical cancer include past or current **chlamydial infection**, in utero DES exposure, and long-term (>5 years) use of oral contraceptives. The risk of cervical cancer in **oral contraceptive pill** (OCP) users returns to normal within 10 years of cessation of OCPs. Women who have **three or more full-term pregnancies** and those who have their first full-term pregnancy before age 17 are twice as likely to develop cervical cancer. Although the etiology is unclear, women with a **family history** (mother or sister) of cervical cancer are two to three times more likely to develop cervical cancer.

CLINICAL MANIFESTATIONS

Even though the Pap test has been proven to be an excellent screening method for cervical dysplasia, some patients still do not get routine Pap tests and occasionally present with advanced stages of cervical cancer. Early disease is usually **asymptomatic**. When symptoms are present, the most common is **postcoital bleeding**. Other signs and symptoms that accompany cervical cancer include any **abnormal vaginal bleeding**, watery discharge, pelvic pain or pressure, and rectal or urinary tract symptoms. On speculum examination, a friable, bleeding cervical lesion or mass may be seen with possible invasion into the upper vagina. In advanced cases, bimanual examination may reveal a cervical mass or invasive lesions in the upper vagina or cul-de-sac.

DIAGNOSTIC EVALUATION

Pap tests are not sufficient to diagnose cancer. Cervical cancer can be diagnosed only with a **tissue biopsy**. If an abnormal Pap test is found, a colposcopy and cervical biopsies should be obtained. Next, a LEEP conization or cold knife conization, is often performed to rule out microinvasive disease (Figs. 28-5 and 28-7). If the physical examination is abnormal, ultrasound or computed tomography (CT) may be performed to confirm the findings and define the extent of disease.

CLINICAL STAGING

Cervical cancer is the only gynecologic cancer that is still **clinically staged** (Table 28-7 and Fig. 28-7) rather than surgically staged. This is due in large part to the fact that it is the leading cause of cancer death in women in developing nations, where many diagnostic tools are not readily available. Clinical

TABLE 28-7. FIGO Staging for Carcinoma of the Cervix Uteri

Stage	Clinical/Pathologic Findings
I	**The carcinoma is strictly confined to the cervix (extension to the corpus should be disregarded)**
Ia	Invasive cancer identified only microscopically. All gross lesions—even with superficial invasion—are stage Ib cancers. Invasion is limited to measured stromal invasion with maximum depth of 5.0 mm and no wider than 7.0 mm[a]
Ia-1	Measured invasion of stroma no greater than 3.0 mm in depth and no wider than 7.0 mm
Ia-2	Measured invasion of stroma greater than 3.0 mm and no greater than 5.0 mm and no wider than 7.0 mm
Ib	Clinical lesions confined to the cervix or preclinical lesions greater than stage Ia
Ib-1	Clinical lesions no greater than 4.0 cm in size
Ib-2	Clinical lesions greater than 4.0 cm in size
II	**The carcinoma extends beyond the cervix but has not extended to the pelvic wall. The carcinoma involves the vagina but not as far as the lower third**
IIa	No obvious parametrial involvement
IIa-1	Clinically visible lesion ≤4.0 cm in greatest dimension
IIa-2	Clinically visible lesion >4.0 cm in greatest dimension
IIb	Obvious parametrial involvement
III	**The carcinoma has extended to the pelvic wall. On rectal examination, there is no cancer-free space between the tumor and the pelvic wall**
	The tumor involves the lower third of the vagina
	All cases with hydronephrosis or nonfunctioning kidney are included unless they are known to be due to other causes
IIIa	No extension to the pelvic wall
IIIb	Extension to the pelvic wall and/or hydronephrosis or nonfunctioning kidney
IV	**The carcinoma has extended beyond the true pelvis or has clinically involved the mucosa of the bladder or rectum. A bullous edema as such does not permit a case to be allotted to stage IV**
IVa	Spread of the growth to adjacent organs
IVb	Spread to distant organs

[a]The depth of invasion should be no more than 5 mm taken from the base of the epithelium, either surface or glandular, from which it originates. Vascular space involvement, either venous or lymphatic, should not alter the staging.

staging involves evaluating the patient for invasion into adjacent structures and metastatic involvement (Figs. 28-7 and 28-8). **Acceptable diagnostic tools** for staging of cervical cancer include examination under anesthesia, chest X-ray, cystoscopy, proctoscopy, intravenous pyelography (IVP), and barium enema. Magnetic resonance imaging and CT may be used to define the extent of the disease, but cannot be used to determine the stage of the disease. Likewise, once the stage has been assigned, it does not change based on intraoperative findings or progression of disease.

Stage I is confined to the cervix (Table 28-7 and Fig. 28-7). Stage II extends beyond the cervix but not to the pelvic sidewalls or the lower third of the vagina. Stage III extends to the pelvic sidewalls or lower third of the vagina. Stage IV is defined as extension beyond the pelvis, invasion into local structures, including the bladder or rectum, or distant metastases.

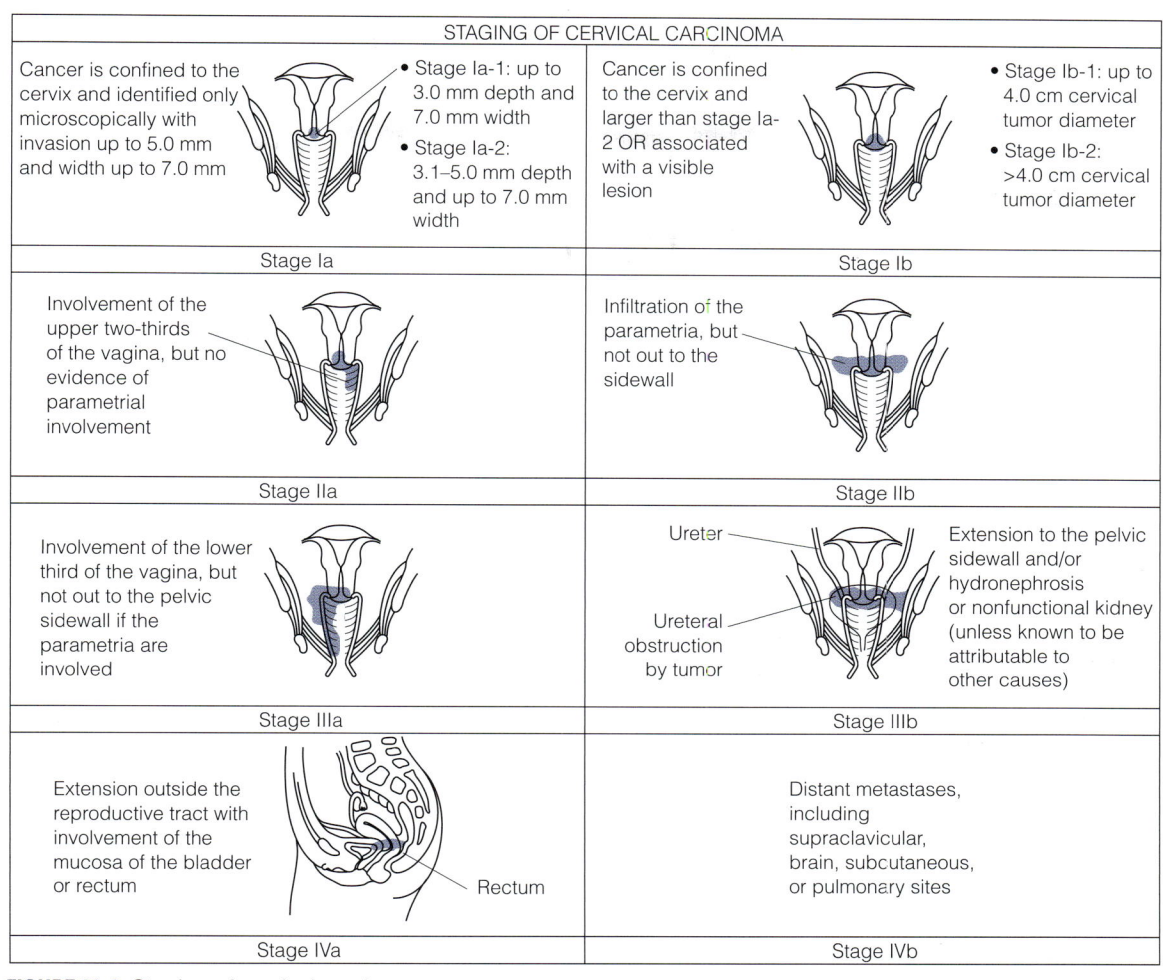

FIGURE 28-8. Staging of cervical carcinoma.

TREATMENT

Microinvasive Disease

In the case of microinvasive carcinoma (stage I to IA1 with no lymphovascular space invasion [LVSI]), the standard of care is **simple hysterectomy**. A cold-knife cone may be adequate therapy if the patient wants to maintain fertility (Table 28-8).

Early Disease

Early disease (stages IA1 with LVSI to IIA2) may be treated with either radiation **therapy or radical hysterectomy** (with bilateral pelvic lymph node dissection) (Table 28-8). In addition to removing the uterus, a radical hysterectomy also removes the parametria, upper vaginal cuff, uterosacral/cardinal ligament complex, and local vascular and lymphatic supplies. For early disease, both radical hysterectomy and radiation therapy have similar recurrence and survival rates. The choice of treatment depends on the patient's age, ability to tolerate surgery, and proximity to radiation facilities. Young patients who are otherwise healthy are often treated with surgery to maintain ovarian function that would be diminished or terminated by radiation therapy.

TABLE 28-8. Treatment of Cervical Cancer by Stage of Disease Invasion

Level	Stage	Treatment
Microinvasion	I to IA1 (no LVSI)	CKC or simple hysterectomy
Early disease	IA1 (with LVSI) to IIA2	Radical hysterectomy or radiation
Advanced disease	IIB to IV	Chemoradiation[a]

[a]External beam radiation, cisplatin-based chemotherapy, and intracavitary radiation.
LVSI, lymphovascular space invasion.

Advanced Disease

For more advanced lesions (stages IIb to IV) that have spread to the pelvic sidewall or beyond (Fig. 28-8), the treatment is **chemoradiation therapy**. Both external beam radiation and intracavitary radiation are used in combination with cisplatin-based chemotherapy. The goals of chemoradiation are to eradicate local disease and prevent metastatic disease. This combined treatment regimen has led to significantly prolonged disease-free survival when compared with radiation therapy alone.

Recurrent Disease

When cervical cancer recurs in a patient initially treated with surgery alone, **radiation** can be used to treat the recurrence. When the cancer recurs in a patient already treated with radiation, surgical treatment with **pelvic exenteration** can be used if the recurrence is centrally located. Exenteration involves removal of all of the pelvic organs including the uterus, tubes, ovaries, vagina, bladder, distal ureters, rectum, sigmoid colon, muscles of the pelvic floor, and the supporting ligaments. The 5-year survival rate after exenteration is about 50%.

TABLE 28-9. Overall 5-Year Survival Rate for Cervical Cancer

Stage	5-Y Survival Rate (%)
0	93
I	80–93
II	58–63
III	32–35
IV	15–16

Palliative Care

Palliative radiation with external beam or intracavitary therapy may be used to control bleeding or for pain management. Cisplatin chemotherapy may also be used for palliative care.

PROGNOSIS

When detected at an early stage, the overall 5-year survival rate for cervical cancer is estimated to be 93% (stage 0 = 93%, stage IA = 93%, stage IB = 80%). However, survival rates drop as the stage at diagnosis advances. Overall survival rates for cervical cancer by stage are presented in Table 28-9.

KEY POINTS

- Cervical cancer is the leading cause of cancer deaths in women in developing nations.
- HPV is the causative agent in CIN and cervical cancer. HPV types 16, 18, 31, and 45 are considered high-risk types.
- HPV testing can be used in the diagnosis and surveillance of CIN and cervical cancer. HPV vaccination can protect against some HPV infections, thereby preventing up to 97% of cervical cancers.
- Regular Pap and high-risk HPV testing can reduce a woman's risk of cervical cancer by 90%.
- Regular Pap testing should begin at age 21 regardless of the onset of sexual activity. Pap tests should then be repeated every 3 years through age 29.
- Screening in women 30 and over should include Pap and HPV testings every 5 years (preferred). If HPV testing is not available, a Pap test alone can be used for screening every 3 years (acceptable).
- For women with no history of CIN II/III or higher, Pap test screening can be stopped after age 65.
- Women with a history of CIN II/III or higher should continue to have routine screening for at least 20 years after the CIN II/III diagnosis and treatment. They can stop routine surveillance at that time or at age 65, whichever comes last.
- Women who have a complete hysterectomy (with removal of the cervix) for benign indications and who have no history of CIN II/III or higher can stop routine Pap screening at the time of hysterectomy.
- Women who have a history of CIN II/III and who undergo a complete hysterectomy should continue to have routine vaginal Pap test surveillance for at least 20 years after the CIN II/III diagnosis and treatment. They can stop routine surveillance at that time or at age 65, whichever comes last.
- Pap tests are classified as negative for intraepithelial lesions and malignancy (NILM), atypical squamous cells (ASC-US and ASC-H), LSIL, HSIL, or SCC.
- ASC-H and HSIL Pap tests should be evaluated with colposcopy and directed biopsies as

- should ASC-US Pap tests that are positive for high-risk types of HPV.
- Women with normal Pap screen but positive for high-risk HPV screen can either have both the Pap and HPV tests repeated in 1 year, or, if available, be subtyped for HPV 16 and 18. If either is present, they should proceed to colposcopy. If both are negative, both the Pap and HPV tests can be repeated in 1 year.
- CIN I reflects abnormalities in the basal one-third of epithelial cells of the cervix. These changes can potentially lead to cancer, but a high number (70%) will spontaneously regress.
- In general, patients with biopsies showing CIN I can be followed with repeat screening in 12 months and 3 years, before returning to routine screening.
- Women with CIN II and CIN III biopsies require treatment with surgical excision, typically with loop/LEEP/LLETZ. Young women with CIN II may be observed with Pap and colposcopy every 6 months for up to 24 months.
- Complications of cervical conization include bleeding and infection and, much less likely, cervical stenosis or cervical insufficiency.
- High-risk HPV is the most important risk factor for cervical cancer. Other major risk factors include smoking and immunosupression.
- Most cervical cancer is asymptomatic. When symptoms are present, they may include postcoital bleeding, pelvic pain and watery vaginal discharge.
- Diagnoses of cervical cancer requires a tissue biopsy. A cervical conization with LEEP or CKC is often done to rule out microinvasion and direct treatment.
- Cervical cancer is clinically staged. Early disease is treated with radiation or radical hysterectomy. Late disease is treated with chemoradiation.
- Five-year survival rates for cervical cancer vary from 80% to 93% for stage I disease, and 15% to 16% for stage IV disease.

CLINICAL VIGNETTES

VIGNETTE 1

A 25-year-old G1P1 female comes to the office for colposcopy because of low-grade squamous intraepithelial lesion (LSIL) pap 1 month prior. Her pap was normal 3 years ago. She began sexual activity at age 16 and has had five partners. She has had Chlamydia and vulvar warts in the past, both of which have been treated and resolved. She is a smoker of approximately 10 cigarettes/day since she was 15. She uses Depo Provera for contraception. Her mother died last year of cervical cancer at age 44.

1. What are her risk factors for CIN?
    a. Age 16 at onset of sexual activity
    b. Five sex partners
    c. Her history of Chlamydia
    d. Smoking 15 cigarettes a day
    e. All of the above
2. You perform colposcopy and see an acetowhite lesion on her cervix with no punctations. The biopsy of the lesion confirms CIN I consistent with HPV changes. What do you recommend for management?
    a. Imiquimod (Aldara)
    b. Loop electrosurgical excision procedure (LEEP) procedure
    c. HPV test in 1 year
    d. Repeat pap in 12 months
    e. Repeat colposcopy in 12 months then return to routine screening
3. She returns in 1 year, and her pap is ASC-US, but her reflex HPV test is positive. She returns for colposcopy, and on examination you see a dense acetowhite area on the anterior cervix in the transformation zone (TZ). You can easily see the entire squamocolumnar junction (SCJ). Biopsy of this lesion returns CIN II. What is your recommendation?
    a. Repeat Pap test in 1 year
    b. Repeat Pap test and colposcopy in 6 months
    c. Excision or ablation of TZ
    d. Cold knife conization
    e. Simple hysterectomy

VIGNETTE 2

A 30-year-old G0 comes in for her annual examination and tells you that she plans to become pregnant sometime in the next year. She had a LEEP procedure 7 years ago at another facility for moderate dysplasia, CIN II. She states her Pap testing has been negative since the LEEP and her last pap was 3 years ago, but you do not have any records documenting these results.

1. What is the recommended cervical cancer screening for this patient, assuming she has given an accurate history?
   a. Pap testing every 6 months
   b. Pap testing and colposcopy every 6 months
   c. Pap testing every 3 years
   d. Pap testing and high-risk HPV testing every 5 years
   e. Colposcopy

2. Her Pap test returns high-grade squamous intraepithelial lesion (HSIL) and she is high-risk HPV positive. You have her return for colposcopy. After the application of acetic acid, you see a large, dense, white area with mosaic vessels encompassing the entire anterior cervix and extending into the endocervical canal. You obtain a biopsy of this area and perform an endocervical curettage. The pathology report for the biopsy and ECC are both CIN III. What treatment do you recommend?
   a. LEEP in office
   b. Cryotherapy in the office
   c. LEEP in OR
   d. Simple hysterectomy
   e. Radical hysterectomy

3. What are the potential complications of surgical excisional procedures of the cervix?
   a. Cervical stenosis, cervical insufficiency, infection, and bleeding
   b. Cervical stenosis, infertility, infection, and bleeding
   c. Cervical insufficiency, cervical polyp infection, and amenorrhea
   d. Vaginitis and bleeding
   e. There are no known complications

VIGNETTE 3
A 21-year-old woman presents to your colposcopy clinic after HSIL, moderate dysplasia was reported on her Pap test at her family medical clinic. She is a heavy smoker with four lifetime sexual partners. She had negative STD testing at her annual examination, and she has no other complaints.

1. What is the recommended management?
   a. Repeat pap with HPV testing have her return to the office at age 21 to repeat the Pap test
   b. Pap test in 1 year
   c. HPV testing in 1 year
   d. Colposcopy with biopsies
   e. Immediate LEEP

2. She has seen a lot of information about HPV infections and cervical cancer in school and in the community, and she wants to know how she can decrease her own risk. You tell her
   a. Take a multivitamin containing folic acid.
   b. Start and complete the HPV vaccine series.
   c. You inform her that the HPV vaccine will not work for her, because she is already sexually active and likely has an HPV infection.
   d. You recommend she stop smoking.
   e. Both b and d.

3. Your colposcopic examination shows minimal abnormalities and the SCJ is seen in its entirety. The biopsy is negative for CIN. What is the next step?
   a. No follow up is needed
   b. Pap test and HPV screen in 1 year
   c. Pap testing with colposcopy every 6 months for 2 years
   d. Diagnostic excisional procedure (LEEP)
   e. Refer to GYN oncology

4. At her 6-month follow-up colposcopy, you see small faint acetowhite epithelial changes at 12 o'clock along her SCJ. There is some punctation, but the edges do not extend into the endocervix. You biopsy the lesion and a diagnosis of CIN 1 returns. Her pap is read as LSIL. What is her recommended follow-up?
   a. LEEP procedure
   b. Pap test in 1 year
   c. Return for an HPV test
   d. Pap test and colposcopy in 6 months

VIGNETTE 4
A 62-year-old woman presents to the office complaining of watery vaginal discharge and bleeding for the last 2 months. She has not had a Pap test in 25 years. She states that she had a mildly abnormal pap in her 30s, but that was treated with cryotherapy. She went through menopause at age 50 and has never been on hormone replacement therapy. She does admit to smoking one-half pack a day for 40 years. Her husband is deceased, and she has not been sexually active in 10 years. Her examination reveals a necrotic cervical mass approximately 4 cm in size. Rectovaginal examination is suspicious for left parametrial involvement. There is no evidence of adnexal masses, but examination of the uterus and adnexa is limited by the patient's body habitus.

You suspect that this may be cervical cancer. You obtain a Pap test and take a biopsy of her cervical abnormality. The Pap test returns with a reading of SCC, and the biopsy confirms cervical cancer. She also received a cystoscopy for hematuria with positive urine cytology. You order a CT scan, which shows a cervical mass measuring $7.7 \times 3 \times 5.0$ cm as well as an enlarged left internal iliac lymph node consistent with locally metastatic disease.

1. What is the International Federation of Gynecology and Obstetrics (FIGO) stage for her cancer?
   a. Stage Ia
   b. Stage IIb
   c. Stage III
   d. Stage IV

2. What do you recommend for the next step in the treatment of her cervical cancer?
   a. Cold-knife cone
   b. Simple hysterectomy
   c. Radiation and chemotherapy
   d. Chemotherapy alone
   e. Palliative care

3. She is treated with chemoradiation, and 3 years later, she has a local recurrence. You proceed with pelvic exenteration for her recurrent cancer. What is her 5-year survival rate after pelvic exenteration?
   a. 5%
   b. 10%
   c. 25%
   d. 50%
   e. 90%

ANSWERS

VIGNETTE 1 Question 1
1. Answer E:
Risk factors for cervical dysplasia include characteristics that predispose patients to multiple and early exposure to HPV (early intercourse, multiple sex partners, early childbearing, "high-risk" partners, low socioeconomic status, sexually transmitted infections, cigarette smoking, immunodeficiency, and multiparity). Most of these behavioral and sexual risk factors are associated with HPV infection rather than independent risk factors in and of themselves.

VIGNETTE 1 Question 2
2. Answer D:
Women with CIN I have high rates of regression to normal. LSIL lesions usually represent a transient infection with HPV, so the majority will regress spontaneously over time. Imiquimod is a treatment for perineal condyloma, but is not indicated for vaginal or cervical HPV. A LEEP procedure should be used for CIN II or CIN III in a woman her age. CIN I can be followed with repeat Pap testing in 1 year. Repeat colposcopy would only be done if the follow up Pap test was abnormal.

VIGNETTE 1 Question 3
3. Answer C:
For young women aged 21 to 24 with CIN II, it is acceptable to offer observation with colposcopy and Pap testing every 6 months for 24 moths because CIN lesions lesions in this age group have a very high rate of spontaneous regression. Repeat Pap testing only is not a recommended follow-up for CIN II in any age group. Treatment with cold-knife cone is unnecessary because her exam is adequate (entire SCJ is visible), and there is no concern for cancer. Excision or ablation of TZ is the recommended treatment for CIN II in a 25-year-old woman. Simple hysterectomy is not indicated and is overly aggressive.

VIGNETTE 2 Question 1
1. Answer D:
Pap testing and high-risk HPV testing every 5 years are routine screening for women aged 30 and above. She does have a history of a prior abnormal pap and LEEP, but with normal follow-up for the 5 years following the LEEP, she can return to routine screening. Screening recommendations for women aged 21 to 29 are to have Pap testing every 3 years. A colposcopy is not indicated unless she has another abnormal Pap test.

VIGNETTE 2 Question 2
2. Answer C:
A result of CIN III needs to be excised and because of the size of the area and the extension into the endocervical canal, an OR procedure is recommended. Cryotherapy is acceptable for small lesions confined to the ectocervix, when LEEP is not available. LEEP in the office is appropriate for focal lesions confined to the ectocervix. Hysterectomy is not indicated, because she does not have cervical cancer.

VIGNETTE 2 Question 3
3. Answer A:
Complications of cervical excision procedures are cervical stenosis, cervical insufficiency, infection, and bleeding. These risks are infrequent. Cervical excision should not cause infertility or cervical polyps.

VIGNETTE 3 Question 1
1. Answer D:
The current recommendation for screening for cervical dysplasia and cancer should begin at age 21 regardless of the onset of sexual activity. The appropriate screening for women from age 21 to 29 is to have a Pap test every 3 years. Routine HPV screening is not indicated in this population. There is no role for low-risk HPV screening in the detection or management of cervical dysplasia and cancer. Although guidelines do not recommend Pap testing at her age, she does now have a high-grade abnormality, and it should be evaluated with colposcopy.

VIGNETTE 3 Question 2
2. Answer E:
There are no data to suggest a multivitamin can reduce the risk of cervical cancer. This patient is at the

appropriate age to receive HPV immunization. HPV vaccination is recommended at age 11 to 12 years old, but may be given from age 9 to 26. Smoking cessation would also decrease her risk of cervical dysplasia and cancer.

VIGNETTE 3 Question 3

3. Answer C:
For women age 21 to 24, an HSIL pap with should be followed with pap testing and colposcopy every 6 months for 2 years as long as no CIN 2 or 3 is seen. The abnormality will likely regress, so LEEP or GYN oncology referral are not indicated. It is possible that the HSIL lesion could progress, however. Therefore, the 2 year follow up with Pap and colposcopy should be completed even if with biopsy shows no CIN. If the HSIL persists for 2 years even with a negative colposcopy, a *diagnostic* excisional procedure would be indicated.

VIGNETTE 3 Question 4

4. Answer D:
Pap test and colposcopy are still the recommended follow-up because the patient had a previous HSIL pap. Although you do not need to treat CIN 1, it does not change your plan of management. HPV testing in young women is likely to be positive and will not alter their management.

VIGNETTE 4 Question 1

1. Answer D:
Cervical cancer is *clinically staged* as opposed to surgically staged. The FIGO staging system is largely based on physical examination. This clinical staging process can include physical examination, examination under anesthesia, cervical biopsy and/or conization, chest X-ray, hysteroscopy, cystoscopy, proctoscopy, and IVP and/or barium enema, if indicated. Other imaging studies, laboratory tests, and surgical procedures are often used to assess for lymph node involvement and metastases. However, these results *do not* alter the FIGO stage.

Stage I disease is confined to the cervix. Stage II involves the upper two-thirds of the vagina and/or involvement of the parametria. Stage III involves the lower vagina, extension to the pelvic side wall, and/or hydronephrosis from ureteral obstruction by the tumor. Stage IV involves extension outside the reproductive tract including involvement of the bladder mucosa and distant metastases.

This patient has a large lesion with likely parametrial involvement. The CT information is not used for FIGO staging, but the cystoscopy showing bladder involvement is. This would place her at stage IV, given involvement of the mucosa of the bladder.

VIGNETTE 4 Question 2

2. Answer C:
For stages I and II of cervical cancer, radial hysterectomy and radiation have similar survival rates. The choice of treatment depends on the patients' age, ability to tolerate surgery, and proximity to radiation facilities. Young patients are often treated with surgery to maintain ovarian function that would be diminished or eliminated by radiation.

More advanced stage III or stage IV disease requires chemoradiation in order to treat local disease and prevent metastatic disease. This typically involves the use of both external beam radiation and intracavitary radiation (brachytherapy) in concert with cisplatin-based chemotherapy.

VIGNETTE 4 Question 3

3. Answer D:
When cervical cancer recurs in a patient initially treated with surgery alone, radiation can be used to treat the recurrence. When the cancer recurs in a patient who has already been treated with radiation, surgical treatment with pelvic exenteration can be used if the recurrence is centrally located (vaginal apex or pelvis without pelvic sidewall involvement), and there is no metastatic disease. Exenteration involves removal of the pelvic organs, including the uterus, tubes, ovaries, vagina, bladder, rectum, sigmoid colon, and muscle and support structures of the pelvic wall. The 5-year survival rate after pelvic exenteration for recurrent cervical cancer is about 50%.

29 | Endometrial Cancer

Endometrial carcinoma is the **fourth most common cancer** in American women, exceeded only by cancer of the breast, bowel, and lung. According to the SEER Cancer Statistics Review, over 60,000 women are diagnosed with this disease each year in the United States alone, accounting for 3.6% of all cancers in women. Although endometrial cancer is the most commonly encountered gynecologic malignancy in the United States, it is associated with a **favorable survival profile** because the majority of disease is diagnosed early. In fact, 72% of women are diagnosed with **stage I disease**, thus rendering the surgical staging itself as curative treatment. Fortunately, early symptoms and accurate diagnostic modalities contribute to the fact that despite being the most common gynecologic cancer, endometrial cancer is only the third most common cause of gynecologic cancer deaths (behind ovarian and cervical cancer). It accounts for 10,470 deaths each year in the United States.

Factors such as obesity, chronic anovulation, nulliparity, late menopause, unopposed estrogen use (i.e., without progesterone), hypertension, and diabetes mellitus lead to an increased risk of endometrial hyperplasia and intraepithelial neoplasia (EIN) (see Table 14-6) as well as endometrial cancer.

PATHOGENESIS

There are two distinct pathogenic etiologies of endometrial cancer. The most common type, **type I (80%) endometrial cancer**, occurs in women with a history of chronic estrogen exposure unopposed by progestin. These are referred to as **estrogen-dependent neoplasms**. These tumors usually start as atypical endometrial hyperplasia or **endometrial intraepithelial neoplasia (EIN)** that progress to carcinomas. The tumors tend to be well differentiated (endometrioid type) with lower grade nuclei and usually have a more favorable prognosis.

Type II (20%) endometrial cancer is believed to be an **estrogen-*in*dependent** neoplasm that is *not* related to unopposed estrogen stimulation or EIN. These tumors often occur within a background of atrophic endometrium or polyps. These cancers often have high-grade nuclear atypia with **serous or clear cell histology**. Many are associated with a mutation in the p53 tumor suppression gene.

Grossly, endometrial cancer itself may appear as a single mass within the endometrium, or it may be spread diffusely throughout the endometrium. Depth of myometrial invasion is an important component in the staging and prognosis of endometrial cancer. The prognosis is dramatically worsened, when the cancer has invaded more than one-half of the thickness of the myometrium.

Endometrial carcinoma has four primary routes of spread. The most common route is **direct extension** of the tumor downward to the cervix or outward through the myometrium and serosa. When there is significant myometrial penetration, cells may spread through the **lymphatic system** to the pelvic and para-aortic lymph nodes. Exfoliated cells may also be shed **transtubally** through the fallopian tubes to the ovaries, parietal peritoneum, and omentum. **Hematogenous spread** occurs less frequently, but can result in metastasis to the liver, lungs, and/or bone.

The most common type of endometrial cancer is **endometrioid adenocarcinoma (75% to 80%)**. Other nonendometrioid tumor types include mucinous carcinomas (5%), clear cell carcinomas (5%), uterine serous carcinomas (4%), and squamous carcinomas (1%). These types are less common but also tend to be more aggressive. Invasive adenocarcinoma usually results from **proliferation of the glandular cells** of the endometrium in a back-to-back fashion without intervening stroma.

TABLE 29-1.	Prognostic Factors for Endometrial Cancer: Histologic Grade—Degree of Differentiation	
Grade	Percentage Solid Growth	Differentiation
Grade 1 (G1)	5% or less of the tumor shows a solid growth pattern	Highly differentiated
Grade 2 (G2)	6%–50% of the tumor shows a solid growth pattern	Moderately differentiated
Grade 3 (G3)	More than 50% of the tumor shows a solid growth pattern	Poorly differentiated

TABLE 29-2. Major Independent Prognostic Factors for Endometrial Cancer
Age
Depth of myometrial invasion
Histologic grade
Histologic type
Surgical stage
Peritoneal cytology
Tumor size
Lymphovascular invasion
Pelvic lymph node metastasis

Histologic grade is the most important prognostic factor for endometrial carcinoma (Table 29-1). Poorly differentiated tumors have a higher grade and a higher percentage of solid (nonglandular) growth. High-grade tumors have a much poorer prognosis because of the likelihood of spread outside of the uterus. The histologic type of carcinoma also affects prognosis. Other prognostic factors are presented in Table 29-2.

EPIDEMIOLOGY

Endometrial cancer occurs in both premenopausal (25%) and postmenopausal (75%) women. Five percent to 10% of those with premenopausal diagnoses are under 40 years old. The **average age of diagnosis is 61**; the largest affected group is between age 50 and 59. Most tumors are caught early when they are of low grade and low stage (Table 29-3); therefore, the **overall prognosis for the disease is good**. Eighty percent of women have Type I endometrial cancer, although 20% have the more aggressive Type II cancers.

TABLE 29-3. Stage at Which Endometrial Cancer Is Diagnosed	
Stage I	72%
Stage II	12%
Stage III	13%
Stage IV	3%

RISK FACTORS

Several risk factors have been identified for Type I endometrial cancer. These include a history of **unopposed estrogen exposure**, obesity, nulliparity, late menopause, chronic anovulation, and tamoxifen use (Table 29-4). Other risk factors include diabetes mellitus; cancer of the breast, ovary, or colon; and a family history of endometrial cancer and/or Lynch Syndrome.

Excess exogenous estrogen exposure can result from unopposed use of **estrogen replacement therapy** (ERT) in the absence of progesterone in a woman with a uterus. Studies show that 20% to 50% of women who are given ERT without progesterone will develop endometrial hyperplasia or endometrial intraepithelial neoplasia within 1 year. Similarly, **tamoxifen**, a selective estrogen receptor modulator, can also act as a source of exogenous estrogen. It is typically used in women with estrogen–progesterone receptor positive breast cancer (see Chapter 32) to competitively inhibit estrogen at the estrogen receptor. Therefore, it works to block stimulation of breast tissue in women with estrogen–progesterone receptor positive breast cancer. However, in endometrial tissue, tamoxifen acts as a **partial agonist/weak estrogen** to stimulate endometrial proliferation.

TABLE 29-4. Risk Factors for Endometrial Cancer	
Risk Factor	Relative Risk
Nulliparity	2–4
Late menopause	2–4
Chronic anovulation (PCOS)	3
Diabetes mellitus	2–8
Tamoxifen use	3–8
Obesity	
21–50 lb overweight	2–4
>50 lb overweight	10
Unopposed estrogen therapy	2–10
PCOS, polycystic ovary syndrome.	

Endometrial cancer can also be caused by prolonged exposure to **excess endogenous estrogen** without concomitant progesterone exposure. This mechanism of action is demonstrated in **obese women**. These women have higher endogenous estrogen levels because of peripheral conversion of androgens to estrone and estradiol in the adipocytes. These women have also lower sex hormone-binding globulin levels. Many are anovulatory as well.

Women with **chronic anovulation** and/or **polycystic ovary syndrome** (PCOS) typically have more central obesity and therefore have more **peripheral conversion** of androgens to estrone and estradiol. Additionally, these patients have a relative lack of progesterone in the luteal phase because of their **anovulatory cycles**. This mechanism of action may also explain the higher rates of endometrial cancer in nulliparous women. These women are thought to be at higher risk of infertility and subfertility secondary to anovulatory cycles. The increased risk of endometrial cancer with **early menarche** and **late menopause** is presumably due to increased lifetime endogenous estrogen exposure.

Diabetes (Type II > Type I) also increases a patient's risk of endometrial cancer. This is partially attributed to the comorbid risk of **obesity** and **chronic anovulation** in this patient population. Even when controlling for these factors, diabetes is still an independent risk factor for endometrial cancer. It is hypothesized that the presence of hyperinsulinemia, insulin resistance, and insulin-like growth factors may lead to **abnormal endometrial proliferation** in these patients.

There is an increased risk of endometrial cancer in women who have at least one **first-degree relative** (mother, sister, or daughter) with uterine cancer. Women with a known family history of **Lynch II syndrome** have an increased risk of endometrial cancer as well. Lynch II syndrome is also known as hereditary nonpolyposis colorectal cancer (HNPCC) and is associated with a genetic predisposition to colorectal, endometrial, ovarian, kidney, stomach and small bowel cancers. Specific **germline gene mutations** are responsible for the cancers in the majority of these women with Lynch II syndrome. Cowden syndrome is associated with multiple noncancerous hamartomas of the mouth, nose, and intestines; and some cancers, including breast, thyroid, and endometrial malignancies. Peutz–Jeghers syndrome (PJS) is a hereditary polyposis syndrome notable for benign hamartomatous polyps in the gastrointestinal tract and brown macules on the lips and oral mucosa. Women with PJS are also at increased risk for certain cancers, including lungs, breast, uterus, and ovaries. Patients with a personal history of breast cancer have also an increased risk of endometrial cancer. This is attributed to the presence of similar risk factors (obesity, nulliparity, and high-fat diet) in both cancers. The presence of *BRCA1* increases the risk of the rare but aggressive serous uterine cancers. This raises concern with leaving the uterus in situ in women with BRCA mutations.

Endometrial **hyperplasia, now known as EIN**, is another risk factor for endometrial cancer. The degree of risk of malignant transformation of endometrial hyperplasia to endometrial cancer depends on the type of hyperplasia (see Table 14-5). Its mildest form, simple hyperplasia *without* atypia, poses a 1% risk of endometrial cancer, whereas its most severe form, complex hyperplasia *with atypia*, poses a 29% risk of developing endometrial cancer if left untreated. Furthermore, women with atypical endometrial hyperplasia may have a coexistent endometrial cancer as often as 17% to 52% of the time.

Despite these known risk factors for Type I endometrial cancer, there are no effective screening mechanisms for endometrial carcinoma. Neither annual Pap smears nor endometrial biopsies have been shown to offer cost-effective screening in asymptomatic patients.

Conversely, **protective factors** include those that decrease lifetime estrogen exposure, including combination oral contraceptive pills (OCPs), progestin-containing contraceptives, and combination estrogen and progesterone hormone-replacement therapy. These patients have a lower rate of endometrial cancer compared with nonusers. The protection conferred on a woman who takes combination OCPs lasts for 15 years after discontinuation. Other protective factors include high parity, pregnancy, physical activity (decreased obesity, favorable immune function, and endogenous hormone levels), and smoking (causes increased hepatic metabolism of estrogen). Women can also lower their risk of endometrial cancer by avoiding obesity, hypertension, and diabetes, and by eating a healthy diet and exercising. Women who exercise regularly have one-half the risk of endometrial cancer because those who do not exercise.

Unfortunately, there are **no identifiable risk factors** for women who may be at risk for Type II endometrial cancer.

CLINICAL MANIFESTATIONS

HISTORY

Ninety percent of women with endometrial cancer have either **postmenopausal bleeding** or some form of **abnormal vaginal bleeding** (heavy or prolonged menstrual bleeding, postcoital spotting, or intermenstrual bleeding). Ten percent of women may also present with a nonbloody vaginal discharge. As a result of these early symptoms, most endometrial cancers are diagnosed at an early stage (Table 29-3). **Pelvic pain**, **pelvic mass**, and **weight loss** are seen in women who present with more advanced disease.

PHYSICAL EXAMINATION

The physical examination may reveal obesity, acanthosis nigricans, hypertension, or stigmata of diabetes. The clinician should look for signs of metastatic disease, including pleural effusion, ascites, hepatosplenomegaly, general lymphadenopathy, and abdominal masses.

Women with endometrial carcinoma typically have a **normal pelvic examination**. In more advanced stages of the disease, the cervical os may be patulous, and the cervix may be firm and expanded. The uterus may be normal size or enlarged. The adnexae should be carefully examined for evidence of extrauterine metastasis and/or coexistent ovarian carcinoma.

DIFFERENTIAL DIAGNOSIS

Most women with endometrial cancer present with a complaint of **abnormal uterine bleeding**. This may include heavy or prolonged menstrual bleeding, intermenstrual bleeding, postcoital spotting, or oligomenorrhea from anovulation. The differential diagnosis for premenopausal bleeding includes uterine fibroids, endometrial polyps, adenomyosis, endometrial hyperplasia, ovarian cysts, and thyroid dysfunction (see Fig. 22-1).

The **differential diagnosis** for **postmenopausal bleeding** is presented in Table 29-5. Note that EIN and endometrial cancer are collectively responsible for 15% to 25% of postmenopausal bleeding. However, the older the patient and the higher the number of years since menopause, the higher the probability of malignancy. The amount of bleeding does not correlate with risk of malignancy.

DIAGNOSTIC EVALUATION

Although dilation and curettage (D&C) was once the gold standard for the evaluation of abnormal bleeding, office **endometrial biopsy** (EMB) has an accuracy of 90% to 98% without the need for anesthesia and operative risks. In postmenopausal women, **transvaginal ultrasound** can be helpful in triaging suspicious lesions from the most common source of postmenopausal bleeding-genitourinary atrophy. An endometrial thickness of 4 mm or less is indicative of low risk for malignancy in postmenopausal women. These women do not require EMB unless their bleeding is persistent/recurrent or they are at high risk for malignancy. Premenopausal women are subject to a high degree of variability in the thickness of the endometrial lining. Therefore, **persistent abnormal bleeding**, even in the setting of normal imaging, warrants a **tissue diagnosis** with EMB for women >45. Women at high risk for malignancy should undergo sampling of the endometrium regardless of age.

If an adequate EMB cannot be performed because of patient discomfort, cervical stenosis, or insufficient tissue sample, **a D&C (± hysteroscopy)** should be done to sample the endometrium. A D&C should also be done if there are suspicious findings (EIN or necrosis) on EMB or if the patient continues to have symptoms after a negative EMB.

In addition to endometrial sampling, the initial workup for a woman with abnormal vaginal bleeding should also include a **thyroid stimulating hormone** (TSH), a **prolactin level** (if oligomenorrheic), and possibly a **follicle stimulating hormone** (FSH) and estradiol level (to distinguish whether the patient may be peri- or postmenopausal). A **complete blood count** (CBC) should be obtained to rule out anemia preoperatively if bleeding is heavy or prolonged. Because very high **CA-125 levels** are suggestive of spread beyond the uterus, a CA-125 level may be drawn if extrauterine spread is suspected. These levels can also be followed postoperatively to assess the effectiveness of treatment.

An up-to-date **Pap test** should also be obtained in women with abnormal bleeding, although only 30% to 40% of patients with endometrial cancer will have an abnormal Pap test. When the Pap cytology shows **endometrial cells** in a woman 40 years or older, an

TABLE 29-5. Differential Diagnosis of Postmenopausal Bleeding

Cause of Bleeding	Frequency (%)
Endometrial atrophy	60–80
Exogenous estrogens/MHT	15–25
Endometrial cancer	10–15
Endometrial or cervical polyps	2–12
Endometrial intraepithelial neoplasia (EIN)	5–10
Miscellaneous	10

MHT, menopausal hormone therapy.

EMB should be considered to rule out endometrial cancer. These cytology reports are particularly concerning when atypical **glandular or atypical endometrial cells** are found.

A **pelvic ultrasound** should also be performed to look for fibroids, adenomyosis, polyps, and endometrial hyperplasia and EIN. Postmenopausal women with an endometrial stripe less than or equal to 4 mm are unlikely to have EIN or cancer. However, even if the endometrial stripe and the remainder of the pelvic ultrasound appear normal, the physician is still obliged to obtain an endometrial sampling via EMB or D&C if the bleeding is persistent. Likewise, even if another potential source of bleeding is identified, the endometrium must still be sampled. If bone pain is present, a chest radiograph, CT, or bone scan can be performed.

More than 60% of women at risk for **Lynch II syndrome** (or HNPCC) will develop endometrial and/or ovarian cancer before developing colon cancer. Given this, these women who carry Lynch II syndrome–associated mutations or who have a family member known to carry such a mutation should undergo yearly EMB beginning at age 35.

TREATMENT

Although endometrial cancer was once clinically staged, in 1988, the International Federation of Gynecology and Obstetrics (FIGO) changed to a **surgical staging system** that more accurately reflects the true degree of disease progression. This system relies on **pathologic confirmation** of the extent of spread of the disease (Table 29-6).

STAGE I AND STAGE II DISEASE

In general, treatment for endometrial carcinoma includes **systematic surgical staging**, including **total hysterectomy** and **bilateral salpingo-oophorectomy** (TH-BSO), pelvic washings, pelvic and para-aortic lymph node (LN) resection, and complete resection of visible tumor for all stages of the disease (Table 29-7). Minimally invasive laparoscopic surgery is increasingly used for staging of endometrial carcinoma. Exceptions to complete surgical staging are young women with Grade I endometrioid carcinoma who desire future fertility or women with a high mortality risk related to surgery. When practical and feasible,

TABLE 29-6. FIGO Surgical Staging of Endometrial Carcinoma

Stages	Extent of Disease
Stage I	
Ia	Limited to the endometrium no myometrial invasion or invasion
Ib	Invasion limited to less than one-half of myometrium
Ic	Invasion is greater than one-half of the myometrium
Stage II	
IIa	Spread to the endocervical glands only
IIb	Invasion of cervical stroma
Stage III	
IIIa	Tumor invades serosa and/or positive peritoneal cytology
IIIb	Vaginal or parametrial metastases
IIIc	Metastases to pelvic and/or para-aortic lymph nodes
IIIc1	Positive pelvic nodes
IIIc2	Positive para-aortic nodes
Stage IV	
IVa	Tumor invasion of bladder and/or bowel mucosa
IVb	Distant metastases including intra-abdominal and/or inguinal lymph nodes

TABLE 29-7. Treatment Recommendations for Endometrial Cancer by Stage

Stage I	TH-BSO, pelvic and para-aortic LN sampling; if high risk[a], then radiation
Stage II	TH-BSO, pelvic and para-aortic LN sampling; if high risk, then radiation, ± chemotherapy
Stage III	TH-BSO, pelvic and para-aortic LN sampling, radiation, ± chemotherapy
Stage IV	TH-BSO, pelvic and para-aortic LN sampling, radiation, ± chemotherapy
Recurrence, pelvic	Radiation, high-dose progestins, chemotherapy
Recurrence, vaginal	Vaginal radiation

TH-BSO, total hysterectomy and bilateral salpingo-oophorectomy.

[a]Grade 3 lesions, Grade 2 lesion greater than 2 cm, lower uterine segment involvement, cervical involvement, poor histologic differentiation, papillary serous or clear cell histology, and greater than one-third myometrial penetration.

TABLE 29-8. High-Risk Features for Endometrial Cancer
>50% Myometrial invasion
Serous or clear cell tumors
Grade 3 tumors (>50% solid growth)
Large tumor (>2 cm or filling cavity)
Spread beyond the uterine fundus (Stages III and IV)
Lymphovascular involvement

referral to a gynecologic oncologist is recommended to facilitate the most appropriate treatment modality.

Patients with greater than 50% myometrial invasion have a poorer prognosis even if they have Stage I or Stage II disease confined to the uterus. These patients and those with other **poor prognostic factors** such as large tumor mass (>2 cm or filling the cavity), Grade 3 tumor type (more than 50% of the tumor is solid); uterine serous, clear cell or carcinosarcoma histologic types; or enlarged lymph nodes may also require radiation therapy ± chemotherapy even if the disease is confined to the uterus.

STAGE III AND STAGE IV DISEASE

When the malignancy has spread to the uterine serosa or beyond it (Stages III and IV disease), patients will require **pelvic radiation therapy ± chemotherapy** after surgical treatment.

ADVANCED AND RECURRENT DISEASE

Chemotherapy or progestin therapy alone may be used to treat advanced extrauterine or recurrent disease, based on histologic subtype and location of tumor spread.

PROGNOSIS

Because most endometrial cancers are Stage I at diagnosis and endometrioid subtype, the overall 5-year survival rate is quite good at 65%. Survival rates for the various stages of endometrial adenocarcinoma are 87% for Stage I, 76% for Stage II, 59% for Stage III, and 18% for Stage IV. The presence of certain high-risk features (Table 29-8) confers a higher risk of recurrence and lower survival rates.

FOLLOW-UP

Follow-up should include a thorough history and physical examination (with speculum and rectovaginal examination) every 3 to 6 months for 2 years, followed by every 6 months for the subsequent 3 years. If without evidence for recurrent disease, the patient can likely be followed annually. Radiologic evaluation should be used only for diagnostic purposes and not for routine surveillance.

Recurrence is influenced by the original treatment received, as well as the patient's previous history of metastasis and the presence of high-risk features (Table 29-8). The risk of recurrence is **greatest within the first 3 years** after treatment. About 50% of all recurrences are local, 30% are distant, and 20% are combined. Treatment options for recurrent disease are radiotherapy (if not previously radiated), chemotherapy, or high-dose progestin therapy (Table 29-7). **Progestin therapies**, typically megestrol (Megace) or medroxyprogesterone (Provera), have been used with a 30% response rate and minimal side effects in low-grade endometrioid-type tumors.

The use of estrogen replacement therapy (ERT) in patients treated for endometrial carcinoma has been controversial. A few preliminary studies suggest that ERT may not affect the rate of recurrence of endometrial cancer. However, at this time, it is usually reserved for those patients with low-risk disease whose cancer was well differentiated and minimally invasive. Even then, it is initiated no sooner than 6 to 12 months after treatment. As with traditional use of hormone replacement, the use of ERT should be initiated only for severe vasomotor symptoms and should be given at the lowest effective dose, for the shortest possible duration in patients <60 years old.

KEY POINTS

- Endometrial cancer is the most common gynecologic cancer, but has the best survival rates because it is associated with early symptoms and easy and accurate diagnostic modalities. It is thus diagnosed and treated early.
- Endometrial cancers are classified as Type I (80%) or Type II (20%). Type I endometrial cancers can be caused by prolonged exposure to exogenous or endogenous estrogen in the absence of progesterone. Endometrial intraepithelial neoplasia (EIN) is the typical precursor to Type I disease.
- Type II endometrial cancers are *not* estrogen-dependent neoplasms. They are not

- generally associated with EIN. They tend to be more aggressive and have a poorer prognosis than Type I cancers.
- The most common type of endometrial cancer (80%) is endometrioid adenocarcinoma. Other types have poorer prognosis, including uterine serous and clear cell carcinomas.
- Endometrioid cancer is diagnosed at a median age of 61, with 25% of patients being diagnosed premenopausally and 75% postmenopausally.
- The major risk factors for Type I endometrial cancer include unopposed estrogen exposure, EIN, obesity, chronic anovulation, nulliparity, and late menopause. Diabetes and family history if Lynch Syndrome are also important risk factors.
- The most common presenting symptom is abnormal uterine bleeding.
- Endometrial biopsy (EMB) is the standard of care for diagnosing endometrial cancer.
- Currently, there are no cost-effective screening tools for endometrial cancer; however, because of abnormal bleeding, most women are diagnosed early, with 75% of lesions being at Stage I at the time of diagnosis.
- Endometrial cancer is surgically staged. Treatment may involve TH-BSO with pelvic and para-aortic lymphadenectomy for low-risk, low-stage disease (Stages I and II).
- In addition to TH-BSO, pelvic and para-aortic lymph node dissection and pelvic radiation ± chemotherapy are used to treat women with Stage III or IV disease and those with high-risk features (including papillary serous or clear cell types, Grade 3 differentiation, large tumor size, lymphovascular invasion, or enlarged lymph nodes).
- Advanced or recurrent disease can be treated with tumor-directed radiation therapy, chemotherapy, or high-dose progestin therapy.
- Overall 5-year survival rate is 65%, with 85% to 100% of recurrences occurring in the first 3 years after treatment.

CLINICAL VIGNETTES

VIGNETTE 1

A 63-year-old G4 P4 woman presents to your office with a chief complaint of vaginal spotting. She reports an isolated episode 1 week prior to presentation that consisted of scant vaginal bleeding. She denies any associated symptoms, including pelvic pain, pressure, or early satiety. She also denies any family history of gynecologic malignancy. Her past medical history is significant for morbid obesity, hypertension, and inflammatory bowel disease.

1. What is the most likely diagnosis?
   a. Atrophic endometrium
   b. Endometrial cancer
   c. Endometrial polyp
   d. Ovarian cancer
   e. Adenomyosis

2. After obtaining a thorough history and performing a physical examination (including a pelvic examination), what is the next best step in evaluation?
   a. CA 125
   b. MRI
   c. Cervical cytology
   d. Transvaginal ultrasound and possible endometrial biopsy (EMB)
   e. Mammography

3. What is the patient's most significant risk factor for endometrial cancer?
   a. Multiparity
   b. History of prior tobacco use
   c. Remote history of oral contraceptive use
   d. Inflammatory bowel disease
   e. Morbid obesity

4. Upon further questioning, the patient's family history is significant for breast and colon cancer. You are considering a referral to genetic counseling for further evaluation. What familial syndrome (gene mutation) is associated with these malignancies?
   a. BRCA
   b. HER 2 NEU
   c. Lynch II syndrome (hereditary nonpolyposis colorectal cancer)
   d. Cowden syndrome
   e. Peutz–Jeghers syndrome (PJS)

VIGNETTE 2

A 30-year-old nulligravid patient presenting for her annual examination reports a family history positive for breast and ovarian cancer. On further discussion, she notes that her mother developed breast cancer at age 39 and her grandmother passed away from ovarian cancer. After having recently watched an episode about hereditary cancers on her favorite medical talk show, she is wondering if she is a candidate for genetic testing.

1. Which of the following should be recommended?
   a. No testing recommended at this time
   b. Schedule an appointment with a genetic counselor
   c. Order a BRCA test yourself
   d. Recommend a risk-reducing bilateral salpingo-oophorectomy
   e. Recommend surveillance with mammograms every 6 months

2. The patient does accept the referral but is hesitant to pursue the appointment secondary to concerns about losing her health insurance if she tests positive for a genetic predisposition. How do you counsel her?
   a. Reassure her that her results can be kept out of her medical record if she pays cash
   b. Tell her that it is a risk that she must be willing to take
   c. Reassure her that current legislation protects against genetic discrimination
   d. Recommend that a different family member undergoes testing instead
   e. Recommend testing in another country

3. The patient undergoes genetic counseling and tests positive for a BRCA mutation. She is most concerned with her risk for ovarian cancer. After considering the limitations of surveillance for ovarian cancer, she is eager to pursue risk-reducing surgery and declines any fertility sparing measures. Which procedure do you offer the patient?
   a. Bilateral oophorectomy only
   b. Exploratory laparotomy, hysterectomy, and bilateral oophorectomy
   c. Laparoscopic ovarian biopsies, with removal of any cysts
   d. Bilateral salpingo-oophorectomy only
   e. Exploratory laparoscopy, pelvic washings, and bilateral salpingo-oophorectomy

VIGNETTE 3

Your patient is a postmenopausal woman who was recently diagnosed with ductal carcinoma in situ of the breast. Her oncologist has initiated treatment with tamoxifen, and she presents to your office for an annual visit. Her oncologist counseled her to report any postmenopausal bleeding immediately, and she makes an inquiry about the significance of this.

1. In this patient, the use of tamoxifen is associated with an increased risk of which of the following?
   a. Endometrial intraepithelial neoplasia (EIN)
   b. Invasive carcinoma
   c. Uterine sarcoma
   d. Endometrial polyps
   e. All of the above

2. After receiving the above information, the patient asks whether she warrants any special testing or treatment. She is otherwise asymptomatic. Which do you recommend?
   a. Routine care with pelvic examination, no additional measures unless bleeding develops
   b. Annual transvaginal ultrasound
   c. Annual EMB
   d. Defer to the recommendation of the prescribing oncologist
   e. Serial CA-125 levels

VIGNETTE 4

A 37-year-old patient reports lifelong oligomenorrhea with limited previous evaluation. Her last menstrual period was 10 months ago. She does bring images and report of a recent outside ultrasound that is negative for any anatomic pathology. Her physical examination is significant for obesity (BMI 43) and moderate facial hirsutism, but no other signs of hyperandrogenism. She does not have any other significant comorbidities.

1. What is the most likely diagnosis?
   a. Congenital adrenal hyperplasia
   b. Androgen producing tumor
   c. Conn syndrome
   d. Polycystic ovary syndrome
   e. Anabolic steroid administration

2. In addition to serum testing, what is your next step in the evaluation of this patient?
   a. EMB
   b. Pelvic MRI
   c. Pelvic angiogram
   d. ACTH stimulation test
   e. Transabdominal ultrasound

ANSWERS

VIGNETTE 1 Question 1
1. Answer A:
Although any vaginal bleeding in a postmenopausal woman warrants a thorough evaluation to rule out endometrial carcinoma, up to 80% of patients will be diagnosed with a benign condition—most commonly endometrial atrophy. The differential diagnosis also includes exogenous estrogens, endometrial or cervical polyps, endometrial intraepithelial neoplasia (EIN), fibroids, ovarian cysts, and endometrial and cervical cancer.

VIGNETTE 1 Question 2
2. Answer D:
Office EMB has an accuracy of 90% to 98% in the detection of endometrial carcinoma. Another option includes transvaginal sonography to assess the thickness of the endometrial lining. An endometrial thickness of 4 mm or less in a postmenopausal woman is indicative of low risk for malignancy. If the endometrial stripe is more than 4 mm or if the patient continues to experience postmenopausal vaginal bleeding, consideration should be given to an EMB or a hysteroscopy, D&C for direct visualization and sampling of the endometrial cavity. Lastly, laboratory studies (TSH, FSH, CBC, prolactin level, and cervical cytology) are commonly included in the evaluation of abnormal bleeding, but in the patient described above, pelvic ultrasound with possible EMB is the next best step.

VIGNETTE 1 Question 3
3. Answer E:
Multiparity, tobacco use, and hormonal contraceptive use are all considered protective factors that decrease the lifetime risk of endometrial cancer. Obesity does confer an increased risk for the development of endometrial cancer, with a relative risk of 10 for those patients who are more than 50 lb overweight. Exogenous unopposed estrogen exposure, nulliparity, late menopause, chronic anovulation (PCOS), and diabetes mellitus are also risk factors for endometrial cancer.

VIGNETTE 1 Question 4
4. Answer C:
More than 50% of women who are identified as "at risk" for Lynch syndrome will develop a gynecologic malignancy (ovarian or endometrial) before they develop colorectal cancer. For known carriers of this mutation, annual EMB is recommended, starting at age 35. Although there is no reliable screening test for ovarian cancer, evaluation with transvaginal ultrasound ± CA 125 is offered at age 30 to 35, or 5 to 10 years earlier than the earliest age of the first diagnosis of these cancers in the family (whichever is earlier). Discussion of prophylactic hysterectomy and salpingo-oophorectomy at around age 35 or at the end of childbearing is appropriate. These patients are not candidates for ovarian preservation if they undergo hysterectomy. Patients who carry the BRCA 1 or 2 germline mutations have an increased risk of breast and ovarian cancer. Patients with Cowden syndrome are at risk for multiple noncancerous hamartomas of the mouth, nose, and intestines. They are also at increased risk for some cancers, including breast, thyroid, and endometrial malignancies. PJS is a hereditary polyposis syndrome notable for benign hamartomatous polyps in the gastrointestinal tract and brown macules on the lips and oral mucosa. Patients with PJS are also at increased risk for certain cancers, including lungs, breast, uterus, and ovaries.

VIGNETTE 2 Question 1
1. Answer B:
Although all patients should be evaluated with a thorough family history, a hereditary cancer risk assessment is best performed by an expert in cancer genetics. These providers have received special training in risk assessment, education, and counseling—and may or may not include genetic testing. Genetic testing may raise several psychological and familial issues; therefore, thorough discussion is merited before obtaining the patient's consent. In general, for patients with a first-degree relative (mother, sister, or daughter) with breast cancer, mammograms start 5 to 10 years before the age at which the earliest diagnosis was made. This patient would start at age 29, 10 years prior to her mom's diagnosis at 39.

VIGNETTE 2 Question 2
2. Answer C:
The Federal Genetic Information Nondiscrimination Act of 2008 protects individuals against health and employment discrimination based on genetic testing. In addition, many state laws protect against the same. However, these laws do *not* apply to other forms of insurance such as life insurance or disability insurance.

VIGNETTE 2 Question 3
3. Answer E:
For risk-reducing procedures, either open or laparoscopic procedures can be performed, although laparoscopy may be preferred secondary to morbidity. For either approach, a thorough inspection of all peritoneal surfaces is warranted, along with pelvic

washings. Any abnormal areas should be biopsied or resected. Because carriers of the BRCA mutation are at increased risk for fallopian tube carcinoma, all ovarian and fallopian tissues should be resected.

VIGNETTE 3 Question 1
1. Answer E:
Postmenopausal women taking tamoxifen are at increased risk for endometrial proliferation, hyperplasia, EIN, polyp formation, invasive endometrial carcinoma, and uterine sarcoma. The risk of developing endometrial cancer is related to dose and duration of tamoxifen use and is greatest in women over 50. A large multicenter study confirmed that the risk of developing endometrial cancer among tamoxifen users was approximately 1.6 per 1,000 person years. But because the use of tamoxifen significantly increased the 5-year survival of patients with breast cancer, the authors concluded that the small risk of developing endometrial cancer is outweighed by the significant survival benefit provided by the drug.

VIGNETTE 3 Question 2
2. Answer A:
Postmenopausal patients on tamoxifen should be vigilant for symptoms of endometrial hyperplasia or cancer; *any* vaginal bleeding, spotting, bloody discharge, or staining should be reported and warrants further evaluation. Routine sonographic evaluation in asymptomatic women has not proven effective, because tamoxifen is known to induce subepithelial stromal hypertrophy (which may not be clinically significant). Similarly, studies have not supported the use of routine EMB for asymptomatic women.

VIGNETTE 4 Question 1
1. Answer D:
In reproductive age women, up to 10% may have hyperandrogenic chronic anovulation (i.e., polycystic ovary syndrome). The clinical hallmarks of this entity are noncyclic menstrual bleeding, hirsutism, and obesity. Adult women with menstrual irregularities should undergo an evaluation that includes TSH, FSH, and prolactin levels. In women with rapid virilization, a tumor can be ruled out by obtaining a pelvic ultrasound and checking levels of testosterone and DHEA-S, and 17-OH progesterone.

VIGNETTE 4 Question 2
2. Answer A:
Although the overall risk of endometrial cancer is very low in women under 45 years, those who are at high risk for EIN and cancer are <45 and present with abnormal uterine bleeding require evaluation. In younger patients with chronic unopposed estrogen exposure, prolonged amenorrhea, or other risk factors for uterine carcinoma, endometrial assessment should be performed regardless of age. In this case, the patient is <45 but is at high risk for hyperplasia and EIN with a prolonged period of amenorrhea. She should undergo laboratory evaluation, transvaginal ultrasound and EMB.

30 | Ovarian and Fallopian Tube Tumors

TUMORS OF THE OVARIES

There are many types of benign and malignant tumors of the ovaries (Table 30-1), each possessing its own characteristics. Fortunately, 80% of ovarian tumors are benign. In the United States, ovarian cancer is the second most common cancer of the female genital tract (Fig. 30-1). Moreover, it is the fifth most common cause of cancer death and the **most common cause of gynecologic cancer death**. Fallopian tube carcinoma is extremely rare, but the incidence is likely underestimated.

Although ovarian carcinoma accounts for **25% of all gynecologic malignancies** (22,280 new cases per year), it is responsible for over **50% of gynecologic cancer deaths** (14,420 deaths per year). This high mortality is due in part to the **lack of effective screening tools** for early diagnosis and **presentation at late stages of disease** when tumors have spread throughout the peritoneal cavity, and the chance for cure is low. Because the overall 5-year survival rate for women with ovarian carcinoma is only 46%, a high degree of suspicion and prompt diagnosis and intervention are critical.

PATHOGENESIS

Tumors of the ovaries are associated with one of the three distinct components of the ovary: the surface epithelium, the ovarian germ cells, or the ovarian stroma (Fig. 30-2). Over 65% of all ovarian tumors and 90% of all ovarian cancers are **epithelial tumors** on the ovary capsule. About 5% to 10% of ovarian cancer is metastatic from other primary tumors in the body, usually from the gastrointestinal tract, known as Krukenberg tumors, or the breast and endometrium.

Ovarian cancer is spread primarily by **direct exfoliation** of malignant cells from the ovaries. As a result, the sites of metastases often follow the broad circulatory path of the peritoneal fluid. **Lymphatic spread** can also occur, most commonly to the retroperitoneal pelvic and para-aortic lymph nodes (Fig. 28-7). **Hematogenous spread** is responsible for more rare and distant metastases to the lung and brain. In advanced disease, intraperitoneal tumor spread leads to accumulation of ascites in the abdomen and encasement of the bowel with tumor. This results in intermittent bowel obstruction known as a **carcinomatous ileus**. In many cases, this progression results in malnutrition, slow starvation, cachexia, and death.

Although the cause of ovarian carcinoma is unclear, it is believed to result from **malignant transformation of ovarian tissue** after prolonged periods of **chronic uninterrupted ovulation**. Ovulation disrupts the epithelium of the ovary and activates the cellular repair mechanism. When ovulation occurs for long periods without interruption, this may provide the opportunity for **somatic gene deletions and mutations** during the cellular repair process. An emerging theory is that serous ovarian cancers originate in the **distal fallopian tube**.

About 10% to 15% of women with ovarian cancer have a **familial cancer syndrome**. Patients with mutations in the **BRCA1 gene** have an 85% chance of developing breast cancer and a 30% to 50% chance of developing ovarian cancer. A smaller proportion of patients with **BRCA2 gene** mutations (25%) also have an increased risk of ovarian cancer. Patients with **Lynch II syndrome** (hereditary nonpolyposis colorectal cancer [HNPCC] syndrome) have a high rate of familial ovarian, colorectal, endometrial kidney, stomach and small bowel cancer. Environmental factors such as talc and asbestos have been proposed, but have not been definitively linked with the pathogenesis of ovarian cancer.

TABLE 30-1. Benign and Malignant Ovarian Tumors

Epithelial tumors

Serous tumors
   Serous cystadenoma
   Borderline serous tumor
   Serous cystadenocarcinoma
   Adenofibroma and cystadenofibroma
Mucinous tumors
   Mucinous cystadenoma
   Borderline mucinous tumor
   Mucinous cystadenocarcinoma
Endometrioid carcinoma
Clear cell adenocarcinoma
Brenner tumor
Undifferentiated carcinoma

Germ cell tumors

Teratoma
Benign (mature, adult)
   Cystic teratoma (dermoid cyst)
   Solid teratoma
Malignant (immature)
   Monodermal or specialized (e.g., carcinoid, struma ovarii) Dysgerminoma
   Endodermal sinus tumor
   Choriocarcinoma
   Embryonal carcinoma
   Polyembryoma
   Mixed germ cell tumors

Sex cord–stromal tumors

Granulosa-theca cell tumors
   Granulosa cell tumor
   Thecoma
   Fibroma
Sertoli–Leydig cell tumor (androblastoma)
Gonadoblastoma

Unclassified

Ex. lipoid-cell tumors and sarcomas

Metastatic tumors

Ex. from GI tract, female genital tract, or breast

Data from Robbins S, Cotran R, Kumar V. *Robbins' Pathologic Basis of Disease*. Philadelphia, PA: WB Saunders; 1995:1158.

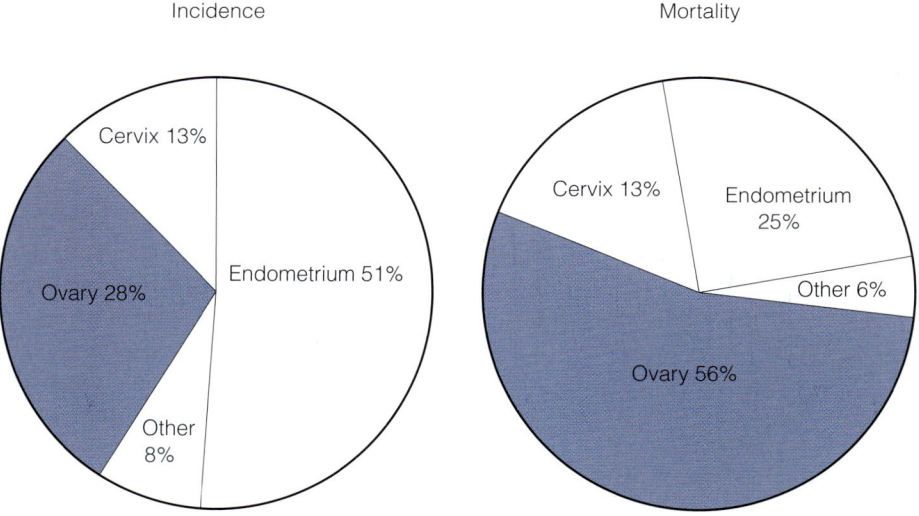

FIGURE 30-1. Relationships of ovarian cancer to other gynecologic cancer for incidence and mortality; United States, 1996. (Modified from Parker SL, Tong T, Bolden S, et al. Cancer statistics. *CA Cancer J Clin.* 46:5–27, 1996.)

EPIDEMIOLOGY

An average woman has a 1 in 70 chance of developing ovarian carcinoma over her lifetime and a 1 in 95 chance of dying from invasive ovarian cancer. The median age of diagnosis is 63 years with two-thirds of women with ovarian cancer being over the age of 55 at the time of diagnosis. Hereditary ovarian cancers typically occur in women who are, on average, 10 years younger than those with nonhereditary ovarian cancer. Nonepithelial ovarian cancers are more common in girls and young women. There is a slightly increased frequency in Caucasian women compared to the incidence in Hispanic, Asian, and African American women.

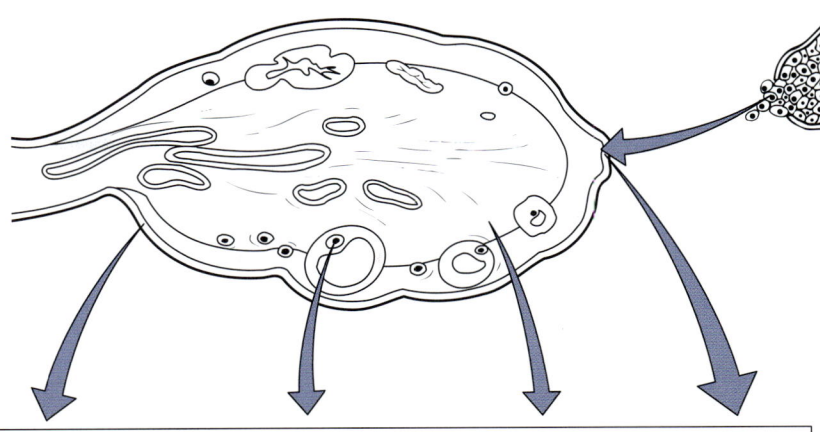

Origin	Surface epithelial cells (common epithelial tumors)	Germ cell	Sex cord–stroma	Metastasis to ovaries
Percent of all ovarian tumors	65%–70%	15%–20%	5%–10%	5%
Age group affected	20+ years	0–25+ years	All ages	Variable
Types	• Serous tumor • Mucinous tumor • Endometrioid tumor • Clear cell tumor • Brenner tumor • Undifferentiated	• Teratoma • Dysgerminoma • Endodermal sinus tumor • Choriocarcinoma • Embryonal carcinoma	• Granulosa–theca cell tumor • Sertoli-Leydig cell tumor • Fibroma	

FIGURE 30-2. Classification of various ovarian neoplasms (benign, borderline, and malignant).

RISK FACTORS

Table 30-2 highlights the major risk factors and protective factors for ovarian cancer. Women with a **familial ovarian cancer syndrome** have a significantly increased risk of ovarian cancer. This includes women with BRCA1 (35% to 70% risk of ovarian cancer), BRCA2 (10% to 30%), and Lynch Syndrome/HNPCC (10% to 50%). Women with a **family history of ovarian cancer** have the next highest risk (5% to 15%). Women with a mother, sister, or daughter with ovarian cancer are at increased risk of developing the disease. The younger the relative is at the time of diagnosis, the higher the risk to first-degree relatives. Similarly, women with **a personal history of breast cancer** have a twofold increase in the incidence of ovarian cancer.

Because the mechanism of ovarian cancer is thought to be linked to mutations occurring during ovulation, women with a history of long periods of **uninterrupted ovulation** (early menarche, infertility, nulliparity, delayed childbearing, and late-onset menopause) are at increased risk of ovarian cancer.

TABLE 30-2. Risk Factors and Protective Factors for Ovarian Cancer

Risk factors
Familial ovarian cancer syndrome
Family history of breast and/or ovarian cancer
Personal history of breast cancer
Increasing age
Early menarche (<12 y)
Infertility
Nulliparity
Late-onset menopause (>50 y)
Obesity (BMI > 30)
Protective factors
Use of OCPs (5+ y)
Multiparity
Breastfeeding
Tubal ligation
Hysterectomy

BMI, body mass index; OCP, oral contraceptive.

For the same reason, **increasing age** is another major risk factor for ovarian cancer. Fifty percent of all women diagnosed with ovarian cancer are 63 years of age or older.

PROTECTIVE FACTORS

Many of the factors found to be protective from ovarian cancer (Table 30-2) are also linked to the **incessant ovulation** hypotheses. This speculates that **ovulation suppression** results in less disruption of the ovarian epithelium and less need for activation of the cellular repair mechanism. Thus, there are fewer opportunities for gene deletions and mutations. **Oral contraceptives** (OCPs) have been found to have a protective effect against ovarian cancer by suppressing ovulation. The use of OCPs for greater than 5 years can reduce the risk of ovarian cancer by 50%. Similarly, **breastfeeding**, **multiparity**, and **chronic anovulation** have also been found to be protective agents that act by interrupting or suppressing ovulation. **Tubal ligation** and **hysterectomy** have been associated with a 67% and 30% reduction in ovarian cancer, respectively, even in patients with a familial cancer syndrome. This may be due to impairment of ovarian blood supply by these procedures and/or decreased migration of carcinogens from the lower genital tract up to the ovaries. Newer theories of ovarian cancer pathogenesis suggest that the etiology of serous carcinomas arises from the distal end of the fallopian tube. Thus, **prophylactic salpingectomy** at the time of routine surgery for benign indications may provide an opportunity to prevent ovarian cancer.

CLINICAL MANIFESTATIONS

History

Patients diagnosed with ovarian cancer are most often **asymptomatic** or have **vague, nonspecific complaints** until the disease has progressed to the advanced stages. Some patients may present with **vague lower abdominal pain**, abdominal distension, bloating, and **early satiety** (Table 30-3). As the tumors progress, other symptoms may develop, including gastrointestinal complaints (nausea, anorexia, and indigestion), urinary frequency, dysuria, and pelvic pressure. Ascites may develop in later stages and cause shortness of breath secondary to pleural effusion. Ventral hernia may also be seen due to increased intra-abdominal pressure.

Physical Examination

There is no evidence to suggest that routine pelvic examination improves the early diagnosis of ovarian cancer. As the disease progresses, the primary findings on examination are a **solid, fixed, irregular pelvic mass** (Table 30-4) that may extend into the upper abdomen along with **ascites** (Fig. 30-3). Ovarian cancer metastasis to the umbilicus is known as **Sister Mary Joseph nodule (SMJN)**. The presence of this hard indurated mass on examination may be the first sign of malignancy, a sign of advanced disease progression or recurrence.

DIAGNOSTIC EVALUATION

Transvaginal pelvic ultrasound is the primary diagnostic tool for investigating an adnexal mass. These sonographic traits help to distinguish between benign and malignant tumors (Table 30-5). Other studies, including **computed tomography** (CT) and **magnetic resonance imaging** of the pelvis and abdomen, can assist in diagnosis and in delineation of the spread of disease. Because malignant cells can spread via direct exfoliation, paracentesis and cyst aspiration should be avoided. Once the diagnosis is made, studies are undertaken to look for **metastatic disease** and to distinguish between primary and secondary ovarian cancer. **Barium enema** and **intravenous pyelography**

TABLE 30-3. Symptoms of Ovarian Cancer

Initial symptoms

Bloating

Early satiety

Dyspepsia

Abdominal pain

Pelvic pain

Later symptoms

Back pain

Urinary frequency/urgency

Constipation

Fatigue

Dyspareunia

Menstrual changes

TABLE 30-4. Evaluation of Pelvic and Abdominal Masses Found on Physical Examination

	Benign	Malignant
Mobility	Mobile	Fixed
Consistency	Cystic	Solid
Tumor surface	Smooth	Irregular
Bilateral or unilateral	Unilateral	Bilateral

FIGURE 30-3. Laparoscopic view of large ovarian mass (*M*), normal uterus (*U*), and ovary (*O*). (From Berek JS. *Berek & Novak's Gynecology*, 14th ed. Philadelphia, PA: Lippincott Williams & Wilkins; 2006.)

TABLE 30-5. Ultrasound Findings in Patients with a Pelvic Mass

	Benign	Malignant
Size	<8 cm	>8 cm
Consistency	Cystic	Solid or cystic and solid
Solid components	Not present	Nodular, papillary
Septations	Not present or singular	Multilocular, thick (>2 mm)
Doppler flow	Not present	Present in solid component
Bilateral or unilateral	Unilateral	Bilateral
Associated features	Calcification, especially Teeth	Ascites, peritoneal masses, lymphadenopathy

are helpful in looking for gastrointestinal (GI) and genital urinary sources of disease. Serum biomarkers CA125 and HE4 are not recommended for routine evaluation of an undiagnosed pelvic mass.

Depending on the type of tumor, ovarian malignancies can be monitored using the **serum tumor markers** CA-125, α-fetoprotein (AFP), lactate dehydrogenase (LDH), and human chorionic gonadotropins (hCG).

SURGICAL STAGING

Ovarian carcinoma is **surgically staged** (Table 30-6). Primary staging includes **total abdominal hysterectomy, bilateral salpingo-oophorectomy (TAHBSO), omentectomy, peritoneal washings,** Pap test of the diaphragm, and **sampling the pelvic and para-aortic lymph nodes**. Because there are no reliable screening tools for ovarian cancer and few early symptoms, nearly **75% of patients present with Stage III or IV.** Subsequently, the 5-year survival is low overall (25% to 45%) and decreases with increasing age. The different types of ovarian cancers are discussed below.

EPITHELIAL TUMORS

PATHOGENESIS

Epithelial cell tumors of the ovaries are derived from **malignant transformation of the epithelium** cells of the surface of the ovary. These cells come from

TABLE 30-6. Staging of Ovarian Carcinoma

Stage I: Growth limited to the ovaries

Ia—one ovary involved

Ib—both ovaries involved

Ic—Ia or Ib and ovarian surface tumor, ruptured capsule, malignant ascites, or peritoneal cytology positive for malignant cells

Stage II: Disease extension from the ovary to the pelvis

IIa—extension to the uterus or fallopian tube

IIb—extension to other pelvic tissues

IIc—IIa or IIb and ovarian surface tumor, ruptured capsule, malignant ascites, or peritoneal cytology positive for malignant cells

Stage III: Disease extension to the abdominal cavity

IIIa—abdominal peritoneal surfaces with microscopic metastases

IIIb—tumor metastases >2 cm in size

IIIc—tumor metastases >2 cm in size or metastatic disease in the pelvic, para-aortic, or inguinal lymph nodes

Stage IV: Distant metastatic disease

Malignant pleural effusion

Pulmonary parenchymal metastases

Liver or splenic parenchymal metastases (not surface implants)

Metastases to the supraclavicular lymph nodes or skin

TABLE 30-7. Gynecologic and Nongynecologic Conditions Associated with Elevated CA-125 Levels

Gynecologic cancers

Epithelial ovarian cancer

Fallopian tube cancer

Endometrial cancer

Endocervical cancer

Nongynecologic cancers

Pancreatic cancer

Lung cancer

Breast cancer

Colon cancer

Benign gynecologic conditions

Normal and ectopic pregnancy

Endometriosis

Fibroids

Pelvic inflammatory disease

Benign nongynecologic conditions

Pancreatitis

Cirrhosis

Peritonitis

Recent laparotomy

---

the primitive mesoderm and are capable of undergoing metaplasia. The six primary types of epithelial tumors are serous, mucinous, endometrioid, clear cell, Brenner, and undifferentiated (Fig. 30-2). The neoplasms in this group range in malignant potential from benign to borderline (tumors of **low malignant potential**) to frankly malignant. **Serous cystadenocarcinomas** are the most common malignant epithelial cell tumors.

Malignant epithelial tumors extend from the surface capsule of the ovary to seed the peritoneal cavity. In more than 75% of patients, tumors have spread beyond the ovary at the time of diagnosis; thus, the prognosis is very poor.

EPIDEMIOLOGY

Epithelial tumors tend to occur in patients who are in their 50s with a **peak incidence from 56 to 60 years of age**. Epithelial cell cancers account for **65% of all ovarian tumors** and **more than 90% of ovarian cancers**. **Serous tumors** (serous cystadenocarcinomas) are the most common type of epithelial ovarian cancer. These tumors are large, cystic, and bilateral 65% of the time.

CLINICAL MANIFESTATIONS

The **serum tumor marker CA-125** is elevated in 80% of epithelial cell cancers. Because CA-125 levels correlate with the progression and regression of these tumors, it has been useful in **tracking the effect of treatment and recurrence of epithelial ovarian carcinoma**. Its value as a screening tool for the detection of ovarian cancer has not yet been established. One reason for this is the high number of benign and malignant gynecologic and nongynecologic conditions associated with an elevated CA-125 level (Table 30-7).

TREATMENT

Surgery is the mainstay of treatment for epithelial cell tumors, including TAHBSO, omentectomy, cytoreduction or "debulking," and bilateral pelvic and para-aortic lymph node sampling. The goal of debulking is to leave behind no visible tumors or tumor nodules not greater than 1 cm. When this is achieved, the patient is said to have undergone **optimal debulking**. When optimal debulking is not achieved, there is a greater chance of recurrent or persistent disease.

After surgery, epithelial ovarian cancer is treated with **combination chemotherapy**, most commonly intravenous carboplatin and paclitaxel (Taxol) or docetaxel (Taxotere). Patients who have had optimal debulking are offered **intraperitoneal cisplatin and paclitaxel chemotherapy** along with intravenous chemotherapy, which not only increases overall survival, but also has more side effects than traditional intravenous chemotherapy.

The tumor marker **CA-125** and the **CAT scan imaging** are most commonly used to evaluate the success of treatment and to diagnose recurrent disease. Unfortunately, tumors **frequently recur** despite aggressive treatment. Recurrent or persistent cancer is treated with chemotherapy. Recurrent ascites is treated with paracentesis.

The overall **5-year survival rate is 20%** for patients with epithelial ovarian cancer (80% to 95% for Stage I, 40% to 70% for Stage II, 30% for Stage III, and <10% for Stage IV disease).

GERM CELL TUMORS

PATHOGENESIS

Germ cell ovarian tumors arise from **primordial germ cells** of the ovary and may be benign (95%) or malignant (5%). These undifferentiated, totipotent germ cells are capable of differentiating into any of the three germ cell layers: yolk sac, placenta, and fetus. This accounts for the various subtypes of germ cell tumors (Fig. 30-4).

The most common type of germ cell tumor is the **benign cystic mature teratoma**, also known as **dermoid cysts**. Dermoids are cystic masses containing mature adult tissue such as skin, hair, and teeth mixed in sebaceous material, giving them a very characteristic appearance (Fig. 30-5). Cystectomy is recommended for definitive diagnosis and to rule out malignancy.

The most common malignant germ cell tumors are **dysgerminomas** (50%), **immature teratomas** (20%), and endodermal sinus (yolk sac) tumors (20%). Embryonal carcinoma (composed of undifferentiated cells), nongestational choriocarcinoma (composed of placental tissue), and mixed germ cell tumors are much less common.

Many germ cell tumors produce **serum tumor markers** that can be useful in the diagnosis of a pelvic mass and in assessing a patient's response to therapy (Table 30-8). Although there is wide variation in the type of serum tumor markers, in general, dysgerminomas produce LDH, endodermal sinus (yolk sac) tumors produce AFP, and choriocarcinomas produce hCG. The undifferentiated embryonal carcinomas that give rise to the more differentiated germ cell tumors produce both AFP and hCG.

In contrast to epithelial tumors, most germ cell tumors **grow rapidly**, are **limited to one ovary**, and are at **Stage I** at the time of diagnosis. The prognosis for germ cell tumors is therefore far better than that for epithelial tumors. In most cases, **these tumors are considered curable**.

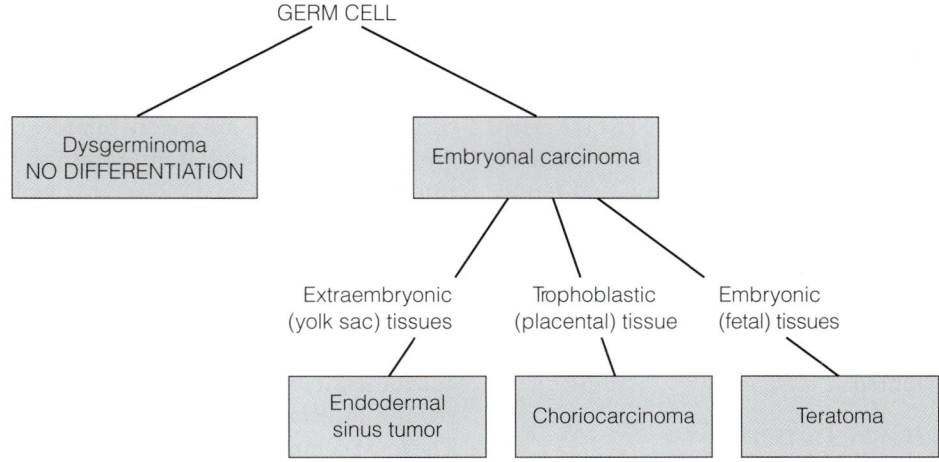

FIGURE 30-4. Histogenesis of tumors of germ cell origin. Because they are totipotent, germ cells may remain undifferentiated, or they may develop into any of the three germ layers: yolk sac or placental or fetal tissue.

FIGURE 30-5. Mature cystic teratoma (dermoid cyst). (From Berek JS. *Berek & Novak's Gynecology*, 14th ed. Philadelphia, PA: Lippincott Williams & Wilkins; 2006.)

TABLE 30-8. Primary Serum Tumor Marker for Germ Cell Cancers

Tumor Type	Primary Tumor Marker
Dysgerminoma	LDH
Immature teratoma	N/A
Endodermal sinus (yolk sac) tumor	AFP
Embryonal carcinoma	AFP and hCG
Choriocarcinoma	hCG

LDH, lactate dehydrogenase; AFP, α-fetoprotein; hCG, human chorionic gonadotropins.

EPIDEMIOLOGY

Germ cell tumors account for 20% to 25% of all ovarian tumors but make up less than 5% of ovarian cancers. Although **95% are benign**, the remaining 5% of germ cell tumors are malignant and found primarily in children and in young women. This makes germ cell tumors the **most common ovarian malignancy in women less than 20 years of age**. Malignant germ cell tumors are three times more common in **Black and Asian women** compared to Caucasian women.

CLINICAL MANIFESTATIONS

Unlike the slow-growing epithelial ovarian cancers, germ cell tumors **grow rapidly**, and thus, cause symptoms leading to earlier diagnosis. Most commonly, distension of the ovarian capsule from rapid growth, **hemorrhage**, and **necrosis** results in acute **pelvic pain**. Patients may also complain of **pressure symptoms** on the bladder or rectum or pain from **torsion or rupture** of the tumor. Eighty-five percent of women will have abdominal pain and a pelvic mass at the time of presentation.

TREATMENT

Women with benign germ cell tumors such as mature teratomas (dermoid cysts) are diagnosed and cured by removing the part of the ovary containing the tumor (ovarian cystectomy) or by removing the entire ovary (oophorectomy).

Because most germ cell cancers are diagnosed in the early stage and are **rarely bilateral**, surgery is typically limited to **unilateral salpingo-oophorectomy** if fertility is desired. However, complete surgical staging should still be performed. If childbearing is complete or if the cancer is bilateral, total abdominal hysterectomy and **bilateral salpingo-oophorectomy** (TAH/BSO) is required along with surgical staging.

With the exception of Stage Ia dysgerminomas and immature teratomas, all germ cell malignancies require **multiagent chemotherapy** after surgery. The most common regimen is bleomycin, etoposide, and cisplatin (Platinol) (BEP). In patients who have elevated **serum tumor markers** prior to treatment, these markers can be used to judge the effectiveness of therapy between chemotherapy cycles.

In the past, **radiation therapy** was used as the primary treatment for **dysgerminomas**, which are exquisitely sensitive to radiation. However, current combination chemotherapy regimens have proved to be as good as or better than radiation therapy. Chemotherapy is also more protective of future fertility, when only one ovary is removed.

Fortunately, most cases of germ cell cancer are considered curable with surgery and chemotherapy. The overall **5-year survival rate is 85%** for dysgerminomas, 70% to 80% for immature teratomas, and 60% to 70% for endodermal sinus tumors.

SEX CORD–STROMAL TUMORS

PATHOGENESIS

Ovarian stromal cell tumors originate from either the cells surrounding the oocyte (before the differentiation into male or female) or from the ovarian stroma (Fig. 30-2). In general, these tumors are **low-grade malignancies**, which can occur at any age. They are **usually unilateral** and **rarely recur**. Granulosa-theca cells are low-grade malignancies and the most common (70%) type of tumor in this group. Sertoli–Leydig tumors are very rare.

Both granulosa-theca cell tumors and Sertoli–Leydig cell tumors are known as **functional tumors** because they are characterized by **hormone production**. Ovarian stroma can develop into an ovary or a testis. As a result, ovarian **granulosa-theca cell tumors** resemble fetal ovaries and produce large amounts of estrogens. Microscopically, the granulosa cells have grooved "coffee-bean" nuclei, and the cells are arranged in small clusters around a central cavity. These histologic configurations are known as **Call–Exner bodies**, which are pathognomonic for granulosa cell tumors. Conversely, ovarian **Sertoli–Leydig cell tumors** resemble fetal testes and produce testosterone and other androgens.

The third type of stromal cell tumor, the ovarian fibroma, is derived from mature fibroblasts and, unlike the other sex cord–stromal tumors, is not a functioning tumor. Occasionally, fibromas are associated with ascites. The triad of an ovarian **tumor**, **ascites**, and **right hydrothorax** is known as **Meigs syndrome**.

EPIDEMIOLOGY

Sex cord–stromal ovarian tumors can affect women of any age but occur most commonly in women between ages **40 and 70**. The mean age at diagnosis is 50. Because of these tumors produce estrogen, 25% to 50% of women with granulosa cell tumors will have **endometrial hyperplasia** or EIN and 5% will have concurrent **endometrial cancer**. Most Sertoli–Leydig tumors occur in women under 40.

CLINICAL MANIFESTATIONS

Granulosa-theca cell tumors often produce **estradiol and inhibin A/B**. The estrogen stimulation can cause feminization, precocious puberty, menstrual irregularities, secondary amenorrhea, or postmenopausal bleeding. This estrogen stimulation can lead to endometrial intraepithelial neoplasia and/or endometrial cancer; therefore, **endometrial sampling** with EMB and/or D&C is very important in this setting. Sertoli–Leydig cell tumors produce **androgens** (testosterone and androstenedione) that can cause **virilizing effects** in 75% of patients, including breast atrophy, hirsutism, deepened voice, acne, clitoromegaly, and receding hairline. Patients may also have oligomenorrhea or amenorrhea.

TREATMENT

Because most sex cord–stromal tumors are low-grade lesions, unilateral, and do not often recur, the usual treatment is **unilateral salpingo-oophorectomy**. In women who have completed their childbearing, total hysterectomy and bilateral salpingo-oophorectomy (TH/BSO) should be performed. Chemotherapy and radiation have no regular role in treating sex cord–stromal cell cancers.

The 5-year survival rate for patients with sex cord–stromal carcinomas is 70% to 90%. However, granulosa cell tumors are slow growing, and late recurrences can be detected 15 to 20 years after the removal of the primary lesion.

CANCER OF THE FALLOPIAN TUBES

PATHOGENESIS

Fallopian tube carcinoma is **extremely rare**, comprising only 0.5% of all cancers of the female genital tract. However, the incidence is likely underestimated. An emerging theory is that the fallopian tube is the source of high-grade serous ovarian, fallopian tube, and primary peritoneal cancers. The disease progression of these tumors is similar to that of ovarian cancer, including wide **peritoneal spread** and ascites accumulation. However, the exact etiology of fallopian cancer is unknown. Most fallopian tube cancers are **adenocarcinomas** arising from the mucosa of the tube. The tube is often hugely dilated, and the lumen is filled with papillary growth of solid tumor. The fimbriated end is closed in 50% of cases. Fallopian cancer is bilateral in 10% of cases and is **often the result of metastasis** from other primary tumors. Sarcomas and mixed tumors are less common.

EPIDEMIOLOGY

Primary fallopian tube carcinoma is very rare. These tumors can occur at any age (18 to 80), but the mean age at diagnosis is 55 to 60. Like epithelial ovarian cancers, fallopian tube cancers occur **more frequently in Caucasian women** when compared with African American women. Risk factors include **familial cancer syndromes** (BRCA1 and BRCA2), **nulliparity**, and **infertility**.

CLINICAL MANIFESTATIONS

Fallopian tube cancer is typically **asymptomatic** and is usually diagnosed during pelvic surgery for other indications. When symptoms do occur, the most common are watery vaginal discharge, intermenstrual uterine bleeding, low abdominal pain, and/or low back pain. **The classic triad of profuse watery discharge, pelvic pain, and pelvic mass is known as Latzko triad**. Although the triad is only seen in <15% of cases, it is considered pathognomonic for fallopian tube carcinoma. Similarly, the classic symptom of **hydrops tubae profluens** is also considered pathognomonic for fallopian tube carcinoma even though it is rarely seen. This phenomenon describes colicky low abdominal pain due to an intermittent hydrosalpinx. The pain is relieved periodically when the hydrosalpinx empties resulting in an intermittent, profuse, watery vaginal discharge.

DIAGNOSIS

The diagnosis of fallopian tube cancer is almost never made preoperatively. **Pelvic ultrasound** may reveal a complex adnexal mass or ascites. The **CA-125** is often elevated in these patients, and **cervical cytology** may rarely show malignant cells with subsequent negative cervical and endometrial biopsy.

TREATMENT

Fallopian tube cancers are **surgically staged**. One-third of patients are Stage I at the time of diagnosis, one-third are Stage II, and one-third are Stage III or IV. The treatment of fallopian tube cancer is the same as that of epithelial ovarian cancer, including TAH/BSO, omentectomy, cytoreduction, peritoneal cytologic studies, and retroperitoneal lymph node sampling and debulking. After surgery, **adjuvant chemotherapy** is given including intravenous chemotherapy with **carboplatin and paclitaxel** (Taxol) or with intraperitoneal and intravenous chemotherapy for optimally debulked advanced stage cancers. CA-125 levels and CT imaging can be used to monitor the effectiveness of treatment.

The prognosis for fallopian tube cancer is reported to be slightly better than that of epithelial ovarian cancer. The overall **5-year survival rate is 45%** (71% for Stage I, 48% for Stage II, 25% for Stage III, and 17% for Stage IV disease).

KEY POINTS

- Epithelial tumors of the ovary account for 90% of ovarian cancers.
- Most patients diagnosed with epithelial tumors of the ovary are diagnosed at Stage III or IV because of the lack of early symptoms and effective screening tools.
- When symptoms are present, they might include low abdominal pain, bloating, early satiety, pelvic mass, and ascites. Pelvic ultrasound and abdominal-pelvic CT often reveal a fixed, solid, nodular mass.
- Epithelial ovarian cancers are staged surgically and treated with surgery (TAHBSO, omentectomy, pelvic and para-aortic lymph node sampling, and cytoreduction) followed by Taxol and carboplatin chemotherapy.
- The tumor marker CA-125 can be used to evaluate the success of treatment and look for recurrence of disease, but is not appropriate to use as a screening tool for ovarian cancer.
- The 5-year survival rate for epithelial ovarian cancer is less than 20%.
- Germ cell tumors arise from totipotential germ cells capable of differentiating into yolk sac, placental or fetal tissue; 95% are benign and 5% are malignant.

- The most common germ cell tumor is the benign mature cystic teratoma (dermoid cyst). The most common malignant germ cell tumors are dysgerminomas (50%) and immature teratomas (20%).
- Germ cell tumors occur primarily in women under age 20, grow rapidly, are usually unilateral, and are diagnosed at early stages. They often produce serum tumor markers (LDH, AFP, and/or hCG) that can be used in the diagnosis of a pelvic mass and to assess response to therapy.
- Most germ cell tumors are treated by removal of the affected ovary, staging, and combination chemotherapy with good 5-year survival rates (60% to 85%), depending on the type of tumor.
- Sex cord–stromal germ cell tumors are derived from the cells surrounding the oocyte that produce steroid hormones or from the ovarian stroma.
- Sex cord–stromal tumors are slow-growing tumors with low malignant potential and are often found only incidentally, usually in women between 40 and 70 years old. Sertoli–Leydig cell tumors are rare and occur most often in women under age 40.
- Granulosa cell tumors are the most common type (70%) of sex cord–stromal tumor. They secrete inhibin and estradiol, resulting in feminization and potentially EIN and/or cancer. Microscopic Call–Exner bodies are pathognomonic for granulosa cell tumors.
- Sertoli–Leydig cell tumors are rare. They secrete androgens causing virilization in patients.
- Ovarian fibromas are derived from mature fibroblasts. These are nonfunctioning tumors. Meigs syndrome consists of the triad of ovarian tumor, ascites, and right hydrothorax.
- The sex cord–stromal tumors are treated surgically, usually with unilateral salpingo-oophorectomy in younger women or TAHBSO in women who have completed their childbearing.
- Sertoli–Leydig cell tumors do not frequently recur, but granulosa cell tumors often have late recurrences 15 to 20 years later.
- Fallopian tube cancers are rare malignancies that can occur at any age. They behave very similar to epithelial ovarian cancers.
- These are usually adenocarcinomas arising from the mucosa or metastases from other primary tumors. Fallopian tube cancers are usually asymptomatic and are rarely diagnosed preoperatively.
- The classic triad of pain, profuse watery discharge (hydrops tubae profluens), and pelvic mass is considered pathognomonic for fallopian tube carcinoma but only occurs in <15% of patients.
- Fallopian tube cancers are treated similar to epithelial ovarian cancers with TAHBSO, omentectomy, cytoreduction, and pelvic lymph node sampling followed by combination chemotherapy.
- The overall 5-year survival rate of fallopian tube cancer is 45%.

CLINICAL VIGNETTES

VIGNETTE 1

1. A 17-year-old Asian teen presents to the ED with left lower quadrant (LLQ) pain. Her pregnancy test, UA, and cervical cultures are all negative. She denies sexual activity. On pelvic ultrasound, she is found to have a unilateral complex ovarian mass. What is the most likely diagnosis?
   a. Serous cystadenocarcinoma
   b. Dysgerminoma
   c. Granulosa-theca cell tumor
   d. Mature teratoma
   e. Any of the above

2. What tumor marker is associated with this type of tumor?
   a. hCG
   b. α-Fetoprotein
   c. CA-125
   d. LDH
   e. All of the above

3. Expected treatment would likely include which of the following?
   a. Unilateral salpingo-oophorectomy plus surgical staging
   b. Bilateral salpingo-oophorectomy plus surgical staging

c. Total abdominal hysterectomy and bilateral salpingo-oophorectomy with surgical staging
d. Chemotherapy only
e. Radiation only

VIGNETTE 2

1. A 56-year-old G3 P2 presents with postmenopausal bleeding. Transvaginal ultrasound reveals a 12-mm endometrial stripe and an 8-cm complex left adnexal mass. An endometrial biopsy reveals endometrial intraepithelial neoplasia (EIN). What characteristics of the mass make it concerning for malignancy?
   a. Fixed, nonmobile location
   b. Internal septations
   c. Surface excrescences
   d. Papillary and nodular solid components
   e. All of the above

2. What is the most likely diagnosis in this patient?
   a. Mucinous cystadenocarcinoma
   b. Benign teratomas
   c. Granulosa-theca cell tumor
   d. Endometrioma
   e. Choriocarcinoma

3. During her preoperative evaluation, she undergoes an abdominal-pelvic CT and chest X-ray for imaging. She is found to have ascites and a right hydrothorax. This combination of adnexal mass, ascites, and hydrothorax is known as:
   a. Latzko triad
   b. Hydrops tubae profluens
   c. Syndrome X
   d. Meigs syndrome
   e. Metabolic syndrome

VIGNETTE 3

1. A 63-year-old G0 presents to you with a complaint of LLQ pain, intermittent nausea, abdominal pressure, and bloating. Her history is notable for mild obesity, right breast cancer, and hypertension. She and her husband desired children but were never able to conceive. Her family history is notable for premenopausal breast cancer in her mother and maternal aunt. She had a pelvic ultrasound showing a normal appearing uterus with a 7-cm left ovarian mass containing internal septations and papillary excrescences. She has moderate ascites and her CA-125 was 719. Which of the following is associated with an increased risk of ovarian cancer?
   a. Personal history of breast cancer
   b. Multiparity
   c. Breastfeeding
   d. Tubal ligation
   e. Hysterectomy

2. She underwent TAH, BSO, collection of pelvic washings, omentectomy, cytoreduction or "debulking," and bilateral pelvic and para-aortic lymph node sampling. The mass had spread beyond the ovary to the omentum, peritoneum, and bowel. She was found to have ascites, and pelvic washings were positive. There did not appear to be any liver or lymph node involvement. There was no visible residual disease left after surgery. What stage of ovarian cancer does she have?
   a. Stage I
   b. Stage II
   c. Stage III
   d. Stage IV
   e. None of the above

3. Postoperative chemotherapy is most likely to include which regimen?
   a. Cisplatin
   b. Taxol
   c. Intraperitoneal and intravenous cisplatin and Taxol
   d. Methotrexate
   e. Methotrexate and actinomycin-D

VIGNETTE 4

A 64-year-old G2 P2 presents for her annual examination. She complains of abdominal bloating and has noted some difficulty zipping her pants despite a recent unplanned 10-lb weight loss. She has also noticed copious watery vaginal discharge, often preceded by a sharp pain in her LLQ.

1. This complex of symptoms is suspicious for what condition?
   a. Epithelial ovarian cancer
   b. Germ cell
   c. Dysgerminoma
   d. Fallopian tube cancer
   e. Endometrial cancer

2. Which of the following is *not* true regarding this patient's cancer?
   a. It is extremely rare
   b. It often results as a metastasis from another site
   c. It is bilateral 90% of the time
   d. It spreads along the circulatory path of the peritoneal fluid
   e. It is associated with an elevated CA-125 and ascites, but rarely with abnormal cervical cytology

3. Fallopian tube cancer behaves most like what other GYN cancer?
   a. Vulvar
   b. Vaginal
   c. Cervical
   d. Endometrial
   e. Ovarian

ANSWERS

VIGNETTE 1 Question 1

1. Answer B:
In a young patient, immature teratomas and dysgerminomas are most common. This patient likely has a dysgerminoma. Eighty-five percent of patients with dysgerminomas present similar to this with abdominal pain and a pelvic mass. These occur most commonly in children and young girls. They are more common in Black and Asian females. They tend to be rapid growing and present with pelvic pain, pressure, and rupture. Serous cystadenocarcinoma is an epithelial ovarian cancer—which makes up 80% of all ovarian cancers. These occur most commonly in the sixth decade and tend to be bilateral.

VIGNETTE 1 Question 2

2. Answer D:
Many ovarian tumors produce serum tumor markers that aid in the diagnosis and clinical monitoring of treatment. Dysgerminomas most commonly produce LDH. hCG secretion is common in embryonal sinus tumors and choriocarcinomas. CA-125 can be found in ovarian neoplasms that are derived from the epithelium of the ovary. The CA-125 tumor marker can also be seen in any number of benign and malignant gynecologic and nongynecologic conditions, such as pancreatic cancer, lung cancer, breast cancer, endometriosis, pregnancy, fibroids, PID, pancreatitis, cirrhosis, and peritonitis.

VIGNETTE 1 Question 3

3. Answer A:
Because most germ cell tumors are diagnosed in the early stages and are rarely bilateral, most can be treated with unilateral salpingo-oophorectomy. However, complete surgical staging should be done. If childbearing is complete or if the cancer is bilateral, total abdominal hysterectomy and bilateral salpingo-oophorectomy should be done along with surgical staging. Dysgerminomas are very sensitive to radiation therapy and chemotherapy. Either can be used after surgical treatment in all but Stage Ia patients.

VIGNETTE 2 Question 1

1. Answer E:
Some characteristic findings on pelvic examination and imaging are concerning for malignancy. On examination, a fixed, solid, irregular, bilateral tumor is more likely to be malignant than a mobile, cystic, smooth, unilateral tumor. Similarly, on imaging, masses that are above 8 cm with solid components, internal septations, surface nodules, or excrescences are more concerning for a malignant process. Associated features such as ascites, peritoneal masses, and lymphadenopathy are more suggestive of a malignant process.

VIGNETTE 2 Question 2

2. Answer C:
Although many of these options are possible, the presentation of the endometrial hyperplasia along with the ovarian mass is more characteristic of a granulosa-theca cell tumor. These sex cord–stromal tumors resemble cells of the fetal ovaries, and thus, produce high amounts of estrogens. They are often unilateral, low-grade, and functional tumors. This endogenous unopposed estrogen production results in stimulation of the endometrium, a thickened endometrial stripe on pelvic ultrasound, and bleeding in this postmenopausal patient. Microscopically, the nuclei of the granulosa cell tumors are grooved and "coffee-bean" shaped, and the cells are arranged in microclusters known as Call–Exner bodies. These are pathognomonic for granulosa cell tumors. Mucinous adenocarcinomas tend to be quite large and may be associated with mucinous tumors of the appendix as well. Benign cystic mature teratomas (dermoid tumors) are the most common type of germ cell tumor. Both dermoids and endometriomas have very characteristic appearances. Dermoids can contain tissue from skin, hair, teeth, bone, and sebaceous material. Endometriomas have a ground glass appearance.

VIGNETTE 2 Question 3

3. Answer D:
Meigs syndrome is the presentation of ascites and hydrothorax along with an ovarian fibroma or other pelvic tumor. Latzko triad is associated with the classic triad of profuse watery discharge (hydrops tubae profluens), pelvic pain, and pelvic mass seen in association with fallopian tube cancers. Hydrops tubae profluens (or intermittent hydrosalpinx) is the phenomenon of spontaneous or pressure-induced release of watery or blood-tinged vaginal discharge resulting in shrinkage of a pelvic mass. This is likewise associated with fallopian tube cancers.

Syndrome X is also known as metabolic syndrome and insulin-resistance syndrome. This syndrome is characterized by hypertension, obesity, insulin resistance, or NIDDM along with hypertriglyceridemia, increased peripheral vascular disease, and elevated catecholamine levels.

VIGNETTE 3 Question 1
1. Answer A:
Risk factors for ovarian cancer include familial ovarian cancer syndromes (Lynch II/hereditary nonpolyposis colon cancer, BRAC1, and BRAC2), family history of breast and/or ovarian cancer, personal history of breast cancer, increasing age, early menarche and late menopause, infertility, nulliparity, and obesity (BMI > 30). Most of these characteristics are associated with prolonged or increased ovulation. Conversely, many of the protective factors for ovarian cancer include those which decrease the lifetime number of ovulations, such as multiparity, breastfeeding, and greater than 5 years of OCP use. Other protective factors include hysterectomy and tubal ligation.

VIGNETTE 3 Question 2
2. Answer C:
Ovarian cancer is surgically staged with TAH, BSO, collection of pelvic washings, omentectomy, cytoreduction or "debulking," and bilateral pelvic and para-aortic lymph node sampling. Stage I ovarian cancer is confined to the ovary or ovaries. Stage II describes disease extending to the pelvis (uterus, fallopian tubes, and peritoneal washings). Stage III disease includes spread to the abdomen, and stage IV includes distant metastases including positive pleural effusion and disease of the liver.

VIGNETTE 3 Question 3
3. Answer B:
The most common chemotherapeutic regime following treatment for epithelial ovarian cancer is intravenous carboplatin with Taxol. The same is used to treat fallopian tube carcinoma. Intraperitoneal and intravenous cisplatin and Taxol can be used to treat Stage III tumors, after optimal debulking, especially with no visible residual disease. Methotrexate has many therapeutic indications, including treatment of ectopic pregnancy and rheumatoid arthritis. Methotrexate or actinomycin-D may be used to treat persistent/invasive molar pregnancies.

VIGNETTE 4 Question 1
1. Answer D:
Symptoms most characteristic of fallopian tube cancer are watery vaginal discharge and intermittent hydrosalpinx. Latzko triad is the classic triad of profuse watery discharge, pelvic pain, and pelvic mass seen in association with fallopian tube cancers. Hydrops tubae profluens (aka intermittent hydrosalpinx) is the phenomenon of spontaneous or pressure-induced discharge of watery or blood-tinged vaginal discharge resulting in shrinkage of a pelvic mass. Both are characteristic of fallopian tube cancers. Epithelial ovarian cancer could present with abdominal pain, bloating, and increasing abdominal girth in the setting of a pelvic mass. However, the watery vaginal discharge and intermittent hydrosalpinx are more commonly associated with fallopian tube cancer. Dysgerminomas occur most commonly in girls and young women and in Asian and African American women. Eighty percent of patients with endometrial cancer present with abnormal uterine bleeding and would not necessarily have a pelvic mass.

VIGNETTE 4 Question 2
2. Answer C:
Fallopian tube adenocarcimonas are extremely rare tumors. Primary disease is rarely picked up preoperatively and most are discovered incidentally, and many result from metastasis from other tumors of the ovaries, endometrium, GI tract, or breast. They are associated with both ascites and elevated CA-125 levels. They are most often unilateral and are only bilateral 10% of the time.

VIGNETTE 4 Question 3
3. Answer E:
Primary fallopian tube cancer is very rare. Like epithelial ovarian cancers, the mean age is 55 to 60, it is more common in Caucasian women, and its risk factors include familial cancer syndromes, nulliparity, and infertility. The treatment for both fallopian tube and epithelial ovarian cancers includes TAH, BSO, omentectomy, debulking, pelvic, and para-aortic lymph node sampling. Likewise, postsurgical chemotherapeutic regime includes carboplatin and Taxol. The prognosis for fallopian tube cancer is slightly better than that of epithelial ovarian cancer.

31 | Gestational Trophoblastic Disease

Gestational trophoblastic disease (GTD) is a diverse group of interrelated diseases resulting in the abnormal proliferation of trophoblastic (placental) tissue. These can be grouped into four major classifications (Table 31-1): **molar pregnancies** (80%), **persistent GTD and invasive moles** (10% to 15%), **gestational choriocarcinoma** (2% to 5%), and very rare **placental site trophoblastic tumors** (PSTTs). These tumors are unique in that the proliferation results from abnormal fetal tissue rather than maternal tissue. These neoplasms also share the ability to produce **human chorionic gonadotropin (hCG)**, which serves both as a tumor marker for diagnosing the disease and as a tool for measuring the effects of treatment. GTD is also extremely **sensitive to chemotherapy** and is therefore the most curable gynecologic malignancy and one of the few that may allow for the preservation of fertility.

BENIGN GESTATIONAL TROPHOBLASTIC DISEASE

Benign GTD consists of molar pregnancies, also known as **hydatidiform moles**. Complete and partial moles account for 80% of all GTD. Ninety percent of molar pregnancies are classified as **classic or complete moles** and are the result of molar degeneration but have no associated fetus. Ten percent of molar pregnancies are classified as **partial or incomplete moles** and are the result of molar degeneration in association with an abnormal fetus. The distinct characteristics of complete and partial molar pregnancies are compared in Table 31-2.

EPIDEMIOLOGY

The incidence of molar pregnancy is about **1 in 1,500 pregnancies** and 1 in 600 therapeutic abortions in the United States. There is a decreased rate of GTD in African American women in the United States. The worldwide incidence of molar pregnancy varies from region to region. Low and intermediate rates are seen in North America and Europe, whereas Latin America and Asia have moderate to high rates. The global rate is **highest among South East Asian women** and women in Japan, where molar pregnancies may occur as often as 1 in 500 pregnancies.

RISK FACTORS

Extremes in age and **prior history of GTD** are two of the most common risk factors for molar pregnancy. There is a slight increase in women under 20 and a significant increase in women over 35 years of age. Women over 35 also have an increased risk of malignant disease. Similarly, women with a history of GTD are at increased risk for having subsequent pregnancies affected by GTD. The baseline risk of GTD in a woman with **no previous history of the disease is 0.1%.** That risk increases to **1% to 2% in women with one prior molar pregnancy** and can be as high as 16% to 28% in a woman with two prior molar pregnancies.

Over 70% of women with GTD have never given birth, making **nulliparity** another important risk factor. Conversely, the rate of GTD seems to decrease with increasing parity. Higher incidences have also been found in geographic areas where the diet is low in β-carotene, folic acid, and animal fat. Other possible associated factors include smoking, infertility, spontaneous abortion, blood group A, and a history of oral contraceptive pill use.

COMPLETE MOLAR PREGNANCIES

PATHOGENESIS

Although the cause of molar pregnancy is unknown, it is believed that most complete moles result from the fertilization of an **enucleate ovum or empty egg,**

TABLE 31-1. Classification of GTD
Benign GTD (80%)
Complete mole (classic mole)
Partial mole (incomplete mole)
Malignant GTD (20%)
Postmolar GTD
Invasive molar pregnancy
Gestational choriocarcinoma
PSTTs
GTD, gestational trophoblastic disease; PSTT, placental site trophoblastic tumors.

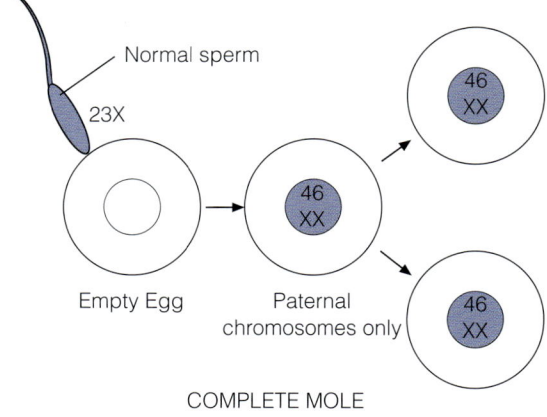

FIGURE 31-1. A complete mole arises from the fertilization of an empty enucleate egg by a normal sperm. The sperm duplicates its own chromosomes, resulting in a 46,XX diploid karyotype; all of the chromosomes are, therefore, of paternal origin. (From Beckmann C, Ling F. *Obstetrics & Gynecology,* 5th ed. Philadelphia, PA: Lippincott Williams & Wilkins; 2006.)

one whose nucleus is missing or nonfunctional, by one normal sperm that then replicates itself (Fig. 31-1). All of the resultant chromosomes are therefore **paternally derived**. The most common chromosomal pattern for complete moles is diploid (**46,XX**). Rarely, a complete mole may be formed by the fertilization of an empty egg by two normal sperm.

TABLE 31-2. Comparison of Characteristics of Complete and Partial Molar Pregnancies		
Features	**Complete (Classic) Mole (90%)**	**Partial (Incomplete) Mole (10%)**
Genetics		
Most common karyotype	46,XX	69,XXY
Chromosomal origin	All paternally derived	Extra paternal set
Pathology		
Coexistent fetus	Absent	Present
Fetal red blood cells	Absent	Present
Chorionic villi	Hydropic (swollen)	Few hydropic
Trophoblasts	Severe hyperplasia	Minimal/no hyperplasia
Clinical presentation		
Associated embryo	None	Present
Symptoms/signs	Abnormal vaginal bleeding	Missed abortion
Classic symptoms[a]	Common	Rare
Uterine size	50% large for dates	Size equals dates
Theca lutein cysts	Present in 15–25%	Rare
hCG levels	High (>100,000 mIU/mL)	Slightly elevated
Malignant potential		
Nonmetastatic malignant GTD	15%–25%	2%–4%
Metastatic malignant GTD	4%	0%
Follow-up		
Weeks to normal hCG	14 wk	8 wk
[a]Hyperemesis gravidarum, early preeclampsia, hyperthyroidism, anemia, and excessive uterine enlargement. hCG, human chorionic gonadotropin.		

FIGURE 31-2. Gross morphology of villi. (**A**) Normal chorionic villi. (**B**) Partial mole with normal villi admixed with swollen ones (case of triploidy, 69,XXY). (**C**) Complete mole with swollen, vesicular villi.

TABLE 31.3. Symptoms Associated with Molar Pregnancy	
Symptoms	**Percent**
Vaginal bleeding	90–97
Passage of molar vesicles	80
Anemia	50
Uterine size greater than dates	30–50
Bilateral theca lutein cysts	15–25
Hyperemesis gravidarum	10–25
Preeclampsia before 20 wk gestation	10–15
Hyperthyroidism	10
Trophoblastic pulmonary embolic	2

The placental abnormality in a complete mole is characterized by **noninvasive trophoblastic proliferation** associated with diffuse swelling of the chorionic villi. This hydropic degeneration gives the complete mole the appearance of **grape-like vesicles** filling the uterus in the **absence of an embryo** (Fig. 31-2).

In complete molar pregnancy, there is abnormal proliferation of the **syncytiotrophoblasts** that produce hCG. This is responsible for the extremely high hCG levels (>100,000 mIU/mL) that can be associated with complete moles, and explain many of the signs and symptoms associated with complete moles. Although the β subunit is unique to hCG, the **α subunit mimics that found in luteinizing hormone (LH), follicle-stimulating hormone (FSH), and thyroid-stimulating hormone (TSH).** Therefore, high hCG levels associated with complete moles can act as a homolog to LH and FSH, resulting in stimulation of large **theca lutein ovarian cysts** (>6 cm). hCG can similarly act as a homolog to TSH, resulting in **hyperthyroidism** in patients with complete moles. **Hyperemesis gravidarum** and **early onset preeclampsia** may also result from the extreme elevation of hCG. Although these symptoms occur infrequently in GTD, when they are diagnosed, it is typically in the first or second trimester.

Although most molar pregnancies are benign, complete moles have a higher malignant potential than do partial moles (Table 31-2).

CLINICAL PRESENTATION
History
The most common presenting symptom of molar pregnancy is **irregular or heavy vaginal bleeding in the setting of a positive pregnancy test (97%)**. The bleeding is caused by separation of the tumor from the underlying decidua, resulting in disruption of the maternal vessels. Table 31-3 lists other sequelae associated with complete molar pregnancy, in descending order of frequency. Many of these symptoms can be attributed to the high hCG levels, including severe nausea and vomiting (from hyperemesis gravidarum); irritability, dizziness, and photophobia (from preeclampsia); or nervousness, anorexia, and tremors (from hyperthyroidism although subclinical hyperthyroidism is more common than overt hyperthyroidism).

Physical Examination
In complete molar pregnancy, the physical examination may show sequelae of **preeclampsia** (hypertension) or **hyperthyroidism** (tachycardia and tachypnea). The **abdominopelvic examination** in molar pregnancy may be remarkable for the **absence of fetal heart sounds** because there is no associated embryo in a complete molar pregnancy. Fifty percent of women with complete molar pregnancies will measure **large for gestational age** because of the presence of large amounts of proliferative tissue, hemorrhage, and/or clot in the uterus. The pelvic examination may reveal

FIGURE 31-3. Ultrasound scan of a complete molar pregnancy demonstrating the classic "snow storm" appearance. Large theca lutein cysts can sometimes be seen on the ovary (hydatidiform mole [HM], theca lutein cyst [TC]).

the expulsion of **grape-like molar clusters** into the vagina or blood in the cervical os. Occasionally, the provider may palpate **large bilateral theca lutein cysts** (Fig. 31-3). Usually, physical examination findings will be somewhat unrevealing, requiring further diagnostics to evaluate what is initially presumed to be a **threatened abortion**.

DIAGNOSTIC EVALUATION

In the presence of a molar pregnancy, **quantitative serum hCG levels** can be extremely high (>100,000 mIU/mL). The hCG level reflects the amount of tumor volume and can be used for diagnosis, risk stratification, and assessment of treatment effectiveness. Suspicion of GTD is usually confirmed using pelvic ultrasound. In the case of a complete mole, no embryo or gestational sac is present. Instead, the intrauterine environment appears as a **"snowstorm" pattern** due to swelling of chorionic villi (Fig. 31-3). The scan may also reveal **bilateral theca lutein cysts** (15% to 25% of cases), which appear as large (>6 cm) multilocular cysts on both ovaries. The definitive diagnosis of molar pregnancy is made on **pathologic examination of the intrauterine tissue** once the uterus is evacuated.

DIFFERENTIAL DIAGNOSIS

The differential diagnosis for GTD includes conditions that can result in abnormally high hCG levels, vaginal bleeding in pregnancy, and/or enlarged placentas, such as multiple gestation pregnancy, erythroblastosis fetalis, intrauterine infection, uterine fibroids, threatened abortion, ectopic pregnancy, or normal intrauterine pregnancy.

TREATMENT

The treatment for molar pregnancy, regardless of the duration of pregnancy, is immediate removal of the uterine contents with suction **dilation and curettage (D&C)**. Prior to evacuation of the uterus, laboratory examination should include a baseline hCG level, a complete blood count (CBC), coagulation studies, along with renal, thyroid, and liver function tests. Maternal blood type and antibody screen should also be obtained to **determine Rh(D) status** and in preparation for the possibility of heavy vaginal bleeding during the procedure. A chest X-ray (CXR) is not routinely necessary, but can be used in the event that metastasis is suspected. If a patient is demonstrating signs of preeclampsia, **antihypertensives** may be used to decrease risk of maternal stroke. Similarly, patients with sequelae of hCG-induced hyperthyroidism benefit from the use of **β blocker** such as propranolol to avoid precipitation of **thyroid storm** by anesthesia and/or stress of the surgical procedure.

Prior to the procedure, cross-matched blood should be made available in case of heavy bleeding, and intravenous (IV) access should be optimized. General anesthesia is typically used, given the risk of hemorrhage and complications such as thyroid storm and trophoblastic embolization. **Suction D&C** is the definitive treatment for most patients with complete molar pregnancy. After the uterine contents have been removed, **uterotonics** can be administered to stimulate uterine contraction and minimize blood loss. Even though no fetal tissue is present, **Rh immunoglobulin (RhoGAM)** should be given to all Rh-negative women. Theca lutein cysts should be managed expectantly. In general, the cysts will spontaneously involute as the hCG levels decrease following the procedure.

In patients who have completed childbearing, hysterectomy is an alternative therapy. Although this will eliminate the risk of local invasion, hysterectomy does not prevent metastasis of the disease.

FOLLOW-UP

The prognosis for molar pregnancy is excellent, with 95% to 100% cure rates after molar evacuation. **Persistent postmolar GTD** will develop in **6% to 32% of patients with complete moles** but <5% of

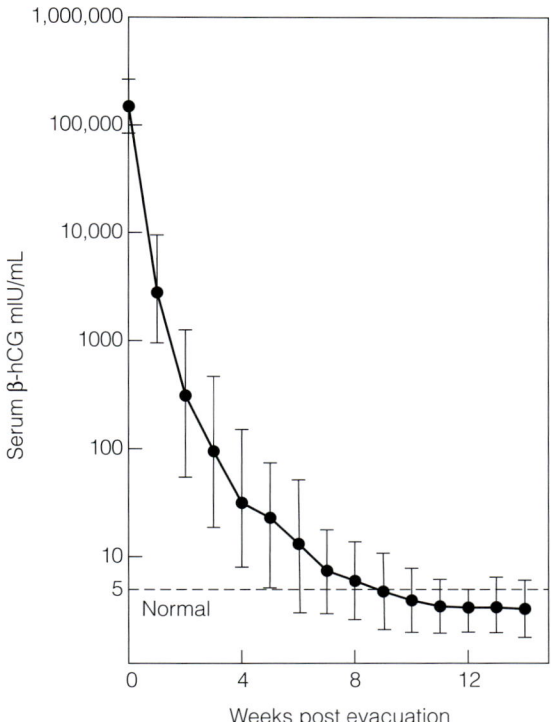

FIGURE 31-4. Normal regression of β-hCG levels after molar evacuation of the uterus. The average time to normalization of levels is 8 to 14 weeks. β-hCG, beta human chorionic gonadotropin.

patients with partial moles. For this reason, close follow-up is essential even after hysterectomy.

After evacuation of a molar pregnancy, **serial hCG surveillance** is necessary to ensure complete resolution of the disease and to watch for development of malignant postmolar GTD. Serum levels are typically measured 48 hours after evacuation and then every 1 to 2 weeks until negative for 3 consecutive weeks. The levels are then followed monthly for an additional 6 months as most persistent disease will occur within 6 months of the evacuation.

Figure 31-4 demonstrates the normal regression of hCG titers after molar evacuation. The average time to normalization of levels is 14 weeks for a complete mole compared with 2 to 4 weeks following a normal pregnancy, miscarriage, or termination. A **plateau or rise in hCG** levels during surveillance or the presence of hCG several weeks to months after the D&C is indicative of **malignant postmolar GTD**.

Patients at highest risk for **persistent trophoblastic disease** are those with β-hCG levels >100,000 mIU/mL, those with ovaries >6 cm, and those with large uterine sizes (14 to 16 weeks). In patients with these "high-risk moles," a single dose of **prophylactic chemotherapy** (with methotrexate and folinic acid or dactinomycin) has been found to greatly lower the rate of persistent GTD without significant increase in morbidity or mortality.

Rarely, a false-positive hCG value may be obtained because of nonspecific heterophilic antibodies in the patient's serum that cross-react with the hCG assay test. This phenomenon is known as a "**phantom hCG**." When phantom hCG is suspected, a negative urine pregnancy test or serial dilutions of the patient's serum hCG aid in the diagnosis. No treatment is required for these false-positive results.

Reliable contraception is recommended during the surveillance period to avoid a new pregnancy that would interfere with interpretation of the hCG levels. **Hormonal contraception** does not interfere with the risk of recurrence nor does it interfere with interpretation of the hCG assay. **IUD** use is generally held until after a normal hCG level has been obtained given the potential for uterine perforation.

Patients who are cured of the disease can have normal pregnancies with no increase in the rate of spontaneous abortion, complications, or congenital malformations. However, all subsequent pregnancies should be closely monitored with early ultrasound to rule out recurrent GTD. Following delivery in a subsequent pregnancy, an hCG level should be checked at the 6-week postpartum visit. It is no longer necessary to send the placenta for pathologic examination, but any tissue obtained from a miscarriage or termination should be evaluated for molar tissue. The risk of developing **recurrent GTD** in a subsequent pregnancy is increased 10-fold in women with a history of one molar pregnancy. Compared with the incidence of 0.1% in women with no history of GTD, the risk of recurrent GTD is 1% to 2% after one molar pregnancy and 16% to 32% after two molar pregnancies. The risk of postmolar GTD is 3% to 5% even after hysterectomy.

PARTIAL MOLAR PREGNANCY

PATHOGENESIS

A partial or incomplete mole is formed when a **normal ovum is fertilized by two sperm simultaneously** (Fig. 31-5). This results in a **triploid karyotype with 69 chromosomes**, of which two sets are paternally derived. The most common karyotype is **69,XXY** (80%). The placental abnormality in a partial mole is characterized by **focal hydropic villi and trophoblastic hyperplasia primarily of the cytotrophoblast**. Because cytotrophoblasts do not

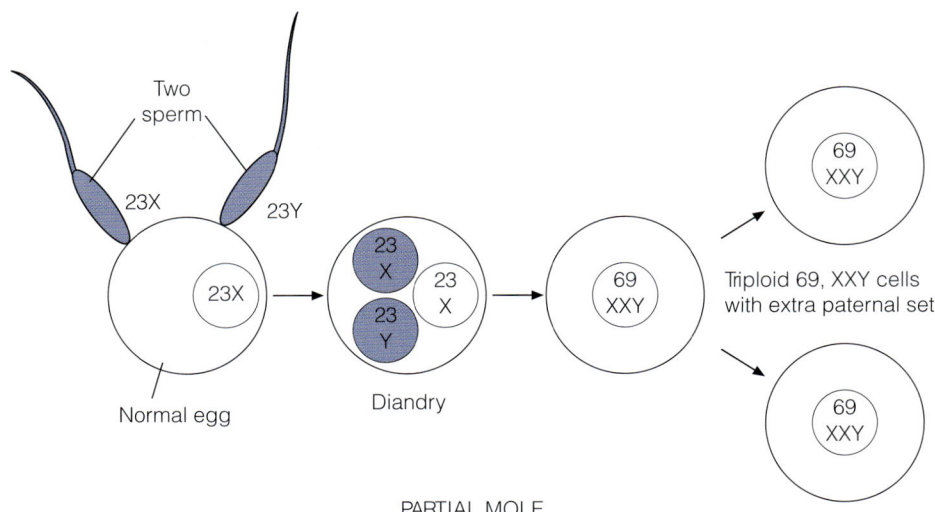

FIGURE 31-5. An incomplete mole arises from the simultaneous fertilization of a normal ovum by two sperm (diandry). The resulting triploid karyotype is most commonly 69,XXY.

produce hCG, levels in partial molar pregnancies are normal or only slightly elevated compared with the extreme elevations seen in complete moles.

Partial moles are the only histologic type of GTD associated with the **presence of an embryo**. In fact, a gestational sac and fetal heart rate may also be present. These embryos often have multiple anomalies such as syndactyly and hydrocephalus and are often growth restricted. Most embryos associated with partial moles survive only several weeks in utero before being spontaneously aborted in the late first or early second trimester. As a result, **partial moles are often misdiagnosed as spontaneous or missed abortions**. Partial moles are almost always benign and have a much **lower malignant potential** than complete moles.

CLINICAL PRESENTATION

History

Similar to complete molar pregnancy, partial molar pregnancy often presents with delayed menses in the setting of a positive pregnancy test. The hCG levels are normal or only slightly elevated. As a result, patients with partial moles may have similar but much less severe symptoms than those with complete molar pregnancy. Ninety percent of patients with partial moles present with **vaginal bleeding from miscarriage or incomplete abortion in late first trimester or early second trimester**. Consequently, partial moles may be diagnosed somewhat later than complete molar pregnancies. **Diagnosis is often made on pathologic examination of the products of conception.**

PHYSICAL EXAMINATION

In partial molar pregnancy, the physical examination is typically normal. Given the relatively normal hCG levels, hyperemesis, hyperthyroidism, and preeclampsia are rarely seen in women with partial moles. **Fetal heart sounds** may be present because there is a **coexistent fetus in** partial molar pregnancies. These pregnancies are often complicated by a uterine size that measures small for gestational age and for intrauterine growth restriction (**IUGR**), especially if the pregnancy reaches the second trimester.

DIAGNOSTIC EVALUATION

Unlike complete molar pregnancy, quantitative **serum hCG levels are likely to be relatively normal** in partial molar pregnancies. Pelvic ultrasound may reveal a fetus with cardiac activity, congenital malformations, and/or IUGR. Amniotic fluid is usually present but reduced, and these patients generally do not have theca lutein cysts associated with complete molar pregnancy. The intrauterine tissue may contain anechoic spaces juxtaposed against chorionic villi, giving the tissue a "**Swiss-cheese**" **appearance**. The definitive diagnosis of partial molar pregnancy is made on **pathologic examination of the intrauterine tissue** once the uterus is evacuated.

TREATMENT

Treatment is immediate removal of the uterine contents via **suction D&C,** as described in the complete molar pregnancy treatment section. Less than 5% of patients with partial moles will develop persistent malignant disease (Table 31-2).

FOLLOW-UP

Surveillance with **serial hCG levels**, as described in the previous section on complete molar pregnancy, is critical to the treatment of this disease. The average time to normalization of levels is **8 weeks** for a partial mole compared with 14 weeks for a complete mole and 2 to 4 weeks following a normal pregnancy, miscarriage, or termination. **Reliable contraception** is also important to prevent pregnancy and allow accurate hCG surveillance.

MALIGNANT GESTATIONAL TROPHOBLASTIC DISEASE

OVERVIEW

Whereas 80% of gestational trophoblastic disease comprises benign molar pregnancies, 20% of patients with GTD are diagnosed with a malignant form of the disease. Malignant GTD is so named because of the potential for **local invasion** into the myometrium and **metastasis** to other parts of the body. Malignant GTD encompasses several different histologic types (Table 31-1). The bulk of these (75%) are either **persistent postmolar pregnancies** or **invasive molar pregnancies**. Other types of malignant GTD include gestational choriocarcinomas (25%) and placental site trophoblastic tumors (rare).

In terms of management and prognosis, the clinical presentation of malignant GTD has a more important impact than the actual histology. The diagnosis of malignant GTD is made most commonly by plateauing or rising hCG levels after molar evacuation. For malignant GTD following nonmolar pregnancies, the most common presentations include abnormal uterine bleeding >6 weeks following pregnancy or more subtle symptoms of metastatic disease in a reproductive-aged woman with an unknown primary cancer.

Table 31-4 demonstrates an **anatomic staging system** for malignant GTD. Using clinical criteria, malignant GTD can be classified as **nonmetastatic** if the disease is confined to the uterus or **metastatic** if the disease has progressed beyond the uterus (Fig. 31-6). Metastatic disease can further be classified as **good prognosis or poor prognosis**, depending on factors such as length of time since antecedent pregnancy, hCG level, presence of brain or liver metastases, type of antecedent pregnancy, and the result of prior chemotherapy trials (Fig. 31-6).

However, this type of system does not adequately predict outcomes. More current systems include the modified World Health Organization Prognostic Index Score and the Revised Federation of International Gynecologists and Obstetricians (FIGO) Staging System. These have been modified to make them **more predictive of outcome** by incorporating clinical patient characteristics (Table 31-5).

During the process of diagnosis and management of malignant GTD, patients should be carefully evaluated with history and physical examination; serum hCG levels; hepatic, renal, and thyroid function tests; and baseline CBC prior to and during therapy. Metastatic workup should include CXR, pelvic ultrasound, CT of abdomen and pelvis, and CT or MRI of the head.

One distinguishing feature of malignant GTD is its **extreme sensitivity to chemotherapy**. Patients with low-risk disease are almost all cured by **single-agent chemotherapy**, whereas patients with high-risk disease require **combination chemotherapy**.

Surgery does not generally play a role in the treatment of malignant GTD except for high-risk patients and those with PSTT. As with benign forms of GTD, serum hCG levels are monitored after treatment of malignant GTD.

TABLE 31-4. FIGO Staging of Malignant GTD

Stage	Extent of Disease[a]
I	Confined to the uterus
II	Metastases to the pelvis
III	Metastases to the lung (with or without pelvic metastases)
IV	Distant metastases (with or without lung metastases)

[a]Metastasis sites in order of frequency are lung, vagina, pelvis, brain, and liver.
GTD, gestational trophoblastic disease.

PERSISTENT POSTMOLAR GTD AND INVASIVE MOLES

PATHOGENESIS

Again, most malignant GTD (75%) occurs after a molar pregnancy. Following molar evacuation, about 15% to 20% of patients will have persistent local disease and 4% will have metastatic disease (mostly gestational choriocarcinoma). Postmolar GTD typically comprises either **noninvasive trophoblastic proliferation** or an **invasive mole**. Less frequently, gestational choriocarcinoma and PSTT can occur. Characteristics that are most frequently associated

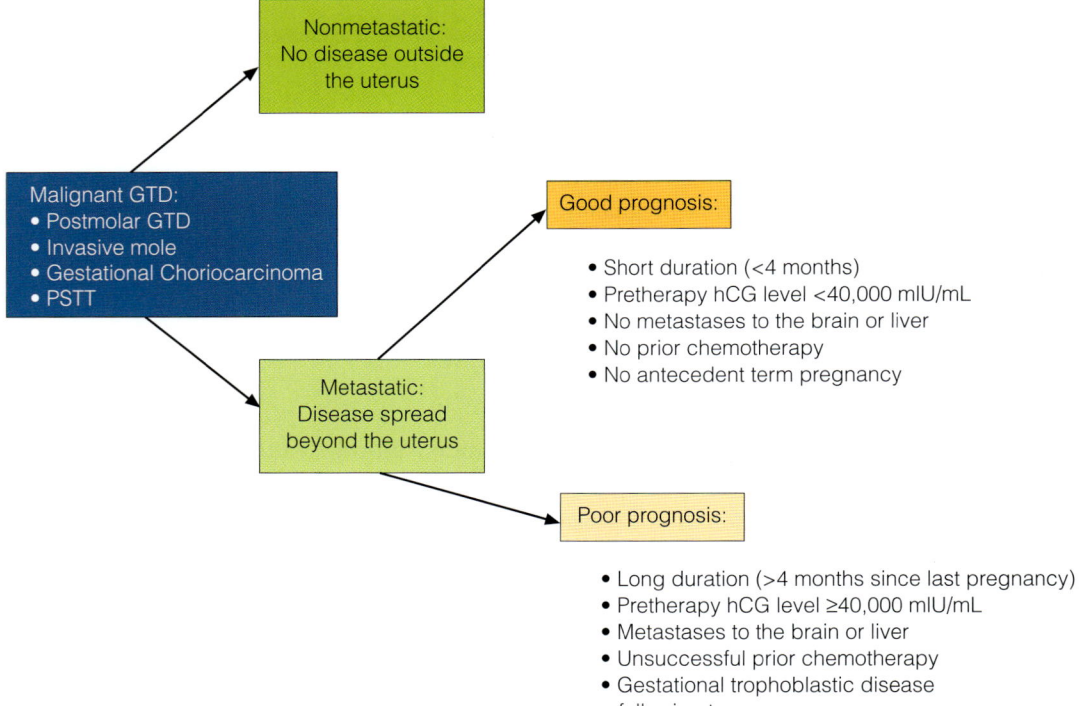

FIGURE 31-6. Classification of malignant GTD. Anatomic spread as well as clinical presentation impacts the prognosis of malignant disease.

TABLE 31-5. Revised FIGO Scoring System for GTD[a]				
Risk Factors	0	1	2	4
Age (y)	≤39	≥40		
Antecedent pregnancy	Mole	Abortion	Term	
Pregnancy event to treatment interval (mo)	<4	4–6	7–12	>12
Pretreatment hCG level (mIU/mL)	<1,000	1,000–10,000	10,000–100,000	>100,000
Number of metastases	0	1–4	4–8	>8
Site of metastases	Lung, vagina	Spleen, kidney	Gatrointestinal tract	Brain, liver
Largest tumor size, including uterine (cm)	3–4	5		
Prior number of failed chemotherapy drugs			Single drug	Two or more drugs

[a]The total score for a patient is obtained by adding the individual scores for each prognostic factor. Total score: 0–6 = low risk; ≥7 = high risk.

GTD, gestational trophoblastic disease.

Modified from American College of Obstetricians and Gynecologists. Diagnosis and treatment of gestational trophoblastic disease (Practice Bulletin No. 53). *Obstet Gynecol* 2004;103:1365–1377, from the original source: Kohorn EI. The new FIGO 2000 staging and risk factor scoring system for gestational trophoblastic disease: description and clinical assessment. *Int J Gynecol Cancer* 2001;11:73–77.

TABLE 31-6. Risk Factors for Persistent Postmolar GTD and Invasive Moles
hCG > 100,000 mIU/mL
Uterine size >14–16 wk
Theca lutein cysts >6cm
Coexistent fetus
GTD, gestational trophoblastic disease, hCG, human chorionic gonadotropin.

with persistent postmolar disease are presented in Table 31-6.

Postmolar GTD and invasive moles are characterized by the penetration of large, swollen (**hydropic**) **chorionic villi** and **trophoblast proliferation** into the myometrium. This proliferation can sometimes extend through the myometrium to the peritoneal cavity to invade the uterine vasculature. In rare cases, persistent postmolar GTD can cause uterine rupture, hemoperitoneum, and severe anemia. Despite this, invasive moles rarely metastasize and are capable of spontaneous regression.

EPIDEMIOLOGY

Persistent postmolar GTD and invasive moles have an overall incidence of 1 in 15,000 pregnancies.

CLINICAL PRESENTATION
History
Most patients with persistent postmolar GTD and invasive moles are identified as a result of **plateauing or rising hCG** after treatment for a molar pregnancy and are usually asymptomatic at the time of diagnosis. The most common symptom is abnormal uterine bleeding.

Physical Examination
The physical examination in patients with invasive moles is similar to that for molar pregnancy. Women with persistent postmolar GTD and invasive moles are more likely to have hCG levels above 100,000 mIU/mL, excessive uterine size for dates, and prominent theca lutein cysts.

DIAGNOSTIC EVALUATION
As with benign forms of GTD, **hCG levels** and **pelvic ultrasound** are the cornerstones of diagnosis. Pelvic ultrasound may also rule out pregnancy as a source of plateauing or rising hCG. Ultrasound may also reveal one or more intrauterine masses with possible invasion of the myometrium. Doppler examination typically shows high vascular flow.

TREATMENT
Persistent postmolar GTD and invasive moles are typically **nonmetastatic** and confined to the uterus. Because they are often invasive, repeat D&C should be avoided given the risk of perforation. Persistent and invasive molar pregnancies respond well to **single-agent chemotherapy**, usually methotrexate or actinomycin-D. When metastases are present, low-risk patients are treated with single-agent chemotherapy, and high-risk patients are treated with **multiagent chemotherapy**.

FOLLOW-UP
As with benign GTD, careful follow-up with **serial hCG levels** as described is critical to demonstrating resolution of the disease (Fig. 31-4). Likewise, **reliable contraception** is critical in order to maintain accurate measurement of hCG levels and verify resolution of the disease.

GESTATIONAL CHORIOCARCINOMA
PATHOGENESIS
Gestational choriocarcinoma is a **malignant necrotizing tumor**. Although 50% of patients with gestational choriocarcinoma are diagnosed after a complete molar pregnancy, 25% develop the disease after a normal-term pregnancy and 25% after miscarriage, abortion, or ectopic pregnancy. Gestational choriocarcinoma should be considered in any reproductive-aged women found to have metastases from an unknown primary cancer.

Gestational choriocarcinoma is a **pure epithelial tumor**. The characteristic histologic pattern of gestational choriocarcinoma includes sheets of **anaplastic cytotrophoblasts and syncytiotrophoblasts** in the absence of chorionic villi. Gestational choriocarcinoma invades the uterine wall and uterine vasculature, causing destruction of uterine tissue, necrosis, and potentially severe hemorrhage. These tumors are often metastatic and usually **spread hematogenously** to the lungs, vagina, pelvis, brain, liver, intestines, and kidneys. These lesions tend to be very vascular and bleed easily.

EPIDEMIOLOGY

Gestational choriocarcinoma is very rare in the United States, where its incidence is only 1 in 20,000 to 40,000 pregnancies, but is more common in women of Asian or African ethnicity.

CLINICAL PRESENTATION

History

Patients with gestational choriocarcinoma often present with **late postpartum bleeding** (beyond 6 to 8 weeks postpartum), but can also present with irregular uterine bleeding years after an antecedent pregnancy. Unlike patients with persistent postmolar or invasive moles, patients with gestational choriocarcinoma often present with **symptoms of metastatic disease**. Metastases to the lungs may cause cough, dyspnea, respiratory distress, or hemoptysis. Central nervous system (CNS) lesions may cause headaches, dizziness, blackouts, or other symptoms common to space-occupying lesions. Hepatic, urologic, and gastrointestinal symptoms are often signs of metastatic disease. Vaginal metastases may cause vaginal bleeding.

PHYSICAL EXAMINATION

Physical examination of patients with gestational choriocarcinoma may reveal signs of metastatic disease, including uterine enlargement, vaginal masses, bilateral theca lutein cysts, and neurologic signs from CNS involvement.

DIAGNOSTIC EVALUATION

The primary workup for gestational choriocarcinoma includes measurement of quantitative **hCG levels** and **assessment for metastasis** to the lungs, liver, kidneys, spleen, and brain. This entails laboratory tests including a CBC, coagulation studies, along with renal and hepatic function tests. **Pelvic ultrasound** may reveal a uterine mass with hemorrhage and necrosis. These tumors are typically highly vascular, as demonstrated by Doppler analysis. Other imaging studies might include a CXR or chest CT to look for lung metastases as well as an **abdominopelvic CT or MRI** to look for metastatic disease if indicated. If vaginal or lung metastases are present, a CT or MRI of the brain should also be obtained. Biopsy of suspected metastases is not typically needed and could result in excessive bleeding.

DIFFERENTIAL DIAGNOSIS

Gestational choriocarcinoma has been found to metastasize to virtually every tissue in the body. It is known as "**the great imitator**," because its signs and symptoms are similar to those of many disease entities. Also, given that gestational choriocarcinoma can occur from weeks to years after any type of gestation and is relatively rare, the diagnosis is often delayed when the disease occurs outside the context of a prior molar pregnancy.

TREATMENT

Classification and treatment of gestational choriocarcinomas mirror those of persistent postmolar GTD and invasive moles (Fig. 31-6). Nonmetastatic and **good-prognosis metastatic disease** may be treated with **single-agent chemotherapy**. **Poor-prognosis metastatic gestational choriocarcinoma** is treated with **multiagent chemotherapy**. The cure rate for good-prognosis disease is 95% to 100%, and the cure rate for poor-prognosis disease is 50% to 70%.

FOLLOW-UP

As with all other forms of malignant GTD, gestational choriocarcinoma requires **close monitoring of hCG levels** in conjunction with **reliable contraception**.

PLACENTAL SITE TROPHOBLASTIC TUMORS

PATHOGENESIS

PSTTs are extremely rare tumors that arise from the **placental implantation site**. In this form of malignant GTD, intermediate cytotrophoblasts from the placental site infiltrate the myometrium and then invade the blood vessels. Histologically, these tumors are characterized by the absence of villi and the proliferation of intermediate trophoblasts and **excessive production of human placental lactogen (hPL)**, as opposed to proliferation of syncytiotrophoblasts and cytotrophoblasts seen in other forms of GTD.

CLINICAL PRESENTATION

Persistent irregular vaginal bleeding is the most common symptom of PSTT and may occur weeks to years after any type of antecedent pregnancy. Physical examination may reveal an enlarged uterus.

DIAGNOSTIC EVALUATION

Unlike other forms of malignant GTD, these tumors produce **chronic low levels of hCG** because the tumors lack proliferation of syncytiotrophoblasts (the placental layer responsible for hCG production). **Serum hPL** may be used as a diagnostic tool. The **pelvic ultrasound** may show a uterine mass, but there is typically less hemorrhage than seen in gestational choriocarcinomas. Both cystic and solid components may be present. As with other forms of malignant GTD, the tumor can invade the uterine wall and surrounding tissues.

TREATMENT

PSTTs are also generally **not sensitive to chemotherapy** but, fortunately, they rarely metastasize beyond the uterus. Therefore, **hysterectomy** is the treatment of choice for PSTT. Multiagent chemotherapy may be considered after surgery to prevent recurrent disease.

KEY POINTS

- GTD is a group of related diseases resulting from abnormal proliferation of trophoblastic (placental) tissue.
- Eighty percent of GTD is benign disease (complete and partial moles), and 20% is malignant disease (persistent postmolar GTD and invasive moles, gestational choriocarcinomas, and PSTTs).
- Of benign GTD, 90% are complete moles. Complete moles result from the fertilization of an empty ovum by one sperm that then duplicates. The most common karyotype is 46,XX—all chromosomes are paternally derived.
- There is no associated embryo in complete molar pregnancy, and patients usually present with irregular vaginal bleeding, an enlarged uterus, or passage of vesicles.
- Complete molar pregnancy can have very high hCG levels (>100,000 mIU/mL), resulting in classic symptoms of hyperemesis gravidarum, preeclampsia before 20 weeks' gestation, hyperthyroidism, and/or large bilateral theca lutein cysts.
- Complete molar pregnancy is diagnosed by hCG levels and pelvic ultrasound showing a "snowstorm" pattern and is treated with immediate suction D&C to empty the uterus. Oxytocin is often given to avoid hemorrhage.
- Complete molar pregnancy requires close follow-up with weekly, then monthly, hCG levels for 6 months. Concurrent reliable contraception is imperative during this time.
- Complete molar pregnancy results in persistent malignant disease in 15% of cases and has a risk of recurrence of 1% to 2% after one molar pregnancy and 16% to 28% after two molar pregnancies.
- Partial moles account for 10% of molar pregnancies and result from the simultaneous fertilization of a normal ovum by two sperm. The most common karyotype is 69,XXY.
- Partial moles have a coexistent abnormal embryo and usually present with vaginal bleeding from spontaneous or incomplete abortion.
- Partial moles are diagnosed by hCG levels and pelvic ultrasound and treated with D&C. Persistent malignant disease develops in only 4% of cases. Follow-up is similar to complete moles with serial hCG levels and reliable contraception.
- Persistent postmolar GTD and invasive moles make up 75% of malignant GTD. They are usually diagnosed by detecting plateauing or rising hCG levels after molar evacuation.
- These moles have an overall incidence of 1 in 15,000 normal pregnancies. They are generally confined to the uterus and respond well to single-agent chemotherapy (95% to 100% cure rate).
- Gestational choriocarcinoma makes up 25% of malignant GTD with an overall incidence of 1 in 20,000 to 40,000 pregnancies in the United States. It is a malignant, necrotizing tumor that can occur weeks to years after any type of gestation.
- Patients can present with signs and symptoms of metastases to the lungs, vagina, liver, brain, or kidneys. Gestational choriocarcinoma is diagnosed by pelvic ultrasound, hCG levels, and a thorough workup for metastatic disease.
- Gestational choriocarcinoma is usually treated with multiagent chemotherapy, depending on the presence of disease outside the uterus and on the disease prognostic category.
- PSTTs are extremely rare tumors that arise from the placental implantation site. They are characterized by the absence of villi and the proliferation of cytotrophoblasts. This results in chronic low levels of hCG (<100 mIU/mL) and elevated levels of hPL.
- PSTTs spread by invasion into the myometrium and blood vessels. Patients most commonly present with vaginal bleeding and persistently low levels of hCG (<100 mIU/mL).
- PSTTs are treated by hysterectomy followed by consideration of chemotherapy to prevent recurrences.

CLINICAL VIGNETTES

VIGNETTE 1

A 40-year-old woman presents to your office with a positive home pregnancy test and a 3-day history of vaginal bleeding. She is concerned that she may be having a miscarriage. On examination, the uterine fundus is at the level of the umbilicus. By her last period, she should be around 12 weeks of gestation. On pelvic examination, there is a moderate amount of blood in the vaginal vault, and the cervix is closed. The laboratory then calls you to say that her serum β-hCG result is greater than 1,000,000 mIU/mL.

1. Which of the following is the best next step in this patient's evaluation?
   a. Surgical intervention (suction curettage)
   b. Methotrexate administration
   c. Determination of Rh status
   d. Schedule a follow-up visit in 2 weeks to recheck a β-hCG level
   e. Complete pelvic ultrasound

2. The patient undergoes an uncomplicated suction D&C. The pathology report is available the next day and is consistent with a complete molar gestation. What is the best next step in the care of this patient's condition.
   a. Radiation therapy
   b. Chemotherapy
   c. Repeat pelvic imaging
   d. Office follow-up in 4 weeks
   e. Serial surveillance of serum β-hCG levels

3. During postoperative surveillance, you meet with her in your office about 3 months after the index visit. Which of the following interventions is most important to emphasize during her follow-up period?
   a. Reliable contraception
   b. Prophylactic antibiotic use during surveillance
   c. No further pregnancies are recommended
   d. Await pregnancy attempt for 2 years
   e. Prophylactic chemotherapy to decrease the risk of persistent and recurrent disease

VIGNETTE 2

A 41-year-old G4 P3 woman presents to your emergency department with a 6-month history of irregular bleeding and a new onset of perfuse vaginal bleeding and coughing up blood. Her history reveals three term vaginal deliveries, her last being approximately 6 months ago. That delivery was uncomplicated. On physical examination, vital signs are stable, her uterus is approximately 10 to 12 weeks' size, and there is a moderate amount of blood in the vaginal vault. CXR shows a new single nodule in the left lower lobe suspicious for a metastatic lesion from unknown location.

1. Which of the following laboratory tests will most likely assist in her diagnosis?
   a. CBC
   b. Fibrinogen
   c. CA 125
   d. Serum β-hCG
   e. Prothrombin time

2. The quantitative serum β-hCG is 108,000 mIU/mL. Which of the following is the most likely diagnosis?
   a. Incomplete molar pregnancy
   b. Gestational choriocarcinoma
   c. Placental site trophoblastic tumor (PSTT)
   d. Complete molar pregnancy
   e. Persistent molar pregnancy

3. The pelvic ultrasound reveals bilateral multicystic ovarian masses along with an enlarged uterus. What is the most likely diagnosis and most appropriate management of this finding?
   a. Theca lutein cysts/conservative surveillance
   b. Primary epithelial ovarian carcinoma/surgical intervention
   c. Metastatic lesions/chemotherapy
   d. Theca lutein cysts/percutaneous drainage
   e. Metastatic lesions/surgical intervention

4. You refer the patient to a gynecologic oncologist for evaluation and management of gestational choriocarcinoma. What is the most likely intervention to be recommended?
   a. Total abdominal hysterectomy
   b. Pulmonary wedge resection
   c. Whole pelvis radiation
   d. Chemotherapy
   e. Serum β-hCG surveillance

VIGNETTE 3

A 17-year-old G1 P0 patient presents to your office with vaginal bleeding at approximately 8 weeks' gestation by her last menstrual period. Her examination is benign with a 10-week-sized uterus, a closed cervical os, and a small amount of blood within the vaginal vault. You order a complete pelvic ultrasound that shows an intrauterine gestational sac containing a fetus measuring approximately 6 weeks' gestation. Doppler sonography is unable to demonstrate any fetal heartbeat. The placenta demonstrates marked thickening and increased echogenicity with scattered cystic spaces within the placenta. A serum β-hCG is 52,000 mIU/mL.

1. What is the most likely diagnosis?
   a. Complete molar pregnancy
   b. Incomplete molar pregnancy
   c. Incomplete abortion
   d. Missed abortion
   e. Inevitable abortion

2. You decide to perform a suction D&C. When giving informed consent, you discuss the risk most commonly encountered in this operation. Which of the following is the most common risk associated with suction D&C?
   a. Uterine perforation
   b. Infection
   c. Damage to the bladder
   d. Uterovaginal bleeding
   e. Need for future surgery

3. After pathology returns, you discuss the findings with your patient in follow-up at your office. Which of the following is most accurate when discussing risk of persistent gestational trophoblastic disease (GTD)?
   a. 2% to 4%
   b. Less than 1%
   c. 6% to 10%
   d. 11% to 15%
   e. Greater than 20%

VIGNETTE 4

A 44-year-old woman presents to your emergency department with profuse vaginal bleeding. Her medical history is unremarkable. She has had two term vaginal deliveries, her last being 10 years ago. An initial workup shows a solid intrauterine mass and a serum β-hCG level of 220 mIU/mL. You decide to proceed with endometrial sampling, which is uncomplicated. Final surgical pathologic diagnosis is consistent with PSTT.

1. Which of the following elevated serum markers is most associated with PSTT?
   a. Prolactin
   b. Human placental lactogen
   c. Inhibin-A
   d. CA-125
   e. Serum β-hCG

2. Which of the following is typically the primary treatment of choice for PSTT?
   a. Systemic chemotherapy
   b. Directed external beam radiation therapy
   c. Hysterectomy
   d. Hysteroscopy, D&C
   e. Serum β-hCG surveillance

3. In the preoperative workup of your patient, a CXR shows bilateral solid masses within the middle lung lobes. According to the FIGO stratification, which stage of the disease does she have?
   a. I
   b. II
   c. III
   d. IV

ANSWERS

VIGNETTE 1 Question 1
1. Answer E:
This patient's vignette is most consistent with GTD, which is a proliferative disorder of trophoblastic placental tissue. The initial workup should include a pelvic ultrasound to determine the exact etiology of the patient's examination and laboratory findings. Rh status would be included in this patient's workup after a diagnosis has been established. Suction D&C is the treatment of choice for GTD and allows for an exact diagnosis to be made but should not be entertained until the sonographic diagnosis has been confirmed. Methotrexate is not generally a treatment of choice in the early diagnosis of GTD. It can be used as adjuvant therapy if malignant GTD is discovered. Conservative management is never an option in patients with suspicion for GTD because the therapy of choice is surgical intervention.

VIGNETTE 1 Question 2
2. Answer E:
Persistent GTD after evacuation of a complete molar gestation can occur in approximately 20% to 30% of patients (compared to a <5% risk in partial incomplete molar gestation). Risk factors for persistence typically include hCG level over 100,000 mIU/mL, the presence of large (>6 cm in diameter) theca lutein cysts, and significant uterine enlargement (all of which are consistent with larger amounts of trophoblastic tissue). Serum β-hCG surveillance, usually lasting

approximately 6 months, proves reliable in confirming that all proliferative trophoblastic cells have disappeared. Conservative management without hCG surveillance is not appropriate in this patient. Chemotherapy would be entertained if persistent GTD was confirmed. However, during the initial surveillance period, it is reasonable to allow the serum β-hCG to decrease spontaneously. Repeat imaging of the pelvis is not indicated at this time.

VIGNETTE 1 Question 3
3. Answer A:
Reliable contraception is paramount during surveillance of serum β-hCG after a molar gestation. This will decrease confusion with the possibility of a new pregnancy during the interval period. Typically, the most common method used is combination oral contraception. Medroxyprogesterone acetate injection is an appropriate alternative. Implants are typically avoided given the high rate of irregular bleeding with these devices. Pregnancy should be avoided during the 6-month surveillance period; however, after persistent GTD has been ruled out, attempt at pregnancy is reasonable. Prophylactic antibiotics and/or prophylactic chemotherapy are not warranted in these cases.

VIGNETTE 2 Question 1
1. Answer D:
This patient's clinical history and physical examination are most consistent with metastatic GTD. A quantitative serum β-hCG is the most important initial diagnostic test that will confirm the presence of proliferative trophoblastic tissues. CA-125 is a very nonspecific laboratory test that is unlikely to assist given this patient's clinical history. Although CBC, prothrombin time, and fibrinogen level are reasonable to order, they will not lead to a diagnosis in this patient.

VIGNETTE 2 Question 2
2. Answer B:
The malignant forms of GTD include persistent/invasive gestational trophoblastic neoplasia (after complete or incomplete molar pregnancy), gestational choriocarcinoma, and PSTT. The most likely diagnosis in this patient is metastatic gestational choriocarcinoma. This is a rare condition occurring most commonly after evacuation of a complete molar gestation (50%), and less commonly after term pregnancies (25%) and spontaneous abortions or ectopic pregnancies (25%). When malignant GTD is encountered after a *nonmolar* pregnancy, the diagnosis is almost always gestational choriocarcinoma and rarely PSTTs. Gestational choriocarcinoma is an aggressive tumor and most commonly presenting with abnormal uterine bleeding. The most common site of metastasis is the lung (80%). Other sites include the vagina (30%), liver and brain (10%). Complete and incomplete molar pregnancies are potentially malignant. If there is evidence of metastasis, malignant GTD is the diagnosis. Invasive or persistent molar pregnancy usually occurs after evacuation of a molar gestation and rarely metastasizes. PSTT is exceedingly rare, associated with a persistent *low* β-hCG levels, and is typically confined to the uterus.

VIGNETTE 2 Question 3
3. Answer A:
Theca lutein cysts result from overstimulation of ovarian parenchyma from high levels of serum hCG. The typical appearance is multiseptated cysts, commonly occurring bilaterally. Conservative management of these cysts is recommended, because they resolve once the hCG has been eliminated. Ovarian metastasis from choriocarcinoma is not common. Epithelial ovarian carcinoma is unlikely in this particular patient.

VIGNETTE 2 Question 4
4. Answer D:
Malignant GTD is extremely sensitive to chemotherapy and is therefore the mainstay of treatment in these patients. Single or multiagent therapies are used, guided by the presence or absence of certain prognostic factors. The International Federation of Gynecology and Obstetrics (FIGO) established a four-tiered staging system based mostly on the location of metastatic lesions. Other risk factors for recurrence include serum β-hCG greater than 100,000 mIU/mL and greater than 6 months from the index pregnancy. Surgical intervention and radiation therapy are typically reserved for tumor that is resistant to initial chemotherapy and/or cerebral tumor involvement, respectively.

VIGNETTE 3 Question 1
1. Answer B:
The combination of findings including an intrauterine fetus, marked thickening and cystic formation within the placenta, and an increased serum β-hCG is highly suggestive of an incomplete (partial) molar pregnancy. Partial molar pregnancies are triploid karyotypes, compared to diploid in complete molar pregnancies. Typically, these pregnancies present and are often confused with missed and/or incomplete abortions. Diagnostic accuracy using pelvic ultrasound is the gold standard in the evaluation of this patient.

VIGNETTE 3 Question 2
2. Answer D:
Vaginal bleeding is commonly encountered during these cases mostly because of the high vascularity of the pregnancy and the abnormal placental tissue. Uterotonics (oxytocin, methylergonivine, misoprostol) are frequently used in these cases to help prevent and minimize excessive bleeding. Other choices are associated risks but are less common.

VIGNETTE 3 Question 3
3. Answer A:
Incomplete (partial) molar gestation is associated with approximately a 2% to 4% risk of persistent disease (compared to approximately 20% risk of persistence with a complete molar pregnancy). The importance of serial β-hCG surveillance is paramount in the management of these patients postoperatively. If levels plateau during surveillance or begin rising, further workup for persistent disease should be initiated.

VIGNETTE 4 Question 1
1. Answer B:
PSTT is a slowly growing malignant tumor that arises from placental cytotrophoblasts. These cells produce low amounts of β-hCG and high amounts of hPL. This can be used in the diagnosis of PSTT. These tumors have persistently low levels of serum β-hCG. The remaining choices are not typically used in this condition.

VIGNETTE 4 Question 2
2. Answer C:
Definitive hysterectomy is typically the treatment of choice for patients with PSTT. This is in contrast to all other forms of malignant GTD, which typically involves treatment of primary disease with systemic chemotherapy.

VIGNETTE 4 Question 3
3. Answer C:
Stage I is defined as persistently elevated serum β-hCG levels with tumor confined to the uterus. Stage II is defined by the presence of tumor outside the uterus, but limited to the vagina and/or pelvis. Stage III is defined as pulmonary metastasis with or without uterine, vaginal, or pelvic tumor metastasis. Stage IV includes all other metastatic lesions most commonly including the brain, liver, kidneys, and the gastrointestinal tract.

32 | Benign Breast Disease and Breast Cancer

Breast cancer is the most common malignancy in women (except for nonmelanoma skin cancers), representing approximately 30% of female cancers and 250,000 new diagnoses annually in the United States. It is also the second most common cause of cancer deaths in women (after lung cancer deaths), accounting for some 40,000 deaths per year. A woman has a **one in eight chance (12%)** of developing invasive breast cancer over her lifetime. Yet, despite its incidence, the cause of breast cancer remains unknown.

In addition to breast cancer, as many as 50% of women will have benign breast lesions over their lifetime. Therefore, understanding the range of benign and malignant breast lesions and their symptoms is enormously important. Obstetrician–gynecologists, primary care providers, and surgeons evaluate breast pain, nipple discharge, and breast masses in addition to screening for breast cancer. The anatomy and physiology of the breast as well as the diagnosis and treatment of breast lesions should be understood by all physicians involved in women's health.

ANATOMY

Breast parenchyma is divided into segments containing **mammary glands** that consist of 20 to 40 lobules drained by **lactiferous ducts** that open individually into the nipple (Fig. 32-1). Fibrous bands—called Cooper suspensory ligaments—span between two fascial layers to support the breast. The breast is divided into four quadrants for ease of description: upper outer quadrant (UOQ), lower outer quadrant (LOQ), upper inner quadrant (UIQ), and lower inner quadrant (LIQ). Notably, breast tissue also extends into the axilla.

The **major blood supply** to the breast is from the **internal mammary** (derived from the internal thoracic artery) and **lateral thoracic arteries** (Fig. 32-2). The medial and central aspects are supplied by the anterior perforators of the internal mammary artery, and the UOQ is supplied by the lateral thoracic arteries. Venous drainage is primarily accomplished via the axillary vein.

The **axillary lymph nodes** drain up to 97% of the ipsilateral breast and secondarily drain the supraclavicular and jugular lymph nodes. These nodes are subdivided into three levels for the purposes of specifying disease progression. The **internal mammary nodes** are responsible for 3% of drainage, mainly of the UIQ and LIQ. The interpectoral nodes (Rotter nodes) lie between the pectoralis major and pectoralis minor muscles and drain to the axillary nodes.

Breast innervation is mostly supplied by the 4th-6th intercostal nerves. Several nerves not primarily involved in breast innervation may be at risk during breast surgeries due to the proximity of their path to

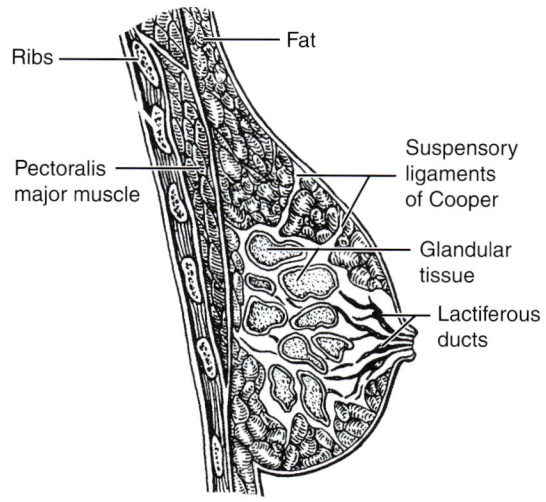

FIGURE 32-1. Clinical anatomy of the female breast and chest wall. (From Beckmann C, Ling F. *Obstetrics & Gynecology*, 5th ed. Philadelphia, PA: Lippincott Williams & Wilkins; 2006.)

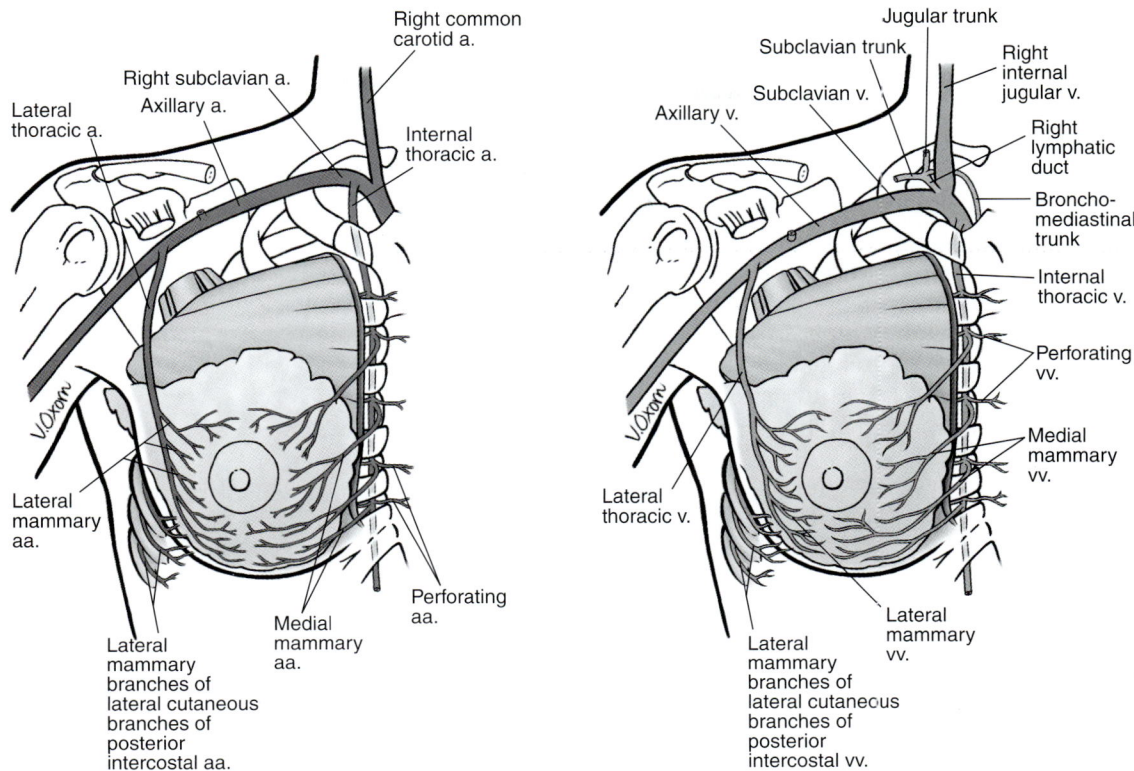

FIGURE 32-2. Arterial and venous blood supply to the breast and chest wall. The breast is supplied primarily by the internal thoracic arteries and the lateral thoracic arteries. (From Moore KL, Agur A. *Essential Clinical Anatomy*, 2nd ed. Philadelphia, PA: Lippincott Williams & Wilkins; 2002.)

key breast anatomy. Nerves at risk of injury include the **intercostobrachial nerve** that transverses the axilla to supply sensation to the upper medial arm; the **long thoracic nerve** (of Bell) of C5 to C7 that innervates the serratus anterior muscle (injury during mastectomy can lead to "winged" scapula); the **thoracodorsal nerve** that innervates the latissimus dorsi muscle; and the lateral pectoral nerve that innervates the pectoralis major and minor muscles.

PHYSIOLOGY

Breast development is classified into **Tanner stages 1 to 5** (see Chapter 20 and Fig. 20-3). The breast responds to cyclic hormones, as well as to changes in pregnancy and menopause. **Estrogen** promotes ductal development and fat deposition, whereas **progesterones** promote the lobular–alveolar (stromal) development that makes lactation possible. **Prolactin** is involved in milk production, whereas **oxytocin** from the posterior pituitary causes milk letdown. In **postmenopausal women**, the hypoestrogenic state is associated with **tissue atrophy**, loss of stroma, and replacement of atrophied lobules with fatty tissue.

EVALUATION OF THE BREAST

ROUTINE EVALUATION—WOMEN AT AVERAGE RISK

There are three major screening components for **women at average population risk** of breast cancer. These include the clinical breast examination by a health care provider, the breast self-examination, and screening mammography. Guidelines for breast cancer screening vary between leading medical organizations, such as the American Cancer Society (ACS), the U.S. Preventive Services Task Force (USPSTF), and the American Congress of Obstetricians and Gynecologists (ACOG).

Most of these organizations support routine **clinician breast evaluation** every 1 to 3 years for all women above age 20. After age 40, clinical breast evaluation by a health care provider should be done annually. Physical examination involves careful **inspection of the skin** for contour changes, color irregularities, dimpling, and retractions. These maneuvers should be performed with the patient in both the upright and supine positions. This is followed by evaluation for lymphadenopathy in the axillary and supraclavicular nodes. The breast, including the axillary tail, is then palpated for evaluation of masses, nipple discharge, pain and other changes.

Most of the leading medical organizations now consider **breast self-examination** for women aged 20 and over to be optional. For those that do support breast self-examination, emphasis has moved from the monthly breast self-examination toward general **"breast self-awareness."** The latter encourages women to become familiar with their breasts and to report any changes from baseline. Breast self-awareness should be reviewed at each annual gynecology visit.

Screening mammography is the third component of routine breast care for the patient at average risk of breast cancer (Fig. 32-3). Although there has been some controversy regarding the frequency of mammograms between ages 40 and 50, current mammography screening guidelines by the ACS include a mammogram every year starting at age 40 and continuing for as long as a woman is in good health. There is no agreed upon consensus of an **upper age limit** at which mammogram screening can be stopped, although the risk of breast cancer continues to increase in women until age 84.

ROUTINE EVALUATION—WOMEN AT HIGH RISK

Women at *highest* risk of breast cancer are those who have a known **BRCA1** or **BRCA2 gene mutation**, a first-degree relative (mother, sister, or daughter)

FIGURE 32-3. Mammogram. (From LifeART image copyright © 2006 Lippincott Williams & Wilkins. All rights reserved.)

with either mutation, and those deemed to be at high risk based on a validated risk assessment tool (e.g., Gail or Claus model). Women at *high* risk of breast cancer include those who underwent radiation to the chest between the ages of 10 and 30 or who have a hereditary syndrome associated with multiple cancer diagnoses (e.g., Li–Fraumeni, Cowden, or Lynch syndrome). Women at *moderate* risk are those deemed to be at moderate risk based on a validated screening tool, those with a personal history of breast cancer or its precursor lesions, or those who have particularly dense breast tissue on mammogram.

Hereditary syndromes associated with multiple cancers, such as Li–Fraumeni, Cowden, or Lynch (HNPCC—hereditary nonpolyposis colorectal cancer) are important considerations. Breast cancer is the most common cancer associated with Cowden syndrome. Patients with Li–Fraumeni syndrome are at a 50% lifetime risk of breast cancer development by age 60. Finally, Lynch syndrome is associated with multiple primary cancers (especially endometrial cancer); however, breast cancer risk also varies with the mutation.

Screening recommendations for these women at high risk vary, but they typically include the teaching of breast self-awareness, clinical breast examination every 6 to 12 months, and annual mammography starting at age 25 *or* 5 to 10 years before the age of the youngest cancer diagnosis in the family. Women at highest or high risk for breast cancer also typically have interval breast MRIs in addition to their annual screening mammogram. Women at moderate risk can consider adding MRI screening to their annual mammography after discussion with their physician.

Other Tools

Breast ultrasonography has been established as a useful addition to mammography. It can be helpful in the evaluation of breast cysts, uncertain mammographic findings in women younger than 40, in women with dense breast tissue, and as a guidance tool for needle breast biopsies. It is also useful in distinguishing a breast cyst from a solid mass during targeted evaluation. If a high-risk patient is unable to undergo MRI imaging, ultrasound may be utilized.

2D digital mammography (as compared with film mammography) has become the standard of care for breast cancer screening and diagnosis. In 2003, the Food and Drug Administration (FDA) approved the first commercial 3D mammography system known as **digital breast tomosynthesis** (or simply "tomo") for breast cancer screening, diagnosis, and intervention. Clinical research regarding tomosynthesis has shown increased cancer detection, decreased callbacks for repeat imaging, and improved characterization of lesions and their margins in both dense and fatty breasts. The exact implications for clinical use are being further defined, and the strategies for decreasing radiation dose are being investigated.

EVALUATION OF BREAST PAIN

Breast pain (mastalgia or mastodynia) is a common complaint (65%) in women and men but is not always reported to a healthcare provider. In men, breast pain is often due to **gynecomastia**. For women, pain is typically **mild** and may be **cyclic** (67%) or **noncyclic** (33%) in nature. For breast pain that is cyclic, it usually occurs bilaterally in the UOQs approximately one week prior to menses. Breast pain can be a normal physiologic response to hormonal fluctuations, or it can be a pathologic response to trauma or malignancy. Mastalgia may be a component of premenstrual syndrome, associated with menopausal hormone therapy (MHT), pregnancy, or caused by menstrual irregularities or fibrocystic change. Only 1% to 7% of women with breast pain will have underlying malignancy.

The patient's **medical history**, including benign or malignant diseases of the breast, is relevant. Clinicians need to establish whether the pain is cyclic or noncyclic, bilateral or unilateral, diffuse or focal. They must also ask about **associated symptoms** (back/neck pain, erythema, and fever) and use of medications such as oral contraceptive pills (OCPs) and MHT. Also relevant are any history of trauma, radiation or surgery to the breast, family history of breast disease, and constitutional symptoms such as weight loss or gain, chest wall pain, or amenorrhea. If the patient is **breastfeeding**, the physician should rule out mastitis or a breast abscess.

The history and physical examination are typically enough to provide **reassurance** to a patient. Focal lesions or areas of trauma can be evaluated with an **ultrasound** in women. Women at high risk of cancer should be evaluated with **mammography**. Nonbreast sources may also refer pain to the breast. These can include underlying pulmonary, cardiac, chest wall, or musculoskeletal causes. The vast majority of breast pain, however, is benign and can be treated with acetaminophen, **nonsteroidal anti-inflammatory drugs** (NSAIDs), a **supportive bra** or sports bra, diet and lifestyle changes (decrease caffeine intake and smoking), the use of warm and cool **compresses** and massage. Many women will require a decreased dose or discontinuation of OCPs or MHT in order to relieve their breast pain. Danazol is the only medication approved by the FDA to treat mastalgia; however, it is associated with significant side effects. Severe mastalgia may be treated with tamoxifen; however, menopausal side effects and increased blood clot risks should be discussed. The data have been inconclusive regarding the effectiveness of vitamin E and evening primrose oil for breast pain. Management of breast pain associated with specific benign and malignant processes is further discussed below.

EVALUATION OF NIPPLE DISCHARGE

As many as 50% to 80% of women will have nipple discharge at some point during their reproductive years. Nipple discharge is primarily due to normal physiologic or benign processes (such as lactation); however, 5% of cases are associated with an underlying malignancy (Table 32-1). The **most concerning** discharge is spontaneous, **bloody** (or serosanguinous), **unilateral**, **persistent**, **from a**

TABLE 32-1. Causes of Nipple Discharge

Etiology Class	Conditions
Benign breast disease	Intraductal papilloma, ductal hyperplasia, duct ectasia, and fibrocystic breast changes
Premalignant and malignant breast disease	Intraductal carcinoma (in situ or invasive) and diffuse papillomatosis
Systemic disease	Hyperprolactinemia, hypothyroidism, pituitary adenomas, sarcoidosis, chronic renal failure, and liver cirrhosis
Medications	Oral contraceptives, phenothiazines, methyldopa, reserpine, imipramine, amphetamines, and metoclopramide
Chest wall lesions	Thoracotomy, chest wall trauma and burns, and herpes zoster
Skin changes mistaken for nipple discharge	Paget disease, insect bites, local infection, and eczema
Chronic breast stimulation	Poorly fitted bra, stimulation by partner, and self-stimulation

single duct, and **associated with a mass**. Bilateral, nonbloody, multiductal secretions that occur with breast manipulation are typically benign regardless of color.

When a patient presents with nipple discharge, it is important to accurately describe the nature of the discharge: **color**, **laterality**, number of **duct openings** involved, and whether it occurs **spontaneously** or with manual expression. The physical examination should look for **skin changes**, associated **masses**, and lymphadenopathy. An attempt should be made to elicit nipple discharge by applying pressure to the base of the areola—either by the provider or by the patient. Bloody or serosanguinous discharge should be tested on a **guaiac card** and sent for **cytologic evaluation**. Routine culture of the fluid is not indicated. Women with associated amenorrhea, menstrual irregularities, headaches, or visual disturbances should have **prolactin and thyroid levels** drawn. Depending on their age, women with associated breast masses should have targeted **ultrasound and/or mammography** evaluation.

The most common cause of bloody nipple discharge is an **intraductal papilloma**, although invasive papillary cancer can also present in this manner. **Galactorrhea** is physiologic nipple discharge outside of pregnancy or breastfeeding that is associated with pituitary adenomas, hypothyroidism, stress, chronic breast stimulation (manipulation), or medications such as OCPs, antihypertensives, and psychotropic drugs. Serous discharge is associated with normal menses, OCPs, fibrocystic change, or early pregnancy. Yellow-tinged discharge is associated with fibrocystic change or galactocele. Green, sticky discharge is associated with duct ectasia. Purulent discharge indicates a superficial mastitis or central breast abscess.

Most nipple discharge is benign and does not require treatment beyond reassurance. When indicated, treatment should be individualized to the specific cause of the discharge.

EVALUATION OF BREAST MASSES

The most common breast masses are benign fibroadenomas and breast cysts. If a patient is found to have a **breast mass** on the clinician's examination or her own self-examination, a thorough history and examination are crucial. Importantly, up to **10% to 15% of new breast cancers are not seen or detected via mammography**; therefore, a suspicious mass should never be dismissed based on a negative or normal mammogram.

When evaluating a breast mass, it is important to ascertain the manner in which it was discovered, associated tenderness, recent trauma, and the relationship of breast changes to the menstrual cycle. Likewise, the location, size, shape, consistency, and mobility should be noted in addition to any overlying skin or nipple changes. Worrisome breast lumps are dominant, discrete, and dense. **Malignant masses are classically single, firm, nontender, and immobile with irregular borders**. Lymph nodes are worrisome if larger than 1 cm, fixed, irregular, firm, or multiple.

Abnormal breast masses should be **evaluated radiographically** as well. For **women younger than 30 years, ultrasound** is the preferred initial method of imaging. Ultrasound is also useful in women of any age to distinguish **solid versus cystic** masses or for additional evaluation of women with dense breast tissue. For **women aged 30 or older, mammography** is used to further evaluate suspicious masses. To standardize mammogram reporting, a collaborative scoring system was devised and published by the American College of Radiology. It is known as the **Breast Imaging Reporting and Database System (BI-RADS).** This system (Table 32-2) categorizes mammographic findings based on radiographic evidence supporting the absence or likelihood of breast cancer. Findings that are most suggestive of malignancy include a spiculated mass; architectural distortion with retraction; asymmetric localized fibrosis; microcalcifications with linear, branched patterns; increased vascularity; or altered subareolar duct pattern (Fig. 32-4).

Any concerning palpable mass or abnormality seen on radiologic imaging should be evaluated with mammography (if not previously performed) and biopsied for a **pathologic diagnosis** (Table 32-3). The goal of tissue biopsy is to obtain an adequate sample using the least invasive sampling technique. If a palpable cystic mass is found on examination and confirmed on ultrasound, it can be drained and sampled for diagnosis using **needle aspiration** (Fig. 32-5). This treats the cyst while providing fluid for cytology if indicated by a turbid or bloody aspirate. The **cyst should be excised** if the fluid is bloody, a mass persists after fluid is removed, the cyst is persistent after two aspirations, or if the fluid reaccumulates within two weeks.

When a **solid mass is palpated** on examination and confirmed with ultrasound or mammography, a tissue sample should be obtained for diagnosis. In women less than 30 years old, **fine-needle aspiration** (FNA) can be used to sample solid masses

TABLE 32-2. BI-RADS for Characterization of Mammogram Findings

Category	Assessment Category	Recommended Action	Risk of Malignancy
0	Incomplete	Additional imaging needed	N/A
1	Negative	Routine follow-up	0%
2	Benign finding(s)	Routine follow-up	0%
3	Probably benign	Short-interval (6 mo) follow-up	≤2%
4	Suspicious of malignancy	Core-needle biopsy ASAP	2%–95%
5	Highly suspicious of malignancy	Core-needle biopsy ASAP	≥95%
6	Known, biopsy-proven malignancy	Definitive treatment ongoing	100%

BI-RADS, Breast Imaging Reporting and Database System.

FIGURE 32-4. A cephalocaudal mammogram film contrasting a small speculated mass carcinoma (*arrow*) versus a well-marginated fibroadenoma (*arrowhead*). (From Beckmann C, Ling F. *Obstetrics & Gynecology*, 5th ed. Philadelphia, PA: Lippincott Williams & Wilkins; 2006.)

TABLE 32-3. Evaluation of Abnormal Breast Masses and Abnormal Mammogram Findings

Abnormal Findings	Appropriate Evaluation
Palpable cystic lesion	→ Needle drainage
Recurrent cyst, bloody fluid	→ Excision
Solid, palpable mass (≤30 y)	→ FNA
Nondiagnostic FNA of solid mass	→ Excisional biopsy
Solid, palpable mass (≥30 y)	→ Core-needle biopsy
Nondiagnostic core-needle biopsy	→ Excisional biopsy
Nonpalpable abnormal mammogram finding	→ Wire-guided excision

FNA, fine-needle aspiration.

(Fig. 32-6). This technique involves an experienced cytopathologist aspirating a syringe while making multiple passes through the mass from different angles using a small needle. Diagnostic accuracy approaches 80% to 90%. An **excisional biopsy** is performed if the FNA does not obtain fluid or tissue. Excisional biopsy is also performed if cytology or histology is not diagnostic. In women aged 30 years or older with a palpable solid mass, a **core-needle biopsy** is recommended.

When a **nonpalpable lesion** is found by mammography, excisional biopsy can also be performed under **needle or wire guidance**. To qualify as a lumpectomy, the abnormal tissue should be excised with a 1-cm rim of normal tissue, thus avoiding the need for repeat surgery if the mass is malignant.

BENIGN BREAST DISEASE

Benign breast symptoms and findings are common and occur in approximately 50% of women, with a higher incidence in younger women. Abnormal breast findings are biopsied for definitive diagnosis based on individual patient risk factors for malignant

FIGURE 32-5. Needle aspiration of a breast cyst. (From LifeART image copyright © 2006 Lippincott Williams & Wilkins. All rights reserved.)

FIGURE 32-6. Fine-needle aspiration of a solid breast mass. (From Beckmann C, Ling F. *Obstetrics & Gynecology*, 5th ed. Philadelphia, PA: Lippincott Williams & Wilkins; 2006.)

disease. Two-thirds of tumors in reproductive-age women are benign; however, half of palpable masses in perimenopausal women and the majority of lesions in postmenopausal women are malignant.

FIBROCYSTIC BREAST CHANGE

Pathophysiology
Fibrocystic change includes a spectrum of clinical findings owing to an **exaggerated stromal response** to hormones and growth factors. It typically presents as **painful, sensitive, often multiple and bilateral breast masses**. There can be rapid fluctuation in the size of the masses. Associated breast changes may include cystic change, nodularity, stromal proliferation, or epithelial hyperplasia. In the absence of atypical hyperplasia, **fibrocystic change is not associated with increased cancer risk**.

Epidemiology
Peak incidence is between ages 30 and 40, but changes can persist throughout a woman's entire life. Fibrocystic changes are rare in postmenopausal women.

Diagnosis

Patients with fibrocystic changes present with breast swelling, pain, and tenderness. Fibrocystic disease may have more focal symptomatic areas, involve both breasts, and vary throughout the menstrual cycle. The pain is commonly worse because the mass size increases during the **premenstrual part of the cycle**. Depending on patient age, evaluation with mammogram, ultrasound, and/or biopsy should be performed for suspicious lesions (such as a dominant mass that does not fluctuate in size).

Treatment

The pain of fibrocystic breast changes can be ameliorated with **reduction of caffeine, tea, and chocolate**, although the role of caffeine reduction is controversial. **Avoiding trauma, wearing a support bra, and use of hot or cold compresses** may also help decrease the pain as will the use of over-the-counter NSAIDs and decreasing MHT or oral contraception dosing. Although the data have been inconsistent, other recognized treatments include **evening primrose oil, vitamins E and B_6, danazol, progestins, bromocriptine, and tamoxifen** (not approved for this indication). Danazol is the only FDA-approved prescription medication for the treatment of breast pain.

HYPERPLASIA (DUCTAL OR LOBULAR)

Pathophysiology

Epithelial hyperplasia is the overgrowth of cells lining the ducts (ductal hyperplasia) or glands (lobular hyperplasia) of the breast. Depending on the pattern of growth, hyperplasia is classified as usual or atypical. In **usual hyperplasia**, the cell growth pattern is close to normal. In **atypical hyperplasia**, the cells are more atypical and distorted.

The risk for subsequent breast cancer after a diagnosis of hyperplasia depends on the type of hyperplasia. Mild usual hyperplasia is not associated with an increased risk of breast cancer. Women diagnosed with moderate to florid hyperplasia of the usual type have a 1.5 to 2 times increased risk of breast cancer compared to women with no breast abnormalities. Both atypical ductal hyperplasia (ADH) and atypical lobular hyperplasia (ALH) carry a 3.5 to 5 times higher risk of breast cancer than women with no breast abnormalities. ADH increases the risk for cancer in the ipsilateral breast, whereas ALH increases the risk of developing cancer in both the ipsilateral and contralateral breasts.

Diagnosis

Hyperplasia is typically asymptomatic but can result in changes on mammogram. Diagnosis is achieved via core biopsy.

Treatment

Standard treatment for women with atypical hyperplasia is close follow-up with clinical breast examination, mammograms, and breast MRIs. Some women with atypical hyperplasia (ductal or lobular) will take selective estrogen receptor modulators (SERMs) (tamoxifen or raloxifene) daily for five years to decrease their risk of developing breast cancer. The use of these medications increase the risk of deep vein thrombosis and pulmonary embolism. Additionally, they can cause menopausal symptoms.

FIBROADENOMA

Pathogenesis

Breast fibroadenomas are benign tumors made up of both glandular breast tissue and stromal connective tissue (Fig. 32-4). Most masses are simple fibroadenomas and measure 1 to 3 cm in diameter at the time of detection. Lesions larger than 5 cm are termed *giant fibroadenomas*. In these cases, cystosarcoma phyllodes should be ruled out. Fibroadenomas are **often solitary** but can be multiple. These are bilateral up to 25% of the time. The etiology is unknown but is likely related to the hormonal milieu, specifically estrogen.

Women with fibroadenomas have a 1.5- to 2-fold greater risk developing breast cancer than do women with no breast changes.

Epidemiology

Fibroadenomas are the **most common benign tumors of the breast**. They can be found at any age but most commonly occur in young women in their 20s and 30s. They are more common than breast cysts in women younger than 25 years. They very rarely occur and often regress after menopause.

Diagnosis

Fibroadenomas are often palpated on physical examination as rubbery, round, well-circumscribed, mobile, firm lesions that are nontender. The patient may report changes in the lesion during the menstrual cycle, pregnancy, and with OCP use. Classic fibroadenoma in a woman less than 30 years old may be the only solid breast mass that does not require tissue diagnosis.

Treatment

A young patient (<30 years old) with classic presentation of a simple fibroadenoma with no adjacent proliferative damage and no family history of breast cancer can be **followed clinically if stable**. Otherwise, FNA for cytology is highly sensitive for detecting cancer or phyllodes tumors. If simple fibroadenoma is confirmed by biopsy and is **asymptomatic, it can be left in place or treated with cryoablation**. If the fibroadenoma is large, growing, or changing in shape, excision is recommended to remove the tumor and establish pathologic diagnosis.

CYSTOSARCOMA PHYLLODES
Pathogenesis
Phyllodes tumors are a **rare variant of fibroadenomas**. They start in the stromal (connective) tissue and involve both epithelial and stromal proliferations.

Epidemiology
These tumors are diagnosed most commonly in premenopausal women in their 30s and 40s, although they can occur at any age. There have been no etiologic or predisposing factors identified, with the exception of Li–Fraumeni syndrome.

Diagnosis
This lesion appears as a painless, **large, bulky, mobile mass**. The overlying skin is warm, erythematous, shiny, and engorged. The mass is generally **large** (4 to 7 cm), smooth, well-circumscribed, and characterized by **rapid growth**. Most lesions are benign; however, some physicians consider cystosarcoma phyllodes a **low-grade malignancy**, and a few tumors do develop true sarcomatous potential. These tumors are worrisome for aggressive malignancies; therefore, pathologic diagnosis must be made. **Core-needle biopsy** is the preferred method for diagnosis, but results should be strongly correlated with clinical suspicion.

Treatment
The clinical course of these tumors is unpredictable because most are benign; however, **10% do contain malignant cells**. Compared to fibroadenomas, these tumors have a high rate of local recurrence after simple excision. Therefore, the recommended treatment is **wide local excision** (with a 1-cm margin) for small tumors or a **simple mastectomy** for large lesions not amenable to wide local excision. Follow-up should involve frequent clinical breast examination and imaging.

INTRADUCTAL PAPILLOMA
Pathogenesis
Intraductal papilloma is a benign solitary lesion that grows in the **epithelial lining of breast ducts**. It is the most common cause of **bloody nipple discharge** in the absence of a concurrent mass. These wart-like growths can also appear as small masses under or adjacent to the nipple.

Diagnosis
Intraductal papilloma usually appears with bloody nipple discharge in premenopausal women. The serosanguinous discharge is **sent for cytology** to rule out invasive papillary carcinoma, which has similar symptoms 25% of the time. Ductograms can be used to identify the papilloma. If the lesion is large enough, a core-needle biopsy can be performed.

Treatment
Definitive diagnosis and treatment is achieved by surgical resection of the papilloma and the portion of the duct in which it is found. No further treatment is warranted after excision if the pathology confirms no evidence of malignancy.

MAMMARY DUCT ECTASIA (PLASMA CELL MASTITIS)
Pathogenesis
The exact cause of ductal ectasia is unknown. However, it is thought to result from normal age-related widening and shortening of the ducts near menopause. These anatomic changes result in inflammation of the duct with subsequent plasma cell infiltration and blockage of the duct. As a result, the duct may produce a thick, sticky, green, or black discharge. The nipple may become red, tender, and inverted, and fibrosis can result in a small lump in the duct.

Epidemiology
This lesion most commonly occurs **at or after menopause**; however, it can also be a cause of breast masses in adolescents.

Diagnosis
Patients present with **nipple discharge**, noncyclic **breast pain**, **nipple retraction**, or subareolar masses. The discharge is multicolored, sticky, originating from multiple ducts, and **often bilateral**. The patient should have a mammogram, and excisional biopsy is indicated to rule out carcinoma if a lump is present.

Treatment
This condition usually **improves without treatment**. If mastitis occurs in the affected duct, warm compresses and antibiotics may be indicated. However, if symptoms persist, definitive treatment is **local excision** of the inflamed area, and extensive subareolar duct excision is sometimes required.

MALIGNANT BREAST DISEASE
Epidemiology
Breast cancer is the most common nonskin malignancy affecting women of any race or ethnicity in the United States. One in every eight American women will develop this disease during her lifetime and will have a 3.5% chance of dying from it. It accounts for 30% of all cancers in women and 20% of women's cancer deaths. Although black women in the United States have a lower incidence of breast cancer, they have a higher mortality rate compared with white women in the United States. This difference in mortality rates is not completely understood.

The risk of getting breast cancer increases with age. Four of every five women with breast cancer are above age 50. Although the incidence of diagnosis is increasing, the death rate had decreased by one-third over the past 25 years. This is likely due to more widespread acceptance of breast cancer screening, earlier detection, and improved therapies. Currently, breast cancer is the leading cause of death in US women aged 40 to 59. The median age of diagnosis is 62.

Risk Factors
Numerous risk factors are associated with breast cancer (Table 32-4). One major risk factor is **increasing age**. For example, an American woman's annual risk of invasive breast cancer increases from 1 in 2,000 by age 30 to 1 in 8 by age 80. Similarly, **a personal history of breast cancer** increases the risk of developing invasive cancer in the contralateral breast. For women with invasive breast cancer, the risk of developing cancer in the contralateral breast is 1% per year for premenopausal women and 0.5% per year for postmenopausal women.

A **family history of gynecologic malignancies** also significantly increases a patient's risk of breast cancer. Having a first-degree relative (parent, sibling, or child) with breast cancer increases a woman's risk greatly, depending on the number of affected relatives, their age at diagnosis, and the bilaterality of their disease. Having one affected first-degree family member increases the patient's risk by nearly two times, and having two first-degree family members increases a patient's risk by nearly three times. Less than 15% of women with breast cancer will have a first degree relative with the disease.

A strong family history is suspicious for a **genetic predisposition**. Although **<15% of women with breast cancer have a family history** of the disease, inherited genetic mutations are still rare. Six familial syndromes have been identified with an increased risk of breast cancer (Table 32-4). The best known of these are the *BRCA1* and *BRCA2* gene mutations. Women who carry the BRCA1 mutation have, on average, a 55% to 65% lifetime risk of breast cancer (range is 55–85%). For BRCA2 mutations the risk is about 45%.

Exposure to ionizing radiation of the chest at a young age (such as used in the treatment of Hodgkin lymphoma), menarche before age 12, menopause after age 55, and consuming 2-5 alcoholic drinks per day all increase the risk of breast cancer. Diagnosis of atypical ductal (ADH) or lobular hyperplasia (ALH) increases risk by a factor of 5. The presence of ductal or lobular carcinoma in situ (LCIS) or noninvasive carcinomas also increases cancer risk.

Importantly, between 0.5% and 4.0% of breast cancer diagnoses are made around **pregnancy or lactation**. Compared to nonpregnant women with breast cancer at a similar stage and age, **survival rates seem equivalent for pregnant or lactating women** with breast cancer. Younger age at menarche, nulliparity, later date of first live birth, and later age at menopause have all been linked with increased risk of breast cancer. This is believed to be due to cumulative **lifetime estrogen exposure**.

The question of whether or not **menopausal hormone therapy (MHT)** changes the risk of breast cancer has been hotly debated. It is now generally believed that patients who use combination MHT for more than 5 years are at a slightly **increased risk** of developing invasive breast cancer. This risk may also be increased in women using estrogen-only hormone therapy (ET for more than 10 years.). Use of oral contraceptives slightly increases the risk of breast cancer but the risk goes back to normal within 10 years of stopping the pills. The use of caffeine, breast implants, electric blankets, bras, and antiperspirants has not been found to increase breast cancer risk.

Prevention
Early pregnancy, prolonged lactation, chemical or surgical sterilization, exercise, abstinence from alcohol, and a low-fat diet may help prevent breast cancer. The studies linking phytoestrogens to a reduction of breast cancer risk have been inconclusive. Phytoestrogens are naturally occurring plant substances similar to estradiol. They are composed primarily of isoflavones and are found in soybeans—a major component of tofu. Similarly, no protective effect has been proven with the use of aspirin and other NSAIDs.

Tamoxifen, a SERM, is effective in suppressing the development of breast cancer. By binding to the estrogen receptor (ER), tamoxifen acts as a **competitive inhibitor to estrogen** thereby blocking stimulation of breast cancer cells. Tamoxifen is used as adjuvant therapy in patients with early stage, surgically treated, ER-positive breast cancer, and it has been shown to

TABLE 32-4. Breast Cancer Risk Factors

Risk Factors	Category at Risk	Comparison Category	Relative Risk
Alcohol intake	Two drinks per day	Nondrinker	1.2
Body mass index	80th percentile, age 55 or greater	20th percentile	1.2
HRT with estrogen and progesterone	Current user for at least 5 y	Never used	1.3
Radiation exposure	Repeated fluoroscopy	No exposure	1.6
	Radiation therapy for Hodgkin disease	No exposure	5.2
Early menarche	Younger than 12 y	Older than 15 y	1.3
Late menopause	Older than 55 y	Younger than 45	1.2–1.5
Age at first childbirth	Nulliparous or first child after 30	First child before 20	1.7–1.9
Current age	65 or older	<65	5.8
Past history of breast cancer	Invasive breast carcinoma	No history of invasive breast carcinoma	6.8
Other histologic findings	LCIS	No abnormality detected	16.4
	DCIS	No abnormality detected	17.3
Breast biopsy	Hyperplasia without atypia[a]	No hyperplasia	1.9
	Hyperplasia with atypia	No hyperplasia	5.3
	Hyperplasia with atypia and positive family history	No hyperplasia, negative family history	11
Cytology (FNA, nipple aspiration fluid)	Proliferation without atypia[a]	No abnormality detected	2.5
	Proliferation with atypia	No abnormality detected	4.9–5
	Proliferation with atypia and positive family history	No abnormality detected	18.1
Family history	First-degree relative 50 y or older with postmenopausal breast cancer	No first- or second-degree relative with breast cancer	1.8
	First-degree relative with premenopausal breast cancer	No first- or second-degree relative with breast cancer	3.3
	Second-degree relative with breast cancer	No first- or second-degree relative with breast cancer	1.5
	Two first-degree relatives with breast cancer	No first- or second-degree relative with breast cancer	3.6
Germline mutation	Heterozygous for BRCA1, age <40	Not heterozygous for BRCA1, age <40	200[b]
	Heterozygous for BRCA1, age 60–69	Not heterozygous for BRCA1, age 60–69	15[b]

[a]There is controversy over whether pathologic hyperplasia detected in breast biopsy samples is directly equivalent to cytologic hyperplasia detected in samples obtained through FNA or nipple aspiration.
[b]Begg has suggested that these relative risks are subject to ascertainment bias and may overestimate the true risk associated with germline mutations in BRCA genes.

decrease the rate of recurrent breast cancer by 40% and breast cancer mortality by 35%.

Diagnosis

The trifecta of routine breast care is **breast self-awareness**, the annual **clinician breast examination**, and annual **mammography** for women aged 40 and over or those who are at high risk for breast cancer. Thirty percent to 50% of breast cancers are diagnosed as a result of an abnormality detected via mammography.

Patients may present clinically with **breast masses**, **skin change**, **nipple discharge**, or symptoms of metastatic disease. **Skin dimpling** can occur due to the tethering of Cooper ligaments from the mass underneath. The skin can appear erythematous and warm, and the **nipples may be retracted** or inverted. Tissue edema, or a **peau d'orange appearance**, may occur due to dermal lymphatic invasion and blockage. The superficial epidermis of the nipple may appear eczematous or ulcerated, as in Paget disease.

Bloody nipple discharge should be evaluated to rule out invasive papillary carcinoma, although the most common cause is benign intraductal papilloma. Palpable masses are often detected by the patient or the partner on self-examination and are frequently nontender, irregular, firm, and immobile. **Fifty percent of tumors occur in the UOQ** (Fig. 32-7). These tumors can be multifocal, multicentric, or bilateral. Mammography is the best tool for early detection, which reduces mortality by 32% to 50%. Recent studies have shown that mammography is less effective in women with dense breast tissue—for example African American women or younger women. Furthermore, up to **20% of new breast cancers are not detectable on mammography**, so any suspicious lesion should be biopsied if clinically indicated, even if the mammogram is normal.

A nonpalpable suspicious lesion found on mammogram requires **localized needle biopsy** or **stereotactic FNA** for pathologic diagnosis.

The evaluation for metastatic disease via thorough history, physical, and diagnostic imaging is also an important part of breast disease management. Breast cancer tends to metastasize to the **bone, liver, lung, pleura, brain,** and **lymph nodes**. Patients may present with constitutional symptoms of weight loss, anorexia, night sweats, and fatigue. They may also have dyspnea, cough, and/or bone pain.

NONINVASIVE DISEASE

Lobular Carcinoma In Situ

Pathogenesis

LCIS, also called lobar neoplasia, is the proliferation of **malignant epithelial cells** contained within the breast lobules (milk producing glands) with no invasion through the walls of the lobules (Fig. 32-8). It is usually multicentric and is bilateral 50% to 90% of the time. It is considered by some to be a premalignant lesion and not a true cancer. However, most agree that LCIS is **an important indicator for subsequent risk of invasive breast cancer** (25% to 30% within 15 years) in one or both breasts.

Epidemiology

The average age at diagnosis is the mid-40s. Patients are typically premenopausal.

Diagnosis

LCIS is usually diagnosed incidentally on biopsy for another finding because it **is not palpable** and often **not visible on mammograms**.

Treatment

The optimal treatment for LCIS is controversial since it doesn't seem to become an invasive cancer even if left untreated. Before deciding on treatment, however, invasive cancer and ductal carcinoma in situ (DCIS) must be ruled out. Once invasive cancers and DCIS are ruled out, there are three options: close **observation without further therapy**, prophylactic chemoprevention with **SERMs** (such as tamoxifen or raloxifene), or bilateral simple mastectomy because LCIS is linked to increased cancer risk in both breasts. SERMs may reduce the risk of subsequent cancer by 50%. Increased cancer risks linked to LCIS include intraductal, invasive ductal, and lobular carcinoma. The subsequent cancer may be in the ipsilateral or contralateral breast.

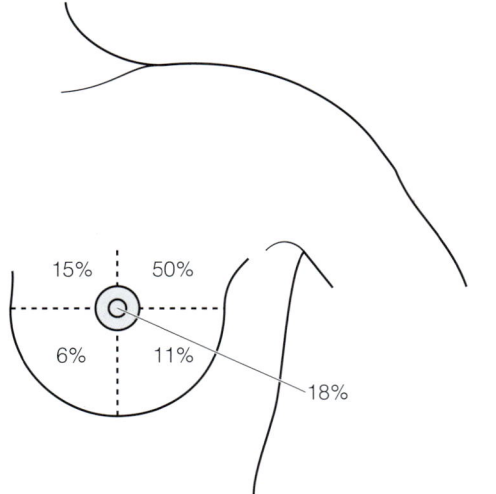

FIGURE 32-7. Most common locations of malignant lesions.

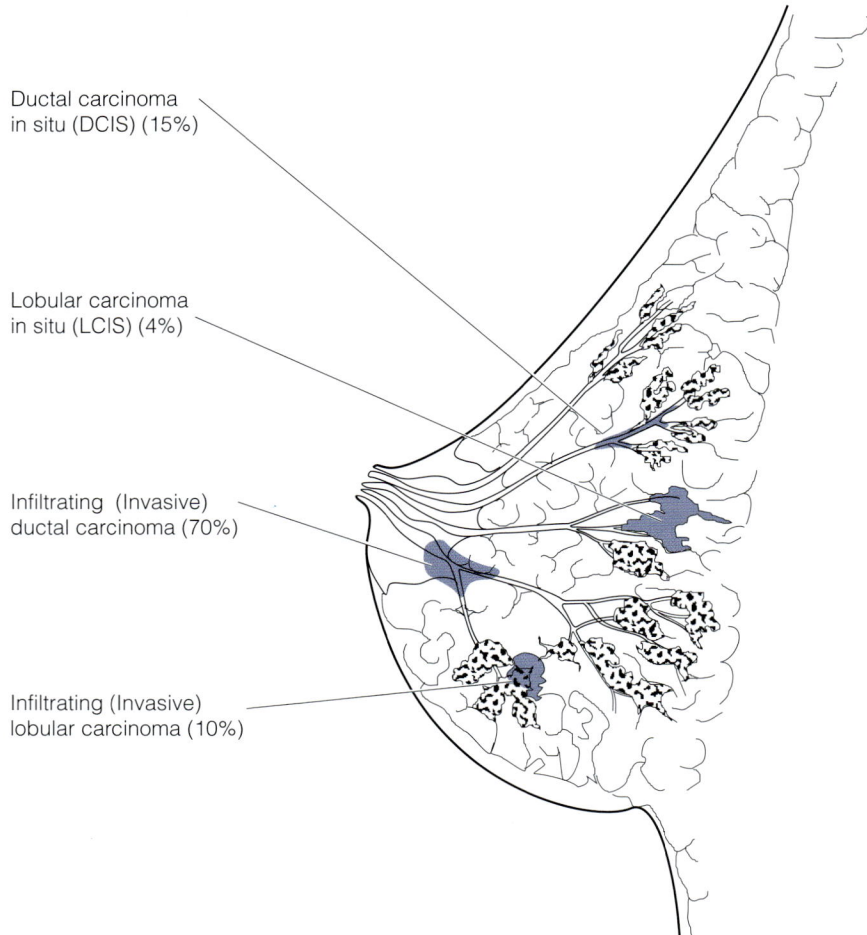

FIGURE 32-8. Subtypes of breast cancer. DCIS is believed to be a precursor to invasive ductal carcinoma; LCIS is, in contrast, more akin to atypical hyperplasia and carries a risk of future ductal or invasive lobular carcinoma anywhere in the breast. Invasive ductal carcinoma is the most common type of breast cancer in women.

Ductal Carcinoma In Situ
Pathogenesis
DCIS—also called intraductal carcinoma—involves proliferation of **malignant epithelial cells** in mammary ducts without spread to the breast stroma (Fig. 32-8). It is more common than LCIS and, if left untreated, has a **higher potential for progression to invasive carcinoma** than LCIS.

Epidemiology
Average age at diagnosis is mid-50s.

Diagnosis
Ninety percent of DCIS is detected by **screening mammography** revealing **clustered microcalcifications**. Ten percent present with a **palpable mass**. Diagnosis can be established by needle localization biopsy or excisional biopsy of a palpable lesion. Thirty-five percent of lesions are multicentric; bilateral disease is rare.

Treatment
Current treatment involves conservative surgical **excision of all microcalcifications with wide margins**. Simple **mastectomy** is occasionally necessary for extensive lesions, but this is considered overly aggressive for the treatment of all women with DCIS. If resection margins are inadequate (<10 mm), **radiation therapy** may be used to reduce the risk of local recurrence without an impact on survival. The risk of subsequent invasive ductal carcinoma or local recurrence of intraductal carcinoma is approximately 5% per year. Of recurrent disease, 50% will be DCIS; the other 50% will be invasive carcinoma.

INVASIVE BREAST CANCERS
Infiltrating Ductal Carcinoma
This is the **most common breast malignancy**, accounting for **76% of all invasive breast cancers**. The tumor arises from the ductal epithelium and

infiltrates the supporting stroma (Fig. 32-8). Less frequent but more favorable subtypes include medullary carcinoma, colloid carcinoma, tubular carcinoma, and papillary carcinoma.

Invasive Lobular Carcinoma
Lobular carcinoma arises from the lobular epithelium and infiltrates the breast stroma (Fig. 32-8). It accounts for 8% of all invasive breast cancers and tends to be bilateral.

Paget Disease of the Nipple
Paget disease accounts for 1% to 3% of all breast malignancies. It is often concomitant with DCIS or invasive carcinoma in the **subareolar area**. The malignant cells enter the **epidermis of the nipple**, causing the classic eczematous changes in the nipple. Examination reveals crusting, scaling, erosion, discharge, and possibly a breast mass.

Inflammatory Breast Carcinoma
This is an **extremely aggressive** malignancy, accounting for 0.5% to 2% of all breast cancers in the United States. It is a poorly differentiated tumor characterized by **dermal lymphatic invasion**. Symptoms include edema, erythema, warmth, and diffuse induration of the skin described as **peau d'orange**. It is usually accompanied by axillary lymphadenopathy and has distant metastases on presentation 17% to 36% of the time.

Strategies for the Treatment of Invasive Breast Cancer
Primary Surgical Treatment
Surgical resection is required in all patients with invasive breast cancer. Historically, radical mastectomy was standard of care; however, currently most patients undergo **breast-conserving therapy** (BCT) (lumpectomy with radiation), or **modified radical mastectomy** with or without reconstruction at the time of surgery.

BCT with **lumpectomy and radiation therapy results in identical survival rates as modified radical mastectomy** in appropriately selected patients. The type of primary treatment depends on the **size and histology** of the cancer as well as the preoperative presence of **palpable lymph nodes**. Large tumors (>5 cm) and those that have spread to the lymph nodes tend to recur more often, so BCT is not recommended. Patients with large tumors benefit from mastectomy coupled with postoperative radiation therapy. Even with these exceptions, **60% to 75% of women will be candidates for BCT** with lumpectomy and radiation.

Breast Reconstruction
Breast reconstruction carries significant **psychosocial benefits** for women with breast cancer. Reconstruction can be achieved with **implants or autogenous tissue** (Fig. 32-9). The need for reconstruction is determined by the type of primary surgery. Notably, BCT does not typically require reconstruction unless a large mass is removed from a small breast. Also, reconstruction can be performed **at the time of initial surgery or deferred** until later without any adverse oncologic impact. In either case, the reconstructive surgeon should be consulted before the initial surgery.

Axillary Lymph Node Evaluation
As **axillary node status** is one of the **most important outcome predictors** of breast cancer, they must always be closely evaluated. In the past, this has been accomplished using full **axillary lymph node dissection** (ALND). ALND has been proven to increase

FIGURE 32-9. Postmastectomy breast reconstruction. (From Georgiade NG, Reifkohl R, Levine LS. *Georgiade Plastic, Maxillofacial and Reconstructive Surgery*, 3rd ed. Baltimore, MD: Lippincott Williams & Wilkins; 1997.)

survival, decrease recurrence, and provide valuable prognostic information. However, it can also result in significant arm morbidity, including edema, seroma formation, loss of sensation, and shoulder dysfunction. As a result, many centers now utilize **sentinel lymph node biopsy** (SLNB) as an alternative to ALND. This less morbid procedure involves intradermal injection of dye or radioactive colloid around the primary tumor prior to surgery to identify the sentinel lymph nodes. These lymph nodes are either sampled prior to the surgical resection of the cancer or sent for frozen section at the time of surgery. If the sentinel nodes are negative for cancer, there is a very low likelihood that the remaining nodes are positive, so the patient can be spared full ALND. If these nodes return positive; however, ALND must be performed.

Radiation Therapy

Due to the risk of recurrence, radiation therapy is necessary for **all patients who undergo conservative therapy**. Radiation therapy has also been indicated for patients who undergo modified radical mastectomy if they are at a **high risk for recurrence**. Factors that indicate a high risk of recurrence include lymph node or blood vessel invasion, a large primary tumor, positive resection margins, and grossly evident extracapsular nodal resection. Some authorities advocate the use of radiation therapy for all patients regardless of node status. The field of radiation therapy should encompass the chest wall, supraclavicular, and infraclavicular regions.

Tumor Receptor Status

The **hormone receptor status** of a tumor has significant implications for **prognosis and treatment** options. To ascertain the status, special assays are run to look for estrogen receptors (ER), progesterone receptors (PR), S-phase analysis (measure of cell growth), and HER2/neu status in the excised tumor. In general, **estrogen and progesterone receptor-positive** (ER1 and PR1) tumors are well differentiated and exhibit a less aggressive clinical behavior, including lower recurrence rates and lower capacity to proliferate. Estrogen and progesterone-positive status, therefore, carries a **more favorable prognosis** than negative hormone receptor status. In addition to estrogen and progesterone receptor status, **HER2/neu status** has become an important assessment for treatment options. Overexpression of HER2/neu indicates more **aggressive tumors**.

Systemic Adjuvant Chemotherapy

Systemic adjuvant therapy with hormonal therapy, chemotherapy, or both may also be indicated based on lymph node status, tumor size, tumor grade, menopausal status, and tumor receptor status (ER, PR, and HER2). Adjuvant chemotherapy significantly **decreases risk of recurrence** and **morbidity**.

Women with **positive lymph node status** are twice as likely to have metastases to other parts of the body, so chemotherapy is indicated. Women with **negative lymph node status but at higher risk** (tumor size >1 cm, high tumor grade) should also undergo chemotherapy with the goal of controlling micrometastases. Various chemotherapy regimens are currently in use. A typical regimen might include a combination of cyclophosphamide (C), methotrexate (M), and 5-fluorouracil (F).

Systemic Adjuvant Hormone Therapy

Systemic hormonal therapy with or without chemotherapy is also utilized for patients with receptor-positive cancers (ER1 and PR1) regardless of the patient's age or menopausal status. **Tamoxifen** is available for women with positive ER and/or PR status. This antiestrogen stops estrogen from stimulating the growth of the cancer cells by competitively binding ERs in mammary tissue. Tamoxifen does, however, have some estrogen agonist activity in other tissues such as the endometrium and bone. It is generally used for 5 years after the primary surgical treatment, and it is currently the first-line postsurgical treatment for premenopausal breast cancer patients and second-line therapy for postmenopausal patients (after aromatase inhibitors). **Fulvestrant** is a new ER antagonist that has no agonist effects. It has been approved by the FDA for use in postmenopausal women with hormone receptor-positive breast cancer and metastases. It also has positive treatment effects on HER2-positive breast cancer.

Aromatase inhibitors such as letrozole, anastrozole, and exemestane are also available for postmenopausal women with receptor-positive cancers. These newer agents have **antiestrogenic** properties and have been shown to have a longer disease-free survival when compared with tamoxifen.

HER2/neu status is another prognostic factor for more aggressive tumors, and monoclonal antibodies such as trastuzumab are used for adjuvant treatment. Trastuzumab works by binding to the HER2/neu receptor and preventing proliferation.

Treatment of Metastatic or Recurrent Disease

ER-negative patients with metastatic or recurrent disease are best treated with combination chemotherapy that may include doxorubicin (Adriamycin [A]) and vincristine (V), in addition to CMF. There is a 75% response to chemotherapy, but this is only temporary

(6 to 8 months) with the average additional survival being 1.5 to 2 years from the time of recurrence.

ER-positive patients with metastatic or recurrent disease benefit most from hormonal therapy rather than chemotherapy. Premenopausal women may be treated with oophorectomy or gonadotropin-releasing hormone (GnRH) antagonists, whereas postmenopausal women are treated with tamoxifen or aromatase inhibitors.

The choice to continue or reenter treatment should balance the impact on survival with the effects on quality of life.

Prognosis

The most reliable predictor for survival is the **stage of breast cancer at the time of diagnosis** (Table 32-5). Staging is determined by the **size** of the primary tumor and the absence or presence of regional **lymph node** involvement and/or distant **metastases**. Other prognostic indicators include lymph node status, hormone receptor status, tumor size, nuclear grade, histologic type, proliferative rate, and oncogene expression. The current overall 5-year survival rate for Stage 0 and stage I breast cancer is near 100%. The 5-year disease-free survival rate is 93% for Stage II, 72% for Stage III, and 22% for Stage IV disease. **Positive estrogen and progesterone receptor status carries a more favorable prognosis as does negative lymph node status.** HER2-positive status carries a less favorable prognosis.

Follow-Up

Follow-up after breast cancer treatment should include a **physical examination** every 3 to 6 months for 3 years, every 6 to 12 months for years 4 and 5, and annually thereafter. In women who received breast-conserving surgery, a **mammogram** is performed 6 months after the completion of lumpectomy and radiation treatment, then annually. Women who had a mastectomy should continue to have **yearly mammograms** on the remaining breast.

Routine CBC, blood chemistries, tumor markers, chest X-ray, CT, and bone scans are not recommended for routine breast cancer follow-up or for asymptomatic patients. These tests have been replaced with **clinical monitoring for metastatic disease** (dry cough, exertional dyspnea, bone and body pains, pleuritic chest pain, etc.). Women taking **tamoxifen** should be followed for irregular bleeding given the possibility of increased endometrial cancer risk with its use. Endometrial biopsy should be performed for abnormal uterine bleeding in these women.

Hormone Use After Breast Cancer Treatment

Some premenopausal patients may wish to become pregnant after breast cancer treatment. Traditionally, this has been discouraged for fear that pregnancy-related estrogens may stimulate dormant cancer cells. Studies now suggest that **there is no difference in survival rates in women who become pregnant after breast cancer treatment**. For women who wish to avoid fertility after cancer treatment, permanent birth control should be considered if childbearing is complete. Highly effective, long-activing reversible contraception is best provided by the copper-containing IUD in women with hormonally mediated breast cancer. A levonorgestrel-containing IUD should be considered first line in women with non-hormonally mediated breast cancer and those taking tamoxifen.

The use of menopausal hormone therapy (MHT) in breast cancer survivors has been widely debated. The median age of diagnosis of breast cancer in the United States is 62, and the majority of breast cancer patients are menopausal. This combined with the often induced menopausal state based on surgical or medical breast cancer treatment means that menopausal symptom management for this population is extremely important. Several well-constructed and long-term studies, such as the Women's Health Initiative, have identified an increased risk of breast cancer in women utilizing combination HRT. For this reason, **MHT use is not recommended in women with a personal history of breast cancer**.

For hormone receptor-positive breast cancer patients with **vasomotor symptoms**, first-line treatment options include the use of nonhormonal medications such as venlafaxine (Effexor), clonidine, and gabapentin. Paroxetine (Paxil) has been found to lower the protective effect of tamoxifen and should not be used in these patients. Lifestyle changes such as the use of fans, cotton clothing, dressing in layers, and acupuncture should also be used to manage hot flashes and night sweats.

Another common concern of breast cancer survivors is naturally occurring or treatment-induced symptomatic vaginal dryness and painful intercourse. This can be uncomfortable and can significantly affect sexual function and satisfaction. This natural occurrence can be exacerbated by the use of aromatase inhibitors and tamoxifen. Traditionally, topical estrogens have been used for vaginal atrophy and dryness; however, there has been concern for use of these medications in women with hormonally-mediated breast cancer. Vaginal lubricants and moisturizers should be the first line of therapy in these women. The American College of Obstetricians and Gynecologists (ACOG) now supports the use of vaginal estrogen in women with a history of estrogen-dependent breast cancer.

TABLE 32-5. TNM Staging of Breast Cancer

Cancer Stages	Primary Tumor Size	Lymph Node Involvement	Distant Metastases
0	T_{is}	N_0	M_0
I	T_1	N_0	M_0
IIa	T_0	N_1	M_0
	T_1	N_1	M_0
	T_2	N_0	M_0
IIb	T_2	N_1	M_0
	T_3	N_0	M_0
IIIa	T_0	N_2	M_0
	T_1	N_2	M_0
	T_2	N_2	M_0
	T_3	N_1	M_0
	T_3	N_2	M_0
IIIb	T_4	Any N	M_0
	Any T	N_3	M_0
IV	Any T	Any N	M_1

Key: TNM classification

T	Primary tumor
T_x	Primary tumor unassessable
T_0	No evidence of primary tumor
T_{is}	Carcinoma in situ; intraductal carcinoma, LCIS, or Paget disease of the nipple with no tumor
T_1	Tumor ≤2 cm in largest dimension

Key: TNM classification

T_{1c}	Tumor <2 cm but >1 cm
T_2	Tumor ≤5 cm but >2 cm in greatest dimension
T_3	Tumor >5 cm in greatest dimension
T_4	Tumor any size extending to chest wall or skin
N	Regional lymph nodes
N_x	Regional lymph nodes cannot be assessed
N_0	No regional lymph node metastases
N_1	Metastasis to mobile ipsilateral axillary lymph node(s)
N_2	Metastasis to the ipsilateral axillary lymph node, fixed and/or internal mammary nodes
N_3	Metastasis to ipsilateral infraclavicular and/or supraclavicular lymph node(s)
M	Distant metastasis
M_x	Presence of distant metastasis cannot be assessed
M_0	No clinical or radiographic evidence of distant metastasis
M_1	Distant metastasis, determined by clinical or radiographic means

LCIS, lobular carcinoma in situ.
Adapted from American Joint Committee on Cancer. *Manual for Staging of Cancer,* 7th ed. (2010).
Modified from American College of Obstetricians and Gynecologists. Diagnosis and management of benign breast disorders (Practice Bulletin No. 164). *Obstet Gynecol* 2016;127:e141–156, from the original source: Sickles EA, D'Orsi CJ, Bassett LW. ACR BI-RADS® mammography. In: *ACR BI-RADS® atlas, Breast Imaging Reporting and Data System.* Reston, VA: American College of Radiology; 2013.

KEY POINTS

- Breast cancer is the most common noncutaneous neoplasm in women, with a lifetime risk of 1 in 8 for women in the United States.
- Clinical breast examination every 1 to 3 years is recommended for all women over age 20. Greater emphasis is placed on overall breast self-awareness.
- Current routine mammogram recommendations include a mammogram annually beginning at age 40. No upper age limit has been identified.
- Women with a strong family history of breast cancer should begin screening mammograms 5 years earlier than the age of diagnosis of the youngest family member with breast cancer; 10 years earlier in the case of premenopausal breast cancer.
- Evaluation of breast masses includes careful physical examination, evaluation with mammography and ultrasound of any abnormal findings, and biopsy of suspicious findings to rule out malignancy.
- Benign breast symptoms and findings are common and occur in approximately 50% of women. The incidence is higher in younger women.
- Two-thirds of breast tumors in reproductive-age women are benign, whereas half of palpable masses in perimenopausal women, and the majority of lesions in postmenopausal women are malignant.
- The most common benign breast conditions are breast cysts and fibroadenomas.
- Patients with fibrocystic change often have cyclic breast pain and masses due to an exaggerated stromal response to hormones and growth factors. Reduction in caffeine, tea, and chocolate, and treatment with vitamins E and B$_6$, progestins, danazol, and tamoxifen have been found to help symptoms.
- Fibroadenomas are benign rubbery breast tumors that are usually solitary. They can be followed with expectant management. When large, they should be biopsied to rule out cystosarcoma phyllodes.
- Benign intraductal papilloma is the most common cause of bloody nipple discharge.
- Numerous risk factors have been identified for breast cancer (increasing age, family history, high-fat diet, ionizing radiation, early menarche, late childbearing, atypical hyperplasia, and prolonged MHT use); however, most patients have no known risk factors.
- Only 5% to 10% of breast cancer is related to genetic predisposition.
- DCIS (15%) is a preinvasive disease and is treated with lumpectomy and radiation therapy. LCIS (4%) is treated with observation and possible use of tamoxifen to prevent subsequent invasive breast cancer.
- Invasive breast disease—including infiltrating ductal carcinoma (76%) and infiltrating lobular carcinoma (8%)—is treated with lumpectomy and radiation or with modified mastectomy with equal risk of recurrence and survival in properly selected patients.
- Breast reconstruction can be an important part of recovering from breast cancer. It can be done during the primary surgery or delayed until later.
- All women with invasive breast disease should have ipsilateral lymph node evaluation with ALND or sentinel node dissection. The resected tumors should also be checked for hormone receptor status and HER2 status.
- The standard adjuvant treatment for women with positive lymph nodes is combination chemotherapy.
- All hormone receptor-positive patients should receive hormone therapy aimed at suppressing estrogen, and thereby suppressing stimulation of cancer cells. This is most commonly achieved with tamoxifen (an estrogen agonist/antagonist) or aromatase inhibitors (e.g., letrozole and anastrozole), which have antiestrogen activity.
- Follow-up for patients with invasive breast cancer includes annual bilateral mammography in women who underwent lumpectomy and radiation, or annual mammography of the contralateral breast in women who underwent mastectomy.
- Frequent physical examination to evaluate for recurrent metastatic disease is also indicated. Other routine blood and imaging studies are not indicated in the asymptomatic patient.
- The use of MHT should be avoided in breast cancer survivors.

CLINICAL VIGNETTES

VIGNETTE 1

A concerned 38-year-old female G0 presents to your office for her annual gynecologic examination. She has just moved to your area, and this is the first time you have seen her. During her history, she reports regular, painful, monthly menses with moderate flow since menarche at 11. Her mother was diagnosed with breast cancer at age 48, and her paternal aunt was diagnosed with breast cancer at age 67. She has no other family history for cancer. She frequently notices pain in both breasts, and she has a clear discharge from both nipples around the time of her menses. Her previous gynecologist diagnosed her with fibrocystic breast change, and this worries her. Her breast examination shows Tanner Stage 5 breasts that are symmetric and without palpable mass or abnormal skin changes. Upon palpation of the nipples of both breasts, a clear discharge is noted.

1. Which element of her history and examination is most associated with an increased risk of breast cancer over the general population?
   a. Mother with breast cancer at age 48
   b. Paternal aunt with breast cancer at age 67
   c. Menarche at age 11
   d. Fibrocystic change
   e. Nipple discharge

2. Which element of her history and examination is most associated with a low risk of breast cancer?
   a. Age
   b. Gravidity and parity
   c. Regular menses
   d. Normal breast examination
   e. Paternal aunt with breast cancer at age 67

3. What is the most appropriate evaluation of the nipple discharge?
   a. Express the discharge and send for culture
   b. Express the discharge, perform guaiac, and send for cytology
   c. Start breast ultrasound
   d. Fine-needle aspiration (FNA)
   e. Expectant management

VIGNETTE 2

A 42-year-old nonpregnant G4P3 female presents to your office with complaint of a new palpable breast mass that she noticed while performing her breast self-examination. After taking her history, you perform a clinical breast examination that reveals a solitary, 3-cm, mobile, nonpainful, rubbery mass, no nipple or skin changes, and no noted nipple discharge with attempted expression.

1. On the basis of her clinical examination, what is most likely her diagnosis?
   a. Fibrocystic breast change
   b. Fibroadenoma
   c. Cystosarcoma phyllodes
   d. Intraductal papilloma
   e. Invasive breast cancer

2. She undergoes the recommended diagnostic tests for a palpable breast mass in her age group. On the biopsy specimen, the pathologist finds epithelial and stromal proliferation consistent with a fibroadenoma; however, she notes few scattered malignant cells. On further discussion, the patient reports that this mass was smaller a few months ago. Her diagnosis is now most consistent with:
   a. Invasive breast cancer
   b. Fibroadenoma
   c. Cystosarcoma phyllodes
   d. Trauma
   e. Intraductal papilloma

3. She returns to your office to discuss the treatment plan. The most appropriate management of her diagnosis is:
   a. Expectant management with serial imaging
   b. Lumpectomy with radiation
   c. Wide local excision with 1-cm margins
   d. Modified radical mastectomy
   e. Bilateral modified radical mastectomy

VIGNETTE 3

A 35-year-old G0 woman presents to your office with complaints of bloody nipple discharge from the left breast. She is most distraught. Her mother was diagnosed with breast cancer at age 45. When asked about breast self-examination, she denies feeling a mass at home but states she is also not very consistent in examining herself. You perform a breast examination, collect some of the discharge, perform a guaiac test, and then send it for cytology.

1. The most likely diagnosis associated with her nipple discharge is:
   a. Physiologic discharge
   b. Fibroadenoma
   c. Cystosarcoma phyllodes
   d. Intraductal papilloma
   e. Invasive papillary carcinoma

2. The cytology shows malignant cells, and you can palpate a breast mass just lateral to the nipple. She is sent for diagnostic imaging. On mammogram, a spiculated mass is identified. Now her most likely diagnosis is:
   a. Fibrocystic breast change
   b. Fibroadenoma
   c. Cystosarcoma phyllodes
   d. Intraductal papilloma
   e. Invasive papillary carcinoma

3. You refer her to a specialist for treatment; however, she is most comfortable talking with you about her concerns. She strongly desires to start her family soon, so what is the most appropriate counseling for this patient?
   a. Breast cancer patients should never become pregnant in the future because of the increased risk of recurrence with a pregnancy
   b. There is no difference in survival among premenopausal patients who become pregnant after treatment and those who do not
   c. If her tumor is ER positive only, she is at increased risk of recurrence if she becomes pregnant
   d. If her tumor is PR positive only, she is at increased risk of recurrence if she becomes pregnant
   e. If her tumor is estrogen *and* progesterone receptor positive, she is at increased risk of recurrence if she becomes pregnant

VIGNETTE 4

A 59-year-old female G4P4 with a history of normal breast imaging in the past presents to her OB/GYN for her annual examination. On her examination, there are no palpable masses, lymphadenopathy, skin changes, nor any nipple changes or discharge. She goes for her routine screening mammogram, and this year the radiologist gives her a score of BI-RADS 4 (suspicious of malignancy). She then undergoes stereotactic FNA for biopsy. The result is infiltrating ductal carcinoma. The tumor is ER1, PR1, and HER2/neu neg. The tumor is less than 4 cm in size.

1. The most appropriate treatment plan for her is:
   a. Bilateral radical mastectomy with full ALND followed by radiation therapy
   b. Wide local excision with periodic surveillance with breast examination and annual mammogram
   c. Modified radical mastectomy with ALND, followed by trastuzumab
   d. BCT with lumpectomy, SLNB, and tamoxifen for 5 years
   e. BCT with lumpectomy, SLNB, breast reconstruction, followed by radiation and letrozole

2. During surgery, the tumor was found to be 4 cm in size, with negative sentinel node biopsy and negative margins after excision. After she undergoes her treatment, she wants to discuss her prognosis with you. The most appropriate counseling regarding her prognosis is:
   a. The current overall 5-year survival rate is 90%; however, the most reliable predictor of survival is the stage of breast cancer at the time of diagnosis
   b. Her tumor's estrogen and progesterone receptor status (both positive) is a marker of poor prognosis and decreased survival
   c. Her tumor's HER2/neu receptor status (negative) is a marker of poor prognosis and decreased survival
   d. Tumor size is not a predictor of prognosis
   e. Because she received radiation anyway, her lymph node status is not a predictor of survival

3. She has completed her treatment and is curious how to follow-up with her doctor. She does not want to miss a recurrence. The most appropriate recommendations for follow-up are:
   a. Physical examination yearly with annual mammogram
   b. Physical examination monthly for 1 year, mammogram every 3 months for 1 year, then annually thereafter for both
   c. Physical examination every 3 to 6 months for 3 years then annually, annual mammogram, tumor markers, and CT scan
   d. Physical examination every 3 to 6 months for 3 years, then every 6 to 12 months for years 4 and 5, with annual mammogram (beginning 6 months after radiation)
   e. Physical examination every year, with CBC, chest X-ray, and tumor markers every 6 months, and annual mammogram

4. Two years later during a routine visit, she shyly mentions that she is suffering from hot flushes and vaginal dryness. These symptoms have disrupted her routine activities and her relationship. She now reports often feeling depressed and tearful. She has been compliant with her routine breast cancer follow-up, and there is no evidence of any new lesions. What is the most appropriate counseling for this patient?
   a. Discuss that mood changes, hot flashes, and depressions symptoms are not disruptive or unsafe, and they take time to improve
   b. Discuss options for initiating antidepressant and vaginal lubrications
   c. Discuss options for initiating HRT for symptom management
   d. Discuss cessation of breast cancer treatments as it has been two years
   e. Discuss that she should increase the soy products in her diet

ANSWERS

VIGNETTE 1 Question 1
1. Answer A:
The risk for breast cancer with a first-degree relative (mother, sister, or daughter) diagnosed before menopause is 1.8–8.8 to 1 (depending on unilaterality or bilaterality of the disease). This risk with having a second-degree relative diagnosed with breast cancer is 1.5 to 1. Early menarche (before age 12) carries a risk of 1.3 to 1. Fibrocystic change is not associated with an increased risk of breast cancer. Only 5% of patients presenting with nipple discharge will have a malignancy, and this is more likely with unilateral or bloody discharge.

VIGNETTE 1 Question 2
2. Answer A:
The median age of breast cancer diagnosis is 62 years, and four of every five women with breast cancer are over age 50; thus, this patient's young age is her most protective quality. Nulliparity is associated with a 3:1 risk of breast cancer compared to parous women. Regular menses, though theoretically protective due to a constant monthly control of estrogen exposure, are not as protective as young age. A normal breast examination is a reassuring clinical sign, but 30% to 50% of breast abnormalities are diagnosed by mammography because a lesion is not palpable. Having a second-degree relative with breast cancer is a risk factor and is not protective against breast cancer.

VIGNETTE 1 Question 3
3. Answer E:
With a normal examination and bilateral clear nipple discharge with expression only, expectant management and reassurance are appropriate. Bloody nipple discharge should be evaluated by testing with a guaiac card and sent for cytology. This helps rule out a bloody component. The most common cause of bloody nipple discharge is benign intraductal papilloma; however, the differential includes potential underlying malignancy. Culture, especially without a foul odor or sign of infection, is not necessary in this case. Ultrasound, mammography, and biopsy are reserved for the evaluation of breast masses.

VIGNETTE 2 Question 1
1. Answer B:
A solitary, mobile, nonpainful, rubbery mass is most likely a fibroadenoma. Fibrocystic breast change is typically multiple, painful, bilateral, and fluctuates throughout the menstrual cycle. Cystosarcoma phyllodes is a rare variant of fibroadenoma that is usually associated with overlying skin changes. Intraductal papilloma usually presents as bloody nipple discharge in the absence of a mass. Invasive breast cancer is not usually mobile and rubbery, but is a firm, fixed mass.

VIGNETTE 2 Question 2
2. Answer C:
Cystosarcoma phyllodes is a rare variant of fibroadenoma that grows quickly and is considered a low-grade malignancy due to a small proportion of malignant cells found on biopsy. Fibrocystic breast change, fibroadenoma, and trauma are not associated with malignant cells. Intraductal papilloma does not present as a mass. Invasive breast cancer would be constituted almost completely of malignant cells.

VIGNETTE 2 Question 3
3. Answer C:
The most appropriate treatment of cystosarcoma phyllodes is wide local excision with 1-cm margins or simple mastectomy. Because it is considered a low-grade malignancy, expectant management is contraindicated. One-centimeter margins are necessary because of the high rate of local recurrence after simple excision. Lumpectomy with radiation and modified radical mastectomy are reserved for treatment of invasive breast cancers.

VIGNETTE 3 Question 1
1. Answer D:
Intraductal papilloma is the most common cause of bloody nipple discharge. The second most common cause is invasive (papillary) breast cancer. Fibrocystic breast change, fibroadenoma, and cystosarcoma phyllodes typically present as painful and nonpainful breast masses. Physiologic discharge is not bloody in appearance.

VIGNETTE 3 Question 2
2. Answer E:
Invasive papillary carcinoma is the second most common cause of bloody nipple discharge, and it is a malignancy (unlike intraductal papilloma). Fibrocystic breast change and fibroadenoma are not malignant. Cystosarcoma phyllodes is not associated with bloody nipple discharge.

VIGNETTE 3 Question 3
3. Answer B:
Studies have shown that there is no difference in survival rates in women who become pregnant after successful breast cancer treatment, regardless of

tumor type or receptor status. However, it is generally recommended that pregnancy be delayed until 2 to 3 years after completion of treatment, not because of any influence of the pregnancy on the malignancy, but rather to defer childbearing until after the period of greatest risk of recurrence.

VIGNETTE 4 Question 1
1. Answer E:
Tumors less than 5 cm in size and with no palpable lymph nodes are candidates for BCT. SLNB or full axillary lymph node biopsy may be considered; however, full axillary lymph node biopsy results in greater morbidity, and many patients can be thoroughly evaluated with sentinel nodes alone. Radiation therapy is necessary for all patients who undergo conservative therapy. Breast reconstruction should be considered, when a large mass is removed from the breast because it carries significant psychosocial benefits. Estrogen/progesterone receptor-positive tumors should be treated with an anti-estrogen agent or aromatase inhibitor following surgical resection. Postmenopausal women (like this patient) with ER+ and PR+ tumors should be first treated with an aromatase inhibitor, like letrozole. Tamoxifen is the first-line hormone therapy for *premenopausal* women. Trastuzumab is a monoclonal antibody for adjuvant treatment in tumors that are HER2/neu positive.

VIGNETTE 4 Question 2
2. Answer A:
Currently, the overall 5-year survival rate is 90%, and the most reliable predictor of survival is the stage of breast cancer at the time of diagnosis. Positive estrogen and progesterone receptor status are favorable prognostic signs. Negative HER2/neu is also a favorable prognostic sign, because HER2/neu positive tumors are more aggressive. Other prognostic indicators are lymph node status, tumor size, nuclear grade, histologic type, proliferative rate, and oncogene expression.

VIGNETTE 4 Question 3
3. Answer D:
Follow-up after breast cancer treatment should include a physical examination every 3 to 6 months for 3 years, every 6 to 12 months for years 4 and 5, and annually thereafter. In women who receive breast-conserving surgery, the first follow-up mammogram is usually performed 6 months after completion of radiation treatment. Unless otherwise indicated, breast cancer patients should have annual mammograms. Women with BCT should have bilateral mammograms, and women who are status postmastectomy should have unilateral mammograms of the contralateral breast. Routine CBC, blood chemistries, tumor markers, chest X-ray, CT, and bone scans are not recommended for routine breast cancer follow-up. They should only be used in symptomatic patients in whom metastasis is suspected.

VIGNETTE 4 Question 4
4. Answer B:
Vasomotor symptoms and atrophic vaginal changes can have significant effects on the daily life and activity of women. These symptoms can be exacerbated by treatment options for breast cancer. These symptoms should be validated and not ignored by the healthcare provider. The use of certain antidepressants and vaginal lubricants is a first-line treatment option. HRT should be avoided in women with a history of breast cancer. Cessation of treatments is not recommended at two years. There is some evidence to support decreasing the amount of soy in the diet.

Questions

1. A 39-year-old woman presents to your emergency department with complaints of irregular vaginal bleeding for the past 1 year. Upon evaluation of her surgical history, she tells you she had a D&C outside of the country for an "abnormal pregnancy" about 1 year ago. She has had no follow-up since then and has not been sexually active since her procedure. On review of systems, she tells you she has been coughing up blood for the past 1 week. Physical examination reveals old blood in the vaginal vault. Your laboratory data are significant for a serum β-hCG of 112,000 mIU/mL. The most likely diagnosis is:
   a. Complete molar pregnancy
   b. Partial molar pregnancy
   c. Metastatic persistent GTD
   d. Placental site trophoblastic tumor
   e. Ectopic pregnancy

2. A 37-year-old woman presents to your office with a 3-month history of intermenstrual bleeding and intermittent pelvic pain. She is sexually active and reports one new sexual partner in the last year. She uses condoms for contraception. A pelvic ultrasound is found to be normal. Subsequently, an endometrial biopsy is performed. The biopsy specimen shows leukocytic infiltrate with plasma cells. Which of the following is the most appropriate course of action?
   a. Doxycycline 100 mg orally twice daily for 14 days
   b. Insertion of a levonorgestrel intrauterine system (LNG-IUS)
   c. Hysteroscopy
   d. Total abdominal hysterectomy
   e. Cefoxitin 2 g IV every 6 hours

3. A 24-year-old G2P0010 presents for an initial prenatal visit. Gestational age by known last menstrual period (LMP) is 22 weeks. This is a desired pregnancy and she shares that she believes she had a miscarriage 6 months ago while traveling abroad. Medical history is complicated by migraine headaches. Bedside ultrasound demonstrates intrauterine pregnancy with fetal heart rate of 154. You order a prenatal laboratory panel and quad screening test for the patient. The prenatal panel reveals that the patient is Rh-negative and antibody positive. You order a titer level on your patient and offer her partner testing. The father of the baby is Rh-positive, making the fetus at risk for fetal hydrops. What is the lowest titer level that you would begin with to be concerned about development of fetal hydrops and start serial MCA Doppler testing?
   a. 1:4
   b. 1:8
   c. 1:16
   d. 1:64
   e. 1:256

4. A 25-year-old woman presents to your office requesting a mammogram immediately. She just found out that her paternal grandmother has breast cancer at age 64, and she is very concerned. She wants to make sure that she does not have breast cancer. What is your most appropriate recommendation for her?
   a. Immediate mammogram
   b. Immediate breast MRI
   c. Immediate breast ultrasound
   d. Reassurance and counseling about risk factors. Collection of a family history and recommendation for breast self-awareness and clinical breast examination every 1 to 3 years until age 39, then annually after that along with annual mammogram starting at age 40.
   e. Counseling about risk factors, BRCA 1 and 2 testing, and then, if negative, follow-up at age 40 for first mammogram

5. Maternal serum screening screens for all of the following conditions, except:
   a. Down syndrome
   b. Trisomy 18
   c. Fragile X syndrome
   d. Abdominal wall defects
   e. Neural tube defects

6. A 36-year-old G4P4004 woman comes to you for contraceptive advice. She had a intrauterine device (IUD) placed last year; however, it was noted to be perforated, so it was removed. She

does not want another IUD. She asks if she is a candidate for the birth control pill. Her medical history is significant for a history of DVT during her last pregnancy. She has a BMI of 42 and Type II diabetes mellitus controlled with an oral agent. She has occasional tension headaches relieved with nonsteroidal anti-inflammatory drugs (NSAIDs). She is a nonsmoker, and otherwise has had only uncomplicated vaginal deliveries and no surgeries. Which of the following is an absolute contraindication to starting combined oral contraceptive pills in this patient?
   a. Age greater than 35 years
   b. History of DVT
   c. Diabetes mellitus
   d. History of tension headaches
   e. Obesity

7. A common complication of both epidural and spinal anesthesia includes:
   a. Maternal hypotension
   b. Maternal hyperventilation
   c. Fetal tachycardia
   d. Tetanic uterine contractions
   e. Chorioamnionitis

8. Which of the following is not a sign of active labor?
   a. Bloody show
   b. Palpable contractions
   c. Nausea and vomiting
   d. Fever and chills
   e. Maternal pain

9. A 36-year-old G3P1103 at 10 weeks 3 days presents to establish prenatal care. In addition to advanced maternal age, her antenatal issues include chronic hypertension and Type 2 diabetes mellitus. She currently smokes approximately one pack of cigarettes/day. Additionally, she reports that her last pregnancy was induced at 35 weeks for severe preeclampsia. Risk factors for the development of preeclampsia include all of the following, except:
   a. Smoking
   b. Diabetes mellitus
   c. History of preeclampsia in a prior pregnancy
   d. Advanced maternal age
   e. Chronic hypertension

10. A 21-year-old woman presents to your office with a complaint of no menses for 2 months. A pregnancy test is positive, and ultrasound confirms an intrauterine pregnancy at 7 weeks of gestation. She and her mother request information regarding termination of pregnancy. What proportion of first-trimester abortions have complications?
    a. 0.3%
    b. 3%
    c. 13%
    d. 30%
    e. 53%

11. A 25-year-old G1P0 at 31 weeks' gestation presents with blood pressure in the 160 to 170/110 to 120 range and a severe headache that does not decrease with acetaminophen treatment. On laboratory testing, her platelets are 72,000; AST is 226; and Creatinine is 1.4. Your plan is:
    a. Betamethasone and expectant management
    b. Hydralazine and expectant management
    c. Magnesium sulfate and expectant management
    d. Immediate delivery
    e. Magnesium sulfate, hydralazine, betamethasone, and immediate delivery

12. A 34-year-old G4P1112 presents at 40 weeks 3 days to labor and delivery with onset of painful contractions 3 hours ago. She denies leaking fluid or vaginal bleeding. Her obstetric history is significant for a prior vaginal delivery at 41 weeks after induction for oligohydramnios. Her second pregnancy was complicated by a placental abruption at 35 weeks after a motor vehicle accident (MVA) and required emergent delivery by cesarean section. This pregnancy has been complicated by low back pain, secondary to her history of MVA. She has chosen a trial of labor after cesarean. Cervical examination on arrival is 4 cm dilation, 80% effaced, and −1 station. Contractions are regular every 3 minutes. The contractions are more painful 2 hours later, and she requests an epidural. Cervical examination at that time is 5 cm dilated, 100% effaced, and zero station. She receives an epidural with good pain relief. You are called to her room 1 hour later because she suddenly developed worsening abdominal pain. The nurse reports that the fetus has had a few deep variable decelerations to the 70s that are new. You lift the sheet to perform a cervical examination and notice bright red blood at the introitus and on the sheets. Cervical examination is still 5 cm dilated, 100% effaced, but is now −3 station. There is a moderate amount of vaginal bleeding now. The fetus is now having a prolonged deceleration. You get the patient's consent for an emergent cesarean section. What do you expect to find at time of fetal delivery?
    a. Placental abruption
    b. Vasa previa
    c. Uterine rupture
    d. Fetal nuchal cord
    e. No abnormality noted

13. A 24-year-old G1P0 at 28 weeks 5 days' gestation presents to routine prenatal care with complaint

of increased discharge today. She first noticed it after going to the bathroom. When she stood up she felt as if a little urine continued to leak out. Throughout the afternoon, she has continued to feel like water is leaking from the vagina. There is no vaginal bleeding or abdominal pain. The discharge is clear and odorless. Her pregnancy has been otherwise uncomplicated. Which of the following is the first step in evaluating this patient?
   a. Amnio dye test/tampon test
   b. Ultrasound to check for Amniotic Fluid Index (AFI)
   c. Sterile speculum examination
   d. AmniSure test
   e. Amniocentesis to rule out chorioamnionitis

14. Your next patient is a 34-year-old who was diagnosed with endometriosis 10 years earlier. She and her husband have been unable to conceive after 1.5 years of unprotected intercourse. Which of the following is most likely to improve their chance of conceiving?
    a. NSAIDs
    b. Oral contraceptive pills
    c. Oral medroxyprogesterone acetate
    d. Depot Lupron with add back therapy
    e. Surgery for lysis of adhesions and fulguration of endometriosis

15. Which of the following is most likely to improve pregnancy outcomes in a patient with preterm premature rupture of membranes (PPROM)?
    a. Tocolysis for 48 hours with nifedipine
    b. Administration of betamethasone
    c. Hospital observation and bed rest
    d. Augmentation of labor

16. A 33-year-old G2P0101 at 34 weeks' gestation is evaluated in fetal ultrasound for fetal size less than dating by fundal height. The fetus has been lagging in growth throughout the pregnancy, but recently the obstetrician did not notice interval growth in the fundal height. Fundal height today measures 31 weeks. She had an ultrasound at 18 weeks, which showed normal anatomy and growth in the 30th percentile. The patient's medical history is complicated by a history of oxycodone abuse, and she is currently taking methadone in pregnancy. She has had negative urine drug screening at each prenatal visit. She delivered her first child vaginally at 36 weeks secondary to PPROM. You are covering for her provider today and are looking at the ultrasound report, which shows that her fetus is small with head and abdominal circumferences at the 5th percentile and femur length less than the 10th percentile. There are abnormal findings with the placenta. Which of the following placental conditions do not increase a fetus's risk of IUGR?
    a. Chronic placental abruption
    b. Placenta previa
    c. Thrombosis
    d. Chorioamnionitis
    e. Marginal cord insertion

17. A 26-year-old G1P0 at 33 weeks 3 days presents for routine prenatal visit. She reports contractions, which have been off and on for the past few weeks but today she notes that they have become regular, occurring every 5 minutes, and uncomfortable. She denies leaking fluid or vaginal bleeding. The baby is very active. Pregnancy is notable for elevated 1-hour glucose tolerance test but a normal 3-hour glucose tolerance test. Upon examination you note that the fundal height measures 37 weeks. You palpate two moderately firm contractions while listening to the fetal heart tones. You decide to send the patient over for evaluation on the labor and delivery ward. Monitoring there reveals contractions every 2 to 3 minutes and Category 1 fetal tracing. Cervical examination is notable for a closed cervix, 25% effacement, and −3 station. Bedside ultrasound demonstrates an AFI of 28 cm, fetus in cephalic presentation and posterior placenta. An hour later you recheck the patient's cervix and it is unchanged. She continues to have contractions but they are now every 5 minutes and less painful. Polyhydramnios is not associated with which of the following conditions?
    a. Gestational diabetes
    b. Congenital anomalies
    c. Multiple gestations
    d. Potter syndrome
    e. Neural tube defects

18. A 19-year-old G1P0 presents to routine prenatal follow-up visit at 35 weeks' gestation. Her blood pressure is 142/88 mm Hg and a urine dip is negative for protein. She has no headache, no visual symptoms, and no right upper quadrant pain. You send preeclamptic labs (CBC, LFTs, Cr, and lactate dehydrogenase [LDH]), which are all within normal limits. What is her diagnosis and plan?
    a. Gestational hypertension—expectant management
    b. Preeclampsia—expectant management
    c. Rule out preeclampsia—send 24-hour urine protein
    d. Gestational hypertension—delivery
    e. Preeclampsia—delivery

19. A 23-year-old G1P0 Caucasian woman at 12 weeks gestational age (GA) presents for a routine prenatal visit. Her medical history is unremarkable. Her temperature is 37.3°C, blood

pressure is 120/84 mm Hg, pulse is 85/min, and respirations are 13/min. BMI is 24. Her best friend was diagnosed with gestational diabetes, and the patient is concerned she may develop it as well. Gestational diabetes is seen at higher rates in all of the following except:
a. Caucasian race
b. Family history of diabetes
c. Hispanic ethnicity
d. Increasing maternal age
e. Native American race

20. A 36-year-old G3P2 woman at 35 weeks' gestation presents for a routine prenatal visit. Her previous two pregnancies 10 and 12 years ago, respectively, resulted in healthy vaginal deliveries. In the past decade, she has gained weight, and her BMI today is 29. She was diagnosed with gestational diabetes a few weeks ago, which is well-controlled with insulin. She asks you about expectations for her delivery management. All of the following would be appropriate steps in her management except:
a. Induce labor at 39 weeks of gestation
b. Offer patient an obstetric ultrasound for estimated fetal weight at 35 weeks
c. Offer patient an elective cesarean birth if EFW is greater than 4,500 g
d. Upon admission, regulate blood glucose levels with insulin and dextrose drips
e. Utilize forceps and vacuum if macrosomia is suspected to assist the mother in delivery

21. A 25-year-old G1 at 9 weeks' GA comes to her initial prenatal visit, and in addition to a series of blood tests, a screening urine culture is obtained. She is asymptomatic and asks why this additional test must be performed. You counsel her that:
a. Even though she is asymptomatic, she is still at risk for STIs and this is one way to screen for those types of infections
b. Asymptomatic bacteriuria if not treated has been associated with higher rates of chorioamnionitis and neonatal sepsis
c. She is at increased risk of having asymptomatic bacteriuria compared to nonpregnant patients
d. Asymptomatic bacteriuria increases her risk of cystitis, pyelonephritis, and preterm birth
e. You are worried that she has pyelonephritis

22. A 34-year-old G3P0020 at 11 weeks GA presents for a follow-up prenatal care visit. You review her screening prenatal labs, which are significant for a positive Hepatitis B surface antigen. She remembers being told she had hepatitis as a child, but has never been symptomatic. She asks how this might affect her pregnancy and you counsel her that her pregnancy and delivery will not be managed any differently.
a. She likely has chronic Hepatitis B, and there is an increased risk of transmission to the neonate around the time of delivery
b. There is no way to tell if this is an acute or chronic infection, so she will need close monitoring during her pregnancy
c. Chronic Hepatitis B has been associated with increased risk of congenital anomalies, and she will need a detailed anatomy ultrasound between 18 and 20 weeks, which includes a fetal echo
d. Reactivation of Hepatitis B is more common during pregnancy and places her at risk for hepatic failure

23. Congenital toxoplasmosis infection is associated with what fetal manifestations?
a. Chorioretinitis, intracranial calcifications, and hydrocephalus
b. Deafness, saber shins, mulberry molar, Hutchinson teeth, and a saddle nose
c. Deafness, cardiac abnormalities, cataracts, and mental retardation
d. Hepatomegaly, splenomegaly, thrombocytopenia, jaundice, cerebral calcifications, and chorioretinitis
e. Disseminated granulomatous lesions with microabscesses, placental lesions, and chorioamnionitis

24. A 23-year-old G2P0101 at 28 weeks GA comes to the office for an urgent visit. She complains of vaginal irritation and increased thin, gray discharge. She denies leakage of fluid, vaginal bleeding, or contractions. The baby is moving well. She is in a monogamous relationship and last had intercourse 2 weeks ago. She has not noticed any dysuria or urinary frequency. She has no history of sexually transmitted infections. You perform a sterile speculum examination (SSE), and there is no evidence of ruptured membranes. You collect a sample of discharge and perform a wet mount and KOH, which shows clue cells, a positive whiff test, and no hyphae. The pH of the discharge is less than 5.0. You diagnose her with bacterial vaginosis. If this had gone untreated, how would it have increased her risk during this pregnancy?
a. Increased risk of neonatal blindness
b. Increased risk of neonatal sepsis and admission to the NICU
c. Increased risk of PPROM
d. Increased risk of placental abruption
e. Increased risk of congenital malformations

25. While working on labor and delivery, you admit a 32-year-old G4P3003 at 40 2/7 weeks GA in active

labor. Her contractions occur every 5 minutes and started 2 hours ago. She denies any leakage of fluid or vaginal bleeding. Her fetal heart tracing is Category 1. During your evaluation, you can find no record of group B *streptococcus* (GBS) testing done at her clinic. You review her obstetrical history and find that she has had three previous vaginal deliveries that were all uncomplicated. What would be an indication to treat her with GBS prophylaxis?
a. Evidence of ruptured membranes
b. Previous history of GBS positive test in prior pregnancy
c. GBS bacteriuria on her initial prenatal urine screening culture
d. If the pregnancy was less than 40 weeks GA
e. Prior infant with *Escherichia coli* sepsis

26. You are paged to the emergency room to see a patient with an early pregnancy. She is an 18-year-old G1P0 at 8 weeks GA by a self-reported LMP. She has not previously been seen in clinic for this pregnancy. She states that since the beginning of her pregnancy, she has had progressive nausea and vomiting. She has not been able to keep anything down for the past 24 hours and has vomited seven times in the past day. She denies diarrhea, but had a normal bowel movement yesterday. She feels very weak and lightheaded, especially when standing. She denies any fevers or chills, dysuria, headaches, or other symptoms. She has had no sick contacts. She is tachycardic, but otherwise her vital signs are normal. Her abdominal examination is benign. You get a urinalysis and it shows a specific gravity of greater than 1.030 and moderate ketonuria. There are no urinary nitrates or leukocyte esterase. A complete metabolic panel is significant for mild hypokalemia and hypochloridemia. The CBC is normal. Her serum β-hCG is 150,000. You plan to admit her for IV fluids, antiemetics, and electrolyte replacement. What should be the next step in her care?
a. Order an obstetric ultrasound
b. Place a nasogastric tube for nutritional supplementation
c. Order blood cultures and a chest X-ray to evaluate for an infectious etiology for her symptoms
d. Consult general surgery, given your concern for a small bowel obstruction
e. Place a PICC line and start total parenteral nutrition

27. A 32-year-old woman comes to your clinic for preconception counseling. She was diagnosed with epilepsy at age 12 and is currently taking phenytoin and carbamazepine. She has been seizure-free for 1½ years. She and her husband are planning to conceive within the next year. What should you advise to decrease the risks for the upcoming pregnancy?
a. Stop all seizure medications
b. Optimize her seizure regimen to include only one medication
c. Start taking a prenatal vitamin and 400 mcg of folic acid
d. Keep the same dose of both medications and start taking 4 mg of folic acid
e. Recommend she transition off both her current medications and start taking valproic acid for monotherapy

28. A 35-year-old G4P0030 presents to the office for her initial prenatal visit. She is 8 weeks pregnant, dated by her last normal menstrual period. Her obstetric history is significant for an elective termination of pregnancy as a teenager, and two losses at 16 weeks' gestation in the past 3 years. With both of her later pregnancy losses, she reports that she presented to the hospital with mild spotting, was found to be 4 to 5 cm dilated, and delivered very shortly thereafter. Genetic analysis of both fetuses was normal. Her medical history is significant for a history of cervical dysplasia leading to a LEEP procedure at age 27. She denies any history of bleeding or clotting disorders. She is in a monogamous relationship, and her current partner is also the father of her two most recent pregnancies. This is a highly desired pregnancy. What recommendation would you give this patient?
a. She and her husband should undergo karyotyping to look for a balanced translocation
b. She should have a hysterosalpingogram after this pregnancy to look for uterine abnormalities
c. She should undergo chorionic villus sampling (CVS) to evaluate the chromosomes of the fetus
d. She should start progesterone supplementation for presumed luteal phase defect
e. She should have a prophylactic cerclage placed between 12 and 14 weeks for presumed cervical incompetence

29. Which of the following treatments are most appropriate for varicose veins that develop in pregnancy?
a. Diuretics
b. Pressure stockings and lower extremity elevation
c. Low sodium diet and fluid restriction
d. Surgical intervention
e. Antihypertensive medication

30. A 39-year-old G1P0 presents at 12 weeks for fetal nuchal translucency (NT) screening. Her medical history is noncontributory. Her family history is unremarkable. After genetic counseling today, the patient states that she desires screening, given her risk of chromosomal disorders associated with advanced maternal age. The patient proceeds with the ultrasound screen, which reveals a thickened NT. What is the most appropriate next step?
    a. Repeat the test in 1 week
    b. Repeat the test in 2 weeks
    c. Offer CVS now
    d. Offer amniocentesis now
    e. Offer termination of the pregnancy

31. A 34-year-old G2P0010 at 39 weeks GA presents to labor and delivery in active labor. Her pregnancy has been complicated by a bicuspid aorta with moderate aortic stenosis. She has had a recent ECHO that shows a normal ejection fraction of greater than 65%, a gradient across the aorta of 30 mm Hg (moderate 25 to 40 mm Hg), and a valve area of 1.4 cm² (moderate 1.0 to 1.5 cm²). She has had no symptoms of heart failure or arrhythmia during this pregnancy. What is the best management plan to minimize her cardiovascular risks during the intrapartum and postpartum period?
    a. Start ampicillin for endocarditis prophylaxis
    b. Monitor strict intake and output, place an early epidural and plan for an assisted vaginal delivery with forceps or vacuum once the fetus is 12 station
    c. Proceed immediately to cesarean delivery to minimize cardiac stress
    d. Admit to the ICU and place a central venous line
    e. To maintain cardiac output give lasix to decrease afterload

32. You are called to see a 21-year-old G3P2002 at 28 weeks GA who has had limited prenatal care. She has diffuse complaints of abdominal pain, cold sweats, anxiety, and insomnia. Upon review of her history, she tells you that she usually has two to three vodka drinks every day. For the past 3 days, she has not been able to afford to purchase any alcohol. She denies any other significant medical or surgical history. You diagnose her with alcohol withdrawal and admit her to the hospital for treatment. What is the most significant long-term complication of alcohol dependence during pregnancy?
    a. Fetal alcohol syndrome
    b. Maternal withdrawal
    c. Neonatal withdrawal
    d. Low fetal birth weight
    e. Neonatal admission to the NICU

33. A patient in your clinic is a 22-year-old G2P1001 at 26 weeks GA. Her pregnancy is complicated by tobacco use, and she is currently smoking one pack per day (PPD). This is down from two PPD at the start of her pregnancy. You continue to counsel her to quit at each visit. Which of the following are not adverse outcomes of maternal tobacco use during pregnancy?
    a. Placental abruption
    b. Decreased birth weight
    c. Cardiac defects
    d. Preterm birth
    e. Spontaneous abortion

34. You are assisting in a gynecologic oncology clinic when you see a 57-year-old G3P3 female patient who is a former nurse. She presents with 6 months of pelvic discomfort, increasing abdominal girth, and early satiety. Physical examination reveals a large abdominopelvic mass. A pelvic ultrasound and CT scan show bilateral ovarian masses, ascites, and studding of the peritoneum. In your discussion with the patient you predict that this most likely represents a malignant ovarian neoplasm. She asks about the primary method of treatment for ovarian carcinoma. You explain that the mainstay of treatment for epithelial ovarian cancer is:
    a. Radiation therapy alone
    b. Surgery alone
    c. Surgery followed by chemotherapy
    d. Surgery followed by radiation therapy
    e. Chemoradiation alone

35. A 20-year-old African American G2P2 is seen in the hospital on postpartum day number 1, after a spontaneous vaginal delivery of a healthy male infant with APGAR score of 8 and 9. Her pregnancy was uncomplicated. Her delivery was complicated only by a second degree perineal laceration that was repaired in standard fashion. Her medical history is significant for having Hepatitis C. She also reports a history of breast augmentation. She received an intramuscular injection of Depo-Provera for postpartum contraception. This morning she appears very tired and although doing well from a physical standpoint is noted to be bottle-feeding her infant. She acknowledges the benefits of breast-feeding but explains that bottle-feeding has its merits as well. Which of the following describes one of the benefits of bottle-feeding over breast-feeding?
    a. She decreases her risk of vertical transmission of Hepatitis C by bottle-feeding
    b. She will be unable to breast-feed because of her history of breast augmentation
    c. Breast-feeding is contraindicated in women receiving Depo-Provera for contraception

d. Bottle-feeding ensures a more adequate supply of milk to her baby during the first few days of life
e. Breast-feeding may not provide enough Vitamin D for some infants compared with that supplemented in formula

36. A 34-year-old Caucasian G3P2002 presents to labor and delivery at 41 weeks and 1 day for induction of labor for postdate pregnancy. Her pregnancy was uncomplicated. Her medical history is significant only for mild intermittent asthma; she denied any history of hypertension. Her surgical history is significant for a cesarean section during her last pregnancy for Stage II arrest. Her induction is started with a Foley bulb for cervical ripening, followed by oxytocin, which succeeds in progressing her to Stage II of labor. She delivers a viable male infant in three pushes with APGAR score of 8 and 9. She subsequently delivers a normal-sized, normal-appearing placenta with membranes intact and a centrally inserted three-vessel cord. She has an intact perineum. Her cervix is intact on examination. She is noted to have continued brisk bleeding from her vagina. Her fundus is noted to be above the umbilicus and boggy despite fundal massage. Which of the following medications would be contraindicated in the management of her hemorrhage?
   a. 10 mg intramuscular oxytocin
   b. 200 mcg intramuscular methylergonovine
   c. 800 mcg rectal misoprostol
   d. 250 mcg carboprost
   e. 20 mg IV oxytocin in 1,000 mL lactated Ringer

37. A 27-year-old Caucasian G1P01001 is seen in the hospital on postpartum day number 2, after a spontaneous vaginal delivery of a healthy female infant with APGAR score of 9 and 9. She reports feeling febrile and has intermittently moderate uterine cramping. She is tolerating a regular diet, breast-feeding without difficulty, voiding spontaneously without discomfort, and having minimal lochia. She has been slow to ambulate, having only recently had her epidural catheter removed. Her pregnancy was complicated solely by her rubella nonimmune status. Her delivery was complicated only by a superficial vaginal laceration that was repaired in standard fashion. Her medical and surgical histories are noncontributory. She is taking an iron supplement and recently received her MMR and TDaP vaccines. Her vitals are significant for a temperature of 38.0°C; her pulse 85, blood pressure 112/72. She is comfortably breathing room air. Her physical examination shows no acute distress, with regular heart rate and rhythm, clear lungs, a soft abdomen with a firm, though mildly tender, uterus, and nontender symmetric lower extremities significant for +1 pitting edema. Which of the following is the most likely cause of her postpartum fever?
   a. Postpartum endometritis
   b. Urinary tract infection
   c. Deep vein thromboembolism
   d. Vaccine reaction
   e. Breast fever

38. A 36-year-old Hispanic American now G6P6006 at 41 weeks and 2 days gestation arrives on labor and delivery and precipitously delivers a viable male infant followed by a large gush of fluid. Her infant was notable for an APGAR score of 8 and 9 and weight of 9 lb. She subsequently delivered a normal-sized, normal-appearing placenta with a centrally inserted three-vessel cord over an intact perineum. Her cervix was intact on examination. Her pregnancy was complicated by A1 gestational diabetes, which was suboptimally controlled. Her medical history is significant for a 2 × 3 × 3 cm intramural fibroid noted in the anterior wall during routine pregnancy ultrasound. She denied any history of asthma or hypertension. Her surgical history is significant for a cesarean section during her last pregnancy for Stage II arrest. Review of her previous pregnancy ultrasounds is significant for a low-lying placenta without previa. During her medical interview conducted postpartum she is noted to have continued brisk bleeding from her vagina. Which of the following is not a risk factor for her postpartum hemorrhage?
   a. Her parity
   b. Her fibroid
   c. Her baby's weight
   d. Her low-lying placenta
   e. All of the above

39. A 21-year-old G0 presents for her first gynecologic examination. She states that she became sexually active 2 months ago for the first time. She has no significant medical history. She has regular menses with some mild dysmenorrhea. During the speculum examination, you observe a small raised 5 mm lesion on her non-tender cervix. It is smooth and light-bluish in color and looks like a bubble under the epithelial surface of the cervix. What is your diagnosis?
   a. Bartholin duct cyst
   b. Cervical dysplasia
   c. Nabothian cyst
   d. Skene gland cyst
   e. Chlamydial cervicitis

40. A 68-year-old woman presents with vulvar pruritus for over 12 months. Her symptoms have increased

over the past few months. She has tried antifungal medications, which seem to help, but the symptoms keep recurring. She went through menopause at age 49 and has not been sexually active for 10 years. She does not use any douching products and is not taking any antibiotics. On physical examination, you note thin white epithelium of the labia minora with red oval-shaped erosions, varying in size from 0.5 to 1.5 cm. How would you proceed?
   a. Culture the vagina and treat with high-dose antifungal
   b. Wide local excision of the lesions
   c. Cryotherapy to eradicate the lesions
   d. Punch biopsy of the vulvar lesions
   e. Prescription of moderate–high potency topical steroids

41. A 40-year-old woman with regular menstruation returns for assessment of vulvar pruritus. She has had itchy vulvar skin for over a year; the symptoms vary in severity over the past 3 months. She has been treated with oral and topical antifungal creams. She has adhered to vulvar skin care guidance. She had a vulvar biopsy 3 months ago showing lichen simplex chronicus without evidence of fungal infection, VIN, or malignancy. She has been applying a low-potency topical steroid since her last visit with you; she says that it helps for a while and then her symptoms recur and she has to use it again. On examination, you note thickened epithelium of the inner labia majora and labia minora, with several small areas of excoriation. What do you recommend?
   a. Punch biopsy of vulvar skin
   b. Topical clobetasol ointment
   c. Laser vaporization of affected area
   d. Prolonged course of antifungals
   e. Topical estrogen cream

42. A 13-year-old girl presents with severe lower abdominal pain of 24 hours' duration. She states that the pain is sharp and constant and that she has had similar pain for several days, approximately every month over the past 4 months. She has no vomiting or diarrhea with the pain, but she is constipated frequently, having a bowel movement about every 3 to 4 days. She feels that her jeans are getting tighter around the waist, although she remains active, playing soccer daily. She has never had a menstrual period and denies ever being sexually active. She has normal vital signs, normal stature, Tanner stage 3 breast development, and Tanner stage 3 pubic hair. Abdominal examination reveals a firm and tender midline mass that is inferior to the umbilicus. The patient refuses a pelvic examination, but agrees to a visualization of the vulva; when parting the labia minora, a tense bulging membrane can be seen. Of the following, the most likely diagnosis is
   a. Pregnancy
   b. Fibroid uterus
   c. Hematocolpos
   d. Endometriosis
   e. Ovarian cyst

43. A 22-year-old G2P1001 at 39 weeks 2 days presents with history of contractions every 3 minutes for the past 2 hours. Her prior pregnancy was induced at 41 weeks and 3 days. Her first stage of labor lasted 9 hours and during her second stage of labor she pushed for 2 hours, resulting in delivery of a male infant weighing 3,800 g. She denies rupture of membranes, vaginal bleeding, or decreased fetal movement. Her initial cervical examination is 2 cm dilation, 50% effacement, and −2 station. Per the records, her cervical examination in the clinic last week was 2 cm, 25% effaced, and −2 station. You decide to have her ambulate and repeat her cervical examination in 2 hours to assess if she is in labor. Two hours later you evaluate the patient and see that she is painfully contracting and requesting epidural placement. Your cervical examination reveals 4 cm dilation, 100% effacement, and −1 station. You admit the patient to labor and delivery for expectant management, and she receives an epidural for pain control. Which of the following findings will cause you to recommend a cesarean delivery at this time?
   a. Fetus in right occiput posterior presentation
   b. Maternal hypotension
   c. Development of vaginal bleeding with change in hematocrit from 33 to 32
   d. Repetitive fetal decelerations to 80 beats per minute with absent variability

44. A healthy 28-year-old G1P0 comes to you for established prenatal care. She has always had regular menstrual cycles, but she was not in the habit of tracking them. This pregnancy was desired but unplanned. An early ultrasound for dating shows that the embryo is in the left horn of a bicornuate uterus. This diagnosis is new to her and she is concerned about the implications for her pregnancy. You explain that the most common pregnancy-related risk associated with a bicornuate uterus is
   a. Infertility
   b. Antepartum bleeding

c. Recurrent first-trimester miscarriage
d. Cervical insufficiency
e. Preterm labor and delivery

45. A 32-year-old G0 comes in for consultation for an enlarged fibroid uterus. She and her husband are planning their first attempt at conception in the next month or two but she wants to have her fibroids treated before she becomes pregnant. A review of her outside medical records reveals a recent transvaginal ultrasound showing a 7-cm uterus with a 2- and 1-cm intramural fibroid. There are no signs of adenomyosis, and the endometrial stripe and ovaries are all normal. She has a history of mild dysmenorrhea but no history of abnormal uterine bleeding, postcoital spotting, or intermenstrual bleeding. Her examination at your visit is unremarkable. What treatment options would you recommend to her for management of her uterine fibroids?
   a. IUD
   b. Endometrial ablation
   c. Hysteroscopic resection
   d. Uterine artery embolization
   e. Expectant management

46. A 48-year-old G3P3 patient comes to see you for a complaint of heavier, longer menses. She is healthy with no major medical problems and a BMI of 27. Her only medication is a daily multivitamin. She has always had regular menstrual periods until recently. She is also experiencing increased pain with her menstrual cycles. Her last pap and high-risk human papillomavirus (HPV) screen were negative less than a year ago. She denies any postcoital spotting but has had a few episodes of intermenstrual bleeding. A transvaginal ultrasound reveals a normal myometrium with an endometrial stripe of 22 mm. An endometrial biopsy reveals proliferative endometrium without evidence of glandular crowding or cytologic atypia. What is the most likely diagnosis?
   a. Fibroids
   b. Adenomyosis
   c. Perimenopause
   d. Endometrial polyp
   e. Endometrial intraepithelial neoplasia (EIN)

47. A new female patient presents to your office on referral from her primary care physician. She is a 62-year-old G2P2. She has been menopausal for more than 10 years and has occasional right lower quadrant discomfort. Ultrasound from the PCP's office showed a 15-cm complex ovarian mass with cystic and solid components, two internal nodules, septations, and increased Doppler flow. A thorough history is taken. Your physical exam is normal except for a mass and a fluid wave on abdominal exam. CT confirms the mass, ascites and post-hysterectomy status. You explain to the patient your assessment and plan. Which of the following is the next best step in the management of this patient?
   a. Surgical evaluation
   b. Repeat ultrasound in 3 months
   c. Colonoscopy
   d. Pregnancy test
   e. Expectant management

48. A 24-year-old G0 Caucasian woman presents to your office with the complaint of worsening dysmenorrhea over the last 6 months. She was recently married and reports stopping her oral contraceptives, which she started as a teenager for severe dysmenorrhea. She also complains of deep dyspareunia. On further questioning, she reports that her mother has a history of endometriosis. You suspect that your patient may also have endometriosis. Which of the following conditions should you counsel her about as potential results of endometriosis?
   a. Pelvic inflammatory disease
   b. Abnormal uterine bleeding
   c. Hirsutism
   d. Infertility
   e. Endometrial cancer

49. A 26-year-old G0 woman presents to your office with complaints of a palpable breast mass discovered by her husband. She has no family history of breast cancer. You perform a clinical breast examination and can palpate the mass as well. The next step in management of this patient would be:
   a. Diagnostic mammogram
   b. Diagnostic ultrasound
   c. Breast MRI
   d. Core-needle biopsy
   e. Excisional biopsy

50. A 27-year-old G1P0010 presents to the clinic for a postoperative visit. Two weeks earlier, she underwent a laparoscopic left salpingostomy for an ectopic pregnancy. A review of her medical history reveals a history of infection with chlamydia 2 years ago. Both she and her partner received a single-dose course of antibiotics. They have been mutually monogamous since that time. She denies any abnormal pap smears. On physical examination, she is afebrile with stable vital signs. Her abdomen is nontender, and she has three well-healed surgical incisions from the laparoscopic port sites. This was a desired pregnancy, and she and her partner hope she becomes pregnant again in the future. What

counseling should you give her regarding her future risk?
a. Her history of chlamydia makes it unlikely that she will ever conceive normally and she should consider in vitro fertilization (IVF)
b. Her risk of a subsequent ectopic pregnancy is 10%
c. Her risk of a subsequent ectopic pregnancy is 25%
d. She should avoid using an IUD for contraception as it increases her risk of ectopic pregnancy
e. She should receive a single dose of methotrexate to ensure that all of the pregnancy tissue has been evacuated

51. A 32-year-old G1P1 woman returns to your clinic for a follow-up visit. She has a history of endometriosis proven by biopsy at the time of laparoscopy years ago. Since then, she has been using a combination oral contraceptive pill in a continuous fashion to manage her cyclic pelvic pain. Over the past several months, she has been experiencing more dyspareunia and cyclic pelvic pain. She would like to know what other medical treatments she can use to manage her symptoms. You explain to her that there are several options, and they include all except which of the following?
a. NSAIDs
b. Oral progestins
c. Selective serotonin reuptake inhibitors (SSRIs)
d. Gonadotropin-releasing hormone (GnRH) agonists
e. Levonorgestrel-releasing intrauterine device

52. A 43-year-old G3P3 presents to your clinic for an annual examination. She is a longtime patient of yours and reports that a friend of hers recently had a hysterectomy for adenomyosis. Your patient is concerned and wonders if she may have adenomyosis. Which finding on history or examination would *not* be suggestive of adenomyosis?
a. Heavy menstrual bleeding
b. Prolonged menstrual bleeding
c. Secondary dysmenorrhea
d. Enlarged, firm uterus with distinct masses on ultrasound
e. Boggy, globular, and tender uterus with indistinct endometrial–myometrial junction

53. A 46-year-old G2P2 returns for follow-up after endometrial biopsy for heavy menstrual bleeding that has developed over the last 6 months. Her biopsy revealed normal secretory endometrium. You suspect that she most likely has adenomyosis. Which of the following most accurately describes the condition?
a. The presence of endometrial cells outside the endometrium with the hallmark of cyclic pelvic pain
b. An extension of endometrial tissue into the uterine myometrium leading to heavy menstrual bleeding and dysmenorrhea
c. Local proliferation of smooth muscle cells within the uterus, often surrounded by a pseudocapsule potentially leading to heavy menstrual bleeding and dysmenorrhea
d. A cystic collection of endometrial cells on the ovary possibly causing pelvic pain and infertility
e. Inflammation or irritation of the lining of the uterus (endometrium), typically caused by infection

54. A 32-year-old woman comes to the gynecologist with 1-week history of vulvar ulcers. She first noticed two red "bumps," which subsequently opened up and are now extremely painful. She is sexually active and reports three new sexual partners in the last month. She reports a remote history of gonorrhea, which was treated. On pelvic examination, there are two 1.5-cm ulcers on the left labia minora. The ulcer bases are erythematous, and the borders are irregular but well demarcated. There is tender inguinal lymph node enlargement on the left side. Bacterial and viral cultures from the ulcer base are negative. Venereal Disease Research Laboratory (VDRL) and herpes simplex virus (HSV) testing are negative. What is the best initial treatment for this patient?
a. Benzathine penicillin G 2.4 million units IM once
b. Ceftriaxone 250 mg IM once
c. Doxycycline 100 mg orally twice daily for 14 days
d. Erythromycin 500 mg orally four times daily for 21 days
e. Acyclovir 200 mg five times daily for 7 days

55. A 25-year-old nulligravid woman comes to the gynecologist for sexually transmitted infection screening. She has been sexually active since age 16 and reports eight new partners in the last year. She is currently asymptomatic. Testing results include Hepatitis B surface antigen negative, rapid plasma reagin (RPR) positive, HIV antibody negative, and nucleic acid amplification test (NAAT) for *Chlamydia* and gonorrhea negative. What is the next best step in the management of this patient?
a. VDRL testing
b. Treatment with benzathine penicillin G 2.4 million units IM once
c. Fluorescent treponemal antibody absorption testing
d. Serial RPR titers

e. Treatment with benzathine penicillin G 2.4 million units IM weekly for three doses

56. A 25-year-old G1P1 woman presents to urgent care with a 4-day history of suprapubic pain, increased urinary frequency, burning with urination, and increased vaginal discharge. She reports a history of similar symptoms 1 month ago when she was treated empirically for a urinary tract infection. All of the following are appropriate in the management except:
    a. Administer trimethoprim-sulfamethoxazole PO twice daily for 3 days
    b. Send urine specimen for urinalysis
    c. Send urine specimen for urine culture
    d. Perform microscopy of the vaginal discharge
    e. Perform NAAT for *Chlamydia* and gonorrhea

57. A 27-year-old woman presents to her gynecologist for evaluation of new vulvar lesions. She first noticed several "bumps" on her outer labia 3 weeks ago. She is otherwise without any associated symptoms. On pelvic examination, there are six flesh-colored, nontender, 1- to 3-mm verrucous papules. Which of the following is the most likely cause of the patient's vulvar lesions?
    a. HPV serotype 16
    b. HSV Type 1
    c. Pox virus
    d. HPV serotype 6
    e. *Haemophilus ducreyi*

58. A 37-year-old G2P1 presents at 12 weeks for prenatal diagnosis. She does not currently have any medical issues and takes no medications. After genetic counseling, the patient states that she wishes to proceed with a CVS. She undergoes CVS, which reveals normal chromosomes. What further prenatal testing do you offer?
    a. Maternal serum α-fetoprotein (AFP)
    b. Amniocentesis
    c. Repeat CVS
    d. Fetal echocardiography
    e. Cordocentesis

59. A 17-year-old nulligravid woman presents to the emergency department with a 2-week history of abdominal pain. The pain started in her lower abdomen, but has become progressively generalized to include her upper abdomen, especially on her right side. The pain is worse with deep breathing, coughing, and movement. She reports intermittent nausea and vomiting for the past day. Six months ago, she was treated for *Neisseria gonorrhoeae* and *Trichomonas vaginalis* infection. She uses a contraceptive implant (Implanon) and reports five new sexual partners in the last year. Her temperature is 38.3°C (100.9°F), pulse is 94/min, respirations are 20/min, and blood pressure is 118/70 mm Hg. Abdominal examination shows diffuse tenderness, especially in the right upper quadrant. On pelvic examination, there is foul smelling frothy discharge. There is tenderness with manipulation of the cervix and uterus. There is no adnexal fullness or tenderness. What is the most likely diagnosis?
    a. Tubo-ovarian abscess
    b. Disseminated gonorrhea
    c. HELLP syndrome
    d. Fitzhugh–Curtis syndrome
    e. Secondary syphilis

60. A 22-year-old woman comes to the emergency department with acute onset of fever, myalgias, abdominal pain, vomiting, and diarrhea. She is sexually active in a monogamous relationship and uses an oral contraceptive pill. Her menses began 3 days prior to onset and she reports using super tampons. Her temperature is 39.5°C (103.1°F), pulse is 124/min, respirations are 26/min, and blood pressure is 80/50 mm Hg. On examination, there is a diffuse, red, macular rash. Her abdomen is tender, slightly distended with guarding. All of the following are included in the diagnostic criteria except:
    a. Positive blood culture
    b. Fever greater than 38.9°C
    c. Hypotension
    d. Multisystem involvement
    e. Diffuse erythematous macular rash

61. A 42-year-old G4P4 woman presents to the gynecologist for an annual examination. She was recently diagnosed with HIV and is receiving treatment with highly active antiretroviral therapy. Her most recent viral load was 12,000 copies/mL and CD4 count 940 cells/mm^3. She is otherwise healthy. She is not currently in a sexual relationship. She denies any history of CIN 2 or CIN 3, and she has had three consecutive negative cervical cytology screening tests. How often should cervical cancer screening be performed?
    a. Pap smear every 6 months
    b. Pap smear annually
    c. Pap smear twice in the first year after diagnosis of HIV and annually thereafter if both are normal
    d. Colposcopy every 6 months
    e. Pap smear every 3 years

62. A 67-year-old patient presents with a chief complaint of pelvic pressure, low back pain, and a vaginal bulge that is worse after prolonged standing or rigorous activity. Your suspicion of pelvic organ prolapse is confirmed on physical examination. All

of the following risk factors may have contributed to this pathologic process except:
a. Genetic predisposition
b. Chronic constipation with a long history of straining to defecate
c. Postmenopausal status
d. Chronic obstructive pulmonary disease
e. Sexual inactivity

63. You are consulted on an 89-year-old inpatient in a nursing facility. Your patient has complete eversion of the vagina. What is another term for this?
a. Procidentia
b. Cystocele
c. Rectocele
d. Urethrocele
e. Enterocele

64. A 45-year-old G5P4 presents for evaluation because her primary care physician has diagnosed her with pelvic organ prolapse. She denies any pelvic pressure, bulge, or difficulty with urination. Her only medical comorbidity is obesity. She is found to have an asymptomatic grade 1 pelvic organ prolapse, what do you recommend?
a. Conservative management with pelvic floor muscle exercises and weight loss
b. Colpocleisis obliterative procedure
c. Gellhorn pessary
d. Round ligament suspension
e. Hysterectomy

65. A postmenopausal woman with symptomatic vaginal vault prolapse after remote hysterectomy elects to proceed with surgical correction. You determine that she is an appropriate candidate for an uterosacral ligament suspension. After completion of the surgery, successful anatomic restoration is noted. Before you conclude the surgery, what additional procedure is indicated?
a. Hysteroscopy
b. Defecography
c. Cystoscopy
d. Episiotomy
e. Anterior colporrhaphy

66. A 62-year-old G2P2 presents to the urogynecology clinic with complaints of urinary incontinence. She has urinary urgency and cannot make it to the bathroom before leaking a large amount of urine. She gets up two to three times per night to urinate. A urinalysis and urine culture done 1 week ago at her PCP's office are both negative. What is the most likely diagnosis and appropriate treatment option for this type of urinary incontinence?
a. Stress incontinence, mid-urethral sling
b. Urgency incontinence, oxybutynin (anticholinergic medication)
c. Overflow incontinence, oxybutynin (anticholinergic medication)
d. Urinary fistula, surgical repair
e. Functional incontinence, bladder suspension

67. A 42-year-old G2P2 complains of urinary leakage when exercising. She recently began jogging for exercise in an effort to lose weight. She does wear a pad when she jogs and reports that it is approximately 75% soaked when she finishes her run. She denies loss of urine at any other time. Urinalysis and urine cultures were negative. Her BMI is 38. Which of the following would you recommend as part of the initial treatment plan for this patient?
a. Mid-urethral sling
b. Detrol LA (anticholinergic medication)
c. Tibial nerve stimulation
d. Pelvic floor muscle exercises
e. Vaginal hysterectomy

68. Urinary incontinence, the involuntary loss of urine is. . .
a. rare, affecting fewer than 3% of women in the United States in 2010
b. common, and expected to affect more than 28 million women in the US by 2050
c. not considered a significant cost burden, because it affects so few women
d. rarely seen in nursing home residents
e. almost always due to urge incontinence

69. Labor is divided into stages and phases. These delineations are used to communicate where patients are in the progress of labor. In particular, the first stage of labor:
a. Begins at the time of full cervical dilation
b. Has a latent phase that ends with dilation exactly at 6 cm
c. Has an active phase that begins with repetitive contractions
d. Has an active phase wherein at least 1.0 cm/hour of dilation is expected in the nulliparous patient
e. Has a latent phase with a rapid rate of cervical change

70. Micturition is voluntary and occurs with relaxation of the urethra and sustained contraction of the bladder until emptying is complete. Sustained contraction of the detrusor muscle of the bladder requires parasympathetic stimulation. Parasympathetic control of the detrusor is supplied by which of the following nerves?
a. Hypogastric nerve
b. Pudendal nerve
c. Peroneal nerve

d. Pelvic nerve
e. Sciatic nerve

71. A long-term patient of yours brings her 14-year-old daughter in to see you for concern over irregular menses. The daughter started menstruating at age 13. Her cycles are irregular in that they may come monthly but she often skips a month. The daughter is of normal weight without any hirsutism, abnormal acne, or acanthosis. Her breast development and height are appropriate for her age. She is a high school soccer player and practices twice a week. She also does yoga and light weight lifting two to three times a week. They want your opinion about how to proceed. How do you counsel them?
    a. You recommend checking follicle stimulating hormone (FSH), LH, estradiol, and progesterone levels to look for the etiology of her menstrual irregularity
    b. You recommend a pelvic ultrasound to verify normal anatomy and to rule out structural abnormalities and polycystic appearing ovaries
    c. You recommend a hysteroscopy to better evaluate the endometrial cavity and lining
    d. You advise expectant management for now with completion of menstrual calendar over the upcoming year
    e. You refer her to a reproductive endocrinologist or pediatric gynecologist because this issue is beyond the scope of your practice

72. A 52-year-old G3P2 comes in to see you for management of her hot flashes and night sweats. She stopped having menses 1.5 years ago and still has her ovaries and uterus in situ. She has been suffering with recurrent hot flashes and night sweats, which interfere with her quality of life. She had hoped to avoid taking hormones but her symptoms have not improved over the past 1.5 years, and she is now ready for treatment. In counseling her about treatment options for her hot flashes and night sweats, which of the following would *not* be an appropriate option?
    a. Oral estrogen and progesterone
    b. Topical estrogen and progesterone patch
    c. Low dose vaginal estrogen cream
    d. An SSRI such as paroxetine (Paxil) or fluoxetine (Prozac)
    e. Oral Gabapentin (neurontin)

73. Your next patient is here with her husband to inquire about attempting pregnancy. She is a 28-year-old G0P0 pulmonary fellow with regular 28- to 30-day menstrual cycles without heavy menses or dysmenorrhea. Her last pap was done 6 months ago and was normal. Both she and her husband are healthy and have no major medical problems. They do not have any children. She is up-to-date on her immunizations and has had a recent flu shot. She has started a prenatal vitamin and takes no other medications. She confesses that she has forgotten a lot about the menstrual cycle since medical school, but is excited to learn when their most fertile time of the month would be. Which of the following is true about ovulation and fertilization?
    a. Fertilization occurs in the uterine cavity
    b. Fertilization of the ovum must occur within 72 hours of ovulation or else it degenerates
    c. Ovulation is triggered by the production of estrogen, which triggers an LH spike from the anterior pituitary
    d. She will be most fertile during the luteal phase of her cycle and they should increase sexual activity during this time
    e. It is impossible to predict the most fertile time period for a given patient

74. A 28-year-old G1P0 woman presents at 10 weeks' gestation for her initial prenatal visit. In addition to the routine prenatal screening tests, she wishes to obtain screening for aneuploidy. The prenatal diagnostic screening modality for Down syndrome that will give the highest sensitivity is:
    a. NT at 11 weeks
    b. Combined screening (NT 1 PAPPA and free β-hCG) at 12 weeks
    c. Maternal serum triple screen (MSAFP 1 estriol 1 β-hCG) at 17 weeks
    d. Second trimester ultrasound
    e. Sequential screening with combined screening in first-trimester and quad screening in the second

75. You are consulted to see a 16-year-old G0 who presented to the emergency department with primary amenorrhea and cyclic abdominal pain. She notes that her symptoms have been worsening over the past 6 months, such that she most recently had to miss school secondary to abdominal pain and now she presents to the emergency room. You are consulted because an ultrasound revealed a normal-appearing uterus with a 4-cm cystic heterogeneous mass in the vagina below the cervix, and bilateral adnexal masses with low level echoes. You perform a physical examination, which reveals normal breast development and normal distribution of pubic hair. She has a tender, but nonacute abdomen, and her vital signs are normal. Pelvic examination reveals a normal-appearing hymenal ring, with no visible cervix. Instead, you visualize a bulging, bluish

purple pouch at the apex of the vagina. What is the most likely diagnosis?
a. Uterine didelphys
b. Uterine agenesis
c. Transverse vaginal septum
d. Imperforate hymen
e. Uterine septum

76. A 32-year-old G0 presents to your office with absent menses for 1 year. She notes that her menses had become closer together over the previous 2 years, and she attributed this to increased stress in her life. She is otherwise healthy, with no prior surgeries, and actually is hoping to get pregnant soon. She and her husband got married a little over a year ago and have been having unprotected intercourse for the past 3 months. She has become increasingly alarmed as she has been reading online about fertility because of her absent menstrual cycles. She does endorse some vague symptoms of "temperature deregulation." You perform a physical examination, which is normal. You perform a series of tests, including a TSH (normal), β-hCG (negative), prolactin (normal), a complete blood count (normal), FSH (elevated), and estradiol (low). What is the next step in your diagnosis?
a. Serum LH to determine if she is ovulating
b. Serum progesterone on Day 21 to determine if she is ovulating
c. Karyotype
d. Pelvic ultrasound and MRI to evaluate for Müllerian anomalies
e. Nothing, you have enough information to determine your diagnosis

77. A 33-year-old G3P2012 woman presents to your office with a complaint of absent menses for the past 6 months. She has a history of tubal ligation, and did a urine pregnancy test earlier that morning, which was negative, and further, she states that she is not sexually active. She has noted that she has been increasingly fatigued lately, and has noted that her hair has become more brittle and coarse, and she seems to be losing more hair than usual in the shower and on her hairbrush. She attributed many of these symptoms to stress at home related to recent separation with her husband as well as feeling exhausted chasing after her two young children. She denies any other medical problems, and other than the tubal ligation has had no surgeries. She does note that she breastfed for 6 months after her most recent child without difficulty. She takes only occasional ibuprofen for a headache and a multivitamin. She denies allergies to medication. On physical examination, you note a heart rate of 58, normal blood pressure. Her skin is notably coarse and dry, but otherwise your examination is unremarkable. You perform a series of laboratory studies including a urine pregnancy test, complete blood count, prolactin, FSH and estradiol, and thyroid function testing. All are normal with the exception of her TSH, which is markedly elevated, and T4, which is low. You recommend treatment with T4 replacement. She is hoping to have another pregnancy sometime in the future and wonders about how the medication will affect her pregnancy. You inform her that:
a. She will need less thyroid medication during pregnancy
b. She will be able to stop her thyroid medication in pregnancy
c. Her thyroid medication will not need adjustment because the fetus autoregulates its own thyroid
d. She will need more medication during her pregnancy
e. The dose of her thyroid medication will be tripled upon confirmation of pregnancy and will continue at the same dose throughout gestation

78. A 29-year-old G2P0020 presents to your office with a chief complaint of irregular menses for the past 6 months. She denies any medical problems and has a history of having her wisdom teeth extracted, but otherwise has had a negative surgical history. She is taking a multivitamin only and is using no contraception at the current time (but she denies sexual activity in the past year). Her two prior pregnancies were therapeutic abortions induced with misoprostol. She previously had normal menses, every month, not too heavy or too painful until 6 months ago. Since then she has only had two periods, the first, which seemed normal, and the second, which was light and during which she spotted for 2 weeks. For the past 2 months, she has not had any menses. She has no history of STDs, and is up-to-date with her Pap smears, all of which have been normal. On review of systems, she denies symptoms of acne or excessive hair growth, but does admit to a small amount of bilateral nipple discharge, and occasional headaches. Physical examination is performed and reveals normal vital signs, and a wholly normal examination with the exception of confirmation of bilateral clear white nipple discharge. You perform an in-office urine pregnancy test, which is negative. What is the next test or series of tests you might perform?
a. Karyotype
b. Urinary LH predictor kit

c. Pelvic ultrasound and pelvic MRI
d. TSH and PRL
e. FSH and serum estradiol

79. Your 38-year-old G4P3 calls for a work-in appointment for worsening pain with her menses. She has had regular menses all of her life with a normal amount and length of flow. She occasionally had mild to moderate cramping, which was easily treated with a dose or two of ibuprofen. Six months ago, she underwent an elective repeat cesarean section that was complicated by endomyometritis. Since the birth of her daughter 6 months ago, she had noticed that her periods are progressively more painful. Most months she finds herself curled up in a ball, using a heating pad and missing work during her cycle. She also finds that she is having pain associated with activities such as intercourse, exercise, and lifting the baby. Her pain is not relieved with NSAIDs or narcotics. On examination, she has a normal-sized uterus, which is nontender, but her pain is exacerbated with movement of her uterus during bimanual pelvic exam. Her Gonorrhea and Chlamydia screens are both negative. You order a pelvic ultrasound and CT, which both show a normal upper abdomen, uterus, tubes, and ovaries. You maximize her pain regimen, but she is still in significant pain with activity and menses. What is the most likely next step?
    a. Tell her you have done all you can, given her negative workup
    b. Start her standing narcotic order
    c. Counsel her for a diagnostic laparoscopy for likely lysis of pelvic adhesions
    d. Counsel her for a hysterectomy
    e. Refer her to the local pain clinic and/or psychiatric evaluation

80. A 34-year-old African American woman and her partner present to their first prenatal visit. She is currently 12 weeks with diamniotic–dichorionic twin gestation. Dating is by sure LMP. The patient has a history of chronic hypertension, which has been poorly controlled. She is currently taking labetalol 200 mg t.i.d., and her blood pressure today is 134/80. She quit smoking prior to conception but used to smoke one-half PPD. Her mother and sister both have diabetes, and she has been told she had prediabetes a few years ago, but has not had any follow-up care or testing. You are counseling her that her pregnancy is at risk for a number of complications due to her twin gestation, history of chronic hypertension, and history of insulin resistance. You explain that she is at increased risk for preterm labor, preterm birth, PPROM, preeclampsia, need for cesarean section, and IUGR. What is the difference between the terms SGA and IUGR?
    a. SGA refers to the fetus, whereas IUGR is specific for neonates
    b. IUGR specifically describes growth disorders related only to placental or maternal disease
    c. SGA refers to growth disturbance owing to chromosomal abnormalities or toxins
    d. SGA refers to a neonate in whom cause of small size is uncertain, whereas IUGR describes the fetus and suggests an intrauterine etiology for growth restriction
    e. IUGR refers to a neonate in whom the cause of growth disruption is not identified, whereas SGA refers to a fetus and suggests a known cause for growth restriction

81. A 45-year-old G3P2 comes to see you with a complaint of 14 months of "irregular bleeding." She previously had regular monthly menses, but over the past 2 years, they have become totally unpredictable. Sometimes she will bleed for 2 to 3 weeks off and on, and then, she may go 2 months without a cycle at all. Her pelvic examination, cervical cytology, Gonorrhea and Chlamydia screening, pregnancy test, TFTs, PRL, and FSH are all within normal limits. She has no hot flashes, night sweats, or vaginal dryness. Her pelvic ultrasound shows a normal uterus and adnexa. Her endometrial biopsy shows proliferative endometrium without hyperplasia, EIN or malignancy. How would you define her bleeding pattern?
    a. AUB-N
    b. Menorrhagia
    c. Menometrorrhagia
    d. Intermenstrual bleeding
    e. Dysfunctional uterine bleeding

82. A mother brings in her 17-year-old G0 daughter to see you for heavy painful periods. Her menarche was at age 13, and she has had fairly regular cycles for the past 2 years. However, her bleeding has often been so heavy that she soaks through a tampon and pad every 2 to 3 hours. She routinely bleeds for 7 to 9 days each cycle. She has been chronically anemic with a hematocrit of 31 despite fair compliance with iron supplementation. She also bruises easily and has a history of gingival bleeding with tooth brushing. She has frequent nosebleeds. Her mother also reports that the patient had a difficult time with persistent bleeding

after her tonsillectomy and again after her wisdom teeth extraction earlier this year. What is the next step in her evaluation?
a. Do a pregnancy test, CBC, TFTs, PRL and, if normal, start her on oral contraceptive pills to decrease her heavy menstrual bleeding
b. Do a pregnancy test, CBC, TFTs, PT, PTT, von Willebrand antigen, ristocetin cofactor, and refer to hematology to rule out bleeding disorder
c. Do a pelvic ultrasound to rule out congenital malformation and fibroids. If normal, recommend a Mirena IUD to control her bleeding
d. Recommend a trial of tranexamic acid (Lysteda) to be taken with each menstrual period
e. Get a saline sonohysterogram to evaluate the endometrial cavity and consider endometrial ablation, given her severe level of bleeding

83. Historically, before the development of the standard pregnancy test, it was diagnosed by history and physical examination. Which of the following is not a sign of pregnancy?
a. Chadwick sign
b. Goodell sign
c. Ladin sign
d. Development of linea nigra
e. Cullen sign

84. A 27-year-old G0 presents to your clinic with irregular menses. She reports 4 to 5 menstrual cycles per year for the past year. She also complains of worsening acne, and having to pluck dark hairs from her upper lip, chin, and abdomen. Your physical examination is remarkable only for the hair and acne she described, as well as obesity. You perform a bedside ultrasound that reveals multiple small follicular cysts on her bilateral ovaries. You correctly diagnose her with polycystic ovary syndrome. PCOS patients are likely to have which of the following physiologic changes?
a. Increased levels of FSH
b. Increased frequency of GnRH pulses
c. Low estradiol concentrations
d. Low free testosterone
e. Low inhibin levels

85. An 18-year-old woman presents to the emergency room with abdominal cramping and vaginal bleeding. Her vital signs are temperature 37.3°C, blood pressure 110/70, pulse 82 beats per minute, and respiratory rate 18 breaths per minute. Abdominal examination reveals mild lower abdominal tenderness to palpation without rebound tenderness or guarding. Pelvic examination reveals a mildly enlarged uterus with right adnexal fullness. A urine pregnancy test is positive. You obtain a quantitative β-hCG, complete blood count, type and screen, complete metabolic panel, and pelvic ultrasound. Her β-hCG level is 9,000 mIU/mL. Her complete blood count and complete metabolic panels are normal. Her blood type is A negative, antibody negative. The pelvic ultrasound reveals an ectopic pregnancy and a moderate amount of fluid in the pelvis. What is the next best step in treating this patient?
a. Multidose methotrexate therapy
b. Emergent laparotomy for evacuation of the ectopic pregnancy
c. Laparoscopic evacuation of the ectopic pregnancy
d. Misoprostol therapy
e. Administer RhoGAM

86. You are covering the postpartum ward and are asked to perform an examination of a 1-day-old female infant. The examination is normal with the exception of an enlarged clitoris, and only one opening other than the anus. What is the most common cause of ambiguous genitalia in females?
a. Polycystic ovary syndrome
b. Müllerian agenesis
c. Transverse vaginal septum
d. Congenital adrenal hyperplasia

87. A 30-year-old patient with polycystic ovary syndrome returns to your clinic for a follow-up visit after starting the oral contraceptive pill to reduce her symptoms of acne and hirsutism. After 6 months of use, she is pleased with the aesthetic improvements to her appearance. She wonders how the birth control pill works to improve her symptoms. You explain that the effects are due to the oral contraceptive causing:
a. Increased 5-α reductase activity in the skin
b. Lower sex hormone-binding globulin, and therefore, lower circulating testosterone
c. Increased sex hormone-binding globulin, and therefore, higher circulating testosterone
d. Increased sex hormone-binding globulin, and therefore, lower circulating testosterone
e. Stimulation of LH production leading to lower circulating testosterone

88. A 20-year-old G1P1001 presents to your clinic for her annual examination. She denies any significant past medical history or surgical history. Her pregnancy, which was 1 year prior, was uncomplicated other than gestational diabetes. She has a family history of Type 2 diabetes mellitus and

hypertension. On physical examination, you note that her BMI is 32, and that she has a gray–brown velvety discoloration on her neck and around her vulva. Her examination is otherwise normal. These findings prompt you to add which test to her health care maintenance testing?
a. Fasting glucose
b. Vulvar biopsy
c. Papanicolaou test
d. Cholesterol screening
e. Mammogram

89. A 27-year-old G1P1001 woman comes to your office 8 months following an uncomplicated vaginal delivery of a healthy male newborn. She and her husband have been trying to conceive a second pregnancy for 3 months, but she has been unsuccessful and is very anxious about this. After a thorough history, you find that she is still breast-feeding her newborn routinely and is not menstruating. Assuming that she has not yet ovulated, what is the likely underlying cause of the findings in this patient?
a. Thyroid hormone suppression of the anterior pituitary
b. Abnormal endometrial regeneration causing failure of implantation
c. Prolactin-induced inhibition of pulsatile GnRH from the hypothalamus
d. Reduced tubal motility secondary to subclinical inflammation after vaginal delivery
e. Pathologically decreased sperm count of the male partner

90. A 24-year-old G3P3003 woman presents to your practice requesting the best contraception that you have available. She has undergone three uncomplicated vaginal deliveries and has no underlying chronic medical conditions. She is agreeable to taking a pill daily and states that she is "very responsible." Which of the following has the highest actual efficacy in preventing pregnancy?
a. Coitus interruptus
b. Combined oral contraceptive pill
c. Diaphragm
d. Progesterone-only pill
e. IUD

91. A 35-year-old woman has been your patient for the past 5 years. You recently placed her on a progestin-only birth control pill given her history of smoking one PPD for nearly 20 years. All of the following are mechanisms of action for progestin-only contraceptive methods except:
a. Suppression of ovulation
b. Thickening of the cervical mucous
c. Making the endometrium unsuitable for implantation
d. Inhibiting sperm motility
e. Stimulating regression of the corpus luteum

92. A 33-year-old G2P1001 woman at 15 weeks EGA presents to your office for a return visit after a fetal diagnosis of Trisomy 18. She desires pregnancy termination. You discuss that options include labor induction and dilation and evacuation (D&E). She opts for labor induction. Which risk below would you *not* include on the consent form?
a. Infection
b. Bleeding
c. Uterine perforation
d. Possible need for additional procedures
e. Transfusion

93. A 15-year-old adolescent female presents to a family planning clinic for termination of pregnancy. Her father accompanies her. Ultrasound confirms that she has an intrauterine gestation of 6 weeks. She was recently diagnosed with chlamydia and has completed treatment. Her medical history is significant for Lupus for which she is taking daily prednisone. She desires medication abortion. Which is a contraindication to medication abortion?
a. Age less than 18
b. Gestational age less than 8 weeks
c. Chronic steroid use
d. Recent diagnosis of chlamydia
e. Teen pregnancy

94. Two weeks ago your partner performed a medical abortion on a 26-year-old G1P0 woman at 6 weeks' gestation. The patient now presents to you for her follow-up appointment and reports that she had light bleeding in the first few days after the procedure and has had no bleeding since then. On examination, she is afebrile and her abdomen is nontender. She has scant blood in the vaginal vault, her cervix is closed and her uterus is nontender. A transvaginal ultrasound shows a gestational sac. The patient is healthy but is on iron for a chronic anemia with a hematocrit of 29%. What is the best next step?
a. Repeat dose of misoprostol
b. Repeat dose of mifepristone
c. Serial ultrasounds
d. Perform a D&C
e. Perform a D&E

95. Which of the following is *not* a major cause of infertility?
a. PCOS
b. Endometriosis
c. PID and pelvic adhesions
d. Uterine fibroids
e. Advanced maternal age

96. Which of the following are potential causes for male factor infertility?
    a. Anabolic steroid use
    b. Erectile dysfunction
    c. Varicocele
    d. a and c
    e. All of the above

97. A 20-year-old G1 at 34 weeks 0 day is being induced for severe preeclampsia. She is receiving magnesium sulfate 2 g/hour IV for seizure prophylaxis. In the fourth hour of her labor induction, she experiences a tonic clonic seizure lasting approximately 2 minutes. After ensuring her airway, breathing, and circulation are intact and normal, the next step in treating this patient is:
    a. Administer hydralazine 5 mg IV push
    b. Deliver the baby immediately via cesarean section
    c. Stop the magnesium infusion and convert to phenytoin
    d. Rebolus magnesium sulfate 2 g IV
    e. Administer furosemide 40 mg IV

98. As part of routine prenatal care, there are a series of tests offered throughout pregnancy. Usually, these tests are delineated by the trimester in which they are offered. Which of the following tests are routinely offered in the second trimester?
    a. GBS
    b. Hematocrit
    c. Amniocentesis
    d. Transvaginal ultrasound for dating
    e. Fern test

99. Which are potential treatments for unexplained infertility?
    a. Ovulation induction with clomiphene citrate (Clomid) and intrauterine insemination
    b. Ovulation induction with injectable gonadotropins and intrauterine insemination
    c. IVF
    d. Expectant management
    e. All of the above

100. A 28-year-old G2P1 woman at 30 weeks GA presents to the clinic for a routine OB visit. She was diagnosed with gestational diabetes 4 weeks ago and was started on a diabetic diet and exercise regimen. She adhered to the recommendations, measured her glucose levels four times a day, and recorded results for the past week. Her average fasting glucose value is 84 mg/dL and 1-hour postprandial values after all three meals range from 135 to 165 mg/dL. What is the best next step in the management of this patient?
    a. Continue diabetic diet plus exercise
    b. Start the patient on Lispro and NPH in the morning and Lispro at dinner
    c. Start the patient on Lispro in the morning, and Lispro and NPH at dinner
    d. Start the patient on Metformin 500 mg PO daily
    e. Start the patient on NPH in the morning and NPH at dinner

101. On the basis of the 2015 ISSVD classification of squamous intraepithelial lesions of the vulva, VIN is divided into three categories. Which of the following are the correct categories?
    a. VIN 1, VIN 2, and VIN 3
    b. Vulvar low-grade squamous intraepithelial lesion (LSIL), vulvar HSIL, and differentiated type VIN
    c. Usual type, differentiated type, and undifferentiated type VIN
    d. Low-risk HPV, high-risk HPV, and non-HPV-related VIN
    e. Benign, premalignant, and malignant VIN

102. A 24-year-old G1P0 patient at 25 weeks GA presents for a routine OB visit. She is sexually active with her boyfriend of 4 years. Her BMI is 29. Physical examination is otherwise unremarkable. She was surprised when you told her she screened positive for diabetes. She is uninsured and prior to this pregnancy, had only utilized Student Health for acute illnesses, but has never been told she had diabetes before. Which of the following are the most likely diagnosis and etiology of her diabetes?
    a. Type 2 diabetes mellitus—Autoimmune destruction of β-islet cells
    b. Type 1 diabetes mellitus—Elevated progesterone levels
    c. Gestational diabetes—Human chorionic somatomammotropin
    d. Type 1 diabetes mellitus—Preexisting peripheral insulin resistance
    e. Gestational diabetes—Recently acquired HCV infection

103. Based on the current knowledge of Paget disease of the vulva, all of the following are true EXCEPT:
    a. It is most commonly seen in postmenopausal Caucasian women
    b. It may present with a concomitant adenocarcinoma
    c. Recurrences may be treated with CO_2 laser ablation
    d. The risk of invasive squamous cell carcinoma is approximately 5%
    e. It can present with chronic vulvar pruritus, red velvety lesions, and white plaques

104. A 76-year-old G0 with morbid obesity, systemic lupus, and renal failure presents to clinic with persistent vulvar pruritis in the same location for several years. She has tried multiple antifungal agents and steroid

creams over the years, but she still has persistent itching. Given this history, you perform a vulvar biopsy that shows a superficially invasive vulvar cancer. She wants to know how this happened. All of the following are risk factors of vulvar cancer except:
   a. Vulvar HSIL
   b. Oncogenic HPV types
   c. Lichen sclerosus
   d. Breast cancer
   e. Cigarette smoking

105. A 23-year-old G0 who has never had a Pap test or pelvic examination comes to the office to start on birth control pills. She tells you her periods are regular but heavy and last 7 days, and she has terrible cramps. She has been sexually active for the past 2 years with three different partners. She uses condoms most of the time. You perform an examination, including STI testing and a Pap test and prescribe a trial of oral contraceptive pills. Her STI testing is negative but her Pap test result is "atypical squamous cells of undetermined significance (ASCUS)" and a reflex HPV test is negative. What is your recommendation for this Pap test result?
   a. Proceed to colposcopy
   b. Repeat the Pap test in 3 months
   c. Repeat the Pap test and HPV test in 3 years
   d. Repeat the HPV test in 1 year
   e. LEEP conization of the cervix

106. A 38-year-old G2P2002 comes for her annual examination and Pap testing. Her periods are very light and infrequent since she had Mirena placed 3 years ago. She is recently divorced and has a new partner. She tells you her last Pap test was normal 3 years ago. Her cytology result is "negative for intraepithelial lesion or malignancy" (NILM), and the HPV test is positive for genotype 16. What do you recommend?
   a. Colposcopy
   b. Repeat Pap test and HPV in 1 year
   c. Repeat Pap test in 3 months
   d. Repeat HPV test only in 1 year
   e. LEEP conization of the cervix

107. A 28-year-old G0 had an LSIL Pap result at age 26 followed by colposcopic examination findings of CIN 1. Twelve months later, her repeat pap was normal, but HPV test was positive and colposcopy was again consistent with CIN 1. Twelve months later, the pap is still normal, but the high-risk HPV test was repeated this year and remains positive. At her colposcopy examination, you see a faintly acetowhite lesion at the squamocolumnar junction (SCJ) and biopsy of the area again returns CIN 1. The examination is satisfactory (the entire SCJ is seen), and the entire lesion is viewed. She is very concerned and would like to know what she should do now. She is a smoker but is otherwise healthy. Which option would *not* be recommended for this patient?
   a. Repeat Pap every 3 months for 1 year
   b. Cryotherapy
   c. Excisional procedure (LEEP)
   d. Repeat Pap and HPV test again in 1 year
   e. Encourage smoking cessation

108. A 16-year-old G0 is accompanied by her mother who requests you to perform STI testing, check a Pap test, and prescribe birth control pills for her daughter. The patient recently told her mother she had been sexually active for the past 2 years. She tells you she has used condoms most of the time but wants to try pills to help control her painful periods. You recommend all of the following EXCEPT
   a. HPV vaccination
   b. Pap testing in 2 years
   c. HIV, chlamydia, and gonorrhea testing
   d. Educational materials on safe sex, contraception, and dysmenorrhea
   e. Pregnancy testing

109. A 73-year-old woman presents with a chief complaint of scant vaginal spotting. She has had no other abnormal bleeding. She has had regular Pap tests her entire life. Her Pap tests have all been normal and her last one was at age 65. After obtaining a thorough history and physical examination, what test would you likely order as your next step in evaluating this patient with postmenopausal bleeding?
   a. FSH level and estradiol level
   b. Transvaginal ultrasound
   c. CA-125
   d. Complete blood count, PT/PTT
   e. Pap smear and HPV screen

110. Staging for endometrial cancer generally entails which of the following?
   a. Clinical staging with physical examination, pyelogram, chest X-ray, and anoscopy
   b. Clinical staging with physical examination, pyelogram, chest X-ray, and CAT scan
   c. Surgical staging with total hysterectomy, BSO, pelvic washings, and possible pelvic and para-aortic lymphadenectomy
   d. Surgical staging with total hysterectomy, BSO, pelvic nodes, pelvic washings, and omentectomy
   e. Surgical staging with hysterectomy only

111. Which of the following is *not* a protective factor against the development of endometrial cancer?
   a. Parity
   b. Smoking
   c. Physical activity
   d. Oral contraceptive use
   e. Tamoxifen use

112. Which of the following is the most commonly diagnosed gynecologic malignancy in the United States?
    a. Endometrial
    b. Cervical
    c. Ovarian
    d. Fallopian tube
    e. Vulvar

113. A 22-year-old G0 presents for routine examination. She is without complaints. Her LMP was 3 weeks ago and was normal. On pelvic examination, you detect a large mobile mass in the right lower quadrant. Her urine pregnancy test is negative. Pelvic ultrasound shows a 8 cm right ovarian mass. The mass is cystic with a focal solid component, calcifications, and teeth. What is the next step in the management of this patient?
    a. Repeat ultrasound in 6 weeks
    b. Exploratory laparotomy, TH/BSO
    c. Right ovarian cystectomy
    d. Removal of the right ovary and tube (RSO)
    e. Expectant management

114. A 37-year-old G2P2 reports irregular menses, intermittent pelvic pain, and a recent increase in facial and body hair. On physical examination, the patient has acne, facial hair, and a 10-cm left adnexal mass. Pelvic ultrasound confirms a solid lobulated 10-cm mass arising from the left ovary. Which of the following serum concentrations were most likely elevated?
    a. LDH
    b. Estradiol and FSH
    c. Testosterone and androstenedione
    d. AFP
    e. CA-125

115. A 20-year-old woman presents to your emergency department for new onset abnormal uterine bleeding. She is found to be pregnant with a serum β-hCG level of 300,000 mIU/mL. Both her heart rate and blood pressure are elevated. On physical examination, you palpate her uterus to be near the umbilicus, whereas her LMP places her at about 8 weeks' gestation. On ultrasound examination, there is a profound amount of vesicular appearing material without an identifiable fetus. Which of the following is *not* part of the immediate initial management plan?
    a. Determination of Rh status
    b. Surgical intervention (Suction curettage)
    c. Methotrexate administration
    d. Evaluation of thyroid status
    e. Complete blood count

116. A 25-year-old G1P0 presents to the emergency room with vaginal bleeding. Her last normal menstrual period was 6 weeks earlier. She reports that she is sexually active with male partners and does not use any hormonal or barrier methods for contraception. On arrival, her temperature is 37°C, blood pressure is 115/80, pulse is 75 beats per minute, respiratory rate is 16 breaths per minute, and she has 100% oxygen saturation on room air. A pelvic examination reveals a small amount of dark blood in the vagina. The external cervical os appears 1 to 2 cm dilated. Her uterus is mildly enlarged, anteverted, and nontender. A urine pregnancy test is positive. A pelvic ultrasound is obtained and shows an intrauterine gestational sac with a yolk sac. No fetal pole or cardiac motion is seen. Bilateral adnexa are normal. What is her diagnosis?
    a. Incomplete abortion
    b. Threatened abortion
    c. Ectopic pregnancy
    d. Missed abortion
    e. Inevitable abortion

117. A 21-year-old woman undergoes hysteroscopy and curettage for persistent irregular uterine bleeding after her term vaginal delivery 8 months ago. Final pathologic findings from the D&C are consistent with choriocarcinoma with invasion into the myometrium. Baseline serum β-hCG is 50,000 mIU/mL. Which of the following is *not* currently indicated?
    a. Imaging for distant metastatic lesions
    b. Surgical intervention with hysterectomy
    c. Chemotherapy
    d. Close surveillance of serum β-hCG
    e. Reliable contraception

118. An 18-year-old G1 sees you in your office and tells you she missed her last period and had a positive home urine pregnancy test. You perform your normal first obstetrical examination and obtain basic prenatal labs as well as a first-trimester viability ultrasound. The radiologist calls you to discuss the findings, which demonstrate a gestational sac with a fetus measuring approximately 8 weeks' gestation. There is no fetal heartbeat demonstrated. The placenta is markedly thickened and echogenic, more than would be expected in the first trimester. There are multiple areas of small cystic spaces within the placenta as well. The most likely diagnosis and corresponding karyotype is:
    a. Complete Mole, 46 XX
    b. Incomplete Mole, 46 XY
    c. Incomplete Mole, 69 XXY
    d. Complete Mole, 69 XXX
    e. Incomplete Mole, 69 XYY

119. A 33-year-old G2P1 woman presents to your office with a complaint of nipple discharge. She states that it is milky in color, comes from both

breasts, and is present even when she does not express it. You perform a breast examination, and express milky-discharge from both breasts. You diagnose her with galactorrhea. Which condition is *not* associated with galactorrhea?
a. Pregnancy
b. Breast abscess
c. Pituitary adenoma
d. Psychotropic medications
e. Hypothyroidism

120. A 42-year-old G1P1 presents to your office with a complaint of bloody nipple discharge. She undergoes excision of the involved duct for an intraductal papilloma. On pathology, she is also noted to have lobular carcinoma in situ. Which of the following statements about this diagnosis is *not* true?
a. LCIS is considered a premalignant lesion (but not a true cancer itself) because it is an indicator for subsequent risk of breast cancer
b. It is not palpable or seen on mammogram
c. The recommended treatment is observation; however, selective estrogen receptor modulators may reduce the risk of subsequent invasive cancer
d. Subsequent cancers are always on the same side as the LCIS
e. Subsequent cancers may be intraductal, invasive ductal, or lobular carcinoma

121. Which of the following would be most reassuring when assessing a fetal heart tracing?
a. Fetal heart rate of 140 with marked variability
b. Fetal heart rate of 100 with minimal variability
c. Fetal heart rate of 150 with moderate variability
d. Fetal heart rate of 90 with absent variability
e. Fetal heart rate of 190 with moderate variability

122. A 30-year-old G2P1 at 30 weeks' gestation is transported to the emergency department (ED) via ambulance after MVA. The accident involved the patient who was driving her car at approximately 40 miles/hour when she was hit on the driver's side by another car going 30 miles/hour. She was restrained by her seatbelt and her airbag deployed. She was found on the scene of the accident by the paramedics to be awake, alert, oriented despite significant pelvic pain, bruises on her abdomen from the seat belt, and a few minor lacerations. She is afebrile, BP 120/70 mm Hg, HR 120 beats per minute, arterial oxygen saturation 100%, and RR 18/min. The OB team arrives in the ED and places the baby on continuous external fetal monitoring. She is noted to have contractions every 2 minutes, and the fetal heart rate is approximately 110 beats per minute with late decelerations noted with every contraction. The paramedics report that they have not noted any vaginal bleeding. On SSE, the cervix appears to be closed with no blood noted in the vaginal vault. On bedside ultrasound, there appears to be a normal AFI and an anterior low-lying placenta and a small retroplacental fluid collection. What is the most likely cause of the late decelerations on the continuous fetal monitoring?
a. Umbilical cord compression
b. Preterm labor
c. Concealed placental abruption
d. Fetal head compression
e. Placenta previa

123. A 25-year-old Hispanic G2P1 at 36 weeks' gestation by 24 weeks ultrasound presents to L&D complaining of painful uterine contractions every 2 to 4 minutes for the last hour. She was late to prenatal care and had her first ultrasound at 28 weeks' gestation. On her ultrasound at 28 weeks, she was noted to have normal fluid and growth, no anomalies, and an anterior placenta with a posterior velamentous cord insertion. When Doppler was used during the ultrasound, it was noted that there appeared to be fetal vessels coursing across the internal os connecting to the posterior velamentous cord insertion. After her last ultrasound, the patient was lost to follow-up until she presented today. The patient denies any leakage of fluid or vaginal bleeding. On SVE, the cervix is noted to be 6 cm/90% effaced/0 station. FHR tracing is reactive with no decels. Which of the following is the most appropriate delivery plan for this patient?
a. Expectant management, vaginal delivery
b. Artificial rupture of membranes with placement of IUPC, vaginal delivery
c. Emergent cesarean section
d. Oxytocin augmentation
e. None of the above

124. In prenatal genetic testing, which of the following is *not* a trait commonly screened for in parents from high-risk populations?
a. Sickle cell disease
b. Cystic fibrosis
c. Thalassemia
d. Prader–Willi
e. Tay–Sachs

125. A 38-year-old African American G1P0 presents to L&D at 34 weeks complaining of painful uterine contractions for the last 2 hours. She denies

leakage of fluid or discharge. She does report vaginal bleeding that started 30 minutes ago. She has no significant PMH but has a past surgical history of a prior abdominal myomectomy in which she had a large anterior fibroid removed. Per the operative report, the endometrial cavity was entered to remove the fibroid. On examination, she is afebrile, vital signs stable. On ultrasound, the fetus is vertex, normal AFI, no evidence of retroplacental clot, and posterior placenta. On SSE, she has approximately 100 cc bright blood in the vaginal vault, no pool, and no ferning. Nitrazine is positive. Her cervix appears to be approximately 3 cm dilated. On the FHR tracing, the FHTs are 120s with moderate variable decelerations down to the 60s with each contraction; on tocometry, she appears to be contracting every 2 to 4 minutes. Which of the following is the most likely etiology of the antepartum hemorrhage in this clinical situation?
a. PPROM
b. Uterine rupture
c. Cervical laceration
d. Placenta previa
e. Vasa previa

126. A 34-year-old Asian woman G4P3003 at 34 weeks' gestation presents to L&D triage complaining of hematuria, dysuria, and occasional contractions for 1 week. She also notes some occasional vaginal spotting over the last 3 days. She denies any leakage of fluid or discharge. She denies back or flank pain but has had some suprapubic discomfort. She had an anatomy ultrasound at 18 weeks, where she was noted to have normal fetal anatomy, normal AFI, and an anterior complete placenta previa. She has no significant PMH. She has surgical history of three previous cesarean sections at term. Her first cesarean section was 8 years ago in China for breech at term. Owing to her social situation, she has not been able to schedule a repeat ultrasound at 30 weeks, as was recommended at the time of her anatomy ultrasound. She has not had recent intercourse. Which of the following is *not* an appropriate initial test to determine the etiology of this patient's hematuria?
a. Urine analysis
b. Urine culture
c. SSE
d. CT scan of abdomen and pelvis
e. Abdominal ultrasound of uterus

127. A 33-year-old G7P1224 at 34 weeks 1 day's gestation, with a history of prior preterm birth at 35 weeks for diamniotic–dichorionic twins and at 33 weeks with a singleton PPROM, presents with sudden onset vaginal bleeding and abdominal pain. Her medical history is significant for ruptured appendectomy requiring emergency surgery at age 19. Social history is complicated. She lives with her mother and older sister in a two-bedroom apartment with her four children. She does not work outside the home and smokes one-half PPD of tobacco. She takes methadone for history of heroin use. Current medications include methadone, prenatal vitamin, and iron supplement. Which of the following is not associated with risk of preterm birth?
a. Socioeconomic status
b. PPROM
c. Placental abruption
d. Her age
e. Her BMI of 18

128. Your next patient is a 62-year-old G2P2 with biopsy proven vulvar HSIL who is returning for discussion of results. While counseling her you explain the risk factors for the development of vulvar intraepithelial neoplasia including
a. Immunosuppression
b. Smoking
c. High-risk HPV infection
d. Asian ethnicity
e. a, b, and c

Answers

1. c (Chapter 31)
Metastatic persistent gestational trophoblastic neoplasia (GTD) most commonly (90%) presents after evacuation of a molar pregnancy given the persistent elevated β-hCG and evidence of metastatic disease. This patient's history is consistent with a suction curettage performed a year ago, probably for molar pregnancy. Most patients with persistent GTD will have localized disease in the uterus (typically due to invasive mole), but rarely, metastasis can occur. Metastatic foci are more associated with choriocarcinoma than invasive molar pregnancy. This patient's symptoms are probably due to spread to the lungs, the most common site for metastasis. The brain, liver, bowel, kidney, and vagina are other potential sites of metastasis. The bloody sputum and high β-hCG level would not be associated with an ectopic pregnancy.

2. a (Chapter 17)
The histologic finding of plasma cells in the endometrial stroma is indicative of chronic endometritis. Both acute and chronic inflammatory cells are often seen histologically. Chronic endometritis is often asymptomatic but can be linked to infertility. Symptomatic women usually present with abnormal uterine bleeding (AUB) and lower abdominal pain or cramping. Doxycycline is the treatment of choice.

b. Insertion of a levonorgestrel-releasing intrauterine system (LNG-IUS) is not a treatment for chronic endometritis. LNG-IUS may be used to treat women with endometrial hyperplasia. Histologic findings of endometrial hyperplasia include proliferation of endometrial glands and an increased gland-to-stroma ratio. Other noncontraceptive uses of the LNG-IUS include treatment of dysmenorrhea, pelvic pain, and menorrhagia.

c. Hysteroscopy is a minimally invasive surgical approach that can be utilized to view the inside of the endometrial cavity. It is used for the evaluation and treatment of a variety of conditions, including AUB, polyps, fibroids, Müllerian anomalies, and infertility. In this case, the patient has already undergone a pelvic ultrasound and endometrial biopsy. No further evaluation is needed because a diagnosis of chronic endometritis has already been made.

d. Chronic endometritis is not an indication for hysterectomy.

e. Cefoxitin is commonly used in the treatment of puerperal endomyometritis.

3. c (Chapter 7)
There is concern for fetal hemolysis when a titer of 1:16 or greater is identified. Once Rh sensitization is discovered, titers should be checked every 4 weeks. You would begin fetal testing between 16 and 20 weeks of gestation when the titer reaches 1:16. Testing used to be performed by serial amniocentesis, and the amniotic fluid was analyzed by a spectrophotometer that measures the light absorption (DOD_{450}) by bilirubin, which will accumulate in the amniotic fluid with increasing fetal hemolysis. The results were plotted on the Liley curve (Fig. 7-5), which predicts the severity of disease. Fetal cells obtained via amniocentesis can also be analyzed for Rh status. If fetal Rh status is negative, Rh incompatibility is no longer a concern for the pregnancy. Over the past decade, fetal anemia in the setting of alloimmunization is screened for with middle cerebral artery (MCA) Doppler measurements. With fetal anemia, the blood is shunted to the fetal brain and the velocity of the blood is faster. Thus, the measurement on MCA Doppler followed is the peak systolic velocity. When this measurement exceeds 1.55 multiples of median, the concern for fetal anemia is high and a percutaneous umbilical blood sampling (PUBS) procedure is performed. A fetal blood transfusion can be performed if anemia is confirmed.

a, b. These describe titer levels that are not concerning. At levels of 1:4 and 1:8, the patient can continue to be monitored but does not require further intervention until the titer reaches 1:16.

d, e. Both these titer levels warrant further testing with MCA Doppler but they are not the lowest answer choices available in this scenario.

4. d (Chapter 32)
Many patients' fears over breast cancer can be alleviated by counseling and discussion of risk factors with them. Genetic counseling and breast center referral are available for patients who require additional reassurance and those who are in high-risk categories. Recommendations for breast cancer screening vary slightly among major national health organizations. The American College of Obstetrics and Gynecology (ACOG) and the American Cancer Society (ACS) agree that overall breast self-awareness is the recommended surveillance for women age 20–39, coupled with clinical breast examination (CBE) every 1 to 3 years. She may participate in breast self-examinations

if she chooses. If a mass is palpated or she turns 40, she is then a candidate for imaging. Women at high risk should include MRI with the screening mammography every year, beginning at age 40. However, she is not in the high-risk category with her history. High-risk groups include women who have a known *BRCA1* or *BRCA2* gene mutation, have a first-degree relative with either mutation, are at high risk based on an evaluation by a validated risk assessment tool, underwent radiation to the chest between the ages of 10 and 30, or have a hereditary syndrome associated with multiple cancer diagnoses (e.g., Lynch syndrome). These women should begin screening at age 30 or 5-10 years before the earliest familial breast cancer diagnosis. Ultrasound is used in the evaluation of uncertain mammographic findings, breast cysts, in women under 40, in women with dense breast tissue, and as a tool to guide a needle for breast biopsies.

5. c (Chapter 3)

Maternal serum screening is both for aneuploidy such as Trisomy 21, 18, or 13 and for neural tube defects via the maternal serum alpha fetoprotein (MSAFP). Of note, an elevated MSAFP screens for fetal abdominal wall defects as well. Fragile X syndrome is an X-linked disorder whose etiology is a triplet repeat. Carriers usually have the premutation with 40 to 49 triplet repeats, which then can expand to a full mutation. Because it is X-linked, women are usually only mildly affected, but women with cognitive disabilities related to the Fragile X mutation have been identified. Fragile X is not screened for with maternal serum screening.

6. b (Chapter 24)

A history of venous thromboembolism (DVT and PE) is an absolute contraindication to using combined oral contraceptives. Other absolute contraindications include history of coronary artery disease, cerebrovascular accident, and a history of breast cancer, endometrial cancer, or other estrogen-dependent cancers. Benign or malignant liver tumors, severe cirrhosis, and uncontrolled hypertension are also absolute contraindications to combined oral contraceptive pill (OCP) use. All of the others listed are relative contraindications. Migraine headaches without aura, instead of tension headaches, are a relative contraindication to use. Migraine headache with vascular compromise or visual aura is generally regarded as absolute contraindication to combined OCP use. Women over 35 who smoke greater than 15 cigarettes/day should not use OCPs. Progestin only contraception would be acceptable in this patient. However, long-acting reversible contraception (LARC) or permanent contraception would be best for a patient with this history. In general, combination OCPs may be used in women with well-controlled hypertension, uncomplicated diabetes, and depression.

7. a (Chapter 4)

Maternal hypotension, secondary to decreased systemic vascular resistance, is a complication associated with both epidural and spinal anesthesia, though it is a bit more common with spinal anesthesia. In severe cases, it can lead to decreased placental perfusion and fetal heart rate decelerations or even bradycardia. Occasionally, if the anesthetic reaches the innervations of the diaphragm, it can cause maternal respiratory depression as opposed to hyperventilation. Increased contraction strength is not associated with either spinal or epidural analgesia, though a decrease in contractions has been seen with both. Finally, chorioamnionitis is not associated with spinal or epidural anesthesia, though increased maternal fever is seen with epidural analgesia, particularly over time.

8. d (Chapter 4)

All of the answer choices are signs of active labor with the exception of fever and chills, which is not normal and could be a sign of infection.

9. a (Chapter 8)

There are a wide range of risk factors for developing preeclampsia, including extremes of maternal age, nulliparity, chronic hypertension, renal disease, diabetes, lupus, African American race, short cohabitation time, history of preeclampsia, molar pregnancy, and so on. However, smoking, while a risk factor for many other problems in pregnancy, has been associated with a decreased risk of preeclampsia in several studies.

10. a (Chapter 25)

First-trimester abortion is very safe. It is important to counsel the patient and her mother on possible risks of the procedure but they can be reassured that the risk of serious complication is very low. The most recent maternal mortality rate for induced abortion in the United States ranges from 0.3 per 100,000 abortions at or <8 weeks of pregnancy to 6 per 100,000 abortions >18 weeks of gestation. This is in comparison to a maternal mortality of 18.5 per 100,000 for completed pregnancy and delivery. The major causes of abortion mortality are complications of hemorrhage and infection, followed by thromboembolism (DVT and PE) and anesthetic complications. In general, maternal morbidity is lowest if abortion is performed before 8 weeks of gestation. Less than 0.05% of abortions performed in the first-trimester result in complications that require hospitalization.

11. e (Chapter 8)

In this setting, there are two indications for immediate delivery. The first is the severe headache that does not resolve with acetaminophen. The second is Hemolysis, Elevated Liver Enzymes, Low Platelets (HELLP) syndrome with markedly elevated liver function tests (LFTs) and platelets less than 100,000. Although expectant management of severe preeclampsia is the standard of care in most settings, severe symptoms and HELLP are two of the reasons to abandon with expectant management. However, one can still give betamethasone as an induction of labor may take 24 hours, and the fetus will get the acute steroid benefits. During the induction, one would control blood pressure, most commonly with IV labetolol or hydralazine, to keep them in the 140 to 150/80 to 100 range not only to minimize risk from severe blood pressure, but also to avoid hypotension as well. Magnesium sulfate would be given for seizure prophylaxis.

12. c (Chapter 6)

This scenario describes a uterine rupture. History of prior cesarean section is a risk factor for uterine rupture. In this case, the patient experienced a sudden change in pain, vaginal bleeding, followed by a change in fetal status, and a change in fetal station with the fetus moving back out of the pelvis. Placental abruption can present with similar findings of vaginal bleeding, abdominal pain, and change in fetal status; however, this scenario is most suggestive of uterine rupture, given the history of prior cesarean section. Vasa previa presents with painless vaginal bleeding and fetal distress, often precipitated by rupture of membranes. Fetal nuchal cord can cause changes in fetal heart rate such as variable decelerations, but generally does not occur until the patient is in the second stage of labor, and is not associated with vaginal bleeding.

13. c (Chapter 6)

Standard evaluation for ruptured membranes includes a sterile speculum examination. Findings of liquid pooling in the vagina, positive nitrazine test, and ferning on microscopy are diagnostic of ruptured membranes. AmniSure, ultrasound, and amnio dye tests are all tests that can be used to diagnose rupture when standard sterile speculum findings are not conclusive. Amniocentesis is helpful if you are concerned about infection, which is suspected based on maternal fever, elevated WBC, or abdominal tenderness.

14. e (Chapter 26)

All of these options will treat pain due to endometriosis. However, in women who are trying to conceive, medical management has no role in decreasing infertility. It is thought that endometrial implants result in infertility by causing disruption of normal tissue, formation of adhesions and fibrosis, and severe inflammation. The resulting adhesions and inflammation can also result in distortion of the fallopian tubes and other anatomic structures. Surgical resection of endometrial implants has been found to increase the fertility rate in women with mild, moderate, and severe endometriosis.

15. b (Chapter 6)

Betamethasone is the only choice that has been shown to improve pregnancy outcomes. Betamethasone, if given 48 hours prior to delivery, reduces neonatal morbidity. Tocolytics can be used for up to 48 hours to administer corticosteroids for fetal well-being. With prolonged ruptured membranes, hospital observation and bed rest are the standard of care due to the risk of development of chorioamnionitis, cord prolapse, and placental abruption, but they do not have as great a benefit as corticosteroids. Lastly, augmentation of labor would not be recommended until after completion of corticosteroids and 34 weeks of gestation unless there was a nonreassuring fetal heart rate tracing or signs of fetal infection.

16. d (Chapter 7)

Chorioamnionitis occurs in approximately 1% to 5% of pregnancies and is generally the result of an ascending infection from organisms normally present in the vaginal flora. Occasionally, it may result from hematogenous dissemination. Young age, low socioeconomic status, nulliparity, prolonged rupture of membranes, and preexisting infection in the genital tract are all risk factors for chorioamnionitis. It is not associated with intrauterine growth restriction (IUGR).

Answers b, c, d, and e are all placental problems that can result in IUGR. Abnormal placental vascular development or disruptions in the vascular network all can lead to growth disruption in the fetus. Chronic placental abruption reduces the functioning surface of the placenta. Placenta previa is believed to increase the risk for IUGR because the placenta is located in the lower uterine segment, which is felt to a suboptimal location for nutrient exchange. Placental thrombosis or infarction decreases the volume of functioning placenta and thereby decreases the nutrient and oxygen exchange interface between the mother and the fetus. Lastly, marginal cord insertion is associated with IUGR because of its abnormal vascular formation and likely effect on nutrient exchange.

17. d (Chapter 7)

Polyhydramnios is associated with gestational diabetes, congenital anomalies, multiple gestations, and neural tube defects. Polyhydramnios is not found in Potter syndrome. In fact, Potter syndrome is characterized by anhydramnios secondary to renal agenesis and therefore decreased production of amniotic fluid.

a. Gestational diabetes is a common cause of mild polyhydramnios presenting later in pregnancy.

b. Congenital anomalies such as esophageal atresia or other intestinal obstructions limit fluid passage uptake in the GI tract and result in polyhydramnios.

c. Twin–twin transfusion syndrome (TTTS) can cause polyhydramnios in the recipient twin. TTTS occurs in monochorionic gestations, where vascular connections exist between the veins and the arteries on the surface of the placenta. The donor twin shunts arterial blood to the recipient via arterial–venous connections. The recipient twin, therefore, sees a larger volume of blood flow and as a result may develop polyhydramnios.

e. Neural tube defects contribute to polyhydramnios by leaking cerebrospinal fluid into the amniotic environment.

18. c (Chapter 8)

This patient has only had one elevated blood pressure, so she does not have a diagnosis yet. To make the diagnosis of gestational hypertension, one must have two elevated blood pressures 6 hours apart. A patient with a mildly elevated blood pressure, no symptoms, and normal labs may go home to do the 24-hour urine protein to bring it back for a recheck of BPs and labs. In some institutions, the initial evaluation would occur entirely in the hospital. Even though she has a negative urine dip for protein, a significant proportion of such patients will have significant proteinuria on a 24-hour collection; thus, it is important to do a 24-hour urine collection. Patients with mild gestational hypertension or preeclampsia are usually managed expectantly until 37 weeks and then delivered.

19. a (Chapter 9)

Between 1% to 12% of pregnant women will develop gestational diabetes, depending on the population. In the United States, the range is between 5% and 8%. Gestational diabetes is seen at higher rates in women of Hispanic/Latina, Native American, and Asian/Pacific Islander descent. GDM is also seen with increasing maternal age, obesity, presence of family history of diabetes, previous stillborn infant, or birth of a previous infant weighing more than 4,000 g. Initial studies found African American women to have higher rates of GDM compared with Caucasians. However, when controlled for maternal body mass index (BMI) in subsequent studies, little difference in incidence was observed between African Americans and Caucasians.

20. e (Chapter 9)

Forceps and vacuum should generally not be used when macrosomia is suspected owing to increased risk of shoulder dystocia, except in the case of true outlet forceps for nonreassuring fetal monitoring.

a. Class A2 gestational diabetics, who by definition are on insulin or a hypoglycemic agent, are generally scheduled to be induced at 39 weeks of gestation.

b. Because of increased risk of macrosomia in A2 GDM patients, they commonly receive an obstetric ultrasound to estimate fetal weight between 34 and 37 weeks of gestation.

c. Patients with an EFW greater than 4,000 g have increased risk of shoulder dystocia. However, elective cesarean delivery is not routinely offered to women until the EFW is greater than 4,500 g.

d. Upon admission to labor and delivery, long-acting hypoglycemics are withheld to closely monitor blood glucose levels. Dextrose and insulin drips are used to maintain blood glucose between 100 and 120 mg/dL. If levels increase above 120 mg/dL, insulin can be increased. If levels drop between 80 and 100 mg/dL, dextrose can be started or increased.

21. d (Chapter 10)

A urine culture is performed at the initial prenatal visit to screen for asymptomatic bacteriuria, defined as greater than 100,000 colony forming units. The rate of asymptomatic bacteriuria during pregnancy is approximately 5% and is the same for nonpregnant women. However, in pregnant women, they are at increased risk of progression to cystitis or pyelonephritis, which has significant morbidity. In addition, the presence of asymptomatic bacteriuria also increases the risk of preterm birth, and this risk can be decreased with appropriate treatment.

a. You can screen for gonorrhea and chlamydia by performing a DNA probe analysis of an unclean urine sample; however, these sexually transmitted infections (STIs) are not detected by urine culture.

b. There are no data to support an association between asymptomatic bacteriuria and chorioamnionitis or neonatal sepsis. During pregnancy, screening for group B streptococcus is performed between 35 and 37 weeks, and if a woman is found to be positive, she is treated during labor with penicillin to decrease her risk of chorioamnionitis and neonatal sepsis.

c. Rates of asymptomatic bacteriuria are the same in pregnant and nonpregnant women. Increased bacterial ascent up the urinary system is thought to be caused by progesterone-induced increased smooth muscle relaxation and ureteral dilation. This leads to an increased risk of cystitis and pyelonephritis compared with nonpregnant women.

e. The patient is clinically well and has no symptoms of pyelonephritis (fever, dysuria, or costovertebral angle tenderness).

22. b (Chapter 10)

Chronic Hepatitis B is diagnosed by serum studies showing persistent Hepatitis B antigen. Pregnancy is generally well-tolerated by these women, and the reactivation of the virus or exacerbation of the disease rarely occurs. The placenta acts as a barrier to the Hepatitis B virus, and as a result intrauterine infection with the virus is exceptionally rare. This patient's main risk is that of vertical transmission at the time of delivery due to exposure to maternal blood. To decrease this risk, the neonate should be given both the Hepatitis B vaccine (HBV) and Hepatitis B antibody at birth. There is no evidence that cesarean delivery decreases vertical transmission and vaginal delivery should be encouraged. Women who have high HBV viral loads may be candidates for treatment with antivirals (e.g. lamivudine) to further decrease rates of vertical transmission.

    a. We would recommend that this patient be referred to a physician that specializes in chronic liver disease. She may be a candidate for serial LFTs based on the duration of her disease and viral load.

    c. Hepatitis B screening is performed by testing for hepatitis surface antigen. The chronic carrier state for HBV is defined by the persistence of HBsAg and the absence of Hepatitis B surface IgG antibody (anti-HBs). Acute infection with hepatitis B is diagnosed by the presence of IgM antibody to the hepatitis B core antigen (IgM anti-HBc), which is then present for approximately 6 months after initial infection.

    d. Chronic Hepatitis B has not been associated with fetal malformations because the virus does not cross the placenta.

    e. See description to answer b.

23.   a (Chapter 10)

The classic triad of congenital toxoplasmosis includes chorioretinitis, intracranial calcifications, and hydrocephalus. Severe congenital infection can involve fevers, seizures, chorioretinitis, hydro- or microcephaly, hepatosplenomegaly, and jaundice.

    b. Although vertical transmission of syphilis can occur at any time during pregnancy and during any stage of disease, because there must be spirochetemia for vertical transmission to occur, approximately half of prenatal transmission occurs in pregnant women with primary or secondary syphilis. If early congenital syphilis is untreated, manifestations of late congenital syphilis can develop, including eighth nerve deafness, saber shins, mulberry molar, Hutchinson teeth, and a saddle nose.

    c. Rubella infection can be transmitted to the fetus and cause congenital rubella infection, which may lead to congenital rubella syndrome (CRS). The maternal–fetal transmission rate is highest during the first trimester, as are the rates of congenital abnormalities. The congenital abnormalities associated with CRS include deafness, cardiac abnormalities, cataracts, and mental retardation. Specifically, if maternal rubella infection occurs during the period of organogenesis, any fetal organ system may be affected.

    d. CMV causes in utero infections in approximately 1% of all newborns. Of these infected infants, approximately 10% will be symptomatic at birth. Infants who are symptomatic can develop cytomegalic inclusion disease manifested by a constellation of findings, including hepatomegaly, splenomegaly, thrombocytopenia, jaundice, cerebral calcifications, chorioretinitis, and interstitial pneumonitis. Affected infants have a high mortality rate of up to 30% and may develop mental retardation, sensorineural hearing loss, and neuromuscular disorders. Of the remaining 90% of asymptomatic infants, 15% will go on to develop late disabilities, whereas 85% will have no sequelae of the infection.

    e. Fetal infection with *Listeria* causes disseminated granulomatous lesions with microabscesses, chorioamnionitis, and placental lesions. The overall mortality from listeriosis is about 25% in reported cases.

24.   c (Chapter 10)

A large Cochrane review has shown that in women with prior preterm birth, similar to this patient, screening and treatment for bacterial vaginosis may decrease the risk of preterm premature rupture of membranes. There have been some studies to suggest that screening and treatment for bacterial vaginosis may decrease preterm birth, but this finding was not seen in the Cochrane meta-analysis. Screening and treating women who are at average risk for preterm birth have not been shown to decrease rates of preterm birth or PPROM.

    a. Untreated gonorrhea at the time of delivery can lead to ophthalmia neonatorum and blindness. In the United States, this is uncommon due to routine screening at the beginning of pregnancy and the application of prophylactic erythromycin eye therapy after delivery.

    b. During pregnancy, screening for group B streptococcus is performed between 35 and 37 weeks, and if a woman is found to be positive, she is treated during labor with penicillin to decrease her risk of chorioamnionitis and neonatal sepsis.

    d. Placental abruption is most commonly due to hypertensive disorders of pregnancy, preterm premature rupture of membranes, trauma, and cocaine or tobacco use, among other etiologies.

    e. Bacterial vaginosis has not been shown to increase risk of congenital malformations. Oral metronidazole is the recommended treatment during pregnancy. A meta-analysis found no evidence that the use of oral metronidazole in the first trimester leads to congenital malformations.

25.   c (Chapter 10)

Group B *Streptococcus* is a major pathogen in neonatal sepsis, which has severe implications. Although early-onset neonatal sepsis occurs in 2 to 3 per 1,000 live births, the mortality rate with group B *Streptococcal* sepsis ranges from 5% to 50%, depending on gestational age at the time of delivery. To protect infants from group B *Streptococcus* infections, widespread screening programs have been implemented utilizing a rectovaginal culture for group B *Strep* colonization between 35 and 37 weeks. Large prospective studies have demonstrated that these screening programs do decrease the rate of neonatal sepsis from group B *Strep*. Women with positive group B *Strep* cultures are subsequently treated with IV penicillin G in labor. Treatment is also recommended on the basis of risk factors for women with an unknown group B *Strep* status and one of the following risk factors: gestational age before 37 weeks, rupture of membranes greater than 18 hours, GBS bacteriuria in the current pregnancy, previous infant with invasive GBS disease, or intrapartum fever greater than 100.4°F.

26. a (Chapter 11)

This patient likely has hyperemesis gravidarum based on clinical symptoms of persistent nausea and vomiting with ketonuria and electrolyte disturbances. This occurs with approximately 0.3% to 2% of pregnancies. Once diagnosed, the main goal is to correct any underlying electrolyte disturbances and admit for IV fluids and antiemetics for symptom control. Your next step should be to order an obstetric ultrasound to confirm an intrauterine pregnancy. Hyperemesis gravidarum is more likely to occur with molar pregnancies and your management would be to proceed with dilation and curettage.

b. The initial goal for treatment of hyperemesis gravidarum is to control symptoms. This often means replacement of IV fluids due to dehydration and IV electrolytes given persistent emesis in addition to IV antiemetics. Most patients will improve with conservative management and begin to tolerate a bland diet. A nasogastric tube is indicated for severe cases that are refractory to all pharmacologic and nonpharmacologic interventions.

c. This patient's clinical presentation is consistent with hyperemesis gravidarum. She is afebrile and has no symptoms concerning an infectious etiology.

d. This patient has had a recent bowel movement and currently has a benign abdominal examination, which is inconsistent with a diagnosis of small bowel obstruction.

e. Initial treatment for hyperemesis gravidarum is to control symptoms. TPN has significant risk of liver dysfunction, lipid abnormalities, and sepsis and should be avoided during pregnancy.

27. b (Chapter 11)

To minimize the risk of congenital malformations, the goal should be to optimize her regimen with a plan to transition to one medication. There is evidence that epileptic women have an increased risk of fetal malformations even without AED use. The data suggest that monotherapy does not increase that baseline risk, and decreasing her regimen to one medication should be the goal to minimize her risk during the upcoming pregnancy. There is evidence that with each additional AED medication, there is an increased incidence of fetal malformations.

a. She should be counseled not to stop her seizure medications because this puts her at risk of increased seizure activity. Women who are seizure-free for 2 to 5 years may want to trial being off all therapy because they have an improved chance of remaining seizure-free when off medications.

c. Women with epilepsy have an increased incidence of neural tube defects, even if not on antiepileptic medication. In a randomized controlled trial, supplementation with 4 mg of folic acid significantly reduced that risk. As a result, women with epilepsy should be counseled to take 4 mg of folic acid, not the standard 400 mcg that all women are counseled to take prenatally.

d. Because this patient has been seizure-free for almost 2 years, she has a good chance of weaning down to one medication. Monotherapy has the lowest rates of fetal malformations, and that should be the goal. Simply increasing the folic acid to 4 mg is not sufficient to decrease her risk.

e. The recommendation is to attempt to transition to monotherapy, but valproic acid would not be the medication of choice, given the increased rates of fetal malformations with this medication.

28. e (Chapter 2)

The patient's reported history of two second-trimester losses with rapid delivery after mild spotting is suggestive of cervical incompetence. Cervical incompetence accounts for 15% of all second-trimester miscarriages. The patient has also had a prior LEEP, which places her at increased risk for cervical incompetence. She should be offered a prophylactic cerclage, which may have as much as a 90% success rate (e). With both of her prior losses, genetic analysis of fetal tissue was normal. Karyotyping and chorionic villus sampling of the patient and her partner are less appropriate first steps (a, c). Although a hysterosalpingogram may reveal a uterine anomaly, this test cannot be performed during pregnancy and thus will not help your patient during her current pregnancy (b). There is no evidence of a luteal phase defect in this patient (d).

29. b (Chapter 1)

Conservative therapy such as lower extremity elevation and pressure stockings during pregnancy can help to minimize existing varicose veins and prevent new ones from forming. If varicose veins do not improve by 6 months postpartum, surgery can be considered, but it is not the first line of treatment. The other answer choices are not indicated for the treatment of varicose veins.

30. c (Chapter 3)

Fetal nuchal translucency (NT) screening in the first trimester offers an evaluation of risk of trisomy 21, 13, and 18 early in pregnancy between 11 and 14 weeks. One of the benefits of this early test is that information is gained early and if it is a positive screen, it can be followed by a diagnostic test. CVS and amniocentesis can both provide diagnostic testing for chromosomal disorders, but CVS can be done much earlier in pregnancy. Offering CVS testing to this patient is the most appropriate next step. Although one would also offer amniocentesis in several weeks as an alternative, it would not be appropriate at the current gestation. It appears that the pregnancy loss risk may be slightly higher with CVS, so some individuals will choose to wait. Repeating the ultrasound is not an appropriate option if the nuchal region of the fetus was adequately seen. Lastly, termination of the pregnancy without definitive diagnostic testing in a desired pregnancy would not be the most appropriate next step.

31. b (Chapter 11)

This patient has a moderate-risk cardiac lesion, and pregnancy is not contraindicated. If she were to come for preconception counseling, a referral to a cardiologist would have been recommended to discuss valve replacement, as that could decrease her risk of complications during this pregnancy. At the time of her presentation to labor and delivery, the most important plan for management is strict fluid monitoring with a goal to maximize afterload to maintain cardiac output. Strict intake and output will allow for appropriate fluid balance to be maintained. In addition, for most cardiac patients, the stress of labor and delivery is minimized with an early epidural to diminish pain response, and possibly an assisted vaginal delivery (using forceps or vacuum) to diminish the effects from Valsalva.

a. This patient does not have a high-risk cardiac lesion, and therefore, it is not recommended that she receive antibiotic prophylaxis against subacute bacterial endocarditis (SBE). The 2007 American Heart Association Guidelines state that routine vaginal delivery and cesarean section are not indications for SBE prophylaxis. SBE prophylaxis may be considered for women with high-risk lesions (mechanical or prosthetic valves, unrepaired cyanotic lesions, etc.) and an infection that could cause bacteremia (chorioamnionitis or pyelonephritis).

c. There have been no clinical benefits shown with cesarean delivery in patients with cardiac lesions. As a result, vaginal delivery is the preferred option to minimize recovery time.

d. Patients with moderate risk cardiac lesions can often be managed on labor and delivery with strict intake and output and close observation. Patients with high-risk lesions or evidence of cardiovascular compromise may be admitted to the ICU for more intensive monitoring.

e. To maintain adequate cardiac output in aortic stenosis, adequate afterload is necessary. Giving lasix would decrease afterload, decrease cardiac output, and may precipitate cardiovascular compromise.

32. a (Chapter 11)

A constellation of abnormalities in the infants born to women who abuse alcohol during pregnancy have been included in the diagnosis of fetal alcohol syndrome (FAS). FAS, which includes growth retardation, CNS effects, and abnormal facies, is estimated to occur in approximately 1 in 2,000 live births. The syndrome has a spectrum of increasing severity in children of women who drink more heavily (two to five drinks/day) during pregnancy. However, there is no safe amount of alcohol in pregnancy that confers no risk. The diagnosis is made by a history of alcohol abuse in the mother combined with the constellation of infant abnormalities. Other teratogenic effects of alcohol include almost every organ system. Cardiac defects are particularly associated with alcohol abuse.

Maternal and neonatal withdrawal, low fetal birth weight, and neonatal admission to the NICU are all complications of alcohol dependence in pregnancy; however, these are self-limited.

33. c (Chapter 11)

Tobacco use during pregnancy has not been shown to increase rates of fetal malformations. In contrast, maternal alcohol use in pregnancy has been shown to increase the risk of cardiac defects and FAS (growth retardation, abnormal facies, and CNS effects).

a, b, d and e. Cigarette smoking in pregnancy has been associated with increased risk of spontaneous abortions, preterm births, abruptio placentae, and decreased birth weight. Further, infants exposed to cigarette smoking in the womb are at an increased risk for sudden infant death syndrome and respiratory illnesses of childhood. A dose–response effect has been noted for many of these outcomes. In the Ontario Perinatal Mortality Study, smokers were divided into less than one pack per day (PPD) and more than one PPD. A 20% increase in the risk of fetal death was found in those pregnancies in which patients smoked less than one PPD and a 35% increase in the more than one PPD group.

34. c (Chapter 30)

The mainstay of treatment for ovarian cancer is surgery with complete surgical staging, including total abdominal hysterectomy, bilateral salpingo-oophorectomy, collection of peritoneal washings, sampling of pelvic and paraaortic lymph nodes, omentectomy, and cytoreduction of any visible tumor. The patient typically then undergoes chemotherapy with paclitaxel or docetaxel combined with carboplatin or cisplatin. For advanced stage disease, if the patient has undergone optimal tumor debulking, a combination of intravenous and intraperitoneal chemotherapy is recommended.

35. e (Chapter 12)

Infants who are not exposed to adequate amounts of sun will not generate sufficient quantities of vitamin D if exclusively breast-feeding. Breast milk alone does not provide adequate amounts of vitamin D (25 IU/L).

Published case reports of rickets in breast-fed infants in the United States exist. Consequently, in 2008, the American Academy of Pediatrics (AAP) published guidelines for the supplementation of breast-feeding infants with 400 IU of vitamin D per day, beginning in the first few days of life. At risk breast-feeding infants include those living at high latitudes, in areas of high pollution or cloud cover, or those using sunscreen or with darker skin.

a. Maternal Hepatitis C is not a contraindication to breast-feeding. Although the virus is transmissible via the breast milk, the rate of infant infection is the same as that seen among bottle-fed infants owing to baseline risk of infection with vaginal delivery (4%). There is similarly no contraindication to breast-feeding among patients with active Hepatitis B so long as their infants receive Hepatitis B IgG passive prophylaxis and vaccine active prophylaxis.

b. Breast augmentation is not a contraindication to breast-feeding, although 65% of women who have undergone augmentation mammoplasty have lactation insufficiency. This is most common among patients who undergo a periareolar approach, which is more likely to sever ducts and damage breast tissue. Although some patients with a history of augmentation may initially have a low supply, there is no reason not to try because it can become sufficient if suckling is continued regularly.

c. Depo-Provera is a progesterone-only method that is compatible with breast-feeding. Methods that may affect breast-feeding include combined methods such as pills, rings, and patches.

d. Many young parents are often concerned about their milk supply during the first days of feeding, resorting to bottle-feeding to satiate their infant. However, parents should be reminded of the small volume of the newborn stomach that needs relatively small amounts initially. Continuous attempts at suckling should be encouraged to stimulate lactation and ultimately ensure an adequate supply in the future.

36. d (Chapter 12)

Carboprost is a synthetic prostaglandin analog of $PGF_{2\alpha}$. As $PGF_{2\alpha}$ is also an inflammatory mediator of bronchial smooth muscle, case reports have been written on the incidence of bronchospasm associated with the use of Carboprost (Hemabate) in asthmatic patients. Given that there are other readily available pharmaceutical options for the treatment of postpartum hemorrhage, including oxytocin, misoprostol, and methergine; the general consensus is that Carboprost should be avoided when possible in patients with any history of asthma.

a. Contraindications to oxytocin in the immediate postpartum period are few. Case reports exist of patients exhibiting severe water intoxication, with convulsions and coma, as a function of slow oxytocin infusion over a 24-hour period. Maternal death has been reported. Acute injection of Oxytocin is considered a safe option and is sometimes routinely used in Stage III of labor for active, expeditious delivery of the placenta.

b. Methylergonovine is an ergot-alkaloid that functions by stimulating blood vessel constriction and smooth muscle contraction. It is frequently used to both prevent and control postpartum hemorrhage. Given its vessel constricting properties, methylergonovine can raise the blood pressure, making it contraindicated in patients with a history of hypertension or preeclampsia.

c. In this patient's case, misoprostol may have been contraindicated in the management of her labor due to an increased risk of uterine rupture with a history of cesarean section; however, in the postpartum period, misoprostol is a valuable medication for postpartum hemorrhage that can be given per oral, sublingual, buccal, or rectum. Although less acutely effective than injectables, misoprostol is a shelf-stable, inexpensive uterotonic that is gaining in popularity, even for the prevention of hemorrhage during cesarean sections.

e. As per response a, Oxytocin is not contraindicated in the treatment of postpartum hemorrhage; however, in a patient who is acutely hemorrhaging, a slow drip of Oxytocin may be less effective than any of the above listed methods.

37. d (Chapter 12)

Fever from a vaccine should be a diagnosis of exclusion, which is the case in this particular vignette, given the patient's lack of signs and symptoms. Mild fever is a common side effect of the measles, mumps, and rubella vaccine, occurring in one in every six recipients, according to the CDC. Recipients may report temporary pain and stiffness in the joints (one in four). A mild rash can also be seen commonly (1 in 20). Severe problems are very rarely encountered, and the vaccine is not contraindicated in breast-feeding.

a. Postpartum endometritis is a bacterial infection of the deciduas that may also extend into the myometrium, in which case it is known as endomyometritis. Classic signs and symptoms include a fever greater than or equal to 38.0°C, uterine tenderness, and sometimes foul-smelling uterine discharge. A boggy uterus is sometimes encountered, which may be accompanied by bleeding. Although this patient has a fever and uterine tenderness, her fundus is firm and the degree of tenderness she reports may be more consistent with that experienced by normal uterine involution postpartum.

b. Although the patient complains of mild pelvic cramps, has fever and a history of Foley catheter use that together point toward a possible urinary tract infection, she is voiding comfortably and denies any urgency. Classic symptoms or signs of urinary tract infection would include dysuria, hematuria, and foul-smelling urine. As multiple vaginal examinations, catheterizations during labor, and obstruction from periurethral edema can be associated with urinary tract infections, it should remain part of the differential diagnosis of postpartum fever.

c. Fever and swelling are two of the classic symptoms of deep vein thrombosis, along with pain and erythema of the involved extremity. For patients who are pregnant and have had epidural catheters and sometimes been immobilized for prolonged periods of time, providers should recognize their increased risk of thromboembolism. In this case, however, the patient's swelling is bilateral, which is more likely to be caused by postpartum fluid shifts than bilateral thrombi. Tenderness to palpation of the patient's calf would be more predictive of a thrombus.

e. Fever is common after the start of lactation, which is often associated with engorgement of the breasts. The fever is transient, self-limited, and often resolves with pumping or manual expression of breast milk. For patients not planning on breast-feeding, suppression of lactation can be facilitated with binding. Pain associated with engorgement can be relieved with ice or nonsteroidal anti-inflammatory medications. Breast fever differs from mastitis in its lack of infection as manifested by erythema, induration, and tachycardia.

38. a (Chapter 12)

Several studies have cited grand multiparity, defined as carriage of the fifth baby, as a risk factor for postpartum hemorrhage. Although parity may be associated with age and accumulation of comorbidities that might predispose a patient to postpartum hemorrhage, the effect of parity has been shown to be independent of such confounders. One possible etiology for postpartum hemorrhage in these patients is their association with precipitous deliveries, where the uterus contracts so forcefully that it becomes hypotonic postpartum, leading to hemorrhage from the placental bed.

b. Hemorrhage is significantly more likely in women with fibroids as they can distort the uterine architecture and interfere with myometrial contractions necessary for the prevention of atony and postpartum hemorrhage. Hemorrhage risk is greater in cases of larger intramural fibroids located behind the placenta.

c. Her baby's weight, in this case meeting the criteria for macrosomia (birth weight of 4,000 to 4,500 g, 8 lb 13 oz to 9 lb 15 oz), increases her risk of postpartum hemorrhage. The suspected mechanism for increased risk is uterine distension by the baby's size and based upon the description of a large fluid gush, likely polyhydramnios associated with poor control of gestational diabetes. Multiple gestations would also increase the risk of hemorrhage by the same mechanism.

d. The lower uterine segment comprises the thinnest layer of myometrium, making it the least contractile. Although this property makes it the ideal region for entry during a cesarean section, its lack of contractility when coincident with a low-lying placenta leads to an inability to adequately constrict a bleeding placental bed, leading to increased risk of postpartum hemorrhage. In patients with a history of cesarean section with incision in the lower uterine segment, placentas are likelier to grow into the wound, also known as accreta, leading to increased risk of retained products and subsequent hemorrhage as well.

39. c (Chapter 13)

The lesion described is most likely a nabothian cyst, a normal variant among menstruating women. Nabothian cysts appear as single or multiple bubbles under the surface of the cervix and are often bluish in color. Cervical dysplasia is diagnosed after colposcopic biopsy of areas showing punctuations, mosaicism or atypical vessels. Similarly, cervical cancer is typically diagnosed with biopsy of colposcopic changes and confirmed with cervical conization with LEEP or cold knife cone. The risk of cervical cancer is extremely low at this patient's age. Only 0.1% of all cervical cancer cases occur before age 20. This represents 1 to 2 cases per year per 1,000,000 females aged 15 to 19. Bartholin duct cysts are found slightly posterior to the opening of the vagina at 4 and 8 o'clock on the introitus. The Bartholin glands produce lubrication for the opening of the vagina. Skene gland cysts (also called periurethral cysts) are located near the urethral meatus not on the cervix. Gartner duct cysts are benign vaginal cysts most commonly found in the upper vagina. Cervicitis typically presents with purulent discharge and cervical motion tenderness.

40. d (Chapter 13)

Vulvar pruritus is a common symptom of many benign and malignant diseases of the vulva. When a postmenopausal patient presents with vulvodynia or vulvar pruritus that is refractory to treatment, a punch biopsy should be performed to identify the lesion and guide the choice of treatment. In this patient, where lichen planus or lichen sclerosus is most likely, biopsy should be performed to confirm the diagnosis and rule out any underlying neoplasia or malignancy (such as VIN, squamous cell cancer, and Paget disease) prior to starting therapy. Surgical therapy is not indicated at this point in the evaluation, because lichen planus or lichen sclerosus can be treated with topical steroids such as clobetasol. Destruction of the lesion(s) with cryotherapy should never be performed without first having a pathologic diagnosis.

41. b (Chapter 13)

The patient history and findings are pathognomonic of lichen simplex chronicus, with thickened skin. The first course of action would be consistent use of high-potency topical steroid clobetasol. The patient should be advised to continue use even when she begins to have improvement in symptoms. This lesion is not associated with a higher risk of squamous cell cancer, and the patient has had a prior biopsy, so repeat biopsy is not necessary. There is no evidence of a current fungal infection. The woman is in her reproductive phase, so estrogen cream would not be indicated. Laser vaporization is not an appropriate intervention for lichen simplex chronicus.

42. c (Chapter 13)

The adolescent described has a clinical history and physical examination compatible with an imperforate hymen, which is the most common obstructive anomaly of the female reproductive tract. The differential also includes transverse vaginal septum, other obstructive malformations, and ovarian tumors. An adolescent patient who has an imperforate hymen may be asymptomatic or may have a history of cyclic abdominal pain that may occur for several years before the diagnosis is made. A bluish, bulging hymen may be seen on genital inspection, and a distended vagina (hematocolpos) causes bulging of the imperforate hymen. It may also have a mass effect in the rectal space including elevation of the distended uterus (hematometra), which may be palpated on rectoabdominal or abdominal examination. If the vagina becomes substantially enlarged with accumulated blood, the patient may experience back pain, pain with defecation that can result in constipation, nausea and vomiting, or difficulty in urinating. Treatment is excision of the hymen, under anesthesia, which allows the retained menses to drain and normal menstruation to commence. Fibroid uterus is very unlikely in this age group. An ovarian cyst or pregnancy might cause an abdominal mass, but they would not cause the vaginal bulging. Endometriosis can cause cyclic and acyclic pain in adolescents but would not cause a palpable mass or bulging vagina.

43. d (Chapter 6)

Cesarean delivery should be considered in any patient with repetitive fetal decelerations not responsive to conservative measures and who is remote from delivery. In the setting of placental abruption, fetal decelerations may indicate worsening of the abruption. Although vaginal bleeding is a clinical sign of placental abruption, concealed bleeding can also exist. Vaginal bleeding and a small change in hematocrit is not a cause for serious concern and recommendation of cesarean delivery unless other mitigating factors are present such as change in maternal or fetal status. If the fetal and maternal statuses are reassuring, serial hematocrits should be checked, two peripheral IVs placed, and active type and screen sent. This patient should be counseled on the change in fetal tolerance of labor and recommendations for cesarean section. Upon transfer to the operating room, the patient should have a repeat cervical examination, because multiparous patients can progress rapidly in labor, and vaginal delivery could then be considered. Fetuses in the ROP position are likely to spontaneously rotate during the birthing process. Therefore, cesarean delivery is not indicated for this reason. Placement of an epidural can cause maternal hypotension, but this usually responds to fluid bolus, repositioning, or vasoactive medications such as ephedrine. If hypotension persists in addition to fetal decelerations, other sources of hypotension should be considered and investigated.

44. e (Chapter 14)

Unlike a uterine septum, a bicornuate uterus is not primarily associated with an increased risk of infertility or recurrent miscarriage. In the case of the uterine septum, the septum is often avascular, and thus, an implanted pregnancy is more likely to be aborted due to the lack of vascularized endometrium on the septum. Because each horn of the bicornuate uterus is smaller than the normal-sized endometrial cavity, there is less room for fetal growth. The first trimester is largely uneventful in a pregnancy complicated by a bicornuate uterus, so there is not an increased risk of first-trimester bleeding or miscarriage. However, as the fetus grows larger in later pregnancy, there is less room for growth. As a result, malpresentation, second-trimester loss, and preterm labor and preterm delivery are more commonly seen in women with bicornuate (and unicornuate) uteri. Cervical insufficiency (CI), on the other hand, is painless; cervical dilation and effacement often seen in the second trimester. CI is associated with a history of in utero DES exposure and with prior history of cervical insufficiency. CI is also associated with cervical trauma and multiple instrumentations of the cervix such as with LEEP, cold knife cone, or obstetric laceration. CI is not more common in women with bicornuate uteri.

45. e (Chapter 14)

This patient does have uterine fibroids, but they are small and asymptomatic. At this time, there is no indication for treatment. Endometrial ablation and uterine artery embolization are not indicated for these small fibroids which are in the myometrium (intramural) but not impinging on the endometrium (submucosal). Furthermore, these two procedures are contraindicated in patients who wish to conceive in the future. Likewise, while hysteroscopic resection is an appropriate treatment option for women with submucosal fibroids, it is not indicated here. Resection of submucosal fibroids has been shown to improve pregnancy rates in women with infertility and submucosal fibroid(s). Intrauterine devices are LARCs and should not be used in a patient planning a pregnancy in the next month or two. The progesterone-containing IUD (Mirena) is sometimes used to treat dysmenorrhea and menorrhagia associated with fibroids. It is not indicated in this situation because the patient wishes to conceive shortly.

46. d (Chapter 14)

Changes in the menstrual cycle are very common as women approach the age of menopause (average age is 51). The differential diagnosis includes each of the options. With a normal myometrium, it is very unlikely that she has fibroids as the etiology of her bleeding. Thyroid disorders and perimenopause can each cause a change in the menstrual cycle, but her thickened endometrial stripe is more indicative of a structural source for her bleeding. The normal endometrial bilayer in a premenopausal woman is typically less than 14 mm depending on the time in the menstrual cycle. At 22 mm, this patient's endometrial lining is significantly thickened and concerning for a mass or other structural issue. The endometrial biopsy reveals normal findings. Although endometrial intraepithelial neoplasia (EIN) is possible, she does not have risk factors for hyperplasia such as obesity, oligomenorrhea, hypertension, diabetes, and PCOS. Furthermore, the lack of glandular crowding and cytologic atypia on endometrial biopsy makes this diagnosis much less likely. The most likely diagnosis is an endometrial polyp. In this case, the diagnosis could be confirmed with a saline sonohysterogram and/or hysteroscopy. Polyps are most commonly benign; however, they can have abnormal cells where the stalk attaches to the endometrial wall. Given this, and the fact that the polyp is large and symptomatic, the recommendation would be for surgical removal.

47. a (Chapter 14)

Any ovarian mass or cyst that contains thick septations, nodularity, solid components, abnormal Doppler flow, cyst wall thickening, or the presence of ascites is concerning for malignancy. Additionally, this patient is postmenopausal which places her at higher risk for cancer.

A follow-up ultrasound is incorrect in this scenario, as well as a pregnancy test and colonoscopy. A CT scan of the abdomen may also be used to evaluate for metastatic disease and lymphadenopathy.

This patient would need to be consented for bilateral salpingo-oophorectomy (removal of both ovaries and fallopian tubes) as well as for ovarian cancer staging, which includes collection of peritoneal washings, removal of omentum and any visible tumor, and sampling of pelvic and periaortic lymph nodes. Expectant management is not an option in this setting.

48. d (Chapter 15)

Some of the common clinical manifestations of endometriosis are cyclic pelvic pain, particularly just prior to menses, dyspareunia, dysmenorrhea, abnormal bleeding, and infertility. An adnexal mass noted on examination is common for women with endometriomas. Also, women with first-degree relatives who have endometriosis are more likely to develop endometriosis themselves. Women with endometriosis are not at higher risk for endometrial cancer.

49. b (Chapter 32)

Women with breast complaints at any age should undergo a CBE. If the CBE and history are indicative, diagnostic breast imaging should be obtained using diagnostic ultrasonography, mammography, or digital tomosynthesis depending on the patient age and clinical suspicion. In general, women less than 30 years of age with a palpable mass should first be evaluated with diagnostic ultrasound. The most likely diagnosis is a simple cyst or fibroadenoma. Initial imaging for a palpable mass in women 30 years and older would be a diagnostic mammogram; often followed by a diagnostic ultrasound. Depending on clinical suspicion or initial imaging, tissue diagnosis may be indicated. Fine-needle aspiration and core needle biopsy are the most common techniques used. They are minimally invasive and inexpensive. These techniques can be guided by palpation or imaging with mammography (stereotactic), ultrasonography, or MRI. Less frequently, excisional biopsy is used for tissue diagnosis in specific scenarios (breast implants, difficult mass location, inconclusive core needle biopsy, concerning imaging characteristics, etc.)

50. b (Chapter 2)

b, c. After one prior ectopic pregnancy, the risk of subsequent ectopic pregnancy is 10%. This increases to 25% after more than one prior ectopic pregnancy.

a. Although an increase in STIs is thought to have contributed to the incidence of ectopic pregnancy, we cannot be certain that this patient will be unable to conceive a normal pregnancy. Given the single-dose treatment, it is more likely that she had a chlamydia cervicitis and not pelvic inflammatory disease. If there was concern for a history of PID or infertility, the patient might be offered a hysterosalpingogram to evaluate tubal patency.

d. A history of one prior ectopic pregnancy does not preclude the use of an IUD for contraception. In fact, an IUD is the most effective type of reversible contraception and decreases the overall risk of pregnancy significantly. It is true that in the case of a contraceptive failure, the rate of ectopic pregnancy is as much as 25% to 50%, but the absolute risk remains exceedingly low.

e. As long as the pathologic report suggests that pregnancy tissue was removed at the time of surgery, there is no indication for additional methotrexate therapy.

51. c (Chapter 15)
NSAIDs, hormonal contraceptives (pill, patch, and ring), oral and IM progestins (Depo Provera, medroxyprogesterone), GnRH agonists (Lupron), danazol, and the LNG-IUS are all potentially effective medical treatments for pelvic pain and dyspareunia associated with endometriosis. Patients with endometriosis may develop depression or anxiety over the chronic pain associated with endometriosis. SSRIs can be used to treat anxiety and depression, but they are not used specifically for the treatment of endometriosis itself. SSRIs have also been shown to be effective in the treatment of PMS, PMDD, and postmenopausal vasomotor symptoms (hot flashes and night sweats).

52. d (Chapter 15)
Increasingly heavy or prolonged menstrual bleeding is common (50% to 60%) in women with adenomyosis. Thirty percent of women with adenomyosis have secondary dysmenorrhea and about 30% are asymptomatic. On examination, the uterus with adenomyosis is often diffusely enlarged, boggy, and may be mildly tender. A classic ultrasound finding for adenomyosis is an indistinct junction between the endometrium and myometrium. An enlarged firm uterus with distinct masses seen on ultrasound is suggestive of fibroids rather than adenomyosis. Women with adenomyosis also have a higher likelihood of also having fibroids and/or endometriosis.

53. b (Chapter 15)
Choice b is the most accurate description of adenomyosis. In the past, it was described as endometriosis interna; however, this nomenclature is not typically used any longer. Choice a most accurately describes endometriosis. Choice c most accurately describes a leiomyoma (fibroid). Choice d most accurately describes an endometrioma. Choice e most accurately describes endometritis.

54. b (Chapter 16)
This patient has chancroid, an STI caused by *Haemophilus ducreyi*. Because it is often difficult to culture *H. ducreyi*, the diagnosis is usually made clinically after ruling out syphilis and genital herpes. There are many treatment options for chancroid, including ceftriaxone 250 mg IM once, azithromycin 1 g orally once, ciprofloxacin 500 mg orally twice a day for 3 days, or erythromycin 500 mg four times a day for 7 days. Sexual partner(s) should receive treatment as well.

   a. Benzathine penicillin G is used to treat primary, secondary, or early latent syphilis. Syphilis is a systemic STI caused by the spirochete *Treponema pallidum*. The hallmark lesion of primary syphilis is known as a chancre, which is characterized by a nontender, red, round, firm ulcer approximately 1 cm in size with raised edges. It is usually associated with lymphadenopathy.

   c. Doxycycline can be used to treat chlamydial infections and is an alternative treatment for primary, secondary, or early latent syphilis in penicillin-allergic patients.

   d. A 21-day regimen of erythromycin is used to treat lymphogranuloma venereum (LGV), which is caused by *Chlamydia trachomatis* L-serotypes L1, L2, or L3. The primary stage of LGV is characterized by nontender papules or shallow ulcers, which heal quickly and often go unnoticed. Painful inguinal lymphadenopathy typically occurs 2 to 6 weeks after the primary lesion.

   e. Acyclovir is used to treat herpes simplex virus (HSV). The first episode of primary genital herpes is often the most severe and described as a painful cluster of small vesicles and ulcers. The lesions are often preceded by systemic flulike symptoms. The diagnosis of HSV should be confirmed with laboratory testing (viral culture, serum HSV antibody testing).

55. c (Chapter 16)
There are two nontreponemal serologic tests for syphilis available: The Venereal Disease Research Laboratory (VDRL) test and the rapid plasma reagin (RPR) test. False-positive nontreponemal tests can occur with various autoimmune conditions, other infections, malignancy, pregnancy, and IV drug use. Therefore, a positive result must be confirmed with specific treponemal antibody studies, such as the fluorescent treponemal antibody absorption test and the *Treponema pallidum* particle agglutination assay.

   a. The VDRL test is another nontreponemal serologic test for syphilis. Only a specific treponemal antibody study can confirm the diagnosis of syphilis.

   b. The diagnosis of syphilis should be confirmed with a specific treponemal antibody study prior to initiating treatment with penicillin. Benzathine penicillin G 2.4 million units IM once is the treatment of choice for primary, secondary, or early latent syphilis.

   d. The treatment of syphilis can be verified by following RPR or VDRL titers at 6, 12, and 24 months. Prior to monitoring titers, the diagnosis of syphilis must be confirmed and treatment initiated.

   e. The diagnosis of syphilis should be confirmed with a specific treponemal antibody study prior to initiating treatment with penicillin. Benzathine penicillin G 2.4 million units IM weekly for three doses is the treatment of choice for late latent or latent of unknown duration syphilis.

56. a (Chapter 16)
In otherwise healthy, nonpregnant women with dysuria, urinary frequency, or suprapubic pain in the absence of vaginal discharge, more than 90% will have a urinary tract infection. In those cases, treatment can be initiated without further workup. For patients with recurrent/frequent symptoms or concurrent vaginal

discharge, it is not appropriate to initiate treatment for a urinary tract infection until further workup has been completed. This workup should include sending the urine specimen for urinalysis and more importantly, a urine culture. In addition, the vaginal discharge should be evaluated to rule out an underlying STI.

57. d (Chapter 16)
The findings are most consistent with genital warts or condyloma acuminata. Approximately 90% are genital warts caused by HPV serotypes 6 and 11.
   a. Cervical cancer is associated with HPV serotypes 16, 18, and 31.
   b. The classic findings of HSV genital lesions are painful clusters of small vesicles and ulcers.
   c. Molluscum contagiosum is caused by a pox virus. The lesions are typically described as small, 1 to 5 mm, domed papules with an umbilicated center.
   e. Haemophilus ducreyi causes chancroid, which is an ulcerated genital lesion. The lesion presents initially as an erythematous papule, which evolves to a pustule and ulcer. The ulcer is painful with an erythematous base and irregular, well-demarcated borders.

58. a (Chapter 3)
The patient's normal karyotype as obtained via CVS is entirely reassuring regarding aneuploidy. However, she still needs a screening test for neural tube defect, so should undergo the MSAFP screen between 15 and 20 weeks' gestation. She does not need to bear the risk of an amniocentesis unless the MSAFP is elevated. Because a second trimester anatomy scan has a high sensitivity for neural tube defects, some clinicians have stopped offering the MSAFP, but in most practices, it is still the standard of care. Fetal echocardiography is to rule out fetal cardiac anomalies in women who are at increased risk for such anomalies (e.g., pregestational diabetes). The CVS does not need to be repeated. A cordocentesis or percutaneous umbilical blood sampling is utilized to obtain fetal cells when getting a karyotype immediately is important or if one needs to know the fetal hematocrit as in Rh-alloimmunization.

59. d (Chapter 17)
Fitzhugh–Curtis syndrome is a perihepatitis from ascending PID infection. It is associated with *Chlamydia* and gonorrhea infections. Fitzhugh–Curtis syndrome should be suspected in women with right upper quadrant pain or pleuritic pain in the context of pelvic inflammatory disease. It can be associated with elevated liver enzymes, but this is less common because the inflammation is usually confined to the liver capsule. Laparoscopy is the gold standard for diagnosis. In practice, the diagnosis is usually made clinically. If laparoscopy is performed, classic "violin-string" adhesions can be seen between the anterior liver capsule and the anterior abdominal wall or diaphragm. Treatment is the same as for PID.
   a. Tubo-ovarian abscess (TOA) is an important sequela of pelvic inflammatory disease (PID). It is estimated that 3% to 16% of PID cases will progress to TOA. The diagnosis of TOA is made clinically in the setting of PID and the appreciation of an adnexal or cul-de-sac mass or fullness. In this case, there is no adnexal fullness, making TOA less likely.
   b. Disseminated gonococcal infections are characterized by fever and erythematous macular skin lesions that proceed to a tenosynovitis and septic arthritis.
   c. HELLP syndrome is a disease specific to pregnancy.
   e. Although secondary syphilis can involve multiple organs (including the liver), the classic presentation includes a maculopapular rash on the palms and soles.

60. a (Chapter 17)
This patient has staphylococcal toxic shock syndrome (TSS). In 1981, the CDC established a case definition, which continues to serve as the criterion for TSS. To meet the case definition for a confirmed case, patients must have a fever greater than 38.9°C, hypotension, diffuse erythematous macular rash, desquamation, and involvement of at least three organ systems. The isolation of *Staphylococcus aureus* is not required for the diagnosis of TSS. In fact, blood cultures are often negative. Although menstrual-related TSS has decreased over time, the use of high-absorbency tampons remains a risk factor.

61. c (Chapter 17)
Owing to the high incidence of cervical cancer in HIV-infected women, more aggressive screening is recommended by the CDC. In this case, a pap smear should be performed at first evaluation and 6 months after. Yearly screening can be performed if both pap smears are normal.
   a. Cervical cancer screening should be done every 6 months in HIV-infected women with prior HPV infection, squamous intraepithelial neoplasia, or symptomatic HIV disease.
   b. Closer interval cervical cancer screening is recommended at initial evaluation.
   d. Routine colposcopy is recommended for HIV-infected women with ASC-US or higher grade cervical cytology abnormality.
   e. Women with HIV infections are not eligible to extend the interval between cervical cancer screenings to more than 1 year.

62. e (Chapter 18)
Many factors have been hypothesized to play a role in the development of pelvic organ prolapse (POP). Genetics, menopausal status and associated lack of estrogen, advancing age, history of pelvic surgery (i.e.,

hysterectomy), and connective tissue disorders (i.e., Ehlers-Danlos) are risk factors for POP. Additional factors may be those that contribute to a state of increased intra-abdominal pressure such as chronic constipation, chronic obstructive pulmonary disease, obesity, and heavy lifting. Parity is also considered a risk factor for the development of prolapse. This includes all aspects of parity—pregnancy, labor, and delivery. Increasing parity and increasing numbers of vagina and operative vaginal deliveries are all associated with increased risk of POP. There are no data to indicate that sexual activity plays any part in the development of prolapse.

63. a (Chapter 18)
Procidentia refers to complete eversion of the vagina, with or without a uterus. Historically, pelvic floor defects were named for the organ presumed to be behind the defect. For example, a rectocele implies herniation of the rectum into the vagina and an enterocele implies herniation of the small bowel into the vagina (typically seen after hysterectomy). Cystocele refers to prolapse of the bladder into the vagina, and urethrocele refers to prolapse of the urethra into the vagina. Because a physical examination cannot definitively identify the organ behind the prolapsed vaginal wall (bladder, urethra, rectum, or small bowel), the current preferred nomenclature describes the defect in broader terms, that is, an anterior wall defect (including cystoceles and urethroceles) or a posterior wall defect (including rectoceles and enteroceles).

64. a (Chapter 18)
POP is considered a benign entity, and treatment is indicated when the patient specifies bother from the condition. With an asymptomatic patient, expectant or conservative management may be offered. Although there are no strong data to support the role of pelvic floor muscle exercises in preventing progression of prolapse, there is evidence that it may improve co-existent issues such as stress urinary incontinence. Similarly, even modest weight loss has been shown to improve pelvic floor prolapse. In a young asymptomatic patient, colpocleisis would likely not be an acceptable option because this involves closing the opening to the vagina. Sexual activity is not possible after colpocleisis, so it is generally reserved for elderly women who do not desire sexual activity and who may not tolerate a more involved surgical procedure for POP. Total colpocleisis is the term used for closing the vaginal opening in women who do not have a uterus. LeFort is the same procedure for women who still have a uterus. Round ligament suspensions are not effective for any types of prolapse. A Gellhorn pessary may be used for conservative management in symptomatic women, often in high-grade prolapse. A hysterectomy, in and of itself, will not correct the prolapse.

65. c (Chapter 18)
Vaginal suspension procedures, such as uterosacral ligament suspension, are associated with many advantages including shorter operative time, faster patient recovery, and overall low complication rates compared with other types of prolapse repairs. Although both short- and long-term complication rates for vaginal suspensions are low, *all* prolapse and incontinence procedures carry a risk of injury to the bladder, ureters, and/or urethra. Intraoperative cystoscopy should be performed to check the integrity of these structures. In particular, ureteral injury rates as high as 11% have been reported with uterosacral ligament suspension. Defecography is sometimes used in the evaluation of posterior vaginal wall defects. Episiotomy can be used to improve access during a vaginal hysterectomy. Anterior colporrhaphy is not indicated with an isolated vault defect, especially if the anatomy has successfully been restored with a vault suspension procedure. Hysteroscopy would not be indicated since she no longer has a uterus.

66. b (Chapter 19)
This patient has symptoms consistent with urgency incontinence. An appropriate treatment choice would be oxybutynin, an anticholinergic medication, which increases bladder filling capacity by blocking acetylcholine release. Stress incontinence presents with leakage of urine on physical exertion (e.g., sporting activities), or increased intra-abdominal pressure (sneezing, laughing, coughing, and lifting). Mid-urethral slings such as tension-free vaginal slings and transobturator slings are common surgical options for stress incontinence. These procedures help to reapproximate the position and function of the hypermobile urethra. Overflow incontinence secondary to urinary retention from an underactive detrusor or bladder outlet obstruction is treated based upon the etiology. Continuous incontinence from a urinary fistula usually requires surgical repair. Functional incontinence is urine loss due to the patient's physical or mental inability to get to a bathroom even if they are aware of their need to urinate.

67. d (Chapter 19)
This patient's history is consistent with stress incontinence. Initial treatment with lifestyle and behavioral modifications should include weight loss, caffeine restriction, fluid management, bladder training, pelvic floor muscle exercises (Kegels), and possibly physical therapy. Both detrol LA (anticholinergic medication) and tibial nerve stimulation are used in the treatment of urgency incontinence. A mid-urethral sling is used in the treatment of stress incontinence, but is usually not considered first line therapy; lifestyle and behavioral modifications should be tried first. Vaginal hysterectomy is not indicated in the treatment of urinary incontinence in most circumstances.

68. b (Chapter 19)
The involuntary loss of urine is common, having affected an estimated 18.3 million American women in 2010, with an expected 55% increase to 28.4 million in 2050. Nearly 50% of all women experience occasional urinary incontinence, and nearly 45% of women over age 75 are affected daily. Urinary incontinence is often a major reason for placing individuals in nursing homes, with some 70% of nursing home residents suffering from urinary incontinence. In a large survey study of noninstitutionalized US women, 50% reported incontinence symptoms, of which 50% reported stress incontinence, 35% reported mixed incontinence, and 15% reported pure urge incontinence. It is estimated that more than $17 billion are spent on the treatment of stress incontinence and $76 billion on the treatment for urgency incontinence and overactive bladder annually.

69. d (Chapter 4)
The first stage of labor includes a latent phase characterized by slow cervical change classically described as 3- to 4-cm dilation, but may persist up to 6-cm dilation. This is followed by an active phase characterized by more rapid cervical change of at least 1.0 cm/hour of dilation in nulliparous women and 1.2 cm/hour dilation in multiparous women. The first stage ends when the cervix is completely dilated.

70. d (Chapter 19)
Normal voiding is voluntary and occurs predominantly through parasympathetic innervations via the pelvic nerve, which originates at levels S2 through S4. Inhibition of the pudendal, a somatic nerve, allows relaxation of the external urethral sphincter during normal voiding. Sympathetic control of the bladder is achieved via the hypogastric nerve originating from T10 to L2 of the spinal cord. The sciatic nerve supplies the skin of the leg, the muscles of the back of the thigh, and the leg and foot. The common peroneal nerve is a branch of the sciatic nerve. These two nerves are important to the gynecologist because they can be injured during patient positioning for surgery; they are not involved in micturition.

71. d (Chapter 20)
You advise expectant management for now with completion of menstrual calendar over the upcoming year. This patient is exhibiting typically developmental changes. She started menstruating at an appropriate age and has been menstruating for 1 year so far. It is very typical for adolescents to have irregular menses for the first 1 to 2 years after menarche. This is reflective of anovulatory cycles. It is very reasonable to follow her cycles with menstrual calendar over the next year. If the irregularity persists, you could then begin looking for other etiologies. A common cause of amenorrhea and delayed menarche in young women is hypothalamic amenorrhea (low GnRH and low or normal FSH/LH) which is seen most frequently in athletes who engage in vigorous daily exercise (such as gymnasts, ice skaters, and long-distance runners) as well as in women with eating disorders and extreme stress. Irregular menses, particularly infrequent cycles can also be seen in teens with polycystic ovarian syndrome. PCOS is often accompanied by signs of androgen access (hirsutism and acne) and insulin resistance (obesity and acanthosis nigricans). Patients with PCOS may also have polycystic appearing ovarian morphology but this is not required for the diagnosis. None of these are present in this patient. Moreover, there is no indication to look for structural anomalies via hysteroscopy or pelvic ultrasound at this point since she has menstrual flow and no cyclic pain.

72. c (Chapter 20)
Vasomotor symptoms, such as hot flashes and night sweats, should be treated when they are moderate or severe and interfere with the patient's quality of life during menopause. All of the treatment options are appropriate for management of the patient's symptoms except vaginal estrogen cream. Low-dose vaginal estrogens (estradiol cream, Vagifem, or Estring) are effective treatments for genitourinary menopausal syndrome. However, vaginal estrogen cream has a localized effect, and the systemic levels of estrogen are very low. Thus, systemic vasomotor symptoms are not treated with low-dose vaginal estrogens. Any of the other options would be appropriate for this patient. She still has a uterus in situ, so both estrogen and progesterone would be needed to protect from unopposed estrogen stimulation which can increase the risk of EIN and endometrial cancer. Both oral and transdermal forms of combined hormone therapy would be appropriate. Both SSRIs and gabapentin (neurontin) have been studied and found to be effective nonhormonal treatments of hot flashes and night sweats. A serotonin and norepinephrine reuptake inhibitor such as venlafaxine (Effexor) is another option.

73. c (Chapter 20)
This patient has a regular menstrual period and should be able to predict her most fertile period for conception. Regardless of cycle length, the fixed portion of the menstrual cycle in an ovulatory patient is the 14 days from ovulation to the start of menses. As the dominant follicle matures during the follicular phase of the menstrual cycle, it produces estrogen and later progesterone that enhances follicular maturation. The increasing estrogen level in the late follicular phase then triggers the release of LH from the anterior pituitary (the LH surge), and this triggers the follicle to rupture and release the mature ovum 36 hours after the surge (ovulation). Fertilization occurs in the fallopian tube, not in the uterine cavity. Fertilization of the ovum must occur within 24 hours of ovulation or else it degenerates. After ovulation, the

luteal phase of the cycle begins and the likelihood of fertilization drops steadily. The peak fertility interval is within 1 to 2 days prior to ovulation. The couple should increase sexual activity to every other day just before ovulation to maximize the likelihood of fertilization.

74. e (Chapter 3)

NT screening with or without first-trimester serum screening and second-trimester maternal serum screening are two accepted strategies for Down syndrome screening among women at low risk for chromosomal abnormalities. When using the combined first-trimester screen using NT plus the serum screens of PAPPA and free β-hCG, 80% sensitivity is reached. The second-trimester triple screen has only about 50% sensitivity in women under age 35, but the quad screen, which is the triple screen plus inhibin A, is approximately 80% as well. Thus, the highest sensitivity would be a test that combines the combined first-trimester test with the second-trimester quad screen, and such testing achieves a sensitivity above 90%. A Level II ultrasound has only about 50% sensitivity for Down syndrome as well, and routine obstetric ultrasounds are probably even less sensitive. Of note, the highest sensitivity screening test for Down syndrome is cell-free DNA (cf DNA). This was not provided as an option because it is not routinely used, and particularly not in women less than age 35.

75. c (Chapter 21)

Because a normal-appearing hymen is visualized upon your examination, you can rule out imperforate hymen and your most likely diagnosis would be a transverse vaginal septum. This is supported by the ultrasound findings, which showed a normal-appearing uterus, with a mass below the cervix: This is hematocolpos from menstrual flow that is unable to egress because of the transverse septum. The bilateral adnexal masses are most likely endometriomas secondary to retrograde menstrual flow.

   a. Uterine didelphys is less likely given the normal uterus on ultrasound, although it is true that MRI is more sensitive in detecting abnormalities than ultrasound.

   b. Uterine agenesis is incorrect as a uterus is noted on ultrasound.

   d. Imperforate hymen is incorrect because you note a normal hymen on physical examination.

   e. A uterine septum may additionally be present, although from the case description the most likely cause of her discomfort is a transverse septum preventing egress of menstrual flow.

76. c (Chapter 21)

A karyotype is indicated given that your concern is for premature ovarian failure. You may also consider screening her for Fragile X by checking for mutations in the *FMR1* gene.

   a, b. Given the absence of menses for the past year, you can assume that she is not ovulating. Therefore, performing a test for LH and/or progesterone would not be clinically useful in determining your diagnosis.

   d. An ultrasound and/or an MRI of the pelvis is not indicated in this case. Because she had normal menses in the past, prior to the past year, you can assume that she does not have a Müllerian anomaly causing her secondary amenorrhea.

   e. Technically, you have enough information with the tests above to make your diagnosis; however, your workup is incomplete prior to confirming that the patient has a normal karyotype, as the results from the karyotype may give you a different answer (e.g., Turner syndrome).

77. d (Chapter 21)

Patients with hypothyroidism typically need to increase their dose during pregnancy, often to as much as 50% of their prepregnancy dose. Patients with hypothyroidism are followed closely with serial testing of TSH to ensure that they are in a euthyroid range, increasing the dose of T4 replacement as needed.

   a, b. It would be highly unusual for a patient to require less thyroid medication during pregnancy, given that normally requirements for T4 are increased.

   c. This statement is false. During the first trimester and well into the second trimester until about 20 weeks, the fetus is able to produce only small amounts of thyroid hormone, and is therefore dependent on maternal production.

   e. Typically, providers increase the dose of T4 medication by 30% in the first trimester, and follow TSH levels every 6 weeks to adjust as necessary. Tripling the dose of thyroid medication would be inappropriate and may lead to side effects of palpitations, anxiety, and nausea.

78. d (Chapter 21)

The positive review of systems revealing galactorrhea and headaches should increase your suspicion for a prolactinoma. You would test a TSH as well, given that derangements in her thyroid may cause her secondary amenorrhea. Should her prolactin come back elevated in this case, you may consider repeating it to confirm hyperprolactinemia, and then proceed with an MRI of the head to evaluate for a prolactinoma.

   a. While a karyotype may be helpful to rule out Turner syndrome, this is less likely the cause of her secondary amenorrhea, given her additional symptoms of galactorrhea and headaches.

   b. The use of urinary LH testing kits is for the most part aimed at detecting an LH surge for timed intercourse in patients experiencing infertility, rather than as a diagnostic test to determine whether the patient is ovulatory. In this case, the patient's oligomenorrhea indicates that she is also oligoovulatory.

c. Pelvic ultrasound and/or MRI might be useful if she was also experiencing pain or had primary amenorrhea.

e. FSH, in the context of serum estradiol, is a test designed to evaluate ovarian reserve and egg quality, and evaluate for premature ovarian failure. Although they would be included in a general infertility workup, they are not the tests that would lead to the diagnosis in this case.

79. c (Chapter 22)

This patient's secondary dysmenorrhea is most likely due to pelvic adhesions. The etiology is most likely the repeat cesarean delivery complicated by additional adhesions from the endomyometritis. The adhesions may be structurally impacting the uterus and adnexa, resulting in pain with menses. Moreover, adhesions often cause pain with activity as well. The fact that the pain is reproduced with movement of the uterus is further evidence that adhesions may be present. Pelvic adhesions are generally not identifiable on imaging such as ultrasound or CT. The evaluation has shown no evidence of other causes of her pain such as cervicitis, fibroids, polyps, adenomyosis, and ovarian cysts. If she had endometriosis she would have most likely had a longstanding history of cyclic pelvic pain, and it would have likely been identified during her cesarean sections. Routine narcotic use is inappropriate, as is expectant management, given the level of her pain. Severe dysmenorrhea may be an indication for hysterectomy, but generally, less invasive treatments should be attempted first. Patients with chronic pelvic pain often benefit from pain management consultation and/or psychiatric therapy. This patient's examination and history point to a structural etiology for her pain, which should be evaluated first.

80. d (Chapter 7)

Small for gestational age refers to a neonate whose birth weight is less than the 10th percentile. It describes neonates who do not reach their growth potential and in whom there is evidence of fetal growth disruption, but where a cause or etiology is not known. The term IUGR describes an intrauterine process of fetal growth restriction owing to maternal, uterine, placental, or fetal disorders. All other answer choices are incorrect.

81. a (Chapter 22)

The normal menstrual cycle is defined as regularly spaced menses ranging from every 21 to 35 days, lasting 3 to 5 days with an average blood loss of 30 to 50 mL/cycle. AUB refers to menstrual bleeding of abnormal quantity, duration, or schedule. Nomenclature for AUB in nongravid reproductive-aged women has changed. The use of terms such as menorrhagia, menometrorrhagia, and dysfunctional uterine bleeding has been discouraged. This patient's bleeding pattern would not be described as intermenstrual bleeding because she is no longer having regular cycles. The new FIGO classification system identifies the type of AUB based on the cause of the bleeding. This is known as the PALM-COEIN (pronounced palm-coin) system of AUB. The system is divided into the most common structural causes of AUB including polyp, adenomyosis, leiomyoma, malignancy/hyperplasia (PALM) and nonstructural causes of AUB including coagulopathy, ovulatory, endometrial, iatrogenic, and not yet classified (COEIN). At this point in her evaluation, the patient's AUB would be classified as AUB-N (not yet classified).

82. b (Chapter 22)

Teenagers who present with heavy menstrual bleeding should be evaluated for a possible underlying bleeding disorder (AUB-C). In this patient, the large ecchymoses, history of surgical bleeding, history of epistaxis, and gingival bleeding further support the diagnosis of a likely bleeding disorder. Further examination of her family history would also be helpful. Some initial coagulation studies and referral to hematology for further evaluation is appropriate. A pregnancy test, TFTs, and PRL are also reasonable as would be a pelvic ultrasound. However, while she may eventually be started on OCPs, tranexamic acid, or even a LNG-IUD to help treat her menorrhagia, she should first be evaluated for a bleeding disorder. Although heavy, her bleeding is not life-threatening and does not require emergent treatment. An endometrial ablation is much too invasive and extreme and should not be performed on anyone who desires future fertility.

83. e (Chapter 1)

Development of linea nigra from pubis to umbilicus, bluish discoloration of vagina and cervix (Chadwick sign), softening and cyanosis of the cervix (Goodell sign), and softening of the uterus (Ladin sign) are all common signs associated with pregnancy. The Cullen sign is pathological and is not associated with pregnancy but may be seen with acute pancreatitis.

84. b (Chapter 23)

Patients with PCOS have been shown to have increased pulsatile frequency of GnRH, which in turn leads to high levels of LH. These elevated LH levels cause the increased production of androgens, leading to hirsutism, acne, and anovulation.

    a. Patients with PCOS typically have normal or low levels of FSH. Patients with decreased ovarian reserve or premature ovarian insufficiency have elevated levels of FSH.

    c. Estrogen levels would be normal in PCOS, not decreased.

    d. Patients with PCOS have elevated levels of free testosterone.

    e. Inhibin is a substance produced by the ovaries that inhibits release of FSH and GnRH from the hypothalamus. It is typically normal or slightly elevated in PCOS patients.

85. c (Chapter 2)
c, b. The patient needs to have surgical evacuation of the pregnancy given the blood in her pelvis, the elevated hCG well above 5,000 mIU/mL. Given that she is hemodynamically stable, it is appropriate to first attempt laparoscopy with conversion to laparotomy only if needed.

a. Multidose methotrexate doses have a higher success rate than single-dose therapy (93% vs. 88%); however, both regimens are generally only indicated if the β-hCG is less than 5,000 mIU/mL.

d. Misoprostol is not indicated for the treatment of ectopic pregnancy.

e. Although the patient should have RhoGAM during her hospitalization for Rh-negative status, this is not the next best step.

86. d (Chapter 23)
Congenital adrenal hyperplasia, most often caused by 21-hydroxylase deficiency, is the most common cause of ambiguous genitalia. Prenatal diagnosis and treatment can prevent the formation of ambiguous genitalia. This infant is at presumed risk for adrenal crisis secondary to inability to produce mineralocorticoids and glucocorticoids, and prophylactic replacement of both compounds is indicated until a definitive diagnosis is made (by measuring the levels of 17-hydroxyprogesterone).

a. Polycystic ovary syndrome does not present in the infant years; rather, it usually presents in adolescence or early 20s. Further, it does not typically cause ambiguous genitalia.

b. Müllerian agenesis leads to abnormalities of the internal Müllërian system, and would not lead to ambiguous external genitalia.

c. A transverse vaginal septum would not lead to ambiguous genitalia and typically presents around the time of menarche with cyclic abdominal pain and hematocolpos.

87. d (Chapter 23)
Testosterone (both free and bound) is elevated in patients with polycystic ovary syndrome, and the use of OCPs to decrease the levels of circulating androgens is effective, especially after 6 to 12 months of treatment. The contraceptive pill suppresses production of ovary-derived androgens by suppressing LH secretion by the pituitary (e). Additionally, they function by increasing circulating levels of sex hormone-binding globulin secondary to the estrogen in the combined OCP. This elevated level leads to lower free androgens (b, c). Finally, the improvements in acne and hirsutism are thought to be secondary to the fact that combined contraceptive pills decrease the activity of 5-alpha reductase in the skin (a).

88. a (Chapter 23)
This patient has multiple risk factors for diabetes mellitus, including her obesity, her family history of diabetes, and her personal history of gestational diabetes. Furthermore, the finding of acanthosis nigricans on her neck and vulva increases your suspicion for insulin resistance and hyperinsulinemia. You correctly suggest a diabetes screening test for her, by way of fasting serum glucose.

b. The velvety brown discoloration around the vulva is acanthosis nigricans, and a biopsy is not necessary.

c. This patient is less than 21 years old; a Papanicolaou test is not indicated.

d. Cholesterol screening is a good suggestion; however, at her age and without a family history, it is less pressing an issue than screening for diabetes.

e. A mammogram is not indicated at the age of 20 without a mass or concerning finding, and without family history.

89. c (Chapter 24)
During breast-feeding, prolactin levels are elevated, causing suppression or inhibition of pulsatile GnRH from the hypothalamus. In fact, lactational amenorrhea is widely used as a form of contraception. Thyroid hormone abnormalities can also cause menstrual irregularities, and subsequently fertility problems; however, this is not primarily suggested by the case presentation but should remain a consideration. There is nothing in her history suggesting subclinical infection or decreased tubal motility. And, given her recent pregnancy, it is not likely that her partner's sperm count is a factor.

90. e (Chapter 24)
Intrauterine device failure rates average between 0.7% and 1.9% with adequate placement and nonexpulsion. Depo Provera and Nexplanon are also highly effective contraceptives. Failure rates with combined contraceptive pills or progesterone-only pills approach 8% or greater, owing to imperfections in actual use and less-than-ideal adherence. The least effective methods are coitus interruptus and the diaphragm.

91. e (Chapter 24)
Progestin-only pills act to suppress ovulation, thicken cervical mucus, create an unsuitable environment for implantation, and inhibit sperm motility. They do not cause regression of the corpus luteum.

92. c (Chapter 25)
Termination of a second-trimester pregnancy, 13 to 24 weeks gestation, can be achieved with D&E (dilation and evacuation) or induction of labor. These methods are often preceded by feticide with intramniotic saline or digoxin or intracardiac KCL injections. Recommended regimens for termination also include mifepristone

followed by prostaglandin analogs or by misoprostol alone. Third line for second-trimester induction of labor is IV Oxytocin. These methods are both safe and effective. Uterine perforation is a risk of surgical D&E, not of labor induction. However, potential complications of induction of labor for second-trimester gestations do include infection, bleeding, uterine rupture, transfusion, and the possible need for additional procedures including D&E if the products of conception do not deliver vaginally.

93. c (Chapter 25)
Concurrent long-term corticosteroid use is a contraindication to medication abortion. These medications may interfere with the immune response and increase the risk of infection. Although a state may require parental consent for ages less than 18, the patient's age itself is not a contraindication for medical abortion. Medical termination can be done up to 49 days' gestation; therefore, her gestational age is appropriate for medication abortion. She has been treated for chlamydia, so this is also not a contraindication.

94. d (Chapter 25)
The presence of a gestational sac indicates an ongoing pregnancy. The patient is stable with no signs of endometritis or hemorrhage. The presence of a gestational sac within 1 to 2 weeks after mifepristone termination does not always necessitate surgical intervention. In this setting, repeat misoprostol (cytotec) and expectant management are options. Most typically, if there is a persistent sac with no evidence of ongoing fetal development or cardiac activity, the sac will be spontaneously expelled in the ensuing weeks. Serial ultrasounds might confirm eventual emptying of the uterus but expectant management also puts her at risk for a large bleed at home. Moreover, vaginal bleeding after medical abortion averages 10 to 17 days. Given that this particular patient has a chronic anemia, surgical intervention with D&C would be the safest route for her. D&E is the term used for uterine evacuation in the second trimester, and this patient is still in her first trimester.

95. d (Chapter 26)
PCOS and advanced maternal age are two of the major causes of ovulatory factor infertility. Both endometriosis and pelvic inflammatory disease are associated with pelvic adhesions, tubal blockage, and infertility. Fibroids are not a significant cause of infertility. In general, women with uterine fibroids are able to conceive without difficulty. Large fibroids can lead to overdistension of the uterus during pregnancy with subsequent risk for preterm labor and/or delivery. Fibroids can also restrict fetal movement in the uterus and result in a higher rate of fetal malpresentation. If fibroids grow rapidly during pregnancy, they can result in degeneration and pain. Women with infertility who have submucosal fibroids that project into the endometrial cavity have increased pregnancy rates when submucosal fibroids are removed or partially resected.

96. e (Chapter 26)
Male factor infertility is responsible for about 35% of infertility cases. The etiologies vary widely but include all of the choices listed. In addition, mumps, antisperm antibodies, and congenital cryptorchidism (undescended testes) can result in an abnormal semen analysis and infertility. Thyroid disease and hypogonadotropic hypogonadism (e.g., from tumors, infection, and Kallmann syndrome) are the primary endocrine abnormalities that result in male factor infertility. Environmental exposures that can result in male factor infertility include radiation, heat, and chemicals. Sexual dysfunction (erectile dysfunction, retrograde ejaculation, and ejaculation failure) and structural factors (varicocele, testicular torsion, and vasectomy) also contribute to causality. Medications such as cimetidine, sulfasalazine, and spironolactone and chemotherapy can all result in impaired male fertility as well.

97. d (Chapter 8)
The seizure prophylaxis of choice for preeclampsia is magnesium sulfate. The assumption is that if a woman seizes while on magnesium sulfate, then the serum level is not high enough. Thus, in this setting, one would rebolus, though not the original 4 or 6 g, but a 2 g rebolus. It is rare that another antiseizure medication such as phenytoin would be used. Hydralazine is used commonly in women with preeclampsia to control severe-range blood pressures, which is not mentioned in this case. It is rare that the fetus requires emergent delivery. Usually, the best approach is to stabilize the mother and follow the fetal heart tracing closely and deliver for fetal indications if necessary. Furosemide generally has little use in the management of severe preeclampsia.

98. c (Chapter 1)
Second trimester tests routinely offered include serum screening for neural tube defects and aneuploidy with the MSAFP and Quad screens, second-trimester screening ultrasound for fetal anatomy, and amniocentesis. Hematocrit is offered in the first and third trimesters. GBS is collected late in the third trimester. The fern test is used to determine whether rupture of membranes has occurred, on the basis of a maternal history of leaking fluid. In the first trimester, a transvaginal ultrasound is commonly performed to confirm dating of the pregnancy.

99. e (Chapter 26)
Of couples who undergo infertility evaluation, as many as 20% will have no identifiable cause for their

infertility despite a full infertility work-up. In these patients, Clomid ovulation induction with intrauterine insemination is a safe, initial approach to management. Ovulation induction with injectable gonadotropins and intrauterine insemination is also a reasonable option as is in vitro fertilization. It is important that during counseling, couples realize that most of the available therapies do not have higher pregnancy success rates when compared with expectant management. Therefore, expectant management is also a very reasonable approach. In this group, 60% will conceive spontaneously in 3 to 5 years. After 5 years of unexplained infertility, however, less than 10% of couples will conceive on their own.

100. b (Chapter 9)

The target range for fasting blood glucose value is less than 90 mg/dL and 1-hour postprandial values less than 140 mg/dL or 2-hour postprandial values less than 120 mg/dL. If more than 25% to 35% of glucose levels are elevated, medication is indicated. These patients are considered class A_2, or medication-controlled gestational diabetics in the White classification of gestational diabetes. Because her average glucose values were elevated, diet and exercise alone are not sufficient to control her diabetes. True gestational diabetics will commonly have normal fasting glucose values with elevated postprandial values. This is due to the pathophysiology being related to metabolism of large carbohydrate boluses rather than carbohydrate boluses at baseline. Therefore, it is appropriate to treat patients with a short-acting insulin (Lispro) to cover breakfast, and intermediate-acting insulin (NPH) to cover lunch. This combined insulin saves the patient a prelunch injection. Then, a short-acting insulin (Lispro) predinner dose will cover evening postprandial values.

If the blood sugar levels were within target range, continuing to adhere to a diabetic diet and exercise regimen would have been appropriate. Such patients are classified as class A_1, or diet-controlled gestational diabetics in the White classification of gestational diabetes. The patient's fasting levels have been normal. Starting the patient on NPH in the evening would cause her to become hypoglycemic in the mornings. Historically, oral hypoglycemics have not been used in pregnancy due to concerns of placental transfer, and subsequently, fetal hypoglycemia. However, recent studies have indicated that adequate glucose control may be achieved with oral hypoglycemics in some patients without harm to the fetus. Insulin, on the other hand, has been shown to be safe in pregnancies, with no placental transfer. There is debate in the literature and among clinical providers regarding the use of oral hypoglycemics, but in this patient it would be unusual to start metformin.

101. b (Chapter 27)

Preinvasive neoplastic disease of the vulva is divided into two categories: squamous (vulvar intraepithelial neoplasia; VIN) and nonsquamous intraepithelial neoplasias (Paget disease, melanoma in situ). The classification for VIN was changed in 2004 and again in 2015. In 2015, the VIN terminology was modified to bring the nomenclature in line with other HPV-associated squamous intraepithelial lesions of the lower genital tract (i.e., CIN). Based on the 2015 terminology, vulvar squamous intraepithelial lesions are classified as vulvar LSIL, vulvar HSIL, and Differentiated type VIN.

(1) Low-grade squamous intraepithelial lesions are now called vulvar LSIL. These lesions were formerly known as VIN 1. They are associated with koilocytic changes, HPV effect, and flat condyloma. (2) High-grade squamous intraepithelial lesions are now known as vulvar HSIL. These lesions were formerly categorized as VIN 2 and VIN 3, and then later termed Usual Type VIN in 2004. They are associated with high-risk carcinogenic HPV genotypes and HPV persistence risk factors such as cigarette smoking and immunocompromise. (3) Differentiated type VIN is not associated with high-risk HPV infection. Instead, it is associated with vulvar dermatologic conditions such as lichen sclerosis (LS). Differentiated type VIN associated with lichen sclerosis is more likely to be associated with squamous cell carcinoma in about 5% of women with LS.

102. c (Chapter 9)

This patient has gestational diabetes (GDM). Insulin resistance in pregnancy stems from placental secretion of diabetogenic hormones, which include human chorionic somatomammotropin (placental lactogen), growth hormone, corticotropin-releasing hormone, and progesterone. These hormones increase with the size of the placenta, and thus, abnormal carbohydrate metabolism is usually not apparent until the late second or early third trimester. Somatomammotropin is lactogenic, preparing mammary gland growth for lactation, in addition to regulating maternal glucose, fat, and protein, so that they are available to the fetus. Many patients with gestational diabetes likely have elevated baseline insulin resistance as well and are at high risk of developing frank Type 2 diabetes mellitus over the ensuing decade.

103. d (Chapter 27)

Paget disease of the vulva is a rare type of skin cancer that arises from glandular cells. It can present with chronic pruritis, red velvety lesions and white plaques. About 75% of the time, Paget disease of the vulva is confined to the vulvar epithelium and is noninvasive. Around 25% of patients with vulvar Paget disease will have an underlying invasive adenocarcinoma. Paget is not known to be associated with invasive squamous cell carcinomas. Given the association with invasive adenocarcinoma, evaluation for malignancy with vulvar biopsy in a symptomatic patient is imperative. The initial treatment recommended for Paget disease is excision. Because the tumor often extends into normal appearing skin, wide local excision is recommended. Because microscopic Paget disease often extends beyond the obvious gross lesions, wide margins should be taken, and excised segments checked in pathology for clean margins. It is also important to rule out underlying adenocarcinoma during pathologic evaluation. Finally, even with clean margins, Paget disease has a high recurrence rate and may require multiple local excisions. It is acceptable to treat recurrences with ablative modalities.

104. d (Chapter 27)
Vulvar cancers make up 5% of all GYN malignancies. They occur most commonly in postmenopausal women with a median age of 65. Risk factors for vulvar cancer are all of those listed except breast cancer. Other risk factors include age >70, HIV infection, and cervical cancer. The association with CIN and cervical cancer is likely related to high-risk HPV which can cause both cervical and vulvar cancer. Breast cancer is not a risk factor for vulvar cancer.

105. c (Chapter 28)
The ASC-US category includes minor changes due to inflammation or injury, but can also indicate the presence of a more severe abnormality. In young women ages 21 to 24 years with an ASC-US pap, repeat cytology in 1 year is preferred. In women ages 24 to 29 years with an ASC-US pap, reflex HPV testing is preferred to triage the ASCUS Pap results in order to help to guide providers in developing a plan of care. If the HPV test is negative, cotesting can be repeated in 3 years. If the HPV test is positive, the patient should be evaluated with colposcopy. In this age group, if HPV testing is not available or not done, an ASC-US pap test should be followed with repeat cytology in 1 year. LEEP conization is reserved for moderate–severe dysplasia (CIN 2 and CIN 3), CIN 1 which has persisted for greater than 2 years, and for patients with a HGSIL Pap smear and greater than a two-step difference in biopsy result.

106. b (Chapter 28)
The recommended cervical cancer screening for women aged 30 and older is cotesting every 5 years or cytology alone every 3 years. In women with a normal pap test that is negative for intraepithelial lesions and malignancy, but a positive high-risk HPV screen options include repeat cotesting in one year or obtaining genotype testing on the HPV. If the HPV is negative for oncogenic Types 16 and 18, the patient should have repeat cotesting in one year. If the HPV is positive for oncogenic Types 16 or 18, the patient should be evaluated with colposcopy. LEEP conization is reserved for moderate–severe dysplasia (CIN 2 and CIN 3), CIN 1 which has persisted for greater than 2 years, and for patients with a HGSIL Pap smear and greater than a two-step difference in biopsy result.

107. a (Chapter 28)
CIN 1 that persists for less than 2 years may continue to be followed with or without treatment. If the patient chooses not to treat the lesion, she should continue to have cytology and HPV testing 12 months after the colposcopy. If the patient chooses treatment, either ablative (e.g., cryotherapy) or excisional procedure is acceptable. Excision is the preferred treatment if the colposcopy is unsatisfactory, the endocervical curettage was positive, or if the patient had been previously treated. Cigarette smoking is a known risk factor for the persistence of HPV. Smoking cessation should be offered in addition to management of her CIN 1.

108. b (Chapter 28)
Cervical cancer screening guidelines recommend testing to start at age 21 years regardless of onset of sexual activity. The one exception to this is young women who are HIV positive. These recommendations are based on the fact that >90% of HPV infections resolve within 3 years in adolescents. Also, the risk of cervical cancer is extremely low at this patient's age. Only 0.1% of all cervical cancer cases occur before age 20. This represents 1 to 2 cases per year per 1,000,000 females age 15 to 19. The HPV vaccination is indicated in this patient and for all girls and women ages 9 to 26 years, regardless of possible prior exposure to HPV or Pap smear history. Because the patient has had unprotected intercourse, pregnancy testing, STI screening, and patient education are all indicated.

109. b (Chapter 29)
The question asks about the evaluation of vaginal bleeding in a postmenopausal woman. The differential diagnosis includes urogenital atrophy, exogenous estrogen exposure, endometrial hyperplasia and intraepithelial neoplasia (EIN), endometrial cancer, and endometrial polyps. Transvaginal ultrasound can help in guiding the evaluation of postmenopausal bleeding. An endometrial thickness of 4 mm or less is indicative of low risk for malignancy. If bleeding is persistent or if the lining appears thickened (>4 mm) or if the lining is not adequately visualized, then further tissue evaluation (i.e., endometrial biopsy, hysteroscopy, dilation and curettage) is recommended. In a 73-year-old woman with no stigmata suggestive of a hormone-producing tumor, there is minimal utility in obtaining an FSH or estradiol level at this point. Both would be expected

to be in the menopausal range. A CA-125 level is most useful in the setting of evaluation of a patient with a concerning ovarian mass. The patient has had scant bleeding and no other evidence of bleeding; so a CBC, PT, and PTT are not indicated as a coagulopathy is highly unlikely. The patient has had adequate Pap smear evaluation and has no history of CIN 2/3, so a Pap smear and HPV screen are also not indicated.

110. c (Chapter 29)

Endometrial cancer is surgically staged with total hysterectomy, which may be done abdominally, vaginally, laparoscopically, or with robotic assistance. Pelvic washings should be collected and both tubes and ovaries should be removed (bilateral salpingo-oophorectomy or BSO). Pelvic and para-aortic lymph node dissections should be performed when there is a histologically high-grade tumor or when the depth of tumor invasion is more than one-third of the myometrial thickness. With endometrial cancer, when indicated, it is important to evaluate *both* pelvic and para-aortic lymph nodes because it is possible to have nodal spread to one group while sparing the other. Nodal status does have significant staging and prognostic implications. Answer choice (d) describes staging for ovarian cancer and (a) describes clinical staging for cervical cancer; the only GYN cancer that is clinically staged.

111. e (Chapter 29)

All of the choices, with the exception of Tamoxifen, are considered protective factors for endometrial cancer and lower the lifetime risk of developing the disease. LNG-IUD use and other hormonal contraceptives (pill, patch, and NuvaRing) also decrease the risk of endometrial cancer. Tamoxifen is a selective estrogen receptor modulator (SERM) and, as such, contains both agonist and antagonist properties. Tamoxifen does promote endometrial proliferation, hyperplasia, polyp formation, carcinoma, and sarcoma, while decreasing the risk of recurrent breast cancer. While there is no recommended endometrial screening for women taking Tamoxifen, any abnormal bleeding while on Tamoxifen warrants further investigation.

112. a (Chapter 29)

Although endometrial cancer is the most commonly encountered gynecologic malignancy in the United States, it is associated with a favorable survival profile because the majority of patients are diagnosed with early stage disease. Seventy-two percent of women are diagnosed with stage I disease, thus rendering the surgical staging itself as curative treatment. Fortunately, early symptoms (i.e., vaginal bleeding) and accurate diagnosis modalities contribute to the fact that endometrial cancer is only the third most common cause of gynecologic cancer deaths worldwide (behind ovarian and cervical cancer). Endometrial cancer accounts for 10,500 deaths each year in the United States. While ovarian cancer occurs less frequently than endometrial cancer in the United States, ovarian cancer has a higher mortality rate. This is because there are no screening modalities for ovarian cancer; as a result, 75% of women present with advanced disease.

113. c (Chapter 30)

These ultrasound findings are consistent with a diagnosis of a benign cystic teratoma or dermoid cyst. Dermoid cysts are the most common type of germ cell tumor. The tumors are typically cystic masses containing mature adult tissue such as skin, hair, and teeth mixed in sebaceous material. This gives them a very characteristic appearance on ultrasound (Fig. 30-5). Cystectomy is recommended for definitive diagnosis and to rule out malignancy. Care should be taken to avoid intra-abdominal spill of the cyst contents as this could result in a chemical peritonitis. In the absence of malignancy, removal of the ovary(s), tube(s), and uterus is not indicated.

114. c (Chapter 30)

Both granulosa-theca cell tumors and Sertoli–Leydig cell tumors are known as functional tumors because they are characterized by hormone production. Ovarian Sertoli–Leydig cell tumors resemble fetal testes and produce androgens (testosterone and androstenedione). These elevated hormone levels can cause virilization in 75% of patients including breast atrophy, hirsutism, deepened voice, acne, clitoromegaly, and receding hairline. Patients may also have oligomenorrhea or amenorrhea. CA-125 levels can be elevated in a number of benign and malignant processes (such as pancreatitis, diverticulitis, endometriosis, and epithelial ovarian cancer), but CA-125 levels are not generally elevated in Sertoli–Leydig cell tumors. LDH and AFP are also tumor markers seen in dysgerminomas of the ovary and endodermal sinus (yolk sac) tumors of the ovary, respectively. LDH is also produced in some lymphomas and melanomas, and AFP is also produced in liver cancer.

115. c (Chapter 31)

The clinical picture is consistent with complete molar pregnancy. Compared with incomplete molar pregnancies, complete molar pregnancies have no coexistent fetus, are more likely to present with abnormal bleeding, and size greater than dates. Complete molar pregnancies have higher β-hCG levels, and therefore, are more likely to have coexistent hyperemesis gravidarum, preeclampsia, hyperthyroidism, and theca lutein cysts. They are also more likely to have persistent GTD (20%) and are at higher risk of metastasis (4%). Molar pregnancies are surgically managed by suction evacuation of the uterine contents. Prior to the operation, Rh(D), thyroid, blood counts, liver, and renal status should be evaluated. Evaluation for theca lutein cysts should also be part of your diagnostic workup prior to proceeding with D&C. Rh(D) negative patients should receive RhoGAM after the D&C is completed. Methotrexate is not part of the initial plan of care in patients with molar pregnancies. Methotrexate is used to treat persistent low-risk gestational trophoblastic disease.

116. e (Chapter 2)
An inevitable abortion is a pregnancy complicated by vaginal bleeding with a dilated cervix such that the pregnancy is likely to pass soon.

    a. An incomplete abortion is partial expulsion of POC prior to 20 weeks. This patient has not had any tissue expelled.

    b. A threatened abortion does present with vaginal bleeding, but in this type of abortion the patient does not have cervical dilation.

    c. This patient has an intrauterine pregnancy, as confirmed by an intrauterine gestational sac and yolk sac.

    d. Missed abortion is the death of an embryo with complete retention of all POCs. If the patient does not pass any tissue spontaneously, a missed abortion may develop. However, this is not the best initial diagnosis.

117. b (Chapter 31)
Gestational choriocarcinoma is a malignant necrotizing tumor that is often metastatic to the lungs, vagina, liver, and brain. It is rare (1 in 20,000 to 40,000 pregnancies) and occurs most often after a preceding normal term pregnancy (25%) but can also occur after a molar pregnancy (50%), or after a miscarriage, termination, or ectopic pregnancy (25%). Choriocarcinoma is a pure epithelial tumor (absent chorionic villi) that is highly sensitive to chemotherapy. This patient will require chemotherapy, single or multiagent, depending on the presence of metastasis and other risk factors. Hysterectomy is an option in selected patients; but given her age and likely desire for future fertility, chemotherapy is a better choice in this clinical situation. Contraception is paramount during hCG surveillance to avoid an unintended pregnancy after treatment.

118. c (Chapter 31)
This patient likely has an incomplete (partial) molar pregnancy based on the ultrasound findings showing a coexistent fetus. The workup and treatment is similar to a complete molar pregnancy. Incomplete molar pregnancies result from the fertilization of normal egg by two sperm, so the most common karyotype is triploid, 69 XXY or 69 XXX (one haploid maternal set and two haploid paternal sets). Compared with complete molar pregnancies, incomplete molar pregnancies are more likely to present as a missed or incomplete abortion with uterine size appropriate or small for dates. Incomplete molar pregnancies have only mild to moderate β-hCG elevations, and therefore, rarely have associated hyperemesis gravidarum, early preeclampsia or hyperthyroidism. Incomplete moles are also at low risk for persistent GTD and rarely metastasize.

119. b (Chapter 32)
Galactorrhea is the persistent or intermittent leakage of milky nipple discharge. The nipple discharge is often spontaneous or can be expressed and typically comes from multiple milk ducts in one or both breasts. Galactorrhea may also present with absent or irregular menses, headaches or vision problems. Galactorrhea is a result of pituitary stimulation most commonly caused by pregnancy, pituitary adenoma, thyroid disorders, chronic renal failure, or psychotropic medications. A breast abscess typically results in a purulent discharge, erythema, and pain and is not generally associated with galactorrhea.

120. d (Chapter 32)
LCIS is a premalignant lesion that carries subsequent increased risk of invasive breast cancer of 25% to 30% within 15 years. The subsequent cancer can occur on either side or in both breasts, and may be any of the types mentioned. LCIS does not require immediate treatment, but the use of an SERM-like Tamoxifen may reduce the risk of subsequent cancer by 50%. LCIS is usually found incidentally on biopsy for another finding because it is not palpable or seen on mammogram.

121. c (Chapter 4)
When assessing fetal heart tracings, the baseline should be in the normal range (110 to 160 beats per minute) with moderate variability. Although minimal variability is not reassuring, it can also be a sign that the fetus is asleep or inactive. Absent variability is always worrisome. Tachycardia can be a sign of maternal fever, fetal infection, fetal anemia, and even fetal arrhythmia.

122. c (Chapter 5)
The classic presentation of placental abruption is third-trimester vaginal bleeding associated with severe abdominal pain and/or frequent, strong contractions. However, in 20% of placental separations, bleeding is confined within the uterine cavity and is referred to as a concealed hemorrhage. In this case, there is a retroplacental clot noted on ultrasound, which is consistent with a relatively large concealed placenta abruption. This is the most likely cause, particularly in the setting of an MVA with a "seat belt sign" (i.e., bruises from the seat belt) as the sudden stop as well as the direct trauma of the seat belt can cause shearing of the placenta from the uterine wall, causing

uteroplacental insufficiency, which is reflected in late decelerations on external fetal monitoring (EFM).

a. The fetal heart rate tracing described is more consistent with uteroplacental insufficiency (recurrent late decelerations) rather than umbilical cord compression. Umbilical cord compression is usually seen on the EFM as recurrent variable decelerations.

b. Although the patient is contracting every 2 minutes, there is no evidence of preterm labor on examination. Additionally, labor itself does not usually cause late decelerations.

d. The fetal heart rate tracing described is more consistent with uteroplacental insufficiency (recurrent late decelerations) rather than fetal head compression. Fetal head compression usually manifests on EFM as early decelerations rather than late. Also, the fetal head must be in the pelvis for compression to occur.

e. Although it is possible to have a placental abruption in the setting of placenta previa, contractions in the setting of placenta previa do not usually cause late decelerations. Furthermore on ultrasound, there is no evidence of placenta previa. This would need to be confirmed on TV US if it was felt that the placenta was close to the internal os of the cervix.

123.　c (Chapter 5)

The most appropriate delivery plan in this case is to proceed with emergent (or at least urgent) cesarean section. Given the ultrasound findings, the patient has a known vasa previa and velamentous cord insertion, so to prevent rupture of the fetal vessels as a result of spontaneous rupture of membranes with labor, it is imperative that the cesarean delivery be done expeditiously.

a. Expectant management with the plan for a vaginal delivery in the setting of a vasa previa is an option but does carry significant risk of rupture of the fetal vessels during labor and with spontaneous rupture of the membranes. The patient should be counseled regarding this risk and that if the fetal vessels rupture, it is a surgical emergency with up to 56% perinatal mortality rate associated. Given the significant risk of perinatal mortality associated with rupture of fetal vessels, most obstetricians proceed with cesarean section in the setting of a known vasa previa.

b. In a patient with a known vasa previa, artificial rupture of membranes is generally considered to be contraindicated because both the amniohook and the actual ruptures of the membranes can cause the fragile fetal vessels to rupture, resulting in fetal hemorrhage and perinatal morbidity/mortality.

d. Although not absolutely contraindicated in this setting of known vasa previa, just as with expectant management, the patient should be counseled regarding the risk of vaginal delivery before either expectant or active management of labor. Oxytocin is more appropriately started when it is apparent that the patient is not continuing to labor on her own.

e. Emergent cesarean section is the most appropriate course of action.

124.　d (Chapter 1)

Of the answer choices listed, only Prader–Willi is not routinely offered for genetic screening in high-risk populations. For the other four traits commonly screened and listed in the question, the traits are recessive. Thus, if both parents are found to be positive carriers, the fetus can be genetically tested through amniocentesis or chorionic villus sampling.

125.　b (Chapter 5)

The clinical presentation of uterine rupture is variable. If there is vaginal bleeding, it can range from spotting to passing large clots. In this case, the patient's risk factor for uterine rupture is her prior abdominal myomectomy. It is possible to have a trial of labor after a myomectomy if the endometrial cavity has not been entered during the surgery as the risk of uterine rupture is low; however, this patient had a large fibroid removed that required entry into the endometrial cavity, which increases her risk for uterine rupture significantly. Typically, patients with a history of myomectomy requiring entry into the cavity, prior classical cesarean section, and other major uterine surgery (e.g., corneal wedge resection for ectopic pregnancy) are counseled to avoid labor because they are at high risk for uterine rupture and are usually scheduled for a cesarean section at 36 to 37 weeks, pending fetal lung maturity testing so as to avoid the patient going into labor.

a. There is no evidence of PPROM in this patient. She had a normal AFI, no pool, and no ferning seen on SSE. The nitrazine test was positive most likely secondary to blood in the vaginal vault.

c. There was no evidence of cervical laceration on examination and no factors concerning for this in the patient's history.

d. The patient's placenta was noted to be posterior. There was no mention of the placenta being close to the internal os on ultrasound, so previa is an unlikely source of the antepartum hemorrhage.

e. Vasa previa is a rare cause of antepartum hemorrhage and usually associated with a succenturiate placental lobe or velamentous cord insertion. There was no evidence of vasa previa on ultrasound.

126.　d (Chapter 5)

A CT scan of the abdomen and pelvis is not an appropriate initial test in this patient. In particular, you are concerned about the risk of accreta or percreta invading into the bladder. Although CT scan would help determine whether nephrolithiasis is the source of the patient's hematuria, it is more appropriate to start with a less invasive test with less radiation if at all possible. If imaging is going to progress beyond ultrasound, MRI is the modality of choice.

a. Urine analysis would be an appropriate initial test to rule out a urinary tract infection as the source of the patient's hematuria. It would also confirm hematuria and determine whether there are RBC or WBC casts.

b. Urine culture would be an appropriate initial test in conjunction with the urine analysis because urinary tract infections can cause hematuria and suprapubic pain.

c. A sterile speculum examination would be an appropriate initial test to determine whether the patient's bleeding is coming from the cervix, urethra, or both. It would also help determine whether the patient has vaginal bleeding as a result of labor/cervical dilation or cervicitis.

d. Abdominal ultrasound of the uterus would be an appropriate initial test because the patient has a history of three previous cesarean sections, had a complete anterior previa on her anatomy ultrasound at 18 weeks, and has not been reassessed with ultrasound to determine whether the previa has resolved. Additionally, if the placenta previa has not resolved, this patient is at increased risk for a placenta accreta, increta, or percreta. This is particularly concerning for placenta percreta with bladder invasion if she does still have a placenta previa.

127. d (Chapter 6)
While extremes of age have some association with preterm birth, age 33 is not at particularly increased risk. In terms of BMI, studies have shown that underweight individuals are at increased risk of PTB. Low socioeconomic status, PROM, placental abruption, and history of abdominal surgery are risk factors for PTB. Other risk factors include chorioamnionitis, multiple gestations, uterine anomalies such as a bicornuate uterus, previous preterm delivery, and other maternal diseases including preeclampsia and infections.

128. e (Chapter 27)
Preinvasive neoplastic disease of the vulva is divided into two categories: squamous (vulvar intraepithelial neoplasia; VIN) and nonsquamous intraepithelial neoplasias (Paget disease, melanoma in situ). The classification for VIN was changed in 2004 and again in 2015. Based on the 2015 terminology, vulvar squamous intraepithelial lesions are classified as Vulvar LSIL, Vulvar HSIL, and Differentiated type VIN. Vulvar LSIL lesions were formerly known as VIN 1. They are associated with koilocytic changes, HPV effect, and flat condyloma. Vulvar HSIL lesions were formerly categorized as VIN 2 and VIN 3, and then later termed Usual Type VIN in 2004. Risk factors for Vulvar HSIL include high-risk carcinogenic HPV genotypes and HPV persistence risk factors such as cigarette smoking, immunodeficiency, and immunosuppression. The incidence of HPV-associated VIN decreases as age increases. There is no racial predisposition to VIN.

Index

Note: Page numbers followed by *t* refer to tables; page numbers followed by *f* refer to figures

A

Abacavir, 284
Abdominal ultrasound, 210, 212
Abnormal bleeding, 251
   uterine, 233, 237, 239, 256, 350, 353–358, 354*t*, 357*t*, 393, 409, 466, 493, 495
   vaginal, 455, 466, 466*t*
Abnormal proliferation of trophoblastic tissue. *See* Gestational trophoblastic disease
ABO blood type, 121
Abortion, 121, 395, 406–412, 406*f*, 407*t*. *See also* Recurrent pregnancy loss; Spontaneous abortion
Abortus, 2, 17
Abruptio placentae. *See* Placental abruption
Abscess
   of Bartholin's duct, 221–223*f*, 222
   tubo-ovarian, 281–282, 282*f*
Abstinence, periodic, 379, 381*f*
Abuse. *See* Substance abuse, during pregnancy
Acanthosis nigricans, 355, 371, 423, 424*f*, 466
Accelerated growth rate, 321
Accreta. *See* Placenta Accreta
ACE (angiotensin-converting enzyme) inhibitors, 184
Acetaminophen, 9, 140, 143, 199
ACOG (American College/Congress of Obstetricians and Gynecologists), 48, 115, 133, 147, 170–171, 237, 241, 285, 354, 517
ACS (American Cancer Society), 455, 503
ACTH (adrenocorticotropic hormone), 367
Actinomycin-D, 484, 486, 495
Active phase of labor, 57, 57*f*
Actonel (risedronate), 331
Acute cystitis syndrome, 158
Acute fatty liver of pregnancy (AFLP), 137
Acute hepatitis B, 171
Acute parvovirus infections, 179
Acute renal failure, 91
Acute respiratory distress syndrome (ARDS), 175, 178
Acyclovir, 163, 164, 165, 263*t*, 267, 273, 275, 277
ADA (American Diabetes Association), 146
Add-back therapy, 254

Adenocarcinoma, 223, 437, 440, 450, 454, 463, 481–482
Adenomyoma, 255, 256*t*
Adenomyosis, 255–257, 255*f*, 256*t*, 356–357, 469
Adenosis, vaginal, 223*f*
ADH (atypical ductal hyperplasia), 509
ADH (antidiuretic hormone), 93
Adhesions
   intrauterine, 340, 343, 343*f*, 344, 345, 347–348, 355, 422
   pelvic, 352, 419*t*, 421, 423, 425
Adnexal masses, 239–242, 240*f*, 241*t*
Adrenal cortex, 367
Adrenal crisis, 375, 378
Adrenal disorders, 369–370
Adrenal gland, 367
Adrenal hyperplasia, 215, 369–370
Adrenal medulla, 367
Adrenarche, 320–321, 334
Adrenocorticotropic hormone (ACTH), 367
Adriamycin, 516
Advanced cervical cancer, 457*t*, 458
AEDs (antiepileptic drugs), 105*t*, 182–184, 183–184*t*, 192–193
AFC (antral follicle count), 424
AFI (amniotic fluid index), 117
AFLP (acute fatty liver of pregnancy), 137
African American heritage, 233, 244, 246
AGC (atypical glandular cells), 450
Agenesis
   gonadal, 337
   renal, 34
   vaginal, 216*f*, 217, 336–337
Alcohol abuse, 191, 427*t*
Aldara (Imiquimod), 269, 277, 436
Aldosterone synthase, 367
Alendronate (Fosamax), 331
ALH (atypical lobular hyperplasia), 509
Allen–Masters windows, 251
Alloimmunization, 118–121, 118*t*, 119*f*, 120*f*
ALND (axillary lymph node dissection), 515–516
α-adrenergic agonists, 314*t*
Alpha-blockers, 138
α-thalassemia, 29
Alprazolam, 353
Ambiguous genitalia, 215
Amenorrhea, 238–239, 326, 362, 365, 394
   lactational, 380–381

primary, 336–339, 337–338*t*, 339*f*, 354*t*
secondary, 339–344, 341–342*t*, 342*f*, 343*f*, 354*t*
American Cancer Society (ACS), 455, 503
American College/Congress of Obstetricians and Gynecologists (ACOG), 48, 115, 133, 147, 170–171, 237, 241, 285, 354, 517
American Diabetes Association (ADA), 146
American Society for Colposcopy and Cervical Pathology (ASCCP), 449
American Urogynecologic Society (AUGS), 311
AMH (anti-Müllerian hormone), 424–425, 432, 433–434
Amniocentesis, 38–39, 129, 131, 178, 198
   risks of, 41, 43
Amniotic fluid disorders, 117–118
Amniotic fluid index (AFI), 117
Amniotomy, 51
Amoxicillin, 171, 175, 176, 177
Amphetamines, 505*t*
Ampicillin, 96, 159, 161, 162, 178, 262, 282
Ampulla, 23, 25
Anaerobic organism, 162
Anal incontinence, 210, 212
Analgesia, 65–66, 66*f*, 185, 200, 257, 267
Anastrozole (Arimidex), 253, 516, 519
Anatomic abnormalities
   of cervix, 215–218, 216–218*f*
   of recurrent pregnancy loss, 21
   of secondary amenorrhea, 340
   of upper genital tract, 229–231, 229*t*, 230–231*f*
Ancef (cefazolin), 159, 161
Androgen insensitivity syndrome (AIS). *See* Testicular feminization
Androgen synthesis, 367–369, 368*f*
Androgenic steroid hormones, 320–321
Androgens, 367, 368*f*, 369, 370, 465, 481
   derivative of, 258, 260
Android pelvis, 96, 97*f*
Androstenedione, 324, 334, 429
Anemia, fetal, 119
Anesthesia, 9, 65–66, 66*f*, 203, 490
Aneuploidy. *See* Chromosomal abnormalities
Anogenital region, external, 263
Anogenital syndrome, 268

572 • Index

Anovulation, 340, 342, 355, 357, 357t, 365, 419, 463, 464, 465, 466
Antacids, 9
Antenatal tests, 13, 155
  of fetal well-being, 10
Antepartum care, for HIV-infected woman, 169–170
Antepartum hemorrhage, 72–84, 72t
  fetal vessel rupture, 82–84
  nonobstetric causes of, 84
  placenta previa, 72–78, 73f, 74–75t, 76f
  placental abruption, 78–81, 78t, 79f, 80t
  uterine rupture, 81–82, 82t
Anterior fontanelle, 49
Anthropoid pelvis, 96, 97f
Anti-D immunoglobulin (Rh IgG), 119–120
Anti-inflammatory medications, 200
Anti-La (SSB), 193, 197
Anti-Mullerian hormone (AMH), 424–425, 432, 433–434
Anti-Ro (SSA), 193, 197
Antiandrogens, 371
Antiarrhythmics, 184
Antibiotic prophylaxis, 159, 279, 386, 408
Antibiotics, 21, 47, 96, 159, 161, 162, 175, 206–207, 221, 222, 262–263, 268, 269, 273, 279–283, 285, 315, 386, 431. *See also* Broad spectrum antibiotics
Anticholinergic agents, 315
Anticholinergic drugs, 311, 314t, 317, 319
Anticoagulation treatment, 203t, 394
Antidepressants, 427t
Antidiuretic hormone (ADH), 93
Antiemetic therapy, 181
Antiemetics, 181, 192, 395
Antiepileptic drugs (AEDs), 105t, 182–184, 183–184t, 192–193
Antifungals, 263, 393, 441
Antihypertensive drugs, 104, 136, 138, 184, 490, 506
Antiphospholipid antibody syndrome (APLS), 21, 114, 134t, 189, 190, 197
Antiprostaglandins, 350
Antipyretics, 266
Antiretroviral therapy, 179
Antiretrovirals, 169, 170, 283, 284
Antisperm antibodies, 399, 427t, 428
Antivirals, 165, 168, 170, 267
Antral follicle count (AFC), 424
APLS. *See* Antiphospholipid antibody syndrome
Apocrine sweat gland cysts, 221
Appendicitis, 287, 289
Apt test, 83
ARDS (acute respiratory distress syndrome), 175, 178
Arimidex (anastrozole), 253, 516, 519
Aromatase inhibitors, 253, 429, 516, 519
ARTs (assisted reproductive technologies), 417–432, 429–431, 429–430f
ASB. *See* Asymptomatic bacteriuria

ASC-US (atypical squamous cells of undetermined significance), 449–450, 449–450t
ASCCP (American Society for Colposcopy and Cervical Pathology), 449
Ascites, 473, 476, 477f, 481
Asherman syndrome, 340, 343, 343f, 344, 345, 347–348, 355
Aspirin, 12, 21, 137, 138, 190, 193, 350, 511
Assisted reproductive technologies (ARTs), 417–432, 429–431, 429–430f
Asymmetric growth, 113
Asymptomatic bacteriuria (ASB), 157, 158, 177
  complication of, 175, 177
Atazanavir, 284
Atony, uterine, 203–204
Atosiban, 94
Atresia, vaginal, 216f, 217, 226, 228, 336–337
Atrophic endometrium, 355
Atrophic vaginitis, 228, 229, 317, 318, 524
Atrophy, 292
  endometrial, 358
  genitourinary, 330, 359, 361, 363
  urogenital, 330, 359, 361, 363
  vaginal, 330, 358
Atypical complex intraepithelial neoplasia, 247
Atypical ductal hyperplasia (ADH), 509
Atypical endometrial hyperplasia, 239, 463, 465
Atypical glandular cells (AGC), 450
Atypical lobular hyperplasia (ALH), 509
Atypical squamous cells of undetermined significance (ASC-US), 449–450, 449–450t
Augmentation cystoplasty, 313
Augmentation of labor, 49–51
AUGS (American Urogynecologic Society), 311
Autoimmune inflammatory disorders, 249
Autonomic system, 304
Autosomal dominant diseases, 27
Autosomal recessive diseases, 27
Axillary lymph node, 502, 503f
Axillary lymph node dissection (ALND), 515–516
Aygestin, 239
Azithromycin, 96, 171, 263t, 264, 267, 273, 276, 277
Azole therapy, 271
Azoospermia, 399, 428
AZT. *See* Zidovudine

B
Baby blues, 209, 211
Back pain, 9
Bacterial vaginosis (BV), 160–161, 270, 270f, 273, 276, 277, 278, 281
Bacteriuria, 157–158, 159
Baden-Walker Halfway Scoring System, 294, 295f, 300
Barbiturates, 191, 390t

Barium enema, 476
Barrier methods of contraception, 381–384, 382f, 383f, 384f
Bartholin's duct cyst, 225, 227
  and abscesses, 221–223f, 222
Basal insulin, 153, 155
Bazedoxifene (BZE), 328
BCT (breast conserving therapy), 515
Benadryl, 104
Benign breast disease, 507–518, 512t, 513–515f, 518t
Benign cystic mature teratoma, 479, 480, 485
Benign cysts, of vulva and vagina, 221
Benign disorders, 507–518, 512t, 513–515f, 518t
  of lower genital tract, 215–225
  of upper genital tract, 229–243
Benign endometrial hyperplasia, 238, 239, 357, 359
Benign gestational trophoblastic disease, 487, 488t
Benign lesions, of vulva, vagina, and cervix, 215, 223–224, 223–224f
Benign tumors, of vulva and vagina, 223
Benzalkonium chloride, 384
Benzathine penicillin, 273
Benzathine penicillin G, 264, 277
Benzodiazepines, 182, 184, 191, 353
Beta-agonists, 94, 102, 162
Beta-blockers, 138, 427t, 490
β-hCG. *See* Beta-human chorionic gonadotropin
β-mimetics, 94
β-thalassemia, 29
β-3 agonist drug, 313
Beta-human chorionic gonadotropin (β-hCG), 1, 4, 16–17, 36–37, 36t, 341, 409
  OTC test for, 12
  quantitative level of, 22, 23, 24, 25, 26
  recommendations for, 22, 25
Betamethasone, 19–20, 81, 93, 137, 186
  administration, 127, 130
Bethanechol, 313
BI-RADS (Breast Imaging Reporting and Database System), 506
Bicornuate uterus, 230f, 231, 232f
Bilateral luteomas, of pregnancy, 373, 375
Bilateral salpingo-oophorectomy (BSO), 254, 282, 359, 467, 477, 480, 481, 483, 485
Bimanual pelvic examination, findings on, 240
Biophysical profiles (BPP), 10, 13, 14
Biopsy, 442, 443
  breast, 506, 507, 509–510, 512t, 513–514, 516, 517
  cervical, 450t, 451–454, 453f, 454t
  of cyst wall, 227
  endometrial, 237, 466
  excisional, 507
  of lymph node, 437, 515
  needle, 513
  vulvar, 220, 220f, 226, 227
Bipolar fulguration, 403
Birth trauma, 115, 116, 127, 130, 314
Bishop score, 47, 47t, 51, 68, 70

Bisphosphonates, 329t, 331, 332, 394t
Black cohosh, 330
Bladder
    chart, 306, 306f
    emptying, 308
    filling, 308
    overdistension of, 313, 313f, 314
    pathophysiology of, 303–304, 303–304f
Bladder outlet obstruction, 313–314
    with overflow urinary incontinence, 316, 318
Bleeding. *See also* Abnormal bleeding; Hemorrhage; Menstrual cycle; Uterine bleeding; Vaginal bleeding
    intermenstrual, 224
    postcoital, 455
    postmenopausal, 358–359, 358t
    postpartum, 496
Bleomycin, 480
Blood. *See* Hematology, during pregnancy
Blood count, complete, 241
Blood pressure. *See* Hypertension
Blood sampling, of fetus, 10, 39
Blood urea nitrogen (BUN), 12, 14
Bloody nipple discharge, 506, 510, 513
BMD (bone mineral density), 331
Bone marrow suppression, 176, 179
Bone mineral density (BMD), 331
Bone mineralization, 394, 394t
Boniva (ibandronate), 331
Botulinum toxin, 313, 317, 319
BPP (biophysical profiles), 10, 13, 14
Brachial plexus injuries, 110
Bradycardia, fetal, 101–102
Braxton Hicks, 67, 69
    contractions, 9, 13, 14
BRCA1 gene mutation, 240, 504, 511
BRCA2 gene mutation, 240, 504, 511
Break-through-bleeding, 358
Breast
    anatomy of, 502–503, 502–503f
    benign breast disease, 507–518, 512t, 513–515f, 518t
    bud development, 321, 333, 334
    care of, 199–200
    development of, 320, 321, 322f, 322t, 337–339
    infection. *See* Mastitis
    invasive breast cancers, 514–517, 514f, 515f, 518t
    malignant breast disease, 511–513, 512t, 513f
    masses of, 506–507, 507–508f, 507t, 513
    nipple discharge of, 505–506, 505t, 510, 520, 522
    noninvasive disease of, 513–514, 514f
    pain evaluation of, 505
    physiology of, 503, 504f
    reconstruction of, 515, 515f
    routine evaluation of, 504–505
    ultrasonography, 504
Breast cancer, 465, 475, 502–507, 502–504f, 505t, 507–508f, 507t
    personal history of, 484, 486
    risk for, 520, 522
    treatment, follow-up after, 521, 523

Breast conserving therapy (BCT), 515
Breast Imaging Reporting and Database System (BI-RADS), 506
Breastfeeding, 170, 177, 179, 180, 199–200, 284, 380, 381
    benefits of, 210, 213
    in HIV-infected woman, 287, 289
Breech delivery, trial of, 107, 110
Breech extraction, of twins, 125
Breech presentation, 48–49, 97–98, 98f, 152, 154
    risk for, 107, 110
Breech vaginal delivery, 69, 98
Brisdelle (paroxetine), 330
Broad spectrum antibiotics, 206, 270, 282, 285
Bromocriptine, 343, 349, 509
Brow presentation, 99, 100f
BSO (bilateral salpingo-oophorectomy), 254, 282, 359, 467, 477, 480, 481, 483, 485
BUN (blood urea nitrogen), 12, 14
Buprenorphine (Subutex), 192
BV (bacterial vaginosis), 160–161, 270, 270f, 273, 276, 277, 278, 281
Bypass (urinary) incontinence, 302–303
BZE (bazedoxifene), 328

C

CA-125, 241, 478, 478t, 479, 482
Cabergoline, 349
Caffeine, 191, 509, 519
CAH (congenital adrenal hyperplasia), 215, 369–370, 374, 377
Calcitonin, 329t, 332
Calcium channel blockers, 93, 105, 138
Calcium chloride, 138
Calcium gluconate, 138, 212
Calcium supplementation, 137, 329t, 331, 331t, 343, 353, 360, 394, 394t
Call–Exner bodies, 481, 485
Campbell De Morgan spots. *See* Cherry hemangiomas
Cancer. *See* Adenocarcinoma; Carcinoma; Squamous cell carcinoma
Candida glabrata, 271
Candidiasis, 263, 270–271, 270f
Carbamazepine, 41, 44, 138, 182–183, 183t, 390t
Carboplatin, 479, 482, 484, 486
Carboprost, 204, 212
Carcinoma, 369. *See also* Squamous cell carcinoma
    of Bartholin's gland, 222
    of breast, 465, 475, 502–518, 502–504f, 505t, 507–508f, 507t, 512t, 513–514f, 518t
    of cervix, 454–458, 454f, 456–458t, 457f
    of endometrium, 463–469, 481
    of fallopian tube, 481–482
    of ovaries, 473–479, 474–478t, 474–475f, 477f
    of vagina, 440, 440t
    of vulva, 437–439, 437f, 438t, 439f
Carcinomatous ileus, 473
Cardiac defects, of fetus, 33–34, 34f

Cardiac disease, maternal, 184–186
Cardiac output, 12, 13
    during pregnancy, 2
Cardinal movements, of labor, 55–56, 56f, 68, 70
Cardiovascular disease, 185
Cardiovascular health, 330, 349
Cardiovascular physiology, of pregnancy, 2
cART (combination antiretroviral therapy), 169, 177, 179, 180, 283, 284, 286, 289
Catecholamines, 374, 377
CBC (complete blood count), 81, 91, 356
CCCT (clomiphene citrate challenge test), 424
CCR5 receptor antagonists, 284
CDC (Centers for Disease Control and Prevention), 165, 391, 417
CDE antigens, 121
CEE (conjugated equine estrogen), 328
Cefazolin (Ancef), 159, 161
Cefixime, 273, 274
Cefotetan, 159, 178, 281, 282, 288
Cefoxitin, 178, 280, 281, 282
Cefoxitin plus doxycycline, 286, 287, 288, 289
Ceftriaxone, 159, 171, 263t, 264, 267, 273, 274, 277, 281, 408
Celebrex (celecoxib), 351
Celecoxib (Celebrex), 351
Celexa (citalopram), 353, 364
Cell-free DNA (cfDNA), 8, 30
    screening test, 38–40, 39f
Cellular atypia, 237
Cellular calcium, magnesium sulfate on, 106, 108
Centers for Disease Control and Prevention (CDC), 165, 391, 417
Central disorders, amenorrhea from, 337–338, 337t
Cephalexin, 158, 159, 262
Cephalohematoma, 69, 71
Cephalopelvic disproportion (CPD), 57, 96–97, 97f
Cephalosporins, 158, 159, 162, 199, 206, 280, 281, 282, 285, 288
Cerclage, 20, 20f
Cervarix, 446, 447
Cervical adenocarcinoma, 450
Cervical biopsy, colposcopy and, 450t, 451–454, 453f, 454t
Cervical cancer, 363, 445, 445f, 454–458, 454f, 456–458t, 457f, 460, 461, 462
    screening for, 447–449, 448f
Cervical cap, 383–384, 384f
Cervical culture, 246
Cervical dysplasia. *See* Cervical intraepithelial neoplasia
Cervical excision procedures, complications of, 460, 461
Cervical factor infertility, 418t, 419t, 422
Cervical incompetence. *See* Cervical insufficiency
Cervical insufficiency, 19f, 19–20, 19t, 20f, 92, 223, 345, 347
Cervical intraepithelial neoplasia (CIN), 446–454, 446t, 446–447f, 448–451t, 452–453f, 454t

Cervical polyps, 224, 224f
Cervical stenosis, 224, 340, 352, 422, 426
Cervicitis, 273, 274, 277, 278, 288, 289
Cervidil (PGE$_2$ pessary), 51, 70
Cervix
  benign lesions of, 215, 223–224, 223–224f
  cancer, 284
  dilation of, 224, 410, 410f
  examination of, 47–48, 47t, 48f, 49f
  infections of, 272
    chlamydia trachomatis, 273
    neisseria gonorrhoeae, 272–273
  lacerations of, 203
  transformation zone of, 446, 447f
Cesarean delivery, 63–64, 64t, 98, 162, 170, 177, 178, 179, 199, 202t, 210–211, 213–214
  risk factor for developing postpartum endomyometritis, 286, 288
Cesarean section, indication of, 110
CF (cystic fibrosis), 27–28
cfDNA. See Cell-free DNA
Chancre, 264, 265f
Chancroid, 263, 263t, 267
Chasteberry, 353
Chemoradiation therapy, 458
Chemotherapeutic agents, 113, 241, 427t, 439, 468, 479, 480, 481, 482, 493, 494f, 495, 496, 516, 519
Chemotherapy, 496, 497, 498, 499, 500, 501
Cherry hemangiomas, 223
Chickenpox. See Varicella zoster virus
Chlamydia test, 401, 403
Chlamydia trachomatis, 171, 262, 273, 280, 281, 288, 355
  L-serotypes (L1, L2, or L3), 277
Chlamydial infections, 171, 276
  NAAT for, 276
  treatment, 277, 278
Chloasma, 4
Chlordiazepoxide, 39t
Chocolate cysts, 240, 252
Cholelithiasis, 143
Cholinergic agents, 313
Chorioamnionitis, 110, 161–162, 175, 287
  antibiotics for, 176, 178
  causative organism for, 176, 178
  complications of, 176, 178, 179
  diagnosis of, 176, 178
Choriocarcinoma
  gestational, 487, 488t, 493, 495–496, 497, 498, 500
  ovarian, 473–474, 475f, 476–479
Chorionic villous sampling (CVS), 39, 42, 45
Choroid plexus cysts, 30–31, 30f
Chromosomal abnormalities, 29–31, 30f, 35–37. See also Sex chromosomal abnormalities; 46,XY chromosomes
Chromosomes, 46,XY, 337
Chronic anovulation, 238–239, 247, 355, 465
Chronic hypertension, 133, 138
  pregnant women with, 140, 141, 142
  with superimposed preeclampsia, 138–139

Chronic renal disease, 198
Cigarettes. See Smoking
Cimetidine, 427t
CIN (cervical intraepithelial neoplasia), 446–454, 446t, 446–447f, 448–451f, 452–453f, 454t
Ciprofloxacin, 177, 267
Circumvallate placenta, 74t
Cisplatin chemotherapy, 458, 462, 479
Citalopram (Celexa), 353, 364
CKC (cold-knife conization), 451–452, 453f, 454f, 455
Clear cell adenocarcinoma, 223, 440, 454
Clindamycin, 161, 162, 270, 276, 277, 278, 279, 281, 282, 283, 285
Clobetasol, 219t, 221, 228
Clomid. See Clomiphene citrate
Clomiphene citrate, 123, 340, 343–344, 365, 376, 424, 425, 426t, 429, 430, 431, 432, 433, 434
Clomiphene citrate challenge test (CCCT), 424
Clonidine, 329t, 330
CMV (cytomegalovirus), 113, 166–168, 167f, 282
Coagulation disorders, 187–189, 188–189f
Coagulopathies, 357
Cocaine, 78t, 79, 84, 191, 192, 427t
Cognitive behavior therapy, 330
Coitus interruptus, 379–380, 401, 403
Cold-knife conization (CKC), 451–452, 453f, 454f, 455
Color Doppler, 83, 88
Colpocleisis, 298, 299, 300, 301
Colpoposcopy, 220
Colposcopy, 443, 450, 459, 460, 461, 462
  cervical biopsy and, 450t, 451–454, 453f, 454f
Combination antiretroviral therapy (cART), 169, 177, 179, 180, 283, 284, 286, 289
Combination estrogen and progesterone contraception, 380t, 388–393, 389f, 390–392t, 392f
Combined oral contraceptive pills (OCPs), 373, 376
Complementary and alternative therapies, 330
Complete abortion, 17
Complete blood count (CBC), 81, 91, 356
Complete breech, 97, 98f
Complete molar pregnancies, 487–491, 488–491f, 489t
Complete previa, 72, 76f
Complex hyperplasia, 237, 238t
Complications. See also Fetal complications
  of diabetes during pregnancy, 148–149t
  of labor and delivery, 92–106
    obstetric emergencies, 101–105, 103–104f, 105t
    obstruction, malpresentation, and malposition, 96–101, 97–100f
    preterm and premature rupture of membranes, 46–47, 47f, 94–96

preterm labor, 18, 92
tocolysis, 92–94, 95f
of oral contraception, 389, 390t
of postpartum care, 202–207, 202–203t, 205f
of preeclampsia, 133, 134t
of pregnancy, 15–22, 181–193
  cervical insufficiency, 19f, 19–20, 19t, 20f
  coagulation disorders, 187–189, 188–189f
  ectopic pregnancy, 15f, 15–17, 15t, 16f, 387
  fetal complications, 112–126
  first-trimester abortion, 18, 18t
  hyperemesis gravidarum, 181–182
  maternal cardiac disease, 184–186
  maternal renal disease, 186–187
  maternal thyroid disease, 189
  recurrent pregnancy loss, 21
  second-trimester abortion, 18–19
  seizures, 104–105, 105t, 137–138, 138t, 182–184, 183–184t
  spontaneous abortion, 17, 17f, 18t
  substance abuse, 191–192
  systemic lupus erythematosus, 189–191, 190t
Compound presentation, 99–100, 100f
Computerized tomography (CT), 241
Concealed hemorrhage, 79, 79f
Conception, 254t, 417t, 418
Condoms, 376, 381–382, 382f, 383f
Condyloma, 446
Condyloma acuminata, 268, 268f
Congenital abnormalities
  of cervix, 223, 223f
  fetal, 31–35, 32–34f, 182, 183t
  of vulva and vagina, 215–218, 216–218f
Congenital adrenal hyperplasia (CAH), 215, 369–370, 374, 377
Congenital herpes virus, 129
Congenital müllerian anomalies, of uterus, 229–231, 229t, 230–232f
Congenital rubella syndrome (CRS), 168
Congenital varicella syndrome, 164, 165f
Conjoined twins, 123, 123f
Conjugated equine estrogen (CEE), 328
Conservative surgical therapy, 254
Constipation, 9
Consumptive coagulopathy, 80–81, 91
Continuous urinary incontinence, 302t, 303, 314–315, 314f
Contraception, 379–400, 380t, 399, 407, 412, 414
  barrier methods and spermicides, 381–384, 382f, 383f, 384f
  emergency, 395–397
  hCG and, 496
  hormonal methods of, 388–395, 389f, 390–392t, 392f, 394t
  intrauterine devices, 201, 384–388, 385f, 386t, 387f, 388t, 396
  natural methods, 379–381, 381f
  postpartum, 200–201
  sterilization, 397–399, 397–399f
Contraceptive services, 324
Contractions, 9
Cooper suspensory ligaments, 502, 502f

Copper-T IUD, 201, 380t, 384, 385f, 386–387, 395, 396, 401, 403, 404, 412, 414, 517
Cord compression, 88, 89, 90
Cord prolapse, 126, 127, 130, 132
Coronary artery disease, 327
Corpus luteum cysts, 239, 240, 322, 334
Corticosteroids, 96, 114, 162, 181, 190, 191, 193, 283, 368f, 371
Cortrosyn, 370
Cotton swab test, 306, 307f
Coumadin, 184, 194, 196
Cowden syndrome, 465, 504
COX-2 inhibitors, 350
CPD (cephalopelvic disproportion), 57, 96–97, 97f
Crab louse. See Phthirus pubis
Cramping. See Dysmenorrhea
Creatinine, 12, 14
Crohn disease, 263
CRS (congenital rubella syndrome), 168
Cryotherapy, 451, 452, 460, 461
CT (computerized tomography), 241
Cushing syndrome, 369
    diagnosis of, 374, 377
    therapeutic option, 374, 377
Cutaneous cysts, causes of, 227
CVS (chorionic villous sampling), 39, 42, 45
Cyclic or continuous estrogen–progestin contraceptives, 252, 257
Cyclic pelvic pain, 226, 227
Cyclophosphamide, 190, 516
Cyclosporin, 371
Cyclosporine, 186
Cystadenoma tumor, 371
Cystic adnexal masses, 239–242, 240f, 241t
Cystic fibrosis (CF), 27–28
Cystitis, 157, 158, 159
Cystocele, 227, 291, 293, 293f, 295, 297t
Cystometrogram, 306
Cystometry, 307f, 308
Cystosarcoma phyllodes, 509–510, 520, 522
Cystoscopy, 85, 87, 88
Cystourethroscopy, 247, 315, 318
Cysts
    of breast, 506, 508f
    of cervix, 223–224, 224f
    chocolate, 252
    choroid plexus, 30, 30f
    ovarian, 239–242, 240f, 241t
    theca lutein, 240, 370, 489, 490, 490f
    of vulva and vagina, 221
Cytologic vaginitis. See Trichomoniasis; Bacterial vaginosis; Yeast infection
Cytomegalovirus (CMV), 113, 166–168, 167f, 282

D

Danazol (Danocrine), 235, 253, 254, 257, 258, 260, 353, 425, 505, 509, 519
Danocrine (danazol), 235, 253, 254, 257, 258, 260, 353, 425, 505, 509, 519
Dating, of pregnancy, 2, 121–122
Day 3 FSH level, measurement of, 424
DCIS (ductal carcinoma in situ), 513, 514, 514f

Death, maternal, 188
Death of fetus. See Abortion
Decelerations, of fetal heart rate, 52, 54f, 101–102
Deep infiltrating endometriosis (DIE), 251–252
Deep vein thrombosis (DVT), 187–188, 328, 390
    diagnosis of, 193–194, 196
    treatment of, 196
Deepest vertical pocket (DVP), 117
Defecatory issues, 293
Definitive hysterectomy, 499, 501
Definitive surgical therapy, 254
Dehydration, 9, 181
Dehydroepiandrosterone (DHEA), 320, 367
Dehydroepiandrosterone sulfate (DHEA-S) level, 320, 367, 371, 372, 373, 375, 376
DeLancey levels of vaginal support, 291, 292t
Delayed puberty, 322
Delivery, 46–67, 46–50f, 47t, 53–57f, 59–64f, 61t, 64t, 65t, 66f
    complications of, 92–106
    for mothers with
        diabetes, 148, 151
        epilepsy, 184
    preferred mode of, 85, 88
    of triplets, 125
    of twins, 125
Demise, of fetus, 121
Denosumab, 332
Depo-Provera (depot medroxyprogesterone acetate), 233, 246, 330, 393, 405
Depo-Provera, 201, 239, 351, 355, 373, 376, 393–394, 394t, 402, 404, 405
Depot medroxyprogesterone acetate (DMPA, Depo-Provera), 233, 246, 330, 393, 405
Depot-medroxyprogesterone acetate, 393–394, 394t, 400
Depression. See Postpartum depression
Dermatologic physiology, during pregnancy, 4
Dermatoses, of vulva and vagina, 218–223, 219t, 220–223f
Dermoid cysts. See Benign cystic mature teratoma
DES (diethylstilbstrol) exposure, 19, 19t, 223, 223f, 229, 231f, 422, 440, 449, 454–455
Detrol LA, 317, 319
Detrusor muscle, 303, 313
Detrusor overactivity. See Urge incontinence
Detrusor underactivity. See Overflow (urinary) incontinence
Developmental age, 2
DEXA scan, 345, 348
Dexamethasone suppression test (DST), 369, 425
Dextrose, 148, 151
DHEA (dehydroepiandrosterone), 320, 367
DHEAS (dehydroepiandrosterone sulfate), 320, 367, 371, 372, 373, 375, 376

DHT (dihydrotestosterone), 367
Di-di twins, 123, 123–124f
Diabetes, 116
    endometrial cancer and, 465
    gestational, 8, 145–148, 146t
    pregestational, 145, 148–151, 148–150t
    during pregnancy, 145–152, 146t, 148–150t
Diabetes mellitus, 404
Diaphragm, 382–383, 383f
Diazepam, 390t
Diazoxide, 371
Dicloxacillin, 207, 210, 213
Didanosine, 284
DIE (deep infiltrating endometriosis), 251–252
Diet, diabetic, 146, 147, 148, 149–150
Diethylstilbestrol (DES) exposure, 19, 19t, 223, 223f, 229, 231f, 422, 440, 449, 454–455
Diflucan, 271
Digital breast tomosynthesis, 504
Digoxin, 186, 411
Dihydrofolate reductase inhibitor, 409
Dihydrotestosterone (DHT), 367
Dilapan, 410
Dilation
    of cervix, 224, 410, 410f
    of vagina, 218
Dilation and curettage (D&C), 24, 26, 204, 407–408f, 408–410, 466, 491, 492, 495
    suction D&C, 490, 499
Dilation and evacuation (D&E), 407f, 410–411, 410f
    maternal mortality rate for, 413, 415
Discharge instructions, 201–202
Disseminated gonorrhea, 275, 277
Diuretics, 184, 186
Dizygotic twins, 122, 123
DMPA (depot medroxyprogesterone acetate), 233, 246, 330, 393, 405
Docetaxel (Taxotere), 479
Dominant follicle, 324
Dopamine agonists, 343, 346, 349, 357t
Dopamine antagonists, 340–341
Doppler sonography, 498
Double bubble-duodenal atresia, 41, 43
Double cervix, 223
Double uterus, 232f
Double vision, 140, 141, 143
Down syndrome, 30, 35–37, 36t
    first-trimester screening for, 42, 44
Doxorubicin, 516–517
Doxycycline, 263t, 264, 268, 273, 276, 280, 281, 282, 408
Droperidol, 181
Drospirenone, 353, 364
Drugs, 371–372
DST (Dexamethasone suppression test), 369, 425
DTR (serial deep tendon reflex) examination, 106, 108
Dual-energy X-ray absorptiometry (DXA), 331
Duavee, 328
Ductal carcinoma in situ (DCIS), 513, 514, 514f

Ductal hyperplasia, 509
Duffy antigen, 121
DVP (Deepest vertical pocket), 117
DVT. *See* Deep vein thrombosis (DVT)
DXA (dual-energy X-ray absorptiometry), 331
Dysfunctional uterine bleeding (DUB). *See* Abnormal bleeding, uterine
Dysgerminomas, 479, 480, 481, 483, 484, 485, 486
Dysmenorrhea, 234, 251, 256, 350–352, 351*f*, 352*f*, 387–388
  treatment for, 362, 364
Dyspareunia, 224, 240, 251, 291
Dystrophy, 218
Dysuria, 326

E

Early cervical cancer, 457, 457*t*
Early deceleration, of fetal heart rate, 52, 54*f*
Early menopause, 333, 335
EBL (estimated blood loss), 91
ECC (endocervical curettage), 442, 443
Echogenic intracardiac focus (EIF), 37, 37*f*
Eclampsia, 108, 110–111, 133, 137–138, 138*t*
Eclamptic seizures, 144
Ectopic pregnancy, 15*f*, 15–17, 15*t*, 16*f*, 245, 247, 287, 288, 289, 387, 399, 421
  common site of, 23, 25
  methotrexate therapy for, 22, 25
  recommendations for, 22, 25
  risk for, 23, 26
EDC (estimated date of confinement), 2
EDD (estimated date of delivery), 2
Edema, 9, 135
Edward syndrome. *See* Trisomy 18
EE (ethinyl estradiol), 389
Efavirenz, 284, 286, 289
Effacement, 47, 48*f*
Effexor (venlafaxine), 330, 353, 517
Efficacy rates, of contraception methods, 379, 380*t*
EIF (echogenic intracardiac focus), 37, 37*f*
EIN. *See* Endometrial intraepithelial neoplasia (EIN)
Eisenmenger syndrome, 185
Electric vacuum aspiration, 408
11β-hydroxylase deficiency, 369
ELISA (enzyme-linked Immunosorbent assay), 174
Ella (ulipristal acetate), 395
EMB (endometrial biopsy), 237, 244, 247, 257, 356, 364, 466, 484
Embolectomy, 194, 196
Embryo, 1
Embryogenesis, 31–32, 32*f*
Emergency contraception, 395–397
EMPD (extramammary Paget disease), 437
Empiric medical therapy, 251
Empty egg, 487, 488, 488*f*
EMS (endometrial thickness), 363
End-organ disorders, 337, 337*t*, 338*t*
Endocervical curettage (ECC), 442, 443

Endocrine function, during pregnancy, 4
Endodermal sinus tumor, 474*t*, 475*f*, 479, 479*f*, 480*t*, 481
Endogenous estrogen, 238
Endometrial abnormalities, 422
Endometrial adenocarcinoma, 450
Endometrial atrophy, 358
Endometrial biopsy (EMB), 237, 244, 247, 257, 356, 364, 466, 484
Endometrial cancer, 328, 355, 358*t*, 359, 363, 469, 471. *See also* Endometrial carcinoma; Endometrial adenocarcinoma
Endometrial carcinoma, 463–469, 464*t*, 466–468*t*, 481. *See also* Endometrial cancer
Endometrial hyperplasia, 237–238, 255, 328, 356, 357, 403, 405, 465, 481
Endometrial intraepithelial neoplasia (EIN), 237–239, 238*t*, 257, 260, 328, 463, 465
  risk factors for, 244–245, 247
Endometrial polyps, 237, 359, 361, 363–364
Endometrial proliferation, 238
Endometrial thickness (EMS), 363
Endometrioid adenocarcinoma, 463
Endometrioma, 240, 241*t*, 247, 249, 251, 251*f*, 252, 252*f*, 254*f*, 256*t*, 258, 260
  continued postoperative management, 258, 260
  genetic factors, 258, 260
Endometriosis, 224, 249–255, 250*f*, 251*f*, 252*f*, 253–254*t*, 254*f*, 256*t*, 418*t*, 419, 421–422, 425–426
Endometriosis interna. See Adenomyosis
Endometritis, 205–206, 211, 213, 279–280
Endometrium, 333, 334
  premalignant disease of, 237–239, 238*t*
Endomyometritis, 285, 286, 287, 288
Endothelial dysfunction, 133
Endotoxin, 159, 178
Enoxaparin. *See* Low-molecular-weight heparin
Enterocele, 291, 292*f*, 293, 296, 297*t*
Enterococcus, 262
Entry inhibitors, 284
Enzyme-linked Immunosorbent assay (ELISA), 174
Ephedrine, 102
Epidermal inclusion cysts, 221
Epidural anesthesia, 66, 67, 162, 314*t*
Epilepsy, 182–184, 184*t*
Epinephrine, 104
Episiotomy, 59–60, 60*f*, 70
Epithelial abnormalities, of cervix, 446, 449, 449*t*
Epithelial hyperplasia, 509
Epithelial ovarian cancer, 249, 486
Epithelial tumors, 477–479, 478*t*
EPT (estrogen and progesterone therapy), 328, 328*t*, 345, 348, 349
Ergonovines, 204
Erosive disorders, 220
ERT (estrogen replacement therapy), 328, 339, 372, 464, 468

Erythema infectiosum. *See* Fifth disease; Parvovirus B19
Erythroblastosis fetalis, 119, 119*f*
Erythromycin, 96, 171, 268, 273
Escherichia coli, 158, 262, 263, 281
  treatment for, 175, 178
Essure (microinsert coils) method, 402, 403–404
Essure tubal occlusion, 398–399
Estimated blood loss (EBL), 91
Estimated date of confinement (EDC), 2
Estimated date of delivery (EDD), 2
Estradiol, 324, 327, 429
Estrogen and progesterone therapy (EPT), 328, 328*t*, 345, 348, 349
Estrogen-dependent neoplasms, 463
Estrogen hormone, 4, 232, 238, 238*t*, 253–254, 320, 321, 322, 323*f*, 324, 326, 368*f*, 503, 516, 517
Estrogen-independent neoplasms, 463
Estrogen-progesterone OCPs, 201, 248, 390*t*
Estrogen receptor positive tumor, 517
Estrogen replacement therapy (ERT), 328, 339, 372, 464, 468
Estrogen therapy, 185, 221, 223, 225, 242, 243, 296, 309, 315, 328–329, 328*t*, 330, 332, 339, 340, 341, 342, 343, 344, 353, 356, 385, 393, 394*t*, 395, 396, 397, 400, 423, 426, 429, 463, 464, 465, 468, 481
Estrogens, 213
  synthesis, 324
Estrone, 429
ET (extended therapy), 329
Ethinyl estradiol (EE), 321, 324, 327, 389, 392, 394
Etonogestrel, 392, 394, 400
Etoposide, 480
Evening primrose oil, 353, 509
Evista, 331
Excisional biopsy, 507
Exemestane, 517
Exercise-induced amenorrhea, 346, 348–349
Exogenous cortisol, 215
Exogenous estrogen, 238
Exogenous hormones, 359, 371–372
Expectant management, 225, 226, 227, 228
Extended therapy (ET), 329
External anogenital region, 263
External electronic monitoring, of fetus during labor, 51–52, 53*f*
External hemorrhage. *See* Revealed hemorrhage
External sphincter, 303, 303*f*
Extramammary Paget disease (EMPD), 437

F

Face presentation, 98–99, 99*f*
Failure rates, of contraception methods, 379, 380*t*
Failure to progress (FTP), 96
Fallopian tube abnormalities, 418–419, 421, 423*f*
Fallopian tube carcinoma, 481–482, 484, 485, 486

Falope ring, 397, 398, 398f, 402, 403
False-positive nontreponemal tests, 264
Famciclovir, 163, 267, 277
Familial ovarian cancer syndrome, 475
Family history of gynecologic malignancies, 511
FAS (fetal alcohol syndrome), 191
Fascia, 291
FDA (Food and Drug Administration), 283, 298, 309, 408, 504
Fecundability, 417, 420
Federal Genetic Information Nondiscrimination Act of 2008, 471
Female condoms, 382–383, 383f
Female factor infertility, 418–427, 419–420t, 419f, 420–424f, 426t, 426f
Femara (letrozole), 253, 340, 425, 426t, 429, 431, 516, 519
Fentanyl, 65
Fern test, 47, 47f
Fertility drugs, 425
Fertilization, 324. See also Assisted reproductive technologies
Fetal alcohol syndrome (FAS), 191
Fetal anemia, 85, 87, 88, 119, 176, 179
Fetal blood sampling, 10, 39
Fetal bradycardia, 101–102, 137
Fetal complications
 of diabetes during pregnancy, 149t
 of preeclampsia, 133, 134t
 of pregnancy, 112–126
  amniotic fluid disorders, 117–118
  fetal demise, 121
  fetal growth disorders, 112–117, 113t, 114f, 115f, 116t
  multiple gestations, 122–125, 123f, 124f
  postterm pregnancies, 1, 116, 121–122
  Rh incompatibility and alloimmunization, 118–121, 118t, 119f, 120f
Fetal demise, 121
Fetal goiter, 198
Fetal growth, 112–117, 113t, 114f, 115f, 116t
 regulation of, 112
Fetal heart rate, 52, 53–54f, 101–102
 evaluation of, 52–53
Fetal heart sounds, 492
Fetal heart tones (FHTs), 86, 90
 test for, 24, 26
Fetal hydrops, 119, 119f, 128, 131. See also Erythroblastosis fetalis
Fetal lie, 46
Fetal macrosomia, 115–117, 116t
 cause of, 127, 130–131
Fetal position, 49, 50f, 69, 96–101, 97–100f
Fetal presentation, 46, 48–49, 50f, 96–101, 97–100f, 125
Fetal scalp electrode (FSE), 52
Fetal scalp electrode, 70
Fetal ultrasound, 126, 127, 129, 130
Fetal vessel rupture, 82–84
Feticidal agents, 411
Fetus, 1
 assessment of, 10–11

congenital abnormalities of, 31–35, 32–34f, 182, 183t
imaging of, 39–40, 39f
infections affecting, 162–174, 164f, 165f, 167f, 172f, 174f
lung maturity of, 11
monitoring of, 51–55, 53–55f, 58, 147–148, 149
FHTs. See Fetal heart tones (FHTs)
Fibrin monomer complexes, 194, 196
Fibro-thecomas, 370
Fibroadenoma, 509–510, 520, 522
Fibrocystic breast change, 508–509
Fibroids, 224, 231–237, 233f, 234–236t, 236f, 256, 256t, 359
 locations, with abnormal vaginal bleeding, 244, 246
Fifth disease, 165, 176, 179
FIGO (International Federation of Gynecology and Obstetrics), 354, 438t, 440t, 456t, 460, 462, 493, 500
Filshie clips, 397, 399f, 402, 403
Final menstrual period (FMP), 324
Finasteride, 371
Fine-needle aspiration (FNA), 506, 507t, 508f, 513
First menses, 333, 334, 336
First stage of labor, 57–58, 57f, 67, 69
First trimester
 abortions, 18, 18t, 407, 408–410, 408f, 410t
 definition, 1
 screening, 35–36, 36f
  for Down syndrome, 42, 44
 visits, 7–8
FISH (fluorescent in situ hybridization), 38, 42, 45
Fistula, urinary, 314–315, 314f
Fitzhugh-Curtis syndrome, 281, 282f
5-fluorouracil (5-FU), 269, 439, 441, 516
5-FU (5-fluorouracil), 269, 439, 441, 516
Fluconazole, 271, 278
Fludrocortisone acetate, 215
Fluorescent in situ hybridization (FISH), 38, 42, 45
Fluorescent treponemal antibody absorption (FTA-ABS), 172, 264
Fluoroquinolones, 262, 281
Fluoxetine, 353
FMP (final menstrual period), 234
FNA (fine-needle aspiration), 506, 507t, 508f, 513
Folate
 to reduce neural tube defects, 11, 13
 supplementation, 149, 154, 183
Folic acid, 42, 44
 supplementation, 32, 174
Follicle phase, of menstrual cycle, 322, 323–324, 323f, 325f
Follicle-stimulating hormone (FSH), 253, 320, 333, 334, 356, 367, 424
Follicular atresia, 326
Follicular cysts, 239–240, 242
Fontanelles, 49, 97
Food and Drug Administration (FDA), 283, 298, 309, 408, 504
Footling breech, 97, 98f, 100
Forceps delivery, 60, 61f, 61t
 not required for, 69, 71

vacuum, 61
Forceps extractors, 69, 70
Forteo (teriparatide), 332
46,XY chromosomes, 337
Fosamax (alendronate), 331
Founder effect, 28
Fox-Fordyce disease, 221
Fracture risk assessment tool (FRAX), 331
Frank breech, 97, 98f
FRAX (fracture risk assessment tool), 331
FSE (fetal scalp electrode), 52
FSH (follicle-stimulating hormone), 253, 320, 333, 334, 356, 367, 424
FTA-ABS (fluorescent treponemal antibody absorption), 172, 264
FTP (failure to progress), 96
Fulvestrant, 516
Functional (urinary) incontinence, 302t, 303, 317, 318
Functional ovarian cysts, 239–240, 245, 247
Functional ovarian disorders, 370–371
Functional tumors, 370–371, 481

G

Gabapentin, 330
Galactorrhea, 340, 341t, 342f, 506
Gardasil, 446–447
Gardnerella, 281
Gardnerella vaginalis, 276
Gartner's duct cysts, 222–223, 227
Gaskin maneuver, 104
Gastroesophageal reflux disease, 9
Gastrointestinal physiology, of pregnancy, 3
Gastroschisis, 41, 43
GBS (Group B *Streptococcus*), 161
General anesthesia, 66, 67, 398, 408, 410, 490
Generalized arteriolar vasoconstriction, 133
Genetic abnormalities, 13, 14
Genetic cancer syndromes, 240, 473, 475, 482, 511
Genetic diseases, prenatal screening for, 27–29
Genetic testing, 471
Genital herpes, 266–267, 266f, 277, 278
Genital ridge, 245
Genital tract. See Lower genital tract, benign disorders of; Upper genital tract, benign disorders of
Genital urinary syndrome of menopause (GSM), 221, 223, 326, 359
Genital urinary tract, anomalies in, 215
Genital warts. See Human papillomavirus
Genitalia, ambiguous, 215
Genitourinary anomalies, 228
Genitourinary atrophy, 221, 223, 326, 330, 359, 361, 263
Gentamicin, 159, 162, 178, 279, 281, 282, 285
Germ cell tumors, 370, 479–481, 479–480f, 480t
German measles, 168
Gestational choriocarcinoma, 487, 488t, 493, 495–496, 497, 498, 500

Gestational diabetes, 8, 127, 128, 130–131, 141–142, 145–148, 146t
Gestational hypertension (GH), 133, 135, 136t
Gestational trophoblastic disease (GTD), 487–497, 488–489t, 488–492f, 493–495t, 494f
  benign, 487, 488t
  malignant, 493, 493–495t, 494f
Gestrinone, 235
GH (gestational hypertension), 133, 135, 136t
Ginger, 181
Ginkgo biloba, 353
Glargine insulin, 150
GLT (glucose loading test), 8
Glucocorticoids, 93, 371
Glucophage, 365
Glucose loading test (GLT), 8
Glucose tolerance test (GTT), 8, 128, 131, 146, 146t
Glyburide, 147, 154, 155
Glycemic control, during pregnancy and delivery, 148, 149
GnRH (gonadotropin-releasing hormone), 320, 321, 344, 425, 426t
GnRH (gonadotropin-releasing hormone) agonists, 235, 253, 254, 256t, 257, 372, 377
GnRH (gonadotropin-releasing hormone) antagonists, 517
Gonadal agenesis, 337
Gonadal dysgenesis, 228, 377
Gonadal estrogen production, 321
Gonadarche, 320–321
Gonadorelin, 426t
Gonadotropin-releasing hormone (GnRH), 320, 321, 344, 425, 426t
Gonadotropin-releasing hormone (GnRH) agonists, 235, 253, 254, 256t, 257, 372, 377
Gonadotropin-releasing hormone (GnRH) antagonists, 517
Gonococcal Isolate Surveillance Project, 273
Gonorrhea, 276, 401, 403. *See also* Neisseria gonorrhoeae
  NAAT for, 276
  treatment, 277
Goserelin acetate, 235
Gradual oocyte depletion, 326
Gram stain, 277
Grand mal seizure, 137
Grand multipara, 2, 203
Granulosa-theca cell tumors, 370, 481, 483, 484, 485
Graves disease, 189
Gravidity, 1–2
Griseofulvin, 390t
Group B *Streptococcus* (GBS), 161
Growth hormone secretion, 321
Growth potential, decrease of, 113, 113t
Growth rate, acceleration in, 321
Growth spurt, 320, 321
GSM (genital urinary syndrome of menopause), 221, 223, 326, 359
GTD. *See* Gestational trophoblastic disease
GTT (glucose tolerance test), 8, 128, 131, 146, 146t
Gummas, 264, 265f
Gynecoid pelvis, 96, 97f
Gynecologic cancer
  cervical cancer, 445f, 454–458, 454f, 456–458t, 457f
  cervical neoplasia, 445–454, 446–447f, 446t, 448–451t, 452–453f, 454t
  endometrial cancer, 463–469, 464t, 466t, 467t, 468t
  gestational trophoblastic disease, 487–497, 488–489t, 488–492f, 493–495t, 494f
  ovarian and fallopian tube tumors, 473–483, 474–478t, 474–475f, 477f, 479–480f, 480t
  vulvar and vaginal neoplasia, 435–441, 435t, 436–437f, 438t, 439f, 440t
Gynecomastia, 505

H

H_2 blocker, 9
HAART (highly active antiretroviral therapy), 284
Habitual abortion. *See* Recurrent pregnancy loss
Haemophilus ducreyi, 267, 274, 277. *See also* Chancroid
Haemophilus influenzae, 281
Haldol, 341
Halobetasol, 219t
Halogenated agents, 205
Hammock theory, 309
HAPO (Hyperglycemia and Pregnancy Outcomes), 146
Hashimoto thyroiditis, 189
Hb Bart, 29
HbH (hemoglobin H disease), 29
hCG. *See* Human chorionic gonadotropin (hCG)
Heart and Estrogen/Progestin Replacement Studies (HERS I and II), 328
Heart defects. *See* Cardiac defects, of fetus
Heart failure, 166, 185, 186
Heart rate, of fetus, 52, 53–54f, 101–102
Heavy menstrual bleeding (HMB), 354–355
HELLP (hemolysis, elevated liver enzymes, low platelet count) syndrome, 133–134, 136–137, 137t, 141, 143
Hemabate, 204
Hemangiomas, 223
Hematocolpos, 217
Hematology, during pregnancy, 3–4
Hematomas, 202–203, 212
Hematometra, 216
Hematuria, 87
Hemoglobin H disease (HbH), 29
Hemolysis, elevated liver enzymes, low platelet count (HELLP) syndrome, 133–134, 136–137, 137t, 141, 143
Hemorrhage
  acute, 358
  antepartum, 72–84, 72t
  fetal vessel rupture, 82–84
  nonobstetric causes of, 84
  placenta previa, 72–78, 73f, 74–75t, 76f
  placental abruption, 78–81, 78t, 79f, 80t
  uterine rupture, 81–82, 82t
  postpartum, 201, 202–205, 203t, 205f
Hemorrhoidal medications, 199
Hemorrhoids, 9
Heparin, 21, 114, 188, 190, 193
Hepatitis B, 171
HER2/neu status, 516
Hereditary nonpolyposis colorectal cancer (HNPCC), 238, 240, 465, 467, 473, 475, 504. *See also* Lynch syndrome
Hereditary ovarian cancer syndrome, 239
Hereditary syndromes, 504
Heroin, 192, 427t
Herpes simplex virus (HSV), 13, 162–164, 164f, 262, 263, 263t, 266–267, 266f
Heterotopic pregnancy, 16
Heterozygote advantage, 28
hex A (hexosaminidase A A), 28–29
hexosaminidase A (hex A), 28–29
HGSIL Pap test, 442, 443
Hidradenitis suppurativa, 221
High-grade squamous intraepithelial lesion (HSIL), 436, 442, 443, 449t, 450, 451, 460, 462
Highly active antiretroviral therapy (HAART), 284
Hirsutism, 367–372, 368f, 371–372
Histologic grade, 464, 464t
HIV (human immunodeficiency virus), 169–171, 283–285, 286, 289, 382, 384, 447, 448t, 449, 455
HMB (heavy menstrual bleeding), 354–355
hMG (human menopausal gonadotropin), 344, 428, 429
HNPCC (hereditary nonpolyposis colorectal cancer), 238, 240, 465, 467, 473, 475, 504
Hormonal contraceptive methods, 388–395, 389f, 390–392t, 392f, 394t, 491. *See also* Oral contraceptive pills
Hormonal options, symptoms of leiomyomas, 235
Hormone replacement therapy (HRT), 237, 254–255, 328, 343, 505, 511, 517
Hot flashes. *See* Vasomotor symptoms
HPGA (hypothalamic–pituitary–gonadal axis), 320, 320f, 355, 419
hPL. *See* Human placental lactogen
HPV (human papillomavirus), 268–269, 273, 284, 285, 408, 435–436, 435t, 438, 439, 440, 445, 446–447, 450–451, 450t, 454, 455
HRT (hormone replacement therapy), 237, 254–255, 328, 343, 505, 511, 517

HSG (hysterosalpingogram), 21, 232f, 244, 246, 398, 402, 404, 423f, 425
HSIL (high-grade squamous intraepithelial lesion), 436, 442, 443, 449t, 450, 451, 460, 462
HSV (herpes simplex virus), 13, 162–164, 164f, 262, 263, 263t, 266–267, 266f
HSV-1 IgG, positive, 275, 277
HSV viral culture, 277
Humalog, 147, 150, 150t, 151
Humalog insulin, 153, 155
Human chorionic gonadotropin (hCG), 12, 14, 324, 333, 334, 483, 485, 487, 488t, 491f, 495, 496–497. *See also* Beta-human chorionic gonadotropin
Human chorionic somatomammotropin. *See* Human placental lactogen
Human immunodeficiency virus (HIV), 169–171, 283–285, 286, 289, 382, 384, 447, 448t, 449, 455
Human menopausal gonadotropin (hMG), 344, 428, 429
Human papillomavirus (HPV), 268–269, 273, 284, 285, 408, 435–436, 435t, 438, 439, 440, 445, 446–447, 450–451, 450t, 454, 455
Human placental lactogen (hPL), 4, 496–497
 function of, 12, 14
Hydatidiform moles. *See* Molar pregnancies
Hydralazine, 137, 139
Hydrocodone, 364
Hydropic degeneration, 489
Hydrops. *See* Erythroblastosis fetalis; Immune hydrops
Hydrops tubae profluens, 482, 483, 485, 486
Hymen, imperforate, 215–216, 216–217f, 226, 228, 336
Hymenal ring, 215
Hyperandrogenism, 342, 421. *See also* Hirsutism
Hypercoagulability of pregnancy, 187, 196
Hyperemesis gravidarum, 3, 12, 14, 181–182, 489
Hyperglycemia and Pregnancy Outcomes (HAPO), 146
Hypergonadotropic hypogonadism, 337, 338t, 339, 340
Hyperinsulinemia, 421
Hypermobile urethra, 308, 309
Hyperosmolar urea, 411
Hyperplasia
 adrenal, 215, 369–370
 ductal or lobular, 509
 endometrial, 255, 328, 356, 357, 465, 481
 stromal, 370
Hyperprolactinemia-associated amenorrhea, 334, 340–341, 341t, 342, 343
Hypertension, 465. *See also* Pulmonary hypertension
 during pregnancy, 133–139, 134t

chronic hypertension, 138
chronic hypertension with superimposed preeclampsia, 138–139
 eclampsia, 133, 137–138, 138t
 preeclampsia, 133–137, 134t, 136–137t, 190, 190t
Hyperthyroidism, 189, 489
Hypertonus, of uterus, 58
Hypofibrinogenemia, 80
Hypogastric nerve, 304
Hypoglycemic agents, 147, 151, 390t
Hypogonadotropic hypogonadism, 338, 339, 341, 341t
Hypomenorrhea, 354t, 355
Hypotension, maternal, 104
Hypothalamic disorders, 337–338
Hypothalamic hypogonadism, 365
Hypothalamic-pituitary axis disruption, 341–344, 341–342t, 342f, 343f
Hypothalamic-pituitary failure, 425, 428
Hypothalamic–pituitary–gonadal axis (HPGA), 320, 320f, 355, 419
Hypothyroidism, 189, 341, 341t, 342, 342t, 343
Hypotonia, 158
Hypovolemic shock, 80
Hypoxia, 184, 188
Hypoxic brain injury, 110
Hysterectomy, 85, 88, 205, 236, 239, 257, 296, 314, 358, 359, 449, 457, 461, 476, 490, 491, 497
Hysterosalpingogram (HSG), 21, 232f, 244, 246, 398, 402, 404, 423f, 425
Hysteroscopy, 239, 356, 359, 426

I

Ibuprofen, 14, 350, 356, 358
ICS (International Continence Society), 304–305, 305t
ICSI (intracytoplasmic sperm injection), 428, 428f, 430–431
Idiopathic urgency incontinence, 311, 319
Imaging, of fetus, 39–40, 39f
IMB (intermenstrual bleeding), 224, 355
Imipramine, 505t
Imiquimod (Aldara), 269, 277, 436
Immature teratoma, 479, 480, 480t, 481
Immune hydrops, 121
Immunizations, 169, 170, 171, 200, 408, 438, 447, 462
Immunodeficiency, 447
Immunosuppression, 186, 447, 455
Imperforate anus, 243, 245
Imperforate hymen, 215–216, 216–217f, 226, 228, 336
Implanon. *See* Nexplanon
Implantable progesterone-only contraception, 394–395
Imuran, 186
In Vitro fertilization (IVF), 122, 345, 348, 349, 425–426, 428, 429, 430–431, 430f
 with gestational carrier, 345, 347, 348
Incompetent cervix. *See* Cervical insufficiency
Incomplete (partial) molar gestation, 487, 488t, 491, 492f, 498, 499, 500, 501

Incomplete abortion, 17, 24, 26
Incomplete breech. *See* Footling breech
Incomplete moles. *See* Partial molar pregnancies
Incontinence. *See* Urinary incontinence
Indigo carmine, 47, 69, 315, 316, 318
Indinavir, 284
Indomethacin, 78, 93–94
Induction
 of labor, 49–51, 122, 141, 144, 407, 407f, 411, 411t
 Bishop score, 68, 70
 of ovulation, 343–344, 426t, 429–430, 429–430f
Inevitable abortion, 17, 26
Infant, 1
Infection. *See also* Sexually transmitted infections; Urinary tract infections
 of lower reproductive tract, 262–274
 during pregnancy, 157–175, 157t
 of upper reproductive tract, 279–285, 280–281f
 of uterine lining, 205
 vaginal, 269–272, 270f, 271f
 of wounds, 206
Inferior vena cava filter, placement of, 196
Infertility, 251, 461
 definition of, 434
 female factor, 418–427, 419–420t, 419f, 420–424f, 426t, 426f
 male factor, 417, 417f, 418t, 426f, 427–428, 427–428t, 428f
 unexplained, 428
Infiltrating ductal carcinoma, 514–515, 514f
Inflammatory breast carcinoma, 515
Inflammatory diseases, 352
Inflammatory reaction, 220
Influenza, during pregnancy, 160
Inguinal lymph node dissection, 438, 439f
Initial prenatal visit, 5–6, 7t
Injectable progesterone-only contraceptives, 393–394, 394t
INR (international normalized ratio), 189
Insertion-related pelvic inflammatory disease, 386
Institutes of Medicine (IOM), 331
Insulin, 147, 148, 150–151, 150t
Insulin resistance, 145, 150, 151, 155, 340, 365, 370, 371, 424f, 485
Insulin resistance syndrome. *See* Syndrome X
Integral theory, 308–309
Integrase inhibitors, 284
Intercostobrachial nerve, 503, 503f
Intermenstrual bleeding (IMB), 224, 355
Internal mammary arteries, 502, 503f
Internal mammary nodes, 502, 503f
Internal sphincter, 303, 303f
International Association of Diabetes in Pregnancy Study Group, 146
International Continence Society (ICS), 304–305, 305t
International Endometrial Collaboration Group diagnostic schema, 237

International Federation of Gynecology and Obstetrics (FIGO), 354, 438t, 440t, 456t, 460, 462, 493, 500
International normalized ratio (INR), 189
International Society for Study of Vulvovaginal Disease (ISVVD), 218
International society for Study of Women's Sexual Health in 2014, 326
International Urogynecological Association (IUGA), 304–305, 305t
Interstitial cystitis, 252, 262
Intra-abdominal pressure, incontinence with, 308
Intracytoplasmic sperm injection (ICSI), 428, 428f, 430–431
Intraductal carcinoma. See Ductal carcinoma in situ
Intraductal papilloma, 510, 520, 522
Intramural fibroids, 246
Intramural leiomyoma, 232
Intrapartum, 286, 289
Intrapartum care, for HIV-infected women, 170
Intraperitoneal chemotherapy, 479
Intraurethral pressure, 303–304, 308
Intrauterine adhesions, 422
Intrauterine devices (IUDs), 15–16, 201, 384–388, 385f, 386t, 387f, 388t, 396
Intrauterine fetal demise. See Fetal demise
Intrauterine growth restriction (IUGR), 92, 112–113, 113t, 115f, 492
Intrauterine insemination (IUI), 425, 428
Intrauterine pregnancy (IUP), 16
  β-hCG level, 23, 26
Intrauterine pressure catheter (IUPC), 51, 53–54, 55f, 68, 70
Intrauterine transfusion (IUT), 120
Intravenous (IV) hyperimmune globulin, 168
Intravenous immune globulin (IVIG), 191, 283
Intravenous pyelography, 476
Intravesical pressure, 303, 308
Intrinsic sphincter deficiency (ISD), 309, 311
Invasive breast cancers, 328–329, 514–517, 514f, 515f, 518t
Invasive lobular carcinoma, 514f, 515
Invasive papillary carcinoma, 520, 521, 522
Inversion, uterine, 204–205, 205f
IOM (Institutes of Medicine), 331
Iron supplementation, 5, 8
Irreversible congenital heart block, 195, 197
Irritable bowel syndrome, 259, 260
Ischemic strokes, 328
ISD (intrinsic sphincter deficiency), 309, 311
ISVVD (International Society for Study of Vulvovaginal Disease), 218
Itch mite. See Sarcoptes scabiei

IUDs (intrauterine devices), 15–16, 201, 384–388, 385f, 386t, 387f, 388t, 396
IUGA (International Urogynecological Association), 304–305, 305t
IUGR (intrauterine growth restriction), 92, 112–113, 113t, 115f, 492
IUI (intrauterine insemination), 425, 428
IUP. See Intrauterine pregnancy
IUPC (intrauterine pressure catheter), 51, 53–54, 55f, 68, 70
IUT (intrauterine transfusion), 120
IV clindamycin, 176, 178
  and gentamicin, 286, 288
IV conscious sedation, 413, 415
IV heparin, 194, 196
IV indigo carmine, 315
IV labetalol, 108, 111
IV oxytocin, 413, 415
Ivermectin, 269
IVF. See In vitro fertilization
IVIG (intravenous immune globulin), 191, 283

J
Jarisch–Herxheimer reaction, 266
Jaundice, 127, 130

K
Kallmann syndrome, 337t, 338t, 432, 433
Kaposi sarcoma, 282
Karyotype, 344, 345, 346, 348
Keflex, 177
Kegel exercises, 296, 309
Kell antigen, 121
Ketonuria, 13, 14
Ketoprofen, 350
"Keyhole" fashion, 227
Kidney development, 34
Kidney infection. See Pyelonephritis
Klebsiella, 262
Kleihauer–Betke test, 77
Klinefelter syndrome, 31
Krukenberg tumors, 371, 473
Kyleena. See Levonorgestrel IUD

L
Labetalol, 136, 137, 138, 140, 142, 143
Labial fusion, 215
Labor, 46–49, 46–50f, 47t
  cardinal movements of, 68, 70
  complications of, 92–106
  induction of, 122, 407, 407f, 411, 411t
  and augmentation, 49–51
  cervical examinations for, 68, 70
  prostaglandins in, contraindication to use, 68, 70
  monitoring fetus during, 51–55, 53–55f, 58
  in mothers with epilepsy, 184
  normal labor, 49–66, 53–57f, 59–64f, 61t, 64t, 65t, 66f
  obstetric analgesia and anesthesia, 65–66, 66f
  oligohydramnios in, 127, 130
  with placenta previa, 90
  progression of, 55–66, 56–57f, 59–64f, 61t, 64t, 65t, 66f

Lacerations
  cervical, 203
  repair of, 62–63, 63–64f
  vaginal, 202–203
Lactate dehydrogenase (LDH), 483, 485
Lactation fever, 210, 213
Lactational amenorrhea, 380–381
Lactiferous ducts, 502, 502f
Lactobacilli, 270, 275, 278, 286, 288
Lamaze method, 70
Lamicel, 410
Laminaria, 352, 410
Lamivudine (3TC), 284
Lamotrigine, 182
Laparoscopic tubal ligation (LTL), 397
LARC (long-acting reversible contraception), 201, 284, 397, 403
Large for gestational age (LGA), 112, 115–117, 116t
Large-loop excision of transformation zone (LLETZ). See Loop electrosurgical excision procedure
Laser ablation, 439, 452
Laser conization, 454t
Laser vaporization, 436, 442, 443, 444
Late deceleration, of fetal heart rate, 52, 54f
Latent phase of labor, 57, 57f
Lateral thoracic arteries, 502, 503f
Latzko triad, 482, 484, 486
Laxatives, 9, 199
LBW (low birth weight) infants, 92
LCIS (lobular carcinoma in situ), 513, 514f
LDH (lactate dehydrogenase), 483, 485
Lecithin, 13, 14
LEEP (loop electrosurgical excision procedure), 451, 452, 453f
Leiomyoma, 224, 231–237, 233f, 234–236f, 236f, 256, 256t, 259, 260, 423
Leiomyomata, 357
Leopold maneuvers, 13, 46, 46f, 48
Letrozole (Femara), 253, 340, 425, 426t, 429, 431, 516, 519
Leukocyte esterase, 14
Leuprolide acetate (Lupron), 253, 254, 353, 425
Levetiracetam, 182
Levonorgestrel (LNG) intrauterine systems, 384
Levonorgestrel IUD, 239, 257, 261, 351, 357, 358, 380t, 384–388, 385f
Levonorgestrel pill (Plan B), 395–396, 400, 402, 403
  side effect of, 402, 404
Levothyroxine (Synthroid), 189, 197, 198
Lewis antigen, 121
LGA (large for gestational age), 112, 115–117, 116t
LGV (lymphogranuloma venereum), 263, 263t, 267–268, 277
LH (luteinizing hormone), 253, 334, 367, 376
Lichen planus, 219, 219t
Lichen sclerosis, 218–219, 219t, 220f, 226, 227, 228
Lichen simplex chronicus, 219t, 220
Li–Fraumeni syndrome, 504, 510

LILETTA. *See* Levonorgestrel IUD
Linea nigra, 4
Linezolid, 283
Lipomas, 223
LLETZ (large-loop excision of transformation zone). *See* Loop electrosurgical excision procedure
Lobular carcinoma in situ (LCIS), 513, 514f
Lobular hyperplasia, 509
Local anesthesia, 66, 399–400
Local excision, 436, 439, 510
Long-acting reversible contraception (LARC), 201, 284, 397, 403
Long thoracic nerve, 503, 503f
Loop electrosurgical excision procedure (LEEP), 451, 452, 453f
Lopinavir, 284
Lorazepam, 105t, 111
Lovenox, 190, 194, 197
Low birth weight (LBW) infants, 92
Low bone density, 107, 327, 449t, 451, 459, 461
Low-grade squamous intraepithelial lesion (LSIL), 451, 461
Low-lying placenta, 72
Low-molecular-weight heparin, 196
Lower extremity DVT, confirmation test to, 193–194, 196
Lower genital tract, benign disorders of, 215–225
Lower reproductive tract, infections of cervix, infections of, 272
   chlamydia trachomatis, 273
   neisseria gonorrhoeae, 272–273
  external anogenital region, 263
   vulvitis, 263
  nonulcerative lesions, 268, 268f
   human papillomavirus, 268–269
   molluscum contagiosum, 269, 269f
   phthirus pubis and sarcoptes scabiei, 269
  ulcerated lesions, 263, 263t
   chancroid, 267
   genital herpes, 266–267, 266f
   lymphogranuloma venereum, 267–268
   syphilis, 263–266, 265f
  urinary tract infections (UTIs), 262–263
  vaginal infections, 269–270, 270f
   bacterial vaginosis, 270, 270f
   trichomonas vaginalis, 271–272, 271f
   yeast infections, 270–271
LSIL (low-grade squamous intraepithelial lesion), 451, 461
LTL (laparoscopic tubal ligation), 397
Lung. *See* Pulmonary physiology, of pregnancy
Lung maturity, of fetus, 11
Lupron (leuprolide acetate), 253, 254, 353, 425
Lupus flares, 190, 190t
Luteal phase
  defect, 21, 422
  of menstrual cycle, 322, 323f, 324, 325f
Luteinizing hormone (LH), 253, 334, 367, 376
Lybrel, 389
Lymph node resection, 467
Lymphogranuloma venereum (LGV), 263, 263t, 267–268, 277
Lynch II syndrome, 238, 465, 467, 473, 486
Lynch syndrome, 240, 464, 471, 475, 504
Lysteda (tranexamic acid), 356, 364

M

Macrodantin, 175, 177
Macrosomia, 115–117, 116t
Macrosomic neonates, risk for jaundice, 127, 130
Magnesium, 184, 353, 360
Magnesium sulfate ($MgSO_4$), 77, 94, 105, 105t, 135, 138, 138t, 139, 140, 141, 143, 144, 203
  on cellular calcium, 106, 108
  side effects of, 108
  test for, 106
  therapy, 108, 110–111
Magnetic-Resonance-Guided Focused Ultrasound Surgery (MRgFUS), 236
Magnetic resonance imaging (MRI), 241, 256, 456, 477
Male condoms, 381–382
Male factor infertility, 417, 417f, 418t, 426f, 427–428, 427–428t, 428f
Malignant breast disease, 511–513, 512t, 513f
Malignant endometrial adenocarcinoma carcinoma, 238
Malignant epithelial cells, 513
Malignant gestational trophoblastic disease, 493, 493–494t, 494f
Malignant masses, 455
Malignant necrotizing tumor, 495
Malposition, of fetus, 96–101, 97–100f
Malpresentation, 96–101, 97–100f
  of vertex, 98–100, 99–100f
Mammary duct ectasia, 510
Mammary glands, 502, 503f
Mammography, 504–506, 504f, 507f, 513, 514, 519
Manual vacuum aspiration, 407, 408–409, 408f
MAO (monoamine oxidase) inhibitors, 212, 341
Marfan syndrome, 186
Marginal previa, 72, 73f
Marijuana, 191–192, 427t
Marsupialization, 222, 223f, 227
Masses of breast. *See* Breast
Mastalgia, 502, 505, 509, 510
Mastectomy, 514, 515
Mastitis, 207
  diagnosis of, 210, 213
Maternal cardiac disease, 184–186
Maternal complications, of diabetes during pregnancy, 148t
Maternal Graves disease, 198
Maternal hypotension, 104
Maternal lupus, neonatal complication of, 195, 197
Maternal obesity, 116
Maternal renal disease, 186–187
Maternal seizure, 104–105, 105t, 137–138, 138t, 182–184, 183–184t
Maternal serum alpha-fetoprotein (MSAFP), 8, 36–37, 36t, 37f, 41, 43
Maternal thyroid disease, 189
Maternal varicella pneumonia, 164
Mature teratoma, 479, 480
Mayer–Rokitansky–Kuster–Hauser (MRKH) syndrome. *See* Müllerian agenesis; Vaginal atresia; Vaginal agenesis
MCA (middle cerebral artery) Doppler, 120
McIndoe procedure, 218, 218f
McRoberts maneuver, 70, 102–103, 103f, 109–110
Measles, mumps, and rubella (MMR) vaccine, 169, 200
Medical abortion, 409, 410t
Medication abortion, 412, 415
  nonsurgical, 407, 408
Medroxyprogesterone, 343, 425, 468
Medroxyprogesterone acetate (Provera), 235, 239, 329, 343, 356, 358, 405, 500
Megace (megestrol acetate), 239, 468
Megestrol acetate (Megace), 239, 468
Meigs syndrome, 481, 484, 485
Melanoma, of vulva, 439
Melasma, 4
Menarche, 320, 321–322, 334
Menfegol, 384
Meningomyelocele, 32f, 43
Menometrorrhagia, 234, 354t, 355
Menopausal hormone therapy (MHT), 328–329, 328t
  contraindications to, 333, 335
  indication for, 334, 335
Menopausal hormones. *See* Hormone replacement therapy; Menopausal hormone therapy (MHT)
Menopause, 292, 326–330, 326t, 327f, 328t, 329t
  diagnosis of, 333, 334
  early, 335
  nonhormonal treatment, 329–330, 329t
  symptoms of, 335
Menorrhagia, 234, 256, 354–355, 354t, 387–388
Menstrual cycle, 322–324, 323f, 325f, 333, 334, 350–360, 351f, 352f, 354t, 357t, 358t
Menstrual suppression with progestins, 252, 257
Menstruation, 323
  time length from breast bud development to, 334
Metabolic syndrome, 340. *See also* Syndrome X
Metanephrines, 374, 377
Metastatic disease, 496, 516–517
Metformin, 154, 155, 340, 425, 426f, 426t, 431
Methadone, 192
Methamphetamine, 79, 84, 191, 192
Methergine (methylergonovine), 204, 209, 212

Methimazole, 189
Methotrexate, 17, 22, 25, 190, 357t, 407, 409, 411, 484, 486, 495, 499, 516
Methyldopa, 390t, 505t
Methylergonovine (Methergine), 204, 209, 212
Metoclopramide, 181, 427t, 505t
Metronidazole, 160, 162, 175, 270, 272, 274, 276, 278, 281, 282
Metrorrhagia, 234, 354t, 355
MHT. See Menopausal hormone therapy
MI (myocardial infarction), 185
Miconazole, 271
Microinvasive cervical carcinoma, 455, 457, 457t
Micturition. See Urinary incontinence
Middle cerebral artery (MCA) Doppler, 120
Midurethral sling, 309, 310f, 316, 318
MIF (Müllerian inhibiting factor), 337
Mifepristone, 395, 396, 407, 409, 410t, 411
Mineralocorticoids, 215
Minipill. See Progesterone-only contraception
Minoxidil, 371
Mirabegron (Myrbetriq), 312t, 313
Mirena (Levonorgestrel) IUD, 201, 235, 239, 356, 387–388, 401, 402, 403, 404, 405
Miscarriage. See Spontaneous abortion
Misoprostol (PGE₁M), 18, 51, 70, 204, 212, 407, 409, 410t, 411
Missed abortion, 17, 24, 26
Mixed (urinary) incontinence, 302, 302t
MMR (measles, mumps, and rubella) vaccine, 169, 200
Molar pregnancies
  complete, 487–491, 488–491f, 489t
  partial, 491–493, 492f
Molluscum contagiosum, 268, 269
Mono-di twins, 122–125, 123f, 124f, 128, 131
Mono-mono twins, 122–125, 123f, 124f
Monoamine oxidase (MAO) inhibitors, 212, 341
Monophasic combination pills, 389, 389f
Monozygotic twins, 122–125, 123f, 124f
Montevideo unit, 54
Morbid obesity, 469
Morning after pill, 395
Morning sickness, 3, 181
Morphine sulfate, 65
Mortality rate, of elective termination of pregnancy, 409, 411
Motile, flagellated protozoans, 274, 276, 277
MRgFUS (Magnetic-Resonance-Guided Focused Ultrasound Surgery), 236
MRI (magnetic resonance imaging), 241, 256, 456, 477
MSAFP (maternal serum alpha-fetoprotein), 8, 36–37, 36t, 37f, 41, 43
Mucocolpos, 215, 228
Müllerian agenesis, 345, 347
Müllerian anomalies, 245–246
Müllerian ducts, 347

Müllerian inhibiting factor (MIF), 337
Müllerian system, 229, 245
Müllerian tubercle, 216–217
Multiphasic combination pills, 389
Multiple gestations, 43, 122–125, 123f, 124f
Muscle relaxants, 9
Musculoskeletal physiology, during pregnancy, 4
Mycobacterium avium-intracellulare, 283
Mycobacterium tuberculosis, 279
Mycoplasma species, 178
Myelomeningocele, 41, 43–44
Myocardial infarction (MI), 185
Myoma, 231–237, 233f, 234–236t, 236f
Myomectomy, 236
Myometrial invasion, 463, 464t, 467t, 468, 468t
Myrbetriq (mirabegron), 312t, 313

N

NAAT. See Nucleic acid amplification test
Nabothian cysts, 223, 224f
Nafarelin (Synarel), 253
Nafarelin acetate, 235
Nafcillin, 283
Nägele rule, 2, 12, 13
NAMS. See North American Menopause Society
Naproxen, 350, 361
Narcotics, 9, 65, 192
NAS (neonatal abstinence syndrome), 192
National Institute of Health (NIH), 53
Natural childbirth, 65
Natural methods of contraception, 379–381, 381f
Nausea, 3, 181
Needle aspiration, 506, 507f, 508f
Needle biopsy, 513
Neisseria gonorrhoeae, 170–171, 222, 262, 272–273, 276, 280, 281, 288
Neonatal abstinence syndrome (NAS), 192
Neonatal herpes, 163
Neonatal lupus, 190–191
Neoplastic disease
  of cervix, 445–454, 446–447f, 446t, 448–451t, 452–453f, 454t
  vulvar and vaginal, 435–441, 435t, 436–437f, 438f, 439f, 440t
Neoplastic ovarian disorders, 370–371
Neovagina, 218, 218f
  creation of, 226, 227, 228
Neural tube defects (NTDs), 32–33, 32–33f, 36, 182
Neuraminidase inhibitors, 160
Neutral protamine Hagedorn (NPH), 147, 150–151, 150t, 153
Nevirapine, 170, 177, 179–180
Newborn, transient tachypnea of, 132
Nexplanon, 201, 351, 356, 365–366, 380t, 390, 394–395, 400, 401, 403
Nifedipine, 93, 105, 108, 138, 141, 142, 143, 144
Night sweats. See Vasomotor symptoms
NIH (National Institute of Health), 53

Nipple discharge
  of breast, 505–506, 505t, 510, 513
  and breast examination, 520
  evaluation of, 520, 522
Nipple, Paget disease of, 515
Nitrates, 158
Nitrazine test, 47
Nitric oxide, 185
Nitrofurans, 427t
Nitrofurantoin, 158, 159, 262
Nitroglycerin, 102, 205
Nitroimidazoles, 276
Non-Hodgkin lymphoma, 282
Nonhormonal options, for symptoms of leiomyomas, 234
Noninvasive breast disease of, 513–514, 514f
Nonneoplastic ovarian disorders, 370
Nonnucleoside reverse transcriptase inhibitors, 284
Nonoxynol-9, 384
Nonreassuring fetal status, signs of, 69, 70
Nonsteroidal anti-inflammatory drugs (NSAIDs), 93, 105, 199, 246, 252, 257, 350, 351, 356, 358, 361, 364, 505, 506, 509, 511
Nonstress test (NST), 10, 13, 14, 127, 128, 130
Nonsurgical abortion, 409–410, 410t
Nonulcerative lesions, of lower reproductive tract, 268, 268f
  human papillomavirus, 268–269
  molluscum contagiosum, 269, 269f
  phthirus pubis and sarcoptes scabiei, 269
Norelgestromin, 39
Norethindrone acetate, 235
Normal labor. See Labor
North American Menopause Society (NAMS), 326
  recommendations for menopausal hormone therapy, 329
NovoLog, 147
NPH (neutral protamine Hagedorn), 147, 150–151, 150t, 153
NSAIDs (nonsteroidal anti-inflammatory drugs), 93, 105, 199, 246, 252, 257, 350, 351, 356, 358, 361, 364, 505, 506, 509, 511
NST (nonstress test), 10, 13, 14, 127, 128, 130
NTDs (neural tube defects), 32–33, 32–33f, 36, 182
Nubain, 65
Nuchal translucency, 35
Nucleic acid amplification test (NAAT), 171, 267
  for chlamydial infection and gonorrhea, 274, 276
Nucleoside analogs, 284, 285
Nulliparity, 247
Nutrition, 4–5, 5t
Nutritional supplements, before pregnancy, 11, 13
NuvaRing, 275, 278, 351, 356, 380t, 392–393, 392f, 400
Nystatin, 271

O

Obesity, 116, 303, 355, 442, 443, 465, 471
Obstetric analgesia and anesthesia, 65–66, 66f
Obstetric conjugate, 96
Obstetric emergencies, 101–105, 103–104f, 105t
Obstetric examination, 46, 46f
Obstructed labor, 314
Obstruction to delivery, 96–101, 97–100f
Occiput posterior position, 69, 100–101
Occiput transverse position, 69, 100–101
OCPs (oral contraceptive pills), 201, 233, 237, 242, 254, 256t, 257, 280, 284, 340, 343, 351, 353, 355, 356, 357t, 358, 360, 372, 373, 376, 388–391, 389f, 390–392t, 395, 400, 402–403, 404, 425, 455, 465, 475t, 476, 505, 505t, 511, 517
Octoxynol-9, 384
Ofloxacin, 408
Oligo-ovulation, 421
Oligohydramnios, 47, 117–118, 177, 178
  in labor, 127, 130
Oligomenorrhea, 354t, 355, 356, 375, 377–378
Omphalocele, 30, 31, 43
Ondansetron, 181
Oocyte aging, 419
Oophorectomy, 480
Operative hysteroscopy, 231, 426
Operative vaginal delivery, 60, 314
Opiates, 191, 192, 341
Opioid agonists, 244, 246
Opioids, 199
Oral and intrauterine progestins, 239
Oral contraceptive pills (OCPs), 201, 233, 237, 242, 254, 256t, 257, 280, 284, 340, 343, 351, 353, 355, 356, 357t, 358, 360, 372, 373, 376, 388–391, 389f, 390–392t, 395, 400, 402–403, 404, 425, 455, 465, 475t, 476, 505, 505t, 511, 517
Oral phenazopyridine, 315
Organogenesis, 31–32, 32f
Ortho Evra patch, 351, 356, 380t, 391–392, 392f, 400, 402, 404
Oseltamivir, 160
Osmotic dilators, 410, 410f
Osteopenia, 327
Osteoporosis, 328, 329, 330–332, 330–331t
  prevention of, 329
OTC (over-the-counter) pregnancy tests, 11, 13
Outflow tract anomalies, 336–337, 337t
Ovarian cancer, 399, 473–479, 474–478t, 474–475f, 477f
  risk factors for, 484, 486
  screening of, 471
  stage of, 484, 486
Ovarian carcinoma. See Ovarian cancer
Ovarian choriocarcinoma, 473–474, 475f, 476–479
Ovarian cyst, 242, 248, 260, 363, 405

and adnexal masses, 239–242, 240f, 241t
  diagnosis of, 245, 247
  size of, 245, 248
  treatment of, 245, 247–248
Ovarian cystectomy, 480
Ovarian disorders, 370–371, 419–421, 420–422f, 420t
Ovarian failure, 326, 340, 343, 343f
Ovarian fibroma, 481, 483, 485
Ovarian follicle, 322
Ovarian follicular depletion, 326
Ovarian hyperstimulation syndrome, 432
Ovarian insufficiency, 337, 338t
Ovarian reserve, 419, 420, 424–425, 431, 432, 433–434
Ovarian torsion, 240, 288, 289
Ovarian tumors, 370–371, 473–479, 474–478t, 474–475f, 477f
Ovaries, streak, 228
Over-the-counter (OTC) pregnancy tests, 11, 13
Overdistended bladder, 313, 313f, 314
Overflow (urinary) incontinence, 302, 302t, 313, 313f, 314t
Ovulation, 323f, 324, 325f, 388, 431, 432, 433, 434
  induction of, 343–344, 426t, 429–430, 429–430f
Ovulation-enhancing drugs, 122
Ovulatory disorders, 357, 419–421, 420–422f, 420t
Ovulatory dysfunction, 423
Ovulatory status, 356
Oxacarbemazepine, 182
Oxacillin, 283
Oxybutynin, 312t, 316, 317
Oxytocin, 18, 22, 51, 61, 62, 64, 67, 70, 81, 82t, 86, 89, 96, 104, 121, 199, 204, 412, 413, 497, 503
Oxytocin antagonists, 94

P

Paclitaxel, 479, 482
PACTG (Pediatric AIDS Clinical Trials Group) protocol 076, 179, 284
Paget disease
  of nipple, 515
  of vulva, 437
Pain evaluation, of breast, 505
Palliative care, of cervical cancer, 458
PALM-COEIN system, of abnormal uterine bleeding, 354, 356, 357
Pap (papanicolaou) test, 355, 359, 439, 442, 443, 455, 459, 460, 461, 462
Pap smear. See Papanicolaou smear
Papanicolaou (Pap) smear, 425, 440, 445, 445f, 447, 447f, 466
  abnormal, 449–450, 449–450t
Papanicolaou (Pap) test, 355, 359, 439, 442, 443, 455, 459, 460, 461, 462
Paracervical block, 408, 410
ParaGard IUD. See Copper-T IUD
Paramesonephric ducts. See also Müllerian ducts
  formation of organs, 243, 245–246
Parasitic fibroids, 246
Parasitic leiomyoma, 232

Parathyroid hormone, 332
Paraurethral gland cysts. See Skene's duct cysts
Parity, 1–2
Paroxetine, 212, 353
Paroxetine sulfate, 330
Partial molar pregnancies, 491–493, 492f
Partial previa, 72
Parvovirus B19, 165–166, 176, 179
Patau syndrome. See Trisomy 13
Patch. See Ortho Evra patch
Paternal gametogenesis, 24, 26
Paxil, 353, 364
PCOS. See Polycystic ovary syndrome
PCR. See Polymerase Chain Reaction
PE. See Pulmonary embolus
Peak growth velocity, 321
Pediatric AIDS Clinical Trials Group (PACTG) protocol 076, 179, 284
Pediculosis, 269
Pelvic adhesions, 352, 419t, 421, 423, 425
Pelvic examination, 13
Pelvic exenteration, 439
Pelvic inflammatory disease (PID), 15, 272, 277, 279, 280–281, 280–281f, 286, 288, 386, 421
  barrier contraceptives, 288–289
  with infertility, 288
Pelvic nerve, 304
Pelvic organ prolapse, 291–298, 291–298f, 292–293t, 295t, 297t, 302
Pelvic Organ Prolapse Quantitative scale (POP-Q), 294, 295f, 296, 298, 299, 300
  staging, 295t
Pelvic pain, 215, 217, 234, 240, 249, 251, 280
Pelvic pressure, 291
Pelvic radiation, 314, 439, 468
Pelvic rest, 85, 87
Pelvic ultrasound, 23, 25, 39, 211, 213, 234, 237, 239, 243, 244, 246, 256, 287, 289, 344, 345, 346, 348, 352, 356, 359, 467, 476, 477t, 490, 492, 495, 498, 499, 500
Pelvic X-ray, 246
Pelvis, maternal, 96–97, 97f
Penicillin, 8–9, 158, 172–173, 263t, 264, 266, 273
Penicillin G, 158, 161, 172, 173, 264
PEPI (postmenopausal estrogen/progestin interventions) Trial, 328
Percutaneous tibial nerve stimulation, 313
Percutaneous umbilical blood sampling (PUBS), 10, 38, 120
Perimenopause, 324, 326, 358
Perinatal transmission, 169, 171
Perineal lacerations, 62, 63f
  treatment of, 209–210
Perineal support, 68, 70
Periodic abstinence, 379, 381f
Periodic ultrasound imaging, 242
Peripartum cardiomyopathy (PPCM), 186
Peripartum hysterectomy, 74
Peritoneal biopsy, 252

Permanent contraception, 397–399, 397–399f
Permethrin, 220–269
Persistent occiput transverse and posterior position, 100–101
Persistent postmolar GTD and invasive moles, 493–495, 495t
Persistent/invasive moles, 494f
Pessaries, 296, 296f, 301, 309, 310f
PET (polyethylene terephthalate) fibers, 398
Peutz–Jeghers syndrome (PJS), 465, 471
PGD (preimplantation genetic diagnosis), 430–431
PGE$_1$M (Misoprostol), 18, 51, 70, 204, 212, 407, 409, 410t, 411
PGE$_2$ (prostaglandin E$_2$) gel, 68, 70
PGE$_2$ pessary (Cervidil), 51, 70
PGF2 (prostaglandin F2α), 204
pH, of fetal scalp, 54–55, 55f
Phenazopyridine, 159
Phenobarbital, 105t, 138, 182, 183, 183t
Phenothiazine, 341, 341t, 390t, 505t
Phenytoin, 105t, 138, 182, 183, 183t, 184, 371, 390t
Phthirus pubis, 268, 269
Phyllodes tumor, 509–510, 520, 522
Physical examination, 413, 415
Pica, 9
PID. *See* Pelvic inflammatory disease
Piperonyl butoxide, 269
Pitocin, 204, 212, 411
Pituitary disorders, 338
PJS (Peutz–Jeghers syndrome), 465, 471
Placenta
 delivery of, 61–62, 62f
 development of, 324
 low-lying, 72
 retained, 62, 63f
Placenta accreta, 74, 74t, 75, 76, 204, 345, 347–348
 diagnosis of, 85, 87
 management plan, 85, 87–88
 precautions of, 85, 87
 risk of, 85, 87
Placenta increta, 74, 74t
Placenta percreta, 74, 74t
Placenta previa, 72–78, 73f, 74–75t, 76f, 85, 86, 87, 88, 90
Placental abruption, 78–81, 78t, 79f, 80t, 85, 86, 88, 89, 90, 91, 140, 142, 144
Placental migration, 72
Placental separation, 69, 70
Placental site trophoblastic tumors (PSTTs), 487, 488t, 493, 494f, 496–497, 499, 500, 501
Plan B. *See* Levonorgestrel pill
Plasma ACTH testing, 377
Plasma cell mastitis. *See* Mammary duct ectasia
Platypelloid pelvis, 96, 97f
PMDD (premenstrual dysphoric disorder), 352–353
PMS. *See* Premenstrual syndrome
PMVB (postmenopausal vaginal bleeding), 358–359
Pneumocystis carinii pneumonia, 283
Pneumoniae, 262
POC (products of conception), 17, 204

Podofilox, 269
Podophyllin, 269
POI (primary ovarian insufficiency), 326, 337, 340, 346, 348, 349, 356, 378, 419, 420
Polycystic ovary syndrome (PCOS), 238, 340, 355, 370, 372, 375, 376, 421, 422f, 423, 465
 test for, 373, 376
Polyethylene terephthalate (PET) fibers, 398
Polyhydramnios, 118
Polyhydramnios-oligohydramnios (polyoli) sequence. *See* Twin-to-twin transfusion syndrome
Polymenorrhea, 354t, 355
Polymerase Chain Reaction (PCR), 163
 test, 266
Polymicrobial infections, 176, 178
Polyps, 356
 cervical, 224, 224f
 endometrial, 237
Pomeroy method, 403–404
Pool test, 47
POP-Q. *See* Pelvic Organ Prolapse Quantitative scale
Position, of fetus, 48–49, 50f, 96–101, 97–100f
Post-coital pill, 395
Post-tubal ligation syndrome, 399
Postcoital bleeding, 455
Posterior arm/shoulder, delivery of, 103
Posterior fontanelle, 49
Postmenopausal bleeding, 237, 358–359, 358t, 465–466, 466t
 diagnosis of, 361, 363
Postmenopausal Estrogen/Progestin Interventions (PEPI) Trial, 328
Postmenopausal vaginal bleeding (PMVB), 358–359
Postmenopausal women, 239
Postmenopause, 326–330, 326t, 327f, 328t, 329t
Postoperative chemotherapy, 484
Postpartum bleeding, 496
Postpartum blues, 211
Postpartum care, 199–208
Postpartum complications, 202–207, 202–203t, 205f
Postpartum contraception, 200–201
Postpartum depression, 207, 208, 209, 211, 212
Postpartum endomyometritis, 286, 287–288
Postpartum hematocrit, 210, 212
Postpartum hemorrhage (PPH), 201, 202–205, 203t, 205f
 cause of, 209, 212
 operative management of, 205
 risk factors for, 209, 212
Postpartum preventative medications, 200
Postpartum sterilization (PPS), 397
Postpartum tubal ligation (PPTL), 200–201, 397, 397f
Postterm pregnancy, 1, 116, 121–122
 associations, 129, 132
 diagnosis of, 127, 128, 129, 132
Postvoid residual (PVR), 306

Potassium chloride, 411
Potter syndrome, 34–35
Power morcellation, 237
PPCM (peripartum cardiomyopathy), 186
PPH. *See* Postpartum hemorrhage
PPROM (preterm and premature rupture of membranes), 94–96
PPS (postpartum sterilization), 397
PPTL (postpartum tubal ligation), 200–201, 397, 397f
Precocious puberty, 322
Preconception counseling, 116, 169
Prednisone, 186, 371
Preeclampsia, 133–137, 134t, 136–137t, 140, 141, 142, 143, 144, 190, 190t, 489
 diagnosis of, 194–195, 197, 198
 without severe features, 135
 with severe features, 135–136, 136t
Pregestational diabetes, 145, 148–151, 148–150t
Pregnancy, 1–5, 1t, 3f, 5t, 339, 341, 355, 356
 antiretroviral therapy in, 179
 bilateral luteomas of, 373, 375
 after breast cancer, 517
 during chronic renal disease, 195, 198
 dating of, 2, 121–122
 diabetes during, 145–152, 146t, 148–150t
 early complications of, 15–22
  cervical insufficiency, 19f, 19–20, 19t, 20f
  ectopic pregnancy, 15f, 15–17, 15t, 16f, 387
  first-trimester abortion, 18, 18t
  recurrent pregnancy loss, 21
  second-trimester abortion, 18–19
  spontaneous abortion, 17, 17f, 18t
 fetal complications of, 112–126
 hypercoagulability of, 196
 hypertension during, 133–139, 134t
  chronic hypertension, 138
  chronic hypertension with superimposed preeclampsia, 138–139
  eclampsia, 133, 137–138, 138t
  preeclampsia, 133–137, 134t, 136–137t, 190, 190t
 infection during, 157–175, 157t
 management during, 194, 197–198
 maternal complication during, 194, 197
 medical complications of, 181–193
  coagulation disorders, 187–189, 188–189f
  hyperemesis gravidarum, 181–182
  maternal cardiac disease, 184–186
  maternal renal disease, 186–187
  maternal thyroid disease, 189
  seizures, 104–105, 105t, 137–138, 138t, 182–184, 183–184t
  substance abuse, 191–192
  systemic lupus erythematosus, 189–191, 190t
 routine problems of, 9–10
 rubella infection, 175, 177

termination of, 406–412, 406–408f, 407t, 410–411t, 410f
White classification of diabetes in, 154–155
Pregnancy-induced hypertension. See Gestational hypertension
Preimplantation genetic diagnosis (PGD), 430–431
Preinvasive neoplastic disease
of cervix, 445–454, 446–447f, 446t, 448–451t, 452–453f, 454t
of vagina, 435–441, 435t, 436–437f, 438t, 439f, 440t, 442, 444
of vulva, 435–441, 435t, 436–437f, 438t, 439f, 440t
Premalignant and malignant disease, 220
Premalignant disease of endometrium, 237–239, 238t
Premalignant endometrial intraepithelial neoplasia, 238
Premature ovarian failure (PMOF). See Primary ovarian insufficiency
Premature rupture of membranes (PROM), 46–47, 47f, 94–96
Prematurity, 134t
Premenstrual dysphoric disorder (PMDD), 352–353
Premenstrual syndrome (PMS), 352–353, 362, 364
etiology of, 364–365
with vitamin supplementation, 362, 364–365
Prenatal care, 5–9, 6t, 10–11
Prenatal diagnosis, 27, 39f
Prenatal screening, 27–40, 35–36t, 36–37f, 41, 43
cell-free DNA screening, 38–40, 39f
for chromosomal abnormalities, 29–31, 30f, 35–37
for fetal congenital abnormalities, 31–35, 32–34f
for genetic diseases, 27–29
prenatal diagnosis, 27, 39f
for sex chromosomal abnormalities, 31
Prenatal treatment. See Prenatal screening
Prenatal vitamins, 5, 5t
Prepregnancy BP, 140, 142
Presentation, of fetus, 46, 48–49, 50f, 96–101, 97–100f, 125
Pressors, 283
Preterm and premature rupture of membranes (PPROM), 94–96
Preterm delivery, 1–2, 92
Preterm labor (PTL), 18–19, 92, 345, 347
Preterm rupture of membranes, 94–96
Previable infant, 1
Primary amenorrhea, 215, 217, 336–339, 337–338t, 339f, 354t
Primary dysmenorrhea, 350–351, 361, 364
Primary ovarian follicle, 322
Primary ovarian insufficiency (POI), 326, 337, 340, 346, 348, 349, 419, 420
diagnosis of, 432, 433, 434

Primary syphilis, 277
Primidone, 182, 183, 183t
Primordial ovarian follicles, 323
Prior classical hysterotomy, 69, 70
PRL (prolactin), 4, 334, 342, 355–356, 503, 506
Probenecid, 266, 281
Procaine penicillin, 266
Prochlorperazine, 181
Procidentia, 294, 294f
Prodromal labor, 49
Products of conception (POC), 17, 204
Progesterone, 13, 301, 334, 431, 432, 434
challenge test, 342, 342t
hormone, 232, 238, 238t, 323, 323f, 324, 503
measurement of, 376
receptor
antagonist, 409
modulators, 396–397
positive tumor, 517
therapy, 21, 185, 238, 328, 328t, 342, 343, 372, 386, 395, 396, 400, 424, 429, 463, 464, 465, 468
Progesterone-eluting IUD, 201, 210, 213, 355
Progesterone OCPs, 201
Progesterone-only contraception, 201, 208, 380t, 393–395, 394t, 400
Progesterone-only minipill, 201
Progestin, 330, 334, 335
administration of, 299, 301
therapy, 239, 254, 256t, 257, 328, 330, 340, 356, 357, 357t, 359, 372, 388–393, 389f, 390–392t, 392f, 395, 396, 400, 463, 465, 468, 469, 509, 519
Progestin implant, 394
Progestin-only contraceptives, 351
Progestin-only oral pill, 402, 404
Progression, of labor, 55–66, 56–57f, 59–64f, 61t, 64t, 65t, 66f
Progressive ovarian failure, 324
Prolactin (PRL), 4, 334, 342, 355–356, 503, 506
Prolactinomas, 349
Prolapse. See Pelvic organ prolapse
Prolapsed uterus, 294
Prolia, 332
Proliferative and secretory phases, in endometrium, 334
Proliferative phase, of menstrual cycle, 322
Prolonged rupture of membranes, 94
PROM (premature rupture of membranes), 46–47, 47f, 94–96
Prometrium, 239
Prophylactic chemotherapy, 491
Prophylactic salpingectomy, 476
Prophylaxis, 13
Propranolol, 490
Propylthiouracil (PTU), 189
Prostaglandin analogs, 409, 411
Prostaglandin E_2 (PGE$_2$) gel, 68, 70
Prostaglandin F2α (PGF2), 204
Prostaglandin inhibitors, 93–94
Prostaglandins, 18, 22, 49, 51, 67, 104, 121, 162, 204, 350, 351, 353, 358, 411

Protease inhibitors, 284, 285
Proteinuria, 133, 134, 135, 136t, 137, 138, 198
Proteus mirabilis, 262
Prothrombin time, 189
Proton pump inhibitors, 9
Provera (medroxyprogesterone acetate), 235, 239, 329, 343, 356, 358, 405, 500
Prozac, 360, 364
Pruritus
vaginal, 441
vulvar, 436, 437, 438
Pseudocapsule, 232–233
Pseudomenopause, 253
Pseudopregnancy, 253
Psoriasis, vulvar, 219, 219t
PSTTs (placental site trophoblastic tumors), 487, 488t, 493, 494f, 496–497, 499, 500, 501
Psychotropic drugs, 506
PTL (preterm labor), 18–19, 92, 345, 347
PTU (propylthiouracil), 189
Pubarche, 320, 321, 322f, 334
Pubertal sequence, normal, 320, 333, 334
Puberty, 320–322, 320t, 320–322f, 322t
breast bud development, 333, 334
Public Health Notice, 298, 309
PUBS (percutaneous umbilical blood sampling), 10, 38, 120
Pudendal block, 65, 66f
Pudendal nerve, 304
Puerperium care. See Postpartum care
Pulmonary angiography, 188, 189f
Pulmonary embolus (PE), 188–189, 188–189f, 328, 390
diagnosis of, 193, 194, 196
Pulmonary hypertension, 185
Pulmonary physiology, of pregnancy, 3, 3f
Pulse oximetry, of fetus during labor, 54–55, 55f
PVR (postvoid residual), 306
Pyelonephritis, 158, 159, 262, 287, 288
complication of, 176, 178
Pyrethrins, 269
Pyrimethamine, 174

Q

Quad screen, 8, 13, 36, 140, 142
Quantitative serum β-hCG, 500

R

Radial hysterectomy, 461, 462
Radiation, 461, 462
Radiation therapy, 441, 457, 468, 481, 515, 516. See also Pelvic radiation
Radical hysterectomy, 457
Radical vulvectomy, 438, 439f, 442, 444
Raloxifene, 330, 331, 509, 513
Rapid plasma reagin (RPR) test, 264
Rash allergy, 161
RDS (respiratory distress syndrome), 11
Reclast, 331
Recommended daily dietary allowances, for pregnant women, 5t
Rectocele, 291, 292f, 293, 294f, 295, 297f, 297t

Recurrence
 of breast cancer, 517
 of cervical cancer, 458
 of endometrial cancer, 468
 of ovarian tumors, 478
Recurrent disease, 516–517
Recurrent pregnancy loss, 21
Regional anesthesia, 408
Reglan, 341
Relaxation, pelvic. See Pelvic organ prolapse
Reliable contraception, 491
Renal agenesis, 34
Renal anomalies, 231
Renal disease, maternal, 186–187
Renal physiology, of pregnancy, 3
Reproductive tract. See Lower reproductive tract, infections of; Upper reproductive tract, infection of
Reserpine, 505t
Respiratory distress syndrome (RDS), 11
Retained placenta, 62, 63f
Retained products of conception, 204
Revealed hemorrhage, 79
Reversal, of tubal sterilization, 399
Rh IgG (anti-D immunoglobulin), 119–120
Rh incompatibility, 118–121, 118t, 119f, 120f
Rh status, 412, 415
RhoGAM, 8, 18, 22, 77, 81, 107, 110, 119–120, 121, 126, 407, 490
Rifampin, 390t
Right-sided ectopic pregnancy, 23, 25–26
Right upper-quadrant (RUQ) pain, question about, 134, 140, 142, 143
Risendronate. See Actonel
Ritodrine, 94
Ritonavir, 284
ROM (rupture of membranes), 46–47, 47f, 49, 84, 161
Rotterdam criteria, 370, 371, 375, 421
Round ligament pain, 9
Routine evaluation, of breast, 504–505
Routine postpartum care, 199–202
Routine prenatal laboratory test screening, 175, 177
Routine prenatal visits, 6–9
Routine sonographic, evaluation of, 472
RPR (rapid plasma reagin) test, 264
Rubella, 113, 168–169
 infection, 175, 177
Rubin maneuver, 103, 104f, 107, 109–110
Rupture
 of fetal vessels, 82–84
 of uterus, 65, 65t, 81–82, 82t, 104, 204
Rupture of membranes (ROM), 46–47, 47f, 49, 84, 161. See also Premature rupture of membranes; Preterm rupture of membranes
 diagnosis of, 67, 69
RUQ (right upper-quadrant) pain, question about, 134, 140, 142, 143

S
Sacral neuromodulation, 313, 317, 318
Salpingectomy, 16, 476. See also Bilateral salpingo-oophorectomy
Salpingostomy, 16
Salt wasting, 374, 377
Saprophyticus, 262
Saquinavir, 284
Sarcoptes scabiei, 268, 269
Savage syndrome, 337, 337t, 338t
SBE (subacute bacterial endocarditis) prophylaxis, 185
Scabies, 269
Scalp electrode, 52
SCC. See Squamous cell carcinoma
Scratch–itch cycle, 220
Screening. See also Prenatal screening
 for cervical cancer, 447–449, 448f
 mammography, 504, 504f
 during pregnancy, 7t, 8, 146, 146t
Seasonale, 389
Seasonique, 389
Sebaceous cysts, 221
Second-degree laceration, 68, 70
Second stage of labor, 58
Second trimester
 abortion, 18–19, 407, 407t, 410–411, 410f, 411t
 definitions, 1
 screening, 36–37, 36t, 37f
 visits, 8
Secondary amenorrhea, 339–344, 341–342t, 342f, 343f, 354t
Secondary dysmenorrhea, 234, 256, 351–352, 351f, 352f
Secretory phase, of menstrual cycle, 322
Sedatives, 65
Seizure, 141, 144
 maternal, 104–105, 105t, 137–138, 138t, 182–184, 183–184t
Selective estrogen receptor modulators (SERMs), 328, 330, 332, 394t, 464, 509, 511, 513
Selective serotonin reuptake inhibitors (SSRIs), 207, 212, 329t, 330, 353, 360
Self-catheterization, 313
Semen analysis, 427–428, 428t
Senile angiomas. See Cherry hemangiomas
Sensitized Rh negative patient, 120, 120f
Sentinel lymph node biopsy (SLNB), 438, 516
Septate uterus, 230f, 244
Septic pelvic thrombophlebitis, 287
Septum, transverse vaginal, 216–217, 216f, 336
Septumste uterus, 229, 232f, 246
Serial deep tendon reflex (DTR) examination, 106, 108
SERMs (selective estrogen receptor modulators), 328, 330, 332, 394t, 464, 509, 511, 513
Serotonin and norepinephrine reuptake inhibitors (SNRIs), 329t, 330, 353
Serous cystadenocarcinomas, 478
Serous discharge, 506
Serous tumors, 478
Sertoli cells, 377
Sertoli–Leydig cell tumors, 370, 372, 375, 481
Sertraline, 212, 353
Serum β-hCG (beta human chorionic gonadotropin), 346, 348, 498, 500
Serum pregnancy test, 241
Serum testosterone, 372, 373, 375
Serum tumor markers, 242, 477, 478, 479, 480, 480t
17-α-hydroxylase, 337
17-OHP (17α-hydroxyprogesterone), 369
17α-hydroxyprogesterone (17-OHP), 369
17,20 desmolase, 337
Severe preeclampsia, 135–136
Sex chromosomal abnormalities, 31
Sex chromosomal aneuploidy, 41, 43
Sex cord-stromal tumors, 481
 of ovary, 370, 375
Sex hormone binding globulin (SHBG), 189, 340, 371, 376, 421, 465
Sex steroids, 320, 321, 367, 368f
Sexual dysfunction, 293
Sexual intercourse, 218
Sexual partners, *Trichomonas* infections in, 276
Sexually transmitted infections (STIs), 15, 382, 384
 screening of, 361, 364
SGA (small for gestational age), 92, 112–115, 113t, 114–115f
SHBG (sex hormone binding globulin), 189, 340, 371, 376, 421, 465
Sheehan syndrome, 341t, 345, 347
Shingles. See Varicella zoster virus
Shoulder dystocia, 102–104, 103f, 104f, 212
 fetal complication of, 107, 110
 maneuver used to, 107, 109–110
 risk for, 107, 109
Shoulder presentation, 100
Sickle cell disease, 28
SILs (squamous intraepithelial lesions), 435, 436
Simple atypical hyperplasia, 237, 238t
Simple hyperplasia, 237, 238t
Simple proliferation, 238
Sinusoidal pattern, on fetal monitoring strip, 85, 88
Sister Mary Joseph nodule, 476
Skene's duct cysts, 221–222, 221f
Skin dimpling, 513
Skin separation, 211, 213–214
Skyla. See Levonorgestrel IUD
SLE (systemic lupus erythematosus), 189–191, 190t
Sleep deprivation, in pregnancy, 182
SLNB (sentinel lymph node biopsy), 438, 516
Small for gestational age (SGA), 92, 112–115, 113t, 114–115f
Smoking, 191, 390, 436, 447, 461, 462
SNRIs (serotonin and norepinephrine reuptake inhibitors), 329t, 330, 353
Society of Urodynamics, Female Pelvic Medicine, and Urogenital Reconstruction (SUFU), 311
Somatic nervous system, 304, 304f

Speculum examination, 88, 90
Spermicide, 381–384, 382f, 383f, 384f, 393, 400
Spina bifida, 32–33, 32–33f
Spinal anesthesia, 66, 70, 314t
Spiral chest CT, 194, 196
Spiramycin, 174
Spironolactone, 371, 377
Splinting, 293
Spontaneous abortion, 17, 17f, 18t, 386
Squamous cell carcinoma (SCC)
  of cervix, 454–458, 454f, 456–458t, 457f
  of vagina, 440, 440t
  of vulva, 437–438, 437f, 438t, 439, 439f, 440
Squamous intraepithelial lesions (SILs), 435, 436
Squamous intraepithelial lesions, 461
SSRIs (selective serotonin reuptake inhibitors), 207, 212, 329t, 330, 353, 360
ST-Analysis, of fetus during labor, 54–55, 55f
St. John wort, 390t
Stadol, 65
Staging, 443, 444
  of cervical cancer, 455–456, 456t, 457f
  of endometrial cancer, 464, 464t, 467, 467t
  of fallopian tube carcinoma, 482
  of gestational trophoblastic disease, 493, 493t
  of labor, 56–66, 57f, 59–64f, 61t, 64t, 65t, 66f
  of ovarian tumors, 477, 478t
  of vaginal cancer, 440, 440t
  of vulvar cancer, 438, 438t
STAN (ST-Analysis of fetal electrocardiogram), 55
Staphylococcus aureus, 213, 222, 282, 383
Staphylococcus saprophyticus, 262
Station, 48, 49f
Status epilepticus, 105t
Stavudine, 284
Stein-Leventhal syndrome. *See* Polycystic ovary syndrome
Stenosis, cervical, 224, 340, 352, 422, 426
Sterile vaginal examination, 89, 90
Sterilization, 397–399, 397–399f
Steroids, 9, 93, 219t, 221, 225, 330t, 371, 427t, 441, 447
  topical high-potency, 226, 228
Stillbirth, prevention of, 153, 156
STIs. *See* Sexually transmitted infections
Stool softeners, 9, 199
Streak ovaries, removal of, 226, 228
Streptococci, 281
Streptococcus. See Group B *Streptococcus*
Streptococcus agalactiae, 161
Stress (urinary) incontinence, 302, 302t, 306, 308–311, 308f, 310–311f, 316, 317–318
Stress, in pregnancy, 182
Stress test, 306

Stromal hyperplasia/hyperthecosis, 370
Study of Women's Health Across the Nation (SWAN), 326
Subacute bacterial endocarditis (SBE) prophylaxis, 185
Submucosal fibroids, 232, 234
Subserosal fibroids, 232, 244, 246
Substance abuse, during pregnancy, 191–192
Suburethral sling, 310f
Subutex (buprenorphine), 192
Succenturiate lobe, 73, 82, 85, 88
Succenturiate placenta, 74t
Suction curettage, 408–409, 408f. *See also* Dilation and curettage
Suction D&C, 490, 499
SUFU (Society of Urodynamics, Female Pelvic Medicine, and Urogenital Reconstruction), 311
Sulfadiazine, 174
Sulfasalazine, 427t
Superficial vein thrombosis (SVT), 187
Superimposed preeclampsia, 138–139
Suprapubic pressure, 103, 103f
Surgical evacuation, 407, 407f
Surgical resection, 440
Surgical sterilization, 397–399, 397–399f
Survival rate
  of breast cancer, 517
  of cervical cancer, 457, 458t
  of endometrial cancer, 468, 468t
  of fallopian tube carcinoma, 482
  of germ cell tumors, 481
  of ovarian tumors, 479
  of vaginal carcinoma, 441
  of vulvar carcinoma, 439
SVT (superficial vein thrombosis), 187
SWAN (Study of Women's Health Across the Nation), 326
Swyer syndrome, 337, 337t, 338t
Symmetric growth, 113
Synarel (nafarelin), 253
Syncytiotrophoblasts, 489
Syndrome X, 484, 485. *See also* Metabolic syndrome
Synthroid (levothyroxine), 189, 197, 198
Synthroid, 193
  dose of, 195, 197
Syphilis, 171–173, 172f, 263–266, 263t, 265f, 273, 276, 277
Systemic adjuvant chemotherapy, 516
Systemic adjuvant hormone therapy, 516
Systemic lupus erythematosus (SLE), 189–191, 190t
Systemic pharmacologic intervention, 65
Systemic vascular resistance, during pregnancy, 2

T

T-Score, osteoporosis, 331
T1DM. *See* Type 1 diabetes mellitus
T2DM. *See* Type 2 diabetes mellitus
Tachysystole, 58
Tacrolimus, 186
TAHBSO (total abdominal hysterectomy and bilateral salpingo-oophorectomy), 467, 467t, 477, 478, 480
Tamoxifen, 237, 238, 238t, 330, 464, 470, 472, 505, 509, 511, 513, 516, 517, 519, 523
Tampon tests, 69, 95
Task Force on Hypertension in Pregnancy, 133
Taxol, 484, 486
Taxotere (docetaxel), 479
Tay–Sachs disease, 28–29
Tdap vaccine, 200
Tenofovir disoproxil fumarate plus emtricitabine, 283
TENS (transcutaneous electrical nerve stimulation), 351
Tension-free transvaginal sling (TVT), 318
Teratogenicity, 183
Teratogens, 31, 113, 113t
Teratoma. *See* Benign cystic mature teratoma
Terbutaline, 58, 94, 102
Terconazole, 271
Teriparatide (Forteo), 332
Term delivery, 1–2
Testicular feminization, 337
Testicular regression, 377
Testosterone, 429
  therapy, 221
Tetracycline, 264, 281
Tetrahydrocannabinol (THC), 191
Thalassemia, 29
THC (tetrahydrocannabinol), 191
Theca lutein cysts, 240, 247, 370, 489, 490, 490f, 498, 499, 500
Thelarche, 320, 321, 322t, 322f, 333, 334
Theophylline, 390t
Third stage of labor, 61–62, 62f
Third trimester
  definitions, 1
  labs, 8–9
  visits, 8
Thoracodorsal nerve, 503, 503f
Threatened abortion, 17, 26
3β-HSD (3β-hydroxysteroid dehydrogenase) deficiency, 369
3β-hydroxysteroid dehydrogenase (3β-HSD) deficiency, 369
Three Ps, 109
3TC (Lamivudine), 284
Thrombocytopenia, 81
Thyroid disease, maternal, 189
Thyroid hormone replacement, 21, 343, 357t
Thyroid-stimulating hormone (TSH), 195, 198, 341, 342, 355, 356
Thyroid storm, 490
Thyrotropin-releasing hormone (TRH), 341
Tigan, 181
Tinidazole, 272, 276
Tissue-specific estrogen complex (TSEC), 328
TLR4 response, 158
TOA (tubo-ovarian abscess), 247, 275, 277, 281–282, 282f, 287, 289, 290
Tobacco abuse, 127, 129–130
Tocolysis, 92–94, 95f

Tocolytics, 19–20, 78, 93–94, 102, 105, 162
TOCs (tubo-ovarian complexes), 281, 289
TOLAC. *See* Trial of labor after cesarean
Tolterodine, 312*t*
Tomosynthesis, 504–505
Topical high-potency, steroids, 226, 228
Topical steroids, 221
Topiramate, 390*t*
TORCH titers, 121, 127, 129
Total abdominal hysterectomy and bilateral salpingo-oophorectomy (TAHBSO), 467, 467*t*, 477, 478, 480
Toxic shock syndrome (TSS), 282–283, 383
Toxoplasma gondii, 173
Toxoplasmosis, 173–174, 174*f*, 283
TPAL designation, 11, 13
TPPA (*Treponema pallidum* particle agglutination assay), 264, 275, 277
Tranexamic acid (Lysteda), 356, 364
Transcutaneous electrical nerve stimulation (TENS), 351
Transdermal contraceptive patch, 391–392
Transdermal estrogen and progestin contraception, 380*t*, 391–392, 392*f*
Transformation zone (TZ), of cervix, 446, 447*f*
Transient tachypnea, of newborn, 132
Transobturator approach midurethral sling, 318
Transvaginal aspiration, 429, 429*f*
Transvaginal mesh, 297–298
Transvaginal pelvic ultrasound, 241
Transvaginal ultrasound, 13, 244, 246, 361, 362, 363, 398, 413, 414, 415
Transverse presentation, 48
Transverse vaginal septum, 216–217, 216*f*, 336
Trastuzumab, 516, 521, 523
Treponema pallidum, 263, 264, 276, 277. *See also* Syphilis
Treponema pallidum particle agglutination assay (TPPA), 264, 275, 277
TRH (thyrotropin-releasing hormone), 341
Trial of labor after cesarean (TOLAC), 65, 65*t*
  contraindication to, 69, 70
  setting of, 86, 89
Trichloroacetic acid, 268, 269
Trichomonas, 281
  infections, 276
Trichomonas vaginalis, 271–272, 271*f*, 276, 277, 278
Trichomoniasis, 276
Tricyclic antidepressants, 341, 390*t*
Trimethadione, 182, 183*t*
Trimethoprim/sulfamethoxazole, 158, 159, 262
Triple I, 162
Triple screen, 8, 36
Triplets, 125

Triploid karyotpyes, 500
Trisomy 13, 31, 36*t*
Trisomy 18, 30–31, 36, 36*t*, 42, 45
Trisomy 21. *See* Down syndrome
Trophoblast, 324
Trophoblastic embolization, 490
TSEC (tissue-specific estrogen complex), 328
TSH (thyroid-stimulating hormone), 195, 198, 341, 342, 355, 356
TSS (toxic shock syndrome), 282–283, 383
TTTS (twin-to-twin transfusion syndrome), 122, 124–125, 128, 131
Tubal factors, 421
Tubal ligation, 476
Tubal occlusion, 397–398, 398*f*, 401, 402, 403, 404
Tubal patency, 246
Tubal pregnancy, implantation in, 25
Tubal sterilization, 397–399, 398*f*
Tubo-ovarian abscess (TOA), 247, 275, 277, 281–282, 282*f*, 287, 289, 290
Tubo-ovarian complexes (TOCs), 281, 289
Tuboplasty, 426
Tumor receptor status, 516
Tumors. *See also* Malignant breast disease
  epithelial, 477–479, 478*t*
  germ cell, 479–481, 479–480*f*, 480*t*
  of ovaries, 370–371, 473–479, 474–478*t*, 474–475*f*, 477*f*
  placental site trophoblastic, 487, 488*t*, 493, 494*f*, 496–497
  serous, 478
  of sex cord-stroma, 481
  of vulva and vagina, 221
Turner syndrome, 31, 43, 337, 337*t*, 338*t*, 348, 423. *See also* Gonadal dysgenesis
TVT (tension-free transvaginal sling), 318
24-hour urine protein collection, 135, 140, 142, 377
Twin-to-twin transfusion syndrome (TTTS), 122, 124–125, 128, 131
Twins. *See* Multiple gestations
Two-cell theory, 324
2-hour glucose tolerance test, performing, 128, 131
Two-gonadotropin theory, 324
2D digital mammography, 504
Tylenol, 12, 14
Type 1 diabetes mellitus (T1DM), 150–151, 150*t*
  congenital anomalies, risk of, 152, 154
  risk, during pregnancy, 152, 154
Type 2 diabetes mellitus (T2DM), 151, 303
  congenital anomalies, risk of, 152, 155
  glucose challenge test, 153, 155
TZ (transformation zone), of cervix, 446, 447*f*
Tzanck smear, 267

U

UAE (uterine artery embolization), 212, 235, 236*f*
Ulcerated lesions, of lower reproductive tract, 263, 263*t*
  chancroid, 267
  genital herpes, 266–267, 266*f*
  lymphogranuloma venereum, 267–268
  syphilis, 263–266, 265*f*
Ulcererations, 220
Ulipristal (*Ella, EllaOne*), 395, 396
Ultrasound, 168. *See also* Pelvic ultrasound
  of cervical insufficiency, 19*f*
  of ectopic pregnancy, 16, 16*f*
  of endometrioma, 252*f*
  of neural tube defects, 32–33*f*
  placenta, location of, 90
  of placenta previa, 76*f*
  for pregnancy dating, 2
  for prenatal fetus assessment, 10
  in prenatal screening, 37*f*, 38–40, 39*f*
  of trisomy, 30–31, 30*f*
  umbilical artery Doppler, 114, 114–115*f*
Underactive detrusor muscle. *See* Overflow (urinary) incontinence
Unilateral salpingo-oophorectomy, 480, 483, 485
Unsensitized Rh negative patient, 119–120
UPI (uteroplacental insufficiency), 117
Upper genital tract, benign disorders of, 229–243
Upper reproductive tract, infection of, 279–285, 280–281*f*
Ureterovaginal fistulas, 314
Urethra anatomy, 303–304, 303–304*f*
Urethral caruncles, 223
Urethral diverticula, 223, 242, 314
Urethral function, 308
Urethral pressure profilometry, 308
Urethral prolapse, 223
Urethrocele, 291, 295
Urethrocystometry, 308
Urethrovesical junction (UVJ), 303, 307*f*
Urge incontinence, 306*f*
Urgency (urinary) incontinence, 302, 302*t*, 311–313, 312*f*, 312*t*
Urinalysis, 306
  with culture and sensitivity, 317, 318
Urinary dribbling, 313
Urinary dysfunction, 293
Urinary fistula, 303, 314–315, 314*f*
Urinary frequency, 9–10
Urinary incontinence, 302–315, 302–303*t*, 303–304*f*, 305*t*, 306–308*f*, 310–314*f*, 312*t*, 314*t*
  bladder outlet obstruction with overflow, 316, 318, 319
  continuous incontinence secondary to urinary fistula, 316, 318–319
Urinary ovulation predictor kits, 373, 376
Urinary retention, 302
Urinary tract infections (UTIs), 157–159, 262–263
Urine culture, 306

Urine drug screen, 91
Urine pregnancy test, 241, 401, 403, 412, 413, 414, 415
Urodynamics, 306
Uroflowmetry, 306, 308
Urogenital atrophy, 221, 223, 326, 330, 359, 361, 363
Urogenital diaphragm, 245
U.S. Preventive Services Task Force (USPSTF), 503
USPSTF (U.S. Preventive Services Task Force), 503
Uterine anomalies, 243, 245
Uterine artery embolization (UAE), 212, 235, 236f
Uterine atony, 203–204
  treatment of, 209, 212
Uterine bleeding, 239, 350, 353–358, 354t, 357t, 409, 466, 495
Uterine factor infertility, 419t, 422
Uterine fibroids
  risk factors for, 244, 246
  test for, 244, 246
Uterine hypertonus, 58
Uterine inversion, 204–205, 205f
Uterine leiomyoma, 231–237, 233f, 234–236t, 236f, 256, 256t
Uterine perforation, 413, 415
Uterine prolapse, 291, 296, 297t
Uterine rupture, 65, 65t, 81–82, 82t, 104, 204, 212
  explanation for, 89, 90
  risk of, 89, 211, 214
Uterine septums, 230f, 231, 246
Uteroplacental insufficiency (UPI), 117
Uterosacral nodularity, on rectovaginal examination, 258, 260
Uterotonics, 205, 490, 500
Uterus
  congenital Müllerian anomalies of, 229–231, 229t, 230–232f
  formation of, 216–217, 216f
UTIs (urinary tract infections), 157–159, 262–263
UVJ (urethrovesical junction), 303, 307f

V

Vacuum extraction, 60
  complication of, 69, 71
Vacuum extractors, 68, 69, 70, 71
Vagina
  adenosis of, 223f
  benign cysts and tumors of, 221
  benign lesions of, 215
  cancer of, 440, 440t
  congenital anomalies of, 215–218, 216–218f
  formation of, 216–217, 216f
  lacerations of, 202–203
  preinvasive disease of, 439
Vaginal agenesis, 217–218, 218f, 336–337
Vaginal atresia, 216f, 217, 226, 228, 336–337
Vaginal atrophy, 330, 358, 517
Vaginal birth after cesarean (VBAC), 65, 65t
Vaginal bleeding, 25, 82, 83, 352f, 440, 466, 466t, 489, 492, 496, 500
  pelvic ultrasound for, 22
  with placenta previa, 75
  with placental abruption, 80
  with spontaneous abortion, 18, 18t
Vaginal cancer, 440
Vaginal carcinoma, 440
Vaginal delivery, 58–59, 59f, 199, 202t
Vaginal dilators, 218, 228
Vaginal dryness, 334, 335, 361, 381, 432, 433, 518
Vaginal estrogen, 228
  and progestin contraception, 392–393, 392f
Vaginal hematoma, 202–203
Vaginal infections, 269–270, 270f
  bacterial vaginosis, 270, 270f
  Trichomonas vaginalis, 271–272, 271f
  yeast infections, 270–271
Vaginal intraepithelial neoplasia (VAIN)
  primary treatment for, 442, 444
  of vagina, 439
Vaginal neoplasia, 435–441, 435t, 436–437f, 438t, 439f, 440t
Vaginal ring, 380t, 392–393, 392f
Vaginal septum, 216–217, 216f, 336
Vaginal vault prolapse, 291, 297, 297t, 298
Vaginitis, 160–161, 226, 227, 228, 229, 261, 270, 271–272, 276, 277, 281
Vaginoplasty, 228
Vaginosis. *See* Bacterial vaginosis
VAIN. *See* Vaginal intraepithelial neoplasia
Valacyclovir, 163, 267
Valproate, 182, 183t, 371
Valproic acid, 41, 44, 182–183
Valvular disease, 185
Vancomycin, 283
Variable deceleration, of fetal heart rate, 52, 54f
Varicella infection, 164
Varicella vaccine (Varivax), 165
Varicella zoster immune globulin (VariZIG), 165
Varicella zoster virus (VZV), 164–165, 165f
Varicocele, 427
Varicose veins, 10
Varivax (varicella vaccine), 165
VariZIG (Varicella zoster immune globulin), 165
Vasa previa, 72, 74t, 82, 85, 86, 88, 90
Vasectomy, 399–400, 399f
Vasodilators, 186
Vasomotor symptoms (VMS), 324, 326, 327, 328, 329, 335, 517, 523
Vasopressin, 223
Vasopressors, 16
VBAC (vaginal birth after cesarean), 65, 65t
VDRL (Venereal Disease Research Laboratory) test, 172, 264
Velamentous cord insertion, 82
Velamentous placenta, 74t
Venereal Disease Research Laboratory (VDRL) test, 172, 264
Venlafaxine (Effexor), 330, 353, 517
Venography, 196
Venous stasis, principal causes for, 197
Venous thromboembolism
  risk factors of, 194, 196–197, 213
Venous thromboembolism (VTE), 201
Ventilation/perfusion scanning, 188, 188f
Vertex position, 69
Vertex presentation, 48, 98–100, 99–100f
Vertical incision, 213
Vesicovaginal fistulas, 314
VIN (vulvar intraepithelial neoplasia), 227, 435–437, 435t, 436f
Vincristine, 516–517
Viral shedding, 163, 267, 275, 277–278
Virilism, 367–372, 368f
Virilization, 367
  of fetus, 373, 375
Vitamin B_6 supplementation, 353, 360, 509
Vitamin B_{12} supplementation, 181
Vitamin D supplementation, 331, 331t, 353, 360, 394, 394t
Vitamin E supplementation, 509
Vitamin K supplementation, 184, 184t
Vitamin supplementation
  for PMS and PMDD, 353
  for pregnant women, 5, 5t
VMS (vasomotor symptoms), 324, 326, 327, 328, 329, 335, 517, 523
Voiding cystourethrogram, 315
Voiding diary, 306, 306f
Vomiting, 3, 181
V/Q scanning. *See* Ventilation/perfusion scanning
VTE (venous thromboembolism), 201
Vulva
  benign cysts and tumors of, 221
  benign lesions of, 215
  cancer of, 437–439, 437f, 438t, 439f
  congenital anomalies of, 215–218, 216–218f
  melanoma of, 439
  Paget disease of, 437
Vulvar and vaginal dermatoses, 218–223, 219t, 220–223f
Vulvar architecture, distortion of, 228
Vulvar biopsy, 220, 220f, 226, 227, 228
Vulvar cancer, 436, 437, 438, 442, 444
Vulvar carcinoma, 444
Vulvar intraepithelial neoplasia (VIN), 227, 435–437, 435t, 436f
Vulvar neoplasia, 435–441, 435t, 436–437f, 438t, 439f, 440t
Vulvar pruritus, 436, 437, 438
Vulvar psoriasis, 219, 219t
Vulvar soriasis, 219
Vulvectomy, 439, 439f
Vulvitis, 263
Vulvodynia, 437
Vulvovaginal atrophy (VVA), 326
Vulvovaginal lichen planus, 219
VVA (vulvovaginal atrophy), 326
VZV (varicella zoster virus), 164–165, 165f

W

Warfarin, 187–188, 189, 196
WBC (white blood cell) test, 141, 143
Weight-bearing exercise, 331

Weight loss, 362, 363, 365
WHI (Women's Health Initiative), 292, 328
WHIMS (Women's Health Initiative Memory Study), 328
White blood cell (WBC) test, 141, 143
White classification of gestational diabetes, 146t, 147, 149
WHO. *See* World Health Organization
Wide local excision, 436, 437, 510
Wide radical local excision, 438
Women's Health Initiative (WHI), 292, 328
Women's Health Initiative Memory Study (WHIMS), 328
Wood corkscrew maneuver, 103, 107, 110
Word catheter, 222, 222f, 225–226, 227
World Health Organization (WHO), 146
   1994 (WHO94) schema, 237
   Prognostic Index Score, 493
Wound complications, 206–207
Wound dehiscence, 199, 206
Wound infections, 206
Wound separations, 206–207

X

X-linked disorders, 27
X-linked dominant syndromes, 27

Y

Yeast infection, 270–271. *See also* Candidiasis; Vaginitis

Z

Z-score, osteoporosis, 331
Zavanelli maneuver, 104, 110
ZDV. *See* Zidovudine
Zidovudine (ZDV, AZT), 170, 177, 179, 284
   during labor and delivery, 287, 289
Zika virus, 174
Zoledronic acid, 331
Zoloft, 353, 360, 364
Zona fasciculata layer, adrenal gland, 367
Zona glomerulosa layer, adrenal gland, 367
Zona reticularis layer, adrenal gland, 367

Cardinal movements: engagement, descent, flexion, internal rotation, extension, external rotation

Amnisure detects placental α-microglobulin 1